MOBILE SENSING IN PSYCHOLOGY

Also Available

Handbook of Research Methods for Studying Daily Life
Edited by Matthias R. Mehl and Tamlin S. Conner

MOBILE SENSING IN PSYCHOLOGY

Methods and Applications

Edited by

Matthias R. Mehl

Michael Eid

Cornelia Wrzus

Gabriella M. Harari

Ulrich W. Ebner-Priemer

Foreword by Thomas Insel

THE GUILFORD PRESS

New York London

A Division of Guilford Publications, Inc.
370 Seventh Avenue, Suite 1200, New York, NY 10001
www.guilford.com

Printed in the United States of America

This book is printed on acid-free paper.

Last digit is print number: 9 8 7 6 5 4 3 2 1

Library of Congress Cataloging-in-Publication Data

Names: Mehl, Matthias R., editor.
Title: Mobile sensing in psychology : methods and applications / edited by Matthias R. Mehl, Michael Eid, Cornelia Wrzus, Gabriella M. Harari, Ulrich W. Ebner-Priemer.
Description: New York, NY : The Guilford Press, [2024] | Includes bibliographical references and index.
Identifiers: LCCN 2023011430 | ISBN 9781462553105 (cloth)
Subjects: LCSH: Psychology—Research. | Social sciences—Methodology.
Classification: LCC BF76.5 .M64 2024 | DDC 150.72—dc23/eng/20230802
LC record available at *https://lccn.loc.gov/2023011430*

Foreword

The topic of mobile sensing in psychology may seem to be a new field powered by recent technology, but the quest for more ecological data to measure mood, behavior, and cognition has been an old one. No doubt, Freud wondered about the relationship of what he observed in the consulting room to what was happening in the real world outside. And both clinicians and scientists since have wished for better insight into the real-world experience of people in psychological distress.

There is a highly apocryphal story about the scientist who devotes her life to creating the ideal mobile sensing tools, only to pass away before seeing these tools adopted in clinical use. The story is that such virtuous work is rewarded by St. Peter who, because of her exemplary dedication to improving the human condition, offers her an audience with God and an opportunity to ask the Almighty a single question. With some trepidation, she pops the question, "Father, will we ever have a mobile sensing device that is adopted by patients and providers?" Allegedly, God responds, "Yes, my child. But not in my lifetime."

At the outset of this important volume on mobile sensing, it's important to realize that the task for mobile sensing is neither easy nor quick. It's really two tasks, both covered extensively in this volume. First is the challenge of validation. Do the signals on a wearable or smartphone provide high-quality data, and can those data be tied to some ground truth? Acquiring high-quality signals in a world of variance, interference, and nonadherence feels like one of those "not in my lifetime" challenges. But several chapters in this book demonstrate that we can collect high-quality data on location, activity, emotion, and more. Smartphones, wearables, and social media provide an unprecedented scale of data, capturing the world outside of the consulting room or psychology lab. Yes, we need to create standards for quality and we need to integrate mobile sensing data with other measures, but already we can see the value of this new world of data for giving us insight into a person's *umwelt*.

The second task, the ground truth problem, is arguably more difficult. For measures of mood or cognition, what constitutes ground truth? Should we train algorithms to self-report scales, to diaries of activity and mood, or to clinical ratings? If we are limited to these measures, is the field of mobile sensing destined to be no better than the subjective tools we've been using for decades? Here the analytic tools may help. As Part II of this book makes clear, increasingly sophisticated analytic approaches may help us refine the signals so that they are more informative than traditional measures and ultimately may offer a new kind of ground truth. But mobile sensing data, in the near term, will be adjunctive and not replacements for more conventional measures, remembering that more objective measures are not inherently more valid measures.

These challenges of data collection and data analysis need to be put into the context of clinical need, as noted in Part III of this book. Beyond the importance of psychological research, we find ourselves in a mental health crisis with rising rates of suicide, drug-overdose deaths, and depression in youth. The world of mental health care is supported by dedicated professionals who generally work in a data-free zone, without objective data on what is happening outside of the clinic. They may ask about sleep, activity, social contact, and mood without any objective data on these highly quantitative variables. Imagine helping someone with diabetes without measuring blood sugar (now trackable with a continuous glucose monitor) or someone with hypertension without measuring blood pressure (now trackable with home monitoring systems).

To be clear, our mental health crisis is not caused by this data desert, but better measurement can be part of the solution. More than half of the population with a mental disorder are not in care. Remote monitoring can detect a problem and connect people to care. For those who receive care, diagnosis is largely based on subjective reports in a single visit. Remote monitoring can provide objective data on how someone is thinking, feeling, and behaving in the real world, leading to more precise diagnosis. And for those in treatment, there is a surprising absence of monitoring progress, what the field calls "measurement-based care." There is a saying in business that we can't manage what we can't measure. For mental health care to begin to resolve the mental health crisis, we will need to bake measurement into all aspects of care. Mobile sensing can help to solve this data desert passively, ecologically, and continuously, at scale.

I stress this clinical need and the promise of remote sensing because we seem to be in a world in which worries about perils can stifle the promises of innovation. Yes, we must be mindful of privacy and data provenance. We need to build "with," not just "for," users. Transparency, integrity, and equity are fundamental concerns and essential for success. But in order for these concerns to be welcomed with creative and compassionate solutions, they must not become threats to the overall enterprise of using innovation to solve a public health crisis. We must remember that we face a formidable mental health challenge, which can be solved only via innovations like mobile sensing.

Will this happen in our lifetimes? Bill Gates famously noted, "We always overestimate the change that will occur in the next 2 years and underestimate the change that will occur in the next 10." With recent advances in sensor technology, artificial intelligence, and image analysis, we may be closer than we think. This timely volume provides a comprehensive picture of just how close we are and what remains to be done.

Thomas Insel, MD
Executive Chair, Vanna Health
Former Director (2002–2015), National Institute of Mental Health
Author of *Healing: Our Path from Mental Illness to Mental Health*

Preface

The rapid developments in the field of modern information technology are opening up possibilities for psychological research that were inconceivable 20 years ago. A small device like the smartphone is capable of recording and storing important information about everyday human experience and behavior in real time. Examples can be seen in many areas of psychology and neighboring disciplines: It is possible to collect information about the location where people currently are, which places they visit, how much and how fast they move, and the extent to which other people are present. Audio, photo, and film recordings can be made and sent or shared (and stored) immediately. Internet, social media, and phone usage behavior can be tracked comprehensively and in real time. Linking the smartphone with other mobile (e.g., wrist-worn) sensors enables physiological measurements outside the lab and tracking, for example, physical activity and sleep patterns. By using specific apps, questionnaires can be easily presented in tandem with the direct mobile phone usage tracking. That way, momentary mood states as well as the subjective perception of and attitudes toward objective events can be captured. Compliance with medical treatments and psychological interventions can be monitored (either directly via phone usage behavior or indirectly via other mobile sensors). Also, experimental studies can be planned and implemented using the smartphone. These research methods can allow for unprecedented ecological validity and can facilitate the empirical evaluation of the generalizability of research findings (across time, settings/contexts, and populations).

Also, mobile sensing opens new paths for psychological assessment. The intensive longitudinal assessment of behavioral acts, inner experiences, and physiological activity in everyday contexts facilitates uncovering individual patterns of psychological attributes and allows comparing them interindividually. This provides personalized multimethod assessment strategies that go far beyond retrospective (or momentary or daily) diary recordings or day reconstruction methods. Individual symptom constellations and their change over time can be identified, which can form the theoretical and methodological basis for development of personalized models of personality and psychopathology.

Modern psychometric approaches for intensive longitudinal data also allow the application of psychometric quality criteria to single-case data to measure individual-specific constructs and to test their generality. By using modern statistical methods for Big Data, predictions of future emotional states and behavioral tendencies can be made based on the richness of data a smartphone and connected mobile sensors can provide. Critical life situations can potentially be anticipated and alerted to in real time, personalized interventions can be adapted to momentary contexts, and individuals can obtain helpful support and advice in their daily lives.

The possibilities mobile sensing opens up for the social, behavioral, biomedical, and life sciences appear almost infinite and are bound to become even more comprehensive in the years to come. However, data collection with new information technology also poses new challenges for research and applied fields. Is everything that is possible also legally allowed? What are the personal and societal consequences of the possible deep insights into very private areas of life for research ethics and the relations between the researchers and those being researched? How can data be stored so that anonymity and privacy are preserved? How can quality criteria be formulated for this new and rapidly developing field of research? And how can we ensure that information and predictions derived from mobile sensing are psychometrically accurate and practically useful as we move from scientific proof-of-concept measurements to medical/clinical measurements that aim at supporting and improving the diagnostic process? To find answers to these questions, the German Data Forum, an independent council that advises the German federal government and the federal states with respect to the research data infrastructure for the empirical social, behavioral, and economic sciences, established a working group of experts in which four of the five editors of this handbook participated. Over the course of the council's activity, the need for a comprehensive handbook that would allow students, researchers, and users of mobile sensing methods to obtain comprehensive and state-of-the-art information about the many opportunities, promises, challenges, and limitations that characterize this new area of social and behavioral sciences became apparent.

This handbook is intended to fill this gap. It is based on the conviction that a profound understanding and the sound application of mobile sensing methods require specific knowledge and competencies:

- Knowledge of the scientific background and the key concepts
- Knowledge of how to generally plan and conduct a mobile sensing study
- Knowledge of the different methods of data collection with mobile sensing, in terms of both the technological know-how and the methodological how-to
- Knowledge of the possibilities and limitations of mobile sensing and of best-practice examples from different areas of application

In order to turn this handbook idea into reality, the original group of initiators not only succeeded in inviting another highly renowned colleague as coeditor, but also managed to convince 79 leading international authors, from a range of disciplines, to participate in the handbook project and contribute their specific mobile sensing expertise in the form of a chapter. Working on the publication of this handbook, we editors have learned a great deal about methods and applications of mobile sensing from the chapters provided by the authors, and we are convinced that readers will as well.

Editing a handbook with 33 chapters and 84 authors (from a broad range of disciplines) is a major challenge and is certainly compounded by the fact that this handbook project grew to fruition over the course of the COVID-19 pandemic, which confronted all authors and editors with a whole new set of professional and private challenges. The loss of a few originally planned and committed chapters is certainly due to these challenges. We are very grateful and acknowledge with high gratitude and esteem that the other authors remained committed to the handbook project and submitted high-quality chapters despite these extraordinary (or, rather, unprecedented) adverse circumstances. When publishing such a comprehensive handbook, one has to rely on supportive help. We would like to take this opportunity to thank from the bottom of our hearts our research assistants, Amelie Spliesgart and Julia Sauer, who critically revised and uniformly formatted the individual chapters as well as supervised the formal aspects of this handbook project. Their help was terrific!

Contents

PART I

Mobile Sensing

BACKGROUND AND KEY CONCEPTS

CHAPTER 1

How to Conduct Mobile Sensing Research

Gabriella M. Harari, Serena Soh, and Lara Kroencke

CHAPTER OVERVIEW

Mobile sensing is a methodological approach that leverages digital devices and platforms to collect data about human behavior. This chapter provides a starting point for researchers interested in conducting mobile sensing research in psychological science by describing how to conduct sensing studies with smartphones. First, we consider a series of questions that will help determine whether mobile sensing is the right methodological approach for a given study, set of research questions, and target sample of research participants. Next, we review a series of considerations that will help shape the specific study implementation, such as the resources available, the platform used for data collection, and some of the basic features of the study design (e.g., study duration, sampling rate, strategies for participant engagement, ethical considerations). Finally, we discuss some recommended practices for data monitoring, data cleaning, and data analysis, while highlighting the need for standardized guidelines and best practices for conducting mobile sensing research.

Introduction

Mobile sensing is a methodological approach that leverages digital devices and platforms to collect data about human behavior. Mobile sensing is used in studies across a broad range of scientific disciplines (e.g., computer science and engineering, psychological science) to answer research questions in both technical and substantive domains. In the technical domain, mobile sensing research often focuses on software development or activity recognition in an effort to improve the capabilities of sensing technologies. In the substantive domain, mobile sensing research often focuses on assessing behaviors and/or environments to understand people's daily lives and psychological experiences.

The goal of this chapter is to provide a starting point for researchers interested in conducting mobile sensing research in psychological science. Our aim here is to provide a roadmap for those who are considering or preparing to launch a mobile sensing study by describing how to conduct sensing studies with smartphones in particular. We focus on smartphones because they are the prototype mobile sensing device and the one most commonly used in mobile sensing research to date. However, many of the considerations outlined here also apply to the design of studies that use other sensing technologies to collect sensing data from participants' wearables (e.g., smartwatches, fitness trackers) and smart home appliances (e.g., smart speakers).

First, we consider a series of questions that will help determine whether mobile sensing is the right methodological approach for a given study, set of research questions, and target sample of research participants. Next, we review a series of considerations that will help shape the specific study implementation, such as the resources available, the platform used for data collection, and some of the basic features of the study design (e.g., study duration, sampling rate, strategies for participant engagement). Finally, we discuss some recommended practices for data monitoring, data cleaning, and data analysis. Overall, this chapter lays the foundation for the more advanced chapters in Part II ("Mobile Sensors: Technological Know-How and Methodological How-To") and Part III ("Analysis of Mobile Sensing Data") by outlining the basic steps involved in conducting mobile sensing research. Figure 1.1 provides an overview of the key steps and considerations that shape mobile sensing studies.

Questions to Consider Before You Get Started

Before getting started with mobile sensing research, it is helpful to consider a series of conceptual questions to determine whether mobile sensing is the best or "right" approach for a given study. As with any method, there are several benefits and costs associated with adoption of mobile sensing in research studies. The benefits of adopting mobile sensing primarily stem from the potential to collect large-scale, fine-grained, real-world naturalistic observations of people's behaviors and environments, and to a lesser extent of people's verbalized thoughts and feelings. This window into the daily lives of research participants provides an unprecedented view that is unparalleled when compared to other methodologies. The costs of adopting mobile sensing stem from the logistical (e.g., resources available) and practical hurdles (e.g., analyzing intensive repeated measures data) that must be overcome to successfully design and conduct a mobile sensing study. Whether the benefits outweigh the costs for any given study will largely depend on the research questions one hopes to address and the characteristics of the target population one hopes to study.

What Are the Research Questions and Target Variables?

The research questions one hopes to address and the phenomenon of interest are two key factors that can help determine whether mobile sensing methods are appropriate. Generally, research questions that have a temporal component and are focused on understanding

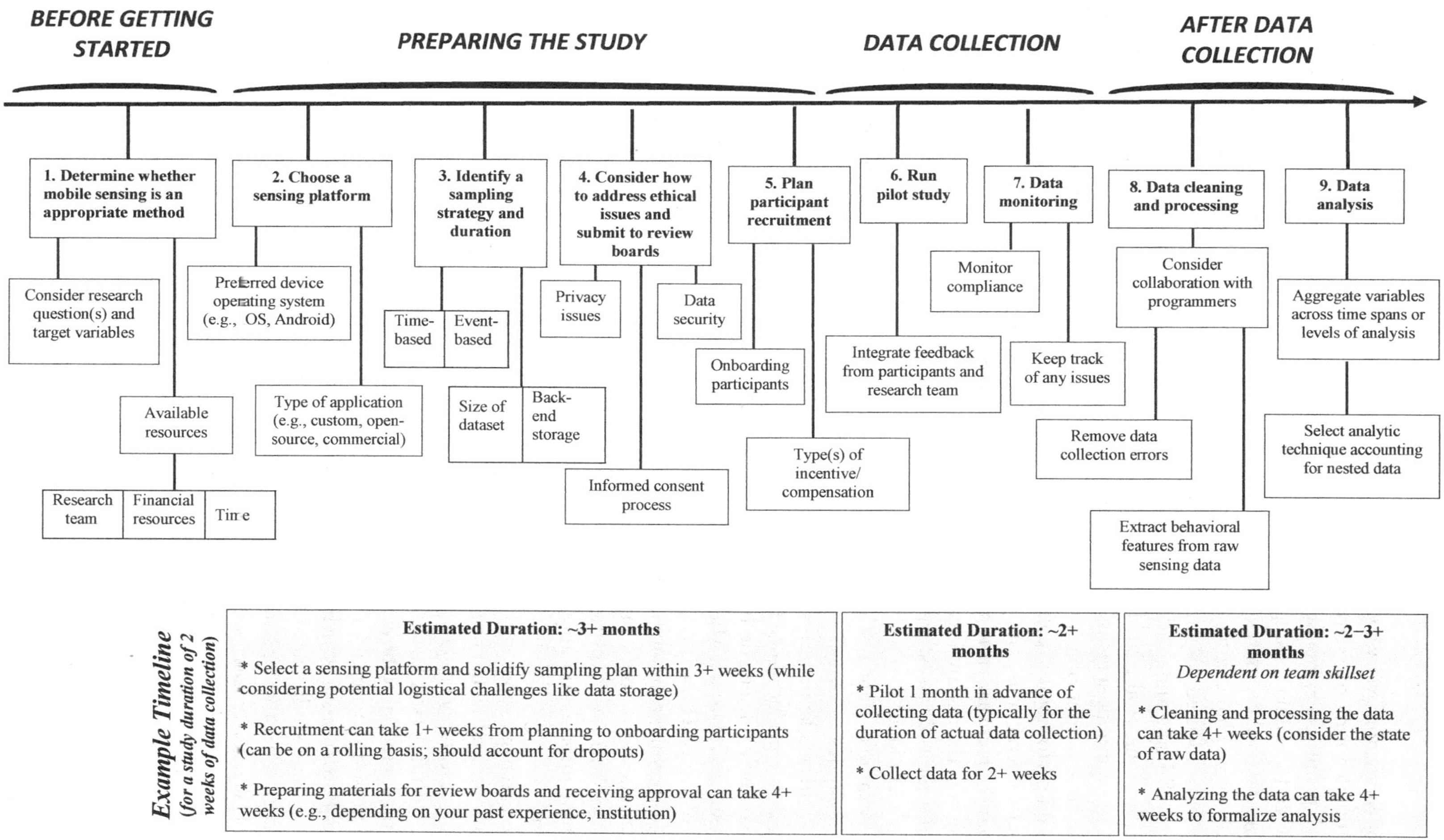

FIGURE 1.1. Overview of steps to consider in mobile sensing research.

some phenomenon over varying units of time (e.g., momentary, hourly, daily, weekly) are most suitable for mobile sensing study design. In addition, any questions about the degree to which people engage in behavior (e.g., frequency or duration of social interactions) are well suited to mobile sensing study design, whereas, at the time of this writing, research questions focused on more subjective aspects of behavior (e.g., quality of social interactions) are more challenging to address with mobile sensing studies. For example, several studies have focused on understanding the behavioral factors associated with college student well-being and academic performance during the academic term (e.g., Doryab et al., 2019; Wang et al., 2014, 2018; Wang, Harari, Hao, Zhou, & Campbell, 2015). In such studies, mobile sensing methods are well suited to addressing the research questions because they permit objective assessments of behaviors that are known to shape well-being and performance, such as the degree to which students engage in physical activity and social interactions, and exhibit certain sleeping patterns. Moreover, the studies benefit from the fact that continuous data are collected to measure the behaviors of interest. This permits the research team to aggregate the timestamped data in different ways and allows for multiple investigations of the research question using different approaches and analytic techniques to obtain a more complete understanding of the phenomena of interest. For example, some research studies have focused on a broad array of student behavior (e.g., physical activity, conversations, studying, partying) at different times of day and across entire academic terms to understand the factors associated with student well-being and academic performance (Wang et al., 2014, 2015). In contrast, other studies focused more narrowly on specific behaviors, such as social behavior (Harari, Müller, Aung, & Rentfrow, 2017; Harari, Müller, Stachl, et al., 2020) or mobility behavior (Müller, Peters, Matz, Wang, & Harari, 2020; Saeb, Lattie, Schueller, Kording, & Mohr, 2016). These examples highlight the opportunities introduced by using mobile sensing for answering research questions about human behavior over time. But it is worth noting that these studies focused on quantified estimates of the behaviors of interest and did not assess qualitative information about the behaviors observed (e.g., quality of social interactions or sleep).

Research questions with a temporal component also include research questions about dynamic intraindividual processes (Kuper, Modersitzki, Phan, & Rauthmann, 2021). For instance, researchers might examine how social behaviors are related to well-being states on the within-person level (i.e., whether individuals feel better after engaging in a conversation compared to how they normally feel) and individual differences therein. These within-person dynamics can best be investigated if the same individuals are observed repeatedly over time, which is typically the case in mobile sensing research. However, mobile sensing studies need not be solely focused on intraindividual processes.

Another area of opportunity presented by mobile sensing data is in understanding and objectively assessing interindividual differences, such as people's characteristic patterns of behaving over time (i.e., dispositional tendencies; Buss & Craik, 1980). If collected over long periods of time in which many types of situations are encountered, researchers can obtain estimates of people's behavioral tendencies by aggregating continuous sensing data at the within-person level over many days, weeks, or months for use in analyses at the between-person level. One point of caution with regard to deriving estimates of behavioral tendencies is that the research team should consider the implicit assumption that participants experienced a representative sampling of situations during the data collection period (e.g., weak and strong situations; Blum, Rauthmann,

Göllner, Lischetzke, & Schmitt, 2018). For example, sensing studies conducted during the COVID-19 pandemic (e.g., Huckins et al., 2020) likely reflect a strong situational effect on social behavior that could affect behavioral estimates of face-to-face interaction and computer-mediated communication. These sensed behavioral tendencies can be used in place of self-reported behavioral tendencies to obtain objective estimates that quantify how a person actually tends to socialize, be physically active, and engage in various daily life activities over time. In past studies adopting this approach, the behavioral tendencies derived from sensing data have been examined in relation to self-reported personality traits (e.g., conversation, calling, texting, and app use tendencies; Harari, Müller, Stachl, et al., 2020; Stachl et al., 2017) and have even been used to predict self-reported personality traits alongside other sensing features (e.g., Mønsted, Mollgaard, & Mathiesen, 2018; Stachl et al., 2020). Chapter 20 provides a review of personality research in this domain.

In terms of target variables of interest, mobile sensing studies can provide information about people's inferred thoughts and feelings, as well as their observed behaviors and surrounding environments. However, they are best suited to providing objective assessments of behavioral and environmental information that can reflect the surrounding situation. The behavioral information that can be obtained from mobile sensing studies includes measures of human movement from accelerometers and Global Positioning System (GPS) data (e.g., physical activity, mobility patterns; see Chapters 4 and 5), social interactions from phone usage data (e.g., call and short messaging service [SMS] logs and app use logs; see Chapters 7 and 8), and various daily activities that are often measured in time use studies (e.g., some of which can be sensed like eating, sleeping, playing games, and listening to music; Harari, Müller, Mishra, et al., 2017; Sonnenberg, Riediger, Wrzus, & Wagner, 2012; White & Dolan, 2009). The environmental information that can be obtained from mobile sensing studies includes measures of ambience (e.g., light, noise, temperature), location (e.g., indoor vs. outdoors, places visited), and proximity to others (e.g., isolation vs. co-location; Harari, Müller, & Gosling, 2020). People's thoughts and feelings can also be inferred to some extent using sensing data, primarily by relying on verbal behavior collected from language data from social media (see Chapter 9) or audio data collected from microphones (see Chapter 10). But given that thoughts and feelings are inherently subjective phenomena, self-report methods may be a more effective and/or convenient assessment approach for research focused on such constructs. Table 1.1 provides an overview of the different target variables of interest that can be derived from sensing data and the data sources needed to obtain them.

Who Are the Research Participants?

Another factor to consider when deciding whether to adopt mobile sensing as a data collection method for one's study is the target research population one plans to recruit. Much of the first wave of mobile sensing research was conducted with college-age young adults, with the aim of understanding the behaviors that shape their well-being. Targeting young adults as research participants in mobile sensing studies comes with several conveniences—they are generally readily available on university campuses where the research is being conducted, they are tech-savvy and already own smartphones, and they may be interested in participating in studies that collect data from their digital devices. For example, one study of student motivations to self-track showed that young adults

TABLE 1.1. Overview of Types of Data in Mobile Sensing Research

		Type of information assessed			
Data types	Description	Thoughts	Feelings	Behaviors	Environment
Mobile sensors					
Accelerometer	Orients the phone display horizontally or vertically; can record duration and degree of physical activity or movement			✓	✓
Bluetooth radio (BT)	Allows the phone to exchange data with other BT-enabled devices; can record the number of unique and repeated interaction partners and devices and co-located individuals			✓	✓
Global Positioning System (GPS) scans	Obtains the phone location from satellites; can record latitude and longitude coordinates			✓	✓
Light sensor	Monitors the brightness of the environment to adjust phone display; can record degree of ambient light or darkness			✓	✓
Microphone	Permits audio for calls; can record duration and frequency of conversations, degree of ambient silence or noise	✓	✓	✓	✓
Wi-Fi scans	Permits the phone to connect to a wireless network; can record location information based on the Wi-Fi network and crowds via the number of unique scans			✓	✓
Other types of data					
Cameras	Records images or video; can take pictures or videos periodically or semicontinuously		✓	✓	✓
Phone use logs	Records usage patterns such as notifications			✓	
App use logs	Records social interactions, entertainment, information-seeking behavior			✓	
Language data	Obtained from text data collected from the keyboard	✓	✓	✓	

Note. The first two columns of this table are adapted from tables presented in Harari et al. (2016) and Harari, Stachl, et al. (2021).

were interested in collecting data from their digital devices (e.g., smartphones, wearables) to improve their productivity and well-being, monitor their mood and daily activities, or improve their social lives (Harari, Müller, Mishra, et al., 2017).

Of course, not all research questions are about the lives of young people or about those young people who happen to be enrolled in universities. In such cases, more thought may need to be given as to how to go about recruiting and incentivizing the target group to participate in the study (see the section "How to Recruit and Incentivize Participants" later in this chapter).

Preparing a Mobile Sensing Study

Having determined that mobile sensing is the right methodology for your research questions and study, the next step is to consider a series of logistical issues that will help shape the design of the study. Mobile sensing studies are generally time and resource intensive, longitudinal in nature, and require careful thought to decisions that can affect the success of the study. Next, we outline how the resources one has available can shape subsequent decisions regarding the key features of the study design, such as the mobile sensing platform used for data collection and whether participants are engaged with the study. Ultimately, the logistical considerations and design decisions made at this step in the research planning will affect the quality of the resulting dataset.

What Resources Are Available?

The resources one has at hand to support the launch and completion of the study are a critical factor in study planning. Three main resources to consider are (1) the individual members and skillsets of the research team, (2) the financial resources available to support the study, and (3) the amount of time available to conduct the research.

The research team is a crucial factor in study planning for mobile sensing studies. The composition of the team and individual skills each member brings to the study will determine how responsibilities are distributed throughout the study period. In general, every sensing study involves several components that require oversight (sometimes simultaneously) and iteratively inform one another (e.g., pilot testing, data monitoring, participant interaction, data processing and analysis), making such studies nearly impossible to conduct by an individual alone. Sensing studies are a team effort, but whether that team is composed of individual students and research assistants or hired staff is a decision to be made early on in the study planning. Students and research assistants may be more motivated and invested in the study success given their likely involvement in the research planning process. However, if accountability is necessary, then hired staff may be a more reliable source of research support. Ultimately, this decision is contingent on the resources available.

In terms of skillsets, it is helpful to have team members who are familiar with the technical aspects of the sensing software being used (whether it be a custom, open-source, or commercial sensing application) and who are experienced in data science and programming to facilitate handling large-scale datasets. In addition, it is important to encourage open communication among the members of the research team throughout the study planning and data collection stages (e.g., via weekly meetings and/or other forms of synchronous and asynchronous interaction).

The financial resources available to help support the study are also important considerations when designing a sensing study. The amount of funding available can influence many of the decisions that must be made during study planning, such as study duration, number of participants to recruit, and type of sensing software used for data collection. For example, the study duration influences the amount of funding needed to pay staff (e.g., graduate students or research assistants hired to work on the project) and the amount of data that is collected, although the latter also depends on the number of participants recruited, the number of sensing data types collected, and the sampling frequency used during data collection. Generally, a study that runs for 1 week and only collects metadata from phone logs (e.g., calls, SMS, and app usage) is going to be less costly than a study that runs for 1 month and frequently collects raw sensor data (e.g., accelerometer, GPS). This is, in part, due to the storage requirements for such data, which drive up costs during data collection and subsequent analyses. The number of participants recruited will also affect the amount of funding needed if individuals are being financially compensated for their participation (see the section "How to Recruit and Incentivize Participants?" for alternative types of compensation). In addition, the decision to use a custom application (specifically developed for the study) or an open-source app (configured based on freely available software) may be a reasonable solution for research teams with the funds to hire people who can handle the more technical aspects of managing sensing software. Using custom or open-source software can permit more flexibility in that features can be customized to the needs of a given study, but this approach simultaneously introduces a great deal of technical complexity and requires more time for preparing and piloting the study to ensure the software is working as it should. Similarly, the decision to use a commercial app may come down to whether one can afford the expenses associated with running a sensing study with a given company. Several commercial sensing apps are available on the market, with each company naturally offering different rates for their services and having their own expenses to consider in providing their services. Some companies charge researchers based on specific study design characteristics, while others charge a flat service fee based on a subscription model (for a brief discussion of academic vs. corporate sensing research, see Chapter 33). In our own work, we have seen commercial companies quote anywhere from several hundred (e.g., ~$500 for a 2-day study collecting experience sampling and GPS data from 200 participants) to tens of thousands of U.S. dollars for sensing studies (e.g., ~$25,000 for a 4-week study collecting experience sampling reports and a full suite of many different types of sensing data from 1,000 participants). Beyond the study duration, the types of data collected and the sampling frequency can also affect the cost of running a study with a commercial company. So, given the variation in pricing we have observed in working with commercial companies, we generally encourage researchers interested in using a commercial app to speak with representatives of several companies to get estimated quotes for the cost of running a study that meets their desired specifications. To illustrate these points with more concrete examples, in Table 1.2 we briefly summarize our recent experiences and approach to conducting two different mobile sensing studies.

Another main resource required to effectively conduct a mobile sensing study is time (see Figure 1.1 for example estimates). Running a mobile sensing study (with any team and set of financial resources) will involve an intensive time commitment during the various stages of the study, from design to data collection to analysis. Thoughtful planning and discussion during the initial stages of the study will be required when the research team is deciding on the study design characteristics, testing and selecting platforms, and preparing materials for ethical review boards. Once the study is designed, the data collection stage is also demanding and can easily become a full-time job for individual members of the research team when accounting for the data monitoring and participant interactions required to ensure high data quality. So, it can be helpful for one or more team members to take the lead on different parts of the study. For example, one person might be responsible for running a pilot study with the research team to test the sensing software before the study launches, another person might be responsible for communicating with and onboarding participants during the study, while another person might be

TABLE 1.2. Study Design Considerations and Examples from Recent Mobile Sensing Studies

	Study names	
Considerations	**COVID-19 Smartphone Sensing Study (Talaifar et al., 2021)**	**Coping with Corona Project (Back et al., 2021)**
Study duration	3 weeks	4 weeks
Recruitment process	Through an online participant recruitment platform (*Prolific*) and university psychology course	Through a university psychology course
Number of participants	300+ students and adults	1,000+ students
Compensation	Course credit or monetary compensation ($10/week) and weekly feedback reports	Course credit and weekly feedback reports
Sensing software	Open-source app (*Beiwe*)	Commercial App (*Ksana Health*)
Sensing data collected	Accelerometer, battery state, Bluetooth, GPS, gyroscope, microphone, phone use logs, screen time, Wi-Fi	Accelerometer, ambient light, battery state, GPS, music, phone use logs
Self-reported data collected	Presurvey; two experience sampling surveys per day at set times; daily audio clip submissions; weekly app usage screenshots	Presurvey; eight experience sampling surveys per day at random times; postsurvey
Members of the research team responsible for data collection	Professors (2); doctoral students (3); undergraduate research assistants (3)	Professor (1); postdoctoral scholar (1); doctoral students (2); undergraduate research assistants (5)
Total cost	~$6,000 (mainly from participant compensation cost and recruitment platform fees)	~$30,000 (mainly from data collection platform fees)

responsible for monitoring the quality of the incoming data during and after the study. Of course, many of the tasks required to efficiently design and conduct sensing studies do ultimately require a collaborative effort. But we have found that many research teams are able to efficiently conduct studies with this kind of delegation of responsibility, so that there is a point of contact for troubleshooting issues that may arise with each aspect of the study.

How to Select a Mobile Sensing Platform?

The selection of a specific mobile sensing platform to use for data collection involves two key factors—the preferred device operating system (e.g., iOS [internet operating system], Android) and the type of application (e.g., custom, open-source, or commercial). The operating system and application selection should be determined based on considerations about the target research participants, the kinds of data needed for the study, and the resources available to the research team.

The selection of operating systems is consequential in that it shapes who can participate in the study and the kinds of sensing data that can be collected. As of 2021, Android and iOS jointly control approximately 99% of the global market share (Statista, 2021);

we therefore limit our discussion to these two mobile operating systems. It is also worth noting that the vast majority of sensing studies to date use applications that run on the iOS and/or Android phones. If participants are expected to use their own smartphones during the study, the research team must also consider the type of operating systems most used by their target sample. Past work has found that iOS users tend to have higher education levels, compared to Android users (Götz, Stieger, & Reips, 2017). But this demographic difference may not necessarily hold in all countries. In fact, Android phones are the most widely used phones around the world, having about a 72% share of the mobile operating system (OS) market (Statista, 2021).

The operating system also influences the kinds of data that can be collected by the sensing application. Generally speaking, iOS is more restrictive than Android in terms of the breadth and granularity of data sources that can be collected. This is in part due to the way that the two OS's allow third-party apps to access and collect data from the user's device. For example, third-party apps on iOS phones are not permitted to access the user's application usage logs at the time of this writing, but these sources of data can be accessed on Android phones (see Chapter 8 for more information about collecting app use data). So if a sensing study is designed to answer questions about the kinds of apps people use, the research team will need to identify a sensing platform that runs on Android phones and focus their recruitment efforts on participants who own Android phones. However, some data sources are commonly collected across both iOS and Android operating systems. These common sources of sensing data include accelerometer sensor data and activity classifications (e.g., stationary, walking, running), as well as GPS data.

The type of application used is also consequential because different sensing applications require different levels of support from the research team. A custom application is one that is designed specifically for and by a research team, and it is typically used in collaboration with computer scientists (e.g., EmotionSense, StudentLife; Rachuri et al., 2010; Wang et al., 2014). An open-source sensing application, such as AWARE[1] (Ferreira, Kostakos, & Dey, 2015) and Beiwe[2] (Torous, Kiang, Lorme, & Onnela, 2016), is one that is freely available for use by researchers. To effectively conduct a mobile sensing study with a custom or open-source application requires technical knowledge about how the sensing software operates. This is because if and when issues arise during data collection, someone on the research team needs to be able to troubleshoot and find a solution to address the issue. In contrast, a commercial sensing application is one that is operated and maintained for profit by a company (e.g., Ethica Data, Ksana Health). Conducting a mobile sensing study with a commercial application requires financial resources, but the benefits can outweigh the costs if the research team is not particularly interested in, skilled, or cares to be responsible for the technical details of how sensing systems operate.

How to Decide on a Sampling Strategy and Study Duration?

When selecting a sampling strategy, researchers must take into account many of the considerations introduced thus far, such as research questions, target variables, populations of interest, and available resources. Sampling strategies in mobile sensing often take the form of time-based sampling, such as continuous or periodic, or event-based data collection. Continuous and periodic sampling refers to schedules that collect data consistently at fixed times or within specifically set intervals, while event-based sampling refers to schedules that collect data contingent on the occurrence of certain events.

Time-based strategies include continuous and periodic sampling, which are often used in mobile sensing research. While continuous collection provides researchers with a wealth of data leading up to, during, and after the occurrence of the phenomenon being studied, periodic sampling enables researchers to decide how often and at what intervals the data are to be collected, depending on the objectives of the study or research question. Although the frequent and consistent nature of mobile sensing methods is considered to be one of its primary benefits, continuous sampling is not necessarily the best option for every study. For example, in the case of GPS data, sampling continuously (e.g., every minute) would lead to large datasets, challenges in data storage, and additional inconvenience to participants due to faster battery drainage. Moreover, participants' locations may not change very frequently during certain hours (e.g., during the work day if they are employed), which means that continuous sampling could result in obtaining redundant information. Rather, collecting GPS data every set interval of minutes within an hour (e.g., every 10 minutes) via periodic sampling may be a more appropriate and appealing option for both researchers and participants. For such reasons, studies like one examining the behavioral trends of college students through smartphones opt to use periodic GPS samples when computing outdoor mobility such as traveled distances (Wang et al., 2014).

Another strategy used in mobile sensing studies is event-based sampling where data collection is triggered by a predefined event. This strategy is most appropriate when examining specific phenomena that do not take place at regularly timed intervals, and it requires researchers to define the events that trigger data collection beforehand. Researchers often apply this strategy when studying smartphone use behaviors through metadata logs, which record events as they occur (e.g., a push notification is logged when it is received; calls and texts are logged as they are made or received). This sampling strategy is also commonly used when collecting movement or location-related data. By setting the events to be significant changes in GPS, the accelerometer, or the Wi-Fi network, data collected in those instances enable researchers to focus on and identify significant patterns in either activity or location changes. For example, this strategy has been observed in a study in which smartphone sensing data were used to predict clinical depression and researchers programmed event-based sampling for iOS users to study location trends by setting distance filters (Farhan et al., 2016). Event-based sampling helps ensure that data collection occurs at necessary times, but researchers must be prepared for the potential technological challenges that may arise. For example, the program may define events too generally and trigger data collection at unintended times, or technological glitches in the software may occur as other types of sampling are simpler in terms of data collection parameters. In the case of using location-related event-based sampling, unintended data collection may occur if data collection is triggered every time a participant is near the target location rather than when they are at the target location. Furthermore, GPS-based sampling can be difficult to program and implement, and additional testing of the location-contingent sampling will be required to identify potential bugs that might unexpectedly hinder data collection. This is why aspects such as ensuring the defined events are specific enough (e.g., precise distance filters for location-related events) and running pilot studies with a smaller pool of participants are especially important to these studies.

Once a sampling strategy is decided on, an appropriate study duration should then be considered given that together they determine the eventual size of the dataset. While mobile sensing studies typically last weeks to months, certain main considerations must be kept in mind when deciding on the length of a study. For instance, researchers must select a length (and sampling frequency) that enables them to answer their research question in terms of whether it examines momentary, hourly, daily, or weekly behavioral trends. If the study revolves around understanding how smartphone use behavior relates to well-being at the momentary level, the study duration can be shorter than a similar study focused on this relation over longer periods of time (e.g., understanding how well-being changes over the academic term). Lastly, from a logistical standpoint, it is important to consider that the combination of sampling rate and study duration determines eventual dataset size and statistical power. Sampling strategies that lead to a high frequency of data collection paired with long study durations, for example, could pose challenges for storing, processing, and analyzing the datasets, which may require the research team to have more advanced technical skills for large-scale analysis. Nonetheless, high sampling frequencies and long study durations have the benefit of increasing the power of the statistical analyses conducted. For example, in a recent 4-week study with ~700 participants, we collected around 4 terabytes of data. Even with an experienced and dedicated research team, we have spent a great deal of effort and time deciding on and implementing a workflow regarding how to aggregate, process, and analyze the data. To this point, the decision on the length of the study should also be made while acknowledging research team bandwidth and resource limitations. Longer durations often require more work on the part of the researchers either in monitoring data collection or analyzing the data afterward, as well as additional resources whether it be the monetary compensation for participants or costs associated with storing, managing, and analyzing large datasets.

How to Address Ethical Issues?

Conducting mobile sensing research introduces a host of new ethical quandaries for the social scientist. How can one respect individual privacy while collecting mobile sensing data from personal devices? How can the data be managed in a secure fashion? How can the study plans be best communicated to ensure appropriate oversight by relevant ethical review boards? As illustrated in the sections above, a great deal of data can be collected that provides detailed information about a person's behaviors (and to some degree, psychological experiences) in context. This is exciting for scientific discovery, while simultaneously concerning with regard to its potential negative effects for the individual participants. In this section we outline some of the main considerations in the ethical domain for getting started with mobile sensing research. However, we point interested readers to Chapter 2 for more detailed discussion of privacy issues and Chapter 3 for discussion of ethical issues as they relate to transparency and reproducibility in this research area.

Privacy issues are one of the most salient ethical concerns with regard to mobile sensing research. This is because sensing methods permit the collection of fine-grained *personal data*, which refers to "any kind of log or sensor data that directly describes an individual" (Wiese, Das, Hong, & Zimmerman, 2017, p. 452). The effects of participation on the individual privacy of the participant depend in large part on (1) the perceptions and concerns of the participants, and (2) the design of the study and the data management and analysis plan established by the research team. With regard to the participants, it is important to consider that people may be uncertain about their privacy preferences and the consequences of their behavior (Acquisti, Brandimarte, & Loewenstein, 2015). For example, participants may be unaware or unsure about the kinds of information they are providing about themselves when they permit collection of GPS data (De Montjoye,

Hidalgo, Verleysen, & Blondel, 2013) or metadata from phone logs (Mayer, Mutchler, & Mitchell, 2016), both of which have been shown to be quite revealing about people's everyday behaviors. With regard to the design, some factors to consider are the types of data being collected, the sampling frequency being adopted, and the format of the data when it is collected. Generally, collecting and analyzing raw data is more sensitive than collecting and analyzing processed data. For example, collecting the *content* of communications is obviously more intrusive of participant privacy than collecting information about the *frequency* of communications. Similarly, raw GPS data (i.e., latitude and longitude coordinates) do not appear particularly sensitive in their raw format, but with additional preprocessing a person's home or work location could be inferred. A more privacy-preserving way of storing such location information would be to store the data as a categorical variable labeling the place a person was in (e.g., indexing a person was "home" or at "work"). In contrast, a threat to participant privacy would occur if such information were stored as the real address of the person's home or workplace. Given that participants may find sensing methods to be potentially invasive, special attention should be paid to facilitating transparency about the data being collected, participant control over personal data, and generally treating informed consent as a process (e.g., Harari, 2020; Kreuter, Haas, Keusch, Bähr, & Trappmann, 2020; Nebeker et al., 2016).

Data security is another aspect of the data management and analysis plan that is important to consider. Ensuring data security in a given study will be somewhat contingent on where the study is taking place (e.g., the institution, country), but some practices are relevant to almost all sensing studies. For example, with regard to the data management and analysis plan, some factors to consider are the people who will have access to the collected data and the strategy for processing and analyzing the data—for instance, ensuring that only key research personnel have access to personally identifying information about participants and that safeguards such as using secure servers for data storage and analysis can minimize potential concerns on behalf of participants and ethical review boards. When submitting mobile sensing research for ethical board review, several key things should be reported to ensure transparency about the design and research plans. In particular, we recommend describing the types of sensing data being collected, the format of the data, the location of where the data are stored, and the personnel who will have access to the files.

How to Recruit and Incentivize Participants?

Participant recruitment and compliance largely depend on the perceived benefits and costs of taking part in the study from the perspectives of the participants as well as their ability to fully participate. Because the cost of participating in a mobile sensing study tends to seem higher than that of other studies and because technologies (e.g., smartphones, wearables) or services (e.g., reliable internet access) are required, incentivizing individuals to make participation more appealing and providing participants with everything they need to actively participate are key to the success of a given study. In general, participant recruitment tends to be more challenging as people typically have concerns regarding privacy, personal data collection, data security, and data storage practices (see Chapter 2). Nevertheless, past mobile sensing studies have successfully recruited research participants from the student population, the general adult and elderly populations (e.g., Rachuri et al., 2010; Röcke, Katana, Fillekes, Martin, & Weibel, 2018; Saeb et al., 2015;

Stieger et al., 2021), and clinical populations (e.g., individuals undergoing chemotherapy, or those diagnosed with schizophrenia or bipolar disorder; Ben-Zeev et al., 2017; Low, 2020; Low et al., 2017; Matthews et al., 2016; Wang et al., 2017). In some cases, additional steps were taken to recruit participants (e.g., from hospitals and treatment centers) and onboard study participants to orient them to the goals and procedure of the study.

Furthermore, as mobile sensing studies require technologies and services that are not accessible to everyone, recruiting participants from rural areas, low-income communities, or developing nations may prove more challenging. According to Pew Research, smartphone adoption is growing in countries around the world, but countries with advanced economies have higher rates of ownership (e.g., in South Korea, Australia, and France, 75–95% of adults own a smartphone), compared to countries with emerging economies (e.g., in India, Indonesia, and South Africa, 24–60% of adults own a smartphone; Silver, 2019). However, with some creative planning in advance of the study launch, there are several ways to work around such constraints. For example, participants can be provided with the devices they need to participate (e.g., smartphones, wearables) and/or the services required for data collection for the study duration period (e.g., data plan for their phone). Providing such devices and services ensures that participants have the basic technical requirements needed to effectively participate in the study. It also can be a way to recruit participants from populations that do not readily have such technologies available to them, and it may help to target non-WEIRD (Western, educated, industrialized, rich, and democratic) samples (Henrich, Heine, & Norenzayan, 2010).

Once the target participants have been recruited into the study, keeping them incentivized and engaged with the study is another factor to consider. Motivations for participating and types of incentives preferred will vary by individual, but past studies have used monetary compensation, university credit, feedback reports, and lottery systems with varying levels of success (Farhan et al., 2016; Harari, Müller, Mishra, et al., 2017; Wang et al., 2014). Given their longitudinal nature and tendency to span weeks or months in duration, many sensing studies suffer from attrition due to participants dropping out over time, which can have negative impacts on the resulting dataset. Additional research is needed to better understand which incentives are most effective in maintaining high compliance rates. However, findings thus far suggest that adjusting self-tracking goals to align with participants' motivations and providing personalized feedback reports as an incentive (in addition to other forms of compensation like course credit, money, or prize lotteries) may help with compliance (Harari, Müller, Mishra, et al., 2017).

To keep attrition rates low, researchers should also consider how to balance study length with participant incentives. The success of the study and data collection efforts are impacted by rates of participation, so research teams have tested out different methods of incentive dispersion to sustain participant interest over time. For example, incentives can be spread out over the duration of the study—every few days, weeks, after every completed task, or all at once poststudy completion (Farhan et al., 2016; Wang et al., 2014). In a smartphone sensing study conducted within the Coping with Corona project in the fall of 2020 and spring of 2021 (Back et al., 2021; described in more detail in Table 1.2), the sample of university students recruited to participate received weekly feedback reports on their psychological states and behavior tendencies based on their sensing data and experience sampling reports. Students also received course credit after participating in each of the three steps in the study (i.e., completing a presurvey, self-tracking for 2 weeks, and reflecting on the study experience in a postsurvey). In a second COVID-19

Smartphone Sensing Study (Talaifar et al., 2021), we used a combination of monetary compensation and feedback reports as incentives for adults recruited from the community, and course credit and feedback reports as incentives for university students. Because adult participants were recruited through an online participant recruitment site, payment disbursements occurred when an individual either decided to no longer participate in the study or at the end of the study. The amount of compensation was dependent on the amount of time the individual spent participating. Feedback reports were also shared with participants weekly and included personalized information on their psychological states and behaviors.

These motivations and incentives should be substantial enough to outweigh the potential burden of participating whether that burden be the need to follow data uploading protocols, deal with app crashes or bugs, and, in some cases, use another device. As is the case with any mobile sensing study, typically participants must consistently follow procedures such as connecting to Wi-Fi and charging one's device regularly to upload their data. Additionally, there is a high likelihood that crashes and bugs in the mobile sensing platforms will arise and require individuals to troubleshoot with the guidance of the research team. These events are generally unavoidable, though they may pose negligible to varying amounts of burden among individuals in the population of interest and influence their decision to continue with the study in different manners. Also, researchers may decide to provide participants with a preprogrammed sensing device (Wang et al., 2014) rather than have them download a mobile sensing app on their personal device. This choice has some benefits, such as greater involvement from participant groups who do not have access to smartphones and services, as well as a standardization in device models or software, which ensures that all participants have devices with the same sensors necessary for some studies. At the same time, having some participants carry around a device second to their personal one may add yet another burden for them and lead to less accurate and missing data (e.g., phone logs; Harari et al., 2016). As providing a device also becomes more difficult with resource limitations and large samples of participants, most research teams opt for having participants use their own device when possible.

Furthermore, participant recruitment and incentives depend heavily on the context and nature of the study, which is why researchers often conduct pilot studies as a smaller-scale, shorter experiment to gauge what works and what does not. For example, based on pilot study recruitment and compliance statistics, researchers have general insight into whether (1) the recruitment strategy is effective, (2) people would be interested in and willing to participate, and (3) the current incentives are adequate. This also provides an opportunity to identify technology-related issues that need immediate attention before involving a large sample of participants or that the research team should be prepared to help troubleshoot.

Recommendations During and After Data Collection

Once the mobile sensing study has been designed, the next set of recommendations is more practical and focuses on the steps involved in conducting the study (e.g., monitoring data quality) and working with the data collected (e.g., data cleaning, processing, and analysis). Next, we outline our key recommendations, but for more detailed information we point interested readers to our past work on this topic (see Harari et al., 2016).

How to Check Participant Compliance and Data Quality?

Data monitoring involves checking compliance and data quality throughout the study. It is particularly important in sensing studies due to the technical demands and the unique challenges of the study design. First, sensing data are typically collected passively (i.e., without participant engagement), so any irregularities might go unnoticed by participants. Second, sensing data are collected continuously (i.e., with a high sampling frequency over uninterrupted periods of time), so problems must be detected quickly to intervene before the data quality is compromised. Third, while there is no need for active engagement with sensing apps in order for them to collect data, there are certain requirements for the app to function properly. For instance, all participants who take part in the sensing study must have their phone turned on and carry their phone with them as often as possible. Moreover, participants are often required to charge their phones and are connected to Wi-Fi regularly so their data can be uploaded. Lastly, some operating systems close apps that run in the background for too long, so participants have to regularly interact with the app to keep it running. In sum, it is important to regularly check the incoming data and to remind participants of the app's requirements.

Data monitoring involves downloading the sensor data and calculating and visualizing summary statistics, such as rates of uploads to the server or number of hours uploaded per day (Harari et al., 2016). Ideally, summary statistics should be calculated separately per sensor, as there may be problems with particular data sources. Some commercial platforms (e.g., Ethica Data, Ksana Health) provide data monitoring dashboards, which display data visualizations to researchers. We recommend checking the incoming data repeatedly throughout the study (e.g., at the end of each day) and contacting participants with missing data.

When monitoring the uploaded data, it is crucial to keep track of any problems that arise during the study. We recommend creating a data monitoring spreadsheet to document any issues that occurred during data collection. A rigorous documentation of problems will help to describe the study procedures later. Moreover, it is a crucial prerequisite for data cleaning.

How to Clean and Process the Data?

Sensing data are typically messy and should be cleaned before analyses. The data cleaning step is sometimes the most difficult step in the analysis, but it is also one of the most important steps. The choice of data cleaning procedures and their ordering can significantly impact the results of further analyses. Therefore, researchers should not use arbitrary data cleaning procedures (e.g., removing outliers when they could be real values) but should carefully think about data cleaning decisions before any analyses are run, and ideally, all decisions should be preregistered when possible.

Different types of data collection errors can compromise the quality of the data. With technically demanding data collections, error often results from technical problems. For instance, the sensing app might crash, or specific sensors might not be working properly (e.g., the GPS signal might be distorted; Müller et al., 2022). Moreover, there may be a lot of missing data if participants turn off their phones or accidentally close the app.

Different techniques are available to identify data collection errors. Unfortunately, only a few guidelines for data cleaning exist, and the decisions will always depend on the unique conditions of the study. Some authors have provided lists of problems they noticed when cleaning their own data and have provided recommendations for how to deal with these problems. For instance, in past work we have recommended removing: inaccurate or unrealistic data points (e.g., when two events occur simultaneously that do not seem possible, such as being in two different locations that are physically far apart within a very short time span); data points with missing timestamps or observations; duplicated data points; outliers (e.g., values above or below three standard deviations from the mean); and days or participants with too little data (e.g., less than 15 hours of data for a given day, or participants with only 1 day of data; Harari, Vaid, et al., 2020; Müller et al., 2022). These papers include relevant R code that provides more information about how one might go about executing these steps. The chapters in Part II and Part III of this handbook should also prove valuable for thinking through data cleaning steps for different types of data and for different analytic techniques.

After data cleaning, the raw sensing data have to be processed before any analysis can be run. The most common data processing process is to extract behavioral features. Feature extraction involves computing psychologically meaningful variables that can be used in further analyses, such as extracting locations visited from GPS data. For instance, in GPS data, psychologically meaningful locations (e.g., an individual's home) are typically represented by many different latitude and longitude coordinates. To extract mobility features for future analyses, researchers first determine key locations for every participant by clustering data points that are in close proximity to each other (for relevant R packages, see Müller et al., 2022). Next, researchers can interpret the locations (e.g., the home is often defined as the cluster where participants spend most of their time during the night) and calculate mobility features, such as the time spent in different locations based on the timestamps (Müller et al., 2022).

As another example, metadata logs (e.g., calls and app usage logs) typically consist of a list of timestamped events, such as when an app is opened or when an incoming call is received. Based on the number of entries and the associated timestamps, researchers can calculate frequencies (e.g., how often participants open an app or receives a phone call) and durations of events (e.g., Harari, Müller, Stachl, et al., 2020). Depending on the research question at hand, the features can be computed for different time intervals (e.g., across days, times of the day, or days of the week). For instance, researchers may calculate the frequency of calls for a given day and then average across days to obtain an estimate representative of a person's typical daily social tendencies (Harari, Müller, Stachl, et al., 2020).

Data from different sensors sometimes have to be combined to derive more complex features that rely on different sources of information (e.g., engaging in conversations in specific places). Sensing data can also be merged with self-report data, such as experience sampling reports. For instance, researchers may use smartphone sensing to obtain objective information about a person's behaviors or situational context, and experience sampling to ask participants about their subjective thoughts or feelings (Harari, Stachl, Müller, & Gosling, 2021). A detailed overview of all available features is beyond the scope of this chapter. However, it should be noted that the datasets are often very large (up to several gigabytes per participant) and that feature extraction requires advanced programming and analytical skills. Therefore, we recommend that psychological researchers interested in working with the unprocessed, raw sensing data refer to the mobile sensing literature for guidance on how to extract the variables of interest. As a starting point, we direct readers to the Reproducible Analysis Pipeline for Data Streams (RAPIDS) website.[3] This comprehensive resource provides an overview of different features and the code needed to compute them.

How to Analyze the Data?

After data cleaning and feature extraction, the data have to be prepared for analysis. Often, researchers have to aggregate their variables across different time spans (e.g., hourly, daily, weekly level) or levels of analysis (e.g., within-person vs. between-person) to answer the research question at hand. After data aggregation, researchers should check the distributions and psychometric properties (e.g., reliability) of all variables and select an appropriate analytic technique.

Because intensive longitudinal datasets consist of repeated observations from the same individuals, the analysis approach has to account for the nested structure of the data. Nested data are often analyzed using multilevel modeling (MLM; also called hierarchical linear modeling or random coefficient modeling; Hox, Moerbeek, & van de Schoot, 2018; Snijders & Bosker, 2012). Multilevel growth curve models (Bolger & Laurenceau, 2013) are one of several techniques to model intraindividual changes in variables across time. By using multilevel growth curve models, researchers can examine how behaviors change across different time spans (e.g., hours of the day, days of the week, or weeks of the academic semester) and examine different forms of change (e.g., linear, curvilinear, discontinuous). Importantly, MLM allows researchers to describe both normative behavior trajectories (e.g., how social behaviors change across the academic semester on average) as well as interindividual differences in these trajectories (to what extent the change trajectories differ between people) and how they are related to other individual difference variables (e.g., whether the differences in trajectories are predicted by personality traits).

In addition to research questions about the effects of time, intensive longitudinal studies are suited for research questions that focus on relationships between momentary states or momentary states and situational variables. Here, MLM allows researchers to disentangle effects on different levels of the analysis (Enders & Tofighi, 2007; Hamaker & Muthén, 2019). Specifically, when multiple measurements are collected from the same individuals, it is possible to analyze effects on both the within- and between-person levels. Within-person effects capture how time-point specific deviations from a person's average tendency in one variable are related to similar deviations in another variable. For instance, in a study that repeatedly assessed individuals' social behaviors (via sensing) and their mood (via the experience sampling method [ESM]), researchers might examine whether a given individual feels better after engaging in a social interaction compared to how they normally feel. Within-person relationships are particularly important when the focus is on intraindividual dynamics and individual differences therein (Kuper et al., 2021).

In addition to within-person relationships, researchers can examine between-person differences in behavioral tendencies. Between-person effects are obtained by aggregating the continuous sensing data on the person level (e.g., how much a person socializes on average) and using the behavioral aggregate instead of a self-report variable in further analyses. These aggregates serve as more objective estimates of how a person actually tends to behave in their everyday lives (as opposed to how they perceive themselves to behave).

Beyond MLM, there are more advanced techniques such as dynamic structural equation modeling, dynamic network analysis, person-centered/ideographic modeling, and machine learning. We point interested readers to Part III of this book for more information on these techniques for mobile sensing research. No matter the analytic technique selected to answer one's research questions, thorough and clear reporting of the data cleaning, processing, and analysis decisions is crucial for enhancing transparency and reproducibility in mobile sensing research (see Chapter 3 for more details).

Conclusions

Mobile sensing holds much promise for improving naturalistic observation in psychological science. The first wave of research studies at the intersection of psychology and computer science has showcased what is possible using these methods. However, a main factor that seems to be impeding the widespread use of these methods in the field more broadly is the lack of know-how regarding the steps involved in conducting a mobile sensing study. This chapter aims to address this knowledge gap by providing a starting point for those interested in or getting ready to launch a sensing study. In the future, more work needs to be done in the field to develop standardized guidelines and best practices for conducting mobile sensing research.

Notes

1. https://awareframework.com.
2. www.beiwe.org.
3. www.rapids.science/1.6.

REFERENCES

Acquisti, A., Brandimarte, L., & Loewenstein, G. (2015). Privacy and human behavior in the age of information. *Science, 347*(6221), 509–514.

Back, M., Bühner, M., Geukes, K., Gosling, S. D., Harari, G. M., Kroencke, L., et al. (2021, December 15). *Coping with Corona (CoCo).* osf.io/2tzp9.

Ben-Zeev, D., Brian, R., Wang, R., Wang, W., Campbell, A. T., Aung, M. S. H., et al. (2017). CrossCheck: Integrating self-report, behavioral sensing, and smartphone use to identify digital indicators of psychotic relapse. *Psychiatric Rehabilitation Journal, 40*(3), 266–275.

Blum, G. S., Rauthmann, J. F., Göllner, R., Lischetzke, T., & Schmitt, M. (2018). The nonlinear interaction of person and situation (NIPS) model: Theory and empirical evidence. *European Journal of Personality, 32*(3), 286–305.

Bolger, N., & Laurenceau, J.-P. (2013). *Intensive longitudinal methods: An introduction to diary and experience sampling research.* Guilford Press.

Buss, D. M., & Craik, K. H. (1980). The frequency concept of disposition: Dominance and prototypically dominant acts. *Journal of Personality, 48*(3), 379–392.

De Montjoye, Y.-A., Hidalgo, C. A., Verleysen, M., & Blondel, V. D. (2013). Unique in the crowd: The privacy bounds of human mobility. *Scientific Reports, 3*, 1–5.

Doryab, A., Villalba, D. K., Chikersal, P., Dutcher, J. M., Tumminia, M., Liu, X., et al. (2019). Identifying behavioral phenotypes of loneliness and social isolation with passive sensing: statistical analysis, data mining and machine learning of smartphone and fitbit data. *JMIR mHealth and uHealth, 7*(7), 1–19.

Enders, C. K., & Tofighi, D. (2007). Centering predictor variables in cross-sectional multilevel models: A new look at an old issue. *Psychological Methods, 12*(2), 121–138.

Farhan, A. A., Yue, C., Morillo, R., Ware, S., Lu, J., Bi, J., et al. (2016). Behavior vs. introspection: Refining prediction of clinical depression via smartphone sensing data. *2016 IEEE Wireless Health (WH)*, pp. 1–8.

Ferreira, D., Kostakos, V., & Dey, A. K. (2015). AWARE: Mobile context instrumentation framework. *Frontiers in ICT, 2*, 1–9.

Götz, F. M., Stieger, S., & Reips, U.-D. (2017). Users of the main smartphone operating systems (iOS, Android) differ only little in personality. *PloS One, 12*(5), 1–18.

Hamaker, E. L., & Muthén, B. (2019). The fixed versus random effects debate and how it relates to centering in multilevel modeling. *Psychological Methods, 25*(3), 365–379.

Harari, G. M. (2020). A process-oriented approach to respecting privacy in the context of mobile phone tracking. *Current Opinion in Psychology, 31*, 141–147.

Harari, G. M., Lane, N. D., Wang, R., Crosier, B. S., Campbell, A. T., & Gosling, S. D. (2016). Using smartphones to collect behavioral data in psychological science: Opportunities, practical considerations, and challenges. *Perspectives on Psychological Science, 11*(6), 838–854.

Harari, G. M., Müller, S. R., Aung, M. S., & Rentfrow, P. J. (2017). Smartphone sensing methods for studying behavior in everyday life. *Current Opinion in Behavioral Sciences, 18*, 83–90.

Harari, G. M., Müller, S. R., & Gosling, S. D. (2020). Naturalistic assessment of situations using mobile sensing methods. In J. F. Rauthmann, R. A. Sherman, & D. C. Funder (Eds.), *The Oxford handbook of psychological situations* (pp. 299–311). Oxford University Press.

Harari, G. M., Müller, S. R., Mishra, V., Wang, R., Campbell, A. T., Rentfrow, P. J., et al. (2017). An evaluation of students' interest in and compliance with self-tracking methods: Recommendations for incentives based on three smartphone sensing studies. *Social Psychological and Personality Science, 8*(5), 479–492.

Harari, G. M., Müller, S. R., Stachl, C., Wang, R., Wang, W., Bühner, M., et al. (2020). Sensing sociability: Individual differences in young adults' conversation, calling, texting, and app use behaviors in daily life. *Journal of Personality and Social Psychology, 119*(1), 204–228.

Harari, G. M., Stachl, C., Müller, S. R., & Gosling, S. D. (2021). Mobile sensing for studying personality dynamics in daily life. In J. F. Rauthmann (Ed.), *The handbook of personality dynamics and processes* (pp. 763–790). Academic Press.

Harari, G. M., Vaid, S. S., Müller, S. R., Stachl, C., Marrero, Z., Schoedel, R., et al. (2020). Personality sensing for theory development and assessment in the digital age. *European Journal of Personality, 34*(5), 649–669.

Henrich, J., Heine, S. J., & Norenzayan, A. (2010). Beyond WEIRD: Towards a broad-based behavioral science. *Behavioral and Brain Sciences, 33*(2–3), 111–135.

Hox, J. J., Moerbeek, M., & van de Schoot, R. (2018). *Multilevel analysis: Techniques and applications* (3rd ed.). Routledge.

Huckins, J. F., DaSilva, A. W., Wang, W., Hedlund, E., Rogers, C., Nepal, S. K., et al. (2020). Mental health and behavior of college students during the early phases of the COVID-19 pandemic: Longitudinal smartphone and ecological momentary assessment study. *Journal of Medical Internet Research, 22*(6), 1–13.

Kreuter, F., Haas, G.-C., Keusch, F., Bähr, S., & Trappmann, M. (2020). Collecting survey and smartphone sensor data with an app: Opportunities and challenges around privacy and informed consent. *Social Science Computer Review, 38*(5), 533–549.

Kuper, N., Modersitzki, N., Phan, L. V., & Rauthmann, J. F. (2021). The dynamics, processes, mechanisms, and functioning of personality: An overview of the field. *British Journal of Psychology, 112*(1), 1–51.

Low, C. A. (2020). Harnessing consumer smartphone and wearable sensors for clinical cancer research. *NPJ Digital Medicine, 3*, 1–7.

Low, C. A., Dey, A. K., Ferreira, D., Kamarck, T., Sun, W., Bae, S., et al. (2017). Estimation of symptom severity during chemotherapy from passively sensed data: Exploratory study. *Journal of Medical Internet Research, 19*(12), 1–11.

Matthews, M., Abdullah, S., Murnane, E., Voida, S., Choudhury, T., Gay, G., et al. (2016). Development and evaluation of a smartphone-based measure of social rhythms for bipolar disorder. *Assessment, 23*(4), 472–483.

Mayer, J., Mutchler, P., & Mitchell, J. C. (2016). Evaluating the privacy properties of telephone metadata. *Proceedings of the National Academy of Sciences, 113*(20), 5536–5541.

Mønsted, B., Mollgaard, A., & Mathiesen, J. (2018). Phone-based metric as a predictor for basic personality traits. *Journal of Research in Personality, 74*, 16–22.

Müller, S. R., Bayer, J. B., Ross, M. Q., Mount, J., Stachl, C., Harari, G. M., et al. (2022). Analyzing GPS data for psychological research: A tutorial. *Advances in Methods and Practices in Psychological Science, 5*(2), 1–11.

Müller, S. R., Peters, H., Matz, S. C., Wang, W., & Harari, G. M. (2020). Investigating the relationships between mobility behaviours and indicators of subjective well-being using smartphone-based experience sampling and GPS tracking. *European Journal of Personality, 34*(5), 714–732.

Nebeker, C., Lagare, T., Takemoto, M., Lewars, B., Crist, K., Bloss, C. S., et al. (2016). Engaging research participants to inform the ethical conduct of mobile imaging, pervasive sensing, and location tracking research. *Translational Behavioral Medicine, 6*(4), 577–586.

Rachuri, K. K., Musolesi, M., Mascolo, C., Rentfrow, P. J., Longworth, C., & Aucinas, A. (2010). EmotionSense: A mobile phones based adaptive platform for experimental social psychology research. In *Proceedings of the 12th ACM International Conference on Ubiquitous Computing* (pp. 281–290).

Röcke, C., Katana, M., Fillekes, M., Martin, M., & Weibel, R. (2018). Mobility, physical activity and social interactions in the daily lives of healthy older adults: The MOASIS project. *Innovation in Aging, 2*(S1), 274.

Saeb, S., Lattie, E. G., Schueller, S. M., Kording, K. P., & Mohr, D. C. (2016). The relationship between mobile phone location sensor data and depressive symptom severity. *PeerJ, 4*, 1–15.

Saeb, S., Zhang, M., Karr, C. J., Schueller, S. M., Corden, M. E., Kording, K. P., et al. (2015). Mobile phone sensor correlates of depressive symptom severity in daily-life behavior: An exploratory study. *Journal of Medical Internet Research, 17*(7), 1–12.

Silver, L. (2019, February 5). *Smartphone ownership is growing rapidly around the world, but not always equally*. www.pewresearch.org/global/2019/02/05/smartphone-ownership-is-growing-rapidly-around-the-world-but-not-always-equally

Snijders, T. A. B., & Bosker, R. (2012). *Multilevel analysis: An introduction to basic and advanced multilevel modeling* (2nd ed.). Sage.

Sonnenberg, B., Riediger, M., Wrzus, C., & Wagner, G. G. (2012). Measuring time use in surveys - How valid are time use questions in surveys?: Concordance of survey and experience sampling measures. *Social Science Research, 41*(5), 1037–1052.

Stachl, C., Au, Q., Schoedel, R., Gosling, S. D., Harari, G. M., Buschek, D., et al. (2020). Predicting personality from patterns of behavior collected with smartphones. *Proceedings of the National Academy of Sciences, 117*(30), 17680–17687.

Stachl, C., Hilbert, S., Au, Q., Buschek, D., De Luca, A., Bischl, B., et al. (2017). Personality traits predict smartphone usage. *European Journal of Personality, 31*(6), 701–722.

Statista. (2021, February 8). *Mobile operating systems' market share worldwide from January 2021 to January 2022*. www.statista.com/statistics/272698/global-market-share-held-by-mobile-operating-systems-since-2009

Stieger, M., Flückiger, C., Rüegger, D., Kowatsch, T., Roberts, B. W., & Allemand, M. (2021). Changing personality traits with the help of a digital personality change intervention. *Proceedings of the National Academy of Sciences, 118*(8), 1–9.

Talaifar, S., Harari, G. M., Marrero, Z., Stachl, C., Vaid, S., & Gosling, S. D. (2021). *Using smartphone sensing to describe behavior during the COVID-19 pandemic*. Presentation at the virtual annual meeting of the Society for Personality and Social Psychology.

Torous, J., Kiang, M. V., Lorme, J., & Onnela, J.-P. (2016). New tools for new research in psychiatry: A scalable and customizable platform to empower data driven smartphone research. *JMIR Mental Health, 3*(2), 1–17.

Wang, R., Chen, F., Chen, Z., Li, T., Harari, G. M., Tignor, S., et al. (2014). StudentLife: Assessing mental health, academic performance and behavioral trends of college students using smartphones. *Proceedings of the 2014 ACM International Joint Conference on Pervasive and Ubiquitous Computing*, pp. 3–14.

Wang, R., Harari, G., Hao, P., Zhou, X., & Campbell, A. T. (2015). SmartGPA: How smartphones can assess and predict academic performance of college students. *Proceedings of the 2015 ACM International Joint Conference on Pervasive and Ubiquitous Computing*, pp. 295–306.

Wang, R., Wang, W., Aung, M. S., Ben-Zeev, D., Brian, R., Campbell, A. T., et al. (2017). Predicting symptom trajectories of schizophrenia using mobile sensing. *Proceedings of the ACM on Interactive, Mobile, Wearable and Ubiquitous Technologies, 1*(3), 1–24.

Wang, R., Wang, W., DaSilva, A., Huckins, J. F., Kelley, W. M., Heatherton, T. F., et al. (2018). Tracking depression dynamics in college students using mobile phone and wearable sensing. *Proceedings of the ACM on Interactive, Mobile, Wearable and Ubiquitous Technologies, 2*(1), 1–26.

White, M. P., & Dolan, P. (2009). Accounting for the richness of daily activities. *Psychological Science, 20*(8), 1000–1008.

Wiese, J., Das, S., Hong, J. I., & Zimmerman, J. (2017). Evolving the ecosystem of personal behavioral data. *Human–Computer Interaction, 32*(5–6), 447–510.

CHAPTER 2

Designing for Privacy in Mobile Sensing Systems

Jason I. Hong

CHAPTER OVERVIEW

Privacy is a complex topic that involves social, legal, market, user experience, and technical issues. This chapter is intended for both researchers and developers of mobile sensing systems, and offers an overview of various definitions of privacy, legal, and pragmatic reasons to care about privacy, and why privacy is hard to achieve in practice. This chapter also covers system design issues, including design methods and frameworks for thinking about privacy, as well as implementation and deployment issues.

Introduction

In recent years, we have seen a Cambrian explosion of mobile devices that weave computation, communication, and sensing into our everyday lives. Today, one can purchase smart watches, fitness trackers, and wireless earbuds from big box retail stores, and smart glasses, smart clothes, and other wearables are not far away. These kinds of mobile sensing devices make it possible to understand human behavior and the world at large at a scale and fidelity never before possible.

There are many exciting opportunities in this space, for example, monitoring for major depression (Doryab, Min, Wiese, Zimmerman, & Hong, 2014; Saeb et al., 2015), measuring sleep quality and quantity (Lane et al., 2014; Min et al., 2014), detecting earthquakes (Kong, Allen, Schreier, & Kwon, 2016), estimating pollution (Devarakonda et al., 2013; Hasenfratz, Saukh, Sturzenegger, & Thiele, 2012), quantifying urban noise (Maisonneuve, Stevens, Niessen, & Steels, 2009), contact tracing, and more. These apps range from fully autonomous sensing to participatory sensing, where users help gather data about the world (Burke et al., 2006). Commercially, fitness apps are perhaps the most prominent applications of mobile sensing, with Fitbit having sold over 100 million devices (Statista, 2020a). Health apps are another rapidly growing area, with the U.S. Food and Drug Administration (FDA) also having recently started to approve smartphone apps for medical use.

A fundamental challenge, however, is that the exact same data can be used in positive ways as well as highly undesirable ways. Typically, these concerns fall under the broad umbrella term of *privacy*. Sharing one's location data can facilitate coordination and awareness between partners, but can also be abused to spy on romantic partners via spouseware or stalkerware software (Federal Trade Commission [FTC], 2019; Franceschi-Bicchierai & Cox, 2017). Some smartphone apps gather data about one's health, which can be used for quantified self, but they have also led to surprising and unwanted ads on social media sites (Reader, 2020; Statt, 2019). Even aggregated and anonymized data poses risks. For example, in 2018, the health fitness app Strava released a data visualization that aggregated the Global Positioning System (GPS) running routes of all of its users, which allowed astute observers to pinpoint the locations of likely U.S. military bases in Syria and Afghanistan (Hern, 2018).

This chapter presents an overview of privacy for mobile sensing, presenting both research in this area and Privacy by Design, that is, how to embed privacy in the design and operation of mobile sensing devices and services (Cavoukian, 2009). For a more general treatment of designing for privacy, see the survey paper by Iachello and Hong (2007). We start out by discussing why researchers and developers of mobile sensing apps should care about privacy. Next, we analyze some constraints and forces at play that make privacy hard to achieve in practice. We continue with a discussion of best practices in designing and deploying mobile sensing systems, looking at some methods and some relevant past findings that may help inform designs. We finish with a discussion of technical issues, including implementation, algorithms, and software architectures.

What Is Privacy?

Privacy is a broad, ill-defined term that captures a wide range of concerns about our relationships with other people and organizations. In fact, there is not a widely agreed-upon definition of privacy that fits all of the cases people care about (Solove, 2008). Some regulations even step around the difficulty of defining privacy by focusing instead on "data protection."

One of the oldest definitions of *privacy* is "the right to be let alone" (Brandeis & Warren, 1890). Later, in the 1960s, as computer databases were becoming commercially available, concerns over the ease with which personal information could be collected and searched led Alan Westin (1967, p. 7) to define privacy as "the claim of individuals, groups, or institutions to determine for themselves when, how, and to what extent information about them is communicated to others."

However, new computer technologies and new uses led to new perspectives on privacy. For example, Bellotti and Sellen (1993), in the context of shared media spaces, centered on end-user control and feedback over one's data. Palen and Dourish (2003), building on social psychology, characterized privacy as a dynamic process of boundary negotiation. Lederer and colleagues (2004) looked at a complementary notion—that an important part of privacy is others seeing you the way you want to be seen—building on Goffman's (1978) ideas of presentation of self in everyday life. Nissenbaum (2004) argued for contextual integrity, emphasizing that uses of data need to conform to political, ethical, and social norms that might evolve over time. The European Union has advanced "the right to be forgotten" as a fundamental privacy right, giving people the option to ask organizations to delete data about them (Daley, 2011). Anonymity is yet another view of privacy and is an especially popular perspective among computer scientists and statisticians because, unlike the other definitions of privacy, it can be quantified and compared against other techniques.

These are just some of the many views and definitions of privacy. One reason for this diversity is that privacy is being encroached on in many ways in modern life. Privacy isn't just about Big Brother, or about corporations collecting lots of data about us. Instead, privacy is about our relationships with all of the individuals and organizations we interact with, each of which poses different issues for privacy and all of which are changing because of advances in technology. For example, with respect to friends and family, some privacy concerns might be overly protective parents or nosy siblings. With employers, the issues might include being constantly monitored at work or workplace discrimination. With governments, the fears might be civil liberties and mass surveillance. With stalkers and hackers, the worries might be one's personal safety or theft of highly personal or potentially embarrassing information.

A key point here is that we need different solutions for the different problems that arise in our different relationships. For example, a common element of privacy laws is notice and consent, which is arguably appropriate for corporations but nonsensical for friends and family. People don't hand their friends a privacy policy before chatting. So while there is no consensus on privacy, these different perspectives helps us focus on specific aspects of privacy. For example, the "right to be let alone" leads to do not call lists and spam filters. The "right to be forgotten" leads to people being able to request that web pages about them be deleted from search engines.

In this chapter, we take a pragmatic view of privacy, loosely defining it as the collection and use of sensitive data in an appropriate and understandable manner.

Security versus Privacy

Security and privacy are two related but distinct concepts. Security was originally defined as confidentiality (unauthorized parties cannot see sensitive data), integrity (unauthorized parties cannot modify that data), and availability (ensuring that data or a service can be used by authorized individuals) (Saltzer & Schroeder, 1975). Today, there are other useful properties to consider for security, for instance, usability (e.g., people can correctly understand and configure security settings) and physical safety (e.g., an autonomous drone will not crash into buildings).

Security is necessary for privacy, but it is not sufficient. For example, Facebook likely has strong security measures, but their data practices still raise many concerns. Also, rather than being a binary state of being secure or not secure, security is more of a spectrum with tradeoffs in terms of cost, complexity, and level of protection. Furthermore, security can be thought of as an ongoing process rather than something you just do once.

These viewpoints on security also apply to privacy in that there is a spectrum of privacy and it is an ongoing process.

In this chapter, we assume reasonable security precautions are in place, and instead we focus on the privacy issues involved with designing, implementing, and deploying mobile sensing apps. Also, note that there are some arguments about fundamental trade-offs between security and privacy. These arguments use a different notion of security, one that is more akin to safety or national security than to computer security. We do not delve into these discussions in this chapter.

Data Privacy versus Personal Privacy

It is also useful to distinguish between data privacy and personal privacy. *Data privacy* is primarily about how organizations collect, use, and protect sensitive data. A major class of sensitive data is Personally Identifiable Information (PII), which the National Institute of Standards and Technology (NIST, 2010) defines as "any information that can be used to distinguish or trace an individual's identity." Examples might include one's name, street address, unique IDs, and pictures. For mobile sensing apps, it might also include behavioral patterns and activities. Data privacy has a strong emphasis on policies and procedures for gathering and using data, many of which are based on Fair Information Practices (FIPs). Many laws embody the FIPs, such as the European Union's General Data Protection Regulation (GDPR) and the U.S. Health Insurance Portability and Accountability Act (HIPAA), Children's Online Privacy Protection Act (COPPA), and Right to Financial Privacy Act. While there are many variations of FIPs, they typically include notice and awareness, choice and consent, access and participation, integrity and security, and enforcement and redress (Cate, 2006; FTC, 1998).

In contrast, *personal privacy* focuses on one's relationships with other individuals, often with an emphasis on managing one's presentation of self to others and negotiating boundaries with others. Examples might include choosing what one shares with friends on social media, opting to put vague information about a sensitive event in a shared online calendar, or switching to invisible mode in an online game to avoid interruptions.

Many products and services need to be designed for both data privacy and personal privacy. Using a mobile sensing fitness app as an example shows that some data privacy concerns include choosing what data are sensed, selecting what data are sent over the network, where that data are stored, securing that data, establishing procedures for how that data are used, making sure users are aware of what data the app collects, offering basic privacy controls, and having good default settings. Some personal privacy concerns might include options for users to add friends and share fitness data with their friends, blocking spammers, and opting in to be part of a global leaderboard.

Note that data privacy tends to be oriented around procedures, in terms of following a set of rules and checking off a set of boxes. In contrast, personal privacy centers more on how users of a system might interact with one another, making sure users feel empowered in understanding and controlling what is shared, as well as minimizing the ways that users can harm others. Privacy tends to be hard to measure in both of these cases, making it difficult to apply quantitative methods to guide the design process or ensure that things are improving over time.

In this chapter, we will discuss issues related to design and implementation in the context of both data privacy and personal privacy.

Why Care about Privacy?

Many books and scholarly articles have framed privacy variously as a moral right, a basic human right, or an essential legal right. The European Union's GDPR Article 1 opens with "This Regulation protects fundamental rights and freedoms of natural persons and in particular their right to the protection of personal data." There is extensive literature advancing these perspectives on privacy and its importance for individuals and society.

We again take a pragmatic perspective on privacy. In particular, the literature suggests that people's privacy concerns are often expressed in specific ways, such as protection from spam (Cranor, Reagle, & Ackerman, 2000) and identity theft (Auxier et al., 2019), the "creepiness" of being tracked by apps (Shklovski, Mainwaring, Skúladóttir, & Borgthorsson, 2014), or wanting to avoid undesired social obligations (Hindus, Mainwaring, Leduc, Hagström, & Bayley, 2001). These attitudes often result in people not adopting technologies viewed as invasive. This last point is especially relevant for mobile sensing apps. A 2015 Pew Research Center survey found that 60% of people chose not to install an app when they discovered how much personal info it required and 43% uninstalled it for the same reason (Olmstead & Atkinson, 2015). A survey by Consumers International (2019) found that 63% of people found connected devices "creepy" in the way they collect data about people, and 28% of people who do not own smart devices were concerned enough to not purchase one in the future. In short, if people have significant privacy concerns, they won't adopt the technologies we research and build.

Failure to address privacy can also lead to serious legal repercussions. For example, the FTC has levied fines on smartphone apps for not informing users what data will be collected and for what purposes (FTC, 2013a, 2013c). There are also new laws—most notably, the European Union's GDPR, the California Online Privacy Protection Act (CalOPPA), and the California Consumer Protection Act (CCPA)—governing notice and consent, with heavy fines for noncompliance. Notably, the FTC has started to require violators to disgorge data. For example, in March 2022, the FTC settled with Weight Watchers over claims of violating children's privacy and required them to delete both improperly collected data and models based on that data (Oberly, Bryan, & Fath, 2022).

In addition, in the United States, there are many different privacy laws, each focused on specific sectors or demographics, such as children, education, finances, and even video and digital rentals. In particular, commercial mobile sensing apps focused on health care in the United States may need to comply with HIPAA as well as FDA regulations. Note that this is one reason why many mobile sensing apps are positioned as fitness or lifestyle apps rather than health care apps, so as to avoid these kinds of health care regulations.

Furthermore, mobile sensing apps that record videos and audios of people may need to comply with local laws. See Chapters 10 ("Behavioral Audio Signal Processing in Mobile Sensing Research") and 11 ("Acquisition and Analysis of Camera Sensor Data [Life Logging]"), this volume, for more details about the range of laws and regulations.

In short, for commercial mobile sensing apps, it may be simpler to avoid recording video and audio if possible. If video and audio are to be recorded, development teams should consult a lawyer about the best ways to comply with various international laws and with any requests for data from law enforcement organizations.

For research-oriented mobile sensing apps, the main requirement is to comply with one's Institutional Review Board (IRB) or equivalent. Some criteria are common to all IRB-approved studies, for example, having clear notice and consent and letting participants stop the study at any time. Some other criteria to consider for mobile sensing apps include keeping data collection to a minimum, preventing potential harms that may arise due to other people seeing the mobile sensing device (e.g., any stigma) as well as any sensed data (e.g., a romantic partner), and minimizing risks to people who might be incidentally recorded (e.g., bystanders). Also, for apps addressing mental well-being, the research team should consider how to handle situations where the gathered data indicate that someone may be at risk of harming themselves or others.

Complementary to legal requirements are social norms and expectations of privacy. In many cases, these norms revolve around privacy for other people rather than the individual using a mobile sensing device. As an example, movie theaters ask moviegoers to turn off their mobile phones so as to not disturb *other* moviegoers. Perhaps the most publicized social pushback against mobile sensing devices was with Google Glass, with people who wore them in public places called "glassholes" (Gross, 2014). A common concern was that people felt they could be surreptitiously monitored at any time (Hong, 2013). These kinds of social reactions can be difficult to predict, and as we discuss in the next section, social norms can change over time. However, the main point here is that privacy needs to consider not just the direct user of a mobile sensing system but also people who may be indirectly impacted.

In summary, mobile sensing devices need to address privacy concerns on a large number of fronts, including individual users, legal and regulatory bodies, and social norms.

Why Is Privacy Hard?

Privacy is a complex topic that intertwines thorny legal, social, market, and technical issues. In this subsection, we look at some of the forces that help shape the privacy landscape. These forces are not a complete list, but we discuss them here to help readers understand some desiderata for privacy as well as constraints on possible solutions.

Technological Capabilities Are Rapidly Growing

Gathering data about people is becoming easier and more pervasive. Everything on the Web is instrumented, making it trivial to collect Web clicks, social media posts, likes, and search terms. A typical smartphone has an array of sensors that can continuously capture data as we go about our daily lives, offering a rich digital portrait of who we are and what we do.

Data storage has also been improving dramatically, making it practical to store, index, and search all of these data. Machine learning is also becoming more powerful and able to infer surprising things about people—for example, using smartphone data to model the onset of major depression (Doryab et al., 2014; Saeb et al., 2015), using one's purchase patterns to deduce pregnancy (Duhigg, 2012), or using one's friends on Facebook to infer sexual orientation (Jernigan & Mistree, 2009). This last example is particularly salient in that an individual might not explicitly disclose sensitive information about themselves, but this information can still be inferred. The other side of the coin is that incorrect inferences can also be made, which can impact an individual in unexpected ways. Overall, these kinds of technical capabilities will only continue to advance, making it harder for people to control the flow of information about themselves.

There Are Strong Incentives for Companies to Collect Data about People

Companies want to collect more data about us because more data mean better machine learning models, which lead to better services, analytics, and ads. Whole industries are now driven entirely by Big Data, such as search engines, speech recognition, image recognition, recommendations, spam filtering, and fraud detection, just to name a few.

Advertising is a particularly voracious consumer of data. An average online ad displayed on a Web page will see clickthrough rates of around 0.05% (SmartInsight, 2020). Anything that can improve those clickthrough rates, even by a small amount, can be worth millions of dollars. As such, more data mean more targeted ads that are more likely to be clicked on.

There are also new kinds of business models for selling hardware based on collecting data about users, known as *postpurchase monetization* (Gilbert, 2019). For example, smart TVs are relatively expensive, and margins are razor thin. One way of improving sales is to lower initial purchase costs, and then use sensors and other tracking to collect rich data about the owners, to sell the data, and to improve targeted advertising. Thus, in addition to simply selling the hardware, a company can also create a continuous revenue stream using sensed data. For example, Vizio, a public company that sells smart TVs, reported that it had profits of about $48 million from selling hardware and about $38 million from selling viewer data and ads (Lawler, 2021).

These incentives for collecting data also lead companies to push back against privacy features. For example, Do Not Track was a Web standard that would let people share tracking preferences with websites. However, the effort ended in 2019 with a note that "there has not been sufficient deployment of these extensions (as defined) to justify further advancement, nor have there been indications of planned support among user agents, third parties, and the ecosystem at large. The working group has therefore decided to conclude its work" (W3C Working Group, 2019).

Companies Get Little Pushback on Privacy

In practice, developers get little negative feedback about privacy from consumers. In an analysis of Google Play reviews, Fu and colleagues (2013) found very few words related to privacy. Similarly, Ha and Wagner (2013) found that only 1% of app reviews mentioned app permissions. Emami-Naeini, Dixon, Agarwal, and Cranor (2019) found similar issues with IoT (Internet of Things) devices; they reported that most consumers did not consider privacy and security prior to their purchase and only became concerned later on because of media reports, comments from friends, or unexpected device behavior. They also found that finding privacy and security information before a purchase was difficult, if any existed at all. This combination of imperfect information and lack of negative feedback leads to what economists call a *market failure* (Hubbard & O'Brien, 2015). Suppose that you want to purchase a Web cam. You can go to your favorite electronics store and compare Web cams based on price, color, and features. However, you can't easily compare these Web cams on privacy (or security, for that matter). As a result, privacy does not strongly influence customer purchases, and so companies are not incentivized to improve privacy.

Several projects have sought to address this problem, all with a common theme of improving transparency. For example, PrivacyGrade.org graded apps based on their privacy (Lin, Liu, Sadeh, & Hong, 2014). Similarly, Emami-Naeini, Agarwal, Cranor, and Hibshi (2020) proposed a privacy nutrition label for IoT devices that would summarize behaviors. Since 2021, Apple has mandated that iOS apps must have a privacy nutrition label that reports what data are used to track users (Morse, 2020). Google has also mandated a new safety section for Android apps highlighting similar information (Frey, 2021). However, a study by Li, Reiman, Agarwal, Cranor, and Hong (2022) suggests that developers face many challenges in filling out these labels correctly. Furthermore, while improving transparency should in theory have a positive effect on privacy, it is unclear how effective they are in practice. For example, as discussed in the next item below, privacy policies aim to improve transparency but have arguably failed in practice.

Developers Have Low Awareness and Knowledge of Privacy Issues and Practices

Studies of smartphone app developers have found that few knew about existing privacy laws or privacy frameworks, what privacy issues they should pay attention to, and how to address them (Balebako, Marsh, Lin, Hong, & Cranor, 2014; Li, Agarwal, & Hong, 2018). Developers also have low awareness of privacy problems with their apps, with many not realizing how much data their app is collecting (Agarwal & Hall, 2013; Balebako et al., 2014; Li et al., 2018). Other studies have examined how developers talk about privacy in online forums. Some developers turn to Stack Overflow for privacy issues, including company requirements (Tahaei, Vaniea, & Saphra, 2020). On a popular Android developer forum, Li, Louie, Dabbish, and Hong (2020) found that developers rarely talked about privacy, and most discussions of privacy were driven by external factors such as changes to smartphone operating systems or app stores.

A major pain point is lack of awareness of the behaviors of third-party libraries. A library is a package of code that offers common functionality and is designed to be easily used by other apps, for example, managing graphics, connecting with social media, or displaying ads. Many third parties offer libraries to connect with their services, for example, Facebook and Twitter. These libraries tend to be used as black boxes. However, in a year-long user study of apps, Chitkara, Gothoskar, Harish, Hong, & Agarwal (2017) found that over 40% of smartphone apps collect sensitive data only because of these libraries. In other words, many apps collect sensitive data and share it with multiple third parties, and their app developers might not even be aware of this behavior.

It's Not Always Clear What the Right Thing to Do Is

Even if a company wants to be respectful of privacy, it's not always clear how to translate that wish into practice. For example, while privacy policies are pervasive, past research has found that few people read them (Auxier et al., 2019, Obar & Oeldorf-Hirsch, 2020). In many respects, not reading these privacy policies is rational. McDonald and Cranor (2008) estimated that it would take 25 full days to read all the privacy policies that one encounters on the Web in a single year.

More broadly, there isn't a widely accepted set of privacy best practices for developers to follow. How can designers best assess what kinds of data uses are and are not acceptable? What is the best way of informing people about data collection practices? What is the best way of storing data? The effectiveness of today's framework of notice and consent is also highly questionable. Cate argues that the Fair Information Practice Principles have failed in practice, stating that "businesses and other data users are burdened with legal obligations while individuals endure an onslaught of notices and opportunities for often limited choice" (Cate, 2006, p. 1).

Similarly, business metrics for privacy are also unclear. Corporations have many metrics such as Customer Acquisition Cost, Year over Year Growth, and Retention Rates. However, it is unclear what the right metrics are for privacy, making it hard to see if progress is being made. Also, as noted earlier, there is a strong incentive to collect data because it impacts the bottom line, and so one could go even further by saying that some business metrics implicitly push against privacy.

The Burden of Privacy on End Users Is Too High

Today, individuals have to make too many decisions about privacy. Does this website have good privacy protections? Should I install this app? What are all the privacy settings I need to know for this device? What are all the terms and conditions for this service? What are trackers, cookies, virtual private networks (VPNs), anonymizers, and incognito mode, and how do I use them to protect my privacy?

Mobile sensing can exacerbate the burden of privacy. SenseCam is a wearable camera developed by Microsoft Research for lifelogging. SenseCam raised many issues about personal privacy; for example, what data are captured and when, and what potential stigmatization may exist since one use of the device was to help people with mental disabilities (King et al., 2013). SenseCam also raised concerns about other people's privacy, for example, incidentally recording other people nearby. To address this problem, the SenseCam researchers designed it to not record audio and made it easy to pause video recording. A study by other researchers found that other people were generally OK with using recorded images for limited purposes, and also wanted notice and consent (Nguyen et al., 2009). However, how to do notice and consent for mobile sensing devices is an open question, let alone how to make it scale if these devices become commonplace. As a counterpoint, in an *in situ* study where participants wore a lifelogging device, bystanders expressed no concerns, and participants wanted to control the capture of images in situ rather than spending time to review images afterward (Hoyle et al., 2014).

In short, the burden of privacy is too high on individual end users, and it will only get worse as technological capabilities advance and mobile sensing devices become more common.

Same Device, Same Data, Very Different Reactions

When new technologies are adopted, they are done so in a specific social and cultural context. Judging whether a given technology or type of data is good or bad for privacy often depends on how it is used within this context. For example, in my dissertation (Hong, 2005), I looked at how nurses used locator badges, which could pinpoint the location of individuals in a hospital. The hospital administration viewed these badges as useful for coordination (e.g., "Where is Alice?") and for protection of individuals from spurious claims (e.g., "The nurse never came to visit me"). However, many nurses felt these badges would be used for surveillance, for example, tracking how long they were in the restroom. In cases where there was clear value for nurses and management was trusted, locator badges were viewed mostly positively. However, if there were existing tensions between the nurses and management, the nurses tended to reject the badges. In other words, the exact same technology was viewed differently depending on external social and cultural factors.

As another example, Foursquare is a social media app that lets people check in to a place and share those check-ins with others. One person took these check-in data and created Girls Around Me, overlaying photos from women's Foursquare profiles on a map (Blue, 2012). The same data are arguably acceptable in one context but with a few slight twists becomes creepy in another.

Complicating matters is the tendency of some users of a system to deliberately try to harm others. For example, the same technology that might be used to streamline coordination in a healthy relationship can facilitate many forms of intimate partner abuse (Matthews et al., 2017).

Woven throughout these examples are power imbalances that can color people's perceptions of privacy. In the case of the nurses, hospital administration can easily fire any single individual. For Girls Around Me, there is potential harm from unknown individuals. For intimate partner violence, there is a strong potential for physical, mental, and emotional harm from a romantic partner. As such, a major challenge in designing mobile sensing systems is understanding the different kinds of social contexts and power dynamics in which one's system might be used, predicting potential misuses and abuses, and designing the system to mitigate these negative scenarios while facilitating positive ones.

Expectations of Privacy Can Change over Time, Sometimes Dramatically So

Over time, people's expectations of privacy can change in ways that are hard to predict. For example, Brandeis and Warren's (1890) famous definition of privacy as "the right to be let alone" came about in part because new cameras in the late 19th century made it possible to take photographs in just several seconds, invading "the sacred precincts of private and domestic life." Today, millions of people choose to share photos on publicly visible social media. Currently, the problem of cameras still exists. The main difference is that our expectations of how these technologies can be used, as well as social norms and laws, have changed over many decades.

Expectations of privacy can also change quite rapidly and dramatically. A good example is the introduction of Facebook's News Feed in 2006 (D'Onfro, 2016; Newcomb, 2018). Before News Feed, one could only see a person's status updates by going to their individual profile pages. What News Feed did was aggregate those updates in a single place. When News Feed was first made public, people's initial reactions were predominantly negative, often viscerally so. Many Facebook groups were formed denouncing News Feed, and Facebook CEO Mark Zuckerberg even publicly responded to all of the negative press. Facebook stayed its course, however, and in a few months, a lot of the criticism died out as people saw value in News Feed and became used to it. Nowadays, it is doubtful that many people would want to give up News Feed.

In summary, people's initial expectations of privacy are fluid and can change quickly but not necessarily in ways that are easy to predict. There have been many failures where product teams have made incorrect assumptions about people's attitudes and behaviors. There have also been examples of product teams facing initial resistance due to privacy concerns, but eventually people have been won over. Furthermore, the research literature also does not offer much guidance in terms of findings or methods for differentiating findings from methods, largely due to the difficulty of studying these kinds of questions in the wild. As such, the best ways of understanding, managing, and influencing people's expectations with respect to privacy remain an open question.

System Design for Privacy

In this section, we examine user-centered design processes for mobile sensing apps, discussing privacy with respect to functionality as well as user interface design. Note that there are some existing guidelines for mobile app privacy. For example, FTC (2013b, 2016) offers advice for mobile apps and for mobile health. Similarly, both Apple (2020a) and Google (2020) offer best practices for app privacy. These are good starting points but are not sufficient because these guidelines are meant more for conventional apps than for rich mobile sensing apps.

Similarly, there are several laws governing the use of sensitive data, notice, and consent, such as HIPAA, GDPR, and CCPA. These laws offer a good start but do not offer much guidance as to design and implementation. Note that GDPR requires a Data Protection Impact Assessment (DPIA) for new projects that pose "a high risk to the rights and freedoms of natural persons" (https://gdpr-info.eu/art-35-gdpr). At a high level, a DPIA involves a description of data processing, an assessment of necessity and proportionality, and an evaluation of risks to rights and freedoms. The GDPR website has a template that can be used to help step through this process (GDPR.eu, n.d.).

Here, we examine four different topics related to design:

1. A privacy risk model, which offers a series of questions to consider about data collection and data use. This kind of risk model is perhaps the most useful thing that researchers and developers can do, as it guides teams into considering what data are being collected, how the data are used, and how the data can be protected.
2. Methods for getting feedback from participants early in the design process while it is still relatively easy to make changes. This kind of feedback can be used to validate and refine the privacy risk model.
3. Optimistic versus pessimistic approaches to privacy.
4. Choosing defaults for privacy settings.

Privacy Risk Models

Development teams need to carefully consider what data will be collected and how that data will be protected. Privacy risk models help development teams think through these issues and their implications. Again, we assume that reasonable security measures are already in place, for example, ensuring that any passwords are secure, that databases with sensitive data are locked down properly, and that strong encryption is used when storing data and when sending it over the network.

Privacy risk models are inspired by the concept of security threat models in computer security. One security researcher describes the importance of security threat models as follows:

> [T]he first rule of security analysis is this: understand your threat model. Experience teaches that if you don't have a clear threat model—a clear idea of what you are trying to prevent and what technical capabilities your adversaries have—then you won't be able to think analytically about how to proceed. The threat model is the starting point of any security analysis. (Felten, 2003)

We call this model a privacy risk rather than a privacy threat model because computer security tends to frame the defense of a system in terms of attackers and adversaries, which does not quite capture the rich range of relationships and privacy concerns we have with other people. For example, a college student might be close with their parents but still not want to share their current location or activity data with their parents. Similarly, some elderly individuals may be OK with sharing their historical activity and fitness data with their children, while others might not. It would be incorrect to label these kinds of relationships as attackers or threats.

Below, we present one privacy risk model for sensor-based systems. This risk model is an updated version developed by Hong, Ng, Lederer, and Landay (2004) and consists of a series of questions to consider. Note that these questions are meant as a starting point for difficult conversations within research and development teams rather than as something that can offer all of the answers. Furthermore, these questions should be validated with potential users of the system, and they should be revisited and refined in parallel with the design and evaluation of early-stage prototypes. We have organized the questions by user experience design, social, organizational, and technical aspects. Note that we do not explicitly consider business concerns here, as that is beyond the scope of this chapter, though they may have significant influence on privacy.

Design Issues

- What kinds of personal information are sensed or gathered (e.g., name, email)?
- How sensitive is the data? If leaked, can the data be easily linked to a specific individual?
- Is there a clear value proposition for end users for sharing their personal data? Is this value proposition clear to end users?
- Does this data collection match people's expectations about the app? For example, it makes sense for a sleep monitor to use a microphone but perhaps not for a food diary app.
- For each type of sensitive information, is it opt-in or opt-out, or do data sharers even have a choice?
- What is the minimal amount of data needed for the mobile device and associated apps? Does the data need to be collected at all?
- What devices and sensors are used to collect personal information? Who has physical control over these devices and sensors?
- What happens if there are sensing or inferencing errors on the data? Is there potential for embarrassment or other mishaps?
- How are data collection and data use practices conveyed to users?
- What kinds of controls and feedback do end users have for managing their personal data? Are these user interfaces easily understandable and accessible?

Social Context

- Who are the data sharers, the people sharing personal information? What kinds of concerns do they have?
- Who are the data observers, other users who might see and use that personal information?
- What kinds of personal data are shared with data observers?
- What are the relationships between data sharers and data observers? What is the level and nature of trust? Is there a power imbalance? What incentives do data observers have to protect data sharers' personal information (or not, as the case may be)?
- Are there potentially malicious data observers (e.g., spammers, stalkers, abusive partners, trolls)? How might they abuse your system?
- What are the social and cultural norms around how personal information will be used?
- What are the data sharers' expectations about how personal information will be used?
- Are there other stakeholders or third parties who might be directly or indirectly impacted by the system, for example, passersby incidentally near a mobile sensing system?

Organizational Context

- What are the policies and procedures for accessing the data by people internal to the organization? What kinds of data and granularities can people internal to the organization see? How will these be enforced? Will accesses be logged and audited?
- Will any collected data be shared with any third parties? Can the data be anonymized before sharing?

Technical Issues

- How are users identified? Is it a device hardware identifier, an app-specific identifier, a user-specified identifier (such as a username or email address), or an advertising identifier (e.g., Apple's IDFA or Google's AAID)? Each has tradeoffs over how much control users have and how much people can be tracked across devices and apps.
- What is the granularity of the information sent or shared, for example, with respect to space (e.g., room, building, street), time (e.g., continuous, every hour, every day), or fidelity (e.g., for identity, is it a specific person, a pseudonym, or anonymous)? How often is information shared? Is it discrete and one time? Is it continuous?
- Can the data be processed entirely on the device? Do the data need to leave the device?
- What sensitive data are sent to the backend? Where are these data stored? Note that there may be legal implications based on in which country the data are stored. Who has access to the data? How long are data retained? What about backups of data?

Note that there are also other models for assessing privacy, including the Privacy Risk Assessment Methodology (PRAM; NIST, 2015) and Privacy Impact Assessment (PIA; Wright & De Hert, 2011). These frameworks are derived from information security and treat privacy in a manner similar to security risks. For example, PRAM asks experts to map out the data processing pipeline within the target system and then catalog contextual factors and data actions that process personal information. Experts then enumerate all potential problems associated with each data action and assign scores to the likelihood and severity of each problem. In this way, development teams can quantify and prioritize privacy risks for the organization (e.g., revenue loss from customer abandonment), and determine appropriate resource allocations to address the risks. Note that both PRAM and PIA focus more on data privacy rather than personal privacy and center more on privacy risks for organizations than end users. Furthermore, neither PRAM nor PIA advocates getting feedback from users about privacy.

Iterative Design and Formative Methods for Probing People's Privacy Concerns

A common best practice in User Experience (UX) design is to design, implement, and evaluate systems as an iterative process rather than a waterfall process. That is, it is better to quickly build cheap mockups and prototypes, put them in front of potential users, get feedback in the early stages of design, and then repeat the whole process with more functional prototypes, rather than linearly trying to do design, implementation, and evaluation just once.

The iterative design process makes it easier to understand people's potential privacy concerns early on and adjust the design as a result. It can also shed light on many of the questions in the privacy risk model (below) and help the development team better understand the tradeoffs involved in the early stages of design, when it is still relatively cheap and easy to make changes.

An important question then is, how can one build mockups and prototypes of mobile sensing apps that are good enough to get feedback? One technique is paratyping (Iachello, Truong, Abowd, Hayes, & Stevens, 2006), which combines experience prototyping with the experience sampling method (ESM). Researchers interact with people as they normally would. At the end of a social encounter, the researcher would hand over a small postcard-sized survey to the other individual, which would explain what data would have been sensed if the mobile sensing device was deployed for real, and ask questions about one's perceptions of privacy in that situation. This survey would come prestamped and could be mailed back to the researchers. For example, Iachello and colleagues (2006) conducted a paratyping study of a Personal Audio Loop, a device that could continuously record audio but only retain the last few minutes. Their survey asked people how important it would be to be aware of the Personal Audio Loop, how important it would be to ask for permission first, how long a conversation should be retained, and so on. This approach lets the researchers investigate people's potential concerns about mobile sensing early in the product concept stage.

Experience sampling can be combined with other formative methods to understand privacy concerns in the early stages of design. For example, Consolvo and colleagues (2005) used a combination of ESM where participants received hypothetical requests from people they knew, a nightly voicemail diary study, questionnaires, and interviews to probe what granularity of location data people are willing to share with their social relations under different circumstances. They found that the most important factors were who was making the request, why the request was being made, and what granularity of location would be most useful to the requester.

Another technique is to use Wizard of Oz to simulate sensors and any underlying artificial intelligence, making it possible for users to get a richer sense as to what a mobile sensing system might be like without building the full system first. Topiary (Li, Hong, & Landay, 2004, 2007) and DART (MacIntyre, Gandy, Dow, & Bolter, 2004) are two examples of rapid prototyping systems that let a designer mock up interactions for location-based services and augmented reality, respectively. However, Wizard of Oz techniques have not been used extensively to gather data about people's perceptions of privacy, and it may be hard to simulate situations that may lead to concerns. As such, while Wizard of Oz techniques are generally accepted as a best practice for UX design, it is still an open question as to the best ways of using it to understand potential privacy concerns.

Surveys and interviews have also been used to probe people's perceptions of privacy. For example, Lin and colleagues (2012) used surveyed people's expectations of privacy with respect to smartphone apps and their use of sensitive data. Emami-Naeini and colleagues (2017) conducted a vignette study with over 1,000 participants, investigating people's preferences over 380 IoT data collection and data usage scenarios. They found that privacy preferences were diverse and context dependent, that participants were more comfortable with data collection in public settings than private ones, and more likely to agree to data collection if there was a clear benefit. In particular, they found that getting help in an emergency or other physical safety was viewed highly positively. Zheng, Apthorpe, Chetty, and Feamster (2018) used interviews to understand people's perceptions of privacy in smart homes. They found that perceived benefit is an important factor for adoption, that users trust device manufacturers to protect their privacy but don't necessarily check that these protections are working as intended, and that there is a lack of awareness of how much can be inferred with even simple IoT devices. These studies are good examples of the diversity of methods for understanding people's needs, and they can be used in early stages of development.

Optimistic versus Pessimistic Approaches to Privacy

Having identified potential privacy issues, we will now consider ways of addressing these problems. Many decisions regarding privacy will require difficult conversations about the tradeoffs involved and how best to protect data and comply with regulations. To a large extent, these are business decisions that need to be guided by ethics, legal requirements, and product-market fit. What we offer here is a discussion of two issues that can have a surprisingly large impact on privacy and adoption, namely, optimistic and pessimistic approaches to privacy and privacy defaults.

At a high level, there are two strategies for addressing privacy issues. *Pessimistic* approaches aim to prevent privacy problems, whereas *optimistic* approaches seek to detect and respond to problems. For example, outside of privacy, a pessimistic approach to people driving over the speed limit might be to require all cars to have speed limiters, which might be automatically adjusted based on one's GPS location. An optimistic approach might be to have highway patrol officers or automated cameras look for people who are speeding and then ticket them.

For privacy, pessimistic approaches might include not collecting data in the first place, proactively deleting older data, and letting end users block specific individuals or allow/disallow sharing of specific types of information. In this scenario, end users often need to take affirmative steps to prevent potential privacy problems. Pessimistic approaches are often useful in cases where the likelihood or cost of a privacy violation is high. However, it can be difficult for developers as well as end users to consider all of the negative cases beforehand. Furthermore, it can be difficult for end users to find, understand, and configure the appropriate privacy controls.

Optimistic approaches work under the assumption that privacy violations are relatively rare or the cost of a violation is not high (Povey, 1999). Optimistic privacy can be useful if trust among people or organizations is high or if access to information is critical (such as hospitals). Examples might include log files, notifications to see who has seen your information, undo functionality, remove access after the fact, or apply social backpressure (such as asking someone not to do something again). For example, smartphone cameras in Japan and Korea emit a loud camera shutter sound that cannot be turned off, making it obvious to everyone nearby that a photo is being taken and deterring voyeuristic shots (Parikh, 2019). Optimistic privacy may also be easier to set up in that there may be fewer things to configure.

Let's use a social fitness app as an example. This app tracks a person's running and can share that person's stats with a global leaderboard and with friends. A more pessimistic design might have nothing shared and require users to opt-in to all possible kinds of sharing. Sensed data might also be processed entirely on the device but at the cost of more battery power and less accurate models. A more optimistic design might have more things shared by default (e.g., assigning people default pseudonyms for the global leaderboard). More sensed data might be collected and processed off the device as well.

Pessimistic and optimistic approaches are not mutually exclusive, but rather a spectrum, and designs will often include elements of both. Pessimistic and optimistic approaches also do not cover the entire space of possible solutions, though we have found them to be a useful tool for thinking about potential ways of addressing people's privacy concerns. Lastly, pessimistic and optimistic approaches can also apply to backend uses of data, such as including access control or adding noise to analytics (pessimistic) or logging all accesses for review (optimistic).

Choosing Default Options for Privacy

Another major design issue centers on what the privacy defaults should be. Palen (1999) found that most people don't change the default settings and that defaults have a significant influence on what is shared and how systems are adopted. Agre and Rotenberg (1997, p. 9) make a similar argument for Caller ID: "If CNID [i.e., Caller ID] is blocked by default, then most subscribers may never turn it on, thus lessening the value of CNID capture systems to marketing organizations; if CNID is unblocked by default and the blocking option is inconvenient or little-known, callers' privacy may not be adequately protected."

Using the social fitness app again, we ask, should people have default profiles? Do these profiles show any personal information by default, such as city or running locations? Are these profiles searchable by other users by default? Is one's running stats visible by others by default? Here, the defaults can range from strongly pessimistic (share nothing) to strongly optimistic (share everything), and the decision for each of these defaults can have a major impact on the user experience of the mobile sensing app, as well as privacy. A challenge here is the lack of enough past research to guide designs. The best advice we can offer here is to use many kinds of early-stage methods, such as rapid prototyping and experience sampling, to understand people's expectations and to get early feedback on how different defaults can balance utility with privacy, and the kinds of defaults that are most attractive for likely early adopters of the system.

User Interface Design for Privacy

There are many challenges in designing user interfaces for privacy for mobile devices, such as devices having small or no displays, slow input speeds, and multiple devices vying for one's attention. While there are some conventions, in general, user interface design for privacy is far from settled. We are still in the early stages of the technological life cycle of mobile sensing, and new kinds of best practices and design patterns are still likely to emerge. As such, this section offers more of an overview on research in user interfaces for privacy rather than best practices.

Multiple studies have found numerous problems with today's privacy user interfaces; for example, these interfaces often lack an explanation of the purposes of data use (Lin et al., 2012) and habituation caused by recurring notifications (Schaub, Balebako, Durity, & Cranor, 2015). Past work has also found that subtle design variations can affect perceived risk and corresponding decisions (Gluck et al., 2016; Habib et al., 2020; Nouwens, Liccardi, Veale, Karger, & Kagal, 2020) and that there are significant individual differences regarding perceptions of privacy notices (Lin et al., 2014; Liu et al., 2016).

Perhaps the most common way to convey privacy issues to users is the privacy policy. Both Apple's App Store and Google Play require apps to have a privacy policy, as do laws such as CalOPPA, CCPA, and GDPR. However, as noted earlier, privacy policies tend to be long, are hard to read, and have a clear cost (one's time) with unclear benefit. Exemplars for how to improve informed consent in the context of research studies include Nebeker and colleagues (2016), Beierle and colleagues (2020), and Kreuter, Haas, Keusch, Bähr, and Trappmann (2020).

There is also growing research examining how to improve the readability and understandability of privacy information. For example, Emami-Naeni and colleagues (2020) developed a privacy nutrition label for IoT devices that can be shown on a Web page or on the box for a device. These labels give consumers relevant privacy information about such things as sensors, data retention, and encryption before purchasing. Layered privacy policies are another proposed format. Users are first presented with condensed information about data collection and its purpose, along with where to go for additional information (Center for Information Policy Leadership, 2005). However, layered privacy policies have not been widely adopted, and at least one study suggests that they are not more understandable than conventional privacy policies (McDonald, Reeder, Kelley, & Cranor, 2009).

User interfaces for mobile sensing systems also need to make it easy for people to understand what sensitive permissions they are granting to an app. Past research has found that Android's permission model presents many usability challenges. For example, mobile users have a poor understanding of permissions (Felt et al., 2012; Kelley, Bresee, Cranor, & Reeder, 2012). They have low attention at install time and cannot correctly understand the permissions they grant; in addition, current permission warnings are not effective in helping users make security decisions. There is also a lack of clarity as to why an app is using sensitive data (Lin et al., 2012). Furthermore, once sensitive data is allowed, it can be used for multiple purposes in an app. Several studies have also examined how people make decisions about whether to install an app, finding that factors such as perceived utility (Good et al., 2005), purpose of use (Lin et al., 2012), or the price of the app (Shklovski et al., 2014) have a strong influence.

Taking a step back, we see that there are roughly four points in time when an app can present privacy-related information to users: before install (e.g., searching for apps); at install time; at runtime while the app is being used; and after an app has been used. Typically, the first two points show the kind of sensitive data an app might access, whereas the latter two show what sensitive data an app is actually accessing. Here, our discussion will focus on designs for runtime, since the majority of research, as well as the design of iOS and now Android, has a strong emphasis on that point of intervention.

Access control gadgets are special kinds of secure user interface elements offered by the operating system that let users grant permission to apps, for example, a button with a camera icon on it to convey that pressing it will access the device's camera (Roesner et al., 2012). Apps can access sensitive data if and only if users interact with these access control gadgets. PERUIM offers a variant idea, analyzing and modifying a smartphone app to overlay the names of permissions that will be accessed if the user interacts with a given graphical user interface (GUI) widget (Li, Guo, & Chen, 2016).

A complementary approach is to help users make better trust decisions. Both Android and iOS recommend that apps include an explanation of why sensitive data are being requested, with iOS offering explicit support for explanation strings. Tan and colleagues (2014) conducted an online survey showing that users are significantly more likely to allow accesses with explanations. Researchers have also investigated experimental designs. One idea is to leverage the wisdom of crowds. For example, when an app requests access to sensitive data, ProtectMyPrivacy shows a dialog box to allow or deny the access, along with what percentage of users chose each option (Agarwal & Hall, 2013). Lin and colleagues (2012) designed an alternative install-time interface that showed what percentage of crowd workers expected an app to use a given type of sensitive data. Another approach is to model user preferences, for example, using such features as time of day and location to predict and possibly automatically grant permissions (Olejnik et al., 2017; Wijesekera et al., 2017). Das, Degeling, Smullen, and Sadeh, (2018) proposed personalized privacy assistants, using predictive models to help inform users about relevant data practices and configure them appropriately.

In addition to controls, researchers have investigated ways of helping users be more aware of what sensitive data an app is using or has used. The conventional design for today's smartphones is to have the operating system show some information on the notification bar indicating that a certain sensor (e.g., GPS or microphone) is currently turned on. iOS also occasionally reminds users of the background location access of a certain app. One variation on these notifications is showing users after the fact how often an app uses sensitive data as a nudge (Almuhimedi et al., 2015). More broadly, researchers have also investigated the design space for just-in-time notifications and have highlighted important features such as timing (if a user should be notified of a sensitive access immediately or later), channel (via the device itself, a secondary device, or a publicly visible device), modality (e.g., visual, aural, haptic), control (how choices are provided), and actionability (making it clear to users what they can do) (Patil, Hoyle, Schlegel, Kapadia, & Lee, 2015; Schaub et al., 2015). Similarly, Feng, Yao, and Sadeh (2021) developed a taxonomy for helping end users make privacy choices, specifying such features as type (e.g., binary or multiple choice), functionality (e.g., presentation or enforcement), timing, channel, and modality.

We close with the observation that, broadly speaking, today's user interfaces for privacy, as well as laws regarding collection and use of sensitive data, all fall under a current framework of notice and consent. Numerous papers have commented on the weaknesses of this approach, for example, that it puts too much burden on individuals, assumes users have fully rational behavior and a great deal of attention and cognitive processing abilities, and that users have a lot of time and desire to understand tradeoffs (Cate, 2006; Hong, 2017; McDonald & Cranor, 2008). However, there is currently no clear alternative to today's notice and consent, and so it still makes sense for future user interfaces for privacy to stay within this framework.

System Implementation Issues

We now examine ways of implementing mobile sensing systems. Here, we offer a brief overview of some of the issues and research related to the front end (the mobile sensing device) and backend (any cloud servers where personal data might also be stored).

One issue regarding the front end is how to handle sensitive data on the mobile device in a safe and secure manner. For example, today's smartphone platforms make it easy to access sensitive data, but there are many other considerations, such as data storage, encryption, identifiers, and where inferencing should be done. Researchers have developed several frameworks and libraries to help, such as AWARE (Ferreira, Kostakos, & Dey, 2015), Funf (Aharony, Pan, Ip, & Pentland, 2010; www.funf.org), PrivacyStreams (https://privacystreams.github.io; see also Li et al., 2017), and mCerebrum (Hossain et al., 2017). These software packages offer a range of functionality, including capturing, inferring, and using sensor data, the experience sampling method, and management of personal identifiers. Note that these frameworks are for smartphones only, have limited technical support, and are oriented toward researchers rather than products. However, these frameworks point out many useful features that developers should consider for their own mobile sensing apps, including support for denaturing data before they egress from one's mobile sensing device, encryption for storing and sending sensitive data, and deidentification of users with codes instead of names or phone numbers.

Researchers have also developed many techniques to identify sensitive data in audio and video streams, as well as selectively degrade the quality or granularity of data (also known as denaturing). For example, a mobile sensing app might only extract and store audio features rather than raw audio, distort audio so that speakers cannot be identified, or scramble the audio so that speakers can be identified but what they are saying cannot (Smith & Hudson, 1995). For images, there are machine learning classifiers to detect bystanders in photos (Hasan et al., 2020), sensitive locations such as a bedroom or bathroom (Templeman, Korayem, Crandall, & Kapadia, 2014), and computer screens in images (Korayem Templeman, Chen, Crandall, & Kapadia, 2016). While these kinds of techniques are promising, it is currently not clear if they would be sufficient from a legal perspective or how well end users might receive them in practice.

With respect to the backend, developers need to consider policies and procedures for accessing and protecting those data. Many potential issues are already presented in the privacy risk model; for example, what data are sent to the backend, where are the data stored, and are data shared with any third parties? This last issue of sharing data is surprisingly complex, given the rise of Big Data and social media. For example, earlier, we mentioned how the health fitness app Strava released a data visualization that aggregated the GPS running routes of all of its users, disclosing the location of likely military bases around the world (Hern, 2018). Although no specific individual could be identified, sensitive data were still leaked due to the sheer quantity of data. The research community has also demonstrated several cases of reidentifying specific individuals in data thought to be anonymized or sufficiently aggregated (Garfinkel, Abowd, & Martindale, 2018; Narayanan & Shmatikov, 2008; Sweeney, 2002). Chapter 3, this volume, has more discussion about the tradeoffs of granting access to raw mobile sensing data to other researchers.

There are also two major considerations for both the front end and the backend. The first is a technique called *differential privacy* (Dwork, 2008), which offers quantifiable guarantees for privacy. The main idea with differential privacy is to add enough noise to queries so that a dedicated attacker cannot tell whether or not a given element is in that data. Perhaps the most notable deployments of differential privacy are telemetry data in the Chrome Web browser (Erlingsson, Pihur, & Korolova, 2014), iOS (Apple, 2020b, 2020c), and the U.S. Census (Mervis, 2019). Differential privacy can be applied both when collecting data on the front end (locally), as is the case with the RAPPOR (Randomized Aggregatable Privacy-Preserving Ordinal Response) system used in Chrome (Erlingsson et al., 2014), or afterward in the backend on queries on raw data (globally). Google has also released several open-source tools to help with differential privacy (Google, n.d.). As of this writing, however, applying differential privacy is still a bit of an art rather than a science.

Development teams also need to consider how best to support the auditing of data practices, on both the front end and backend. This auditing needs to go beyond the immediate development team, and, depending on the size of the organization, might include lawyers, privacy engineers, chief privacy officers, and chief information security officers. This kind of auditing should make it clear to nontechnical people what kinds of data are being collected and when, how those data are used, and what control and feedback end users have over this data collection and data usage. The audit should also examine how the app's behavior is conveyed in the app's privacy policy and whether the app fully complies with what is stated in the privacy policy.

Some Open Research Questions about Privacy

In this section, we pose some open questions about privacy for the research community. First, can we do better than today's framework of notice and consent? Presently, end users bear a great deal of burden in managing their own privacy, which is becoming increasingly untenable due to the growing number of devices and services that people interact with, the increasing amount of data collection and inferences, and the knowledge and skill needed to protect one's data.

Second, can we create better tools and methods to help product teams with privacy in the early stages of design? Presently, product teams have to make a lot of guesses about privacy when they are developing new products. Feedback from surveys, paper prototypes, and experience sampling methods are useful but might not fully reflect how people feel about a product later on. Getting feedback late in the process makes it difficult and expensive to make major changes in design. Better tools and methods in the early stages of design could also help product teams quickly and cheaply explore more design alternatives that match people's expectations and preferences. For example, Lean Privacy Review (Jin, Shen, Jain, Kumar, & Hong, 2021) seeks to combine crowdsourcing with a form of heuristic evaluation for privacy, making it possible for teams to get fast feedback. However, it has not yet been validated at large scale or in the wild.

Third, can we develop better tools to support developers throughout the entire software development life cycle? For example, Li, Neundorfer, Agarwal, and Hong (2021) proposed using developer-provided annotations about data being collected to semiautomatically generate high-quality user interfaces for privacy. Tools to help with auditing across the entire life cycle of data might also be useful, helping nontechnical people trace what data are being collected, where the data came from, where the data are stored, and how the data are being used.

Fourth, are there major cultural differences with respect to personal privacy? Similarly, do things like the Fair Information Practices make sense in other cultural contexts? Mobile devices and services are being adopted worldwide. However, the vast majority of research on privacy is situated in North America and Western Europe. It is currently unclear if there are significant differences, and if there are, how to account for those differences in a design.

Conclusion

Mobile sensing technologies offer tremendous opportunities in terms of health care, safety, sustainability, education, and more. But this vision is possible only if we can find ways of legitimately addressing people's privacy concerns, if we can foster trust that the systems we build can respect people as individuals, and if these systems do what people expect them to do.

Privacy is a complex topic that is still rapidly evolving, and designing for privacy requires a great deal of thought and care across all elements of the system. While there is no one size fits all approach to privacy, in this chapter, we offered an overview of some of the social, legal, market, UX design, and technical issues involved in building mobile sensing systems that can offer tangible value while also respecting people's privacy.

ACKNOWLEDGMENTS

The ideas in this chapter have been refined over many years through numerous discussions with many collaborators, including faculty members Yuvraj Agarwal, Lorrie Cranor, Laura Dabbish, Matt Fredrikson, and Norman Sadeh; graduate researchers Shahriyar Amini, Gokhan Bal, Rebecca Balebako, Fanglin Chen, Saksham Chitkara, Cori Faklaris, Haojian Jin, Su Mon Kywe, Tianshi Li, Yuanchun Li, Jialiu Lin, Minxing Liu, Haoyu Wang; and many staff, master's students, and undergrad students that helped with our work, including Mike Czapik, Shawn Hanna, Swarup Sahoo, Judy Chun, Won-Woo Chung, Aniruddh Iyer, Ally Liu, Shen Lu, Rituparna Roychoudhury, Qian Wang, Shan Wang, Siqi Wang, Vida Zhang, Jessica Zhao, Yuan Jiang, Haojian Jin, Sam Kim, Evelyn Kuo, Tianshi Li, Jinping Liu, Yile Liu, and Robert Zhang. Also, special thanks to members of the staff at Google and Apple who have given us feedback over the years, as well as members of the DARPA Brandeis Mobile Collaborative Research Team for many insightful discussions and incredibly useful feedback over the years.

Our research team's work on privacy has also been supported over the years by the National Science Foundation, Air Force Research Lab, Google, and NQ Mobile. The views and conclusions contained herein are those of the authors and should not be interpreted as necessarily representing the official policies or endorsements, either expressed or implied, of these entities.

REFERENCES

Agarwal, Y., & Hall, M. (2013). ProtectMyPrivacy: Detecting and mitigating privacy leaks on iOS devices using crowdsourcing. *Conference on Mobile Systems, Applications, and Services. Mobisys '13*, pp. 97–110.

Agre, P. E., & Rotenberg, M. (1997). *Technology and privacy: The new landscape.*. MIT Press.

Aharony, N., Pan, W., Ip, C., & Pentland, A. (2010). *Tracing mobile phone app installations in the "friends and family" study.* Workshop on Information in Networks (WIN '10).

Almuhimedi, H., Schaub, F., Sadeh, N., Adjerid, I., Acquisti, A., Gluck, J., et al. (2015). Your location has been shared 5,398 times!: A field study on mobile app privacy nudging. *Conference on Human Factors in Computing Systems (CHI 2015)*, pp. 787–796.

Altman, I. (1975). *The environment and social behavior: Privacy, personal space, territory, and crowding.* Brooks/Cole.

Apple. (2020a, March 4). *App store review guidelines.* https://developer.apple.com/app-store/review/guidelines/#privacy.

Apple. (2020b). *Differential privacy.* www.apple.com/privacy/docs/Differential_Privacy_Overview.pdf.

Apple. (2020c). *This is how we protect your privacy.* www.apple.com/nz/privacy/approach-to-privacy

Auxier, B., Rainie, L., Anderson, M., Perrin, A., Kumar, M., &Turner, E. (2019, November 15). *Americans and privacy: Concerned, confused and feeling lack of control over their personal information.* Pew Research Center. www.pewresearch.org/internet/2019/11/15/americans-attitudes-and-experiences-with-privacy-policies-and-laws.

Balebako, R., Marsh, A., Lin, J., Hong, J. I., & Cranor, L. F. (2014). *The privacy and security behaviors of smartphone app developers.* Workshop on Usable Security (USEC 2014).

Beierle, F., Tran, V. T., Allemand, M., Neff, P., Schlee, W., Probst, T., et al. (2020). What data are smartphone users willing to share with researchers? *Journal of Ambient Intelligence and Humanized Computing, 11*(6), 2277–2289.

Bellotti, V., & Sellen, A. (1993). *Design for privacy in ubiquitous computing environments.* European Conference on Computer-Supported Cooperative Work (ECSCW '93).

Blue, V. (2012, March 30). *Stalker app Girls Around Me hunts women via Facebook, Foursquare.* ZDNet. www.zdnet.com/article/stalker-app-girls-around-me-hunts-women-via-facebook-foursquare

Bonné, B., Peddinti, S. T., Bilogrevic, I., and Taft, N. (2017). Exploring decision making with Android's runtime permission dialogs using in-context surveys. *Symposium on Usable Privacy and Security (SOUPS 2017)*, pp. 195–210.

Brandeis, L., & Warren, S. (1890). The right to privacy. *Harvard Law Review, 4*(5), 193–220.

Burke, J. A., Estrin, D., Hansen, M., Parker, A., Ramanathan, N., Reddy, S., & Srivastava, M. B. (2006). Participatory sensing. *Proceedings of ACM SenSys Workshop on World-Sensor-Web.*

Cate, F. H. (2006). *The failure of fair information practice principles. Consumer protection in the age of the information economy.* https://papers.ssrn.com/sol3/papers.cfm?abstract_id=1156972

Cavoukian, A. (2009). *Privacy by design: The 7 foundational principles.* https://www.ipc.on.ca/wp-content/uploads/resources/7foundationalprinciples.pdf

Center for Information Policy Leadership. (2005). *Multi-layered notices explained.* http://mddb.apec.org/documents/2005/ECSG/DPM1/05_ecsg_dpm1_003.pdf

Chitkara, S., Gothoskar, N., Harish, S., Hong, J. I., & Agarwal, Y. (2017). Does this app really need my location?: Context-aware privacy management for smartphones. *Interactive,*

Mobile, Wearable and Ubiquitous Technologies, 1(3), 42.
Cisco. (2012). *Gen Y: New dawn for work, play, identity.* www.cisco.com/c/dam/en/us/solutions/enterprise/connected-world-technology-report/2012-CCWTR-Chapter1-Global-Results.pdf
Consolvo, S., Smith, I. E., Matthews, T., LaMarca, A., Tabert, J., & Powledge, P. (2005). Location disclosure to social relations: Why, when, and what people want to share. *Conference on Human Factors in Computing Systems* (CHI 2005), pp. 81–90.
Consumers International. (2019) *The trust opportunity: Exploring consumers' attitudes to the Internet of Things.* www.consumersinternational.org/media/261950/thetrustopportunity-jointresearch.pdf
Cranor, L. F., Reagle, J., & Ackerman, M. S. (2000). Beyond concern: Understanding net users' attitudes about online privacy. In I. Vogelsang & B. M. Compaine (Eds.), *The internet upheaval: Raising questions, seeking answers in communications policy* (pp. 47–70). MIT Press.
Daley, S. (2011, August 9). Europe takes its own path on internet privacy. *New York Times.* www.nytimes.com/2011/08/10/world/europe/10spain.html
Das, A., Degeling, M., Smullen, D., & Sadeh, N. (2018). Personalized privacy assistants for the internet of things: Providing users with notice and choice. *IEEE Pervasive Computing, 17*(3), 35–46.
Devarakonda, S., Sevusu, P., Liu, H., Liu, R., Iftode, L., & Nath, B. (2013). Real-time air quality monitoring through mobile sensing in metropolitan areas. *ACM SIGKDD International Workshop on Urban Computing,* pp. 1–8.
D'Onfro, J. (2016, September 6). 10 years ago Facebook had "the most inglorious launch moment in history" but it changed everything. *Business Insider.* https://www.businessinsider.in/10-years-ago-FB-had-the-most-inglorious-launch-moment-in-history160but-it-changed-everything/articleshow/54039367.cms
Doryab, A., Min, J. K., Wiese, J., Zimmerman, J., & Hong, J. (2014). *Detection of behavior change in people with depression.* Workshops at the Twenty-Eighth AAAI Conference on Artificial Intelligence.
Duhigg, C. (2009). What does your credit-card company know about you. *New York Times.* www.nytimes.com/2009/05/17/magazine/17credit-t.html
Duhigg, C. (2012, February). How companies learn your secrets. *New York Times.* www.nytimes.com/2012/02/19/magazine/shopping-habits.html
Dwork, C. (2008). Differential privacy: A survey of results. *International Conference on Theory and Applications of Models of Computation,* pp. 1–19.
Emami-Naeini, P., Agarwal, Y., Cranor, L. F., & Hibshi, H. (2020). *Ask the experts: What should be on an IoT privacy and security label?* IEEE Symposium on Security and Privacy.
Emami-Naeini, P., Bhagavatula, S., Habib, H., Degeling, M., Bauer, L., Cranor, L. F., & Sadeh, N. (2017). Privacy expectations and preferences in an IoT world. *Symposium on Usable Privacy and Security* (SOUPS 2017), pp. 399–412.
Emami-Naeini, P., Dixon, H., Agarwal, Y., & Cranor, L. F. (2019). Exploring how privacy and security factor into IoT device purchase behavior. *Conference on Human Factors in Computing Systems* (CHI 2019), pp.1–12.
Erlingsson, Ú., Pihur, V., & Korolova, A. (2014). Rappor: Randomized aggregatable privacy-preserving ordinal response. *ACM SIGSAC Conference on Computer and Communications Security* (CCS 2014), pp. 1054–1067.
Federal Trade Commission. (1998). *Privacy online: A report to Congress.* www.ftc.gov/sites/default/files/documents/reports/privacy-online-report-congress/priv-23a.pdf
Federal Trade Commission. (2013a, December 5). *Android Flashlight app developer settles, FTC charges it deceived consumers.* www.ftc.gov/news-events/press-releases/2013/12/android-flashlight-app-developer-settles-ftc-charges-it-deceived
Federal Trade Commission. (2013b). *Mobile privacy disclosures: Building trust through transparency.* www.ftc.gov/reports/mobile-privacy-disclosures-building-trust-through-transparency-federal-trade-commission
Federal Trade Commission. (2013c, February 1). *Path social networking app settles FTC charges it deceived consumers and improperly collected personal information from users' mobile address books.* www.ftc.gov/news-events/press-releases/2013/02/path-social-networking-app-settles-ftc-charges-it-deceived

Federal Trade Commission. (2016). *Mobile health app developers: FTC best practices.* www.ftc.gov/tips-advice/business-center/guidance/mobile-health-app-developers-ftc-best-practices

Federal Trade Commission. (2019, October 22). *FTC brings first case against developers of "stalking" apps.* www.ftc.gov/news-events/press-releases/2019/10/ftc-brings-first-case-against-developers-stalking-apps

Felt, A. P., Ha, E., Egelman, S., Haney, A., Chin, E., & Wagner, D. (2012). *Android permissions: User attention, comprehension, and behavior.* Symposium on Usable Privacy and Security (SOUPS 2012).

Felten, E. (2003). *DRM, and the first rule of security analysis.* https://freedom-to-tinker.com/2003/03/19/drm-and-first-rule-security-analysis/

Feng, Y., Yao, Y., & Sadeh, N. (2021). A design space for privacy choices: Towards meaningful privacy control in the internet of things. *Conference on Human Factors in Computing Systems* (CHI 2021), pp. 1–16.

Ferreira, D., Kostakos, V., & Dey, A. K. (2015). AWARE: Mobile context instrumentation framework. *Frontiers in ICT, 2*, 6.

Franceschi-Bicchierai, L., & Cox, J. (2017, April 18). *Inside the "Stalkerware" surveillance market, where ordinary people tap each other's phones.* Vice. www.vice.com/en_us/article/53vm7n/inside-stalkerware-surveillance-market-flexispy-retina-x

Frey, S. (2021, July 28) *Preparing for Google Play's new safety section.* Android developers blog. https://android-developers.googleblog.com/2021/07/new-google-play-safety-section.html

Fu, B., Lin, J., Li, L., Faloutsos, C., Hong, J., & Sadeh, N. (2013). Why people hate your app: Making sense of user feedback in a mobile app store. *International Conference on Knowledge Discovery and Data Mining* (KDD 2013), pp. 1276–1284.

Garfinkel, S., Abowd, J. M., & Martindale, C. (2018). Understanding database reconstruction attacks on public data: These attacks on statistical databases are no longer a theoretical danger. *ACM Queue*, 16(5), 28–53.

GDPR.eu. *Data Protection Impact Assessment (DPIA).* https://gdpr.eu/data-protection-impact-assessment-template

Gilbert, B. (2019, April 15). There's a simple reason your new smart TV was so affordable: It's collecting and selling your data, and serving you ads. *Business Insider.* www.businessinsider.com/smart-tv-data-collection-advertising-2019-1

Gluck, J., Schaub, F., Friedman, A., Habib, H., Sadeh, N., Cranor, L. F., & Agarwal, Y. (2016). How short is too short?: Implications of length and framing on the effectiveness of privacy notices. *Symposium on Usable Privacy and Security* (SOUPS 2016), pp. 321–340.

Goffman, E. (1978). *The presentation of self in everyday life.* Harmondsworth.

Good, N., Dhamija, R., Grossklags, J., Thaw, D., Aronowitz, S., Mulligan, D., & Konstan, J. (2005, July). Stopping spyware at the gate: A user study of privacy, notice and spyware. *Symposium on Usable Privacy and Security* (SOUPS 2016), pp. 43–52.

Google. (2020, June 29). *Privacy best practices.* https://developer.android.com/privacy/best-practices

Google. (n.d.). *Differential privacy.* https://github.com/google/differential-privacy

Gross, D. (2014, February 24). *Google: How not to be a "Glasshole."* CNN. www.cnn.com/2014/02/19/tech/mobile/google-glasshole/index.html

Ha, E., & Wagner, D. (2013, January). Do Android users write about electric sheep? Examining consumer reviews in Google Play. *IEEE 10th Consumer Communications and Networking Conference* (CCNC), pp. 149–157.

Habib, H., Pearman, S., Wang, J., Zou, Y., Acquisti, A., Cranor, L. F., et al. (2020). "It's a scavenger hunt": Usability of websites' Opt-Out and Data Deletion Choices. *Conference on Human Factors in Computing Systems* (CHI 2020), pp. 1–12.

Hasan, R., Crandall, D., Fritz, M., & Kapadia, A. (2020). *Automatically detecting bystanders in photos to reduce privacy risks.* IEEE Symposium on Security and Privacy.

Hasenfratz, D., Saukh, O., Sturzenegger, S., & Thiele, L. (2012). Participatory air pollution monitoring using smartphones. *Mobile Sensing, 1*, 1–5.

Hern, A. (2018, January 20). Fitness tracking app Strava gives away location of secret US army bases. *The Guardian.* www.theguardian.com/world/2018/jan/28/fitness-tracking-app-gives-away-location-of-secret-us-army-bases

Hindus, D., Mainwaring, S. D., Leduc, N., Hagström, A. E., & Bayley, O. (2001). Casablanca: Designing social communication devices for the home. *Conference on Human Factors in Computing Systems* (CHI 2001), pp. 325–332.

Hong, J. (2005). *An architecture for privacy-sensitive ubiquitous computing*. Unpublished doctoral dissertation.

Hong, J. (2013). Considering privacy issues in the context of Google glass. *Communications of the ACM, 56*(11), 10–11.

Hong, J. (2017). The privacy landscape of pervasive computing. *IEEE Pervasive Computing, 16*(3), 40–48.

Hong, J. I., Ng, J. D., Lederer, S., & Landay, J. A. (2004). Privacy risk models for designing privacy-sensitive ubiquitous computing systems. *Designing Interactive Systems* (DIS 2004), (pp. 91–100).

Hossain, S. M., Hnat, T., Saleheen, N., Nasrin, N. J., Noor, J., Ho, B. J., et al. (2017). mCerebrum: A mobile sensing software platform for development and validation of digital biomarkers and interventions. *Conference on Embedded Network Sensor Systems* pp. 1–14.

Hoyle, R., Templeman, R., Armes, S., Anthony, D., Crandall, D., & Kapadia, A. (2014). Privacy behaviors of lifeloggers using wearable cameras. *International Joint Conference on Pervasive and Ubiquitous Computing* (Ubicomp 2014), pp. 571–582.

Hubbard, G. P., & O'Brien, A. P. (2015). *Economics: Global edition*. Pearson.

Iachello, G., & Hong, J. (2007). End-user privacy in human-computer interaction. *Foundations and Trends, 1*(1), 1–137.

Iachello, G., Truong, K. N., Abowd, G. D., Hayes, G. R., & Stevens, M. (2006). Prototyping and sampling experience to evaluate ubiquitous computing privacy in the real world. *Conference on Human Factors in Computing Systems* (CHI 2006), pp. 1009–1018.

International Association of Privacy Professionals. (2018, April 24). *How do the rules on audio recording change under the GDPR?* https://iapp.org/news/a/how-do-the-rules-on-audio-recording-change-under-the-gdpr/

Jernigan, C., & Mistree, B. F. (2009). Gaydar: Facebook friendships expose sexual orientation. *First Monday, 14*(10). https://firstmonday.org/ojs/index.php/fm/article/view/2611

Jin, H., Shen, H., Jain, M., Kumar, S., & Hong, J. I. (2021). Lean privacy review: Collecting users' privacy concerns of data practices at a low cost. *ACM Transactions on Computer-Human Interaction (TOCHI), 28*(5), 1–55.

Kelley, P. G., Bresee, J., Cranor, L. F., & Reeder, R. W. (2009). *A nutrition label for privacy*. Symposium on Usable Privacy and Security.

Kharpal, A (2020, February 6). *Apple Watch outsold the entire Swiss watch industry in 2019*. CNBC. https://www.cnbc.com/2020/02/06/apple-watch-outsold-the-entire-swiss-watch-industry-in-2019.html

King, M., Hu, F., McHugh, J., Murphy, E., Newman, E., Irving, K., & Smeaton, A. F. (2013). Visibility of wearable sensors as measured using eye tracking glasses. *International Joint Conference on Ambient Intelligence*, pp. 23–32.

Kong, Q., Allen, R. M., Schreier, L., & Kwon, Y. W. (2016). MyShake: A smartphone seismic network for earthquake early warning and beyond. *Science Advances, 2*(2), e1501055.

Korayem, M., Templeman, R., Chen, D., Crandall, D., & Kapadia, A. (2016). Enhancing lifelogging privacy by detecting screens. *Conference on Human Factors in Computing Systems* (CHI 2016), pp. 4309–4314.

Kreuter, F., Haas, G.-C., Keusch, F., Bähr, S., & Trappmann, M. (2020). Collecting survey and smartphone sensor data with an app: Opportunities and challenges around privacy and informed consent. *Social Science Computer Review, 38*, 533–549.

Kumar, S., Nguyen, L. T., Zeng, M., Liu, K., & Zhang, J. (2015). Sound shredding: Privacy preserved audio sensing. *International Workshop on Mobile Computing Systems and Applications* (HotMobile 2015), pp. 135–140.

Lane, N. D., Lin, M., Mohammod, M., Yang, X., Lu, H., Cardone, G., et al. (2014). Bewell: Sensing sleep, physical activities and social interactions to promote wellbeing. *Mobile Networks and Applications, 19*(3), 345–359.

Lawler, R. (2021, May 12). *Vizio makes nearly as much money from ads and data as it does from TVs*. Engadget. www.engadget.com/vizio-q1-earnings-inscape-013937337.html

Lederer, S., Hong, J. I., Dey, A. K., & Landay, J. A. (2004). Personal privacy through understanding and action: five pitfalls for designers. *Personal and Ubiquitous Computing, 8*(6), 440–454.

Li, T., Agarwal, Y., & Hong, J. I. (2018). Coconut: An IDE plugin for developing privacy-friendly apps. *Interactive, Mobile, Wearable and Ubiquitous Technologies, 2*(4), 1–27.

Li, T., Louie, E., Dabbish, L., Hong, J. I. (2020). *How developers talk about personal data and what it means for user privacy: A case study of a developer forum on Reddit.* Conference on Computer Supported Cooperative Work (CSCW 2020).

Li, T., Neundorfer, E., Agarwal, Y., Hong, J. I. (2021). Honeysuckle: Annotation-guided code generation of in-app privacy notices. *Interactive, Mobile, Wearable and Ubiquitous Technologies*, 1–27.

Li, T., Reiman, K., Agarwal, Y., Cranor, L. F., Hong, J. I. (2022). *Understanding challenges for developers to create accurate privacy nutrition labels.* Conference on Human Factors in Computing Systems (CHI 2022).

Li, Y., Chen, F., Li, T. J. J., Guo, Y., Huang, G., Fredrikson, M., et al. (2017). PrivacyStreams: Enabling transparency in personal data processing for mobile apps. *Interactive, Mobile, Wearable and Ubiquitous Technologies, 1*(3).

Li, Y., Guo, Y., & Chen, X. (2016). Peruim: Understanding mobile application privacy with permission-UI Mapping. *International Joint Conference on Pervasive and Ubiquitous Computing* (Ubicomp 2016), pp. 682–693.

Li, Y., Hong, J. I., & Landay, J. A. (2004). Topiary: A tool for prototyping location-enhanced applications. *Symposium on User Interface Software and Technology*, pp. 217–226.

Li, Y., Hong, J. I., & Landay, J. A. (2007). Design challenges and principles for Wizard of Oz testing of location-enhanced applications. *IEEE Pervasive Computing, 6*(2), 70–75.

Lin, J., Amini, S., Hong, J. I., Sadeh, N., Lindqvist, J., & Zhang, J. (2012). Expectation and purpose: Understanding users' mental models of mobile app privacy through crowdsourcing. *International Conference on Ubiquitous Computing* (Ubicomp 2012), pp. 501–510.

Lin, J., Liu, B., Sadeh, N., & Hong, J. I. (2014). Modeling users' mobile app privacy preferences: Restoring usability in a sea of permission settings. *Symposium on Usable Privacy and Security* (SOUPS 2014), pp. 199–212.

Liu, B., Andersen, M. S., Schaub, F., Almuhimedi, H., Zhang, S. A., Sadeh, N., et al. (2016). Follow my recommendations: A personalized privacy assistant for mobile app permissions. *Symposium on Usable Privacy and Security* (SOUPS 2016), pp. 27–41.

MacIntyre, B., Gandy, M., Dow, S., & Bolter, J. D. (2004). DART: A toolkit for rapid design exploration of augmented reality experiences. *Symposium on User Interface Software and Technology* (UIST 2004), pp. 197–206.

Maisonneuve, N., Stevens, M., Niessen, M. E., & Steels, L. (2009). NoiseTube: Measuring and mapping noise pollution with mobile phones. *Information Technologies in Environmental Engineering*, pp. 215–228.

Matthews, T., O'Leary, K., Turner, A., Sleeper, M., Woelfer, J. P., Shelton, M., et al. (2017). Stories from survivors: Privacy and security practices when coping with intimate partner abuse. *Conference on Human Factors in Computing Systems* (CHI 2017), pp. 2189–2201.

McDonald, A. M., & Cranor, L. F. (2008). The cost of reading privacy policies. *I/S: A Journal of Law and Policy for the Information Society, 4*, 543.

McDonald, A. M., Reeder, R. W., Kelley, P. G., & Cranor, L. F. (2009). A comparative study of online privacy policies and formats. *Privacy Enhancing Technologies Symposium* (PETS 2009), pp. 37–55

Mervis, J. (2019, January 4). Can a set of equations keep U.S. census data private? *Science.* https://www.science.org/content/article/can-set-equations-keep-us-census-data-private

Min, J. K., Doryab, A., Wiese, J., Amini, S., Zimmerman, J., & Hong, J. I. (2014). Toss'n'turn: smartphone as sleep and sleep quality detector. *Conference on Human Factors in Computing Systems* (CHI 2014), pp. 477–486.

Morse, J. (2020, June 23) Apple's privacy-focused 'nutrition labels' for apps are only a start. *Mashable.* https://mashable.com/article/apple-privacy-nutrition-labels-ios14

Narayanan, A., & Shmatikov, V. (2008). Robust de-anonymization of large sparse datasets. *IEEE Symposium on Security and Privacy*, pp. 111–125.

National Institute of Standards and Technology. (2010). *Guide to protecting the confidentiality of personally identifiable information (PII).* https://doi.org/10.6028/NIST.SP.800–122

National Institute of Standards and Technology. (2015). *Draft NISTIR 8062: An introduction to privacy engineering and risk management in federal systems.* https://csrc.nist.gov/csrc/media/publications/nistir/8062/draft/documents/nistir_8062_draft.pdf

Nebeker, C., Lagare, T., Takemoto, M., Lewars, B., Crist, K., Bloss, C. S., & Kerr, J. (2016). Engaging research participants to inform the ethical conduct of mobile imaging, pervasive sensing, and location tracking research. *Translational Behavioral Medicine, 6*, 577–586.

Newcomb, A. (2018, March 24). *A timeline of Facebook's privacy issues—and its responses.* NBC News. https://www.nbcnews.com/tech/social-media/timeline-facebook-s-privacy-issues-its-responses-n859651

Nguyen, D. H., Marcu, G., Hayes, G. R., Truong, K. N., Scott, J., Langheinrich, M., & Roduner, C. (2009). Encountering SenseCam: Personal recording technologies in everyday life. *International Conference on Ubiquitous Computing* (Ubicomp 2009), pp. 165–174.

Nissenbaum, H. (2004). Privacy as contextual integrity. *Washington Law Review, 79*, 119.

Nouwens, M., Liccardi, I., Veale, M., Karger, D., & Kagal, L. (2020). *Dark patterns after the GDPR: Scraping consent pop-ups and demonstrating their influence.* Conference on Human Factors in Computing Systems (CHI 2020).

Obar, J. A., & Oeldorf-Hirsch, A. (2020). The biggest lie on the internet: Ignoring the privacy policies and terms of service policies of social networking services. *Information, Communication and Society, 23*(1), 128–147.

Oberly, D., Bryan, K. & Fath, K. (March 20, 2022). *Recent FTC settlement highlights Agency's focus on children's privacy and use of disgorgement remedy including in AI context.* Consumer Privacy World. www.consumerprivacyworld.com/2022/03/recent-ftc-settlement-highlights-agencys-focus-on-childrens-privacy-use-of-disgorgement-remedy-including-in-ai-context

Olejnik, K., Dacosta, I., Machado, J. S., Huguenin, K., Khan, M. E., & Hubaux, J. P. (2017). Smarper: Context-aware and automatic runtime-permissions for mobile devices. *IEEE Symposium on Security and Privacy*, pp. 1058–1076.

Olmstead, K., & Atkinson, M. (2015). *Apps permissions in the Google Play store.* Pew Research Center. www.pewresearch.org/internet/2015/11/10/apps-permissions-in-the-google-play-store

Organization for Economic Co-operation and Development. (1980). *Guidelines on the protection of privacy and transborder flows of personal data* [Technical report]. https://legalinstruments.oecd.org/en/instruments/OECD-LEGAL-0188

Palen, L. (1999). Social, individual and technological issues for groupware calendar systems. *Conference on Human Factors in Computing Systems* (CHI 1999), pp. 17–24.

Palen, L., & Dourish, P. (2003). Unpacking "privacy" for a networked world. *Conference on Human Factors in Computing Systems* (CHI 2003), pp. 129–136.

Parikh, P. (2019, May 29). *Here's why the camera shutter sound can't be turned off in Japan and Korea.* https://eoto.tech/camera-shutter-sound

Patil, S., Hoyle, R., Schlegel, R., Kapadia, A., & Lee, A. J. (2015). Interrupt now or inform later? Comparing immediate and delayed privacy feedback. *Conference on Human Factors in Computing Systems* (CHI 2015), pp. 1415–1418.

Povey, D. (1999). Optimistic security: A new access control paradigm. *Workshop on New Security Paradigms*, pp. 40–45.

Reader, R. (2020, March 4). 65 health apps on my phone let Facebook know when I used them. *Fast Company.* https://www.fastcompany.com/90457638/65-health-apps-on-my-phone-let-facebook-know-when-i-used-them

Roesner, F., Kohno, T., Moshchuk, A., Parno, B., Wang, H. J., & Cowan, C. (2012). User-driven access control: Rethinking permission granting in modern operating systems. *IEEE Symposium on Security and Privacy*, pp. 224–238.

Saeb, S., Zhang, M., Karr, C. J., Schueller, S. M., Corden, M. E., Kording, K. P., & Mohr, D. C. (2015). Mobile phone sensor correlates of depressive symptom severity in daily-life behavior: An exploratory study. *Journal of Medical Internet Research, 17*(7), e175.

Saltzer, J. H., & Schroeder, M. D. (1975). The protection of information in computer systems. *Proceedings of the IEEE, 63*(9), 1278–1308.

Schaub, F., Balebako, R., Durity, A. L., & Cranor, L. F. (2015). A design space for effective privacy notices. *Symposium on Usable Privacy and Security* (SOUPS 2015), pp. 1–17.

Shaban, H. (2019, January 17). Airbnb refunds guest who found indoor cameras during his family's stay. *Washington Post.* www.washingtonpost.com/technology/2019/01/17/airbnb-refunds-guest-who-found-indoor-cameras-during-his-familys-stay

Shaban, H. (2018, May 24). An Amazon Echo recorded a family's conversation, then sent it to a random person in their contacts, report says. *Washington Post.* https://www.washingtonpost.com/news/the-switch/wp/2018/05/24/an-amazon-echo-recorded-a-familys-conversation-then-sent-it-to-a-random-person-in-their-contacts-report-says

Shklovski, I., Mainwaring, S. D., Skúladóttir, H. H., & Borgthorsson, H. (2014). Leakiness and creepiness in app space: Perceptions of privacy and mobile app use. *Conference on Human Factors in Computing Systems* (CHI 2014), pp. 2347–2356.

SmartInsight. (2020). *Average display advertising clickthrough rates.* https://www.smartinsights.com/internet-advertising/internet-advertising-analytics/display-advertising-clickthrough-rates

Smith, I., & Hudson, S. E. (1995). Low disturbance audio for awareness and privacy in media space applications. *ACM International Conference on Multimedia*, pp. 91–97.

Solove, D. J. (2008). *Understanding privacy.* Harvard University Press.

Statista. (2020a). *Number of Fitbit devices sold worldwide from 2010 to 2019.* https://www.statista.com/statistics/472591/fitbit-devices-sold

Statt, N. (2019, February 22) App makers are sharing sensitive personal information with Facebook but not telling users. *The Verge.* https://www.theverge.com/2019/2/22/18236398/facebook-mobile-apps-data-sharing-ads-health-fitness-privacy-violation

Sweeney, L. (2002). k-anonymity: A model for protecting privacy. *International Journal of Uncertainty, Fuzziness and Knowledge-Based Systems, 10*(5), 557–570.

Tabassum, M., Alqhatani, A., Aldossari, M., & Lipford, H. R. (2018). *Increasing user attention with a comic-based policy.* Conference on Human Factors in Computing Systems (CHI 2018).

Tahaei, M., Ramokapane, K. M., Li, T., Hong, J. I., & Rashid, A. (2022) *Charting app developers' journey through privacy regulation features in ad networks.* Privacy Enhancing Technologies Symposium (PETS 2022).

Tahaei, M., Vaniea, K., & Saphra, N. (2020). *Understanding privacy-related questions on stack overflow.* Conference on Human Factors in Computing Systems (CHI 2020).

Tan, J., Nguyen, K., Theodorides, M., Negrón-Arroyo, H., Thompson, C., Egelman, S., & Wagner, D. (2014). The effect of developer-specified explanations for permission requests on smartphone user behavior. *Conference on Human Factors in Computing Systems* (CHI 2014), pp. 91–100.

Templeman, R., Korayem, M., Crandall, D. J., & Kapadia, A. (2014). PlaceAvoider: Steering first-person cameras away from sensitive spaces. *Network and Distributed System Security Symposium*, pp. 23–26.

W3C Working Group. (2019, January). *Tracking preference expression (DNT).* https://w3c.github.io/dnt/drafts/tracking-dnt.html

Westin, A. F. (1967). *Privacy and freedom.* Scribner.

Wijesekera, P., Baokar, A., Tsai, L., Reardon, J., Egelman, S., Wagner, D., & Beznosov, K. (2017). The feasibility of dynamically granted permissions: Aligning mobile privacy with user preferences. *IEEE Symposium on Security and Privacy*, pp. 1077–1093.

Wright, D., & De Hert, P. (Eds.). (2011). *Privacy impact assessment.* Springer Science + Business Media.

Zheng, S., Apthorpe, N., Chetty, M., & Feamster, N. (2018). User perceptions of smart home IoT privacy. *Proceedings of the ACM on Human-Computer Interaction,* 2 (CSCW), pp. 1–20.

CHAPTER 3

Transparency and Reproducibility in Mobile Sensing Research

Cornelia Wrzus and Ramona Schoedel

CHAPTER OVERVIEW

Researchers have to decide on a multitude of topics during planning, preparing, and conducting mobile sensing studies, and then analyzing the resulting data. These decisions can alter the answers to a given research question substantially and thus need to be communicated transparently, thereby allowing others to evaluate the scientific evidence and to replicate the research. This chapter outlines critical issues of transparent research along the steps of conducting a mobile sensing study. In summarizing the transparency-relevant issues of each step, the chapter provides suggestions on how to preregister and transparently report mobile sensing studies. Because not everything can be known and decided before the data collection, preregistration might be incomplete, and transparent reporting in an article can compensate for missing details in preregistration. The chapter's final section discusses conditions that can undermine replicability despite transparency. Throughout, we point to potential conflicts and tradeoffs between transparency and privacy, that is, data protection.

Introduction

Around the same time that the smartphone revolution occurred (Miller, 2012) and mobile sensing started in psychology and other fields (Aharony, Pan, Ip, Khayal, & Pentland, 2011; Eagle, Pentland, & Lazer, 2009)—that is, around 2010—psychology experienced another revolution, labeled as the "replication crisis" or alternatively as the "credibility revolution" (Simmons, Nelson, & Simonsohn, 2011). Unreported flexibility in data collection and analyses could substantially increase false-positive findings and thus undermine the replicability and credibility of psychological results (Nosek et al., 2015;

Simmons et al., 2011). To limit harmful flexibility such as deleting observations and/or variables to obtain significant results as well as questionable, actually out-of-question practices such as phrasing hypotheses after obtaining results, guidelines for open and transparent science have been proposed and now adopted in major scientific journals (American Psychological Association, 2021; Nosek et al., 2015; Simmons et al., 2011). *Transparency in open science* means disclosure of the research process—that is, making theoretical considerations, study planning, materials, analyses, and data available to others. It intends to openly communicate all decisions associated with the research process to comprehend whether and to what extent the interpretation of results depends on these decisions (Klein, Hardwicke, et al., 2018). This chapter examines how guidelines derived for psychological experiments and questionnaire studies can be transferred and adapted to mobile sensing research.

At first glance, it may seem that mobile sensing methods are less susceptible to questionable research practices as mobile sensing data appear *objective*. However, researchers have to make many *subjective* choices during planning, preparing, conducting, and analyzing mobile sensing studies. To ensure transparency and replicability, these choices need to be documented and reported, ideally largely before conducting the mobile sensing study and in a standardized way (i.e., in a preregistration of the study). Preregistration and transparent reporting allow other researchers to reproduce the results with the original data and to replicate studies as well as findings with new data. *Reproducibility* (or *verification*) is often understood as using the original raw data and analysis scripts to compute the results again (Clemens, 2017), whereas *replicability* refers to "repeating the methodology of a previous study and obtaining the same result" in an independent sample of participants/observations (Nosek & Errington, 2017, p. 1; see also Steiner, Wong, & Anglin, 2019).

Mobile sensing, especially in psychology, is a relatively young and also complex research field in which transparency standards are still under development. Complexity arises from the multiplicity of available information from many channels and time points (e.g., momentary or aggregated app use, microphone data over several days and weeks), as well as the almost infinite number of ways of analyzing and combining this information. The data complexity, that is, the "unprecedented collection coverage, the invisibility of the collection process, the amount of data collected, and the envisioned system interconnectivity" (Spiekermann & Langheinrich, 2009, p. 389), leads to concerns regarding privacy and misuse, which complicate yet do not preclude transparency.

Ideally, a fully transparent mobile sensing study would openly preregister hypotheses, study design (including sampling, procedures, and materials together with software), and a complete data analysis plan (e.g., Nosek et al., 2015). At the moment, this might be difficult to achieve in mobile sensing, and the greatest challenges arise in specifying the preprocessing and analyses before the data collection. The complexity of the workflow in mobile sensing studies, in comparison to questionnaire-based research and research with few experimental conditions, often impede the detailed, a priori specification of all processing and analytic steps. Also, some decisions can only be made after prior analyses (e.g., when applying machine learning algorithms, selection of variables and algorithms partly depend on how different algorithms perform during the analyses). Furthermore, due to the wide variety of data types available in mobile sensing, it is quite feasible to formulate hypotheses at a conceptual level, but it is much more difficult to establish a precise and specific operationalization of theoretical constructs in advance. For example, a study on communication behaviors can examine indicators of frequency, duration, and perhaps quality of calls, video calls, text messages, voice messages, communication in different apps, personal contact (e.g., based on Bluetooth inferred physical proximity or sound snippets), and many more.

After explaining necessary decisions and challenges at each step of mobile sensing studies (see Figure 3.1), we summarize suggestions for preregistration (Table 3.1 on page 73) and transparent reporting (Table 3.2 on pages 74–75) at different levels of specificity. We encourage researchers to apply a two-step procedure:

1. Define as many preregistration decisions as precisely as possible, for example, based on piloting.
2. Report all decisions made over the course of data collection and processing transparently for parts or cases where preregistration was not possible.

Importantly, we also encourage reviewers and readers of mobile sensing studies to acknowledge the efforts and to consider that appropriate standards are still developing.

Workflow of Transparent Mobile Sensing Studies

The general workflow of a mobile sensing study has steps similar to most other empirical studies in the behavioral sciences (Figure 3.1). Differences arise within each step and during onboard processing and preprocessing of data. In addition, transparency of data and code (i.e., open data, open code) might be highly privacy-sensitive because of potential (commercial) misuse of the super-rich data. These data are more informative than electroencephalograms, or even the browser history of stationary computers, because the captured information is potentially so comprehensive (i.e., breadth of domains such as communication, location, physical activity) and complete (i.e., covering most to all of an individual's daily life).

Research Questions and Hypotheses

Research employing mobile sensing usually falls into one of two areas: The first addresses mobile sensing as a research topic in itself. For example, do samples of people or situations differ from samples in other research approaches (e.g., people might differ in age, digital literacy; situations might differ in intimacy; Beierle et al., 2019; Mehl & Holleran, 2007); how well can mood and daily routines be inferred from smartphone usage (e.g., Servia-Rodríguez et al., 2017); how valid is information on people's physical activity based on smartphone tracking vs. body-attached sensors (e.g., Thomson et al., 2019)? The second kind of research uses mobile sensing as just another, potentially more objective approach to measure behavior and psychological phenomena. For example, how do differences in trait extraversion manifest in daily social behavior (Harari et al., 2020); do people show reliable inter- and intraindividual differences in daily day–night activity patterns (Schoedel et al., 2020)?

For the latter content-focused research questions, it usually will be possible to specify hypotheses in preregistration based on previous theoretical and empirical work

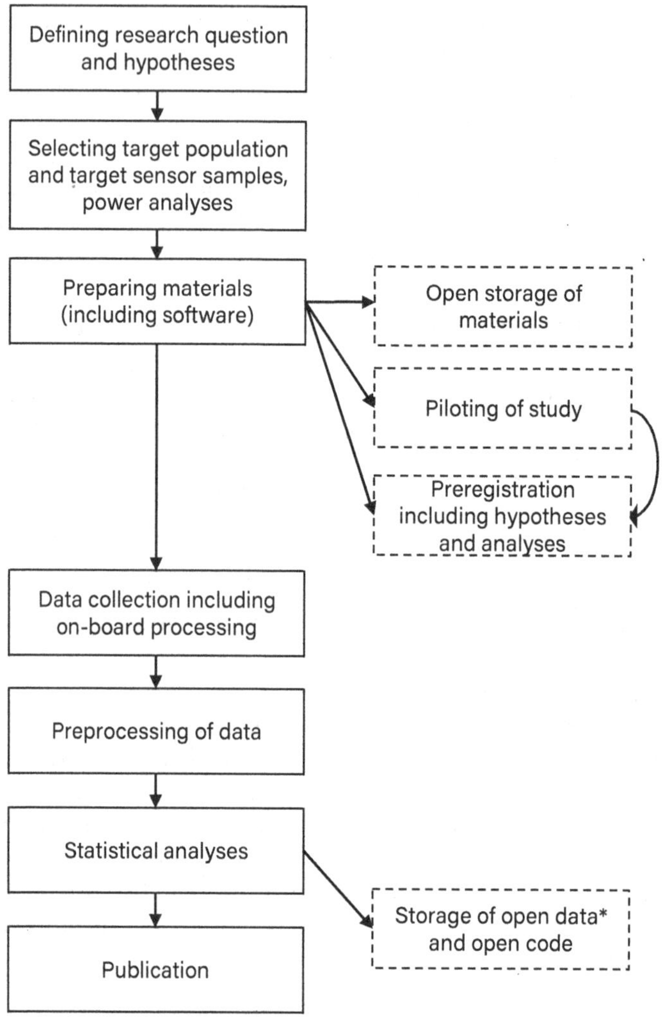

FIGURE 3.1. Steps of conducting mobile sensing studies. *Note:* Boxes with dashed frames indicate optional steps, with open storage and preregistration being strongly recommended for transparent mobile sensing studies. *Contingent on the study, data, review board, confidentiality agreement, and country.

(Table 3.1). As in other research areas, specific hypotheses will be helpful during data analyses when unexpected, even counterintuitive findings emerge, and post-hoc explanations seem all too plausible (Kerr, 1998). At the point of hypothesis specification, the hypotheses are stated on the construct level, for example "direct interpersonal contact." It is not necessary to name the specific parameters derived from the smartphone sensors already in the hypotheses because measurements and parameters are specified separately in preregistrations as variables or indicators of the respective constructs. One would assume effects on the level of the latent construct instead of the measure or indicator. To clarify, one would also not expect the effects of sleep deprivation on cognitive performance to vary substantially among comparable cognitive tests. Still, it is plausible that the mapping of a construct to specific sensor-based indicators is somewhat more complex than that in other studies because no clear standards are available at the moment. For example, does the number of different apps, the number of starting different apps, the total app usage time, or yet another parameter indicate excessive app usage best? At the same time, the hypotheses should be as specific as possible if conceptually distinct information can be derived from the multitude of available smartphone information (e.g., social contact vs. personal contact such as direct, synchronous contact such as calls vs. indirect, asynchronous contact through text or voice messages). Specific, unambiguous hypotheses are also necessary to be able to identify conditions for rejecting hypotheses (Roberts & Pashler, 2000).

Regarding research on mobile sensing itself, for example, its reliability and validity, researchers will often find themselves in situations when stating clear hypotheses is impossible. Instead, exploratory research questions will be posed. Exploratory analyses can be addressed in the project at any time—and labeled as such (Wagenmakers, Wetzels, Borsboom, van der Maas, & Kievit, 2012)—and sometimes ideas for research questions arise after the preregistration during the data collection and analyses. In our opinion, specific indicators can but do not have to be specified in exploratory research, since examining and comparing different indicators can be addressed during multiverse analyses, sensitivity analyses, or cross-validation (Brandmaier, Chapter 17, this volume; Kass & Raftery, 1995; Steegen, Tuerlinckx, Gelman, & Vanpaemel, 2016; see also the section "Statistical Analysis"). As discussed by other scholars, both confirmatory and exploratory analyses possess distinct advantages and yet allow different conclusions regarding the obtained findings, and need to be labeled as such (Wagenmakers et al., 2012; Table 3.2). One project can entail both, and we argue that preregistration of exploratory research questions can still be helpful to minimize the "file-drawer" problem: Until a study and its results are accepted for publication in a scientific journal, or even if they are not accepted, the study and its research questions will still be documented, and other researchers will be able to search for this work. Ideally, the results or a preprint are added to the project later or stored on specific preprint servers (e.g., PsyArXiv) after the data collection and linked with the preregistration.

In our experience, it is helpful to think about how potential publications should be structured already during the preregistration process. Mobile sensing data gathered in one study can often be used to address several distinct questions because the assessed data are often quite complex and comprehensive; for example, data on phone usage, app use, communication, activity, and location are often assessed in one study (Aharony et al., 2011; Stachl, Au, et al., 2020). Specifying all hypotheses that researchers can think of in one large preregistration can lead to one of two problems: Reporting all preregistered yet theoretically unrelated hypotheses in one manuscript might lead to conceptual fuzziness and a lack of focus, thus hampering clarity. Alternatively, selecting a subset of the preregistered hypotheses that belongs to a specific research question for a manuscript and leaving out other hypotheses might evoke the impression of cherry-picking. Both problems can be avoided by either specifying subsections for separate manuscripts (i.e., research questions) in one preregistration or preregistering different manuscripts (i.e., research questions) separately. Registered reports can further help to solve this dilemma because such reports include the theoretical background and methods for a specific research question and are submitted before the data collection starts.

Despite the recommendations described for preregistration of mobile sensing studies prior to data collection, it will not be possible (with reasonable effort) to preregister all potential hypotheses in advance because of the wide variety of data types and their usefulness for a broad range of research topics and domains (e.g., how does app usage vary with personality characteristics, gender, age, socioeconomic status, time of day, mood? . . .). But research projects can still be preregistered *after* the data collection and should also be given high priority in mobile sensing. They help the researcher to approach a research question in a structured manner and to specify the hypotheses, operationalization, and analyses given the abundance of data. The occurrence of questionable research practices, such as a quick screening of data to adjust hypotheses, should be less likely in mobile sensing studies, since raw data must be preprocessed elaborately to extract the variables needed for the hypotheses. Of course, researchers must decide responsibly whether they already know the raw data so well that preregistration is no longer appropriate.

Target Population and Target Sensor Samples

While planning and preparing the mobile sensing study, researchers have to decide on two crucial sampling issues: participants and behaviors. Interestingly, the software/app to conduct the mobile sensing study and the underlying operating system such as Android or iOS can affect both the targeted population and targeted behavior samples.

Target Population

In 2020, about 66% of all humans owned a mobile phone, two-thirds of which were smartphones (Statista, 2020a). In Western countries, such as the United Kingdom, Germany, or the United States, about 80% of the population owned a smartphone (Statista, 2020b). In general, Android-operated smartphones exceeded iOS-based smartphones (86% vs. 14%; Statista, 2020c). In some countries with high gross domestic product (GDP) per capita, the more expensive iPhones were somewhat more common; for example, iOS operated on 38% of U.K. phones and on 41% of U.S. phones (Statista, 2020c). Some studies have reported iOS users to have higher education and income compared to Android users, yet such effects are usually small and inconsistent (Götz, Stieger, & Reips, 2017; Shaw, Ellis, Kendrick, Ziegler, & Wiseman, 2016; Wang et al., 2018). Small differences between iOS and Android users might also be due to smartphone samples being selective in general, that is, not representing the entire population or containing larger proportions of a certain group. For example, recent smartphone studies have consisted mainly of young adults—with a higher sampling probability of men if participants were recruited online (Beierle et al., 2019; Chittaranjan, Blom, & Gatica-Perez, 2013, Montag et al., 2015) compared to participants recruited from college courses (Harari et al., 2020). Notably, the online samples are often still more diverse with respect to age and education compared to student samples (Beierle et al., 2019; Gosling & Mason, 2015; Montag et al., 2015). Regarding the transparency of samples, potential sources of selectivity should be considered carefully and addressed transparently in the preregistration and the published report (Keusch, Struminskaya, Antoun, Couper, & Kreuter, 2019; Kreuter, Haas, Keusch, Bähr, & Trappmann, 2020). This includes where participants are/were recruited, how they are/were incentivized (Harari et al., 2016), and which information on sociodemographic and other characteristics is assessed to later describe the sample and compare it to the target population (Tables 3.1 and 3.2).

In addition to the selectivity of the initial sample, researchers should anticipate hidden dropout, which leads to selective continuation of data collection. For example, participants might use their phones differently than usual due to technical errors, battery consumption of the sensing app, or awareness of being monitored. Also, participants might leave the study earlier or temporarily. Missing days in openly available sensing data (Aharony et al., 2011) hint toward hidden dropout and technical problems. Person characteristics might covary with hidden dropout: For example, in one study, the more conscientious participants were, the more reliably they wore wrist sensors, and they thus produced less missing/hidden dropout (Wiernik et al., 2020). The anticipated dropout should be included in power estimations of intended sample sizes. For example, if power analyses suggest a required sample size of 300 for the expected effects, and a dropout rate of 10% is estimated based on previous research, 333 participants need to be recruited. In general, power analyses are needed for preparing and registering the study and can be done based on the sample sizes and effect sizes of previous comparable research. Often no previous effect sizes are available because the exact same research question has not been examined before, and it is unknown whether the effects for one personal characteristic, for example extraversion, can be adopted for a related characteristic, such as the affiliation motive. In addition, one has to keep in mind that effect sizes might be small if mobile sensing data are linked to other data sources (e.g., questionnaire data) because there is no shared method variance. The latter is positive but influences the size of effects and thus the necessary sample size—both regarding participants and observations per participant. In an additional approach, simulation studies can also estimate complex models. In both cases, the steps and decisions are documented through referring to previous studies and the obtained effect sizes and through providing the (ideally annotated) scripts for the simulation studies (Table 3.1).

Selectivity, that is, individual differences in willingness to share data, might also depend on the study topic, the provided information, and the technical and data protection literacy (Beierle et al., 2019; Keusch et al., 2019; Nebeker et al., 2016). In general, women, and somewhat surprisingly, young adults have been shown to be less willing to share mobile sensing data (but see Kreuter et al., 2020), while no effects of education or personality traits have been found (Beierle et al., 2019; Kreuter et al., 2020; Nebeker et al., 2016). In this respect, transparency also extends to the information provided to participants before and during the study implementation. Although one would assume that providing more information increases transparency, one has to keep in mind that truly informed consent can be achieved only if the provided information is adapted to the technical literacy of participants. If the study is conducted solely online without personal contact with participants, researchers need to ensure that participants read and understand the consent document. Study information might be presented in videos instead of written text, as most participants spend too little time on screens with consent information to actually read the information (Beierle et al., 2019; Kreuter et al., 2020). One could speculate that issues of selectivity will diminish when smartphone data remain completely on people's smartphones and participants share only summary statistics of their phone usage and sensor information. Interesting ideas have been proposed on how to analyze data anonymously on the smartphone using predefined algorithms (Dennis et al., 2019). At the same time, average app usage such as Facebook versus TikTok (at the moment) already offers substantial information on users' age, gender, and personality traits (e.g., Stachl, Au, et al., 2020). Hence, willingness to participate and thus sample selectivity will always be also a question of data protection. Anticipating issues of sample selectivity in the preregistrations and transparently assessing and reporting sample characteristics and dropout (Table 3.2) will facilitate progress on these questions.

Target Time and Behavior

Collecting mobile sensing data is generally effortless to researchers and participants because the app "silently" collects information on phone use and environmental information without additional work for participants (i.e., passive ambulatory assessment). As a result, it is tempting to collect as much information for as long as possible. For example, one of the first mobile sensing studies—the Friends and Family Study (conducted at MIT)—collected information on app use, calls, texting, acceleration, and battery status for several months up to over one year (Aharony et al., 2011). We state the obvious when we suggest that researchers confine themselves to the information that is necessary for the research question and to constrain the duration to the shortest useful period. This is in line with EU data protection guidelines, which advise data parsimony and allow the collection of only the data that are necessary for the intended purpose (GDPR, Art. 5, §1a, https://gdpr-info.eu/art-5-gdpr). Accordingly, researchers have to specify assessed parameters/sensors, assessment times, duration, and sampling frequency. At the same time, shorter periods cover a restricted, perhaps selective part of daily life and may lead to less reliable assessments, potentially compromising the replicability of results at other times.

An alternative thought could be to collect maximally comprehensive data once and to reuse the data. Again, this seems very tempting and economical but entails the risk of too much linked information (e.g., location, social activity, health behavior; Servia-Rodríguez et al., 2017), which is critical from a privacy and data protection perspective, especially regarding sharing (raw) data (see also Chapter 2, "Designing for Privacy in Mobile Sensing Systems"). Furthermore, long time periods potentially increase researchers' degrees of freedom if specific periods of the collected data are analyzed separately (e.g., deleting the first "familiarization" day, excluding holidays). We believe that this does not constitute a major problem because such analytic decisions would have to be preregistered or reported transparently.

Some information will be collected using event-based sampling, that is, when something changes. For example, calls, text messages, and opening/using an app are logged when this action occurs together with the time of occurrence. Other information is available continuously (e.g., position and acceleration of phone, light sensor information), and sampling frequencies have to be determined—basically researchers decide how much they are willing to miss. Importantly, sampling frequencies will vary between studies and with different sensors (e.g., GPS vs. acceleration). For example, determining the GPS- and cell-tower-based position every minute for 2 seconds will result in high-density location information with up to 86,400 location points per day. Researchers may decide that during most periods of the day positions will not change that much—GPS having a precision of 3–10 meters (or 10–30 feet) outdoors—and decide on less frequent sampling. In contrast, researchers might want to assess smartphone acceleration as an indicator of physical activity almost continuously instead of only for a few seconds once per minute to capture most of the movement of the smartphone, that is, its owner. Preprocessing of data (e.g., averaging activity per minute; see the section "Preprocessing of Data") will reduce data bulk. Similarly, researchers could skip or reduce data collection during predefined night hours. As mentioned before, highly dense data will affect privacy issues strongly (Mendes, Cunha, & Vilela, 2020). For example, continuous sound sampling over the course of a day will record complete conversations and thus corrupt privacy. In contrast, random sampling of sounds, including words, for 30 seconds a few times per hour, for instance, offers rich information on social interactions, daily activities, or depressive symptoms, but it still ensures privacy (Mehl, 2017; Mehl, Gosling, & Pennebaker, 2006; Tackman et al., 2019). Any such decisions are plausible and depend on the research question, and they just have to be specified in preregistrations or reported transparently after the data collection. In summary, theoretical considerations and previous work, including pilot studies, are necessary to decide on the best suited sampling frequency and duration. Because duration and sampling frequency have to be specified for the app in any case, they are easily preregistered (Table 3.1).

Preparing Materials Transparently

Materials and Informed Consent

In our view, the greatest challenges for preparing materials transparently apply to the details in and comprehensiveness of the informed consent for participants and in the materials provided in repositories for other researchers.

As outlined in the previous section, to be truly informative for participants, study information has to be not only complete but also adapted to the technical knowledge of the participants. Several guidelines on how to construct informed consent provide valuable advice (Beierle et al., 2019; Nebeker et al., 2016) and yet have to be adapted to specific research projects. In general, suggestions are to provide understandable summaries together with detailed study information, to offer examples of what collected data look like; to ask for permission when it is needed (instead of presenting a long, comprehensive list in the beginning); to have opt-out options for separate features/functions of the app/study; and to describe the secured storage and data transfer (Beierle et al., 2019; Kreuter et al., 2020; Nebeker et al., 2016).

Currently, there is no standard for how to store and document mobile sensing research materials, and researchers face the challenge of preparing documentation that is both accurate and understandable, especially for those researchers who are not too familiar with this kind of research. The general aim of open materials is that other researchers can understand and replicate the research. Again, we assume that this can be achieved at different levels of specificity (Tables 3.1 and 3.2).

As in other study designs, with minimum effort, a complete list of measures of both self-reports and mobile sensors (sensing-derived parameters might be decided on later during the process and can be added later) can be provided, together with the software and hardware used to collect data. This list will also provide a helpful overview, if more details are provided (Tables 3.1 and 3.2). When storing items and software code in open repositories, researchers have to be aware of copyright regulations around items and software. In addition, two obstacles for storing software code should be kept in mind. First, sensing apps often use information already provided by the native operating system of the mobile phone (e.g., Android, iOS). The operating systems and their various versions can differ in how information is collected and preprocessed from sensors (Harari et al., 2016;

Wang et al., 2018). Also, the specific algorithm is often not available from the operating system developers. Second, storing code openly entails the risk of unauthorized (commercial) usage of code and in the worst case provides information for hackers on how to introduce malware into the app and/or steal data (Scott, Richards, & Adhikari, 2015). One helpful solution could be to assess the specific mobile phone types and their operating systems and later report it. This is similar to describing the apparatus for conducting electroencephalography (EEG) or functional magnetic resonance imaging (fMRI) studies together with the software version running on the apparatus.

Piloting the Mobile Sensing Materials

Researchers conducting technology-based studies are well advised to pilot the study setup and materials before collecting data from dozens or hundreds of people. This is equally true for mobile sensing studies because many errors can occur during data collection, such as excessive battery drain, incorrect data storage, or data loss (Harari et al., 2016). In addition to being able to test that the software and mobile phones function properly, piloting can facilitate preregistration. Pilot data, even from a few people over a few days, offer information on the data structure, necessary preprocessing steps, and reliability and validity of measures and indicators, if they are combined with other information, such as demographic information, questionnaire answers, or time of day.

Data Collection

Study Onboarding

Data collection in mobile sensing studies begins with the installation of the tracking app. Researchers can choose among several scenarios for this onboarding procedure. The first decision concerns whether participants are provided with smartphones or are asked to use their own (e.g., Harari et al., 2016). Second, researchers have to choose between online or face-to-face onboarding (e.g., Harari et al., 2020; Schuwerk, Kaltefleiter, Au, Hoesl, & Stachl, 2019). In the first case, participants download the tracking app from online stores or private distribution platforms and install the app on their own. The app can be free or restricted by a study code provided during recruitment. In the second case, participants come to the lab to install the app together with the investigator (e.g., Stachl et al., 2017). Finally, researchers have to decide whether to start data collection simultaneously for all participants or gradually over a specified period.

These decisions about the design of the onboarding scenario are an important source of sampling biases in mobile sensing studies, which we illustrate with a few examples here. First, the specific onboarding scenario might attract people with different traits and therefore be associated with a self-selection bias. For example, more introverted persons might be more likely to decide to participate if the onboarding can be carried out in an uncomplicated way online without further social obligations. However, more suspicious persons might find it more pleasant to have personal contact with the investigator before participating in data-intensive mobile sensing studies. The chosen onboarding procedure might additionally affect dropout. Participants are likely to have a commitment to continue the study until the end if they have already invested time to come to the lab and established a personal relationship with the research staff. Installing the tracking app from an online app store just as any other app might be associated with a higher feeling of anonymity, and therefore dropping out of the study could be a less significant hurdle. So far, these assumptions are speculative because previous mobile sensing studies examining sample selectivity still use the same onboarding scenario for all participants and thus cannot offer results about which participants' characteristics are linked to different onboarding options (e.g., in-person with direct researcher guidance, independently by downloading the app; Beierle et al., 2019; Kreuter et al., 2020; Ludwigs, Lucas, Veenhoven, Richter, & Arends, 2019). For example, from other demanding or privacy sensitive studies, we know that compliance with the study protocol is higher if participants had direct contact with researchers or research assistants—perhaps because they met the persons behind the study. Also, people who download research apps might differ from people who invest the effort to visit research labs. Thus, the chosen onboarding procedure might affect replicability of the study in future samples, if diverse onboarding procedures are used, and thus it should be reported transparently (Table 3.2).

Data Quality Monitoring

After the tracking app installation, the continuous data logging begins. Several challenges arise from the longitudinal data collection and technical character of the study. Because data collection occurs in people's daily life in the absence of research staff, problems that arise during data collection will likely not be detected immediately but have to be inferred later on, often leading to missing data.

During the data collection, participants interact with their smartphones as usual. In doing so, participants sometimes (un-)intentionally revoke permissions that are required by the tracking app. Depending on the study duration, some participants may change their smartphones and reinstall the tracking app on a new device. Besides these user behavior-related challenges, technical incidents can also occur. Despite careful preparation by extensively testing the tracking app in advance, software issues are sometimes only discovered during the study when a large variety of different smartphones and operating systems use the tracking app. Depending on the frequency of occurrence and the severity of the software bugs, they may need to be fixed during the study period, prompting participants to update the tracking app and potentially changing the data collection procedure.

All these cases affect data quality as they result in *systematically missing data*. An example for user-initiated systematically missing data is that participants revoke their permission to track GPS data on weekends because they do not want to be tracked where they are traveling in their free time for privacy reasons. In this context, researchers should also think about including a "pause button" to enable participants to consciously pause data collection (Buschek, Bisinger, & Alt, 2018).

Concerning software-related missing data, it might become apparent only during the study that, for example, the tracking app does not log certain smartphone events for older operating system versions, leading to missing data only for participants with older devices. Finally, missing data can also systematically occur between parts of the study. For example, during the course of the study, researchers notice from the complaints of the participants that the high sampling frequency of physical sensor data (e.g., ambient brightness and noise) leads to high battery consumption. To avoid a high dropout rate, a change to a more battery-friendly sampling frequency may need to be made during the study. In summary, researchers need to assess and document such cases of user- or software-induced missing data so that they will be able to report it transparently without generating the impression of selective exclusion of data.

Onboard Processing

Mobile sensing data can be captured in raw form, that is, as unprocessed technical data, such as those from sensors or other apps. But they can also be processed immediately during data acquisition. For example, instead of collecting GPS raw data (longitude and latitude) to be sorted by location type after the data collection phase (Mehrotra et al., 2017), the application programming interfaces (APIs) of external providers such as the Google Places API[1] could be used to directly extract and store relevant information (in this example, location types such as airport, bar, and church). Meanwhile, many freely available plug-ins for onboard processing are available, for example, for conversation detection (see Harari et al., 2020) or activity recognition (Ferreira, Kostakos, & Dey, 2015).

One benefit of onboard processing is the reduced storage and reduced data preprocessing *after* the data collection (see the section "Preprocessing of Data"). Moreover, from a data protection point of view, this method has the great advantage of not having to store the raw data, which usually contain more sensitive information. However, one challenge is the evaluation of the performance of the onboard processing algorithms and the *validity* and *reliability* of the resulting variables (RatSWD, 2020). Depending on the onboard processing software, algorithms and their performance measures are often not published, especially for those from commercial suppliers. For example, instead of storing raw GPS and physical sensor data, an activity onboard recognition algorithm could be used to extract the users' activities (e.g., steps, doing sports, driving, sleeping). If performance measures for the onboard processing are unknown, researchers have no information about how well the classification algorithm worked (i.e., with what accuracy the respective activities were detected on the basis of the raw sensor data). Even with open-source algorithms, it might be very difficult for researchers to figure out precisely how the algorithm transforms raw data in, for example, steps per day. When no or limited information on the reliability and validity of the classification of activities is available, subsequent results of the data analysis can be interpreted only to a limited extent. Possible solutions could be to validate onboard processing algorithms through pilot studies, which can have the additional benefit of testing the algorithm under the conditions and in the population later examined in the main study—as many algorithms are validated as proof-of-concept, that is, under laboratory conditions with only a few selected people, sometimes the developers themselves. At the very least, it is important to document and report the exact version number of software and, if possible, the software code (Table 3.2), for the later comparison and replication of results.

Preprocessing of Data

Alternatively, or in addition to onboard processing, further processing takes place after the data collection phase. This offline preprocessing comprises any steps related to the extraction of variables that can be used for statistical analyses afterward. If not specified in detail in the preregistration or documented and reported comprehensively, it can impede research transparency severely because so many steps are involved in preprocessing. Usually, raw mobile sensing data are tabular data. That means each row represents a logging event specified by different features represented by the columns. For example, if a participant uses the Facebook messenger app at 11:03 A.M., a new row containing the usage event (app usage), the name of the app (Facebook Messenger), the time of occurrence (11:03), and further specifications is created in the database. Across the whole study period, this results in thousands of rows per (!) participant. However, researchers are usually not interested in raw logging events for statistical modeling but in meaningful variables (e.g., the average daily duration of social interaction). To convert the raw mobile sensing data into meaningful variables, researchers have to make numerous decisions (Hoffmann et al., 2021; Schoedel et al., 2020), which might affect reproducibility and replicability, and should be specified before the data collection (Table 3.1). Some of the decisions depend on the data properties (e.g., distribution, extent of missing data and outliers, and value range of events to be classified, such as package names of apps used by participants). These decisions can only be made after the data collection (i.e., not preregistered) and should thus be documented and reported transparently (Table 3.2).

The preprocessing decisions always include procedures for handling *missing data*. For example, researchers have to think about how many hours per day data must be logged to ensure the validity of study days (e.g., Harari et al., 2020). Based on this information, the question arises as to when researchers exclude invalid study days and how many valid study days are necessary per participant to be included in the sample (e.g., Wang et al., 2018).

In addition, researchers have to define the *temporal characteristics* of their variables. For example, if social interactions are investigated, the researcher has to define what "weekend" means: Do Friday nights already count as a weekend because the next day is usually free and participants are freer to decide how they want to spend their time? Or do Friday evenings belong to the working week because the participants are tired of the working week and therefore behave differently than on Saturday and Sunday? Accordingly, researchers also have to decide which times define day and night (e.g., Stachl, Au, et al., 2020) and whether the day should be considered as a whole or in intervals such as morning, afternoon, evening, and night (e.g., Harari et al., 2020; Wang et al., 2018).

Additionally, *content characteristics* have to be defined. For example, research questions usually do not refer to variables that reflect the usage of a specific app (e.g., Facebook Messenger app), but rather to broader behavioral categories of app usage such as communication, entertainment, or gaming. Therefore, researchers have to decide which apps belong to which categories (e.g., Stachl et al., 2017). Furthermore, researchers have to think about the granularity of the extracted variables. For example, social interaction could be operationalized by simply extracting communication app usage. However, it would also be possible to distinguish between communication app usage in dyadic versus group interactions, or with frequent versus unique interaction partners.

Finally, quantification *metrics* have to be determined. The logging data collected over the entire study period are often aggregated to summarized variables. Regarding measures of central tendency (e.g., the daily average communication app usage), researchers can aggregate the raw data using the median, the arithmetic mean, or the robust mean, depending on the nature of the logging data (e.g., Mønsted, Mollgaard, & Stachl, 2018; Montag et al., 2014). Researchers can choose between the standard deviation and robust estimates for measures of dispersion (e.g., daily variation in the communication app usage; e.g., Mønsted et al., 2018). Other measures, such as the minimum, the maximum, or change over time, can be applied to quantify the distribution of smartphone usage events (e.g., Schoedel et al., 2020).

In summary, researchers have to make many subjective decisions in the process of variable extraction (Hoffmann et al., 2021). Initial work indicates that these seemingly small subjective decisions in data preprocessing affect statistical results based on mobile sensing data (Schoedel et al., 2020). As discussed before, sensed variables can be extracted depending on the part of the week (weekend vs. week; e.g., Harari et al., 2020). But how do researchers actually define the weekend? From Saturday to Sunday or from Friday night to Monday morning because these nights are part of the weekend? For example, the associations between age, gender, conscientiousness, and the duration of nighttime smartphone nonuse on weekends varied depending on how the weekend was coded (Schoedel et al., 2020; see Figure 3.2). Consequently, the degrees of freedom in mobile sensing research imply the risk of *selective reporting* and, as a consequence, false-positive findings (Simmons et al., 2011). This means that researchers might try out different specifications in the variable extraction process and only report on those variable variants for which desired analysis results emerge (Gelman & Loken, 2014). This procedure, in turn, results in a lack of robustness of findings across studies. Tables 3.1 and 3.2 offer suggestions on preregistering some of these decisions before the data collection and on transparently reporting the decisions to facilitate replicability in mobile sensing research. Briefly reporting information in the manuscript and in supplementary materials about multiverse analyses or sensitivity analyses (Kass & Raftery, 1995; Leamer, 1985; Steegen et al., 2016), which demonstrate how findings vary (or not) depending on different specifications during the data preprocessing, would offer readers the necessary information to evaluate the interpretation of the authors (e.g., Schoedel et al., 2020).

Statistical Analysis

After the extraction of meaningful variables, statistical analyses can be performed. As with any other analysis workflow, researchers get a first overview of the variables of interest by looking at descriptive characteristics and visualizing distributions. In comparison to research with questionnaire data, technical data in mobile sensing research are often susceptible to logging errors. Although some of these can be considered already during data preprocessing (e.g., as presented under "Preprocessing of Data"), by using robust aggregation measures, outliers and missing values are often present in the extracted variables. Because there is no "one-size-fits-all" solution for handling them, researchers are again faced with many options for transforming the extracted dataset into a version suitable for statistical modeling. These processing steps include primarily data exclusion, handling of outliers and missing values, and the transformation of variables. With data from pilot studies, rules for identifying and handling outlier, missing, or non-normally distributed data can largely be specified in the preregistration (Table 3.1).

As already mentioned, previous studies have shown that the degrees of freedom in data preparation lead to differences in statistical results (Simonsohn, Simmons, & Nelson, 2015; Steegen et al., 2016) and are thus a risk factor for the nonreplicability of research results (Hoffmann et al., 2021). Traditionally, computer science might be less prone to selective reporting because generally results based on different parameters (e.g., features extracted from sensing data) and algorithms (e.g., kNN, SVM, LDA; Brandmaier, Chapter 17, this volume) are reported in parallel (e.g., Chittaranjan et al., 2013; Kambham, Stanley, & Bell, 2018). To avoid practices such as selective reporting, various statistical analysis techniques have been proposed. They all follow the general principle of performing statistical analysis on the multitude of plausible alternatives for data processing decisions, thereby illustrating the robustness of the results in terms of researchers' data processing decisions (Hoffmann et al., 2021). For example, multiverse analyses (Steegen et al., 2016) require reporting transparently on all processing steps and thinking about plausible alternatives for each decision. Originally, the multiverse approach referred to exclusion criteria for outliers and was then applied to other preprocessing decisions in questionnaire-based research as well (Steegen et al., 2016). In the interest of robust science, it is recommended that the principle of multiverse analyses is applied to mobile sensing research as well, but currently no standards exist. For example, the number of preprocessing steps in mobile sensing is much larger than that in research with questionnaire data, and, even with much effort and expense, researchers will only be able to map a selection of preprocessing decisions in a multiverse analysis. By combining arbitrary decision alternatives, many slightly different datasets are created and then used individually to perform statistical analyses. Finally, the range of results of all analyses is presented descriptively or visualized in overview plots (see Figure 3.2 as an example). Such graphical overviews of results allow readers to evaluate deviations in results based on somewhat different analyses or subsets of data and thus to judge the robustness of the results at a glance—for example, regarding the associations between age, gender, conscientiousness and the duration of nighttime smartphone nonuse on weekends (Schoedel et al., 2020).

In the section "Research Questions and Hypotheses," we discuss why hypothesis-based, preregistered statistical analyses in mobile sensing research will be useful and necessary in future research. In the first steps of mobile sensing research, however, many explorative analyses are carried out (e.g., Montag et al., 2014; Stachl et al., 2017). One reason for this exploratory analysis strategy is certainly that mobile sensing offers a much greater variety of possibilities for operationalizing behavioral variables compared to previous self-report-based research, and thus allows more researchers' degrees of freedom. For example, the variable *interpersonal contact* can be operationalized in many ways: (1) communication app usage, (2) social media app usage, (3) (video-)calls, (4) text messages, (5) voice messages, and (6) in-person contact each regarding frequency, duration, or the number of unique contacts—already leading to 18 options with this incomplete list. Direct behavioral equivalents are often missing in the previous literature, which is why researchers prefer to remain vague by formulating explorative questions.

In line with this observation, predictive approaches, that is, the use of machine learning techniques, have become established in mobile sensing research (e.g., Mønsted et al., 2018; Stachl, Pargent, et al., 2020; Wang et al., 2018). An advantage of machine learning methods is that they can handle a large number of predictors in relation to a criterion to condense information (Brandmaier, Chapter 17, this volume). This means that a large number of different operationalizations for one construct can be included in the model without the researcher having to decide in advance on one of the many plausible alternatives.

However, it should be considered that similar variables usually strongly correlate. A well-known problem in explanation-oriented models in psychology also applies to machine learning models: Correlated variables complicate interpretation of the results.

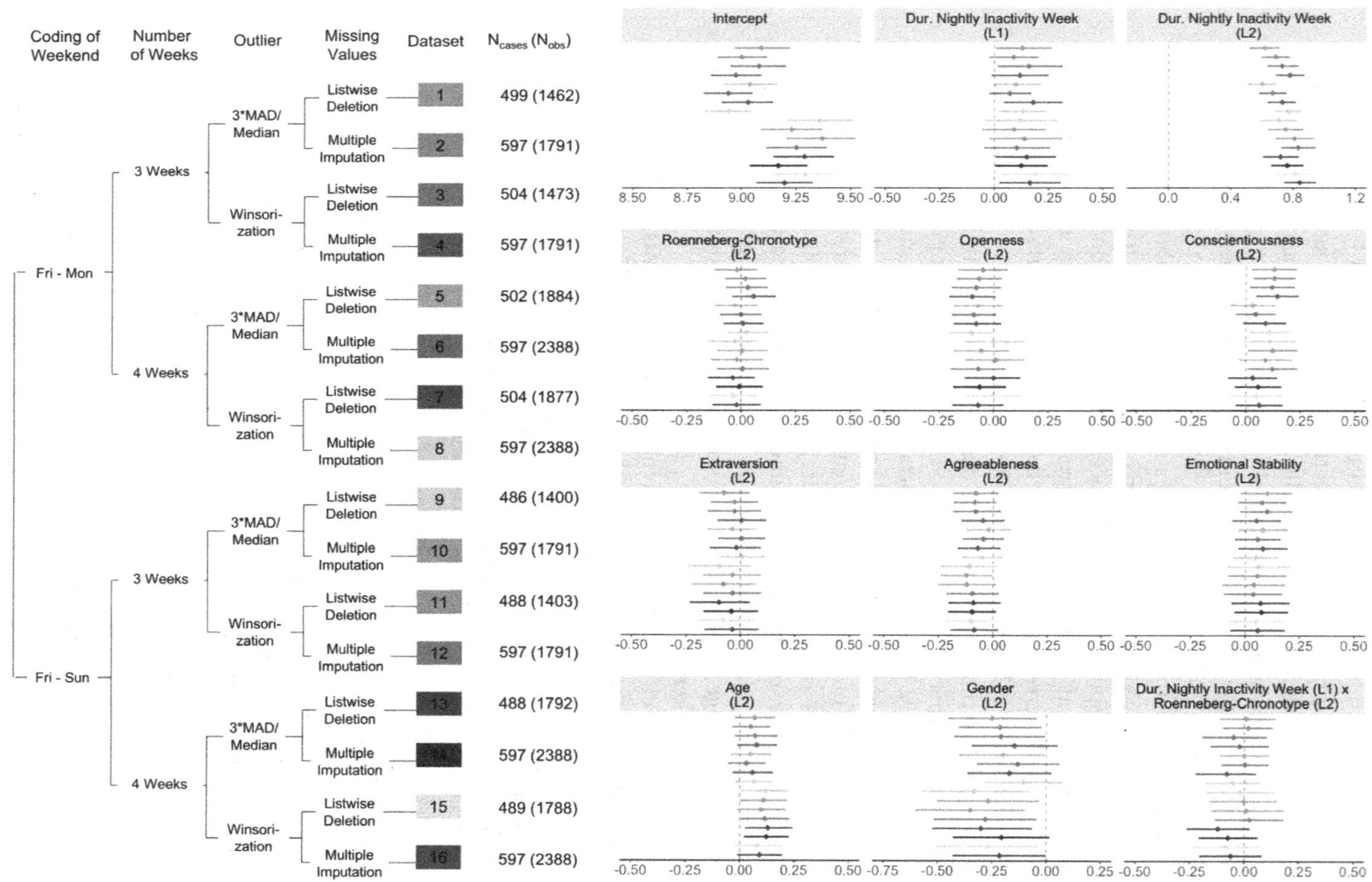

FIGURE 3.2. Illustration of a multiverse analysis in mobile sensing by Schoedel et al. (2020). *Note:* The decision tree on the left gives an overview of the decisions made during preprocessing and shows which different datasets (symbolized by different colors in the original) result from their combination. Each panel on the right maps the coefficients and confidence intervals per predictor of the multilevel model calculated in this example across all different datasets (colors in the original). Figure from Schoedel et al. (2020), published under open access.

To understand the prediction performance, methods of interpretable machine learning are often used to screen the most important variables (Stachl, Pargent, et al., 2020). For example, using lasso penalized regression with correlated variables, the algorithm simply selects one of the correlating variables randomly (Zou & Hastie, 2005). Nonlinear models such as the random forest also provide biased variable importance measures, if predictors are correlated (Strobl, Boulesteix, Zeileis, & Hothorn, 2007). As a consequence, if the rigid ranking of individual variables is interpreted from one study, replication studies might fail to identify the (ranking of) exact same important variables. Therefore, the results of machine learning models should not be interpreted strictly, but rather groups of meaning-related variables should be considered to formulate ideas for future hypothesis-driven confirmatory research (e.g., Brandmaier, Chapter 17, this volume; Schoedel et al., 2018). The groups of variables considered may be defined based on theoretical considerations and previous literature, or they may be data-driven (e.g., considering the variables before a noticeable drop in variable importance measures occurs). To be able to consider several variables for future research, results should be reported as comprehensively as possible, yet without compromising clarity (e.g., Table 1 in de Montjoye, Quoidbach, Robic, & Pentland, 2013, or Figure 2 in Stachl, Au, et al., 2020).

Storage of Open Data and Open Code

In general, (protected) sharing of data and code is imperative in science and will facilitate scientific and often also individual progress in any area of psychology and beyond (Joel, Eastwick, & Finkel, 2018; Van Horn & Ishai, 2007). Also, both scientific associations and funding agencies emphasize data sharing and provide guidelines to do so (e.g., American Psychological Association, German Research Foundation, NSF, Wellcome Trust; see Houtkoop et al., 2018; Schönbrodt, Gollwitzer, & Abele-Brehm, 2017).

Making data and analytic code *openly* accessible has several pros and cons. On the pro side, with both open data and open code, study results can be easily confirmed by independent others without having to rely on authors sending the data. Also, additional analyses (e.g., alternative analytic approaches) can be conducted, which might further strengthen the conclusions presented in the manuscript. In addition, other researchers might learn directly how to conduct certain analyses. Importantly, the software versions that are deployed have to be documented diligently because newer versions might use different commands and estimating procedures, which might compromise exact reproduction of the results with the available code and data. Specific suggestions exist on how to organize files, software versions, and code to achieve cross-platform and long-term computational reproducibility (Peikert & Brandmaier, 2019; see also Table 3.2).

One minor concern about open code relates to the statistical software deployed and the level of documentation. At this point in time, it seems too early to ask researchers to use a specific (open) software, such as R. As a consequence, others not familiar with the software or the specific analyses (e.g., random-forest structural equation modeling, Brandmaier, Prindle, McArdle, & Lindenberger, 2016) will not be able to understand or repeat the code easily. Thus, the challenge of transparent code is the level of description of often quite complex code; in part this also applies to other methods (e.g., preprocessing electroencephalogram data: Pedroni, Bahreini, & Langer, 2019; functional magnetic imaging data: Van Horn & Ishai, 2007).

In our opinion, the largest consideration is necessary regarding open data and privacy (see Chapter 2, "Designing for Privacy in Mobile Sensing Systems"). Mobile sensing data potentially include very dense, very private information regarding third persons, finances, health, and (illegal) activities. Accordingly, mobile sensing data should be strongly protected to ensure the privacy of participants and to prevent misuse.

Psychologists, including the authors themselves, have only begun to understand how to protect the privacy of participants. Until recently, anonymization—that is, assigning a random identifier that can be matched with a person through a separately saved key file—seemed viable. Current advancements in data reengineering and machine learning have demonstrated that individuals are identifiable with little information, such as demographic attributes (Rocher, Hendrickx, & De Montjove, 2019). One alternative could be the sharing of aggregated data, such as means, standard deviations, and covariance matrices, which are sufficient to reproduce certain SEM-based analyses (Muthén & Muthén, 2023). A second alternative could be to store data in repositories with restricted access and allow computation only on the computers of the repository with logging of activities and without the possibility to copy the data—as is the case with the Secure Data Access Center (in French, CASD, www.casd.eu). A third possibility uses differential privacy, where random noise is added to data (Fang, Zeng, & Yang, 2020; Gong, Pan, Xie, Qin, & Tang, 2020). This alternative impedes identification of individuals, yet retains contained information on a sample level. Not all of these options will be equally suitable for all research projects, although different access/security classes of data can be implemented (e.g., Level 0 open data to Level 3 secure data; Schönbrodt et al., 2017). Furthermore, a few years from now the possibilities to store and share sensitive data both securely and easily might have increased (see also Joel et al., 2018).

Providing aggregated data precludes the reproducibility of preprocessing to extract variables, but it ensures the reproducibility of main analyses based on the extracted variables. Openly available preprocessing code makes this preprocessing step at least transparent. Still, to enable other researchers to sustainably reuse mobile sensing data for new analyses and therefore to fulfill the claim of Open Data, it will also be necessary in the long term to find data protection friendly and easy-to-implement solutions for sharing the raw data. This, in turn, will require a change in research infrastructure over the next few years.

At the risk of being too cautious, even depersonalized data entail the risk of misuse—and especially so if transparent accompanying meta-information is reported to a greater degree. For example, data on political opinions, health problems, or financial information might be used to do harm during elections or when individuals enroll in an insurance plan, if the time and location (e.g., city, region) of data collection is reported (Granville, 2018). In summary, storing code will often be unproblematic (Table 3.2), but the storing of data and the related access options should be considered carefully to ensure data protection, privacy, and to guard against misuse.

Publication

Most of the thoughts presented in this section are not specific to mobile sensing studies. Accordingly, we keep it brief. What might be specific is that, at the moment, missing knowledge and existing stereotypes regarding mobile sensing studies might bias the publication process toward one of two directions. First, reviewers, editors, and readers might be enthusiastic, yet relatively uninformed about mobile sensing studies. This might result in an uncritical review process, and it entails the risk of publishing flawed mobile sensing studies or studies with too little information on all the steps outlined before. Second, and likely more common, reviewers, editors, and readers might be overly skeptical about mobile sensing studies because they do not trust the sensors or software, question the multitude of available options when preprocessing and analyzing the data, or are overwhelmed by technical details. In addition, reviewers and editors might underestimate how time-consuming it is to rerun analyses (e.g., extracting variables with somewhat changed specifications), and therefore they may suggest analyses that cannot easily be carried out during typical review phases. Standards from traditional survey research are often applied, which the mobile sensing field cannot yet achieve because it is still in its infancy (e.g., standards regarding validation studies for behavioral measures with several hundred participants). This will likely result in wrongful rejection, delay of the publication, or "file-drawer problems" (Simonsohn et al., 2015).

We do *not* claim that a more substantiated psychometric approach to mobile sensing-based studies is unnecessary. However, at the moment some open-mindedness regarding data preprocessing approaches and analyses might be necessary—provided that choices are made consciously and named transparently—so that mobile sensing can gradually establish itself as a paradigm in the broad field of psychological research. Both being overly enthusiastic and overly critical can be easily prevented by gaining knowledge of mobile sensing procedures, analyses, and standards, as well as by applying rigorous yet realistic standards to mobile sensing studies (e.g., regarding the level of specificity when preregistering analyses).

To embrace open science fully and to avoid rejection and file-drawer problems, researchers might decide to publish their findings solely via open access (e.g., preprint servers such as PsyArXiv or ArXiv) and without structured review processes.[2] This allows other researchers with limited access to academic journals, and also journalists and the general public, to access the study findings. In general, storing the manuscript on preprint servers and/or linked to the preregistration seems unproblematic. Also, several high-quality open-access journals and "classical" journals with open-access options exist that ensure a quality check of the work before publication. At the same time, thousands of questionable journals exist that publish anything, including fabricated results (Bohannon, 2013).

In our opinion, despite the limitations of review processes (Marsh, Jayasinghe, & Bond, 2008), scientific findings should be carefully reviewed—always, but especially, when they are openly accessible to a broad public—to ensure that the study procedures follow the standards of the field and that results are trustworthy. As a side note, publishing results as open access should not depend on the budget of researchers or their university. Thus, offering options to authors whose manuscripts pass the review process but who cannot cover the publication costs, would be highly desirable to advance open science (e.g., Collabra, www.collabra.org/about/faq). Needless to say, in preparing the manuscripts that report on mobile sensing studies, researchers should follow the guidelines of transparent reporting that also apply to any other scientific study (Appelbaum et al., 2018; Simmons et al., 2011), and additionally describe the necessary information specific to mobile sensing. If too much technical information would distract readers from the substantial research questions and contribution, such details can now easily be communicated in supplementary material directly linked to the article or presented in open repositories (see, e.g., Stachl, Au, et al., 2020).

Overview and Tentative Guidelines for Preregistration and Transparent Reporting in Mobile Sensing Studies

To increase transparency and thus replicability, preregistrations have been established in psychological research (Nosek & Lindsay, 2018). Preregistration of hypotheses counteract hindsight bias (Kerr, 1998), and preregistration of planned analyses works against confirmation biases (e.g., Gelman & Loken, 2014; Wagenmakers et al., 2012; Wagenmakers & Dutilh, 2016)—both together aiming at minimizing questionable research practices (e.g., Simmons et al., 2011). Accordingly, preregistrations are also highly recommended in the field of mobile sensing. Due to the complexity of the workflow in mobile sensing studies in comparison to questionnaire-based research, it is often difficult to consider and describe all processing and analytic steps in sufficient detail in advance. We therefore encourage researchers in the field of mobile sensing to apply a two-step procedure:

1. Define as many preregistration decisions as precisely as possible. Again, data from pilot studies will help to achieve this task.
2. For parts or cases when preregistration is not fully possible, report all decisions made in the course of data processing in a transparent way.

Throughout this chapter, we pointed to issues relevant for preregistration and reporting in mobile sensing studies. We summarized these points and described different levels of specificity in Tables 3.1 and 3.2. The different levels partly/largely overlap with levels proposed in Nosek and colleagues (2015). We again state the obvious: A higher level of transparency is generally better—we cannot think of a counterexample. Still, different standards can be necessary for highly sensitive data (e.g., raw GPS data) or sensitive samples (e.g., identifiable patients or public people). Also, one project can follow different levels for the different tasks, for example, openly reporting materials but offering access to sensitive data only to authorized researchers. The achievable level of transparency will depend on the field and research topic and will not necessarily rely solely on the willingness of the researcher. Furthermore, when using commercial/industrial libraries/packages (e.g., Google Maps), information on validation may not be available to researchers.

Threats to Reproducibility and Replicability Despite Transparency

In the beginning, we stated that transparency in mobile sensing research is needed for these studies to be reproduced and findings to be replicated. In this section, we want to raise the awareness that transparency is a necessary but not sufficient condition for replicating findings. Accordingly, even if researchers follow the suggested preregistration and reporting standards presented in the previous section, several threats to reproducibility and replicability exist.

TABLE 3.1. Suggestions for Preregistration Standards in Mobile Sensing Studies

Topic	Level of specificity 0	Level of specificity 1	Level of specificity 2	Level of specificity 3
Research question and hypotheses	Neither research questions nor hypotheses are preregistered.	Preregister exploratory research questions.	Preregister some research questions and directed hypotheses.	Preregister directed hypotheses and specify effect sizes.
Target population: Selectivity	No consideration of recruitment options and how they might affect selectivity of the sample.	Consider basic sources of sample selectivity (e.g., technical ones: specific operating systems or smartphone models).	Consider various recruitment strategies associated with self-selection bias of participants (e.g., where and how are they recruited?).	Preregister quota (e.g., demographics) according to which recruitment takes place to control for selectivity effects.
Target population: Power analyses	Power analyses are not conducted.	Conduct power estimations based on effect sizes reported in previous publications.	Conduct power estimations based on effect sizes reported in previous publications. Explain all decisions and annotate code.	Conduct power analyses based on simulation studies. Explain all decisions and annotate code.
Target sensor samples	Chosen assessment schedules are not explained.	Specify basic assessment schedule (e.g., study period).	Specify target behaviors (e.g., dates such as days of the week or time of the year, time windows, and sampling frequencies).	Same as Level 2.
Materials	Materials are not preregistered.	Provide list of constructs together with number of items, parameters derived in mobile sensing, and units of mobile sensing parameters.	Describe complete materials in repository together with items (if not protected by copyright). Describe algorithms to specify how mobile sensing parameters are determined.	Store and explain/ annotate materials in repository. Store code for data collection in a maximally generic way.
Preprocessing and statistical analyses	(Pre)processing and data analyses are not preregistered.	Specify basic (pre-processing decisions (e.g., definition of daytimes, handling of outliers or missing values) and describe analyses.	Make required decisions about data (pre)processing in advance to reduce researcher degrees of freedom. Check for any theoretical considerations or any earlier work which can be relied on. Describe data analyses.	Store (pre-) processing and analyses code (e.g., based on pilot study) before data collection.

Note. Different levels of specificity (LS) of preregistration standards are presented. LS 0 is shown for comparison and describes scenarios that do not meet any standard. The levels LS 1 to LS 3 are arranged in ascending order, describing the lowest to the highest level of specificity of transparent preregistration. For some topics, only fine differences exist between levels.

TABLE 3.2. Suggestions for Reporting Standards in Mobile Sensing Studies

Topic	Level of specificity 0	Level of specificity 1	Level of specificity 2	Level of specificity 3
Research questions and hypotheses	Exploratory and/or confirmatory analyses are reported, but not labeled differently.	Report exploratory research questions and label as such.	Report on nondirected hypotheses and, if necessary, on exploratory analyses and label them as such.	Report on directed hypotheses and, if necessary, on exploratory analyses and label them as such.
Target population	Recruitment and resulting sample are not described.	Report basic information on how participants were recruited.	Describe recruitment strategy and report descriptive information on sociodemographics of sample.	Describe recruitment strategy, dropouts, and sample characteristics. Compare sample with target population group.
Target sensor samples	Assessment schedules are not explained.	Report basic assessment schedule (e.g., study period, time of the year).	Describe target behaviors (e.g., dates such as days of the week or time of the year, time windows, and sampling frequencies).	Same as Level 2.
Data collection: Onboarding and quality monitoring	Data collection procedures are not reported.	Include overview of data collection procedures in the manuscript.	Extensively describe data collection procedures as supplemental material of the manuscript (e.g., changes to software or specific incidents during the study).	Store and explain/annotate all materials for data collection in open repository.
Data collection: Onboard processing	Onboard processing software is mentioned without further specifications.	Report exact version number of the software.	Describe onboard processing algorithms and, if available from the manufacturer/developer/author, provide measures of validity and reliability.	Describe onboard processing algorithms and report validation measures from own pilot testing.
Preprocessing	Preprocessing decisions are not reported.	Give an overview of preprocessing decisions in the manuscript.	Report on final preprocessing decisions and any changes compared to the preregistered steps. Be aware of the uncertainty implied by researcher degrees of freedom and state them as a limitation of work (Hoffmann et al., 2021).	Integrate alternative preprocessing decisions in the statistical analysis by systematically reporting results and robustness analysis (e.g., multiverse analysis).
Open code	Data processing, analyses, and results are reported in the manuscript.	Publish code without further documentation/explanation.	Publish well-documented code (e.g., codebook describing variables and their abbreviations used in the analysis code; describe preprocessing steps).	Facilitate reproducibility by providing well-documented code/results by using software management tools (e.g., Docker, Packrat, GitHub; see Epskamp, 2019; Peikert & Brandmaier, 2019).

(continued)

TABLE 3.2. *(continued)*

Topic	Level of specificity 0	Level of specificity 1	Level of specificity 2	Level of specificity 3
Open publication	Not openly accessible.	Publish article on preprint server without structured prepublication peer review.	Publish article in peer-reviewed journal with open access.	Publish article in peer-reviewed open-access journal scoring well on the TOP guidelines (www.topfactor.org).

Note. Different levels of specificity (LS) of reporting standards are presented. LS 0 is shown for comparison and describes scenarios that do not meet any standard. The levels LS 1 to LS 3 are arranged in ascending order describing the lowest to the highest level of specificity of transparent reporting. For some topics, only fine differences exist between levels.

Reproducibility (or verification) is often understood as using the original raw data and analysis scripts to compute the results again (Clemens, 2017). Replication often refers to "repeating the methodology of a previous study and obtaining the same result" (i.e., method-focused replication, Nosek & Errington, 2017, p. 1) in an independent sample of participants/observations. Yet replication should mean a research design that tests whether two (or more) studies produce the same causal effect within the limits of sampling error (i.e., causal effect-focused replication; Steiner et al., 2019, p. 281). The differences between reproducibility, method-focused replication, and causal effect-focused replication become apparent when examining the specifics of mobile sensing.

Mobile sensing data often rely heavily on feature extraction and preprocessing of sensor data, for example, determining sleep–wake phases through machine learning algorithms that utilize phone usage and physical sensor data (Min et al., 2014). When implementing third-party software packages for feature extraction, preprocessing, and analysis of data, newer versions of the same packages might result in (slightly) altered results, unknown to the researcher. One solution could be to build dynamic workflows that manage software versions and changes (i.e., containerization, dependence management, and version management; Peikert & Brandmaier, 2019). Yet reproduction of results becomes even more complicated when creating algorithms from original data. For example, machine learning methods such as deep neural networks (DNNs) build their algorithms (i.e., feature weights) partly autonomously from researchers based on training data and optimization procedures (e.g., to predict sleep phases based on physical activity and other sensor information). When repeating the building of DNNs, differences in algorithms might arise, simply due to how DNNs work (Hartley & Olsson, 2020). At the very least, researchers aiming to reproduce results from original data should be aware that different (versions of) algorithms might lead to (somewhat) different results. The same applies to replication attempts, when previously published algorithms do not function the same on new versions of the operating systems: For example, early apps were allowed to read contacts and access the microphone, whereas some new Android versions restrict such access heavily.

Method-focused replication, that is, direct replications with new data (i.e., participants, observations) aim at adhering closely to the published original work (e.g., Klein, Vianello, et al., 2018). Transparent reporting as described in Table 3.2 facilitates direct replications, thus identifying, estimating, and reporting the same effects in both the original and the replication study (Nosek & Lakens, 2014; Steiner et al., 2019). Still, two crucial assumptions necessary for successful replications are not always met in direct, post-hoc replications (i.e., replicating after results are published). Failing to fulfill these assumptions threatens the replicability of results from mobile sensing (and other) studies.

The first assumption is that the treatment (or predictors) and the outcomes are stable across studies (Steiner et al., 2019). On the phenomenological level, the assumption of stability seems implausible because smartphone functions change so rapidly. Certain apps (or functions) might no longer be available or might be replaced by a different app, so that observing usage in a specific population is not possible a few months or years after the original study. Even the meaning of the same behavior might change quickly; for example, using text messaging on the smartphone 40 times per day might have indicated excessive usage in 2015 (Harari et al., 2020), yet this frequency is currently about average (Stachl, Au, et al., 2020). On the level of measurement, one requirement for direct, method-focused replication might be to hold sensing software constant across studies. Yet different research groups use various software solutions, which might differ in their technical implementations. In addition, even if the same sensing app were to be used across studies, operating systems today change rapidly, making it impossible to keep measures constant across time. For example, freely available onboard processing algorithms (e.g., classifying activity data as standing versus moving) are updated, but providers do not necessarily make transparent how and which parts of the software change.

The second crucial assumption for successful replications is that the real-world process causing the effect must be constant across studies (Steiner et al., 2019). Previous research hints that digital behaviors and the underlying processes are temporally stable only across short periods. For example, communication patterns using smartphones changed even over 4 years (Stachl, Pargent, et al., 2020): People used fewer text messages, but more social media and communication apps. Subsequently the associations of specific communication channels with the trait extraversion also changed over time. Thus, along with rapid technological advances, the meaning of narrow digital behaviors (e.g., usage patterns, available apps) might change quickly, and previous results will not be replicable a few years later. Broader and more stable digital behavioral dimensions might be a possible solution to define outcomes, which are replicable over time (Stachl, Pargent, et al., 2020). This proposal is also in line with the idea of causal effect-focused replications, which means to replicate studies focusing on the same theoretical variables but allowing different measures and study procedures (Nosek & Lakens, 2014; Steiner et al., 2019). For example, if the association between extraversion and social behavior is to be replicated, this can be done in a variety of ways operationalized via mobile sensing. For example, social behavior could be equally operationalized as communication app usage, social media app usage, sensed conversations, or call activities (Harari et al., 2020). The progression of the field will reveal whether the principle behind causal effect replications are more appropriate in mobile sensing research.

To summarize, mobile sensing research will likely face direct replication failures despite transparent reporting, due to rapidly changing digital behavior and technical solutions. Paradoxically, replication failures underline the importance of transparency even more. According to Steiner and colleagues (2019, p. 281) "replication failure is not inherently a problem as long as the researcher is able to understand why the result was not reproduced." We argue that transparency in mobile sensing studies can help to foster this understanding.

Conclusion

Mobile sensing in psychology (and beyond) is a quickly developing and complex field. Transparency, both during preregistration and in the later reporting of studies, will help the paradigm to prosper because researchers can evaluate and learn from transparent studies as well as derive standards for conducting mobile sensing studies. The availability of standards, which are again transparently communicated, will facilitate placing mobile sensing research solidly within the method repertoire of behavioral research—similar to EEG, fMRI, or EMA (ecological momentary assessment; Mehl & Connor, 2012)—and thus allow for the easy and valid study of human behavior within the context that matters most, that is, daily life.

In our opinion, one of the major unresolved conflicts in mobile sensing research is still the compromise between achieving a sufficient level of transparency and respecting the data privacy of the participants. To achieve both goals responsibly, we hope that our chapter will encourage interdisciplinary research teams to work together on appropriate technical solutions.

Notes

1. https://developers.google.com/maps/documentation/places.
2. We fully acknowledge that several high-quality open-access journals exist that review manuscripts carefully before publication. For these journals, the same reviewing biases as in "classical" journals—overly enthusiastic or critical—can occur and thus need to be considered.

REFERENCES

Aharony, N., Pan, W., Ip, C., Khayal, I., & Pentland, A. (2011). Social fMRI: Investigating and shaping social mechanisms in the real world. *Pervasive and Mobile Computing, 7,* 643–659.

American Psychological Association. (2021, September 1). *Transparency and openness promotion (TOP) guidelines at APA journals.* www.apa.org/pubs/journals/resources/top-guidelines-journal-flyer.pdf

Appelbaum, M., Cooper, H., Kline, R. B., Mayo-Wilson, E., Nezu, A. M., & Rao, S. M. (2018). Journal article reporting standards for quantitative research in psychology: The APA Publications and Communications Board task force report. *American Psychologist, 73,* 3–25.

Beierle, F., Tran, V. T., Allemand, M., Neff, P., Schlee, W., Probst, T., et al. (2019). What data are smartphone users willing to share with researchers? *Journal of Ambient Intelligence and Humanized Computing,* 1–13.

Bohannon, J. (2013). Who's afraid of peer review? *Science, 342*(6154), 60–65.

Brandmaier, A. M., Prindle, J. J., McArdle, J. J., & Lindenberger, U. (2016). Theory-guided exploration with structural equation model forests. *Psychological Methods, 21,* 566–582.

Buschek, D., Bisinger, B., & Alt, F. (2018). ResearchIME: A mobile keyboard application for studying free typing behaviour in the wild. *Proceedings of the 2018 CHI Conference on Human Factors in Computing Systems,* pp. 1–14.

Chittaranjan, G., Blom, J., & Gatica-Perez, D. (2013). Mining large-scale smartphone data for personality studies. *Personal and Ubiquitous Computing, 17,* 433–450.

Clemens, M. A. (2017). The meaning of failed replications: A review and proposal. *Journal of Economic Surveys, 31,* 326–342.

de Montjoye, Y.-A., Quoidbach, J., Robic, F., & Pentland, A. S. (2013). Predicting personality using novel mobile phone-based metrics. In J. Salerno, S. J. Yang, D. Nau & S.-K. Chai (Eds.), *Social computing, behavioral-cultural modeling and prediction* (pp. 48–55). Berlin: Springer.

Dennis, S., Garrett, P., Yim, H., Hamm, J., Osth, A. F., Sreekumar, V., & Stone, B. (2019). Privacy versus open science. *Behavior Research Methods, 51*, 1839–1848.

Eagle, N., Pentland, A., & Lazer, D. (2009). Inferring friendship network structure by using mobile phone data. *Proceedings of the National Academy of Sciences of the United States of America, 106*(36), 15274–15278.

Epskamp, S. (2019). Reproducibility and replicability in a fast-paced methodological world. *Advances in Methods and Practices in Psychological Science, 2*(2), 145–155.

Fang, X., Zeng, Q., & Yang, G. (2020). Local differential privacy for human-centered computing. *EURASIP Journal on Wireless Communications and Networking, 2020*, 1–12.

Ferreira, D., Kostakos, V., & Dey, A. K. (2015). AWARE: Mobile context instrumentation framework. *Frontiers in ICT, 2*, 6.

Gelman, A., & Loken, E. (2014). The statistical crisis in science. *American Scientist, 102*, 460–465.

Gong, M., Pan, K., Xie, Y., Qin, A. K., & Tang, Z. (2020). Preserving differential privacy in deep neural networks with relevance-based adaptive noise imposition. *Neural Networks, 125*, 131–141.

Gosling, S. D., & Mason, W. (2015). Internet research in psychology. *Annual Review of Psychology, 66*, 877–902.

Götz, F. M., Stieger, S., & Reips, U.-D. (2017) Users of the main smartphone operating systems (iOS, Android) differ only little in personality. *PLoS One, 12*(5), e0176921.

Granville, K. (2018, March 19). Facebook and Cambridge Analytica: What you need to know as fallout widens. *New York Times*. www.nytimes.com/2018/03/19/technology/facebook-cambridge-analytica-explained.html

Harari, G. M., Lane, N. D., Wang, R., Crosier, B. S., Campbell, A. T., & Gosling, S. D. (2016). Using smartphones to collect behavioral data in psychological science: Opportunities, practical considerations, and challenges. *Perspectives on Psychological Science, 11*, 838–854.

Harari, G. M., Müller, S. R., Stachl, C., Wang, R., Wang, W., Bühner, M., et al. (2020). Sensing sociability: Individual differences in young adults' conversation, calling, texting, and app use behaviors in daily life. *Journal of Personality and Social Psychology, 119*, 204–228.

Hartley, M., & Olsson, T. S. (2020). dtoolAI: Reproducibility for deep learning. *Patterns, 1*(5), 100073.

Hoffmann, S., Schönbrodt, F. D., Elsas, R., Wilson, R., Strasser, U., & Boulesteix, A. (2021). The multiplicity of analysis strategies jeopardizes replicability: Lessons learned across disciplines. *Royal Society Open Science, 8*(4), 201925.

Houtkoop, B. L., Chambers, C., Macleod, M., Bishop, D. V., Nichols, T. E., & Wagenmakers, E.-J. (2018). Data sharing in psychology: A survey on barriers and preconditions. *Advances in Methods and Practices in Psychological Science, 1*, 70–85.

Joel, S., Eastwick, P. W., & Finkel, E. J. (2018). Open sharing of data on close relationships and other sensitive social psychological topics: Challenges, tools, and future directions. *Advances in Methods and Practices in Psychological Science, 1*(1), 86–94.

Kambham, N. K., Stanley, K. G., & Bell, S. (2018). Predicting personality traits using smartphone sensor data and app usage data. *Proceedings of the 9th Annual Information Technology, Electronics and Mobile Communication Conference (IEEE IEMCON)*, pp. 125–132.

Kass, R. E., & Raftery, A. E. (1995). Bayes factors. *Journal of the American Statistical Association, 90*, 773–795.

Kerr, N. L. (1998). HARKing: Hypothesizing after the results are known. *Personality and Social Psychology Review, 2*, 196–217.

Keusch, F., Struminskaya, B., Antoun, C., Couper, M. P., & Kreuter, F. (2019). Willingness to participate in passive mobile data collection. *Public Opinion Quarterly, 83*, 210–235.

Klein, O., Hardwicke, T. E., Aust, F., Breuer, J., Danielsson, H., Mohr, A. H., et al. (2018). A practical guide for transparency in psychological science. *Collabra: Psychology, 4*(1), 20.

Klein, R. A., Vianello, M., Hasselman, F., Adams, B. G., Adams, R. B., Jr., Alper, S., et al. (2018). Many Labs 2: Investigating variation in replicability across samples and settings. *Advances in Methods and Practices in Psychological Science, 1*, 443–490.

Kreuter, F., Haas, G.-C., Keusch, F., Bähr, S., & Trappmann, M. (2020). Collecting survey and smartphone sensor data with an app: Opportunities and challenges around privacy and informed consent. *Social Science Computer Review, 38*, 533–549.

Leamer, E. E. (1985). Sensitivity analyses would help. *American Economic Review, 75*, 308–313.

Ludwigs, K., Lucas, R., Veenhoven, R., Richter, D., & Arends, L. (2019). Can happiness apps generate nationally representative datasets?—A case study collecting data on people's happiness using the German socio-economic panel. *Applied Research in Quality of Life, 15*, 1135–1149.

Marsh, H. W., Jayasinghe, U. W., & Bond, N. W. (2008). Improving the peer-review process for grant applications: reliability, validity, bias, and generalizability. *American Psychologist, 63*, 160.

Mehl, M. R. (2017). The Electronically Activated Recorder (EAR): A method for the naturalistic observation of daily social behavior. *Current Directions in Psychological Science, 26*, 184–190.

Mehl, M. R., & Conner, T. (Eds.). (2012). *Handbook of research methods for studying daily life*. Guilford Press.

Mehl, M. R., Gosling, S. D., & Pennebaker, J. W. (2006). Personality in its natural habitat: Manifestations and implicit folk theories of personality in daily life. *Journal of Personality and Social Psychology, 90*, 862–877.

Mehl, M. R., & Holleran, S. E. (2007). An empirical analysis of the obtrusiveness of and participants' compliance with the Electronically Activated Recorder (EAR). *European Journal of Psychological Assessment, 23*(4), 248–257.

Mehrotra, A., Müller, S. R., Harari, G. M., Gosling, S. D., Mascolo, C., Musolesi, M., et al. (2017). Understanding the role of places and activities on mobile phone interaction and usage patterns. *Proceedings of the ACM on Interactive, Mobile, Wearable and Ubiquitous Technologies, 1*(3), 1–22.

Mendes, R., Cunha, M., & Vilela, J. P. (2020). Impact of frequency of location reports on the privacy level of geo-indistinguishability. *Proceedings on Privacy Enhancing Technologies, 2020*(2), 379–396.

Miller, G. (2012). The smartphone psychology manifesto. *Perspectives on Psychological Science, 7*, 221–237.

Min, J. K., Doryab, A., Wiese, J., Amini, S., Zimmerman, J., & Hong, J. I. (2014, April). Toss'n'turn: Smartphone as sleep and sleep quality detector. *Proceedings of the SIGCHI Conference on Human Factors in Computing Systems*, pp. 477–486.

Montag, C., Błaszkiewicz, K., Lachmann, B., Andone, I., Sariyska, R., Trendafilov, B., et al. (2014). Correlating personality and actual phone usage. *Journal of Individual Differences, 35*,158–165.

Montag, C., Błaszkiewicz, K., Sariyska, R., Lachmann, B., Andone, I., Trendafilov, B., et al. (2015). Smartphone usage in the 21st century: Who is active on WhatsApp? *BMC Research Notes, 8*, 331–337.

Mønsted, B., Mollgaard, A., & Mathiesen, J. (2018). Phone-based metric as a predictor for basic personality traits. *Journal of Research in Personality, 74*, 16–22.

Muthén, L. K., & Muthén, B. O. (2023). M*plus* (Version 8) [Computer software]. Los Angeles: Muthén & Muthén.

Nebeker, C., Lagare, T., Takemoto, M., Lewars, B., Crist, K., Bloss, C. S., et al. (2016). Engaging research participants to inform the ethical conduct of mobile imaging, pervasive sensing, and location tracking research. *Translational Behavioral Medicine, 6*, 577–586.

Nosek, B. A., Alter, G., Banks, G. C., Borsboom, D., Bowman, S. D., Breckler, S. J., et al. (2015). Promoting an open research culture. *Science, 348*(6242), 1422–1425.

Nosek, B. A., & Errington, T. M. (2017). Making sense of replications. *ELife*, 6, e23383.

Nosek, B. A., & Lakens, D. (2014). Registered reports: A method to increase the credibility of published results. *Social Psychology, 45*, 137–141.

Nosek, B. A., & Lindsay, D. S. (2018, February 18). Preregistration becoming the norm in psychological science. *APS Observer*. https://www.psychologicalscience.org/observer/preregistration-becoming-the-norm-in-psychological-science

Pedroni, A., Bahreini, A., & Langer, N. (2019). Automagic: Standardized preprocessing of big EEG data. *NeuroImage, 200*, 460–473.

Peikert, A., & Brandmaier, A. M. (2021). A reproducible data analysis workflow with R Markdown, Git, Make, and Docker. *Quantitative and Computational Methods in Behavioral Sciences, 1*(1).

RatSWD [Rat für Sozial und Wirtschaftsdaten] (2020): Datenerhebung mit neuer Informationstechnologie. Empfehlungen zu Datenqualität und management, Forschungsethik und Datenschutz [Data collection using novel IT: Guidelines for data quality, data management, research ethics, and data security]. *RatSWD Output, 6*(6). Rat für Sozial und Wirtschaftsdaten (RatSWD).

Roberts, S., & Pashler, H. (2000). How persuasive is a good fit? A comment on theory testing. *Psychological Review, 107*, 358–367.

Rocher, L., Hendrickx, J. M., & De Montjoye, Y. A. (2019). Estimating the success of re-identifications in incomplete datasets using generative models. *Nature Communications, 10*(1), 1–9.

Schoedel, R., Au, Q., Völkel, S. T., Lehmann, F., Becker, D., Bühner, M., et al. (2018). Digital footprints of sensation seeking: A traditional concept in the big data era. *Zeitschrift Für Psychologie, 226*, 232–245.

Schoedel, R., Pargent, F., Au, Q., Völkel, S. T., Schuwerk, T., Bühner, M., et al. (2020). To challenge the morning lark and the night owl: Using smartphone sensing data to investigate day–night behaviour patterns. *European Journal of Personality, 34*, 733–752.

Schönbrodt, F., Gollwitzer, M., & Abele-Brehm, A. (2017). Der Umgang mit Forschungsdaten im Fach Psychologie: Konkretisierung der DFG-Leitlinien [Handling of research data in psychology: Specification of the guidelines from the German Research Foundation]. *Psychologische Rundschau, 68*, 20–35

Schuwerk, T., Kaltefleiter, L. J., Au, J. Q., Hoesl, A., & Stachl, C. (2019). Enter the wild: Autistic traits and their relationship to mentalizing and social interaction in everyday life. *Journal of Autism and Developmental Disorders, 49*(10), 4193–4208.

Scott, K., Richards, D., & Adhikari, R. (2015). A review and comparative analysis of security risks and safety measures of mobile health apps. *Australasian Journal of Information Systems, 19.*

Servia-Rodríguez, S., Rachuri, K. K., Mascolo, C., Rentfrow, P. J., Lathia, N., & Sandstrom, G. M. (2017). Mobile sensing at the service of mental well-being: A large-scale longitudinal study. *Proceedings of the 26th International Conference on World Wide Web*, pp. 103–111.

Shaw, H., Ellis, D. A., Kendrick, L. R., Ziegler, F., & Wiseman, R. (2016). Predicting smartphone operating system from personality and individual differences. *Cyberpsychology, Behavior, and Social Networking, 19*(12), 727–732.

Simmons, J. P., Nelson, L. D., & Simonsohn, U. (2011). False-positive psychology: Undisclosed flexibility in data collection and analysis allows presenting anything as significant. *Psychological Science, 22*, 1359–1366.

Simonsohn, U., Simmons, J. P., & Nelson, L. D. (2015). *Specification curve: Descriptive and inferential statistics on all reasonable specifications.* http://dx.doi.org/10.2139/ssrn.2694998

Spiekermann, S., & Langheinrich, M. (2009). An update on privacy in ubiquitous computing. *Personal and Ubiquitous Computing, 13*, 389–390.

Stachl, C., Au, Q., Schoedel, R., Gosling, S. D., Harari, G. M., Buschek, D., et al. (2020). Predicting personality from patterns of behavior collected with smartphones. *Proceedings of the National Academy of Sciences, 117*, 17680–17687.

Stachl, C., Hilbert, S., Au, J. Q., Buschek, D., De Luca, A., Bischl, B., et al. (2017). Personality traits predict smartphone usage. *European Journal of Personality, 31*, 701–722.

Stachl, C., Pargent, F., Hilbert, S., Harari, G. M., Schoedel, R., Vaid, S., et al. (2020). Personality research and assessment in the era of machine learning. *European Journal of Personality, 34*(5), 613–631.

Statista. (2020a). *Global smartphone penetration rate as share of population from 2016 to 2020.* www.statista.com/statistics/203734/global-smartphone-penetration-per-capita-since-2005

Statista. (2020b). *Number of smartphone users by country as of September 2019.* www.statista.com/statistics/748053/worldwide-top-countries-smartphone-users

Statista. (2020c). *Share of global smartphone shipments by operating system from 2014 to 2023*. https://www.statista.com/statistics/272307/market-share-forecast-for-smartphone-operating-systems

Steegen, S., Tuerlinckx, F., Gelman, A., & Vanpaemel, W. (2016). Increasing transparency through a multiverse analysis. *Perspectives on Psychological Science, 11*, 702–712.

Steiner, P. M., Wong, V. C., & Anglin, K. (2019). A causal replication framework for designing and assessing replication efforts. *Zeitschrift für Psychologie, 227*(4), 280–292.

Strobl, C., Boulesteix, A. L., Zeileis, A., & Hothorn, T. (2007). Bias in random forest variable importance measures: Illustrations, sources and a solution. *BMC bioinformatics, 8*, 25.

Tackman, A. M., Sbarra, D. A., Carey, A. L., Donnellan, M. B., Horn, A. B., Holtzman, N. S., et al. (2019). Depression, negative emotionality, and self-referential language: A multi-lab, multi-measure, and multi-language-task research synthesis. *Journal of Personality and Social Psychology, 116*, 817–834.

Thomson, N. K., McMichan, L., Macrae, E., Baker, J., Muggeridge, D., & Easton, C. (2019). The accuracy of a smartphone to measure laboratory and free-living physical activity. *Medicine and Science in Sports and Exercise, 51*, 372–373.

Van Horn, J. D., & Ishai, A. (2007). Mapping the human brain: New insights from fMRI data sharing. *Neuroinformatics, 5*, 146–153.

Wagenmakers, E. J., & Dutilh, G. (2016, October 31). Seven selfish reasons for preregistration. *APS Observer*. https://www.psychologicalscience.org/observer/seven-selfish-reasons-for-preregistration

Wagenmakers, E.-J., Wetzels, R., Borsboom, D., van der Maas, H. L. J., & Kievit, R. A. (2012). An agenda for purely confirmatory research. *Perspectives on Psychological Science, 7*, 632–638.

Wang, W., Harari, G. M., Wang, R., Müller, S. R., Mirjafari, S., Masaba, K., et al. (2018). Sensing behavioral change over time: Using within-person variability features from mobile sensing to predict personality traits. *Proceedings of the ACM on Interactive, Mobile, Wearable and Ubiquitous Technologies, 2*(3), 1–21.

Wiernik, B. M., Ones, D. S., Marlin, B. M., Giordano, C., Dilchert, S., Mercado, B. K., et al. (2020). Using mobile sensors to study personality dynamics. *European Journal of Psychological Assessment, 36*(6), 935–937.

Zou, H., & Hastie, T. (2005). Regularization and variable selection via the elastic net. *Journal of the Royal Statistical Society: Series B (Statistical Methodology), 67*(2), 301–320.

PART II

Mobile Sensors

TECHNOLOGICAL KNOW-HOW AND METHODICAL HOW-TO

CHAPTER 4

Acquisition and Analysis of Location Data

Sven Lautenbach, Sarah Lohr, and Markus Reichert

CHAPTER OVERVIEW

Humans' moods, thoughts, and their behavior do not result solely from their genetic background, their learning experience, and other factors, but they are also critically shaped by the context people are exposed to. For example, humans feel and act differently when they are alone compared to spending time with others (Gan et al., 2021), at work compared to being at home, at a funeral compared to having a party, or exposed to a city environment compared to walking in a forest (e.g., Reichert et al., 2021; Tost et al., 2019). The definition of *context* clearly depends on the discipline (e.g., geography vs. computer science). This term is used in various ways (e.g., Corr & Matthews, 2020), and the psychological literature often refers to contextual influences in manifold ways—for example, with respect to time of day and social and environmental factors (e.g., Reichert, Giurgiu, et al., 2020). In this chapter, we want to operationalize context as factors that characterize the geolocation where humans are located at a certain point in time (such as city vs. rural environment, the degree of nature environment, population density, and air pollution).

Contextual influences impact the general population, that is, both healthy subjects but also vulnerable populations that are prone to mental disorders. Therefore, scientific and clinical interest in contextual influences on psychological outcomes is high. Fortunately, we are living in a century of geospatial data and location-based services where vast amounts of geodata (such as weather data, traffic noise data, distance to urban green space, points of interests) are available, offering important context information for psychological analysis. A rich suite of tools from geoinformatics is available to connect these data with georeferenced information from psychological research (e.g., Reichert, Giurgiu, et al., 2020). These data are often acquired by smartphone sensing via the Global Positioning System (GPS) and can be merged to other data sources that have been repeatedly assessed in the everyday life of participants—for example, ratings of psychological outcomes such as mood in electronic diaries and physiological signals from mobile sensors (e.g., electrocardiography, accelerometry).

In this chapter, we highlight a few examples of such research to illustrate how these method combinations have been applied thus far. There have already been very promising research endeavors combining geodata with mobile sensing information to investigate contextual impacts on psychological outcomes.

Almost two decades ago, Froehlich, Chen, Smith, and Potter (2006) assessed location via mobile phone data and related it to personal experience. In 2014, Epstein and colleagues followed 27 polydrug users by tracking geolocation data, stress, mood, and drug-craving ratings across 16 weeks. Interestingly, and opposed to their initial hypothesis, drug-users' mood was increased in shabbier compared to tidy neighborhoods, while their drug craving and stress was decreased. Although this work is of an observational character and thus precludes any causal conclusions, it interestingly points toward the potential role of the discrepancy between participant health status and environment (tidy neighborhoods) for their psychological well-being.

Another study in the field of drug abuse (Gustafson et al., 2014) implemented real-time feedback on smartphones (also called ecological momentary interventions [EMIs], ambulatory assessment interventions [AAIs], and just-in-time adaptive interventions [JITAIs]; e.g., Heron & Smyth, 2010; Nahum-Shani et al., 2018). These studies comprised real-time tracking and analyses of patients' location triggering assistance when participants approached their favorite drinking spots.

In our recent study (Tost et al., 2019), we combined methods from epidemiology, ambulatory assessment, neuroscience, and geoinformatics, aiming to investigate how inner-city nature environments may impact affective well-being. We recruited 33 city dwellers and equipped them with smartphones for assessing time-stamped geolocations. We asked those participants to additionally provide repeated affective valence ratings (on smartphone diaries) and to wear accelerometers for physical activity measurement (via) in their everyday life. After the data acquisition, we quantified the participants' relative exposure to green space immediately prior to the e-diary ratings of affective valence. Multilevel analyses showed that momentary exposure to inner-city green space significantly enhanced affective valence. In an independent sample of 52 adult city dwellers, we replicated this finding (Tost et al., 2019). In this group of participants, we additionally acquired functional magnetic resonance imaging (fMRI) data and found that prefrontal cortex activation during the processing of negative emotional stimuli in an fMRI emotion regulation paradigm was less pronounced in participants exhibiting larger affective benefits from real-life green space compared to low-responsive participants. Interestingly, further geoinformatic analyses revealed that those high-responsive participants spent more time in city neighborhoods that were green-deprived and that were characterized by a heightened incidence of mental disorders. This led us to the conclusion that momentary exposure to inner-city green space can serve as a resilience factor that can compensate for reduced prefrontal resources in the city dweller's everyday life (Tost et al., 2019).

Just recently, Müller, Peters, Matz, Wang, and Harari (2020) used impressive longitudinal Big Data from smartphones to relate geolocation movement patterns (such as distance traveled and irregularity), as well as experience sampling reports on places visited (such as home and social places) to psychological well-being. In this highly interesting work, they showed the associations of distance traveled to stress, anxiety, and affect, relationships of irregularity to loneliness and depression, and a negative connection of time spent in social places to loneliness.

The findings exemplified above demonstrate which kind of in-depth insights can be expected in the coming years and show how investigations on contextual influences can benefit psychological research. Therefore, in this chapter, we aim to introduce readers to basic geoinformatic methods that enable researchers to acquire and analyze geolocation data.

Different Ways to Acquire Location Data

Spatial Coordinate Systems

To be able to connect measurement data from ecological momentary assessments with existing spatial information, it is important to georeference the measurement data. Put differently, it is important to attach coordinates to the measurements. A common way to specify coordinates on earth is to use latitude, longitude, and altitude/elevation. The irregular shape of the earth (the so-called geoid) can be approximated by a spheroid. While there are subtleties—such as that the earth is flattened at the poles, thereby requiring an ellipsoid instead of a sphere for more exact representation of a global navigation satellite system of concern for geodesy, cartography, and geography—here it is fine to think of our coordinate system as a sphere with a fixed radius.

Positions on the surface of the sphere are defined by angles such as 49.41° N 8.716° E (which is located in Heidelberg, Germany, Heidelberg Castle; see Figure 4.1). The latitude of a point is the angle between the equatorial plane and the straight line that passes

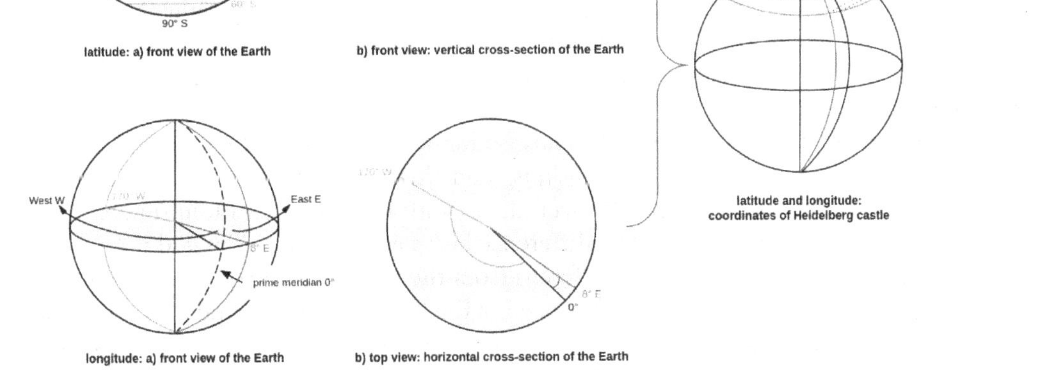

FIGURE 4.1. An example of how positions on the surface of the sphere are defined by angles, here using the location of the Heidelberg Castle, Germany (latitude and longitude: 49.41° and 8.716°).

through that point and the center of the earth. The longitude of a point is the angle east or west of a reference meridian to another point that passes through that point. A meridian is the half of a so-called great circle on the earth's surface that passes through the North Pole and the South Pole; the great circle is thereby split at the poles. The prime or reference meridian is set by convention; nowadays it is common to use the meridian that passes through Greenwich in southeast London, England. Together with the distance to the center, latitude and longitude specify a unique position on the sphere. If just longitude and latitude are given, we are assuming that the location is at the surface of the earth.

Given a common geographic coordinate system, the question that arises is how to measure our position (or the position of a location of interest such as the place where a participant in our experiment is currently located).

Global Navigation Satellite Systems

A global navigation satellite system (GNSS) allows the determination of the location in a geographic coordinate system based on time signals transmitted by satellites. The United States' Global Positioning System (GPS) is the best known GNSS, and GPS is often used—imprecisely—as synonymous to GNSS. Other systems include Russia's GLONASS, China's BDS, and the European Union's Galileo (Madry, 2015).

The underlying idea of satellite positioning is to measure the position of the receiver (e.g., a GPS chip built into smartphones) relative to the known position of several satellites. The distance to the satellites is calculated based on the time it took the signal from the sender (the satellite) to the receiver (e.g., the GPS chip of a smartphone). To estimate latitude, longitude, and altitude by triangulation, it is necessary to receive signals from at least four satellites. Ideally, the satellites would be distributed evenly across the sky; when clustered, position accuracy distinctly degrades.

Since the signal is transmitted by a radio signal, it is necessary to have a clear line of sight between receiver and satellites. If this is not the case, as in one example, since the receiver is located in dense forest, a deep canyon, or indoors, positioning may not be performed or positioning accuracy may be degraded. Environments full of obstacles such as large buildings, road infrastructure, and foliage impose challenges for standard GNSS signals (Madry, 2015): in addition to blockage or attenuation of the signal, the receiver might receive reflections of the signal or might be affected by other non-GNSS signals in nearby frequency bands. Blockage by building fronts or other obstacles might also lead to an unfavorable distribution of available satellites since signals can only be received from a limited part of the sky. We will expand on how one can deal with these challenges in the following sections.

The accuracy of a GNSS signal depends on many factors, including satellite geometry, signal blocking, atmospheric conditions, and the features/quality of the receiver; GPS-enabled smartphones are typically accurate to within a 4.9-meter radius under open sky (van Diggelen & Ende, 2015). The difference between true and estimated position is referred to as the user accuracy; it is different from the user range error (URE) reported by GNSS providers (e.g., Renfro, 2017) since URE is focused on the sender and not the receiver of the GNSS signal (GPS.gov, 2021). With the help of additional systems such as wide-area augmentation systems (WAAS) or dual-frequency receivers, a precision of between 2 meters and 5 meters can be achieved (GPS.gov, 2021). Commercial WAAS are available for North and Central America, Europe, and North Africa as well as for South and East Asia and might be an option if higher precision of location recordings is sought for the intended analysis. An additional source of uncertainty involves the GNSS receiver. As Zandbergen (2009) has shown, a smartphone receiver might produce less accurate results than regular autonomous GNSS receivers.

GNSS can be used to estimate positions, for example, using the smartphones of study participants. Smartphones are not suitable, however, in indoor settings (see below). Care should be taken with respect to the accuracy of the estimated position, especially in areas with a high density of obstacles such as large buildings, road infrastructure, and foliage: Positions are recorded with an attached uncertainty. If one wants, for example, to distinguish between recordings inside or outside of buildings, this might result in recordings that cannot safely be put in one or the other category. Therefore, uncertainty can be included in statistical analysis (e.g., as a dimensional variable), or positions might be filtered to exclude recordings with uncertain assignment (inside/outside). Critical observations can be identified by buffering participants' locations and intersecting those buffers with building footprints (see the subsections below for details on those geoprocessing routines; building footprint data can be freely accessed via OpenStreetMap, or in some countries such as the United States, by open administrative data). Moreover, indoor and outdoor positions can be distinguished based on an intersection of position recordings with building footprints.

Indoor Positioning by Wi-Fi

Studies that focus on indoor settings cannot rely on GNSS to require location data. Examples of such studies involve analysis of the behavioral and psychological symptoms of dementia in a nursing home setting (Wang et al., 2019) or analysis of factors influencing walking distance estimation (Iosa, Fusco, Morone, & Paolucci, 2012).

GNSS is not suitable for indoor positioning because builtup environments do not allow for a reliable connection between receiver and GNSS satellites. While GNSS can receive signals in certain indoor environments, it is not able to provide room-level or sub-room-level location. Indoor positioning must therefore rely on alternative technologies. This requires the setup of a network of sensors that allow triangulation of the positioning of the receiver. Most frequently Wi-Fi is used for indoor navigation and positioning (Loveday, Sherar, Sanders, Sanderson, & Esliger, 2015). Other technologies involve Bluetooth, ZigBee, RFID, UWB, visible light, acoustic signals, and ultrasound (Zafari, Gkelias, & Leung, 2019).

The underlying idea of Wi-FI positioning systems is to triangulate the position of the receiver by employing characteristics of wireless local area network hot spots and other wireless access points. The most commonly used approach relies on measuring the strength of the Wi-Fi signal (received signal strength indication [RSSI]) and identifying the access points. If the position of the access point is known in addition to the dampening of the system with distance to the access point, one can triangulate the position of the receiver from the received signal strength from several receivers. Identification of the different access points is based on parameters such as the Service Set Identifier and media access control address. Precision of the estimation can be improved by an initial calibration of the system—the so-called scene analysis or fingerprinting. Thereby, it is possible to account for the variability of the dampening of the signal due to a heterogeneous environment (variability in building material, furniture, etc.). A statistical model is then used to infer the position of the receiver. Any change of the setup (e.g., by moving furniture) is likely to influence the accuracy of the position estimation.

A median positioning accuracy of 0.6 meters has been reported for systems based on RSSI and fingerprinting (Kotaru, Joshi, Bharadia, & Katti, 2015). If higher accuracy is needed, alternative approaches such as Angle of Arrival, Time of Flight, Time Difference of Arrival, or Return Time of Flight can be used (Dargie & Poellabauer, 2010; Nguyen, Luo, Li, & Watkins, 2020). These alternative approaches are more demanding with respect to the technology used for the receiver and/or the sender (Zafari et al., 2019). Some of those approaches in addition require a line-of-sight connection, which might not be suitable for all environments (Zafari et al., 2019). In addition to its use for indoor positioning, WiFi can also enhance the accuracy of the GNSS-based positioning by using RSSI of WiFi access points (e.g., Stumpp, 2014).

Global System for Mobile Communications

If the focus of the analysis is on larger groups without the need to identify individual users and if requirements on position tracking are lower, Global System for Mobile Communications (GSM) may be an alternative. Based on triangulation between cell towers and signal strength, position accuracy depends heavily on the distribution of cell towers. In urban areas, an accuracy of 50 meters might be achievable, but accuracy will be lower in rural areas. Accessing the data requires cooperation with the service provider and triggers privacy issues in most countries, adding another layer of complexity to the analysis.

Overview/Summary

In most situations, GNSS-based positioning will be the most suitable choice since receiver chips are comparably cheap and available on most mobile devices. Whether participants will be asked to use their own devices or will be equipped with additional devices is a matter of choice that involves nonspatial aspects such as data privacy and trust, in addition to the comparability of different devices. Another factor to consider is battery use by the GNSS sensor, which might impose additional constraints if the participants' devices (e.g., smartphones) should be used. If higher positional accuracy is needed, it might be worthwhile to pay for the use of wide-area augmentation systems. If the experimental design involves indoor settings, GNSS is not suitable, but it has to be substituted or complemented by other systems such as Wi-Fi-based positioning. In any case, one should be aware of the uncertainty associated with the different positioning systems and the factors that influence uncertainty. Ignoring the uncertainty of the location allocation method used might affect subsequent spatial analysis steps (Wan, Kan, & Wilson, 2017).

Analysis of Location Data

The Power of GIScience: Fusing Information to Coordinates

The above-named techniques make it possible to track locations of study participants through time and space by repeated recording of the position. These coordinates can then, for example, be used to analyze the movement patterns of participants. If combined with ambulatory assessment (AA), psychological variables can be recorded together with the location. This allows assessment of how psychological variables (e.g., stress, mood, rumination) change through time and in space. In addition, it is possible to enrich measurements of a study participant with information on the environment and thereby to interpret the measurement in its environmental context, which has proven to be a non-negligible factor when it comes to understanding, for example, psychiatric risk. For instance, in an analysis of subjectively perceived stress, it might be of interest to find the underlying environmental factors surrounding the person's location that either cause or prevent a feeling of being stressed. These might be factors such as the proximity to streets, noise, crowdedness, or even the district's known crime rates. Instead, positive stimuli such as green space or water might help one to recover from stress. In other words, in order to assess the dynamic reactions of humans to their environment, it is not only valuable but also necessary to combine the recorded geometrical location data with factual (also called attribute) data, which is enabled through geoinformatic approaches.

The process of analyzing recorded point location data can be structured into three steps: (1) data acquisition, (2) data processing, and (3) interpretation and visual representation of the results.

Acquisition of Geographic Data

After the location data are recorded, the first step of their contextual analysis is usually the acquisition of geographic data on the environmental factors of interest. Depending on the research question, it might be useful to include several geographic data sources in the analysis; some common sources will be presented in the following.

It is well known that the social composition of an environment affects individuals. For example, the perceived well-being of a person suffering from social anxiety will most likely be low in crowded places. In order to get information on the *social vibrancy* of a place, researchers often use data sources from social media such as Twitter or Weibo posts (e.g., Chen, Hui, Wu, Lang, & Li, 2019). Georeferenced posts, that is, posts with attached spatial coordinates, can be analyzed with respect to their frequency over time and density in space, providing information on the crowdedness or emptiness at different times of a day, week, or year (e.g., Ullah et al., 2019). Furthermore, text mining tools allow extraction of information from the message text that can be used to assign prevalent positive or negative sentiments to a place (Li, Westerholt, & Zipf, 2018; Sykora, Jackson, O'Brien, & Elayan, 2013). Heller and colleagues (2020) showed that novelty and experiential diversity of physical locations and positive affect are bidirectionally linked. They showed that a sociodemographically heterogeneous district can have an activating effect, leading to "upward spirals." Information on *sociodemographic* and *socioeconomic* factors can be obtained, for example, from official census data. For example, the American Housing Survey (AHS, 2021) provides rich information on socioeconomic indicators such as median household income, percentage of inhabitants living alone, or the percentage of age classes at the census tract level. Other countries provide less-open data access by restricting data access to higher-level administrative units. Commercial geodata providers might fill that gap by offering finer scale information. Frequently, such information on finer scales originate from model-based downscaling and not from finer scale data. For administrative units, which might be necessary to extract the region of interest, several sources, such as the Database of Global Administrative Units,[1] are available.

Apart from social factors, the built or natural elements of the environment influence humans and their experiences, such as the density of buildings, the proximity to streets, and noise or air pollution, but also the share of green space or blue space (lakes, rivers). For this purpose, official data about environmental attributes can be used, such as TIGER[2] or INSPIRE,[3] or global crowd-sourced data, such as OpenStreetMap,[4] which can be downloaded (e.g., from Geofabrik[5]). OpenStreetMap offers a large set of attributes that further describe map features (e.g., building types, points of interest such as shops, bars and restaurants, amenity types, street types). For a more detailed assessment, 3D data can also be used, such as 3D city models or LiDAR data, which even allow for identification of single objects such as buildings or trees.

A first characterization of a location at a broader scale can be based on information on its land use or land cover. On the one hand, *land cover* represents the physical properties of the surface (e.g., vegetated, buildup, water body) and can be derived based on satellite or aerial imagery. *Land use,* on the other hand, describes how the land is used (e.g., residential, recreational, industrial, agricultural). The relationship between land use and land cover can be complex since the same land cover (e.g., forest) can be used in different ways (e.g., recreation, forestry, protected area), and the same land use (e.g. recreation) can be linked to different land cover (e.g., recreation can be realized on built-up areas such as Disneyland, at a beach, or in a forest).

Studies show, for example, that inhabitants of areas with larger shares of tree canopy, are on average healthier than those living in areas with comparatively higher shares of grassland (Astell-Burt & Feng, 2019). Exposure to urban green space has been shown to affect the mental well-being of city dwellers in their everyday life (Tost et al., 2019).

Several sources, such as CORINE Land Cover[6] or Urban Atlas[7] for Europe, the National Land Cover Database for the United States,[8] or global datasets such as OSMlanduse,[9] the Copernicus Global Land Service,[10] or AVHRR Global Land Cover Classification[11] provide information on *land cover.* The INSPIRE geoportal, for example, offers several datasets on the built and natural environment for the European Union.

Satellite imagery allows further assessment of these areas through their *reflectance ratios.* The U.S. Geological Survey (USGS) EarthExplorer[12] provides free access to different satellite images for different spatial and temporal units. For example, one commonly used measure to assess the vitality of plants is the Normalized Difference Vegetation Index (NDVI; Carlson & Ripley, 1997; Cihlar, Laurent, & Dyer, 1991), which can be used as a proxy for vegetation cover if land cover information is missing. The NDVI ranges from –1 to 1 and represents water as negative values, built areas and barren lands as low positive numbers, and larger positive numbers as healthier vegetation. Digital *elevation* or digital surface models derived from remote sensing—such as ASTER (Advanced Spaceborne Thermal Emission and Reflection Radiometer) (Tachikawa et al., 2011) or STRM (Shuttle Radar Topography Mission) (Rabus, Eineder, Roth, & Bamler, 2003)—can further provide information on the elevation of a measurement and can therefore be used to calculate the visual field of a person. Terrain information, together with three-dimensional city models (Biljecki, Stoter, Ledoux, Zlatanova, & Çöltekin, 2015) and information on trees, can, for example, be used to calculate the shadiness of a place at a given time. Thermal comfort at a location might affect mood and well-being and could also act as an explanatory factor for the attractiveness of a location.

A large amount of geodata are available as open data. However, data availability differs between countries. While coarser scale information is regularly available, data at higher spatial or temporal resolution might not be available or might involve costs for access. Also, not every dataset might be suitable for the planned analysis. Criteria to be considered to assess the fitness for purpose are the spatial and temporal resolution, the recording date, costs, and data quality indicators. Data provided by agencies or research information come together with the required metadata (data about the data), which allows such an assessment. Volunteered Geographic Information such as OpenStreetMap or data derived from social media tend to be of spatially varying data quality, and therefore they require additional consideration (e.g., Barron, Neis, & Zipf, 2014; Mocnik et al., 2019). In addition, spatial phenomena might be represented in different ways, which affects how data can be further analyzed. Therefore, the next section provides a brief overview on geoinformatic systems and geoinformatic data models, prior to the presentation of common geoinformatic functions.

Processing and Analyzing Geographic Data

Geographic information systems (GIS) are software programs that offer a wide range of tools to work with spatial data (Neteler & Mitasova, 2008). A wide set of GIS and other tools for data processing are available, ranging from commercial systems, such as ArcGIS,[13] ENVI,[14] open-source systems such as QGIS[15] (Menke, 2019), GRASS GIS,[16] GeoDa[17] (Anselin & Rey, 2014), to programming languages with geographic modules, such as Python[18] or R[19] (Brunsdon & Comber, 2016), or spatial databases such as PostgreSQL/PostGIS (Obe & Hsu, 2011) or Oracle Spatial.[20] While the technical skills required to use such systems differ, all systems share common concepts. They all allow combining different spatial datasets by means of an overlay or feature planes technique (*layer concept*); one can think of several layers of information that cover the same place (cf. Figure 4.2). This concept is different from that of joins in conventional relational database systems which rely on common key fields to link data from different datasets. If

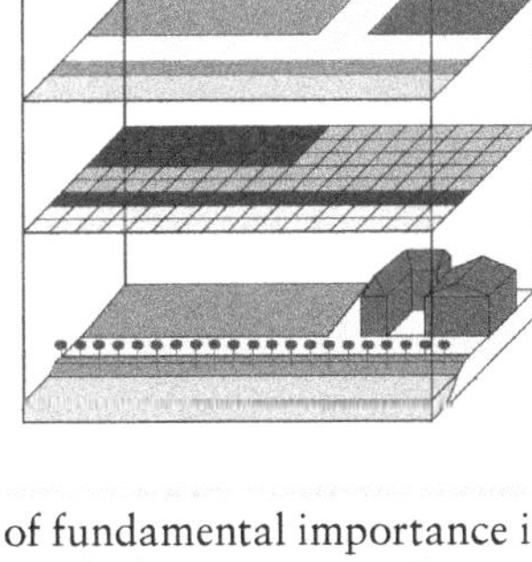

FIGURE 4.2. The *layer concept* is of fundamental importance in spatial information processing. It enables working in different layers with their respective data models and visualizing different data sources at once. The complex reality (bottom layer) is represented either as vector or raster data. Here, the top layers provide information on GPS positions of participants and trees, represented as vector points. The middle layers represent buildings and land use (water, green space, streets, residential) as polygons, while the fifth layer from the top is a raster layer containing NDVI values. Based on coordinates, information from the different layers can be related using geoprocessing approaches.

the positions of participants are enriched by geographic coordinates, links to information from other spatial datasets such as land use, temperature, distance to points of interest, and visibility of green space can be established.

Geographic Data Models

The type of analysis that can be used to further process the geodata depends on its representation, that is, its data type. *Geographic information* is characterized by the clear assignment of each object and its information to a geographical location. Depending on the phenomenon, this information can be continuous (e.g., population density) or discrete in space (e.g., the location of a building). Moreover, the phenomena might change relatively smoothly in space (e.g., air temperature in flat terrain outside of builtup areas) or roughly (e.g., land-use or vegetation cover in residential areas).

When continuous information is not represented as a function, it is discretized to a tessellation of the space that can consist, for example, of regular *raster cells* (cf. Figure 4.3). Each cell of the tessellation provides information about the space it covers. In the case of satellite images, one raster cell might give information on the elevation, temperature, or reflectance per cell. Discrete information, such as a coordinate pair and its attributes, is usually represented as *vector data*.

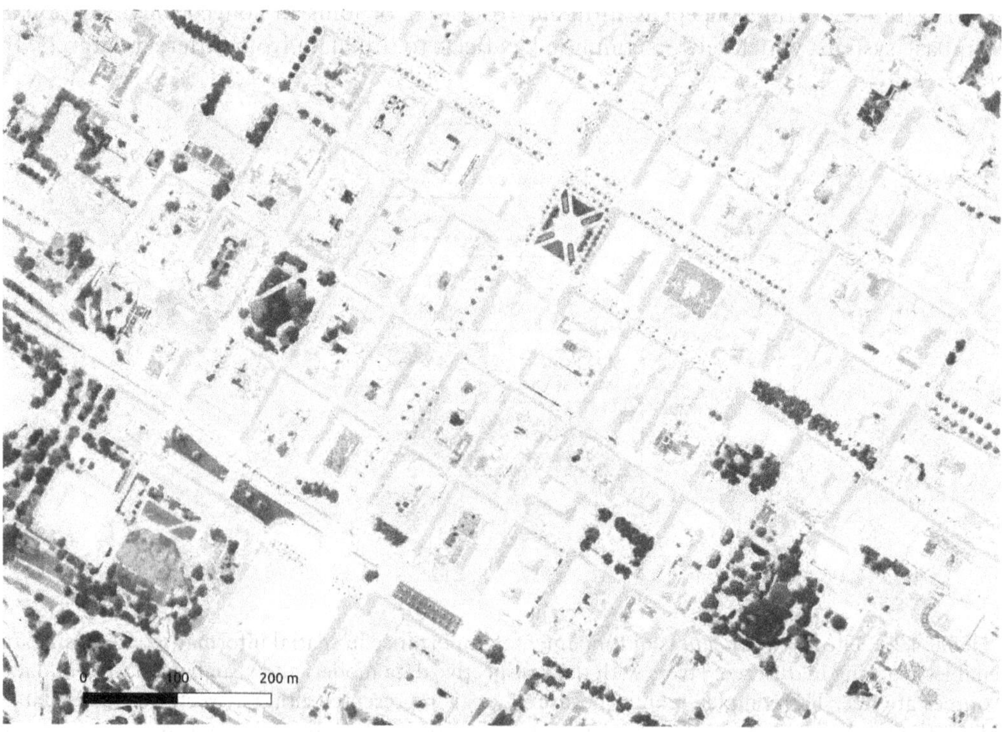

FIGURE 4.3. *Example raster data.* The maps show the amount of green present in the city center of Mannheim, Germany. The data are stored in a raster format. Each cell contains a value that represents the amount of vegetation (NDVI).

Depending on the data type, spatial objects have geometrical, topological and usually thematic properties and can be further enriched by temporal properties (e.g., date of recording), meta-information (e.g., recording method, coordinate system), and object identifiers that allow a well-defined access.

In the two-dimensional space, *vector data* can be *geometrically* represented as point (e.g., a position of a participant, a single trees), line (e.g., rivers, streets, the trajectory of a participant), or polygon features (e.g., parks, administrative areas, the activity space of a participant), all of which rely on points, with each point representing an x- and y-coordinate pair. While a point is stored as a single coordinate pair, a line consists of at least two points, and a polygon is a closed line consisting of at least three points. A set of location points of one person could therefore be combined to a line feature if required. If positions of multiple participants are present in a recording, it will be necessary to group the measurements first by participant and afterward by time before creating line objects. It is also possible to create new features based on existing features: One might be interested in identifying the activity space of a participant based on the individual measurement positions. A simple way to construct the activity space would be to calculate the convex hull of the activity space and use that for further analysis. The convex hull of a feature set is the minimum convex polygon that covers all features; convex in this context implies that all straight-line connections between any two points on the border of the polygon are completely within the polygon. It would also be possible to construct activity spaces for different times of the day (e.g., work, home) or days of the week (workdays and weekdays).

Spatial features can also be described by their position relative to other features. An observation might be inside a building, next to a bakery, or on the eastern side of a major road. These so-called topological relations can be used to link different features. Important *topological* relations between two objects are "disjoint," "contains," "overlap," "meet," "inside," "covers," "covered," and "equal." A possible spatial query using data on a set of trees (point features) and one park (polygon feature) could be to find all the trees or bushes contained by this park. Many studies have already shown that urban green spaces with a higher biodiversity promote more positive emotions in humans (e.g., Cameron et al., 2020; Fuller et al., 2007). As trees or bushes offer habitats to many species, it might be worthy to include them in an analysis. Apart from that, they influence their environment by providing relevant ecosystem services and contributing to a pleasant micro-climate. One might be further interested in identifying participant measurements that were located inside a park, outside of a building, or in a distance of 50 meters from a bar. Or one might be interested in identifying all the urban green spaces or alcohol-selling places inside the activity space of a person.

Raster data are geometrically represented as pixels (e.g., satellite imagery, orthophotos), which are aligned matrix-like in rows and columns and therefore provide topological information through neighboring cells (cf. Figure 4.3). Compared to vector data, only the origin of the matrix must be stored, as the location of each cell can easily be computed due to their regular shape. Information commonly represented by raster data are elevation (digital elevation models, DEM) or information derived from satellite imagery such as vegetation indices, land cover information, or surface temperature. It is best suited for continuous data such as surface temperature or noise, while vector data are best suited for clearly defined objects such as buildings. Instead of representing the activity space of a person as a polygon with distinct borders, one might also represent the activity space by

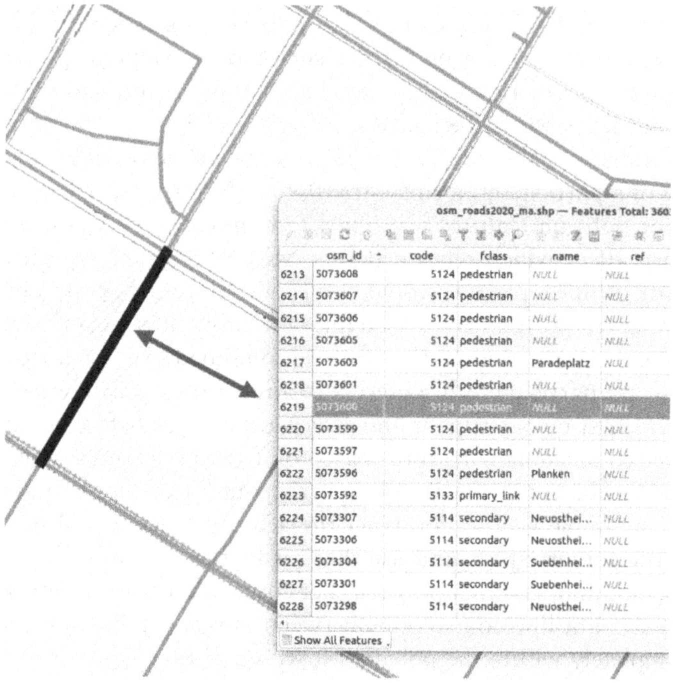

FIGURE 4.4. *Link between geometry and attribute information.* Each geometry object in a feature layer is linked to an attribute table with associated information. The example shows a road network with information on neighboring street segments and the average daily traffic volume at the road segment. The selected road segment in the map is highlighted in black, the corresponding row in the attribute table is highlighted in gray.

a raster in which each cell represents the probability that the cell belongs to the activity space. This allows a fuzzier representation of the information.

A spatial object can provide *thematic* information in the form of attributes that further describe the object (cf. Figure 4.4), such as the answers a participant gave in an e-diary rating at a specific location, together with the time of the recording and the participant ID, the tree species, the height of a building, the air temperature recorded by a sensor, along with the timestamp or the number of lanes of a street. Frequently, geodata already contain attribute data. If additional information is available as tabular data (e.g., comma-separated values, dBase files, Excel sheets, database tables), it is necessary to attach the table to the spatial objects. If spatial objects and tabular data join a common key field, they can easily be combined by a (nonspatial) join of the two tables. For point data, it is also possible to provide coordinates for the individual objects in the table and to import the data directly into the GIS.

Common Geoinformatic Functions

A GIS allows for a deeper understanding of spatial information and its interactions through different possibilities of data modifications, explorations, and analyses (cf. Table 4.1). Functionality to work with spatial data can be broadly categorized as follows (Cromley & McLafferty, 2012):

- Measurement (e.g., distance, area)
- Topology (e.g., adjacency, overlay)
- Network and location analysis (e.g., shortest path routing, accessibility)
- Surface analysis (e.g., viewshed and visibility analysis)
- Statistical analysis (e.g., spatial sampling, spatial autocorrelation, spatial interpolation)

In the following, we provide an overview of spatial operations. We aim here at fundamental operations that might be most suitable in psychological research and related domains without intimidating the reader with variants and special applications.

To prepare data for the region of interest, a common procedure might be to *clip* the data (e.g., the measurements) to the extent of the region of interest. Similar to this spatial filter, the acquired data points can also be *filtered* based on their attribute information, such as the accuracy of the measured location. Depending on the purpose, it could be useful to geometrically modify vector data by *combining*, for example, a set of points to a line. In this way, tracking the points of one person during one day can be united to a path. It might also be necessary to *merge* two datasets of the same attribute if none of them fully covers the study area (e.g., data of two different administrative regions).

A useful function to examine the surroundings of a vector object is the *buffer* function. It can be adequate if the object influences its environment or, more generally stated, the object interacts with its environment through space. Streets influence their surroundings in terms of pollution and noise, and a visual field of a person walking through a city can be modeled by a buffer around the person's location or the person's path. Another possible application is to use a buffer function in order to find all neighboring points of the same person within a certain time frame in order to downsample the data when a person stayed for a long time in the same place, but different GPS locations were stored due to the limits of accuracy of the GPS signal. Another approach, in some sense similar to the buffer, is using *networks* in order to calculate a certain catchment area. For example, for a hospital, a network of streets could be used to find all the buildings which in terms of distance on the streets are closer to the respective hospital than to other hospitals.

Different datasets can also be *intersected*. It may be of interest to intersect a person's visual field at a given location with a layer containing green space polygons. In this way, the percentage of green space exposure of the environment can be calculated.

Geo information systems (GIS) also allow for calculation of *distance* and *area*. This could be the area of an urban green space, the distance of a person's location to the next street, or even the velocity of a person's movement. However, to measure lengths and areas, it is necessary to use a metric coordinate system; therefore, it might be necessary to first reproject your data. Information on the current coordinate system can be found in the meta information.

With geographic data, *spatial statistics* can also be assessed to get an understanding of the spatial distribution of the elements. The point density of GPS measurements can be calculated for different areas to find out more or less visited areas, or, when dealing with location data of a heterogeneous group, differences in spatial behavior can be assessed for the subgroups. For discrete point events, point pattern analysis offers a rich set of statistical approaches to study the distributional pattern, compare it between groups and against theoretical distributions, as well as to include covariates in the analysis (Baddeley,

TABLE 4.1. Elementary Spatial Functions with Examples

Function	Input data	Output	Description
Merge	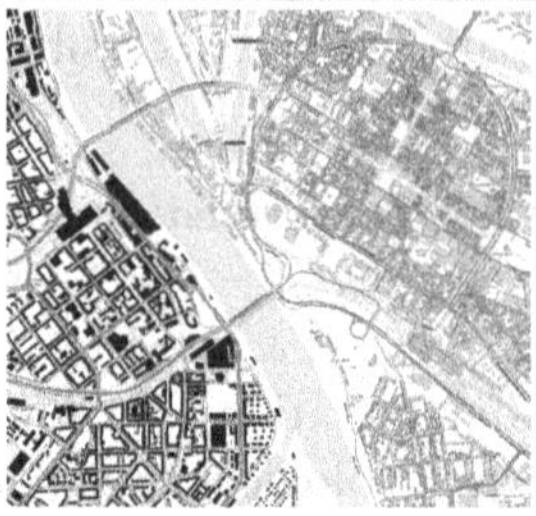	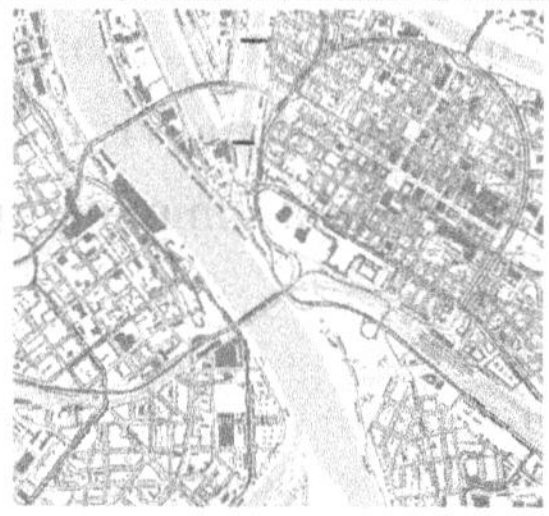	In this example, buildings of two administrative areas (black and gray) are merged to one (dark gray) building layer.
Clip (select by location)	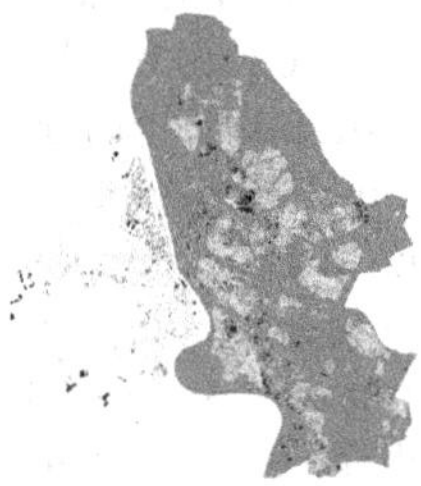	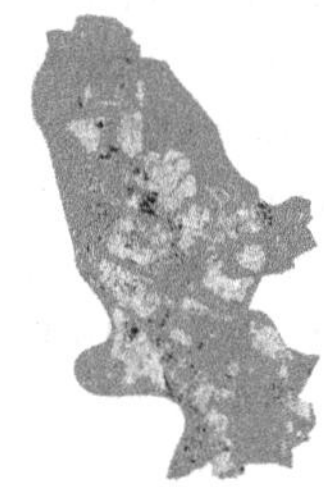	Here, a building layer is clipped to the region of interest (dark gray area).
Select by attribute	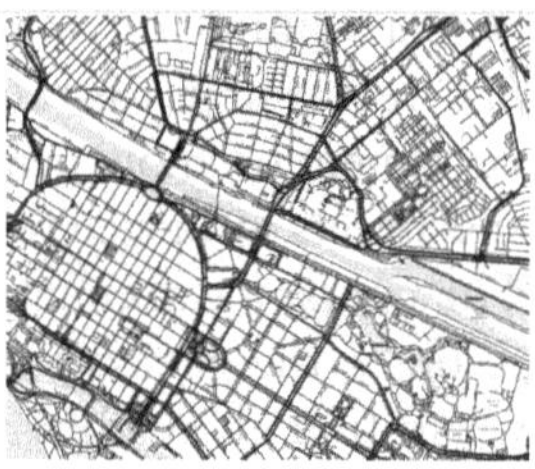	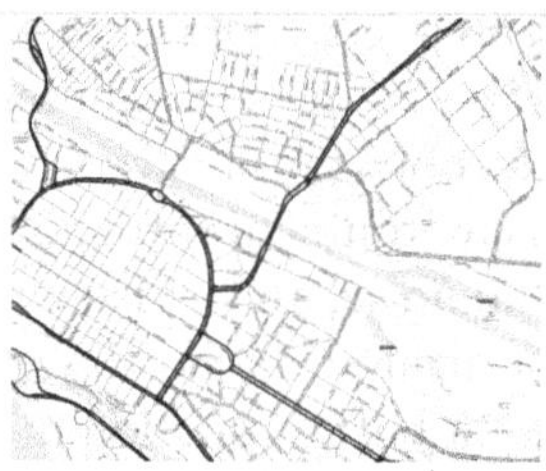	In this case, all the primary roads (black) were selected from a layer containing all types of roads (black).
Buffer	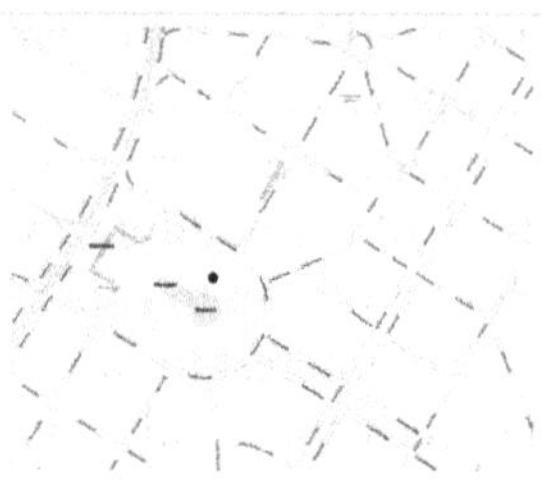	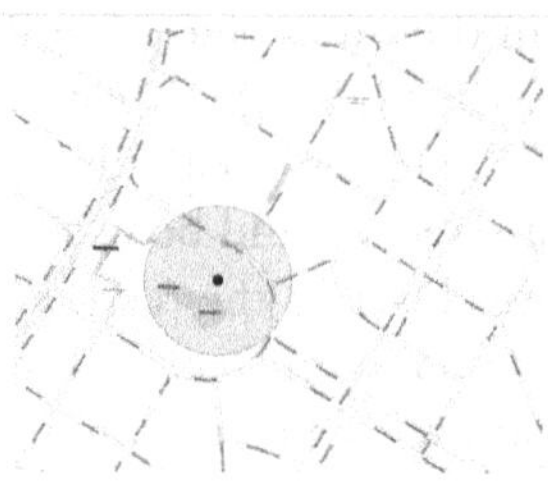	As an approximation of the surroundings of a person at a specific location (black dot), a buffer of 100 meters (gray) was created.
Intersection	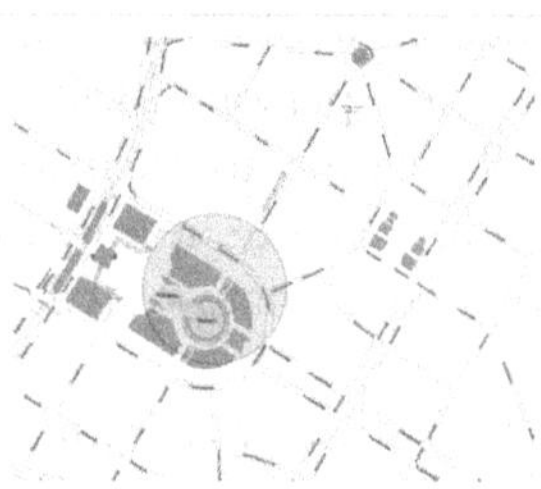	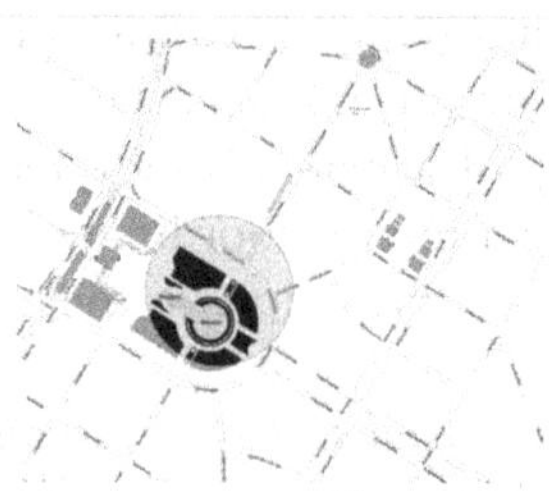	A buffer around a location was intersected with all land-use polygons tagged as grass to obtain the grass areas within the person's environment.

Note. Data source: OpenStreetMap (2020, https://www.openstreetmap.org).

Rubak, & Turner, 2016). Another way to analyze, for example, patterns in spatial or spatiotemporal movement patterns is using specialized cluster analysis (Besag & Newell, 1991; Kulldorf & Nagarwalla, 1995; Zhang, Assunção, & Kulldorff, 2010).

Spatial data might also trigger additional challenges. One of the biggest challenges posed by spatial data is spatial autocorrelation. According to Tobler's first "law" of geography: "Everything is related to everything else, but near things are more related than distant things" (Tobler, 1970, p. 236). If the data points are spatially autocorrelated after the structural component of the model has been considered, the usual assumption of independence of the data points is violated, which might lead to biased estimates and standard errors. To take this nuisance into account, a rich set of statistical methods is available that involve but are not restricted to spatial filtering and spatial eigenvector mapping (Griffith, Chun, & Li, 2019), autoregressive models, generalized estimating equations, wavelets (Carl, Dormann, & Kühn, 2008), and spatial Bayesian approaches (Haining & Li, 2020). These methods vary by complexity, applicable error models, and computational burden (Dormann et al., 2007).

If *temporal information* exists, it can also be assessed in the temporal dimension to assess not only how a *spatial pattern* looks like, but also if a trend or differences in time exist. For these cases, a *grid* that covers the region of interest with symmetrical cells could also be useful. For each cell, parameters such as the number of measurements of the percentage of a certain land cover type (through intersecting the land cover layer with each cell) can be calculated, which could later be displayed as a heat map.

Potential Nuisance: Different Spatial Coordinate Systems

All functions described above require that information is using the same spatial coordinate system. Unfortunately, different geographic coordinate systems are used in different parts of the world because different geographic coordinate systems are better suited to represent the geoid in different parts of the world. In addition, many operations are performed on a plane in cartesian coordinates. This requires projection of the coordinates from the sphere or ellipsoid to the plane and leads to projected coordinate systems. Projected coordinate systems differ in the distortion that is introduced when projecting the 3D surface to a plane. Distortions depend on scale: For small areas such as cities, their effect should be small compared to the errors of positioning by GNSS and other techniques. It is possible to transform data between different geographic and projected coordinate systems; some tools even perform this function automatically. However, it is necessary that the coordinate system of the data is known. Nowadays, this information should be present in most datasets you encounter. Data acquired by GNSS or indoor location systems will typically be stored in the world geodetic system 1984 (WGS84) as long as this is not changed on purpose. Further details on geographic and projected coordinate systems are, for example, provided by Jenny, Šavrič, Arnold, Marston, and Preppernau (2017), Kessler and Battersby (2019), and Snyder (1987).

Cartography: Visualization of Geographic Data

Especially when working with geographic data, maps can be useful not only as a cartographic representation of the results, but can also be part of the analysis process and the interpretation of the results themselves. In comparison to a table, a histogram, or other methods of data visualization, a map can show the underlying spatial patterns at one glance. However, creating good maps is a field in itself, as scale, projection, map symbols, and their visual variables (such as shape, size, hue, gray tone value, texture) can also lead to misleading interpretation or even user manipulation when used inappropriately. Cartography with its old history therefore provides a wide range of literature with guidelines for map making. Good starting points for further studies in cartography are Darkes and Spence (2017), MacEacheren (1995), Monmonier (2018), and Peterson (2015).

Using Spatial Data to Create Experiments

Spatial information can be used not only to analyze and explain the behavior of a person depending on the environment, but also to design experiments. For example, to understand how environmental factors such as availability of green space, noise level, or air pollution influence the well-being and mood of a study participant, one could either passively follow the path of the person through space or actively route the participant to locations that provide a specific exposure. All that is needed is the location of the participant, spatial information about the relevant exposure factors—to identify locations to which the person should be directed—and a routing service. Commercial and open-source routing services typically provide an interface that requires the start and the end coordinates and return the route to the destination. Specialized services allow selection of different criteria of the envisioned route, such as a green or less noisy route (e.g., Novack, Wang, & Zipf, 2018). This, for example, allows extending the analysis of Bratman, Hamilton, Hahn, Daily, and Gross (2015), which assigned participants to fixed routes with different green spaces. Here, the route assigned to a participant could be derived based on the current location of the participant. It is thereby possible to integrate possible interventions easier into the everyday life of participants.

Conclusion

Spatial context matters in everyday behavior. It can be seen as a confounding factor that needs to be controlled for or as an interesting study field on its own. Spatial analysis in psychological research seems to be still in its infancy, which might be more due to lack of knowledge than to lack of interesting research questions. The spatial turn in other disciplines has led to the availability of a rich set of tools to collect, manage, analyze, and visualize spatial data. Spatial data are increasingly publicly available and can be combined with location data of participants. While working with spatial data is not free of challenges, a rich set of tools and expertise is available to address those challenges.

How to Continue

While we have covered the basic concepts of location data analyses here, it will presumably be challenging to start with a real-life data analysis from scratch. How to continue depends on your requirements and on your available resources. If it is sufficient for you to understand the basic concepts, but you lack the time to dig deeper into the practical aspects of spatial data analysis, it might be an option to involve a partner with a GIScience background into your projects. GIS and spatial data analysis are commonly part of geography study programs, so it may be worth it to investigate possibilities at a nearby university. Potentially, they are interested in becoming a partner in new, inspiring research projects. Alternatively, you could hire a consultant to plan and perform the necessary steps for you. Participating in a project with partners experienced in spatial data analysis will help to better understand concepts and challenges of spatial analysis as a first step. If you have the capacity to invest more time and the interest to dive deeper into the topic on your own, free online resources are available both for commercial software as ArcGis and for free software as QGIS. Since commercial GIS software comes at a substantial cost, it might be worth testing a free tool first; with respect to functionality, differences are usually neglectable. While commercial software comes with extended documentation, community resources for open GIS software are often sufficient. For QGIS, a good starting point could be www.qgistutorials.com/en/docs/learning_resources.html. But it is also worthwhile to check the availability of massive online courses offered by many universities and to check out some of the books listed in the references of this chapter. However, be prepared to realize that many examples in applications will (still) be outside of your domain since business and environmental topics are dominant. However, the concepts should be easily transferable to your domain. Similar to other domains, to avoid frustration, at first it is good not to be too ambitious.

Notes

1. https://gadm.org
2. www.census.gov/programs-surveys/geography/guidance/tiger-data-products-guide.html
3. https://inspire-geoportal.ec.europa.eu
4. https://openstreetmap.org
5. https://geofabrik.de
6. https://land.copernicus.eu/pan-european/corine-land-cover
7. land.copernicus.eu/local/urban-atlas
8. https://mrlc.gov
9. https://osmlanduse.org
10. https://land.copernicus.eu/global/products/lc
11. http://prettymap.mooncoder.com/maps/metadata/data.html
12. https://earthexplorer.usgs.gov
13. https://arcgis.com
14. https://nv5geospatial.com/Products/ENVI
15. https://qgis.org
16. https://grass.osgeo.org
17. https://geoda.software.informer.com
18. https://python.org

19. https://R-project.org

20. https://docs.oracle.com/cd/B28359_01/appdev.111/b28400/sdo_intro.htm

REFERENCES

American Housing Survey. (2021). *American Household Survey.* www.census.gov/programs-surveys/ahs.html

Anselin, L., & Rey, S. J. (2014). *Modern spatial econometrics in practice.* GeoDa Press

Astell-Burt T., & Feng, X. (2019). Association of urban green space with mental health and general health among adults in Australia. *JAMA Network Open, 2*(7), e198209.

Baddeley, A., Rubak, E., & Turner, R. (2016). *Spatial point patterns—Methodology and applications with R.* CRC Press.

Barron, C., Neis, P., & Zipf, A. (2014). A comprehensive framework for intrinsic OpenStreetMap quality analysis. *Transactions in GIS, 18*(6), 877–895.

Besag, J., & Newell, J. (1991). The detection of clusters in rare diseases. *Journal of the Royal Statistical Society: Series A (Statistics in Society), 154*(1), 143–155.

Biljecki, F., Stoter, J., Ledoux, H., Zlatanova, S., & Çöltekin, A. (2015). Applications of 3D city models: State of the art review. *ISPRS International Journal of Geo-Information, 4*(4), 2842–2889.

Bratman, G. N., Hamilton, J. P., Hahn, K. S., Daily, G. C., & Gross, J. J. (2015). Nature experience reduces rumination and subgenual prefrontal cortex activation. *Proceedings of the National Academy of Sciences, 112*(28), 8567–8572.

Brunsdon, C., & Comber, L. (2016). *An introduction to R for spatial analysis and mapping.* SAGE.

Cameron, R. W., Brindley, P., Mears, M., McEwan, K., Ferguson, F., Sheffield, D., et al. (2020). Where the wild things are! Do urban green spaces with greater avian biodiversity promote more positive emotions in humans? *Urban Ecosystems, 23*(2), 301–317.

Carl, G., Dormann, C. F., & Kühn, I. (2008). A wavelet-based method to remove spatial autocorrelation in the analysis of species distributional data. *Web Ecology, 8*(1), 22–29.

Carlson, T. N., & Ripley, D. A. (1997). On the relation between NDVI, fractional vegetation cover, and leaf area index. *Remote Sensing of Environment, 62*(3), 241–252.

Chen, T., Hui, E. C., Wu, J., Lang, W., & Li, X. (2019). Identifying urban spatial structure and urban vibrancy in highly dense cities using georeferenced social media data. *Habitat International, 89*, 102005.

Cihlar, J., Laurent, L. S., & Dyer, J. A. (1991). Relation between the normalized difference vegetation index and ecological variables. *Remote Sensing of Environment, 35*(2–3), 279–298.

Corr, P., & Matthews, G. (Eds.). (2020). *The Cambridge handbook of personality psychology.* Cambridge University Press.

Cromley, E. K., & McLafferty, S. L. (2012). *GIS and public health* (2nd ed.). Guilford Press.

Dargie, W., & Poellabauer, C. (2010). *Fundamentals of wireless sensor networks: Theory and practice.* Wiley.

Darkes, G., & Spence, M. (2017): *Cartography: An introduction.* British Cartographic Society.

Dormann, C. F., McPherson, J. M., Araújo, M. B., Bivand, R., Bolliger, J., Carl, G., et al. (2007). Methods to account for spatial autocorrelation in the analysis of species distributional data: A review. *Ecography, 30*(5), 609–628.

Epstein, D. H., Tyburski, M., Craig, I. M., Phillips, K. A., Jobes, M. L., Vahabzadeh, M., et al. (2014). Real-time tracking of neighborhood surroundings and mood in urban drug misusers: Application of a new method to study behavior in its geographical context. *Drug and Alcohol Dependence, 134*, 22–29.

Froehlich, J., Chen, M. Y., Smith, I. E., & Potter, F. (2006, September). Voting with your feet: An investigative study of the relationship between place visit behavior and preference. In *International conference on ubiquitous computing* (pp. 333–350). Springer.

Fuller, R. A., Irvine, K. N., Devine-Wright, P., Warren, P. H., & Gaston K. J. (2007). Psychological benefits of greenspace increase with biodiversity. *Cellular and Molecular Biology Letters, 3*(4), 390–394.

Gan, G., Ma, R., Reichert, M., Giurgiu, M., Ebner-Priemer, U. W., Meyer-Lindenberg, A., et al. (2021). Neural correlates of affective benefit from real-life social contact and implications for psychiatric resilience. *JAMA Psychiatry, 78*(7), 790–792.

GPS.gov. (2021). *GPS accuracy*. www.gps.gov/systems/gps/performance/accuracy.

Griffith, D. A., Chun, Y., & Li, B. (2019). *Spatial regression analysis using eigenvector filtering*. CRC Press.

Gustafson, D. H., McTavish, F. M., Chih, M. Y., Atwood, A. K., Johnson, R. A., Boyle, M. G., et al. (2014). A smartphone application to support recovery from alcoholism: A randomized clinical trial. *JAMA Psychiatry, 71*(5), 566–572.

Haining, R. P., & Li, G. (2020). *Modelling spatial and spatial-temporal data: A Bayesian approach*. CRC Press.

Heller, A. S., Shi, T. C., Ezie, C. E., Reneau, T. R., Baez, L. M., Gibbons, C. J., et al. (2020). Association between real-world experiential diversity and positive affect relates to hippocampal–striatal functional connectivity. *Nature neuroscience, 23*(7), 800–804.

Heron, K. E., & Smyth, J. M. (2010). Ecological momentary interventions: Incorporating mobile technology into psychosocial and health behaviour treatments. *British Journal of Health Psychology, 15*(1), 1–39.

Iosa, M., Fusco, A., Morone, G., & Paolucci, S. (2012). Walking there: Environmental influence on walking-distance estimation. *Behavioural Brain Research, 226*(1), 124–132.

Jenny, B., Šavrič, B., Arnold, N. D., Marston, B. E., & Preppernau, C. A. (2017). A guide to selecting map projections for world and hemisphere maps. In M. Lapaine & E. L. Usery (Eds.), *Choosing a map projection* (pp. 213–228). Springer.

Kessler, F., & Battersby, S. (2019). *Working with map projections: A guide to their selection*. Routledge & CRC Press.

Kotaru, M., Joshi, K., Bharadia, D., & Katti, S. (2015, August). Spotfi: Decimeter level localization using wifi. *Proceedings of the 2015 ACM Conference on Special Interest Group on Data Communication*, pp. 269–282.

Kulldorff, M., & Nagarwalla, N. (1995). Spatial disease clusters: Detection and inference. *Statistics in Medicine, 14*(8), 799–810.

Li, M., Westerholt, R., & Zipf, A. (2018). Do people communicate about their whereabouts? Investigating the relation between user-generated text messages and Foursquare check-in places. *Geo-Spatial Information Science, 21*(3), 159–172.

Loveday, A., Sherar, L. B., Sanders, J. P., Sanderson, P. W., & Esliger, D. W. (2015). Technologies that assess the location of physical activity and sedentary behavior: A systematic review. *Journal of Medical Internet Research, 17*(8), e192.

MacEachren, A. M. (1995). *How maps work: Representation, visualization, and design*. Guilford Press.

Madry, S. (2015). *Global navigation satellite systems and their applications*. Springer.

Menke, K. (2019). *Discover QGIS 3.x—A workbook for classroom or independent study*. Locate Press.

Mocnik, F. B., Ludwig, C., Grinberger, A. Y., Jacobs, C., Klonner, C., & Raifer, M. (2019). Shared data sources in the geographical domain—A classification schema and corresponding visualization techniques. *ISPRS International Journal of Geo-information, 8*(5), 242.

Monmonier, M. (2018): *How to lie with maps* (3rd ed.). University of Chicago Press.

Müller, S. R., Peters, H., Matz, S. C., Wang, W., & Harari, G. M. (2020). Investigating the relationships between mobility behaviours and indicators of subjective well-being using smartphone-based experience sampling and GPS tracking. *European Journal of Personality, 34*(5), 714–732.

Nahum-Shani, I., Smith, S. N., Spring, B. J., Collins, L. M., Witkiewitz, K., Tewari, A., et al. (2018). Just-in-Time Adaptive Interventions (JITAIs) in mobile health: Key components and design principles for ongoing health behavior support. *Annals of Behavioral Medicine: A Publication of the Society of Behavioral Medicine, 52*(6), 446–462.

Neteler, M., & Mitasova, H. (2008). *Open source GIS: A GRASS GIS approach*. Springer.

Nguyen, K. A., Luo, Z., Li, G., & Watkins, C. (2020). *A review of smartphones based indoor positioning: Challenges and applications*. http://arxiv.org/abs/2006.02251

Novack, T., Wang, Z., & Zipf, A. (2018). A system for generating customized pleasant pedestrian routes based on OpenStreetMap Data. *Sensors, 18*, 3794.

Obe, R. O., & Hsu, L. S. (2011). *PostGIS in Action*. Manning.

Peterson, G. N. (2015). *GIS cartography—A guide to effective map design*. CRC Press.

Rabus, B., Eineder, M., Roth, A., & Bamler, R. (2003). The shuttle radar topography mission—A new class of digital elevation models acquired by spaceborne radar. *ISPRS Journal of Photogrammetry and Remote Sensing, 57*(4), 241–262.

Reichert, M., Braun, U., Lautenbach, S., Zipf, A., Ebner-Priemer, U., Tost, H., et al. (2020). Studying the impact of built environments on human mental health in everyday life: Methodological developments, state-of-the-art and technological frontiers. *Current Opinion in Psychology, 32*, 158–164.

Reichert, M., Gan, G., Renz, M., Braun, U., Brüßler, S., Timm, I., et al. (2021). Ambulatory assessment for precision psychiatry: Foundations, current developments and future avenues. *Experimental Neurology, 345*, 113807.

Reichert, M., Giurgiu, M., Koch, E., Wieland, L. M., Lautenbach, S., Neubauer, A. B., et al. (2020). Ambulatory assessment for physical activity research: State of the science, best practices and future directions. *Psychology of Sport and Exercise, 50*, 101742.

Renfro, B. A., Stein, M., Boeker, N., & Terry, A. (2017). *An analysis of Global Positioning System (GPS) Standard Positioning Service (SPS) performance for 2017* (TR-SGL-18-02). Space and Geophysics Laboratory Applied Research Laboratories, The University of Texas at Austin.

Snyder, J. P. (1987). *Map projections—A working manual* (Vol. 1395). U.S. Government Printing Office.

Stumpp, J. (2014). *Platform for interactive ambulatory psychophysiological assessment*. Unpublished doctoral dissertation, Karlsruhe Institute of Technology.

Sykora, M., Jackson, T. W., O'Brien, A., & Elayan, S. (2013). Emotive Ontology: Extracting fine-grained information from terse, informal messages. *IADIS International Conference Intelligent Systems and Agents*, pp. 19–26.

Tachikawa, T., Kaku, M., Iwasaki, A., Gesch, D. B., Oimoen, M. J., Zhang, Z., et al. (2011). *ASTER global digital elevation model version 2-summary of validation results*. NASA.

Tobler, W. (1970). A computer movie simulating urban growth in the Detroit region. *Economic Geography*, 46, 234–240.

Tost, H., Reichert, M., Braun, U., Reinhard, I., Peters, R., Lautenbach, S., et al. (2019). Neural correlates of individual differences in affective benefit of real-life urban green space exposure. *Nature Neuroscience, 22*(9), 1389–1393.

Ullah, H., Wan, W., Ali Haidery, S., Khan, N. U., Ebrahimpour, Z., & Luo, T. (2019). Analyzing the spatiotemporal patterns in green spaces for urban studies using location-based social media data. *ISPRS International Journal of Geo-Information, 8*(11), 506.

van Diggelen, F., & Enge, P. (2015, September). The World's first GPS MOOC and Worldwide Laboratory using Smartphones. *Proceedings of the 28th International Technical Meeting of the Satellite Division of the Institute of Navigation (ION GNSS+ 2015*, pp. 361–369.

Wan, N., Kan, G. L., & Wilson, G. (2017). Addressing location uncertainties in GPS-based activity monitoring: A methodological framework. *Transactions in GIS, 21*(4), 764–781.

Wang, G., Albayrak, A., Cabo, A., Goossens, R., Mol, J., Wijnand, B., et al. (2019). A mixed methods study to understand behavioral and psychological symptoms of dementia: A research protocol. In T. P. Cotrim, F. Serranheira, P. Sousa, S. Hignett, S. Albolino, & R. Tartaglia (Eds.), *Health and social care systems of the future: demographic changes, digital age and human factors* (pp. 109–117). Springer.

Zafari, F., Gkelias, A., & Leung, K. K. (2019). A survey of indoor localization systems and technologies. *IEEE Communications Surveys Tutorials, 21*(3), 2568–2599.

Zandbergen, P. A. (2009). Accuracy of iPhone locations: A comparison of assisted GPS, WiFi and cellular positioning. *Transactions in GIS, 13*(s1), 5–25.

Zhang, Z., Assunção, R., & Kulldorff, M. (2010). Spatial scan statistics adjusted for multiple clusters. *Journal of Probability and Statistics*, Article No. 642379.

CHAPTER 5

Acquisition and Analysis of Physical Behavior Data

Marco Giurgiu and J. B. J. (Hans) Bussmann

CHAPTER OVERVIEW

Physical behavior is defined as the observable physical behaviors (PBs; activities, postures, and movements) that people perform in their regular daily life. It is an umbrella term covering the constructs physical activity, sedentary behavior, and sleep. These constructs are to a large extent similar in measurement methods but with different health effects, and their outcomes partly depend on each other; for example, the longer a person sleeps, the less time remains for physical and sedentary activities. However, at the same time, they are independent of each other and have their own relevance, clinical background, and research platforms. In this chapter, we will focus on physical activity and sedentary behavior; sleep will be discussed mainly from the perspective of its dependency on physical and sedentary behavior. Subsequently, we will address the background, categories and relevance of PBs; discuss issues of measurement, data processing, and metrics; provide an example from psychology; and end with recommendations and future perspectives.

Introduction

Why Measure PB?

Physical behavior—the observable physical behaviors (PBs; activities, postures, and movements) that people perform in their regular daily life—is an umbrella term covering the constructs physical activity, sedentary behavior, and sleep.

Physical activity (PA), defined as any bodily movement produced by skeletal muscles that require energy expenditure (Caspersen, Powell, & Christenson, 1985), is beneficial for physical and mental health outcomes (Warburton & Bredin, 2017). In particular, being regularly physically active is associated with reduced risk for many noncommunicable diseases such as cardiovascular heart disease, hypertension, diabetes, cancer, and all-cause mortality (Lee et al., 2012), and it can contribute to the maintenance of healthy weight (World Health Organization, 2010). Furthermore, being physically active has benefits for mental health (e.g., lower prevalence of depressive symptoms and anxiety or improved self-esteem; Schuch et al., 2016), delays the onset of dementia (Livingston et al., 2017), and contributes to general well-being (Das & Horton, 2012). In simple words, PA is a well-known protective factor for preventing and managing diseases across the lifespan.

Although there is strong evidence that PA is beneficial for physical and mental health, many people are not sufficiently active. For example, researchers have reported that approximately 80% of U.S. adults and adolescents are insufficiently active, which means that they do not meet current PA recommendations, for example, being moderately physically active for 150 minutes throughout the week (Piercy et al., 2018; Tremblay et al., 2017). Technological and social changes in domestic, environmental, and occupational settings have led to an increasingly inactive lifestyle among different cultures and countries (Church et al., 2011). Especially in wealthier countries (e.g., high-income Western countries), the transition toward more inactive occupations and personal motorized transportation contributes to a high physical inactivity level. Tremblay describes the current situation as follows: "People sleep less, sit more, walk less frequently, drive more regularly, and do less PA than they used to." (Guthold, Stevens, Riley, & Bull, 2020).

From a health perspective, it is not only PA and exercise that are essential. Epidemiological studies and laboratory studies using sophisticated biology and medical chemistry methodologies identified unique mechanisms that are distinct from the biological base of PA and exercising (Hamilton, Healy, Dunstan, Zderic, & Owen, 2008). In this context, the construct of *sedentary behavior* (SB) should be discussed, that is, any waking behavior characterized by an energy expenditure ≤ 1.5 metabolic equivalents (METs; 1 MET equals the amount of energy needed while sitting at rest) while in a sitting, reclining, or lying posture (Tremblay et al., 2017). The definition involves two parts: a postural and an intensity part. SB is increasingly recognized as a serious, worldwide public health concern. Researchers have found that SB is negatively associated with cardiovascular diseases, diabetes, cancer, depression, and other physiological and mental health outcomes (Ekelund et al., 2016; Gilchrist et al., 2020; Huang et al., 2020). However, there is an ongoing discussion about the independence of SB effects on health; in other words, can sufficient PA counter the adverse health effects of SB? Previous studies have emerged, offering contradictory findings regarding this issue (Biswas et al., 2015; Ekelund et al., 2016). Even though the dependency between both behaviors is not explicit, SB is an omnipresent behavior in everyday life (Gardner et al., 2019). In particular, previous studies have shown that adults spend most of their waking moments (i.e., about 8–11 hours per day) in a sedentary position (Diaz et al., 2016).

Sleep, completing the 24-hour day, is also well known as a health-related behavior. Sleep is a naturally recurring and easily reversible state characterized by reduced or absent consciousness, perceptual disengagement, immobility, and the adoption of a characteristic sleeping posture. According to the Consensus Statement of the American Academy of Sleep Medicine and the Sleep Research Society, sleep is related to several aspects of human health (Watson et al., 2015). For instance, sleep is critically involved in systematic physiology such as metabolism (Magee & Hale, 2012), cardiovascular systems (Wan Xi, Liu, Zhang, & Fu, 2012), mood regulation (Minkel et al., 2012), brain functions, including neurobehavioral, cognitive and safety-related performance (van Dongen, Maislin, Mullington, & Dinges, 2003), and many other health-related outcomes (Watson et al., 2015).

In summary, the components of PB are one of the most important lifestyle factors related to several mental and physical health conditions. Measurement of it is crucial, among other things, for understanding the relationships with these health conditions, identifying people at risk, and evaluating interventions that aim at optimizing PB.

Categorization of PB

We have already stated that PB is an umbrella term. The distinction between the components PA, SB, and sleep is, however, just one of the possible categorizations. For example, PB can also be studied from the perspective of the duration of intensity categories, such as the subcategories sedentary, light, moderate, and vigorous. In each case and independent of the categorization used, behaviors can be analyzed relative to each other rather than as individual entities (Dumuid et al., 2020). The so-called compositional data analysis (CoDA) offers an advanced approach to take the co-dependencies between PB categories into account. However, time or duration is not the only relevant aspect of PB. For example, sedentary periods can vary in length (e.g., short or long sedentary bouts). Especially longer bouts, that is, periods of uninterrupted sedentary time (Tremblay et al., 2017), reached higher attention. Previous studies reported that longer sedentary bouts such as ≥ 30 minutes may lead to detrimental health effects (Dempsey et al., 2018). In summary, the relevance of PB outcomes depends not only on the duration, but also on other aspects such as intensity, frequency, and type.

So far, these subcategories have been discussed from the perspective of health, but other perspectives and factors can be relevant as well, such as the purpose or context of an activity. To give an example: PB can be assessed from its context, such as house holding, commuting, leisure activities, work, and sports. From a physical health perspective, the purpose or context of PA might not be most crucial, but from the perspective of meaning for a person or mental health, or when a personalized advice is needed, it surely is important. So far, we mainly focus on PA and SB, but the same principles can be applied to sleep. The sleep pattern involves the differentiation between the major sleep period (at night) compared to naps and daytime sleep. Moreover, additional parameters such as sleep (onset) latency, sleep quality, or sleep efficiency are also relevant aspects to describe a sleep pattern and are most used in sleep research (Ancoli-Israel et al., 2015; Fekedulegn et al., 2020). Table 5.1 provides an overview of different operationalization dimensions for each aspect of PB. Since researchers are increasingly interested in all aspects of PB by focusing on the interrelatedness of sleep, PA, and SB (Rosenberger et al., 2019), some research endeavors might be interested in assessing all facets simultaneously and in differentiating them during statistical analysis.

One Aim and Many Devices

The technological process has developed new ways to capture human movement and nonmovement. Nowadays, activity monitors such as *accelerometers* have become the

TABLE 5.1. Overview of Different Operationalization Dimensions for Each Aspect of Physical Behavior

	Sleep	Physical activity	Sedentary behavior
Definition	A naturally recurring and easily reversible state characterized by reduced or absent consciousness, perceptual disengagement, immobility, and the adoption of a characteristic sleeping posture	Any voluntary movement produced by skeletal muscles that results in energy expenditure	Any waking behavior characterized by an energy expenditure of 1.5 metabolic equivalents (METs; 1 MET = energy expenditure in rest), while in a sitting, reclining, or lying posture
Biological state	Sleep	Awake	Awake
Type	Sleep at night, nap	Activity of daily life, exercise	Screen-based sedentary activities and non-screen-based activities
Domain	At home, not at home	Work, home, leisure, transportation	Work, home, leisure, transportation
Energy expenditure	~1 MET	>1.5 METs (light, moderate, vigorous)	≤1.5 METs
Posture	Sitting, reclining, lying	Sitting, reclining, lying, standing, other	Sitting, reclining, lying
Bout length	Short, moderate, long	Short, moderate, long	Short, moderate, long
Parameters (examples)	Sleep time, sleep latency, wake after sleep onset, number of awakenings	Duration, intensity, amount of PA (e.g., expressed in counts), energy expenditure, number of steps	Sedentary time, sedentary bouts, sedentary breaks

preferred method due to their portability, affordability, low cost, small size, low power consumption, and opportunity to obtain large amounts of dense information (Bassett, 2012). Accelerometers are small, wearable devices that record and store acceleration in gravitational units on one or more axes at sampling rates of typically 20–100 Hz. Acceleration signals are then processed to various outcomes (e.g., intensity, energy expenditure, body postures, or movement quality parameter such as smoothness) within a lower resolution (e.g., seconds) and/or expressed per epoch of 5 seconds, 15 seconds, 30 seconds, 1 minute, and the like. The use of accelerometers to assess PB in daily life has increased significantly over the last decade (Burchartz et al., 2020). Multidisciplinary research groups are using accelerometers in a manifold way in different study settings—for example, in national surveillance (Troiano et al., 2008) or in clinical studies (Schasfoort et al., 2018). Parallel to the number of studies, the number of research and consumer devices with different outcomes has increased as well (Wijndaele et al., 2015). Most importantly, outcome parameters from different devices are highly dependent on the used algorithm and processing steps. Mueller, Chimenti, Merkle, and Frey-Law (2020) found large and inconsistent differences between previously validated scoring methods. Therefore, although all of these devices have the same aim, that is, to assess and provide accurate information of PB, the increasing number of scientific and consumer wearables results in several challenges that merit further remarks.

First, since the number of available scientific and consumer devices increased markedly (Lamkin, 2018), the data's parametrization also increasingly varied from device to device. In particular, because of differences in hardware, software, sets of algorithms, or data processing steps (e.g., filters, epoch-length, non-wear-time definition), it has become impossible to compare and pool data. Second, in line with the variety of devices, algorithms, and data processing techniques, there is an ongoing discussion about how the raw data should be processed optimally and harmoniously, which means in a similar way. In particular, different possibilities of processing accelerometer raw data into metrics are presented in the literature—for example, counts (Yang & Hsu, 2010), movement acceleration intensity (van Someren, Lazeron, Vonk, Mirmiran, & Swaab, 1996), euclidian norm minus one (van Hees et al., 2013), or mean amplitude deviation (Vähä-Ypyä et al., 2015). Third, the use of different data collection protocols may also lead to a lack of standardization. In particular, several decisions such as monitoring period, sensor placement, or processing steps (e.g., defining a valid day) often vary from study to study and thus reduce the comparability between study results. Fourth, some studies have shown that consumer wearables have reasonable validity for estimating PB parameters such as energy expenditure (Bai et al., 2016), whereas other studies revealed moderate to substantial differences for PA parameters (e.g., step-count, activity energy expenditure) when comparing outputs from consumer and research devices (Mikkelsen et al., 2020). This results in a controversial discussion about applying consumer wearables for research purposes. For example, Scott (2020) argued that the most significant barrier to using consumer wearables in research and clinical settings is a lack of independent validation. A further main point is that researchers often do not have access to raw data of consumer wearables and that they don't have access to the "black-boxed" algorithms either. In line with this issue, it should be noted that the pace at which technology is evolving in optimizing algorithms far exceeds the pace of published validation research. In general, there is a remarkably shorter product life cycle today, which might be a restriction for longitudinal cohort studies. Fifth, based on the current lack of standardization, applying proprietary algorithms should always be replicable. Thus, open-source methods are needed, which are more flexible to use and allow algorithms to be applied to different devices.

Measurement, Data Processing, and Metrics

Why Signal Processing of Acceleration Data Is Necessary and How It Works

It is not possible to do meaningful analyses with acceleration data before some type of signal processing has been done. Rectifying, one significant part of signal processing, may serve as an instructional example. Rectifying means converting the signal's negative acceleration (deceleration) to its absolute (positive) value. Normal human movement—even when walking at a fixed speed—is characterized by body segments (e.g., trunk, waist, or leg) that are continuously accelerating/decelerating in repeating patterns per step of stride. The amplitudes of acceleration/deceleration depend on the intensity of movement. For example, walking fast will result in more and higher amplitudes than walking slow, while during quiet standing the amplitudes will be minimal. To get meaningful metrics, signal processing is necessary, and this will be explained in detail.

There are many types of acceleration signal processing. Two important aims of signal processing are (1) to calculate movement intensity and, subsequently, to estimate energy expenditure and (2) to estimate the orientation of the sensor and, therefore, the orientation of the body segment the sensor is attached to. For these purposes, frequently applied types of signal processing are (1) eliminating the low-frequency gravitational acceleration, (2) reducing or eliminating high-frequency noise (artifacts, i.e., accelerations not related to movements of interest), and (3) extracting the lower frequency part of the signal to get an estimate of the gravitational component of the signal. For example, for the calculation of movement intensity, the acceleration signal is subsequently high-pass filtered (to eliminate the gravitational component), rectified, low-pass filtered (to eliminate noise), and then averaged over defined time intervals. Often, the movement intensity and/or gravitational information of the different axes of the sensors are combined and converted. Eventually, outcomes from these features are calculated, including type of activity (e.g., walking, standing, sitting), energy cost, and steps.

The results of the different steps of signal processing are shown in the example presented in Figure 5.1. Most accelerometers measure acceleration in three axes. In Figure 5.1A, the raw acceleration data of a three-axis accelerometer is shown (see *y*-axis, "raw acceleration"). The signal is measured in *g* (1 *g* = 9.81 m/sec^2) with the acceleration sensor's sampling frequency (e.g., 50 Hz). The measured signal contains the dynamic changes of the acceleration due to the movement of the device as well as the acceleration due to gravitation. The inertial component is the oscillating part in Figure 5.1A (starting at approximately 50 seconds), whereas the gravitational part is depicted by the level differences (static offset of the gravitational acceleration) that are evident over all 120 seconds but most clearly in seconds 1 to 50 (e.g., *y*-axis with a value of –1 *g*). In other words, the level differences between axes *x*, *y*, and *z* in Figure 5.1A describe how the device is held (placed in a three-dimensional space) but not how it is moved. Accordingly, as a first step, the signal is high-pass filtered to remove the static offset of the gravitational acceleration (see Figure 5.1B with *y*-axis "filtered raw acceleration").

In a second step, higher frequent noise (artifacts; e.g., electronic noise, vibrations when cycling on a rough road surface, shocks of the sensor) has to be removed. The filter used for this process influences the outcome of subsequent steps and therefore has to be designed carefully to eliminate all undesired frequencies without influencing the signal in the frequency range that should be measured. Human movements, for example, show a frequency range of 0.25–11 Hz (van Someren et al., 1996). Accordingly, an ideal filter would leave all movement/motion relevant frequencies in the signal (i.e., it should have a constant filter characteristic in this frequency range) but would cut off all other frequencies (in this case above 11 Hz). After filtering the signal, noises with higher frequencies are eliminated, as shown in Figure 5.2. An acceleration signal during walking (gravitational offset already eliminated) is shown in both the time domain (Figure 5.2A) and the frequency domain (Figure 5.2B). The measured signal contains frequency components up to 32 Hz. High-frequency parts of the signal, above 11 Hz, would be defined as non-physiological and would be filtered. Figures 5.2C and 5.2D show the same data with an additional 11-Hz low-pass filter. Compared to the non-low-pass filtered signal, the time domain signal is smoothed (comparing Figure 5.2A to 5.2C), and the frequency components above 11 Hz are eliminated (comparing Figure 5.2B to 5.2D).

As a third step, the vector magnitude is computed (see the equation below). In detail, the square of the signal is calculated, which automatically includes the necessary step of rectifying the signal. The three axes are then converted into one signal by summing and square rooting.

$$\text{Movement Acceleration Intensity (MovAccInt)} = \sqrt{\left(ax^2 + ay^2 + az^2\right)}$$

The result of building the vector magnitude can be seen in Figure 5.1C (see *y*-axis, "Movement Acceleration Intensity"), where only one signal is left that contains only positive values. In the last step of signal processing, the MovAccInt is averaged to epochs of a defined length, such as 30 seconds or a defined activity episode (e.g., going to school). Figure 5.1D shows the averaged MovAccInt signal. In our example, averaging was performed at 30-second intervals. The outcome of this last step of signal processing can then be used for statistical analysis of the assessed data using standard statistical software packages. However, the presented process accounts for only a one-movement intensity metric of many.

PB Metrics

Generally, PB metrics are the results of algorithms, which use aggregated raw acceleration signals as input. In other words, the sensor captures and stores the acceleration of a person during wear time, which will then be processed by using, for example, a bandpass filter (see the previous section). Given the high variability of research and consumer wearables, the number of different PB metrics increased measurably. Unfortunately, there are no internationally accepted standards for signal processing steps, and thus outcome metrics cannot be compared across devices (Chen & Bassett, 2005). For example, just to calculate movement intensity, the literature describes several types of signal processing: mean amplitude deviation (Vähä-Ypyä et al., 2015), Euclidian norm minus one (van Hees et al., 2013), high-pass filtered Euclidean norm (van Hees et al., 2013), high-pass filtered Euclidean norm plus (van Hees et al., 2013), proportional integrating measure (Jean-Louis, Kripke, Mason, Elliott, & Youngstedt, 2001), zero crossing method (Acebo et al., 1999), and time above threshold (Fekedulegn et al., 2020).

The most promising solution to increase comparability between metrics is to provide open access to raw data and applied algorithms. However, manufacturers are often not willing to reveal all details. Thus, recently researchers' efforts have been aimed at increasing the comparability between metrics by using identical software for different types of accelerometers. A study by Rowlands and colleagues (2018) has shown that identically processed metrics derived from different devices were largely equivalent. Similar results were published by Crowley and colleagues (2019), who showed that pooling and identically harmonizing accelerometer data lead to a negligible difference between different accelerometers.

A further difficulty encountered in comparing PB metrics centers on the different and, in some cases, "dimensionless" units. A possible solution might be to transfer PB metrics into commonly used estimations of energy expenditure. Notably, an additional "formula" is needed to estimate energy expenditure. This potentially leads to even less comparability, because the formula behind this calculation is frequently a "black box" as well as device-dependent. Thus, the prerequisite to enabling comparability is possible only when the converting algorithm from metrics into energy expenditure estimations is available for the public (e.g., open-access code). If the converting algorithm might be

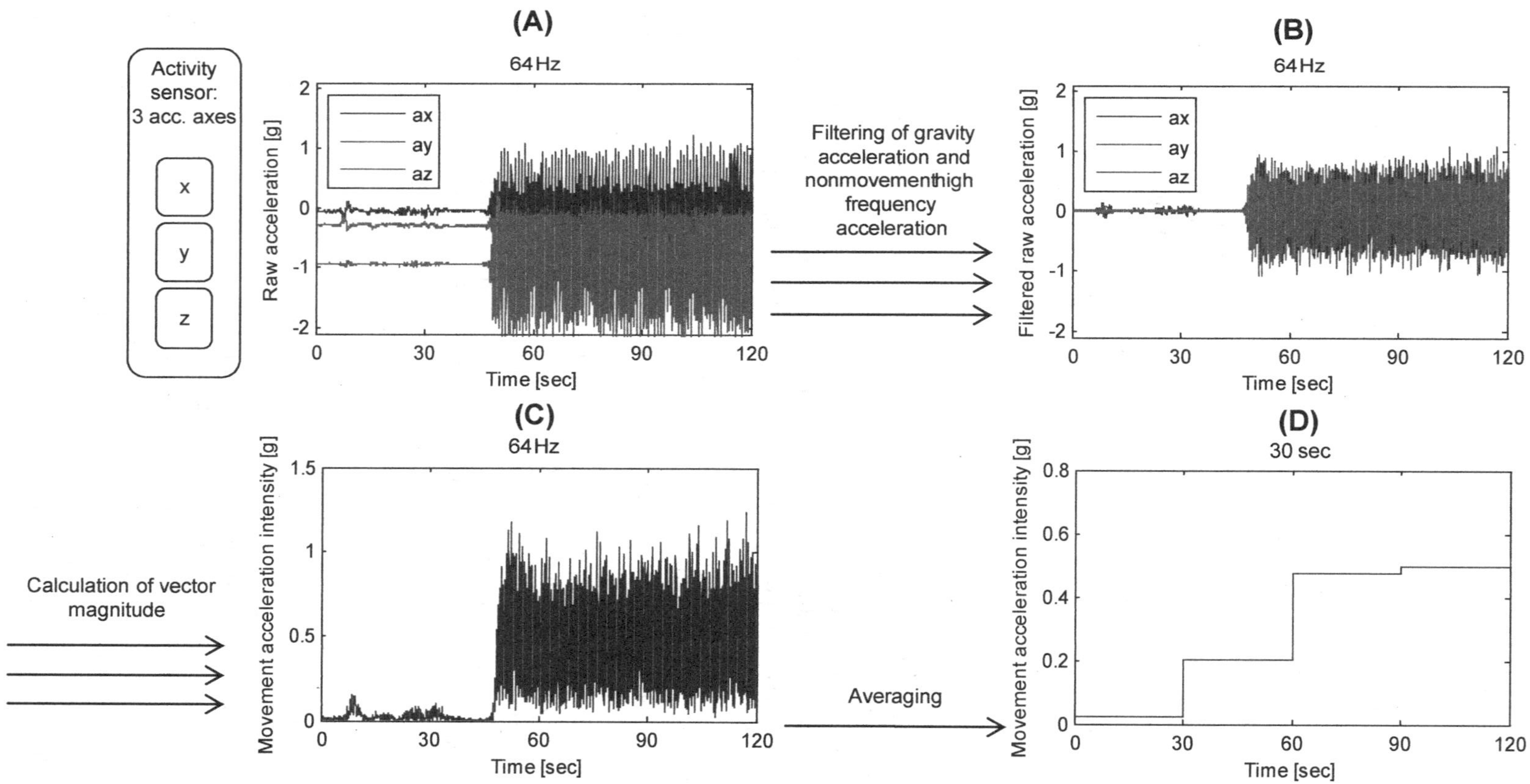

FIGURE 5.1. Outcome of the different steps of signal processing in the analysis of acceleration signals.

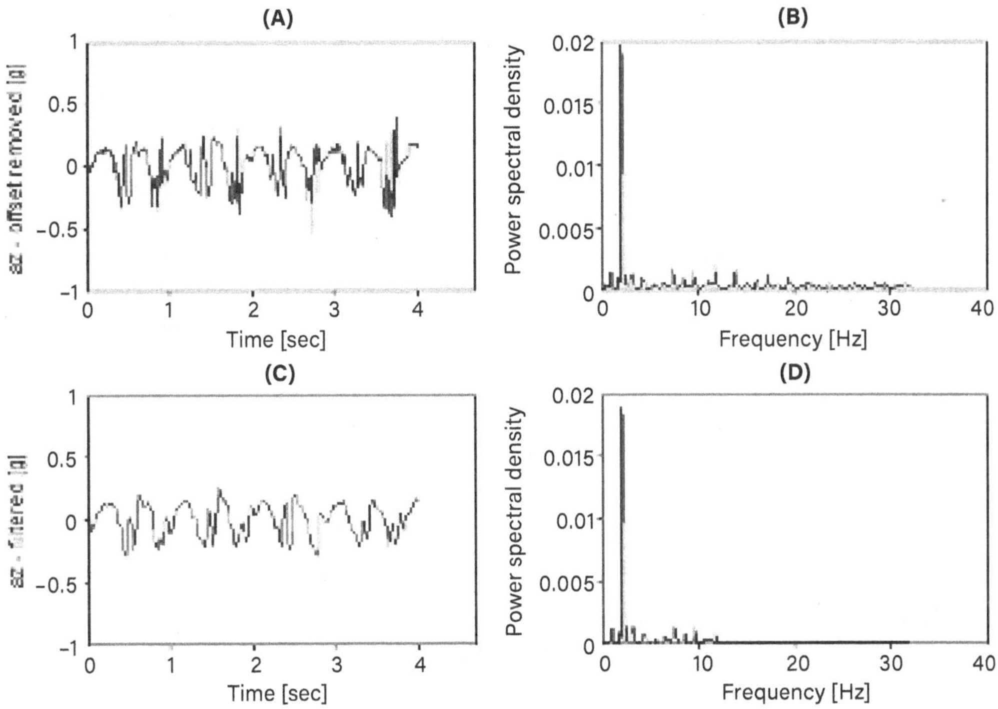

FIGURE 5.2. Effect of low-pass filtering on the acceleration signal.

available for the public, researchers can more easily assess, compare, and validate methods and outcomes.

A growing body of epidemiological literature has shown that SB might be an independent risk factor for all-cause mortality and cardiometabolic diseases (Lee & Shiroma, 2014). As a result, the urgency to differentiate between PA and SB during data assessment has increased greatly (Katzmarzyk et al., 2019). However, the first generation of accelerometers was built to measure the intensity of PA through changes in acceleration. Thus, even though an accelerometer can indicate the absence of movement, this does not automatically mean that they can distinguish between body postures such as sitting and standing, which may increase the intangible risk of an over- or underestimation of SB (Kang & Rowe, 2015). For instance, standing still and sitting still at the bus stop cannot be distinguished, whereas, by definition, sitting still is an SB activity and standing still is non-SB. With regard to the previous part of data processing, applying low-pass filtering to "remove" movement and to retain the gravitational component overcomes this gap. Thus, depending on the sensor location, it is possible to estimate the angular orientation of the sensor and to detect body postures accurately (Janssen & Cliff, 2015). So far, research shows that attachment of an accelerometer to the thigh is the most logical position to provide body posture data. With innovative data analytical techniques, body posture data can also be derived from waist-worn or wrist-worn devices, although so far with lower levels of reliability/validity.

The fast development of technical features may affect the future of data assessment and the processing of PB via wearables. In particular, supervised learning approaches (e.g., machine learning or deep-learning algorithms) gained more and more popularity (see Chapters 17 and 18, this volume). In particular, combined with advances in signal processing techniques and machine learning algorithms, this paved the way to developing methods capable of automatically identifying postures or types of PA from raw acceleration signals (Bastian et al., 2015; Willetts, Hollowell, Aslett, Holmes, & Doherty, 2018). Previous studies suggested that promising automatic posture and activity recognition tools that developed from data acquired in highly controlled environments (i.e., in the laboratory) may not perform as well when applied to real-life data (Gyllensten & Bonomi, 2011). In contrast, other study results demonstrate a superior performance of PA-type classification algorithms compared with traditional approaches (Ellis, Kerr, Godbole, Staudenmayer, & Lanckriet, 2016). Similar results have shown that a deep-learning model performs significantly better in assessing sleep than existing conventional algorithms (Haghayegh, Khoshnevis, Smolensky, & Diller, 2020). To sum up, the uptake of supervised learning approaches has been slow in health behavior research, which may change in the coming years (Trost, 2020).

Scientific Quality Standards

High-quality measurement of PB is essential to draw a conclusion about their influence on health outcomes. Moreover, the selection of an optimal device is necessary since measurement error can be high. In particular, the sources of error can occur in different stages of data collection and interpretation (Kang & Rowe, 2015). To give just a few examples, when collecting raw data, researchers may select the wrong device placement or use a device with inappropriate sampling frequency. Moreover, as mentioned earlier, the lack of transparency and validity of "black-boxed" algorithms may hinder researchers from drawing valid conclusions. Thus, one key argument for the selection process is to consider scientific quality standards (see Chapter 17, this volume). In line with the Consensus-based Standards for the selection of health Measurement INstruments (COSMIN; Mokkink et al., 2010) several standards should be noted: (1) validity (the degree to which an instrument truly measures the construct it purports to measure); (2) reliability (the proportion of the total variance in the measurements, because of "true" differences among participants); (3) responsiveness (the ability of the instrument to detect change over time in the construct); (4) interpretability (e.g., the qualitative meaning of the obtained scores); and (5) feasibility, ease of analysis, economy, measurement invariance, and cultural adaptability (Sylvia, Bernstein, Hubbard, Keating, & Anderson, 2014). In the following paragraphs, we discuss the first two points in depth and address the issue of reactivity.

Validity

To determine the validity of a device is one of the most critical issues. Researchers interested in validating accelerometers have to consider several aspects, such as selecting the appropriate reference method or conceptualizing an adequate study protocol. Whenever possible, accelerometer outcome should be validated against the gold-standard method. For example, if the primary outcome of interest is energy expenditure during free-living activities, it might be reasonable to use portable systems (e.g., indirect calorimetry) as a reference method. When researchers are interested in validating body postures, it is advisable to use video recording as the criterion measure, or if sleep parameters are of primary interest, researchers may use polysomnography as the reference method. Moreover, validation of accelerometers in different samples is recommended.

According to a framework published by Keadle, Lyden, Strath, Staudenmayer, and Freedson (2019), the following five phases should be considered during the validation process. The initial step (Phase 0) relies on bench testing and refining the monitor's technical reliability. In particular, this phase includes mechanical testing of the sensor signal in a controlled and artificial environment to test the within- and between-device reliability and validity of the underlying signals. Especially in the early stages of the application of accelerometers, the sensors were unstable in terms of mechanical drift and robustness. This topic has still to be considered and is less important.

The next steps reflect monitor calibration or the development of algorithms to estimate activity energy expenditure, body postures, or metrics from the device signals under controlled laboratory conditions. Phase I testing includes selected activities of daily living using fixed start/stop times. Phase II testing extends the earlier phase and includes implementing semi-free-living protocols, including transitions between activities to develop algorithms further and refine them. Criterion measures are integral to monitoring the calibration process, and these data are often used to provide initial validity information about new devices or prediction algorithms. Phase III of the development process involves a rigorous independent validation under real-world conditions compared with gold-standard measures (i.e., indirect calorimetry, direct observation, doubly labeled water, polysomnography) in different study samples by using appropriate statistics. Unfortunately, most studies do not surpass Phase I or Phase II. However, some validation studies can be mentioned as examples. Toth and colleagues (2018) evaluated the validity of step counts from various devices compared to direct video observation. In contrast, Valenti, Camps, Verhoef, Bonomi, and Westerterp (2014) validated energy expenditure from an accelerometer outcome, whereas total energy expenditure was measured simultaneously with doubly labeled water under free-living conditions. Phase IV, the final phase of the development process, involves applying and disseminating algorithms that have successfully progressed through previous phases. Thus, aiming to provide open-source code and instructions for implementing algorithms allows other researchers to use those methods in surveillance, experimental, clinical trials, or observational studies.

An important aspect of the validity of accelerometers is *reactivity*. A reactive behavior results when participants become more active simply because they are wearing a monitoring device. In other words, reactivity occurs when participants alter their behavior due to being monitored, the novelty of a new device, or social desirability. In fact, reactivity is a serious issue that reveals a potential source of error. Based on earlier studies, researchers expected reactivity to be a time issue, which means participants may change their behavior at the beginning of the monitoring period and later return to a more stable pattern (Rowe, Mahar, Raedeke, & Lore, 2004). Empirical evidence supports these expectations. In particular, Clemes, Matchett, and Wane (2008) compared the step counts of participants under two conditions: comparing those who knew they were being tracked with those who did not know (Clemes et al., 2008). The authors found a significant increase in the first condition. In contrast, Behrens and Dinger (2007) found no reactivity effect in a sample of young healthy adults (Behrens & Dinger, 2007). To avoid potential sources of reactivity, researchers might be aware of the following points: First, devices that display/provide feedback about PB may enhance the reactivity effect and motivate participants to change their behavior. Second, it is recommended that little information be given about the outcome measure. Third, measurement periods over a longer time period and the exclusion of the first monitoring day, for instance, may counteract bias due to reactivity (Dössegger et al., 2014).

Reliability

The reliability criterion refers to the consistency of a response either across multiple tests within a single assessment (i.e., internal consistency) or across various assessments (i.e., stability reliability, test–retest reliability, or between-day variability; Patterson, 2000). When transferred to accelerometer research, reliability can refer to measurement-related factors (e.g., technological stability of the sensors, inconsistencies of the data acquisition and processing, placement of the device) or behavior-related factors (e.g., variability in PB between days or between seasons). In the early stages of accelerometry, technological stability (e.g., drift of the accelerometer signal) was a main issue, but it is less important nowadays. Current research focuses more on the differences or agreement between placement of the same sensor on different body parts (e.g., wrist vs. hip) or on the effects of undesired placement errors. For example, Stanton, Guertler, Duncan, and Vandelanotte (2016) have shown that changing the accelerometer placement to 2 cm above and below the thigh's midpoint does not produce statistically significant differences.

If researchers are unsure about whether they should select a self-report or a device-based instrument, the results of studies comparing instruments might be helpful. In particular, a systematic review indicates that the volume of PA assessment between questionnaires and devices is low to moderately correlated (Prince et al., 2008). In particular, participants tend to overestimate the amount of PA. Notable differences were also found when comparing instruments for assessment of SB. Prince and colleagues (2020) compared self-reported and device-based assessment of SB, including 185 unique studies in a meta-analysis. The results revealed that self-reported measures underestimated sedentary time by ~ 1.74 hours/day compared to device measures.

A Prototypical Example from Psychology

In psychological research, the usage of accelerometers is applied regularly. Some researchers are interested in the within-subject association between PB and psychological constructs such as mood, stress, or anxiety in real time and real life by using ambulatory assessment (AA; Liao, Shonkoff, & Dunton, 2015; Reichert et al., 2020). To present an example of an AA study, including device-based assessment of PB, we describe the published article by Giurgiu, Koch, Plotnikoff, Ebner-Priemer, and Reichert (2020) in more detail. In particular, we would like to focus on the technical realization; that is, what does the path from data processing to data analysis look like?

Giurgiu, Koch, and colleagues (2020) compared the influence of different break patterns (i.e., variations in frequency, intensity, type, duration, and context) on mood in a healthy sample of university employees ($N = 92$). Over the study period of 5 days (3 working and 2 weekend days), participants carried accelerometers and a smartphone during their daily lives. The smartphone prompted the participants via an acoustic, visual, and vibration signal every 40 to 100 minutes within the 7:30 A.M. to 9:30 P.M.

period. In total, participants answered mood questions approximately 10 times per day. To assess mood, they used the short version of the multidimensional mood questionnaire (MDMQ; Wilhelm & Schoebi, 2007). Giurgiu and colleagues used a mix-sampling strategy—random triggers at various times combined with a sedentary triggered algorithm. In particular, the thigh sensor analyzed and transferred data on body position (sitting/lying or upright) via Bluetooth Low Energy (BLE) to the smartphone in real time. Each time a participant spent more than 30 minutes sitting/lying, the e-diary triggered mood ratings. This approach was implemented to optimize the assessment of the associations between SB and mood. As main predictors, the authors defined different break patterns such as duration (uninterrupted sedentary time), frequency (number of sedentary interruptions), intensity (metabolic equivalent of the break), and context (at home or work). The information about duration, frequency, and intensity was derived from the accelerometer, whereas context information was assessed via electronic diaries. In the process of analyzing data, the following nine steps were described (Giurgiu, Koch, et al., 2020) (see also Figure 5.3).

First, the sampling scheme and forms (e.g., questions about mood and context) were created by using the online platform movisensXS (movisens Ltd., 2021). This step included all setup, such as selecting study duration, specification of the trigger option (e.g., triggering after 20 minutes or 30 minutes of sitting/lying), and implementing time-out triggers. Second, immediately before data collection, the study smartphone was connected to the online platform movisensXS by using the movisensXS-App to download the sampling scheme and forms via an individual participant code. Third, the chosen trigger option (e.g., triggering after 30 minutes of sitting) was calibrated to the selected body position (i.e., lateral aspect of the right thigh) and connected to the smartphone via BLE by using the movisensXS-App. Fourth, after data collection, the recorded raw acceleration data were processed in 1-minute intervals by using the manufacturers' software DataAnalyzer (v.1.13.5) (movisens Ltd.). During this step, a band-pass filter (0.25 to 11 Hz) automatically eliminated gravitational components or artifacts (e.g., vibrations when cycling on a rough road surface or sensor shocks). This resulted in an Excel sheet with a self-selected choice of parameters such as body position, movement acceleration intensity (MAI), metabolic equivalents or activity class. Fifth, the smartphone entries from the participants were downloaded from the online platform movisensXS. Sixth, all accelerometer and ecological momentary assessment (EMA) files from different participants were time-synchronized and combined into a single data file by using DataMerger (v.1.8.0). Seventh, before the analyses, sedentary break-specific variables such as frequency, duration, and intensity were parametrized while calculating the cumulated sum of the dichotomous variable body position (1 = sitting/lying; 0 = upright). Eight, participants were excluded from the dataset if they did not fulfill the wear-time criteria of at least 2 valid days, that is, 10 hours of wear time per day (Troiano et al., 2008).

To analyze whether different break characteristics influence mood dimensions in different ways, Giurgiu, Koch, and colleagues (2020) conducted multilevel analyses of the state-of-the-art procedure in analyzing intensive longitudinal data (Bolger & Laurenceau, 2013). Multilevel analysis has several advantages, notably (1) the analysis of within- and between-subject effects simultaneously in one statistical model, (2) the analysis of hierarchically structured data (i.e., multiple mood assessments nested within participants), and (3) robustness concerning missing data points (Hoffman, 2015).

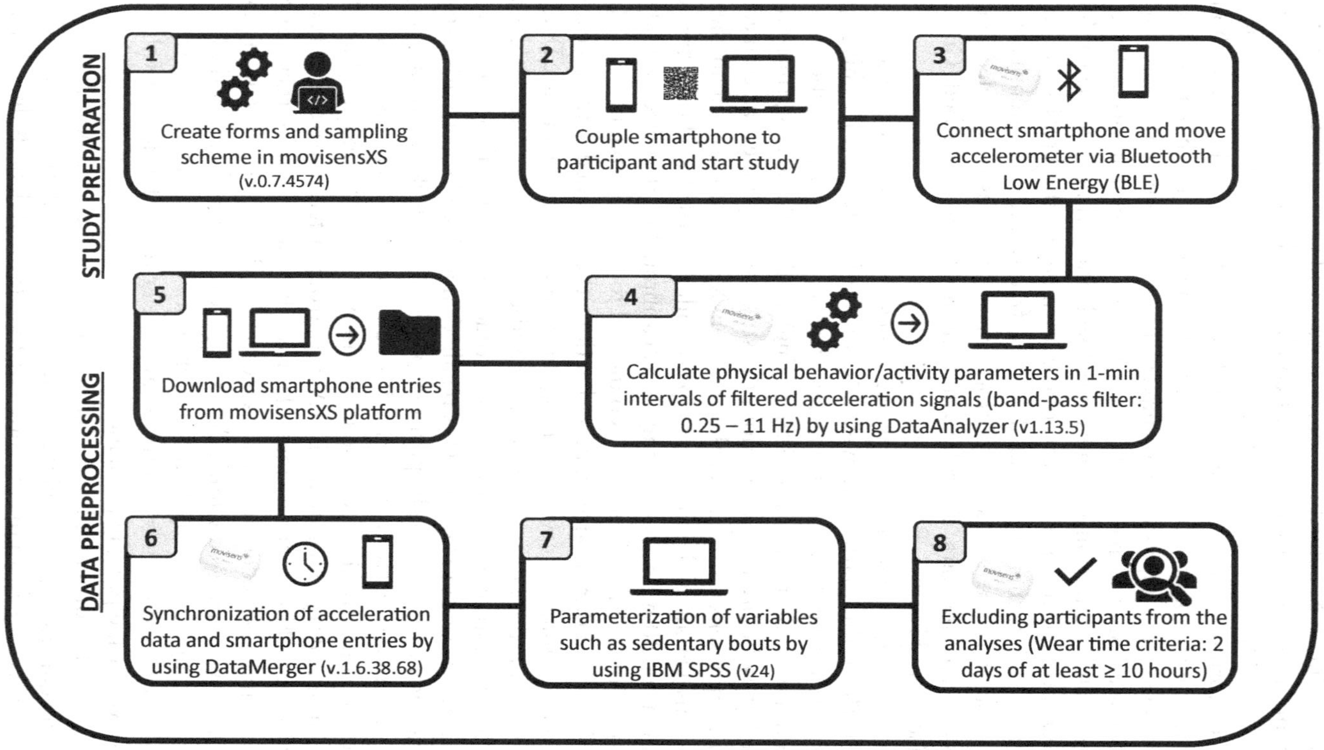

FIGURE 5.3. Process of study preparation and data preprocessing.

The study results indicated that sedentary breaks were associated with mood among healthy adults in daily life. In particular, break intensity was associated with an enhancement in all three mood dimensions, and break frequency was related to enhancement in two of three mood dimensions (valence and energetic arousal). But break duration was not significantly associated with mood at all. Exploratory analyses revealed that the effects of break frequency on energetic arousal, as well as the effect of break intensity on energetic arousal, were significantly higher in the home than in the workplace. The authors concluded that individuals should break up their SB as frequently as possible within an hour through at least moderate-intensity activities, such as slow walking; ideally, this practice would take place in any context.

Recommendations

Using accelerometers in health behavior studies and interventions offers huge possibilities, but at the same time, some challenges merit further consideration. A comprehensive assessment of a 24-hour-cycle of PB requires the acquisition of various information, including biological state (i.e., sleep, awake), movement intensity or energy expenditure, posture classification, and qualitative aspects (e.g., context and type of behavior). Thus, the simultaneous acquisition of all aspects of PB reveals a challenging task, and it might not be possible to select the optimal device and study protocol, which comprises all aspects. Therefore, as a general recommendation and according to the scientific statement from the American Heart Association (AHA; Strath et al., 2013), the following decision matrix might be a helpful guide during the selection process for suitable devices and study protocol. In particular, the decision matrix considers five areas:

1. Study outcomes—for example, What is your primary outcome variable of interest, and what do you want to describe (e.g., PA, SB, sleep, or the whole 24-hour-cycle)?
2. Feasibility and practicality of the device—How many people do you want to measure?
3. What is the patient/participant burden? What are assessment time considerations?
4. Available resources—What are the cost considerations, and are personnel available? and
5. Study administration—What are the data processing, data transfer and data summarization requirements?

The last part of the chapter is reserved for recommendations and future trends for researchers interested in using accelerometers to assess PB. Because of the multilayered perspectives, we focused on different points of view and integrated both technical and conceptual perspectives. Accordingly, recommendations are in line with expert consensus on aspects such as the utilization and harmonization of accelerometry data (Wijndaele et al., 2015) or the conceptualization of study protocols (Migueles et al., 2017; Troiano et al., 2008).

- *Data acquisition.* The way data are acquired in terms of sensor placement, sample frequency, and non-wear algorithms highly influences study results and, therefore, comparability between studies. Therefore, to compare the results from different accelerometer outcomes, researchers should apply standardized procedures whenever possible.

- *Signal processing.* See the previous point.

- *Raw data versus preprocessed summary data.* Due to limited storage possibilities, in the past acceleration data were preprocessed in real time and converted into summary data that were stored. Nowadays, this point is less relevant, and therefore measurement of raw data is strongly recommended.

- *Reporting and replicability.* All information about the study protocol and data processing must be reported, including processing characteristics such as filtering or protocol information such as sensor placement or measurement days. For example, concealing key elements of data processing is not in accordance with good scientific practice and hinders replication (Keil et al., 2014; Open Science Collaboration, 2015).

- *Number of measurement days.* Given the inherent variation in behavior over time, an essential aspect of accelerometer measurement is how many days should be considered to obtain reliable results. The results of studies have shown that necessary days for a reliable assessment vary from 3 to 5 days in adults and 4 to 9 days in children (Donaldson, Montoye, Tuttle, & Kaminsky, 2016; Sasaki et al., 2018; Trost, McIver, & Pate, 2005); from three 24-hour periods to 10 days or 2 weeks (Aadland & Ylvisaker, 2015). An internationally accepted recommendation emphasizes the recording of 7 days (Pedisic & Bauman, 2015; Trost et al., 2005). Moreover, researchers should be aware that behavior varies between weekend and weekdays; thus, at least one weekend day is required (Trost et al., 2005). The primary outcome of interest could also influence the selection of the monitoring period. For example, to assess differences between weekday and weekend sleep patterns, a 14-day recording that captures two weekends is preferred (Acebo et al., 1999). A further issue that is related to the monitoring period comprises reproducibility. Researchers have shown that different PB metrics have a considerable amount of random error from one 7-day monitoring period (Saint-Maurice et al., 2020). It should be realized that the number of measurement days not only depends on the research question, but also on the outcome of interest and the population. For example, the literature indicates that people with disabilities and low levels of PA show less between-day variability than people without disabilities and higher levels of PA.

- *Seasonal variation.* Most studies select a monitoring period of 7 days, intending to assess habitual PB patterns. However, researchers should consider that PB might be influenced by seasonal variation. Empirical data revealed that light PA was significantly higher in summer and spring, whereas SB and time spent in bed were higher in winter (O'Connell, Griffiths, & Clemes, 2014).

- *Single- or multisensor system.* How many accelerometers should be used? Most studies used a single wrist or hip-worn accelerometer, which were recommended for population-based PB research (Sievanen & Kujala, 2017). As of now the hip-worn position has proved to be the best single location for the assessment of different physical activities (Cleland et al., 2013). However, growing interest over the past decade in SB research indicated that the hip position increases the risk of misclassification between a sitting and a standing body position (Kang & Rowe, 2015). In line with point 1 from the AHA matrix, it depends on the primary outcome of interest. An accelerometer measures the movement/orientation of the segment to which it is attached, and so no information on the movement/orientation of other segments can be assessed. A multisensor system (e.g., attached at the thigh and wrist position) offers more data and information, while at the same time a further sensor increases participants' burden. Therefore, researchers may decide if the additional gain is needed and/or is of sufficient added value.

- *Sensor position.* In line with the previous point, selecting the body position largely depends on the primary outcome of interest. In particular, the position of choice for sleep assessment is the nondominant wrist because it optimizes the recording of small movements that occur at the distal extremities when the individual is supine (Ancoli-Israel et al., 2015; Quante et al., 2015). In some populations such as infants, researchers attach the accelerometer to the ankle rather than the wrist to limit the child's engagement with the device and to promote safety. Moreover, a thigh-worn accelerometer enables differentiation between body postures and separates PA from SB (Giurgiu, Bussmann, et al., 2020). Underlining the importance of sensor placement, Edwardson and colleagues (2016) have shown that irrespective of the device brand, thigh-worn accelerometers were highly accurate in differentiating body postures.

- *Addition of extra data sources.* For some research purposes, it might be reasonable to combine accelerometers with further data sources. For example, if sleep is the primary outcome, it might help to add the information from a light sensor to detect whether a person is sleeping or awake. Some manufacturers have already combined light sensors and PB monitoring within a single device (Ancoli-Israel et al., 2015). Another example is integrating a barometric pressure sensor to differentiate between sitting and standing postures during daily activities (Masse, Bourke, Chardonnens, Paraschiv-Ionescu, & Aminian, 2014).

- *Qualitative information:* Since accelerometers are limited to assess qualitative aspects of PB such as context or smoothness, researchers may combine self-reported instruments such as electronic diaries (e.g., application on a smartphone) or questionnaires. In fact, a combination of tools is likely to be the most promising way of assessing PB if researchers would like to assess a comprehensive picture of a behavior (Skender et al., 2016). This implies that a mixed-methods approach that combines device-based and self-reported techniques (e.g., ambulatory assessment) is generally assumed to be most appropriate.

- *Identifying missing data:* One of the most common issues concerning accelerometers is to identify non-wear periods. This issue is further complicated by the fact that there is a large variability between methods and non-wear algorithms, and also different algorithms within one device. Some researchers defined non-wear times based on predetermined thresholds (e.g., zero counts for 60 minutes; Oliver, Badland, Schofield, & Shepherd, 2011). In contrast, other researchers used multiple indicators, such as heart rate and intensity markers. In general, this is a critical aspect since less movement over a predetermined period is only a rough estimation to differentiate wear from non-wear time. Applying such a recommendation may increase the substantial risk of misclassifying sitting and sleep periods as non-wear times. Optimally, an algorithm can detect "real" non-wear times (e.g., during water activities, if the sensor is not waterproof). However, this depends largely on the accuracy of non-wear time algorithms. Thus, a general suggestion is to encourage participants to fill out a non-wear time diary, including time and activities during which the sensor was removed during the day.

- *Identifying a valid day.* In line with the previous point, there is a large variability between existing procedures. Suppose an algorithm can distinguish between wear and non-wear time. This leads to the issue of how many hours of wear time are necessary to define a valid day. The most common recommendations emphasize at least 10 hours of wear time as a precondition for a valid day (Mâsse et al., 2005). For some populations (e.g., toddlers or children) the required wear time can be reduced. In case of a large number of invalid days, it is possible to apply imputation approaches. For example, a multiple imputation approach relied on time-based, sociodemographic, and health information (Borghese, Borgundvaag, McIsaac, & Janssen, 2019).

- *Epoch length.* After data processing, most of the required software packages can calculate output parameters (e.g., PB metrics, energy expenditure or body postures) in different time intervals (i.e., epoch lengths). The selection of the epoch lengths affects the outcome, while most optimal epoch length depends on the primary outcome of interest. For example, most validated and commonly used epoch lengths are 30 seconds and 1 minute. However, some researchers favor using lower epoch lengths (e.g., 15 seconds) because they better capture the quick changes in patterns compared to longer epochs (Janssen & Cliff, 2015). This point should be noted if sit-to-stand transitions are of particular research interest. Furthermore, epoch length should also be considered when comparing data from different studies. In young people (e.g., preschoolers), shorter epochs (1–15 seconds) are recommended to capture the short bouts of activity that frequently occur in these age groups (Migueles et al., 2017).

The Future of the Field

The field of assessing PB via wearables is undergoing fast technological change. Devices that were up to date a moment ago will be obsolete tomorrow. So, what could the near future bring? We would like to look ahead with some example expectations.

First, technical development will influence hardware and data infrastructure. In particular, the size of sensors will decrease, the devices will be able to store more data locally, the technical infrastructure will be improved through, for example, more powerful processors or less power consumption, which will enable longer measurement periods, or data transfer possibilities will increase such as a 5G network, Wi-Fi connections, or data cloud options. But it is not only technical possibilities that may change; the opportunity of wearing wearables as a textile or an implantable sensor might also be an option in the future.

Second, we expect that the current distinction between research-grade and consumer-grade devices will become less significant. Furthermore, the use of consumer-grade devices, such as commercial fitness trackers, smartphones, or smartwatches, will increase, as will their acceptance. This will lower the barriers of the application of activity monitoring.

Third, from an analytic perspective, we expect that future research endeavors will result in a better understanding of the underlying mechanisms and determinants of PB.

Big Data, for example, from surveillance studies, will increasingly become available, together with advanced data analysis techniques (e.g., applying deep learning).

Fourth, we expect that privacy, safety, data protection, and data ownership will be more dominant issues on the agenda. Think, for example, about the General Data Protection Regulation and the role of companies such as Apple, FitBit, and Google, which still have access to an enormous amount of data.

Finally, we expect that technical elements will be an integral part of health care systems—for example, more common assessment of PB in hospital and rehabilitation centers, remote contact with therapist, automated personalized feedback, or remote health measurement (e.g., ECG, blood pressure, PB).

REFERENCES

Aadland, E., & Ylvisaker, E. (2015). Reliability of objectively measured sedentary time and physical activity in adults. *PloS One, 10*(7), e0133296.

Acebo, C., Sadeh, A, Seifer, R., Tzischinsky, O., Wolfson, A. R., Hafer, A., et al. (1999). Estimating sleep patterns with activity monitoring in children and adolescents: How many nights are necessary for reliable measures? *Sleep, 22*(1), 95–103.

Ancoli-Israel, S., Martin, J. L., Blackwell, T., Buenaver, L., Liu, L., Meltzer, L. J., et al. (2015). The SBSM guide to actigraphy monitoring: Clinical and research applications. *Behavioral Sleep Medicine, 13*(Suppl. 1), S4–S38.

Bai, Y., Welk, G. J., Nam, Y. H., Lee, J. A., Lee, J.-M., Kim, Y., et al. (2016). Comparison of consumer and research monitors under semistructured settings. *Medicine and Science in Sports and Exercise, 48*(1), 151–158.

Bassett, D. R. (2012). Device-based monitoring in physical activity and public health research. *Physiological Measurement, 33*(11), 1769–1783.

Bastian, T., Maire, A., Dugas, J., Ataya, A., Villars, C., Gris, F., et al. (2015). Automatic identification of physical activity types and sedentary behaviors from triaxial accelerometer: Laboratory-based calibrations are not enough. *Journal of Applied Physiology, 118*(6), 716–722.

Behrens, T. K., & Dinger, M. K. (2007). Motion sensor reactivity in physically active young adults. *Research Quarterly for Exercise and Sport, 78*(2), 1–8.

Biswas, A., Oh, P. I., Faulkner, G. E., Bajaj, R. R., Silver, M. A., Mitchell, M. S., et al. (2015). Sedentary time and its association with risk for disease incidence, mortality, and hospitalization in adults: A systematic review and meta-analysis. *Annals of Internal Medicine, 162*(2), 123–132.

Bolger, N., & Laurenceau, J. P. (2013). *Intensive longitudinal methods*. Guilford Press.

Borghese, M. M., Borgundvaag, E., McIsaac, M. A., & Janssen, I. (2019). Imputing accelerometer nonwear time in children influences estimates of sedentary time and its associations with cardiometabolic risk. *International Journal of Behavioral Nutrition and Physical Activity, 16*(1), 7.

Burchartz, A., Anedda, B., Auerswald, T., Giurgiu, M., Hill, H., Ketelhut, S., et al. (2020). Assessing physical behavior through accelerometry—State of the science, best practices and future directions. *Psychology of Sport and Exercise, 49*, 101703.

Caspersen, C. J., Powell, K. E., & Christenson, G. M. (1985). Physical activity, exercise, and physical fitness: Definitions and distinctions for health-related research. *Public Health Reports, 100*(2), 126.

Chen, K. Y., & Bassett, D. R. (2005). The technology of accelerometry-based activity monitors: Current and future. *Medicine and Science in Sports and Exercise, 37*(11 Suppl.), S490–500.

Church, T. S., Thomas, D. M., Tudor-Locke, C., Katzmarzyk, P. T., Earnest, C. P., Rodarte, R. Q., et al. (2011). Trends over 5 decades in U.S. occupation-related physical activity and their associations with obesity. *PloS One, 6*(5), e19657.

Cleland, I., Kikhia, B., Nugent, C., Boytsov, A., Hallberg, J., Synnes, K., et al. (2013). Optimal placement of accelerometers for the detection of everyday activities. *Sensors, 13*(7), 9183–9200.

Clemes, S. A., Matchett, N., & Wane, S. L. (2008). Reactivity: An issue for short-term pedometer studies? *British Journal of Sports Medicine, 42*(1), 68–70.

Crowley, P., Skotte, J., Stamatakis, E., Hamer, M., Aadahl, M., Stevens, M. L., et al. (2019). Comparison of physical behavior estimates from three different thigh-worn accelerometers brands: A proof-of-concept for the Prospective Physical Activity, Sitting, and Sleep consortium (ProPASS). *International Journal of Behavioral Nutrition and Physical Activity, 16*(1), 65.

Das, P., & Horton, R. (2012). Rethinking our approach to physical activity. *Lancet, 380*(9838), 189–190.

Dempsey, P. C., Dunstan, D. W., Larsen, R. N., Lambert, G. W., Kingwell, B. A., & Owen, N. (2018). Prolonged uninterrupted sitting increases fatigue in type 2 diabetes. *Diabetes Research and Clinical Practice, 135*, 128–133.

Diaz, K. M., Howard, V. J., Hutto, B., Colabianchi, N., Vena, J. E., Blair, S. N., et al. (2016). Patterns of sedentary behavior in US middle-age and older adults: The REGARDS Study. *Medicine and Science in Sports and Exercise, 48*(3), 430–438.

Donaldson, S. C., Montoye, A. H. K., Tuttle, M. S., & Kaminsky, L. A. (2016). Variability of objectively measured sedentary behavior. *Medicine and Science in Sports and Exercise, 48*(4), 755–761.

Dössegger, A., Ruch, N., Jimmy, G., Braun-Fahrländer, C., Mäder, U., Hänggi, J., et al. (2014). Reactivity to accelerometer measurement of children and adolescents. *Medicine and Science in Sports and Exercise, 46*(6), 1140–1146.

Dumuid, D., Pedišić, Ž., Palarea-Albaladejo, J., Martín-Fernández, J. A., Hron, K., & Olds, T. (2020). Compositional data analysis in time-use epidemiology: What, why, how. *International Journal of Environmental Research and Public Health, 17*(7).

Edwardson, C. L., Rowlands, A. V., Bunnewell, S., Sanders, J. P., Esliger, D., Gorely, T., . . . Yates, T. E. (2016). Accuracy of posture allocation algorithms for thigh-and waist-worn accelerometers. *Medicine and Science in Sports and Exercise, 48*(6), 1085–1090.

Ekelund, U., Steene-Johannessen, J., Brown, W. J., Fagerland, M. W., Owen, N., Powell, K. E., et al. (2016). Does physical activity attenuate, or even eliminate, the detrimental association of sitting time with mortality?: A harmonised meta-analysis of data from more than 1 million men and women. *Lancet, 388*(10051), 1302–1310.

Ellis, K., Kerr, J., Godbole, S., Staudenmayer, J., & Lanckriet, G. (2016). Hip and wrist accelerometer algorithms for free-living behavior classification. *Medicine and Science in Sports and Exercise, 48*(5), 933–940.

Fekedulegn, D., Andrew, M. E., Shi, M., Violanti, J. M., Knox, S., & Innes, K. E. (2020). Actigraphy-based assessment of sleep parameters. *Annals of Work Exposures and Health, 64*(4), 350–367.

Gardner, B., Flint, S., Rebar, A. L., Dewitt, S., Quail, S. K., Whall, H., et al. (2019). Is sitting invisible? Exploring how people mentally represent sitting. *International Journal of Behavioral Nutrition and Physical Activity, 16*(1), 85.

Gilchrist, S. C., Howard, V. J., Akinyemiju, T., Judd, S. E., Cushman, M., Hooker, S. P., et al. (2020). Association of sedentary behavior with cancer mortality in middle-aged and older US adults. *JAMA Oncology, 6*(8), 1210–1217.

Giurgiu, M., Bussmann, J. B., Hill, H., Anedda, B., Kronenwett, M., Koch, E. D., et al. (2020). Validating accelerometers for the assessment of body position and sedentary behavior. *Journal for the Measurement of Physical Behavior, 3*(3), 253–263.

Giurgiu, M., Koch, E. D., Plotnikoff, R. C., Ebner-Priemer, U. W., & Reichert, M. (2020). Breaking up sedentary behavior optimally to enhance mood. *Medicine and Science in Sports and Exercise, 52*(2), 457–465.

Guthold, R., Stevens, G. A., Riley, L. M., & Bull, F. C. (2020). Global trends in insufficient physical activity among adolescents: A pooled analysis of 298 population-based surveys with 1·6 million participants. *Lancet Child and Adolescent Health, 4*(1), 23–35.

Gyllensten, I. C., & Bonomi, A. G. (2011). Identifying types of physical activity with a single accelerometer: Evaluating laboratory-trained algorithms in daily life. *IEEE Transactions on Bio-Medical Engineering, 58*(9), 2656–2663.

Haghayegh, S., Khoshnevis, S., Smolensky, M. H., & Diller, K. R. (2020). Application of deep learning to improve sleep scoring of wrist actigraphy. *Sleep Medicine, 74*, 235–241.

Hamilton, M. T., Healy, G. N., Dunstan, D. W., Zderic, T. W., & Owen, N. (2008). Too little exercise and too much sitting: Inactivity physiology and the need for new recommendations on sedentary behavior. *Current Cardiovascular Risk Reports, 2*(4), 292–298.

Hoffman, L. (2015). *Longitudinal analysis: Modeling within-person fluctuation and change*. Routledge.

Huang, Y., Li, L., Gan, Y., Wang, C., Jiang, H., Cao, S., et al. (2020). Sedentary behaviors and risk of depression: A meta-analysis of prospective studies. *Translational Psychiatry, 10*(1), 26.

Janssen, X., & Cliff, D. P. (2015). Issues related to measuring and interpreting objectively measured sedentary behavior data. *Measurement in Physical Education and Exercise Science, 19*(3), 116–124.

Jean-Louis, G., Kripke, D., Mason, W. J., Elliott, J. A., & Youngstedt, S. D. (2001). Sleep estimation from wrist movement quantified by different actigraphic modalities. *Journal of Neuroscience Methods, 105*(2), 185–191.

Kang, M., & Rowe, D. A. (2015). Issues and challenges in sedentary behavior measurement. *Measurement in Physical Education and Exercise Science, 19*(3), 105–115.

Katzmarzyk, P. T., Powell, K. E., Jakicic, J. M., Troiano, R. P., Piercy, K., & Tennant, B. (2019). Sedentary behavior and health: Update from the 2018 Physical Activity Guidelines Advisory Committee. *Medicine and Science in Sports and Exercise, 51*(6), 1227–1241.

Keadle, S. K., Lyden, K. A., Strath, S. J., Staudenmayer, J. W., & Freedson, P. S. (2019). A framework to evaluate devices that assess physical behavior. *Exercise and Sport Sciences Reviews, 47*(4), 206–214.

Keil, A., Debener, S., Gratton, G., Junghöfer, M., Kappenman, E. S., Luck, S. J., et al. (2014). Committee report: Publication guidelines and recommendations for studies using electroencephalography and magnetoencephalography. *Psychophysiology, 51*(1), 1–21.

Lamkin, P. (2018, February 22). Smartwatch popularity booms with fitness trackers on the slide. *Forbes*. www.forbes.com/sites/paullamkin/2018/02/22/smartwatch-popularity-booms-with-fitness-trackers-on-the-slide/?sh=6d15268b7d96

Lee, I.-M., & Shiroma, E. J. (2014). Using accelerometers to measure physical activity in large-scale epidemiological studies: Issues and challenges. *British Journal of Sports Medicine, 48*(3), 197–201.

Lee, I.-M., Shiroma, E. J., Lobelo, F., Puska, P., Blair, S. N., & Katzmarzyk, P. T. (2012). Effect of physical inactivity on major non-communicable diseases worldwide: an analysis of burden of disease and life expectancy. *Lancet, 380*(9838), 219–229.

Liao, Y., Shonkoff, E. T., & Dunton, G. F. (2015). The acute relationships between affect, physical feeling states, and physical activity in daily life: A review of current evidence. *Frontiers in Psychology, 6*, 1975.

Livingston, G., Sommerlad, A., Orgeta, V., Costafreda, S. G., Huntley, J., Ames, D., et al. (2017). Dementia prevention, intervention, and care. *Lancet, 390*(10113), 2673–2734.

Magee, L., & Hale, L. (2012). Longitudinal associations between sleep duration and subsequent weight gain: A systematic review. *Sleep Medicine Reviews, 16*(3), 231–241.

Mâsse, F., Bourke, A. K., Chardonnens, J., Paraschiv-Ionescu, A., & Aminian, K. (2014). Suitability of commercial barometric pressure sensors to distinguish sitting and standing activities for wearable monitoring. *Medical Engineering and Physics, 36*(6), 739–744.

Mâsse, L. C., Fuemmeler, B. F., Anderson, C. B., Matthews, C. E., Trost, S. G., Catellier, D., et al. (2005). Accelerometer data reduction: A comparison of four reduction algorithms on select outcome variables. *Medicine and Science in Sports and Exercise, 37*(11), S544.

Migueles, J. H., Cadenas-Sanchez, C., Ekelund, U., Delisle Nyström, C., Mora-Gonzalez, J., Löf, M., et al. (2017). Accelerometer data collection and processing criteria to assess physical activity and other outcomes: A systematic review and practical considerations. *Sports Medicine, 47*(9), 1821–1845.

Mikkelsen, M.-L. K., Berg-Beckhoff, G., Frederiksen, P., Horgan, G., O'Driscoll, R., Palmeira, A. L., et al. (2020). Estimating physical activity and sedentary behavior in a free-living environment: A comparative study between Fitbit Charge 2 and Actigraph GT3X. *PloS One, 15*(6), e0234426.

Minkel, J. D., Banks, S., Htaik, O., Moreta, M.

C., Jones, C. W., McGlinchey, E. L., et al. (2012). Sleep deprivation and stressors: Evidence for elevated negative affect in response to mild stressors when sleep deprived. *Emotion, 12*(5), 1015–1020.

Mokkink, L. B., Terwee, C. B., Patrick, D. L., Alonso, J., Stratford, P. W., Knol, D. L., et al. (2010). The COSMIN checklist for assessing the methodological quality of studies on measurement properties of health status measurement instruments: An international Delphi study. *Quality of Life Research: An International Journal of Quality of Life Aspects of Treatment, Care and Rehabilitation, 19*(4), 539–549.

movisens Ltd. (n.d.). *DataAnalyzer—Sensor data analysis.* www.movisens.com/de/produkte/dataanalyzer

movisens Ltd. (2021). *Experience sampling measure emotions in everyday life.* www.movisens.com/de/produkte/movisensxs

Mueller, M., Chimenti, R., Merkle, S., & Frey-Law, L. (2020). Accelerometry analysis options produce large differences in lifestyle physical activity measurement. *Physiological Measurement, 41*(6), 65006.

O'Connell, S. E., Griffiths, P. L., & Clemes, S. A. (2014). Seasonal variation in physical activity, sedentary behavior and sleep in a sample of UK adults. *Annals of Human Biology, 41*(1), 1–8.

Oliver, M., Badland, H. M., Schofield, G. M., & Shepherd, J. (2011). Identification of accelerometer nonwear time and sedentary behavior. *Research Quarterly for Exercise and Sport, 82*(4), 779–783.

Open Science Collaboration. (2015). Estimating the reproducibility of psychological science. *Science, 349*(6251), aac4716.

Patterson, P. (2000). Reliability, validity, and methodological response to the assessment of physical activity via self-report. *Research Quarterly for Exercise and Sport, 71* (Suppl. 2), 15–20.

Pedisic, Z., & Bauman, A. (2015). Accelerometer-based measures in physical activity surveillance: Current practices and issues. *British Journal of Sports Medicine, 49*(4), 219–223.

Piercy, K. L., Troiano, R. P., Ballard, R. M., Carlson, S. A., Fulton, J. E., Galuska, D. A., et al. (2018). The physical activity guidelines for Americans. *Journal of the American Medical Association, 320*(19), 2020–2028.

Prince, A., Adamo, K. B., Hamel, M. E., Hardt, J., Connor Gorber, S., & Tremblay, M. (2008). A comparison of direct versus self-report measures for assessing physical activity in adults: A systematic review. *International Journal of Behavioral Nutrition and Physical Activity, 5*, 56.

Prince, S. A., Cardilli, L., Reed, J. L., Saunders, T. J., Kite, C., Douillette, K., et al. (2020). A comparison of self-reported and device measured sedentary behavior in adults: A systematic review and meta-analysis. *International Journal of Behavioral Nutrition and Physical Activity, 17*(1), 31.

Quante, M., Kaplan, E. R., Rueschman, M., Cailler, M., Buxton, O. M., & Redline, S. (2015). Practical considerations in using accelerometers to assess physical activity, sedentary behavior, and sleep. *Sleep Health, 1*(4), 275–284.

Reichert, M., Giurgiu, M., Koch, E., Wieland, L. M., Lautenbach, S., Neubauer, A. B., et al. (2020). Ambulatory assessment for physical activity research: State of the science, best practices and future directions. *Psychology of Sport and Exercise, 50*, 101742.

Rosenberger, M. E., Fulton, J. E., Buman, M. P., Troiano, R. P., Grandner, M. A., Buchner, D. M., et al. (2019). The 24-hour activity cycle: A new paradigm for physical activity. *Medicine and Science in Sports and Exercise, 51*(3), 454–464.

Rowe, D. A., Mahar, M. T., Raedeke, T. D., & Lore, J. (2004). Measuring physical activity in children with pedometers: Reliability, reactivity, and replacement of missing data. *Pediatric Exercise Science, 16*(4), 343–354.

Rowlands, A. V., Mirkes, E. M., Yates, T., Clemes, S., Davies, M., Khunti, K., et al. (2018). Accelerometer-assessed physical activity in epidemiology: Are monitors equivalent? *Medicine and Science in Sports and Exercise, 50*(2), 257–265.

Saint-Maurice, P. F., Sampson, J. N., Keadle, S. K., Willis, E. A., Troiano, R. P., & Matthews, C. E. (2020). Reproducibility of accelerometer and posture-derived measures of physical activity. *Medicine and Science in Sports and Exercise, 52*(4), 876–883.

Sasaki, J. E., Júnior, J. H., Meneguci, J., Tribess, S., Marocolo Júnior, M., Stabelini Neto, A., et al. (2018). Number of days required for reliably estimating physical activity and sedentary behavior from accelerometer data in older adults. *Journal of Sports Sciences, 36*(14), 1572–1577.

Schasfoort, F., Dallmeijer, A., Pangalila, R., Catsman, C., Stam, H., Becher, J., et al. (2018). Value of botulinum toxin injections preceding a comprehensive rehabilitation period for children with spastic cerebral palsy: A cost-effectiveness study. *Journal of Rehabilitation Medicine, 50*(1), 22–29.

Schuch, F. B., Vancampfort, D., Richards, J., Rosenbaum, S., Ward, P. B., & Stubbs, B. (2016). Exercise as a treatment for depression: A meta-analysis adjusting for publication bias. *Journal of Psychiatric Research, 77*, 42–51.

Scott, H. (2020). Sleep and circadian wearable technologies: Considerations toward device validation and application. *Sleep, 43*(12), zsaa163.

Sievanen, H., & Kujala, U. M. (2017). Accelerometry-simple, but challenging. *Scandinavian Journal of Medicine and Science in Sports, 27*(6), 574–578.

Skender, S., Ose, J., Chang-Claude, J., Paskow, M., Bruhmann, B., Siegel, E. M., et al. (2016). Accelerometry and physical activity questionnaires—a systematic review. *BMC Public Health, 16*, 515.

Stanton, R., Guertler, D., Duncan, M. J., & Vandelanotte, C. (2016). Agreement between activPAL3c accelerometers placed at different thigh positions. *Gait and Posture, 48*, 230–236.

Strath, S. J., Kaminsky, L. A., Ainsworth, B. E., Ekelund, U., Freedson, P. S., Gary, R. A., et al. (2013). Guide to the assessment of physical activity: Clinical and research applications: A scientific statement from the American Heart Association. *Circulation, 128*(20), 2259–2279.

Sylvia, L. G., Bernstein, E. E., Hubbard, J. L., Keating, L., & Anderson, E. J. (2014). Practical guide to measuring physical activity. *Journal of the Academy of Nutrition and Dietetics, 114*(2), 199–208.

Toth, L. P., Park, S., Springer, C. M., Feyerabend, M. D., Steeves, J. A., & Bassett, D. R. (2018). Video-recorded validation of wearable step counters under free-living conditions. *Medicine and Science in Sports and Exercise, 50*(6), 1315–1322.

Tremblay, M. S., Aubert, S., Barnes, J. D., Saunders, T. J., Carson, V., Latimer-Cheung, A. E., et al. (2017). Sedentary Behavior Research Network (SBRN)—Terminology Consensus Project process and outcome. *International Journal of Behavioral Nutrition and Physical Activity, 14*(1), 75.

Troiano, R. P., Berrigan, D., Dodd, K. W., Mâsse, L. C., Tilert, T., & McDowell, M. (2008). Physical activity in the United States measured by accelerometer. *Medicine and Science in Sports and Exercise, 40*(1), 181–188.

Trost, S. G. (2020). Population-level physical activity surveillance in young people: Are accelerometer-based measures ready for prime time? *International Journal of Behavioral Nutrition and Physical Activity, 17*(1), 28.

Trost, S. G., McIver, K. L., & Pate, R. R. (2005). Conducting accelerometer-based activity assessments in field-based research. *Medicine and Science in Sports and Exercise, 37*(Supplement), S531–S543.

Vähä-Ypyä, H., Vasankari, T., Husu, P., Mänttäri, A., Vuorimaa, T., Suni, J., et al. (2015). Validation of cut-points for evaluating the intensity of physical activity with accelerometry-based mean amplitude deviation (MAD). *PloS One, 10*(8), e0134813.

Valenti, G., Camps, S., Verhoef, S., Bonomi, A. G., & Westerterp, K. R. (2014). Validating measures of free-living physical activity in overweight and obese subjects using an accelerometer. *International Journal of Obesity, 38*(7), 1011–1014.

van Dongen, H., Maislin, G., Mullington, J. M., & Dinges, D. F. (2003). The cumulative cost of additional wakefulness: Dose-response effects on neurobehavioral functions and sleep physiology from chronic sleep restriction and total sleep deprivation. *Sleep, 26*(2), 117–126.

van Hees, V. T., Gorzelniak, L., Dean León, E. C., Eder, M., Pias, M., Taherian, S., et al. (2013). Separating movement and gravity components in an acceleration signal and implications for the assessment of human daily physical activity. *PloS One, 8*(4), e61691.

van Someren, E. J., Lazeron, R. H., Vonk, B. F., Mirmiran, M., & Swaab, D. F. (1996). Gravitational artefact in frequency spectra of movement acceleration: implications for actigraphy in young and elderly subjects. *Journal of Neuroscience Methods, 65*, 55–62.

Wang, Q., Xi, B., Liu, M., Zhang, Y., & Fu, M. (2012). Short sleep duration is associated with hypertension risk among adults: A systematic review and meta-analysis. *Hypertension Research, 35*(10), 1012–1018.

Warburton, D. E. R., & Bredin, S. S. D. (2017). Health benefits of physical activity: A systematic review of current systematic reviews. *Current Opinion in Cardiology, 32*(5), 541–556.

Watson, N. F., Badr, M. S., Belenky, G., Bliwise, D. L., Buxton, O. M., Buysse, D., et al. (2015). Joint consensus statement of the American Academy of Sleep Medicine and Sleep Research Society on the recommended amount of sleep for a healthy Adult: Methodology and discussion. *Sleep, 38*(8), 1161–1183.

Wijndaele, K., Westgate, K., Stephens, S. K., Blair, S. N., Bull, F. C., Chastin, S. F. M., et al. (2015). Utilization and harmonization of adult accelerometry data: Review and expert consensus. *Medicine and Science in Sports and Exercise, 47*(10), 2129–2139.

Wilhelm, P., & Schoebi, D. (2007). Assessing mood in daily life. *European Journal of Psychological Assessment, 23*(4), 258–267.

Willetts, M., Hollowell, S., Aslett, L., Holmes, C., & Doherty, A. (2018). Statistical machine learning of sleep and physical activity phenotypes from sensor data in 96,220 UK Biobank participants. *Scientific Reports, 8*(1), 7961.

World Health Organization. (2010). *Global recommendations on physical activity for health.* https://www.who.int/publications/i/item/9789241599979

Yang, C.-C., & Hsu, Y.-L. (2010). A review of accelerometry-based wearable motion detectors for physical activity monitoring. *Sensors, 10*(8), 7772–7788.

CHAPTER 6

Acquisition and Analysis of Ambulatory Autonomic Nervous System Data

Eco J. C. de Geus and Martin J. Gevonden

CHAPTER OVERVIEW

This chapter presents an overview of the biology of the autonomic nervous system (ANS) and the noninvasive ambulatory measurement strategies that can be used to study its activity in daily life settings. Heart rate variability in the respiratory frequency range (RSA) is identified as the measure of choice to index parasympathetic nervous system (PNS) activity, while pre-ejection period (PEP) and nonspecific skin conductance response (nsSCRs) are the measures of choice to index sympathetic nervous system (SNS) activity. Valid recording techniques for these measures that are currently available are tolerated for a number of days at best. To progress to prolonged ambulatory monitoring of ANS activity across multiple weeks or even months, major improvements in technology are required that greatly reduce participant burden without compromising validity. Future contribution of ambulatory assessment to behavioral science, however, does not simply hinge on technological progress; correct interpretation of the ambulatory measures of ANS activity is at least as important. This will require detailed co-registration of the psychosocial context of the individual as well as of the many nonpsychological determinants of ANS activity, most prominently physical activity, respiration, and postural changes. Only ambulatory recordings that allow the separation of the nonpsychological and psychological determinants of ANS activity will move the field forward.

Introduction: Moving Stress Research into Daily Life

Because of its high sensitivity to psychosocial stress, the ANS plays a key role in almost all models in biobehavioral medicine that try to account for the well-known effect of chronic stress exposure on cardiovascular disease (CVD) outcomes (Esler, 2017; Pieper, LaCroix, & Karasek, 1989; Rosengren et al., 2004; Steptoe & Kivimaki, 2012). A vast body of studies on ANS reactivity to stress has shown that frequency, amplitude, patterning, and duration of such reactivity are strongly personalized in nature, meaning that the same contextual psychosocial factors can evoke entirely different responses depending on personal resilience and vulnerability characteristics. Sadly, almost all of this wealth of prior research used short-lasting experiments in the laboratory, with subjects volunteering to be exposed for relatively brief periods of time to artificial stressors (e.g., using speeded reaction time tasks, the Trier social stress test, or their equivalents).

It is likely that the psychological and physiological processes induced by laboratory conditions are only a poor reflection of the actual processes in everyday real-life situations. One-time assessment of historic or current exposure to stressors does not do justice to the complex dynamics of the stress exposures in daily life. Lab stress will often be of insufficient intensity and duration to trigger the full set of physiological responses that come into play when stress is "for real" (Busscher, Spinhoven, & de Geus, 2015). It will thus fail to reveal the slower counter-regulatory responses as well as allostatic adaptations that occur on a time scale of days or weeks. An example is the gradual buildup in resting blood pressure over the course of a stressful work week that subsides in the weekend (Vrijkotte, van Doornen, & de Geus, 2000, 2004).

Laboratory studies also preclude examination of the activities that may have the largest clinical relevance, such as job-related strain, marital conflict, child care or, at the other end of the spectrum, restful sleep. This may jeopardize the predictive validity of the physiological recordings, either basal levels or reactivity for later mental and physical health. In keeping with this idea, superior predictive validity for long-term cardiovascular health has already been shown for ambulatory blood pressure, where full 24-hour recordings proved better predictors for cardiovascular morbidity and mortality than laboratory or office measurements (Hansen, Jeppesen, Rasmussen, Ibsen, & Torp-Pedersen, 2006; Mallion, Baguet, Siche, Tremel, & de Gaudemaris, 1999; Niiranen, Hanninen, Johansson, Reunanen, & Jula, 2010; Palatini & Julius, 2004; Pickering & Devereux, 1987; Verdecchia, 2001; Verdecchia et al., 1994; Ward, Takahashi, Stevens, & Heneghan, 2012).

In short, the dynamics of the physiological stress response, the interaction of its components over time across longer time scales of days, weeks, or months, simply cannot be detected without moving stress research out of the lab and into daily life. This requires dedicated wearables that may be connected to a smartphone but provide continuous, more extensive, and higher quality data than built-in smartphone sensors (e.g., using the camera for intermittent plethysmography). Fortuitously, ongoing technological innovation in such wearables provides unique opportunities for implementation of ambulatory and ecologically valid stress measures over extended periods in daily life. In the past decades, portable lightweight and relatively cheap biosensors and data-logging devices have become available for noninvasive ambulatory assessment of autonomic nervous system activity. Various listings of these devices have been published (Ebner-Priemer & Kubiak, 2007; Fahrenberg, Myrtek, Pawlik, & Perrez, 2007; Houtveen & de Geus, 2009; Peake, Kerr, & Sullivan, 2018), but these listings are typically fated to be outdated when they appear in print. Table 6.1, which lists a selection of the devices focusing on measures informative about ANS activity, therefore neither claims to be up to date nor suggests

TABLE 6.1. Selection of Research, Clinical, and Consumer-Oriented Wearables for ANS Recording

Manufacturer	Device name	Availability	Purpose	Wearable type	Location Sensors	ECG	ICG	EMG	PPG	Respiration	EDA	BP	Accelerometer	Temp	Highest level of Validation Evidence
A&D	TM-2441	Current	Clinical	Box	Arm							X	X	X	internal, peer-reviewed
Affectiva	Affectiva Q	Discontinued	Clinical	Watch	Wrist						X		X		no validation found
Beneware	24h-ABPM	Current	Clinical	Box	Arm							X			external, peer reviewed favorable
Empatica	Embrace	Current	Clinical	Watch	Wrist						X		X	X	FDA approved
Finapres Medical Systems	Portapres	Discontinued	Clinical	Box	Hand				X			X			external, peer reviewed favorable
Fukuda Denshi	FM-970	Current	Clinical	Box	Arm	X						X			no validation found
iRhythm technologies	Zio	Current	Clinical	Patch	Torso	X									external, peer reviewed favorable
Meditech	ABPM-06	Current	Clinical	Box	Arm							X			FDA approved
Petr Telegin	BPLab Compact 2	Current	Clinical	Box	Arm							X	X		external, peer reviewed favorable
ProCare	Physioflow Enduro	Current	Clinical	Box	Torso	X	X			X					external, peer reviewed favorable
Spacelabs Healthcare	LifeCard CF	Current	Clinical	Box	Torso	X									internal, peer-reviewed
Spacelabs Healthcare	90217a	Current	Clinical	Box	Arm							X			Hypertension Society Approval
Temec	Vitaport/ REMbo HST-234	Current	Clinical	Box	Multiple	X		X	X	X			X		external, peer reviewed favorable
VitalJacket	VitalJacket Holter	Current	Clinical	Shirt	Torso	X									external, peer reviewed unfavorable

(continued)

TABLE 6.1. *(continued)*

Manufacturer	Device name	Availability	Purpose	Wearable type	Location Sensors	ECG	ICG	EMG	PPG	Respiration	EDA	BP	Accelerometer	Temp	Highest level of Validation Evidence
Apple	Apple Watch 6	Current	Consumer	Watch	Wrist				X				X		external, peer reviewed unfavorable
Firstbeat	Firstbeat Bodyguard 2	Current	Consumer	Patch	Torso	X							X		external, peer reviewed
Fitbit	Sense	Current	Consumer	Watch	Wrist				X	X			X	X	FDA approved (ECG app)
Fitbit	Fitbit Charge 3	Current	Consumer	Watch	Wrist				X				X		external, peer reviewed unfavorable
Garmin	Vívosmart series	Current	Consumer	Watch	Wrist				X				X		external, peer reviewed unfavorable
Garmin	Forerunner series	Current	Consumer	Watch	Wrist				X				X		external, peer reviewed unfavorable
Hexoskin	Hexoskin	Current	Consumer	Shirt	Torso	X				X			X		external, peer reviewed favorable
Microsoft	Band 2	Dis-continued	Consumer	Watch	Wrist				X		X		X		external, peer reviewed unfavorable
Mio	Alpha 2	Dis-continued	Consumer	Watch	Wrist				X				X		external, peer reviewed unfavorable
Polar	V800	Current	Consumer	Strap/Box	Torso	X							X		external, peer reviewed (once)
Polar	OH1	Current	Consumer	Watch	Wrist, Arm				X				X		external, peer reviewed favorable
Wahoo	TickrX	Current	Consumer	Strap/Box	Torso	X							X		no validation found
Wahoo	TickrFit	Current	Consumer	Strap/Box	Arm				X						no validation found
Withings	ScanWatch	Current	Consumer	Watch	Wrist				X				X		no validation found
Bio-Impedance Technology, Inc.	AIM	Dis-continued	Research	Box	Torso	X	X			X			X		external, peer reviewed favorable

Biopac	Bioharness	Current	Research	Strap	Torso	X				X			X		no validation found
Empatica	E4	Current	Research	Watch	Wrist				X		X		X	X	external, peer reviewed unfavorable
Hexoskin	Astroskin	Current	Research	Shirt	Torso	X			X	X			X	X	external, peer reviewed favorable
MindWare Technologies	MindWare Mobile	Current	Research	Box	Torso	X	X	X	X	X	X		X		internal, peer-reviewed
Movisens	EcgMove 4	Current	Research	Strap/Box	Torso	X							X	X	external, peer reviewed favorable
Movisens	EdaMove 4	Current	Research	Box	Palm, Ankle						X		X	X	external, peer reviewed favorable
Plux	CardioBAN	Current	Research	Strap	Torso	X							X		no validation found
Plux	RespiBAN	Current	Research	Strap	Torso					X			X		no validation found
Shimmer	Shimmer3 ECG	Current	Research	Box	Torso	X				X			X		external, peer reviewed favorable
Shimmer	Shimmer3 GSR+	Current	Research	Box	Wrist				X		X		X		external, peer reviewed favorable
SomnoMedics	Somnotouch NIBP	Current	Research	Watch	Torso, Finger	X			X			X	X		internal, peer-reviewed
VitaMove Research	VitaMove	Current	Research	Box	Multi	X		X		X			X		no validation found (only for activity part)
Vivometrics	Lifeshirt	Dis-continued	Research	Shirt	Torso	X				X			X	X	external, peer reviewed favorable
Vrije Universiteit	VU-AMS 5fs	Current	Research	Box	Torso	X	X			X	X		X		external, peer reviewed favorable
Zephyr (Medtronic)	Bioharness	Current	Research	Shirt	Torso	X				X			X	X	external, peer reviewed favorable

Note: The selection of wearables listed is neither complete nor systematic. It is meant as an illustration of this booming technology only.

that these are the "best" devices for the signal they purport to record. This table mainly serves to illustrate four key features:

1. This is an active field, with many solutions being created to measure a host of peripheral signals influenced by ANS activity.
2. Devices tend to be research-oriented, medical care-oriented, or consumer-oriented.
3. Not all devices have been independently validated.
4. Not all devices stand the test of time even when they have been extensively used or validated.

In the remainder of this chapter, we address some of the neuroanatomical, measurement, and interpretational issues that researchers need to be aware of when they acquire and analyze ambulatory ANS data with current or future wearable devices.

The Biology of the ANS

The term *autonomic nervous system* was coined by John Langley in 1898. Unlike the skeletal motor system, which governs the voluntary action of striated muscles, the autonomic nervous system governs the automated responses of the body's smooth muscle organs and glands. Based on anatomical and functional criteria, Langley divided the ANS into three separate branches: the parasympathetic nervous system (PNS); the sympathetic nervous system (SNS), including the adrenal medulla; and the enteric nervous system. The enteric system, a collection of neurons embedded within the wall of the entire gastrointestinal tract that control gastrointestinal motility and secretions, is often discarded in stress research. Therefore, ANS activity discussed below will refer only to the activity of the sympathetic and parasympathetic branches.

Functions of the SNS and PNS

Activity of the SNS causes, among other problems, an increase in heart rate, contractility, blood pressure, breathing rate, bronchodilation, sweat production, epinephrine secretion, and a redistribution of blood flow favoring the muscles. The SNS is therefore often labeled as the "fight–flight" branch of the ANS. The PNS, on the other hand, promotes maintenance of the body by acquiring energy from food and getting rid of wastes. Its activity causes slowing of the heart, constriction of the pupils, stimulation of the gut and salivary glands, and other responses that help restore energy. The PNS is therefore often labeled as the "rest and digest" branch of the ANS.

The main function of the ANS is coordinating bodily functions to ensure homeostasis and performing adaptive responses when faced with changes in the external and internal environment, (e.g., due to physical activity, posture change, food consumption, or hemorrhage). In addition, the ANS is capable of substantial heterostatic action; it can prepare the body for anticipated threats to homeostasis even in the absence of actual changes in bodily activity. The best-known example is the anticipatory response that prepares the body for physical activity in response to a vast range of stressors that can be purely symbolic in nature and are often not followed by actual physical activity (i.e., fight or flight) or changes in internal environment (i.e., through blood loss, undernutrition, hypothermia, or infection). This response is called the physiological stress response.

Independence of SNS and PNS

For a long time it was assumed that SNS and PNS work in reciprocal ways; indeed, many studies of the physiological stress response have capitalized on the occurrence of a reciprocal increase in SNS activity and decrease in PNS activity during stress. Such a pattern gives rise to increases in heart rate (HR) and blood pressure (BP), and HR and BP reactivity have become the most used variables to indicate changes in ANS activity. Because of their immediate clinical relevance (both are established risk factors for future CVD; see Bohm et al., 2010; Mallion et al., 1999; Palatini & Julius, 2004), ambulatory recording of HR and BP remains extremely valuable. However, a disadvantage of these variables is that they represent an unknown mix of sympathetic and parasympathetic effects when the assumption of complete reciprocity does not hold. HR and BP go up when SNS activity increases, but they likewise increase when PNS activity decreases. Without measurement of either SNS or PNS, there is no telling their relative contributions to any given change in HR or BP.

It has been shown that the classical reciprocal pattern of sympathetic activation with parasympathetic deactivation describes only a limited part of the total autonomic space and that the sympathetic and parasympathetic branches can be activated and deactivated independently (Berntson, Cacioppo, & Quigley, 1991). Different patterns of coactivation, reciprocal activation, and co-inhibition are found across individuals performing the same task or within individuals performing different tasks. For example, dental phobia patients engaged in a stressful mental arithmetic task showed an increase in their SNS activity with decreased PNS activity, but when exposed to phobic stimuli the same subjects showed increased SNS activity with *increased* PNS activity (Bosch, de Geus, Veerman, & Amerongen, 2000). Most importantly, the health outcomes of sympathetic hyperreactivity need not be the same as those of exaggerated parasympathetic withdrawal. Hyperactivity of the SNS has been mostly associated with an increased risk for hypertension, the metabolic syndrome, and left ventricular failure (Brotman, Golden, & Wittstein, 2007; Esler, 2000, 2017; Lambert & Lambert, 2011; Lambert, Schlaich, Lambert, Dawood, & Esler, 2010), while withdrawal of PNS activity causes a reduction in the electrical stability of the heart (Vanoli et al., 1991) and may play a key role in the pro-inflammatory state (Hu, Penninx, et al., 2018; Tracey, 2009).

Inasmuch that the antecedents and consequences of SNS and PNS activity are different, studies in the past two decades began indexing sympathetic and parasympathetic activity separately. In this chapter, we follow this lead and focus on ambulatory measures of "pure" sympathetic or "pure" parasympathetic activity.

Measurements of ANS Activity

Anatomy of the ANS

In keeping with many other figures of the ANS, the central nervous system component of ANS regulation shown in Figure 6.1 is simply summarized by a graphic rendering of the brain. Whereas we acknowledge that this does no justice to the complexity of the

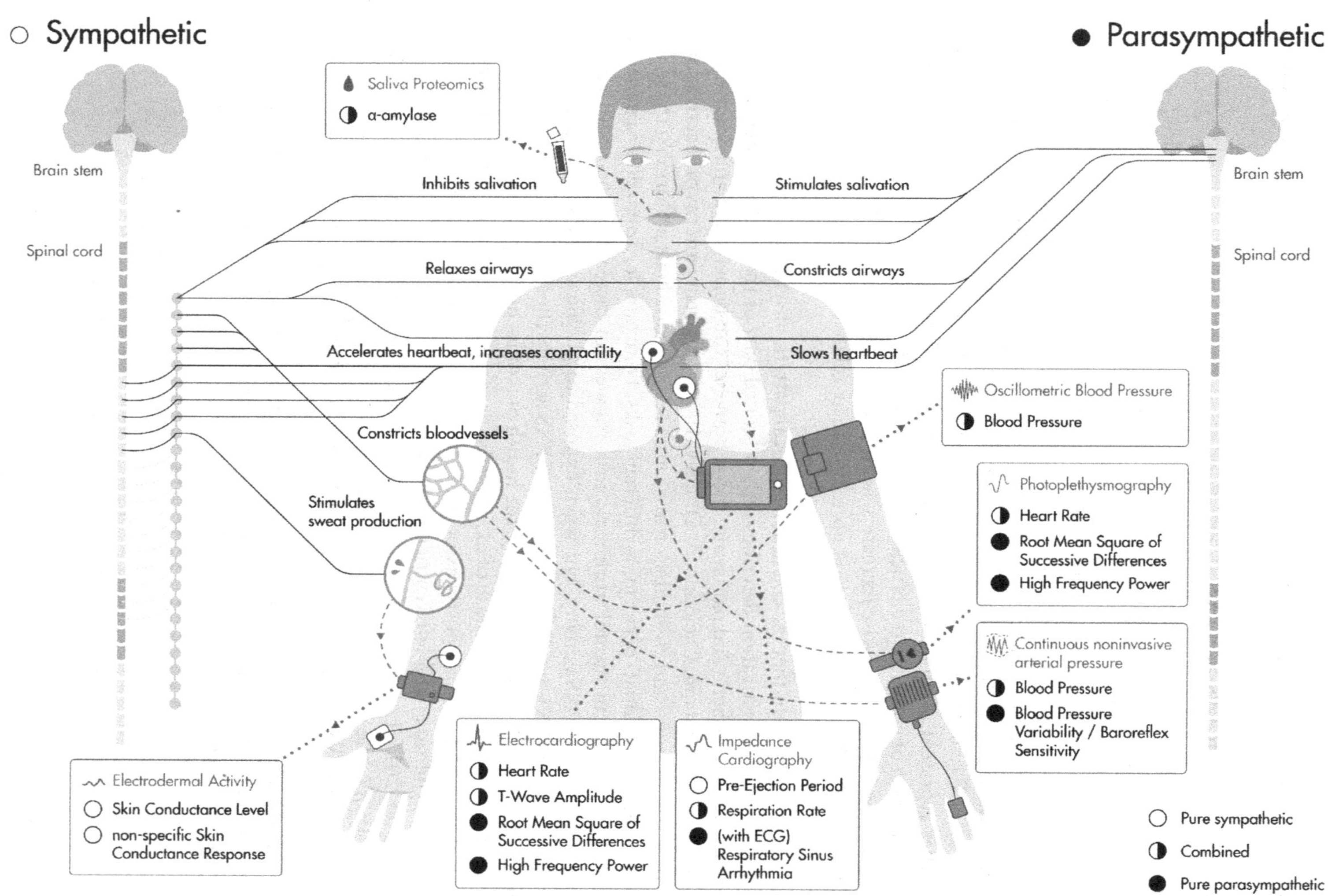

FIGURE 6.1. Mapping of the effects of ANS activity on organ systems and how they can be measured by ambulatory devices.

ways ANS activity originates in the brain (Beissner, Meissner, Bar, & Napadow, 2013; Berntson, Bechara, Damasio, Tranel, & Cacioppo, 2007; Koenig, 2020; Lovallo, 2005), this chapter will focus on the peripheral nerves and the organ systems that are used as a read-out in ambulatory recordings. Figure 6.1 links the innervation of the organs by the ANS to the main measures and the measurement strategies in the ambulatory assessment described in this chapter.

Parasympathetic Nerves

Cranial nerve VII (facial) carries preganglionic axons of the superior salivatory nucleus and controls the lacrimal glands and the submaxillary and sublingual salivary glands, measurable by changes in salivary flow rate and protein composition (e.g., α-amylase). Cranial nerve IX (glossopharyngeal) carries preganglionic axons of the inferior salivatory nucleus, which control the fluid secretion by salivary glands. Preganglionic motor neurons of the dorsal motor nucleus of the tenth cranial nerve (vagus) carry motor fibers of a special visceral nucleus, the nucleus ambiguus, which controls the striated muscles of the pharynx, larynx, esophagus, and the cardiac muscle of the heart.

The preganglionic parasympathetic nerves terminate in parasympathetic ganglia, which lie within or very close to the organs innervated by the short postganglionic neurons. The pre-ganglionic neurons employ acetylcholine (ACh) as the primary neurotransmitter, which binds to a nicotinic receptor subtype on the postganglionic neurons in the ganglia. Postganglionic parasympathetic fibers also employ acetylcholine as a primary neurotransmitter, but the receptor subtypes on the target organ are commonly muscarinic. For instance, the parasympathetic postganglionic receptors in the sinoatrial (SA) node of the heart are type 2 muscarinic (M2), and their activation slows the spontaneous depolarization of pacemaker cells and hence reduces heart rate.

Sympathetic Nerves

The preganglionic nerves from neurons in the interomediolateral column leave the spinal cord at the thoracic and lumbar regions. Most axons synapse onto a chain of sympathetic ganglia that lie close to the spinal cord known as the sympathetic trunk, employing acetylcholine as the primary neurotransmitter. The most rostral ganglion, the superior cervical ganglion, supplies the head and neck, including the salivary glands excreting α-amylase. The middle cervical ganglion and stellate ganglion supply the heart, lungs, and bronchi. The celiac, aorticorenal, superior mesenteric, and inferior mesenteric ganglia—named after their associated arteries, innervate, among others, the kidney and its adrenal glands.

The postganglionic neurons from these sympathetic ganglia to the organs employ norepinephrine as the primary neurotransmitter, which can act on alpha-1-adrenergic (e.g., in arterioles) or beta-1- and beta-2-adrenergic receptors (e.g., on the heart). Stimulation of the alpha-1-adrenergic receptors causes vasoconstriction by acting on the smooth muscles in the medial layer of the blood vessels. Stimulation of the cardiac beta-adrenergic receptors by norepinephrine released from the cardiac sympathetic nerves (accelerans nerves) increases the pacemaker frequency of the SA node, thus increasing heart rate, and in parallel it increases the contractility of the ventricles. Together, vasoconstriction and increased cardiac performance account for the increase in blood pressure seen during sympathetic nervous system activity.

A first exception to the use of norepinephrine as the final effector in the SNS is found in the sympathetic innervation of eccrine sweat glands, which is cholinergic rather than adrenergic. A second exception is a set of preganglionic neurons that end in a special ganglion, namely, the adrenal medulla. Neurons of this medullary ganglion, rather than issuing axons to innervate target organs, function as a neuroendocrine organ. Upon activation by preganglionic neurons, they release norepinephrine (NE), which is rapidly converted to epinephrine (E), and both are released as hormones into the bloodstream in an approximate ratio of 5:1 (E:NE). Circulating epinephrine preferentially binds to beta-2 receptors in the vessels and on the heart, causing vasodilatation (mostly in muscle tissue) and increases in heart rate and contractility.

Direct Measurement of ANS Activity via Action Potentials

The ideal measurement strategy for ANS activity is to probe the actual bursts of action potentials in the sympathetic and parasympathetic nerves to a specific organ or tissue. This can be done in animal studies by using surgically inserted microelectrodes (Ottaviani, Wright, Dawood, & Macefield, 2020; Vallbo, 2018) or by assessing the changes in ACh and NE concentration in the SA node by microdialysis (Shimizu et al., 2009, 2010). For a long time, the feasibility of microneurographic recording in humans was limited to the superficial sympathetic nerves. Direct recordings of sympathetic activity to the skin and the blood vessels in the muscle can be made from Tungsten electrodes in nerves innervating the skeletal muscle or the skin (Hagbarth, Hallin, Wallin, Torebjork, & Hongell, 1972; Wallin, 1984, 2004). Recently, a safe and feasible way was developed to perform microneurography of the vagus nerve at the level of the neck using ultrasound guidance (Ottaviani et al., 2020). Although the vagus is primarily a sensory nerve and its motor components run to multiple other organs than the heart, repeated probing using careful correlation of nerve activity to variation in the cardiac cycle was used to specifically isolate efferent fibers to the sinoatrial node and record their activity.

Indirect Measurement of ANS Activity via Neurotransmitter Spillover

Unfortunately, these "gold-standard" measures are too invasive to be routinely used in research with humans. The alternative is to measure the spillover of ACh or NE from the presynaptic terminals of (para)sympathetic nerves into the bloodstream, as this would theoretically scale with nerve activity. However, for ACh this is not feasible because of the rapid and extensive clearance of the transmitter in the synaptic space by acetylcholinesterase. In contrast, norepinephrine does spill over into the bloodstream and can be used to assess sympathetic nerve activity. By using radioactive tracers, norepinephrine spillover can even be measured on an organ-to-organ basis (Eisenhofer, 2005; Esler et al., 1988; Esler & Kaye, 2000; Kingwell et al., 1994), but this is again an invasive procedure that has been largely abandoned.

Much less invasive measurements of norepinephrine and/or its metabolites in antecubital venous blood are possible by venapuncture or by assessing the excretion of norepinephrine and/or metabolites in urine. These methods have major drawbacks, however, because only a very small proportion of norepinephrine released from sympathetic nerves reaches the bloodstream. Differences in intraneuronal vesicular storage and leakage, reuptake, extraneuronal clearance, and urinary filtration/secretion may (severely) distort the relation between actual sympathetic nervous system activity and plasma and urine norepinephrine concentrations (Eisenhofer, Kopin, & Goldstein, 2004; Esler et al., 1990).

Indirect Measurement of ANS Control via Effects on Innervated Organs

Because direct measurement of activity is not amenable to ambulatory recording and indirect measurements come with substantial methodological concerns, most human studies of autonomic activity in real-life settings have focused on the *effects* of parasympathetic and sympathetic activity on the innervated organs rather than on activity per se. For ambulatory recording of parasympathetic activity, the only organ considered so far is the heart. For sympathetic activity, the heart, sweat glands, salivary glands, and adrenal glands have all been employed in ambulatory recordings. The change from measurement of activity to measurement of effects should be reflected in the terminology, such that "sympathetic control" is used rather than "sympathetic activity." However, we ourselves have sinned against this principle—often by request of reviewers or editors who find the term *activity* more accessible for the readership.

Importantly, relative changes in nerve activity within a single subject will be highly correlated with the organ effects, but this is not true for absolute differences in nerve activity between subjects. Between subjects, the individual differences in the anatomical features (heart size, number of sweat glands), adrenergic and muscarinergic receptor sensitivity, or efficiency of the postsynaptic machinery translating receptor activation into organ effects will substantially reduce the correlation between absolute ANS activity and the observable organ response. The takeaway message is that *studies aiming to assess ANS activity by recording organ responses fare much better in within-subject designs than in between-subject designs.*

Validation of Indirect ANS Measures

Because ambulatory assessment of ANS activity is limited in practice to noninvasive and indirect measurement of its effects on organ systems, validation of such measurements against direct nerve recording or neurotransmitter spillover is essential. An acceptable alternative strategy to these invasive gold standards to show that the noninvasive measure truly detects (only) sympathetic or parasympathetic effects is the use of pharmacological blockade. SNS effects can be measured by blocking either alpha-1 receptors (e.g., phentolamine), beta-adrenergic receptors (e.g., propranolol), or specific classes of these receptors, like beta 1 (e.g., metoprolol) or beta-2 (ICI 118–551) receptors. This has been most extensively done for the assessment of cardiac autonomic activity. Cardiac parasympathetic activity, for instance, can be measured in a dose–response way during infusion of muscarinic receptor antagonists like atropine or glycopyrrolate, effectively removing all vagal effects on the heart. A putative noninvasive measure of cardiac vagal activity should therefore gradually reduce to zero during such blockade and be seen to return to baseline levels during washout (Penttila et al., 2001). Cardiac sympathetic measures, in turn, should be gradually diminished during β-receptor blockade (Berntson, Cacioppo, Binkley, et al., 1994; Cacioppo et al., 1994).

Reliability and Temporal Stability of Indirect ANS Measures

Apart from validation against invasive measures or pharmacological manipulations, it is important to establish the short-term test–retest reliability and long-term temporal stability of ambulatory measures of ANS activity. Whereas we expect substantial variability in ANS activity in response to daily events, we at the same time expect the average levels of ANS activity in real-life settings to be a reasonable stable trait. This expectation is reinforced by a large literature showing substantial heritability of validated measures of ANS activity at rest with heritability estimates even further increasing under conditions of stress (de Geus, Kupper, Boomsma, & Snieder, 2007; de Geus, van Lien, Neijts, & Willemsen, 2015; Neijts et al., 2015). We would, therefore, not only expect high test–retest validity across two comparable days within a single week, but we also expect any valid measure of ANS activity to show at least moderate temporal stability across repeated assessments spanning years. These expectations are particularly strong when we retest ANS activity across comparable activities like sleep, work, or leisure time. When we find low test–retest and/or temporal stability for an ambulatory ANS measure, this may be reflective of poor reliability of the measurement technology or the measure chosen.

Parasympathetic Measures in Ambulatory Assessment

Respiratory Sinus Arrhythmia

The current dominant strategy for ambulatory recording of parasympathetic activity is through time- or frequency-domain indices of heart rate variability in the respiratory frequency range, also called respiratory sinus arrhythmia (RSA). RSA is the difference in heart period during the inspiration and expiration phases of the respiratory cycle caused by respiratory "gating" (Eckberg, 2003) of the tonic firing of the cholinergic motor neurons in the nucleus ambiguus that innervate the sinoatrial node. Although cardiac sympathetic nerve traffic is gated in a similar way, the effect of the respiratory-related changes in vagal activity on heart rate variability is much more prominent than the effect of the respiratory-related changes in sympathetic activity. This is due to the differential filter characteristics of the muscarinergic acetylcholine receptors and adrenergic receptors (Berntson, Cacioppo, & Quigley, 1993). RSA shows relatively little sensitivity to sympathetic blockade but is affected in a dose–response way by muscarinergic blockers in humans (Grossman & Taylor, 2007; Martinmaki, Rusko, Kooistra, Kettunen, & Saalasti, 2006) or vagal cooling in animals (Katona & Jih, 1975). This has led to the use of RSA as a validated proxy for vagal cardiac activity (de Geus, Gianaros, Brindle, Jennings, & Berntson, 2019), although it is acknowledged that change in respiratory behavior (Grossman & Kollai, 1993; Grossman, Wilhelm, & Spoerle, 2004; Ritz & Dahme, 2006) is an important confounder.

Ambulatory Measurement Strategy for RSA

The measurement of RSA requires the continuously recorded time series of the interval between two beats, the heart period. The heart period is most reliably detected as the distance between two R-waves in the electrocardiogram (ECG). Ambulatory devices that give access to a full recording of the ECG are preferable to devices that extract and store a beat-to-beat heart period time series and do not store the raw signal. Full ECGs allow more researchers degrees of freedom to recognize and deal with artifacts of technical or physiological origin. Technical artifacts can arise from poor electrode contact, faulty conduction by lead wires, extraneous magnetic or powerline noise, excessive movement, muscle activity, hardware/software errors, and experimenter-induced data processing errors. Deviance of physiological origin occurs when heartbeats are not generated by the SA pacemaker cells. Such beats do not arise from the normal sinus rhythm generation, typically represent a few percent of the total number of beats, and are referred to as premature, or ectopic, beats. Two common sources of premature beats are the atria and ventricles, which can prompt an atrial premature contraction (APC) and ventricular premature contraction (VPC), respectively. Ectopic beats, other arrhythmic events, and missing data through technical errors may introduce strong bias in RSA estimation.

Full ECG recording requires the attachment of at least one electrode on the chest and a ground electrode, or a patch or chest band with two permanent points of contact to the skin. A disadvantage of continuous skin contact-based ECG recording is that it can be tolerated for a few days only but is harder to maintain when recordings last over weeks or months. An alternative to ECG for obtaining the heart period time series is to detect the distance between two consecutive peaks in a photoplethysmogram (PPG). The PPG is obtained by using a pulse oximeter which illuminates the skin and measures changes in light absorption. This has the great advantage of being minimally invasive and is easy to incorporate into wrist-worn devices that can be worn for prolonged periods of time. Unfortunately, the reliability of PPG-derived heart period is not as good as that of ECG, although reliability may be acceptable in conditions with little physical activity (Georgiou et al., 2018). The reasons for lower quality of PPG-derived chronometrics are manifold, but two factors stand out. First, the blunt peak in the PPG waveform representing distal blood flow is inherently less suited to detect interbeat intervals with millisecond precision than the sharp R-peak in the ECG waveform representing electrical activity generated in the ventricle. Second, the PPG method has a much lower signal-to-noise ratio than the ECG, and this difference is strongly amplified during physical activity.

When the respiratory signal is co-registered with the heart periods, RSA can be derived by peak-valley estimation (pvRSA). Estimates of pvRSA are obtained by subtracting the shortest heart period during heart rate acceleration in the inspiration phase from the longest heart period during heart rate deceleration in the expiration phase (Grossman & Taylor, 2007; Katona & Jih, 1975). This is illustrated for heart period and respiration signals extracted from combined ECG and respiratory plethysmography recording in Figure 6.2.

RSA can also be derived from ECG or PPG recordings only, without an additional respiration signal. PNS effects are reflected in time-domain measures such as the root mean square of successive differences (RMSSD) between successive heart periods (Goedhart, van der Sluis, Houtveen, Willemsen, & de Geus, 2007) or frequency-domain measures obtained by Fourier analysis (Akselrod et al., 1981), Wavelet analysis (Houtveen & Molenaar, 2001), or autoregressive (AR) modeling of the heart periods time series (Cerutti, Bianchi, & Mainardi, 2001). Frequency analyses describe the mean amplitudes of the periodic oscillations of the heart period at different frequencies and provide information on the amount of their relative contribution to the total variance in the heart period (also termed power) across the 0–0.5 Hz frequency range. Spectral power in the respiratory frequency range of 0.15–0.40 Hz can be used to specifically index RSA. This range is also called the high frequency range, and spectral analysis derived RSA is typically labeled

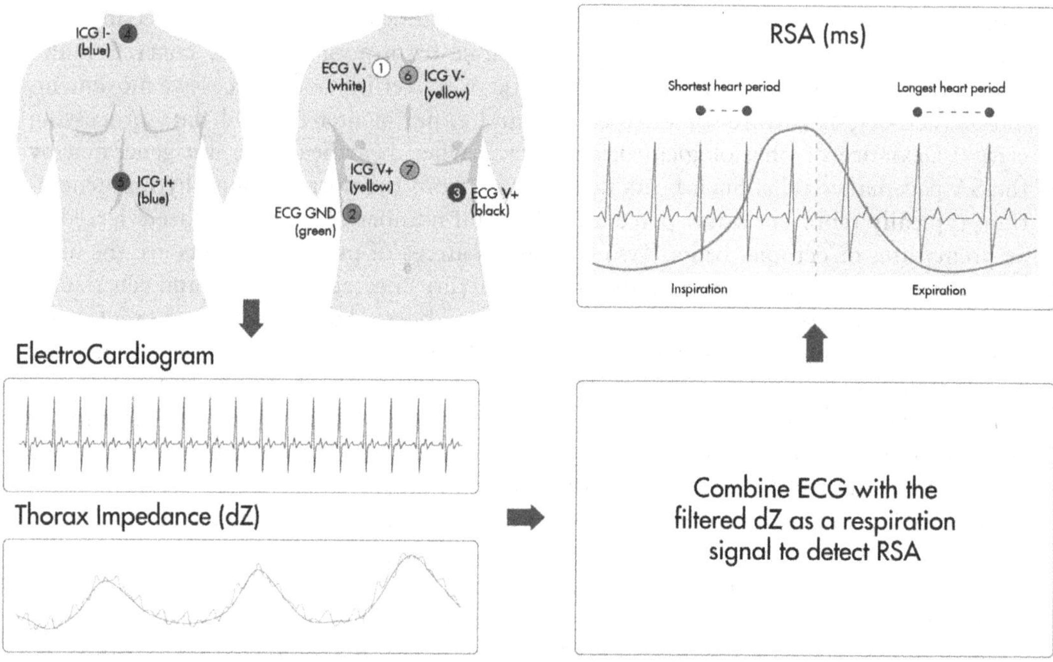

FIGURE 6.2. RSA computed using the peak-valley method from the ECG and a respiration signal derived from the thorax impedance signal.

HF or HF-HRV. Many guidelines are available to extract time- or frequency-domain RSA measures from heart period time series (Grossman, van Beek, & Wientjes, 1990); an often-used software package is Kubios (Tarvainen, Niskanen, Lipponen, Ranta-aho, & Karjalainen, 2014).

Reliability and Temporal Stability of Ambulatory RSA Measures

During a 24-hour ambulatory recording, the different time- and frequency-domain measures of RSA (e.g., RMSSD, HF, pvRSA) were highly correlated across a wide range of values for respiration rate and heart rate (Goedhart, van der Sluis, et al., 2007). Out of these three, RMSSD is the easiest to compute and therefore commonly reported, but it can include variance in HR in the higher frequency ranges, that is, outside of the actual respiratory frequency range and not representing parasympathetic activity. HF, unlike pvRSA, does not need additional recording of a respiration signal, but co-recording of respiration itself has clear advantages when dealing with momentary within-subject confounding. For the average 24-hour levels of RMSSD and HF, high test–retest correlations were found across a few days (Bigger, Fleiss, Rolnitzky, & Steinman, 1992; Bjelakovic et al., 2017; Sztajzel, Jung, & de Luna, 2008; Vrijkotte et al., 2001). In addition, good long-term temporal stability for 24-hour levels of pvRSA, HF and RMSSD has been shown over periods of 7 months to 6 years (Goedhart, van der Sluis, et al., 2007; Pitzalis et al., 1996).

Sympathetic Measures in Ambulatory Assessment

In contrast to ambulatory PNS recording, which is focused entirely on the heart, multiple organs can be used as a read-out for SNS activity. Importantly, the notion of a single emergency SNS response that affects all organs to the same extent has proven to be untenable. In some circumstances, like dynamic whole-body exercise, the SNS acts more or less as a "unitary system," but in many other situations it is capable of differentiated regulation of its activity to separate organs to a substantial degree (Folkow, 2000; Grassi & Esler, 1999; Hjemdahl, Freyschuss, Juhlin-Dannfelt, & Linde, 1984). For example, Goedhart, Willemsen, and DeGeus (2007) show only a modest correlation between the effects of increased SNS activation on the heart and the sweat glands. Even within the same organ, responsivity to SNS activation can differ based on the specific biological function assessed. For example, van Lien, Neijts, Willemsen, and de Geus (2015) found only a modest correlation between SNS effects on ventricular contractility and ventricular repolarization. Therefore, to provide a more complete picture, ambulatory recording of SNS effects on multiple organ functions should be used whenever possible.

Electrodermal Activity

Recording the activity of the skin as an index of pure sympathetic activity dates back to the 1880s (Neumann & Blanton, 1970). Because of its ease of use and low cost, despite not yet being fully understood, electrodermal activity (EDA) recording became a staple in the psychophysiological toolbox, with highly visible field applications such as the lie detector test. Different terminology was historically used, often specific to the applied measurement technique, most notably the galvanic skin response (GSR). We follow the modern-day convention with EDA as the umbrella term for all electrodermal phenomena, independent of measurement technique (Boucsein, 2012).

In laboratory recordings, wet Ag/AgCl("gel") electrodes are the norm, where conductivity is improved by electrolyte cream or gel, and they are held in place with adhesives. The most used "exosomatic" technique measures the (changes in) conductivity of the skin to a direct current (DC) applied through a pair of skin electrodes. Concerns have been voiced about possible electrode polarization with this method, and the use of alternating current (AC) has been demonstrated to be a viable alternative to avoid potential problems related to polarization (Pabst, Tronstad, Grimnes, Fowles, & Martinsen, 2017). Because sweat glands are at the highest density in palmar and plantar regions, approximately 400/mm^2, it is recommended that two electrodes be used at these sites, typically on the fingers (Boucsein et al., 2012).

Electrodermal activity incorporates both slow tonic shifts in basal skin conductance level (SCL) and more rapid phasic transient events (see Figure 6.3). Such skin conductance responses (SCRs) are observed in response to experimental stimuli, often tones or bursts of white noise in classic laboratory paradigms, and their occurrence, latency, rise time, and amplitude are metrics (Boucsein, 2012; Dawson, Schell, & Filion, 2000; Fowles, 1986). SCRs also occur without a clear external event as a trigger. The frequency of such nonspecific SCRs (nsSCRs) per minute, sometimes termed *electrodermal lability* (Mundy-Castle & McKiever, 1953), is thought to reflect SNS activity. Both SCL and nsSCR frequency have been shown to be influenced by emotional stress (Boucsein, 2012),

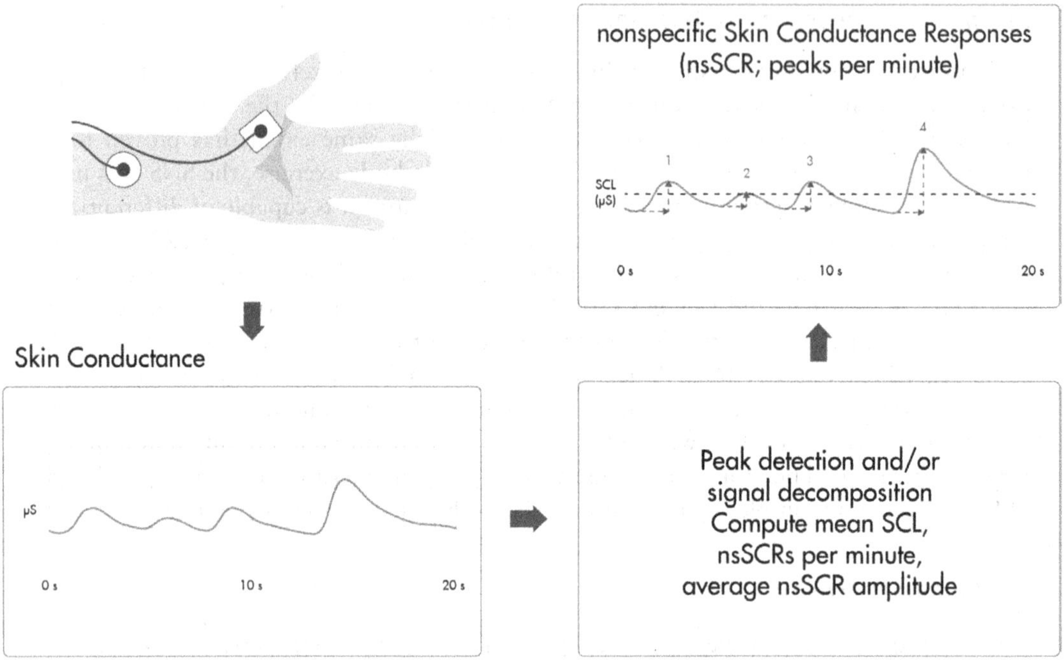

FIGURE 6.3. SCL and nsSCRs extracted from a palmar recording of electrodermal activity using an ambulatory device with the reference electrode placed at a nonobtrusive location.

making them attractive outcome measures for ambulatory studies. A host of quantification strategies are available to extract them from longer recordings (Posada-Quintero & Chon, 2020).

EDA is considered a pure measure of SNS effects because it directly captures the activity of the eccrine sweat glands. These glands are not innervated by the parasympathetic nervous system, but the sympathetic nervous system only. Acetylcholine release from the preganglionic sympathetic nerves increases the activity of the sweat glands, excreting more fluid, which in turn increases the electrical conductivity across the skin (Foster & Weiner, 1970; Fowles, 1986). This finding is supported by studies measuring burst of activity directly in the sympathetic nerve, observing subsequent sweat secretion in associated individual sweat glands (Nishiyama, Sugenoya, Matsumoto, Iwase, & Mano, 2001) and highly correlated electrodermal responses (Wallin, 1981). Furthermore, blockade of preganglionic sympathetic nerves to the skin strongly depresses or abolishes these responses (Bengtsson, Lofstrom, & Malmqvist, 1985).

Ambulatory Measurement Strategies for EDA

When measuring EDA in ambulatory studies the exosomatic DC method is the standard, but different choices are made from those in the lab regarding electrode type and electrode placement. Gel electrodes work well in short ambulatory recordings (24 hour), but in longer ambulatory studies, the electrodes can dry out or fall off, and may not be easy to reapply by the participant. At the cost of general lower signal levels and potentially more movement artifacts and signal loss, longer ambulatory studies may opt for the ease of use and tolerability of dry electrodes. The guiding principle for electrode placement is that they should not interfere with daily activities to the point that it hurts ecological validity, while still yielding a signal of acceptable quality for the research question at hand. Placement should take care to minimize instances of pressure on the electrodes as these are associated with a local change in conductance called Ebbecke waves, an important source of movement artifact (Boucsein, 2012). Since the fingers are involved in the bulk of everyday activity, other parts of the palmar surface with similarly high sweat gland density are the primary alternative.

Electrode placement on the thenar and hypothenar eminences of the hand allows for substantial hand use, although they hinder gripping motions and need to be connected by cable to a measurement device on the arm or elsewhere on the body. Cable and electrode interference may be mitigated further by retaining only a single active electrode on the hand and placing a ground electrode on a less obtrusive location at the ventromedial forearm approximately 15 cm below the hand electrode (van der Mee, Duivestein, Gevonden, Westerink, & de Geus, 2020). Lightly abrading the reference site reduces resistance, and using different electrodes for the active and reference sites further optimizes signal quality. On the thenar eminence, the typical EDA pre-gelled electrodes with isotonic gel (Ag/AgCl contact, wet liquid gel [0.5% chloride salt] electrolyte, 11-mm-diameter contact area) can be used, whereas standard ECG electrodes suffice for the ventromedial forearm. For ECG recording, EDA is considered an artifact; therefore, ECG electrodes contain a layer of gel designed to short-circuit the skin and minimize skin resistance. In terms of minimizing discomfort and interference by movement, ambulatory EDA is typically measured on the side of the nondominant hand. It should be noted that while EDA on the left and on the right fingers are strongly correlated, there is evidence for potential functional asymmetry (Kasos et al., 2020).

By far the most user-friendly location for ambulatory assessment of EDA is the wrist, even though the electrodermal responsiveness here is limited because of lower sweat gland density, with generally lower signal levels and fewer responses than on the fingers, as expressed in moderate to low correlations (Kasos et al., 2020; van Dooren, de Vries, & Janssen, 2012). Thermoregulatory sweating also seems more prominent on the wrist than emotional sweating. Still, the ease of accessibility and participant acceptance of wearing a sensor on the wrist have resulted in commercially available devices that measure there, either on the volar side to maximize electrode contact with sweat glands or on the dorsal side, to further capitalize on having the electrodes integrated within a wristwatch-style device (Westerink et al., 2009).

Reliability and Temporal Stability of Ambulatory EDA Measures

Detailed testing of the reliability and validity of ambulatory EDA in bigger samples is still sparse (Doberenz, Roth, Wollburg, Breuninger, & Kim, 2010; Hoehn-Saric, McLeod, Funderburk, & Kowalski, 2004; Westerink et al., 2009). Several authors have stated the urgent need for such testing and have suggested standardized protocols to do so (Kleckner, Feldman, Goodwin, & Quigley, 2021; Sagl et al., 2019; van Lier et al., 2020). Tools have been developed to aid these efforts (Gersak & Drnovsek, 2020). Validation studies of

24-hour finger-based recording (Boucsein, Schaefer, & Sommer, 2001; Doberenz, Roth, Wollburg, Maslowski, & Kim, 2011) found sufficient signal stability over time. Validation studies of ambulatory wrist-based, dry electrode recording against wet electrode finger or palm-based measures have not always been encouraging. A study comparing a now discontinued Microsoft wrist-based device to finger-based measures in a stationary laboratory paradigm (cold pressor) found no correlation between both SCL measures (Konstantinou et al., 2020). A laboratory study including ambulatory daily life activities investigating the only currently available dry wrist-based device reported neither correlation nor visual resemblance with finger-based EDA (Menghini et al., 2019).

In our discussion, we may come across as overly critical of this nascent technology. This assessment should not be misread as an underappreciation of the pioneering work done so far or as our reluctance to endorse ambulatory assessment of EDA as a good way forward in stress research. On the contrary, we strongly encourage further ambulatory research that delineates the appropriate signals, study designs, and analytical methods.

Cardiac Contractility

In humans, cardiac contractility is influenced predominantly by the sympathetic branch of the ANS. Whereas vagal innervation of the ventricle is sparse and largely nonfunctional, an abundance of beta-adrenergic receptors exert strong inotropic effects on the cardiac muscle through the opening of calcium channels in the membrane as well as the T-tubules of the muscle fibers. The calcium influx increases contractile force and contraction speed of the ventricle. This increased contractility is reflected in a larger ejection fraction of the left ventricle, which is the ratio between the stroke volume and the end-diastolic volume. The ejection fraction can be obtained from recordings of end-diastolic and end-systolic volumes (the difference equals the stroke volume) by echocardiography or magnetic resonance imaging (Malm, Frigstad, Sagberg, Larsson, & Skjaerpe, 2004). Neither of these techniques is amenable to ambulatory recording. Fortunately, changes in contractility can also be measured noninvasively through use of impedance cardiography.

In impedance cardiography, a high-frequency alternating current is introduced across the thorax by electrodes at the level of the neck and the belly (Sherwood et al., 1990). Electrodes at the level of the top and bottom of the sternum measure the changes in the impedance (dZ) of the enclosed thorax column. The first derivative of the pulsatile changes in transthoracic impedance (dZ/dt) is called the impedance cardiogram (ICG), and it reflects the momentary changes in aortic blood flow during the systolic phase. From the combined ECG and ICG, the pre-ejection period (PEP, in milliseconds [ms]) can be derived as the time interval between the onset of ventricular depolarization (QRST-onset) and the opening of the semilunar aortic valves (sharp upstroke in the dZ/dt), as depicted in Figure 6.4. PEP derived from the ICG correlates well with PEP derived from echocardiography (Nederend, Ten Harkel, Blom, Berntson, & de Geus, 2017; Noda et al., 2017), which is another noninvasive method to detect aortic valve opening.

Increases in contractility through increased SNS activity will lead to a shortening of the PEP, which can be reduced from 110 ms at rest to 100 ms during stress and as low as 60 ms during intense exercise (Goedhart, Willemsen, et al., 2007; van der Mee et al., 2020; van Lien, Schutte, Meijer, & de Geus, 2013). Within-subject changes in the PEP validly index changes in β-adrenergic drive to the left ventricle during manipulations known to increase cardiac sympathetic activity like epinephrine infusion, amyl nitrite

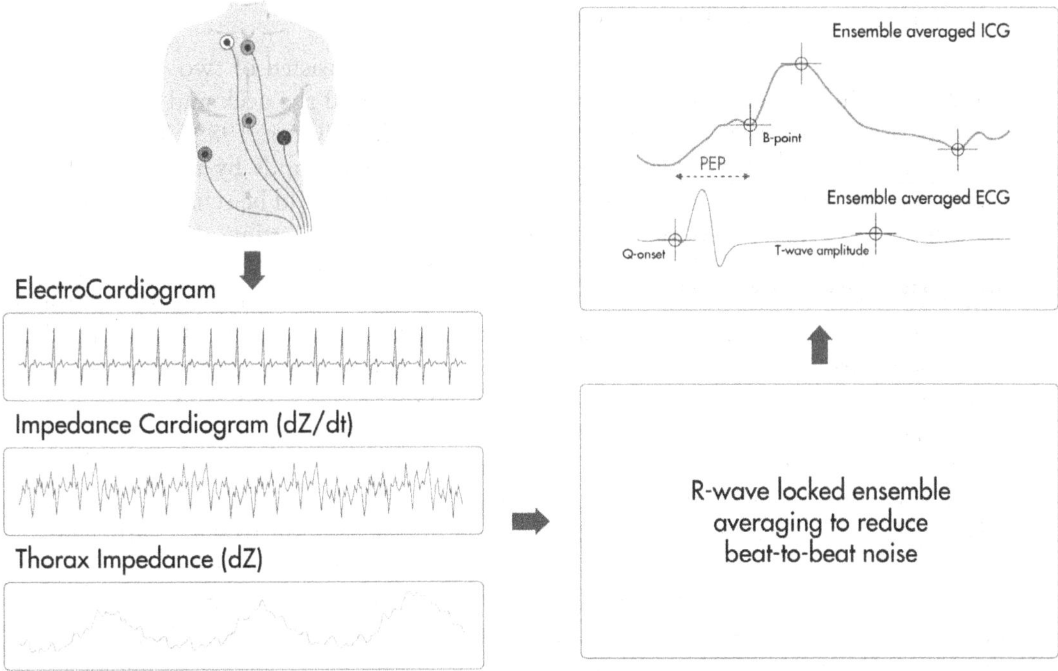

FIGURE 6.4. PEP and TWA computed from the combined ECG and the ICG signals after R-wave locked ensemble averaging.

inhalation, mental stress, and exercise. These manipulations systematically shorten the PEP (Houtveen, Groot, & de Geus, 2005; Krzeminski et al., 2000; Mezzacappa, Kelsey, & Katkin, 1999; Nelesen, Shaw, Ziegler, & Dimsdale, 1999; Richter & Gendolla, 2009; Schachinger, Weinbacher, Kiss, Ritz, & Langewitz, 2001; Svedenhag, Martinsson, Ekblom, & Hjemdahl, 1986). In addition, pharmacological blockade of cardiac sympathetic effects results in the expected lengthening of the PEP (Berntson, Cacioppo, & Quigley, 1994; Cacioppo et al., 1994; Schachinger et al., 2001), whereas the PEP is hardly affected by blockade of cardiac vagal effects (Berntson et al., 1994; Cacioppo et al., 1994; Martinsson, Larsson, & Hjemdahl, 1987).

It is important to again stress that the within-subject changes in PEP closely track changes in cardiac SNS activity (provided that there are no major posture changes; see below) but that between-subject differences in the PEP reflect the extent to which subjects differ in the degree of sympathetic *effects* on their cardiac contractility. These effects are correlated with differences in sympathetic activity, but the correlation is likely to be imperfect. Inotropic responses to norepinephrine and circulating epinephrine will be modulated by individual differences in the effectiveness of the cardiac β_1- and β_2-adrenergic receptors. Density, affinity, and distribution of these receptors may show large individual differences (Liggett, 1995; Liggett et al., 2006). A reassuringly high between-subject correlation (0.82) was found between PEP levels and cardiac sympathetic effects as assessed in healthy subjects (Cacioppo et al., 1994), but the relationship might be weaker in patients with high levels of cardiac sympathetic nerve activity who have very low ventricular beta-receptor densities.

Ambulatory Measurement Strategies for Cardiac Contractility

Originally, the current and measurement ICG electrodes consisted of two 10-cm-wide tetrapolar aluminium band electrode systems that ran around the neck and around the lower part of the thorax of participants (van Doornen & de Geus, 1989). However, it soon became clear that the replacement of the cumbersome bands by four spot electrodes still produced a good ICG signal from which the PEP could be reliably extracted (Boomsma, de Vries, & Orlebeke, 1989). Feasibility of miniaturization of the electronic circuitry needed to generate the AC current for thorax impedance recording and signal storage on memory chips allowed Willemsen, de Geus, Klaver, van Doornen, and Carroll (1996) to successfully pioneer use of the PEP in a 24-hour ambulatory thorax impedance recording using the Vrije Universiteit Ambulatory Monitoring System (VU-AMS). A number of other ambulatory devices similarly showed that reliable and valid PEP recording was feasible in naturalistic settings (Cybulski, 2000; Nakonezny et al., 2001; Panagiotou et al., 2018; Sherwood, McFetridge, & Hutcheson, 1998).

The major limitation of ambulatory ICG is that neither the hybrid tetrapolar spot-band electrode configuration nor a configuration with seven skin electrodes is sufficiently comfortable and inconspicuous to be worn across multiple days, let alone weeks, not in the least because of the (long) electrode cables connected to the recording device (see left upper corner of Figure 6.4). However, the number of electrodes can be reduced to five without loss of signal quality (van der Mee et al., 2020). Moreover, ongoing technological advances may allow the devices to be reduced in size, permitting the device to be worn on a chest strap (not unlike the many wearables for the ECG), greatly reducing electrode cable lengths.

Reliability and Temporal Stability of Cardiac Contractility Measures

High test–retest correlation (>.90) has been found for ambulatory recordings of the PEP within a single day (van Lien et al., 2015) or even across 2 work days of the same work week (Vrijkotte, van Doornen, & de Geus, 2004). That ambulatory PEP acts as a stable trait was further confirmed by demonstrating significant heritability during all periods of a representative work day, of a magnitude (~40%) comparable even to that for resting or stress levels attained under controlled laboratory conditions (Neijts et al., 2015). In addition, good long-term temporal stability ($r > .66$) of 24-hour measurements has been observed (Goedhart, Kupper, Willemsen, Boomsma, & de Geus, 2006), which is again as good as the stability of the pre-ejection period obtained under standardized laboratory conditions (Burleson et al., 2003; Hu, Lamers, Penninx, & de Geus, 2017).

Other Measures of Ambulatory SNS Activity in Use

Low- to High-Frequency Ratio of Heart Rate Variability

Various metrics based on the low-frequency (LF) component of heart rate variability (0.04–0.15 Hz) have been proposed as putative measures of SNS activity. Heart rate variability in the LF band partly arises from the so-called Mayer waves, which are periodic oscillations in arterial blood pressure around the 0.1-Hz frequency (Julien, 2006). To keep blood pressure constant, these changes are countered by rapid cardiac vagal activity but also by slower cardiac and vascular effects of SNS activity. In the late 1980s, Pagani and coworkers advanced the notion that a single ratio, the power in the LF band divided by the power in the high-frequency (HF) band, may capture cardiac sympathetic activity even if imperfectly (Montano et al., 1994; Pagani et al., 1986; Pagani & Malliani, 2000). Although its use as an SNS index has become widespread, the LF/HF ratio is rather controversial (Billman, 2013; Reyes Del Paso, Langewitz, Mulder, van Roon, & Duschek, 2013). It does not compare well against invasive measures of sympathetic activity (Grassi & Esler, 1999) or the PEP (Goedhart, Willemsen, Houtveen, Boomsma, & de Geus, 2008), and stress, exercise, or beta-adrenergic blockade do not systematically induce the expected changes in the LF/HF ratio that one expects from an SNS index (Ahmed, Kadish, Parker, & Goldberger, 1994; Jokkel, Bonyhay, & Kollai, 1995).

The ECG-Derived T-Wave Amplitude

The T wave is the asymmetrical wave in the ECG that comes after the QRS complex and typically lasts approximately 150 milliseconds. The T-wave amplitude (TWA, in μV) is defined as the difference between the peak of the T wave and an isoelectric baseline when only a negligible number of fibers in the cardiac conduction system are depolarizing (Furedy, Heslegrave, & Scher, 1984; Kline, Ginsburg, & Johnston, 1998). Changes in TWA reflect changes in ventricular repolarization (Abildskov, Burgess, Urie, Lux, & Wyatt, 1977; Haarmark et al., 2010) in which the sympathetic nerves play an important role as shown by pharmacological manipulations and direct nerve stimulation studies (Abildskov, 1985). In humans, a TWA decrease is seen after administration of the nonselective beta-agonist isoproterenol (Contrada et al., 1989), which is reversed by beta-blockade with propanolol (Contrada et al., 1989; Furberg, 1968). However, pharmacological evidence is not unanimous. The clear sympathomimetic effects of tricyclic antidepressants and serotonin and norepinephrine reuptake inhibitors on the PEP were not seen for the TWA (Hu, Lamers, Penninx, & de Geus, 2018).

Using 24-hour ambulatory monitoring and ensemble-averaging of the PEP and the TWA in a sample of 564 healthy adults, it was shown that the TWA showed a monotonic decrease from nighttime sleep to daytime sitting and more physically active behaviors (van Lien et al., 2015). Within-participant changes in TWA were significantly but modestly correlated with changes in the PEP across the 24-hour period (mean $r = .35$). However, the TWA proved very sensitive to the mean heart period (mean within-person $r = .71$), invalidating TWA as an exclusive cardiac SNS measure. Van Lien and colleagues (2015) concluded that ambulatory TWA, though far easier to measure as it requires just the ECG, should not replace the PEP, which requires both ICG and ECG. Simultaneous reporting on TWA and PEP does have added value, however, as it provides a more comprehensive picture of changes in cardiac SNS activity in real-life settings without requiring an extra signal to be recorded.

Salivary Alpha-Amylase Secretion

The salivary glands are also innervated by the ANS and the secretion of salivary alpha-amylase (sAA), a digestive enzyme that breaks down insoluble starch into soluble maltose and dextrin and has been suggested as a noninvasive marker for SNS activity (Nater & Rohleder, 2009). The attraction of sAA for stress researchers is that it can be measured from the same salivary samples required to measure the stress hormone cortisol, which is already being widely applied to assess the activity of the hypothalamic–pituitary–adrenocortical (HPA) axis in real-life settings (Schlotz, 2019).

Indeed, increasing central nervous system norepinephrine levels by blocking its reuptake by atomoxetine nearly doubled sAA secretion (Warren, van den Brink, Nieuwenhuis, & Bosch, 2017). Furthermore, exposure to stressors known to evoke sympathetic activation uniformly increase the amount of sAA secreted per unit of time, including stressful academic examination (Bosch, de Geus, Ring, Nieuw Amerongen, & Stowell, 2004; Chatterton, Vogelsong, Lu, Ellman, & Hudgens, 1996), stressful computer games (Skosnik, Chatterton, Swisher, & Park, 2000; Takai et al., 2004), watching a stressful video (Bosch, de Geus, Veerman, Hoogstraten, & Nieuw Amerongen, 2003), the mental arithmetic test (Noto, Sato, Kudo, Kurata, & Hirota, 2005), cold pressor test (van Stegeren, Wolf, & Kindt, 2008), and the Trier Social Stress Test (Rohleder, Nater, Wolf, Ehlert, & Kirschbaum, 2004). Administration of the beta-adrenergic antagonists reduces sAA concentration (Nederfors & Dahlöf, 1992) and attenuates the stress-induced increases in sAA concentration (van Stegeren, Rohleder, Everaerd, & Wolf, 2006).

Nonetheless, various reasons cause us to express concern about the use of sAA as an ambulatory index of SNS activity. First, the salivary glands are innervated by both branches of the ANS, not just the sympathetic branch (Proctor & Carpenter, 2001, 2007). Second, the sampling density that can be realized by sAA measurements is by necessity an order of magnitude less dense than that of wearable devices measuring continuous signals. During a single day of recording, at most two samples per hour would be feasible, but that would already be a major burden on participants. Also, sampling cannot take place during the nighttime. Third, serious methodological concerns have been voiced about the co-collection of sAA with cortisol using the same chewing-on-cotton-swabs procedure among others because this does not allow a correction for salivary flow rate (Bosch, Veerman, de Geus, & Proctor, 2011).

Recommendations for Ambulatory Recording of the ANS

In summary, we prioritize skin-electrode ECG-based RSA, RMSSD, or HF as the preferred noninvasive method to measure PNS activity in ambulatory assessment studies. For ambulatory SNS activity, we prioritize the PEP and palm- or finger-based SCL and nsSCR. For reasons outlined above, we advise against the use of LF/HF as an SNS index. We also see little merit in using SAA concentration from the cotton swabs used to detect diurnal cortisol patterns, at least not as a measure of peripheral SNS nerve activity. Coregistration of the TWA with the PEP seems useful as it only requires the ECG recording that is already needed for the PEP anyway. To increase user acceptance and the feasibility of prolonged recording while reducing the risk of changes in the participants' daily routines due to the measurement procedures, wrist-based PPG and EDA recording are seen as promising alternatives for ambulatory PNS and SNS activity recording, respectively. At the current stage of technology, however, these methods may generate substantially less reliable signals.

Apart from recording the purer SNS and PNS measures, it remains valuable to perform ambulatory recording of the heart rate as a general index of arousal. Heart rate comes "for free" whenever a PPG or ECG signal needs to be recorded to obtain a cardiac SNS or PNS measure. As long as it is understood that heart rate is a mixed bag of SNS and PNS activity, its clinical relevance justifies its reporting in any ambulatory study that records it. Likewise, the clinical importance of blood pressure makes it a valuable parameter in research on ANS activity, particularly when co-recorded with purer cardiac SNS or PNS measures.

The difficult tradeoff facing today's researcher in selecting an instrument from Table 6.1 for their ambulatory assessment research is that the correlation between device reliability/validity and end-user acceptance seems to be sharply negative. Research-oriented devices generally fare best when it comes to validity, but relying on academic groups to make innovative technology user-friendly and widely available at low cost seems naive at best. The long-term viability of research devices is also not necessarily higher than those of commercial companies, the demise of the LifeShirt and Portapres devices being a case in point. These well-validated devices are no longer produced even if the existing versions are still in high demand.

The contrast between research- and consumer-oriented devices is compounded by the lack of empirical evidence on how the balance between measurement error and much longer recording times (= more repeated measurements) affects the ability of ambulatory recording to elucidate the within-subject associations between the ANS and psychological states in daily life. It is also unknown how well the prolonged measurements can compensate for a larger measurement error when it comes to the predictive validity of ANS activity for disease outcomes. We hope and expect that the distinction in user-acceptance of research-oriented, medical application-oriented, and consumer-oriented devices will increasingly blur and that the demands for demonstrated device reliability/validity will sharply increase for all three categories.

Interpretational Issues

The availability of (future) wearable technology that is reliable and well validated does not automatically lead to appropriate scientific interpretation of the measurements generated. It is at least as important to have a good grasp on the social and psychological events that lead to the generation of changes in ANS activity. This requires the careful co-registration in daily life of changes in subjective emotional state (Busscher, Spinhoven, van Gerwen, & de Geus, 2013; Daly, Delaney, Doran, Harmon, & MacLachlan, 2010; Gentili et al., 2017; Kimhy et al., 2017), anxiety-disorder related symptoms (Dennis et al., 2016; Pfaltz et al., 2015), cognitive functioning (Riediger et al., 2014), components of work stress like job demand and decisional control (Kamarck, Schwartz, Janicki, Shiffman, & Raynor, 2003), negative social interactions, including marital conflict (Baucom et al., 2018), cognitive appraisals (Carnevali, Thayer, Brosschot, & Ottaviani, 2018; Gerteis & Schwerdtfeger, 2016), and behavioral coping strategies (Burg et al., 2017)—to name but a few of the psychological constructs that have been linked to ambulatory ANS activity. Many chapters in this handbook are devoted to measurement of such psychological factors using either ecological momentary assessment (EMA) or passive sensing technology, and we point the reader to the excellent strategies outlined there to co-register the relevant contextual and psychological factors that are typically of interest to the behavioral scientist.

However, even with careful characterization of the daily-life contextual and psychological factors impacting on ANS activity, an important component of the optimal ambulatory assessment strategy for ANS is still missing. The high ecological validity of measuring in a daily-life setting comes at a steep price. The organ systems we use as read-outs for ANS activity were not primarily devised by evolution to serve as "psychologist tools." They serve homeostatic functions meant to keep, among others, blood gas concentrations, pH, blood pressure, core temperature, and energy substrate availability within strict boundaries. The heart is a pump, not a stress-o-meter. The strongest sources of within-subject variability in ANS activity are nonpsychological in nature and are often (though not always) outside of the domain of interest of behavioral studies.

The impact of physical activity on cardiac signals, for example, is so pervasive that many ambulatory researchers have defaulted to asking participants to refrain from intensive physical activity such as leisure-time sports or (prolonged) dancing on recording days. In addition, a deliberate selection is made of only those fragments of the recording days where physical activity is stationary across a longer time period, and often selection sternly retains only those recordings when people are either sitting or lying down (sleep) and engaged in sedentary or low physical activity (e.g., sitting in a meeting, using a smartphone or PC). Since many modern-day jobs are predominantly sedentary, this captures about 85% of a normal work day (Vrijkotte et al., 2001). However, for jobs like nursing or manual labor, this strategy would remove large chunks of data. Having to restrain from sports and exercise further compromises ecological validity. One strategy to circumvent these limitations is to carefully establish the transfer function between physical activity and the physiological measure of interest during periods of low psychosocial stress and then mathematically correct the physiological signal obtained during stress for the co-registered physical activity. When applied to heart rate, this strategy yields the concept of "additional heart rate" (Brouwer, van Dame, van Erp, Spangler, & Brooks, 2018; Ebner-Priemer et al., 2007; Myrtek et al., 1988; Myrtek & Foester, 2001; Pfaltz et al., 2015; Verkuil, Brosschot, Tollenaar, Lane, & Thayer, 2016; Wilhelm, Pfaltz, Grossman, & Roth, 2006). In this method, one first regresses increasing levels of physical activity operationalized as oxygen consumption, minute ventilation, or accelerometer output on the heart rate. Based on the regression parameters, the observed heart rate is compared to the expected heart rate based on oxygen consumption, minute ventilation, or accelerometer output during the real-life exposures of interest. The difference is the additional heart rate. "Additional" here literally means that part of the heart rate that cannot be simply explained by physical activity and therefore must be attributed to psychological factors.

Apart from the strong effects of physical activity, ANS activity is also sensitive to postural change, caloric intake, fluid consumption, smoking, alcohol or other substance use, and fluctuations due to circadian rhythms or the menstrual cycle. Some of these may be correlated to the psychological factors of interest, yielding complex patterns of confounding on ANS activity (Sperry, Kwapil, Eddington, & Silvia, 2018). In addition, various factors that only weakly influence SNS and PNS activity themselves can nonetheless strongly impact on the measures we use to index such activity. For example, respiratory behavior strongly impacts on RSA measures independent of vagal activity, and temperature and humidity impact on EDA measures through thermoregulatory rather than emotional sweating.

Co-Registration of Momentary Within-Person Confounders

Physical Activity, Posture, Respiration, Temperature

Many confounders can be controlled in a laboratory setting by design, for instance, by measuring all study participants in a no physical activity, supine position between 9 and 10 A.M. while their respiration rate is paced and after they have abstained from smoking or drinking coffee in the morning before the experiment. Ambulatory assessment, in contrast, aims to make the behavior of the study participants as naturalistic as possible. This invites a multitude of nonpsychological factors to influence ANS physiology that are no longer under the control of the experimenter and so must be co-recorded and dealt with analytically. In Table 6.2, we summarize how the four most important of these factors impact the ANS and the methods to systematically co-record them.

Various Other Within-Subject Factors Can Affect the ANS

After physical activity and posture, the wake–sleep transition is the factor explaining most of the variance in 24-hour recordings of cardiac variables, with sharp changes in SNS and PNS at bedtime and awakening (Kupper et al., 2005). These abrupt transitions reflect a combination of changes in posture and arousal levels, the latter often occurring on top of a more general sinusoid pattern of diurnal variation in ANS activity (Eekelen, Houtveen, & Kerkhof, 2004). This pattern is visible in the gradual increase in PEP and

TABLE 6.2. The Effects of Physical Activity, Posture, Respiration, and Temperature on ANS Measures and Methods to Systematically Co-Record Them by Ambulatory Devices

		Co-recording needed		
Confounder	**ANS effects**	**Concepts**	**Strategies**	**References**
Physical activity	HR (++), BP (++), RSA, RMSSD, HF (++), PEP (++), SCL (++), nsSCR (++), TWA (++)	Type of activities; energy expenditure	EMA-based self-report; accelerometer; minute ventilation	Aminian et al. (1999); Bussmann, Ebner-Priemer, & Fahrenberg (2009); Hendelman, Miller, Bagget, Debold, & Freedson (2000); Pfaltz et al. (2015)
Posture	HR (+), BP (+), RSA/RMSSD/ HF (+), PEP (++), SCL (~), nsSCR (~), TWA (+)	Posture	EMA-based self-report; accelerometer (+ gyroscope)	Berlin & Van Laerhoven (2012); Bussmann et al. (2009); Lawal & Bano (2020); Mannini & Sabatini (2010); Mathie, Coster, Lovell, & Celler (2004); Yen & Lin (2020)
Respiration	HR (~), BP (~), RSA, RMSSD, HF (++), PEP (~), SCL (~), nsSCR (~), TWA ([illegible])	Respiration rate; tidal volume	Respiratory inductance plethysmography; impedance plethysmography; HF component in ECG or PPG; morphological changes in the ECG	Houtveen, Groot, & de Geus (2006); Kent et al. (2008, 2009); Liu, Allen, Zheng, & Chen (2019); Varon et al. (2020)
Temperature	HR (~), BP (~), RSA, RMSSD, HF (~), PEP (~), SCL (++), nsSCR (++), TWA (~)	Ambient temperature; skin temperature; core temperature	Weather/thermostat data; sensor on clothing; thermal infrared imaging; sensor on skin; ingestible sensor	Engert et al. (2014); Kinugasa & Hirayanagi (1999); Low, Keller, Wingo, Brothers, & Crandall (2011); Ren et al. (2011); Turpin, Shine, & Lader (1983)

Note. ~, +, and ++ indicate the relative strength of impact on ANS measures.

RSA in the course of the night reflecting decreasing SNS and increasing PNS activity, although short-term increases in SNS activity in REM sleep have been reported (de Zambotti, Trinder, Silvani, Colrain, & Baker, 2018). The total pattern of 24-hour fluctuations in ANS activity derives from a combination of endogenous circadian rhythms and time-related behavioral variation, including wake–sleep, meals, and work–leisure effects.

During waking hours, the consumption of food and drinks (Adam & Epel, 2007), noise exposure (Morrison, Haas, Shaffner, Garrett, & Fackler, 2003), smoking (Hayano et al., 1990; Lucini, Bertocchi, Malliani, & Pagani, 1996; Ohta et al., 2016), alcohol use (Schwabe, Dickinson, & Wolf, 2011) or other substances (Kennedy et al., 2015; Schmid, Schonlebe, Drexler, & Mueck-Weymann, 2010) are known to affect ANS activity. A female-specific factor that needs to be recorded is the phase of the menstrual cycle (von Holzen, Capaldo, Wilhelm, & Stute, 2016).

Time of day is automatically recorded by almost all devices, but specific co-recording of the time-to-bed and waking-time, as well as the consumption of food and drinks or substance use can be done by EMA-based self-report. Increasingly, passive sensing is being used to detect these behaviors (Berlin & Van Laerhoven, 2012; Harari, Muller, Aung, & Rentfrow, 2017). Noise exposure can be reasonably approximated by sampling incoming noise to the smartphone microphone, but this depends on where and how the phone is carried. Studies specifically focused on stress generated by listening effort (e.g., in the hearing impaired) are using more advanced dual audio recorders placed on a pair of glasses close to the ears (Kowalk, Kissner, von Gablenz, Holube, & Bitzer, 2018).

Between-Subjects Factors

Ambulatory studies of ANS activity do not differ from a typical psychophysiological experimental setting in the laboratory in that many stable between-subject confounders can impact on the mean and variance of ANS measures. Many studies have examined individual differences in ANS activity related to age (Hu, Lamers, Penninx, et al., 2017), sex (Taylor, Arnold, Fu, & Shibao, 2020), body mass index (BMI; Hu, Lamers, Penninx, et al., 2017), genetics (de Geus, Neijts, & Willemsen, 2015), ethnicity (Hill et al., 2015), socioeconomic status (SES; Hemingway et al., 2005), chronic pain (Generaal et al., 2017), disease status, medication use (Licht, Penninx, & de Geus, 2012), habitual alcohol use (Boschloo et al., 2011), smoking (Hu, Lamers, Penninx, et al., 2017), physical activity habits (Hu, Lamers, de Geus, & Penninx, 2017), general sleep quality (Tobaldini et al., 2017), and physical fitness (de Geus, van Doornen, de Visser, & Orlebeke, 1990). Although the reported associations with ANS measures are not always uniform in significance or direction across all studies, it seems prudent to record such factors whenever possible. A complete review is outside of the scope of this chapter, but the minimum person-specific characteristics that we recommend to be measured in any study using ambulatory assessment of the ANS are age, sex, ethnicity, physical activity habits, SES, disease status, and current medication use.

Analytical Strategy

In a typical ambulatory ANS study, repeated observations of variables are nested within persons. As explained above, a set of variables should be selected that captures (1) psychophysiological measures of interest, (2) the psychosocial context, and (3) the time-varying confounders. The ideal strategy is to align the time-axis of sampling for all three sets of variables, but this is not always feasible. To enforce time alignment, researchers often use selection. For instance, if EMA is used to detect the number of cigarettes smoked across the last hour and current positive and negative mood states, the continuous physiological recording of RSA could be restricted to average of RSA in the 5 minutes before or after the EMA beep. This would yield an hourly set of variables reflecting mood, recent cigarettes smoked, and a 5-minute averaged RSA value. Temporal resolution could be greatly improved by successful use of passive sensing and machine learning to estimate emotional state through analysis of speech snippets, smartphone use, and location data. Likewise, automated smoking detection from wrist-worn accelerometers could yield a signal every 60 seconds indicating whether the person is smoking. In that case, the repeated measures structure for all variables would expand to a minute-by-minute basis.

As amply demonstrated elsewhere in this book, multilevel modeling has been shown to be a powerful approach for analyzing within-person repeated measures data. They can be used for analyzing more complex nested data structures, that is, minutes, within days, days within weeks, and so on, and graciously handle unequal numbers of observations across individuals (missings) or even data left at unequally spaced time intervals (Hox, Moerbeek, & van de Schoot, 2017). By simultaneously modeling the effects of the psychosocial context on ANS measures, with the effects of confounders such as time of day, posture, respiration, and physical activity (or other confounders) on these measures, one effectively creates a series of partial regression slopes, describing for each subject the extent to which their ANS activity tends to increase when psychosocial demands increase, after adjustment for the effects of confounders. Note that when such a model is used for the parallel effects of stress and physical activity on heart rate, it effectively recaptures the strategy of computing the additional heart rate that was mentioned previously in this chapter.

Multilevel models for ambulatory ANS data have the added advantage of allowing the temporal structure of cross-variable regressions to be person-specific by modeling the slopes as a random factor. That is, if the effect of stair-climbing on RSA is suspected to be less strong in a well-trained individual, then individual differences in vigorous exercise habits can be added as a level 2 factor.

Conclusion

Ambulatory monitoring of PNS activity through RSA, RMSSD, HF, ambulatory monitoring of SNS activity through PEP, SCL, nSCRs, and indirect monitoring of SNS and PNS activity through ambulatory heart rate and BP provides higher ecological validity and higher predictive validity for clinical outcomes than laboratory studies. The added validity of an ambulatory psychophysiological study, however, does come with the strong requirement of solid co-registration of the psychosocial context *and* a host of confounding influences on the ANS. By far the most important of these influences are physical activity and the wake–sleep cycle for all ANS measures, postural changes for the PEP, respiratory behavior (including speech) for all heart-rate variability measures, and temperature and humidity for the EDA-based measures. Provided there is valid registration of these confounders, solid strategies are available in the data analysis phase to take them into account. These range from simple post-hoc selection of periods where the levels of the confounders are highly comparable, to full modeling of the complex dependency of the ECG, ICG, and EDA signals on the confounders and regressing these out when computing the relevant ANS measures.

Whereas large improvements in the ambulatory assessment toolkit are still needed, technology will not be the Achilles' heel of our understanding of the psychological effects on ANS regulation in daily life. The more fearsome enemies are the overestimation of the validity of the measures used and the underappreciation of the complexity of their underlying biology.

REFERENCES

Abildskov, J. A. (1985). Neural mechanisms involved in the regulation of ventricular repolarization. *European Heart Journal, 6*(Suppl. D), 31–39.

Abildskov, J. A., Burgess, M. J., Urie, P. M., Lux, R. L., & Wyatt, R. F. (1977). The unidentified information content of the electrocardiogram. *Circulation Research, 40*(1), 3–7.

Adam, T. C., & Epel, E. S. (2007). Stress, eating and the reward system. *Physiology and Behavior, 91*(4), 449–458.

Ahmed, M. W., Kadish, A. H., Parker, M. A., & Goldberger, J. J. (1994). Effect of physiological and pharmacological adrenergic-stimulation on heart-rate-variability. *Journal of the American College of Cardiology, 24*(4), 1082–1090.

Akselrod, S., Gordon, D., Ubel, F. A., Shannon, D. C., Berger, A. C., & Cohen, R. J. (1981). Power spectrum analysis of heart rate fluctuation: A quantitative probe of beat-to-beat cardiovascular control. *Science, 213*(4504), 220–222.

Aminian, K., Robert, P., Buchser, E. E., Rutschmann, B., Hayoz, D., & Depairon, M. (1999). Physical activity monitoring based on accelerometry: Validation and comparison with video observation. *Medical and Biological Engineering and Computing, 37*(3), 304–308.

Baucom, B. R. W., Baucom, K. J. W., Hogan, J. N., Crenshaw, A. O., Bourne, S. V., Crowell, S. E., et al. (2018). Cardiovascular reactivity during marital conflict in laboratory and naturalistic settings: Differential associations with relationship and individual functioning across contexts. *Family Process, 57*(3), 662–678.

Beissner, F., Meissner, K., Bar, K. J., & Napadow, V. (2013). The autonomic brain: An activation likelihood estimation meta-analysis for central processing of autonomic function. *Journal of Neuroscience, 33*(25), 10503–10511.

Bengtsson, M., Lofstrom, J. B., & Malmqvist, L. A. (1985). Skin-conductance responses during spinal analgesia. *Acta Anaesthesiologica Scandinavica, 29*(1), 67–71.

Berlin, E., & Van Laerhoven, K. (2012, September). *Detecting leisure activities with dense motif discovery.* Paper presented at the 2012 ACM Conference on Ubiquitous Computing, Pittsburgh, PA.

Berntson, G. G., Bechara, A., Damasio, H., Tranel, D., & Cacioppo, J. T. (2007). Amygdala contribution to selective dimensions of emotion. *Social Cognitive and Affective Neuroscience, 2*(2), 123–129.

Berntson, G. G., Cacioppo, J. T., Binkley, P. F., Uchino, B. N., Quigley, K. S., & Fieldstone, A. (1994). Autonomic cardiac control. III. Psychological stress and cardiac response in autonomic space as revealed by pharmacological blockades. *Psychophysiology, 31*(6), 599–608.

Berntson, G. G., Cacioppo, J. T., & Quigley, K. S. (1991). Autonomic determinism: The modes of autonomic control, the doctrine of autonomic space, and the laws of autonomic constraint. *Psychological Review, 98*(4), 459–487.

Berntson, G. G., Cacioppo, J. T., & Quigley, K. S. (1993). Respiratory sinus arrhythmia: autonomic origins, physiological mechanisms, and psychophysiological implications. *Psychophysiology, 30*(2), 183–196.

Berntson, G. G., Cacioppo, J. T., & Quigley, K. S. (1994). Autonomic cardiac control. I. Estimation and validation from pharmacological blockades. *Psychophysiology, 31*(6), 572–585.

Bigger, J. T., Jr., Fleiss, J. L., Rolnitzky, L. M., & Steinman, R. C. (1992). Stability over time of heart period variability in patients with previous myocardial infarction and ventricular arrhythmias. The CAPS and ESVEM investigators. *American Journal of Cardiology, 69*(8), 718–723.

Billman, G. E. (2013). The LF/HF ratio does not accurately measure cardiac sympatho-vagal balance. *Frontiers in Physiology, 4*.

Bjelakovic, B., Ilic, D., Lukic, S., Vukomanovic, V., Zarko, C., Stankovic, Z., & Marko, J. (2017). Reproducibility of 24-h heart rate variability in children. *Clinical Autonomic Research, 27*(4), 273–278.

Bohm, M., Swedberg, K., Komajda, M., Borer, J. S., Ford, I., Dubost-Brama, A., et al. (2010). Heart rate as a risk factor in chronic heart failure (SHIFT): The association between heart rate and outcomes in a randomised placebo-controlled trial. *Lancet, 376*(9744), 886–894.

Boomsma, D. I., de Vries, J., & Orlebeke, J. F. (1989). Comparison of spot and band impedance cardiogram electrodes across different tasks. *Psychophysiology, 26*(6), 695–699.

Bosch, J. A., de Geus, E. E., Ring, C., Nieuw Amerongen, A. V., & Stowell, J. R. (2004). Academic examinations and immunity: Academic stress or examination stress? *Psychosomatic Medicine, 66*(4), 625–626.

Bosch, J. A., de Geus, E. J. C., Veerman, E. C. I., & Amerongen, A. V. N. (2000). Innate secretory immunity in response to laboratory stressors that evoke distinct patterns of cardiac autonomic activity. *Psychosomatic Medicine, 62*(1), 1276.

Bosch, J. A., de Geus, E. J., Veerman, E. C., Hoogstraten, J., & Nieuw Amerongen, A. V. (2003). Innate secretory immunity in response to laboratory stressors that evoke distinct patterns of cardiac autonomic activity. *Psychosomatic Medicine, 65*(2), 245–258.

Bosch, J. A., Veerman, E. C., de Geus, E. J., & Proctor, G. B. (2011). Alpha-amylase as a reliable and convenient measure of sympathetic activity: Don't start salivating just yet! *Psychoneuroendocrinology, 36*(4), 449–453.

Boschloo, L., Vogelzangs, N., Licht, C. M., Vreeburg, S. A., Smit, J. H., van den Brink, W., et al. (2011). Heavy alcohol use, rather than alcohol dependence, is associated with dysregulation of the hypothalamic-pituitary-adrenal axis and the autonomic nervous system. *Drug and Alcohol Dependence, 116*(1–3), 170–176.

Boucsein, W. (2012). *Electrodermal activity* (2nd ed.). Springer.

Boucsein, W., Fowles, D. C., Grimnes, S., Ben-Shakhar, G., Roth, W. T., Dawson, M. E., et al. (2012). Publication recommendations for electrodermal measurements. *Psychophysiology, 49*(8), 1017–1034.

Boucsein, W., Schaefer, F., & Sommer, T. (2001). Electrodermal long-term monitoring in everyday life. In J. Fahrenberg & M. Myrtek (Eds.), *Progress in ambulatory assessment: Computer-assisted psychological and psychophysiological methods in monitoring and field studies* (pp. 549–560). Hogrefe & Huber.

Brotman, D. J., Golden, S. H., & Wittstein, I. S. (2007). The cardiovascular toll of stress. *Lancet, 370*(9592), 1089–1100.

Brouwer, A. M., van Dame, E., van Erp, J. B. F., Spangler, D. P., & Brooks, J. R. (2018). Improving real-life estimates of emotion based on heart rate: A perspective on taking metabolic heart rate into account. *Frontiers in Human Neuroscience, 12*, 045008.

Burg, M. M., Schwartz, J. E., Kronish, I. M., Diaz, K. M., Alcantara, C., Duer-Hefele, J., & Davidson, K. W. (2017). Does stress result in you exercising less? Or does exercising result in you being less stressed? Or is it both? Testing the bi-directional stress–exercise association at the group and person (*N* of 1) level. *Annals of Behavioral Medicine, 51*(6), 799–809.

Burleson, M. H., Poehlmann, K. M., Hawkley, L. C., Ernst, J. M., Berntson, G. G., Malarkey, W. B., et al. (2003). Neuroendocrine and cardiovascular reactivity to stress in mid-aged and older women: Long-term temporal consistency of individual differences. *Psychophysiology, 40*(3), 358–369.

Busscher, B., Spinhoven, P., & de Geus, E. J. (2015). Psychological distress and physiological reactivity during in vivo exposure in people with aviophobia. *Psychosomatic Medicine, 77*(7), 762–774.

Busscher, B., Spinhoven, P., van Gerwen, L. J., & de Geus, E. J. (2013). Anxiety sensitivity moderates the relationship of changes in physiological arousal with flight anxiety during in vivo exposure therapy. *Behaviour Research and Therapy, 51*(2), 98–105.

Bussmann, J. B., Ebner-Priemer, U. W., & Fahrenberg, J. (2009). Ambulatory activity monitoring: Progress in measurement of activity, posture, and specific motion patterns in daily life. *European Psychologist, 14*(2), 142.

Cacioppo, J. T., Berntson, G. G., Binkley, P. F., Quigley, K. S., Uchino, B. N., & Fieldstone, A. (1994). Autonomic cardiac control. II. Noninvasive indices and basal response as revealed by autonomic blockades. *Psychophysiology, 31*(6), 586–598.

Carnevali, L., Thayer, J. F., Brosschot, J. F., & Ottaviani, C. (2018). Heart rate variability mediates the link between rumination and depressive symptoms: A longitudinal study. *International Journal of Psychophysiology, 131*, 131–138.

Cerutti, S., Bianchi, A. M., & Mainardi, L. T. (2001). Advanced spectral methods for detecting dynamic behaviour. *Autonomic Neuroscience, 90*(1–2), 3–12.

Chatterton, R. T., Jr., Vogelsong, K. M., Lu, Y. C., Ellman, A. B., & Hudgens, G. A. (1996). Salivary alpha-amylase as a measure of endogenous adrenergic activity. *Clinical Physiology, 16*(4), 433–448.

Contrada, R. J., Krantz, D. S., Durel, L. A., Levy, L., LaRiccia, P. J., Anderson, J. R., & Weiss, T. (1989). Effects of beta-adrenergic activity on T-wave amplitude. *Psychophysiology, 26*(4), 488–492.

Cybulski, G. (2000). Ambulatory impedance cardiography: New possibilities. *Journal of Applied Physiology, 88*(4), 1509–1510.

Daly, M., Delaney, L., Doran, P. P., Harmon, C., & MacLachlan, M. (2010). Naturalistic monitoring of the affect-heart rate relationship: A day reconstruction study. *Health Psychology, 29*(2), 186–195.

Dawson, M. E., Schell, A. M., & Filion, D. L. (2000). The electrodermal system. In J. T. Cacioppo, L. G. Tassinary, & G. G. Berntson (Eds.), *Handbook of psychophysiology* (pp. 200–223). Cambridge University Press.

de Geus, E. J. C., Gianaros, P. J., Brindle, R. C., Jennings, J. R., & Berntson, G. G. (2019). Should heart rate variability be "corrected" for heart rate?: Biological, quantitative, and interpretive considerations. *Psychophysiology, 56*(2), e13287.

de Geus, E. J. C., Kupper, N., Boomsma, D. I., & Snieder, H. (2007). Bivariate genetic modeling of cardiovascular stress reactivity: Does stress uncover genetic variance? *Psychosomatic Medicine, 69*(4), 356–364.

de Geus, E. J. C., van Doornen, L. J., de Visser, D. C., & Orlebeke, J. F. (1990). Existing and training induced differences in aerobic fitness: Their relationship to physiological response patterns during different types of stress. *Psychophysiology, 27*(4), 457–478.

de Geus, E., van Lien, R., Neijts, M., & Willemsen, G. (2015). Genetics of autonomic nervous system activity. In T. Canli (Ed.), *The Oxford handbook of molecular psychology* (pp. 357–390). Oxford University Press.

de Zambotti, M., Trinder, J., Silvani, A., Colrain, I. M., & Baker, F. C. (2018). Dynamic coupling between the central and autonomic nervous systems during sleep: A review. *Neuroscience and Biobehavioral Reviews, 90*, 84–103.

Dennis, P. A., Dedert, E. A., Van Voorhees, E. E., Watkins, L. L., Hayano, J., Calhoun, P. S., et al. (2016). Examining the crux of autonomic dysfunction in posttraumatic stress disorder: Whether chronic or situational distress underlies elevated heart rate and attenuated heart rate variability. *Psychosomatic Medicine, 78*(7), 805–809.

Doberenz, S., Roth, W. T., Wollburg, E., Breuninger, C., & Kim, S. (2010). Twenty-four hour skin conductance in panic disorder. *Journal of Psychiatric Research, 44*(16), 1137–1147.

Doberenz, S., Roth, W. T., Wollburg, E., Maslowski, N. I., & Kim, S. (2011). Methodological considerations in ambulatory skin conductance monitoring. *International Journal of Psychophysiology, 80*(2), 87–95.

Ebner-Priemer, U. W., & Kubiak, T. (2007). Psychological and psychophysiological ambulatory monitoring—A review of hardware and software solutions. *European Journal of Psychological Assessment, 23*(4), 214–226.

Ebner-Priemer, U. W., Welch, S. S., Grossman, P., Reisch, T., Linehan, M. M., & Bohus, M. (2007). Psychophysiological ambulatory assessment of affective dysregulation in borderline personality disorder. *Psychiatry Research, 150*(3), 265–275.

Eckberg, D. L. (2003). The human respiratory gate. *Journal of Physiology, 548*(2), 339–352.

Eekelen, A. P. v., Houtveen, J. H., & Kerkhof, G. A. (2004). Circadian variation in base rate measures of cardiac autonomic activity. *European Journal of Applied Physiology, 93*(1), 39–46.

Eisenhofer, G. (2005). Sympathetic nerve function: Assessment by radioisotope dilution analysis. *Clinical Autonomic Research, 15*(4), 264–283.

Eisenhofer, G., Kopin, I. J., & Goldstein, D. S. (2004). Catecholamine metabolism: A contemporary view with implications for physiology and medicine. *Pharmacological Reviews, 56*(3), 331–349.

Engert, V., Merla, A., Grant, J. A., Cardone, D., Tusche, A., & Singer, T. (2014). Exploring the use of thermal infrared imaging in human stress research. *PloS One, 9*(3), e90782.

Esler, M. (2000). The sympathetic system in essential hypertension. *Revista Portuguesa de Cardiologia, 19*(Suppl. 2), II9–II14.

Esler, M. (2017). Mental stress and human cardiovascular disease. *Neuroscience and Biobehavioral Reviews, 74*, 269–276.

Esler, M., Jennings, G., Korner, P., Willett, I., Dudley, F., Hasking, G., et al. (1988). Assessment of human sympathetic nervous system activity from measurements of norepinephrine turnover. *Hypertension, 11*, 3–20.

Esler, M., Jennings, G., Lambert, G., Meredith, I., Horne, M., & Eisenhofer, G. (1990). Overflow of catecholamine neurotransmitters to the circulation: Source, fate, and functions. *Physiological Reviews, 70*(4), 963–985.

Esler, M., & Kaye, D. (2000). Measurement of sympathetic nervous system activity in heart failure: The role of norepinephrine kinetics. *Heart Failure Reviews, 5*(1), 17–25.

Fahrenberg, J., Myrtek, M., Pawlik, K., & Perrez, M. (2007). Ambulatory assessment—Monitoring behavior in daily life settings—A behavioral-scientific challenge for psychology. *European Journal of Psychological Assessment, 23*(4), 206–213.

Folkow, B. (2000). Perspectives on the integrative functions of the "sympatho-adrenomedullary system." *Autonomic Neuroscience, 83*(3), 101–115.

Foster, K. G., & Weiner, J. S. (1970). Effects of cholinergic and adrenergic blocking agents on activity of eccrine sweat glands. *Journal of Physiology, 210*(4), 883–895.

Fowles, D. C. (1986). The eccrine system and electrodermal activity. In M. G. H. Coles, E. Donchin, & S. W. Porges (Eds.), *Psychophysiology: Systems processes and applications.* (pp. 51–96). Guilford Press.

Furberg, C. (1968). Effects of repeated work tests and adrenergic beta-blockade on electrocardiographic ST and T changes. *Acta Medica Scandinavica, 183*(1–2), 153–161.

Furedy, J. J., Heslegrave, R. J., & Scher, H. (1984). Psychophysiological and physiological aspects of T-wave amplitude in the objective study of behavior. *Pavlovian Journal of Biological Science, 19*(4), 182–194.

Generaal, E., Vogelzangs, N., Macfarlane, G. J., Geenen, R., Smit, J. H., de Geus, E. J., et al. (2017). Biological stress systems, adverse life events, and the improvement of chronic multisite musculoskeletal pain across a 6-year follow-up. *Journal of Pain, 18*(2), 155–165.

Gentili, C., Messerotti Benvenuti, S., Palomba, D., Greco, A., Scilingo, E. P., & Valenza, G. (2017). Assessing mood symptoms through heartbeat dynamics: An HRV study on cardiosurgical patients. *Journal of Psychiatric Research, 95*, 179–188.

Georgiou, K., Larentzakis, A. V., Khamis, N. N., Alsuhaibani, G. I., Alaska, Y. A., & Giallafos, E. J. (2018). Can wearable devices accurately measure heart rate variability? A systematicrReview. *Folia Medica (Plovdiv.), 60*(1), 7–20.

Gersak, G., & Drnovsek, J. (2020). Electrodermal activity patient simulator. *PloS One, 15*(2), e0228949.

Gerteis, A. K. S., & Schwerdtfeger, A. R. (2016). When rumination counts: Perceived social support and heart rate variability in daily life. *Psychophysiology, 53*(7), 1034–1043.

Goedhart, A. D., Kupper, N., Willemsen, G., Boomsma, D. I., & de Geus, E. J. (2006). Temporal stability of ambulatory stroke volume and cardiac output measured by impedance cardiography. *Biological Psychology, 72*(1), 110–117.

Goedhart, A. D., van der Sluis, S., Houtveen, J. H., Willemsen, G., & de Geus, E. J. (2007). Comparison of time and frequency domain measures of RSA in ambulatory recordings. *Psychophysiology, 44*(2), 203–215.

Goedhart, A. D., Willemsen, A. H. M., & DeGeus, E. J. C. (2007). Sympathetic nervous system activity in the heart and the skin: comparable measures? In M. Kaneko (Ed.),

Sympathetic nervous system research developments (pp. 147–165). Nova Science.

Goedhart, A. D., Willemsen, G., Houtveen, J. H., Boomsma, D. I., & de Geus, E. J. (2008). Comparing low frequency heart rate variability and preejection period: two sides of a different coin. *Psychophysiology, 45*(6), 1086–1090.

Grassi, G., & Esler, M. (1999). How to assess sympathetic activity in humans. *Journal of Hypertension, 17*(6), 719–734.

Grossman, P., & Kollai, M. (1993). Respiratory sinus arrhythmia, cardiac vagal tone, and respiration: Within- and between-individual relations. *Psychophysiology, 30*(5), 486–495.

Grossman, P., & Taylor, E. W. (2007). Toward understanding respiratory sinus arrhythmia: relations to cardiac vagal tone, evolution and biobehavioral functions. *Biological Psychology, 74*(2), 263–285.

Grossman, P., van Beek, J., & Wientjes, C. (1990). A comparison of three quantification methods for estimation of respiratory sinus arrhythmia. *Psychophysiology, 27*(6), 702–714.

Grossman, P., Wilhelm, F. H., & Spoerle, M. (2004). Respiratory sinus arrhythmia, cardiac vagal control, and daily activity. *American Journal of Physiology-Heart and Circulatory Physiology, 287*(2), H728–H734.

Haarmark, C., Graff, C., Andersen, M. P., Hardahl, T., Struijk, J. J., Toft, E., et al. (2010). Reference values of electrocardiogram repolarization variables in a healthy population. *Journal of Electrocardiology, 43*(1), 31–39.

Hagbarth, K. E., Hallin, R. G., Wallin, B. G., Torebjork, H., & Hongell, A. (1972). General characteristics of sympathetic activity in human skin nerves. *Acta Physiologica Scandinavica, 84*(1), 65–81.

Hansen, T. W., Jeppesen, J., Rasmussen, S., Ibsen, H., & Torp-Pedersen, C. (2006). Ambulatory blood pressure monitoring and risk of cardiovascular disease: A population based study. *American Journal of Hypertension, 19*(3), 243–250.

Harari, G. M., Muller, S. R., Aung, M. S. H., & Rentfrow, P. J. (2017). Smartphone sensing methods for studying behavior in everyday life. *Current Opinion in Behavioral Sciences, 18*, 83–90.

Hayano, J., Yamada, M., Sakakibara, Y., Fujinami, T., Yokoyama, K., Watanabe, Y., et al. (1990). Short-term and long-term effects of cigarette-smoking on heart-rate-variability. *American Journal of Cardiology, 65*(1), 84–88.

Hemingway, H., Shipley, M., Brunner, E., Britton, A., Malik, M., & Marmot, M. (2005). Does autonomic function link social position to coronary risk?: The Whitehall II study. *Circulation, 111*(23), 3071–3077.

Hendelman, D., Miller, K., Bagget, C., Debold, E., & Freedson, P. (2000). Validity of accelerometry for the assessment of moderate intensity physical activity in the field. *Medicine and Science in Sports and Exercise, 32*(9), S442–S449.

Hill, L. K., Hu, D. D., Koenig, J., Sollers, J. J., III, Kapuku, G., Wang, X., et al. (2015). Ethnic differences in resting heart rate variability: A systematic review and meta-analysis. *Psychosomatic Medicine, 77*(1), 16–25.

Hjemdahl, P., Freyschuss, U., Juhlin-Dannfelt, A., & Linde, B. (1984). differentiated sympathetic activation during mental stress evoked by the Stroop test. *Acta Physiologica Scandinavica, 527*, 25–29.

Hoehn-Saric, R., McLeod, D. R., Funderburk, F., & Kowalski, P. (2004). Somatic symptoms and physiologic responses in generalized anxiety disorder and panic disorder—An ambulatory monitor study. *Archives of General Psychiatry, 61*(9), 913–921.

Houtveen, J. H., & de Geus, E. J. C. (2009). Noninvasive psychophysiological ambulatory recordings: Study design and data analysis strategies. *European Psychologist, 14*(2), 132–132.

Houtveen, J. H., Groot, P. F., & de Geus, E. J. (2005). Effects of variation in posture and respiration on RSA and pre-ejection period. *Psychophysiology, 42*(6), 713–719.

Houtveen, J. H., Groot, P. F., & de Geus, E. J. (2006). Validation of the thoracic impedance derived respiratory signal using multilevel analysis. *International Journal of Psychophysiology, 59*(2), 97–106.

Houtveen, J. H., & Molenaar, P. C. (2001). Comparison between the Fourier and Wavelet methods of spectral analysis applied to stationary and nonstationary heart period data. *Psychophysiology, 38*(5), 729–735.

Hox, J. J., Moerbeek, M. & van de Schoot, R. (2017). *Multilevel analysis: Techniques and applications* (3rd ed.). Taylor & Francis.

Hu, M. X., Lamers, F., de Geus, E. J., & Penninx, B. W. (2017). Influences of lifestyle factors on cardiac autonomic nervous system activity over time. *Preventive Medicine, 94*, 12–19.

Hu, M. X., Lamers, F., Penninx, B., & de Geus, E. J. C. (2017). Temporal stability and drivers of change in cardiac autonomic nervous system activity. *Autonomic Neuroscience, 208*, 117–125.

Hu, M. X., Lamers, F., Penninx, B. W. J. H., & de Geus, E. J. C. (2018). Association between depression, anxiety, and antidepressant use with T-Wave amplitude and QT-interval. *Frontiers in Neuroscience, 12*.

Hu, M. X., Penninx, B. W. J. H., de Geus, E. J. C., Lamers, F., Kuan, D. C. H., Wright, A. G. C., et al. (2018). Associations of immunometabolic risk factors with symptoms of depression and anxiety: The role of cardiac vagal activity. *Brain Behavior and Immunity, 73*, 493–503.

Jokkel, G., Bonyhay, I., & Kollai, M. (1995). Heart rate variability after complete autonomic blockade in man. *Journal of the Autonomic Nervous System, 51*(1), 85–89.

Julien, C. (2006). The enigma of Mayer waves: Facts and models. *Cardiovascular Research, 70*(1), 12–21.

Kamarck, T. W., Schwartz, J. E., Janicki, D. L., Shiffman, S., & Raynor, D. A. (2003). Correspondence between laboratory and ambulatory measures of cardiovascular reactivity: A multilevel modeling approach. *Psychophysiology, 40*(5), 675–683.

Kasos, K., Kekecs, Z., Csirmaz, L., Zimonyi, S., Vikor, F., Kasos, E., et al. (2020). Bilateral comparison of traditional and alternate electrodermal measurement sites. *Psychophysiology*, e13645.

Katona, P. G., & Jih, F. (1975). Respiratory sinus arrhythmia: Noninvasive measure of parasympathetic cardiac control. *Journal of Physiology, 39*, 801–805.

Kennedy, A. P., Epstein, D. H., Jobes, M. L., Agage, D., Tyburski, M., Phillips, K. A., et al. (2015). Continuous in-the-field measurement of heart rate: Correlates of drug use, craving, stress, and mood in polydrug users. *Drug and Alcohol Dependence, 151*, 159–166.

Kent, L., Bradley, J. M., O'Neill, B., Davison, G. W., Nevill, A. M., Derchak, P. A., & Elborn, J. S (2008). Validity and reliability of ventilation measured by the Lifeshirt: A potential outcome measure for clinical trials. *Thorax, 63*, A126–A127.

Kent, L., O'Neill, B., Davison, G., Nevill, A., Elborn, J. S., & Bradley, J. M. (2009). Validity and reliability of cardiorespiratory measurements recorded by the LifeShirt during exercise tests. *Respiratory Physiology and Neurobiology, 167*(2), 162–167.

Kimhy, D., Wall, M. M., Hansen, M. C., Vakhrusheva, J., Choi, C. J., Delespaul, P., et al. (2017). Autonomic regulation and auditory hallucinations in individuals with schizophrenia. *Schizophrenia Bulletin, 43*(4), 754–763.

Kingwell, B. A., Thompson, J. M., Kaye, D. M., Mcpherson, G. A., Jennings, G. L., & Esler, M. D. (1994). Heart-rate spectral-analysis, cardiac norepinephrine spillover, and muscle sympathetic-nerve activity during human sympathetic nervous activation and failure. *Circulation, 90*(1), 234–240.

Kinugasa, H., & Hirayanagi, K. (1999). Effects of skin surface cooling and heating on autonomic nervous activity and baroreflex sensitivity in humans. *Experimental Physiology, 84*(2), 369–377.

Kleckner, I. R., Feldman, M. J., Goodwin, M. S., & Quigley, K. S. (2021). Framework for selecting and benchmarking mobile devices in psychophysiological research. *Behavior Research Methods, 53*(2): 518–535.

Kline, K. P., Ginsburg, G. P., & Johnston, J. R. (1998). T-wave amplitude: Relationships to phasic RSA and heart period changes. *International Journal of Psychophysiology, 29*(3), 291–301.

Koenig, J. (2020). Neurovisceral regulatory circuits of affective resilience in youth: Principal outline of a dynamic model of neurovisceral integration in development. *Psychophysiology, 57*(5), e13568.

Konstantinou, P., Trigeorgi, A., Georgiou, C., Gloster, A. T., Panayiotou, G., & Karekla, M. (2020). Comparing apples and oranges or different types of citrus fruits?: Using wearable versus stationary devices to analyze psychophysiological data. *Psychophysiology, 57*(5), e13551.

Kowalk, U., Kissner, S., von Gablenz, P., Holube, I., & Bitzer, J. (2018). An improved privacy-aware system for objective and subjective ecological momentary assessment. *Proceedings of the International Symposium on Auditory and Audiological Research, 6*, 25–30B.

Krzeminski, K., Kruk, B., Nazar, K., Ziemba, A. W., Cybulski, G., & Niewiadomski, W. (2000). Cardiovascular, metabolic and plasma catecholamine responses to passive and active exercises. *Journal of Physiological Pharmacology, 51*(2), 267–278.

Kupper, N., de Geus, E. J., van den Berg, M., Kirschbaum, C., Boomsma, D. I., & Willemsen, G. (2005). Familial influences on basal salivary cortisol in an adult population. *Psychoneuroendocrinology, 30*(9), 857–868.

Lambert, E. A., & Lambert, G. W. (2011). Stress and its role in sympathetic nervous system activation in hypertension and the metabolic syndrome. *Current Hypertension Reports, 13*, 244–248.

Lambert, G., Schlaich, M., Lambert, E., Dawood, T., & Esler, M. (2010). Stress reactivity and its association with increased cardiovascular risk: A role for the sympathetic nervous system? *Hypertension, 55*(6), e20.

Langley, J. (1898). On the union of cranial autonomic (visceral) fibres with nerve cells of the superior cervical ganglion. *Journal of Physiology, 23*, 240–270.

Lawal, I. A., & Bano, S. (2020). Deep human activity recognition with localisation of wearable sensors. *IEEE Access, 8*, 155060–155070.

Licht, C. M., Penninx, B. W., & de Geus, E. J. (2012). Effects of antidepressants, but not psychopathology, on cardiac sympathetic control: A longitudinal study. *Neuropsychopharmacology, 37*(11), 2487–2495.

Liggett, S. (1995). Functional properties of human beta(2)-adrenergic receptor polymorphisms. *News in Physiological Sciences, 10*, 265–273.

Liggett, S. B., Mialet-Perez, J., Thaneemit-Chen, S., Weber, S. A., Greene, S. M., Hodne, D., et al. (2006). A polymorphism within a conserved beta1-adrenergic receptor motif alters cardiac function and {beta}-blocker response in human heart failure. *Proceedings of the National Academy of Sciences of the United States of America, 103*(30), 11288–11293.

Liu, H. P., Allen, J., Zheng, D. C., & Chen, F. (2019). Recent development of respiratory rate measurement technologies. *Physiological Measurement, 40*(7), 07TR01.

Lovallo, W. R. (2005). *Stress and Health: Biological and Psychological Interactions* (2nd ed.). Sage.

Low, D. A., Keller, D. M., Wingo, J. E., Brothers, R. M., & Crandall, C. G. (2011). Sympathetic nerve activity and whole body heat stress in humans. *Journal of Applied Physiology, 111*(5), 1329–1334.

Lucini, D., Bertocchi, F., Malliani, A., & Pagani, M. (1996). A controlled study of the autonomic changes produced by habitual cigarette smoking in healthy subjects. *Cardiovascular Research, 31*(4), 633–639.

Mallion, J. M., Baguet, J. P., Siche, J. P., Tremel, F., & de Gaudemaris, R. (1999). Clinical value of ambulatory blood pressure monitoring. *Journal of Hypertension, 17*(5), 585–595.

Malm, S., Frigstad, S., Sagberg, E., Larsson, H., & Skjaerpe, T. (2004). Accurate and reproducible measurement of left ventricular volume and ejection fraction by contrast echocardiography: A comparison with magnetic resonance imaging. *Journal of the American College of Cardiology, 44*(5), 1030–1035.

Mannini, A., & Sabatini, A. M. (2010). Machine learning methods for classifying human physical activity from on-body accelerometers. *Sensors, 10*(2), 1154–1175.

Martinmaki, K., Rusko, H., Kooistra, L., Kettunen, J., & Saalasti, S. (2006). Intraindividual validation of heart rate variability indexes to measure vagal effects on hearts. *AJP—Heart and Circulatory Physiology, 290*(2), H640–H647.

Martinsson, A., Larsson, K., & Hjemdahl, P. (1987). Studies in vivo and in vitro of terbutaline-induced beta-adrenoceptor desensitization in healthy subjects. *Clinical Science, 72*, 47–54.

Mathie, M. J., Coster, A. C. F., Lovell, N. H., & Celler, B. G. (2004). Accelerometry: providing an integrated, practical method for long-term, ambulatory monitoring of human movement. *Physiological Measurement, 25*(2), R1–R20.

Menghini, L., Gianfranchi, E., Cellini, N., Patron, E., Tagliabue, M., & Sarlo, M. (2019). Stressing the accuracy: Wrist-worn wearable sensor validation over different conditions. *Psychophysiology, 56*(11), e1344.

Mezzacappa, E. S., Kelsey, R. M., & Katkin, E. S. (1999). The effects of epinephrine administration on impedance cardiographic measures of cardiovascular function. *International Journal of Psychophysiology, 31*(3), 189–196.

Montano, N., Ruscone, T. G., Porta, A., Lombardi, F., Pagani, M., & Malliani, A. (1994).

Power spectrum analysis of heart-rate-variability to assess the changes in sympathovagal balance during graded orthostatic tilt. *Circulation, 90*(4), 1826–1831.

Morrison, W. E., Haas, E. C., Shaffner, D. H., Garrett, E. S., & Fackler, J. C. (2003). Noise, stress, and annoyance in a pediatric intensive care unit. *Critical Care Medicine, 31*(1), 113–119.

Mundy-Castle, A. C., & McKiever, B. I. (1953). The psychophysiological significance of the Galvanic skin response. *Journal of Experimental Psychology, 46*(1), 15–24.

Myrtek, M., Bruegner, G., Fichtler, A., Konig, K., Muller, W., Foerster, F., & Hoppner, V. (1988). Detection of emotionally induced ECG changes and their behavioural correlates: A new method for ambulatory monitoring. *European Heart Journal, 9*(Suppl. N), 55–60.

Myrtek, M., & Foester, F. (2001). On-line measurement of additional heart rate. Methodology and application. In J. Fahrenberg & M. Myrtek (Eds.), *Progress in ambulatory assessment: Computer-assisted psychological and psychophysiological methods in monitoring and field studies* (pp. 399–414). Hogrefe & Huber.

Nakonezny, P. A., Kowalewski, R. B., Ernst, J. M., Hawkley, L. C., Lozano, D. L., Litvack, D. A., et al. (2001). New ambulatory impedance cardiograph validated against the Minnesota Impedance Cardiograph. *Psychophysiology, 38*(3), 465–473.

Nater, U. M., & Rohleder, N. (2009). Salivary alpha-amylase as a non-invasive biomarker for the sympathetic nervous system: Current state of research. *Psychoneuroendocrinology, 34*(4), 486–496.

Nederend, I., Ten Harkel, A. D. J., Blom, N. A., Berntson, G. G., & de Geus, E. J. C. (2017). Impedance cardiography in healthy children and children with congenital heart disease: Improving stroke volume assessment. *International Journal of Psychophysiology, 120*, 136–147.

Nederfors, T., & Dahlöf, C. (1992). Effects of the [beta]-adrenoceptor antagonists atenolol and propranolol on human whole saliva flow rate and composition. *Archives of Oral Biology, 37*(7), 579–584.

Neijts, M., van Lien, R., Kupper, N., Boomsma, D., Willemsen, G., & de Geus, E. J. (2015). Heritability and temporal stability of ambulatory autonomic stress reactivity in unstructured 24-hour recordings. *Psychosomatic Medicine, 77*(8), 870–881.

Nelesen, R. A., Shaw, R., Ziegler, M. G., & Dimsdale, J. E. (1999). Impedance cardiography-derived hemodynamic responses during baroreceptor testing with amyl nitrite and phenylephrine: A validity and reliability study. *Psychophysiology, 36*(1), 105–108.

Neumann, E., & Blanton, R. (1970). The early history of electrodermal research. *Psychophysiology, 6*(4), 453–475.

Niiranen, T., Hanninen, M. R., Johansson, J., Reunanen, A., & Jula, A. (2010). Home-measured blood pressure is a stronger predictor of cardiovascular risk than office blood pressure: The Finn-Home study. *Journal of Hypertension, 28*, E13–E13.

Nishiyama, T., Sugenoya, J., Matsumoto, T., Iwase, S., & Mano, T. (2001). Irregular activation of individual sweat glands in human sole observed by a videomicroscopy. *Autonomic Neuroscience—Basic and Clinical, 88*(1–2), 117–126.

Noda, K., Endo, H., Kadosaka, T., Nakata, T., Watanabe, T., Terui, Y., et al. (2017). Comparison of the measured pre-ejection periods and left ventricular ejection times between echocardiography and impedance cardiography for optimizing cardiac resynchronization therapy. *Journal of Arrhythmia, 33*(2), 130–133.

Noto, Y., Sato, T., Kudo, M., Kurata, K., & Hirota, K. (2005). The relationship between salivary biomarkers and state-trait anxiety inventory score under mental arithmetic stress: A pilot study. *Anesthesia and Analgesia, 101*(6), 1873–1876.

Ohta, Y., Kawano, Y., Hayashi, S., Iwashima, Y., Yoshihara, F., & Nakamura, S. (2016). Effects of cigarette smoking on ambulatory blood pressure, heart rate, and heart rate variability in treated hypertensive patients. *Clinical and Experimental Hypertension, 38*(6), 510–513.

Ottaviani, M. M., Wright, L., Dawood, T., & Macefield, V. G. (2020). In vivo recordings from the human vagus nerve using ultrasound-guided microneurography. *Journal of Physiology, 598*(17), 3569–3576.

Pabst, O., Tronstad, C., Grimnes, S., Fowles, D., & Martinsen, O. G. (2017). Comparison between the AC and DC measurement of electrodermal activity. *Psychophysiology, 54*(3), 374–385.

Pagani, M., Lombardi, F., Guzzetti, S., Rimoldi, O., Furlan, R., Pizzinelli, P., et al. (1986). Power spectral analysis of heart rate and arterial pressure variabilities as a marker of sympatho-vagal interaction in man and conscious dog. *Circulation Research, 59*(2), 178–193.

Pagani, M., & Malliani, A. (2000). Interpreting oscillations of muscle sympathetic nerve activity and heart rate variability. *Journal of Hypertension, 18*(12), 1709–1719.

Palatini, P., & Julius, S. (2004). Elevated heart rate: A major risk factor for cardiovascular disease. *Clinical and Experimental Hypertension, 26*(7–8), 637–644.

Panagiotou, M., Vogiatzis, I., Jayasekera, G., Louvaris, Z., Mackenzie, A., Mcglinchey, N., et al. (2018). Validation of impedance cardiography in pulmonary arterial hypertension. *Clinical Physiology and Functional Imaging, 38*(2), 254–260.

Peake, J. M., Kerr, G., & Sullivan, J. P. (2018). A critical review of consumer wearables, mobile applications, and equipment for providing biofeedback, monitoring stress, and sleep in physically active populations. *Frontiers in Physiology, 9*, 743.

Penttila, J., Helminen, A., Jartti, T., Kuusela, T., Huikuri, H. V., Tulppo, M. P., et al. (2001). Time domain, geometrical and frequency domain analysis of cardiac vagal outflow: Effects of various respiratory patterns. *Clinical Physiology, 21*(3), 365–376.

Pfaltz, M. C., Kolodyazhniy, V., Blechert, J., Margraf, J., Grossman, P., & Wilhelm, F. H. (2015). Metabolic decoupling in daily life in patients with panic disorder and agoraphobia. *Journal of Psychiatric Research, 68*, 377–383.

Pickering, T. G., & Devereux, R. B. (1987). Ambulatory monitoring of blood pressure as a predictor of cardiovascular risk. *American Heart Journal, 114*(4 Pt 2), 925–928.

Pieper, C., LaCroix, A. Z., & Karasek, R. A. (1989). The relation of psychosocial dimensions of work with coronary heart disease factors: A meta-analysis of five United States data bases. *American Journal of Epidemiology, 129*, 483–494.

Pitzalis, M. V., Mastropasqua, F., Massari, F., Forleo, C., Di Maggio, M., Passantino, A., et al. (1996). Short- and long-term reproducibility of time and frequency domain heart rate variability measurements in normal subjects. *Cardiovascular Research, 32*(2), 226–233.

Posada-Quintero, H. F., & Chon, K. H. (2020). Innovations in electrodermal activity data collection and signal processing: A systematic review. *Sensors, 20*(2), 479.

Proctor, G. B., & Carpenter, G. H. (2001). Chewing stimulates secretion of human salivary secretory immunoglobulin A. *Journal of Dental Research, 80*(3), 909–913.

Proctor, G. B., & Carpenter, G. H. (2007). Regulation of salivary gland function by autonomic nerves. *Autonomic Neuroscience, 133*(1), 3–18.

Ren, C. Z., O'Neill, M. S., Park, S. K., Sparrow, D., Vokonas, P., & Schwartz, J. (2011). Ambient temperature, air pollution, and heart rate variability in an aging population. *American Journal of Epidemiology, 173*(9), 1013–1021.

Reyes Del Paso, G. A., Langewitz, W., Mulder, L. J., van Roon, A., & Duschek, S. (2013). The utility of low frequency heart rate variability as an index of sympathetic cardiac tone: A review with emphasis on a reanalysis of previous studies. *Psychophysiology, 50*(5), 477–487.

Richter, M., & Gendolla, G. H. (2009). The heart contracts to reward: Monetary incentives and preejection period. *Psychophysiology, 46*(3), 451–457.

Riediger, M., Wrzus, C., Klipker, K., Muller, V., Schmiedek, F., & Wagner, G. G. (2014). Outside of the Laboratory: Associations of working-memory performance with psychological and physiological arousal vary with age. *Psychology and Aging, 29*(1), 103–114.

Ritz, T., & Dahme, B. (2006). Implementation and interpretation of respiratory sinus arrhythmia measures in psychosomatic medicine: Practice against better evidence? *Psychosomatic Medicine, 68*(4), 617–627.

Rohleder, N., Nater, U. M., Wolf, J. M., Ehlert, U., & Kirschbaum, C. (2004). Psychosocial stress-induced activation of salivary alpha-amylase: An indicator of sympathetic activity? *Annals of the New York Academy of Sciences, 1032*, 258–263.

Rosengren, A., Hawken, S., Ounpuu, S., Sliwa, K., Zubaid, M., Almahmeed, W. A., et al. (2004). Association of psychosocial risk factors with risk of acute myocardial infarction in 11,119 cases and 13,648 controls from 52 countries (the INTERHEART study): Case-control study. *Lancet, 364*(9438), 953–962.

Sagl, G., Resch, B., Petutschnig, A., Kyriakou, K., Liedlgruber, M., & Wilhelm, F. H. (2019). Wearables and the quantified self: Systematic benchmarking of physiological sensors. *Sensors, 19*(20), 4448.

Schachinger, H., Weinbacher, M., Kiss, A., Ritz, R., & Langewitz, W. (2001). Cardiovascular indices of peripheral and central sympathetic activation. *Psychosomatic Medicine, 63*(5), 788–796.

Schlotz, W. (2019). Investigating associations between momentary stress and cortisol in daily life: What have we learned so far? *Psychoneuroendocrinology, 105*, 105–116.

Schmid, K., Schonlebe, J., Drexler, H., & Mueck-Weymann, M. (2010). The effects of cannabis on heart rate variability and well-being in young men. *Pharmacopsychiatry, 43*(4), 147–150.

Schwabe, L., Dickinson, A., & Wolf, O. T. (2011). Stress, habits, and drug addiction: A psychoneuroendocrinological perspective. *Experimental and Clinical Psychopharmacology, 19*(1), 53–63.

Sherwood, A., Allen, M. T., Fahrenberg, J., Kelsey, R. M., Lovallo, W. R., & van Doornen, L. J. (1990). Methodological guidelines for impedance cardiography. *Psychophysiology, 27*(1), 1–23.

Sherwood, A., McFetridge, J., & Hutcheson, J. S. (1998). Ambulatory impedance cardiography: A feasibility study. *Journal of Applied Physiology, 85*(6), 2365–2369.

Shimizu, S., Akiyama, T., Kawada, T., Shishido, T., Mizuno, M., Kamiya, A., et al. (2010). In vivo direct monitoring of interstitial norepinephrine levels at the sinoatrial node. *Autonomic Neuroscience, 152*(1–2), 115–118.

Shimizu, S., Akiyama, T., Kawada, T., Shishido, T., Yamazaki, T., Kamiya, A., et al. (2009). In vivo direct monitoring of vagal acetylcholine release to the sinoatrial node. *Autonomic Neuroscience, 148*(1–2), 44–49.

Skosnik, P. D., Chatterton, R. T., Jr., Swisher, T., & Park, S. (2000). Modulation of attentional inhibition by norepinephrine and cortisol after psychological stress. *International Journal of Psychophysiology, 36*(1), 59–68.

Sperry, S. H., Kwapil, T. R., Eddington, K. M., & Silvia, P. J. (2018). Psychopathology, everyday behaviors, and autonomic activity in daily life: An ambulatory impedance cardiography study of depression, anxiety, and hypomanic traits. *International Journal of Psychophysiology, 129*, 67–75.

Steptoe, A., & Kivimaki, M. (2012). Stress and cardiovascular disease. *Nature Reviews: Cardiology, 9*(6), 360–370.

Svedenhag, J., Martinsson, A., Ekblom, B., & Hjemdahl, P. (1986). Altered cardiovascular responsiveness to adrenaline in endurance-trained subjects. *Acta Physiologica Scandinavica, 126*(4), 539–550.

Sztajzel, J., Jung, M., & de Luna, A. B. (2008). Reproducibility and gender-related differences of heart rate variability during all-day activity in young men and women. *Annals of Noninvasive Electrocardiology, 13*(3), 270–277.

Takai, N., Yamaguchi, M., Aragaki, T., Eto, K., Uchihashi, K., & Nishikawa, Y. (2004). Effect of psychological stress on the salivary cortisol and amylase levels in healthy young adults. *Archives of Oral Biology, 49*(12), 963–968.

Tarvainen, M. P., Niskanen, J. P., Lipponen, J. A., Ranta-aho, P. O., & Karjalainen, P. A. (2014). Kubios HRV—Heart rate variability analysis software. *Computer Methods and Programs in Biomedicine, 113*(1), 210–220.

Taylor, C. E., Arnold, A. C., Fu, Q., & Shibao, C. A. (2020). Sex differences in cardiovascular autonomic control: Introduction to the special issue. *Clinical Autonomic Research, 30*, 365–367.

Tobaldini, E., Costantino, G., Solbiati, M., Cogliati, C., Kara, T., Nobili, L., & Montano, N. (2017). Sleep, sleep deprivation, autonomic nervous system and cardiovascular diseases. *Neuroscience and Biobehavioral Reviews, 74*, 321–329.

Tracey, K. J. (2009). Reflex control of immunity. *Nature Review Immunology, 9*, 418–428.

Turpin, G., Shine, P., & Lader, M. (1983). Ambulatory electrodermal monitoring: Effects of ambient temperature, general activity, electrolyte media, and length of recording. *Psychophysiology, 20*(2), 219–224.

Vallbo, A. B. (2018). Microneurography: How it started and how it works. *Journal of Neurophysiology, 120*(3), 1415–1427.

van der Mee, D. J., Duivestein, Q., Gevonden, M. J., Westerink, J., & de Geus, E. J. C. (2020). The short Sing-a-Song Stress Test: A practical and valid test of autonomic responses induced by social-evaluative stress. *Autonomic Neuroscience, 224*, 102612.

van Dooren, M., de Vries, J. J. G., & Janssen, J. H. (2012). Emotional sweating across the body: Comparing 16 different skin conductance measurement locations. *Physiology and Behavior, 106*(2), 298–304.

van Doornen, L. J., & de Geus, E. J. (1989). Aerobic fitness and the cardiovascular response to stress. *Psychophysiology, 26*(1), 17–28.

van Lien, R., Neijts, M., Willemsen, G., & de Geus, E. J. (2015). Ambulatory measurement of the ECG T-wave amplitude. *Psychophysiology, 52*(2), 225–237.

van Lien, R., Schutte, N. M., Meijer, J. H., & de Geus, E. J. (2013). Estimated preejection period (PEP) based on the detection of the R-wave and dZ/dt-min peaks does not adequately reflect the actual PEP across a wide range of laboratory and ambulatory conditions. *International Journal of Psychophysiology, 87*(1), 60–69.

van Lier, H. G., Pieterse, M. E., Garde, A., Postel, M. G., de Haan, H. A., Vollenbroek-Hutten, M. M. R., et al. (2020). A standardized validity assessment protocol for physiological signals from wearable technology: Methodological underpinnings and an application to the E4 biosensor. *Behavior Research Methods, 52*(2), 607–629.

van Stegeren, A., Rohleder, N., Everaerd, W., & Wolf, O. T. (2006). Salivary alpha amylase as marker for adrenergic activity during stress: Effect of beta blockade. *Psychoneuroendocrinology, 31*(1), 137–141.

van Stegeren, A. H., Wolf, O. T., & Kindt, M. (2008). Salivary alpha amylase and cortisol responses to different stress tasks: Impact of sex. *International Journal of Psychophysiology, 69*(1), 33–40.

Vanoli, E., De Ferrari, G. M., Stramba-Badiale, M., Hull, S. S., Jr., Foreman, R. D., & Schwartz, P. J. (1991). Vagal stimulation and prevention of sudden death in conscious dogs with a healed myocardial infarction. *Circulation Research, 68*(5), 1471–1481.

Varon, C., Morales, J., Lazaro, J., Orini, M., Deviaene, M., Kontaxis, S., et al. (2020). A comparative study of ECG-derived respiration in ambulatory monitoring using the single-lead ECG. *Scientific Reports, 10*(1), 5704.

Verdecchia, P. (2001). Using out of office blood pressure monitoring in the management of hypertension. *Current Hypertension Reports, 3*(5), 400–405.

Verdecchia, P., Porcellati, C., Schillaci, G., Borgioni, C., Ciucci, A., Battistelli, M., et al. (1994). Ambulatory blood pressure: An independent predictor of prognosis in essential hypertension. *Hypertension, 24*(6), 793–801.

Verkuil, B., Brosschot, J. F., Tollenaar, M. S., Lane, R. D., & Thayer, J. F. (2016). Prolonged non-metabolic heart rate variability reduction as a physiological marker of psychological stress in daily life. *Annals of Behavioral Medicine, 50*(5), 704–714.

von Holzen, J. J., Capaldo, G., Wilhelm, M., & Stute, P. (2016). Impact of endo- and exogenous estrogens on heart rate variability in women: A review. *Climacteric, 19*(3), 222–228.

Vrijkotte, T. G. M., Riese, H., & de Geus, E. J. C. (2001). Cardiovascular reactivity to work stress assessed by ambulatory blood pressure, heart rate, and heart rate variability. In J. Fahrenberg & M. Myrtek (Eds.), *Progress in ambulatory assessment. Computer assisted psychological and psychophysiological methods in monitoring and field studies* (pp. 345–360). Hogrefe & Huber.

Vrijkotte, T. G. M., van Doornen, L. J. P., & de Geus, E. J. C. (2000). Effects of work stress on ambulatory blood pressure, heart rate, and heart rate variability. *Hypertension, 35*(4), 880–886.

Vrijkotte, T. G., van Doornen, L. J., & de Geus, E. J. (2004). Overcommitment to work is associated with changes in cardiac sympathetic regulation. *Psychosomatic Medicine, 66*(5), 656–663.

Wallin, B. G. (1981). Sympathetic-nerve activity underlying electrodermal and cardiovascular reactions in man. *Psychophysiology, 18*(4), 470–476.

Wallin, B. G. (1984). Sympathetic activity in human extremity nerves and its relationship to plasma norepinephrine. In M. G. Ziegler & C. R. Lake (Eds.), *Norepinephrine* (Frontiers of Clinical Neuroscience, Vol. 2, pp. 431–438). Williams & Wilkins.

Wallin, B. G. (2004). Microneurographic assessment of sympathetic nerve traffic. *Supplements to Clinical Neurophysiology, 57*, 345–351.

Ward, A. M., Takahashi, O., Stevens, R., & Heneghan, C. (2012). Home measurement of blood pressure and cardiovascular disease:

Systematic review and meta-analysis of prospective studies. *Journal of Hypertension, 30*(3), 449–456.

Warren, C. M., van den Brink, R. L., Nieuwenhuis, S., & Bosch, J. A. (2017). Norepinephrine transporter blocker atomoxetine increases salivary alpha amylase. *Psychoneuroendocrinology, 78*, 233–236.

Westerink, J. H. D. M., Ouwerkerk, M., de Vries, J. J. G., De Waele, S., van den Eerenbeemd, J., & van Boven, M. (2009, September). *Emotion measurement platform for daily life situations.* Paper presented at the International Conference on Affective Computing and Intelligent Interaction, ACII, Amsterdam, The Netherlands.

Wilhelm, F. H., Pfaltz, M. C., Grossman, P., & Roth, W. T. (2006). Distinguishing emotional from physical activation in ambulatory psychophysiological monitoring. *Biomedical Sciences Instrumentation, 42*, 458–463.

Willemsen, G. H., de Geus, E. J., Klaver, C. H., van Doornen, L. J., & Carroll, D. (1996). Ambulatory monitoring of the impedance cardiogram. *Psychophysiology, 33*(2), 184–193.

Yen, C. T., & Lin, J. D. (2022). Human body activity recognition using wearable inertial sensors integrated with a feature extraction-based machine-learning classification algorithm. *Proceedings of the Institution of Mechanical Engineers Part B-Journal of Engineering Manufacture, 236*(14), 1820–1827.

CHAPTER 7

Analysis of Phone Logs and Phone Usage Patterns

Sandrine R. Müller, Aaron Cohen,
Marcel Enge, and John F. Rauthmann

CHAPTER OVERVIEW

This chapter provides an introduction for researchers working with phone log and screen usage data. We describe the different data sources related to phone calls, text messages, and screen use, including example data structures and differences between data under the iOS and Android operating systems. We discuss ethical and practical considerations when planning a smartphone study containing these data. Steps to consider when cleaning and computing features from such data are described in detail, including psychometric considerations and suggestions for data visualization. Finally, we describe limitations and future directions for passively collected phone log and screen usage data as well as other phone metadata sources.

Introduction

Phone logs and phone usage patterns have been referred to as *organic data*, that is, "data that are generated without any explicit research design elements and are continuously documented by digital devices" (Xu, Zhang, & Zhou, 2020, p. 1257). Organic data reflect everyday activities based on natural interactions with technological devices or platforms (Groves, 2011). Examples of organic data continuously generated by the phone include logs of sent and received text messages (i.e., short messaging service [SMS]), logs of outgoing and incoming phone calls, as well as high-level screen activity (i.e., is the screen turned on or off), and what the battery status is. This stands in contrast to data resulting from planned investigations (e.g., in-app responses to ecological momentary assessment surveys). In this chapter, we focus on phone logs (calls and messages, specifically) as well as phone (screen) usage patterns because they represent some of the most basic, natural interactions with smartphones, therefore making them particularly relevant and valuable in psychological research. We will describe the different steps to analyze phone log and screen usage data following Xu and colleagues' (2020) workflow of studies, using organic data to organize this chapter.

As listed in Figure 7.1, data sources described in this chapter consist of call and text logs as well as screen usage. When planning a study using or assessing such data, factors to consider include user demographics, information on the devices participants are using (as the specific technology may vary between different brands and models), as well as environmental factors (e.g., economics, politics, culture). Once the study design has been established and the data have been collected or accessed, preprocessing entails cleaning the data, followed by computing any relevant metric for analysis. In addition to data analysis, it is usually helpful to visualize the data and results. Doing so allows for a comprehensive interpretation of the results, revealing unique insights as well as potential avenues for future research.

Data Sources

While it is usually possible for phone users to access and export some of their own historic data (such as call and text logs), this will usually involve many manual steps. In the context of a research study, this can put an additional burden on the participants and will likely require detailed instructions or even supervision to be accomplished successfully. Downloading a smartphone app (see Chapter 1, "How to Conduct Mobile Sensing Research," this volume) will almost always be more convenient for the participants and the researchers involved. In addition, an app can guide participants through the process of enabling any required settings (e.g., switching on screen time tracking on Android, which is disabled by default) and allow collection of data in real time (e.g., via an API) that otherwise does not get stored on the device.

Commonly used open-source apps include the AWARE framework and Funf, while two notable commercial apps are Metricwire and Ksana Health. Notably, Beiwe includes both commercial and open-source options. Table 7.1 provides an overview of accessible

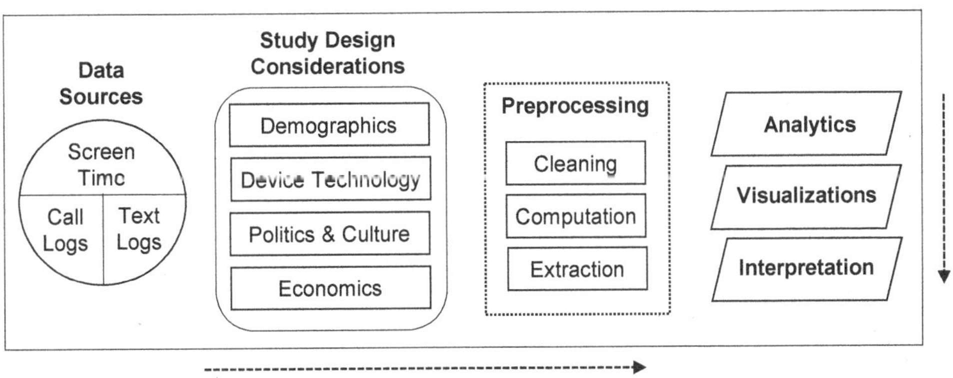

FIGURE 7.1. Conceptual overview of the analysis of phone logs and phone usage patterns.

TABLE 7.1. Overview of Accessible Phone Log and Screen Time Data across iOS and Android Operating Systems

	iOS	Android
Text logs	To a sensing app, no text logs are accessible under iOS. To the user, the entirety of the historic records, including both SMS and iMessages, are accessible if the phone is set to "keep messages forever" (other options are 1 year and 30 days), and messages have not been deleted by the user.	To both the user and a sensing app, the entirety of the historic records is accessible as long as those have not been deleted by the user.
Call logs	The last 1,000 calls are available, yet only 100 are accessible via an iPhone (Bradford, 2021). This means that to look back into one's call history, one would need to delete an equivalent number of recent calls. Furthermore, iCloud must be active to retain the call history; if it is turned off, all data are stored for 180 days and are then deleted.	Entirety of the historic records as long as those have not been deleted by the user.
Screen time	The following screen events can be recorded in real time by a sensing app (e.g., Aware): screen being turned on, turned off, locked, or unlocked. Detailed screen activity is not available (e.g., app usage). Some apps employ work-arounds such as routing all traffic through a VPN (e.g., Qustodio) or extracting the contents of screenshots users take of the iOS Screen Time tracking feature in the phone's settings (e.g., Moment), but iOS will not allow an app direct access to these data. The iOS Screen Time tracking feature stores and displays screen time for up to 7 days only.	The following screen events can be recorded in real time by a sensing app (e.g., Aware): screen being turned on, turned off, locked, or unlocked. Detailed screen activity is switched off by default, but if tracking is enabled by the user, the data are accessible. Tracking can be disabled, and the data deleted anytime.

phone log and screen time data across the iOS and Android operating systems. As of this writing, phone logs and phone usage data are generally more easily available on Android phones (see www.apple.com/privacy for further information on iOS data collection practices).

In particular, historic data are accessible on Android phones with little to no restrictions; that is, an app running on a participant's phone accessing phone and call logs will be able to access the entirety of the records as long as those have not been deleted by the user. For iOS, the last 1,000 calls are available, yet only 100 are accessible via an iPhone (Bradford, 2021). This means that to look back into their own call history, a user will need to delete an equivalent number of recent calls. For example, a person could delete the last 50 calls up to 20 times depending on how many calls they have made until the call record is empty. Furthermore, iCloud must be active to retain the call history; if it is turned off, all data are stored for 180 days and are then deleted.[1] However, Apple does offer an option to request call log data, which is emailed via spreadsheets and takes up to 7 days to process.

Regarding screen use, a sensing app (e.g., AWARE Framework; see https://awareframework.com/screen) will be able to record when the device's screen is being turned on (i.e., wake mode), turned off (i.e., sleep mode), locked, or unlocked for both iOS and Android.

While not the topic of this chapter, it is worth mentioning that detailed screen activity such as app usage is more difficult to access. On Android devices, the recording of detailed screen activity is switched off by default, but if tracking is enabled by the user, the data get recorded and are in theory accessible to a sensing app. Tracking can be disabled, and the data can be deleted anytime.

For iOS, Apple's support site states that "you can see a summary of your device use for the current day or the past week" using the Screen Time app. The iOS Screen Time tracking feature stores and displays screen time—which includes app usage—for up to 7 days only. However, iOS will not allow other apps on the device to directly access these data. Some apps employ work-arounds such as routing all traffic through a virtual private network (VPN; e.g., Qustodio) or extracting the contents of screenshots users take of the iOS Screen Time tracking feature in the phone's settings (e.g., Moment).

Given that (as of writing this chapter) accessibility of log data are more limited under iOS, there may in many instances be greater opportunities for research afforded using Android devices. In the remainder of this chapter, where possible, we will point out differences with iOS (for further information, see the "Feature Computation" section as well as https://developer.apple.com).

Call and Text Logs

Call logs contain data about the temporal calling patterns of smartphone users, including the frequency and duration of calls placed and received as well as the recipients of such calls across various contexts (Lee, Seo, & Lee, 2010). Text logs contain similar temporal records for messages that were received and sent via the device's Messages app. They typically contain the number of characters and words allowing for potentially more robust analyses (Battestini, Setlur, & Sohn, 2010). Importantly, neither call nor text logs record the contents of the call or text message (such as via an audio file or storing the text sent). Also, note that call and text logs will not include records of calls or messages through other apps with calling or messaging functionality (such as WhatsApp and Facebook Messenger). Depending on the population studied, the preferred communication channels of the participants enrolled in the study might prevent call and text logs from providing an accurate (or approximated) representation of their communication patterns. For example, researchers wishing to study the communication behaviors of students might find that at a specific university, students primarily use WhatsApp and Facebook Messenger for their communication, but a consistent percentage of students' communication goes through the Messages app on their phones. This makes the frequency of messaging a useful relative indicator for identifying more and less social students (even if they are not providing a reliable approximation of their overall communication frequency). On the other hand, it is also imaginable that groups among the student population systematically behave differently (e.g., international students heavily using apps that are popular in their home countries). Cross-cultural differences within as well as between groups can introduce biases related to measurement, construct, sample, device-type user practices, and environmental factors when conducting smartphone sensing research (see Phan, Modersitzki, Gloystein, & Müller, 2022, for in an-depth discussion of this topic). Based on such considerations, researchers might want to consider introducing a prescreen when enrolling participants in a study related to communication patterns.

As of this writing, message data are only available for Android. While call data are available for both iOS and Android, there are some differences. For example, iOS call records create unique traces for each contact even if the user has been in touch with the same contact repeatedly, preventing the computation of metrics such as the number of distinct contacts or amount of interaction with the most frequently called contact. We point the interested reader planning to collect, or already in possession of, data spanning across those two operating systems to the Android and iOS developer documentation (https://developer.android.com and https://developer.apple.com), as well as the documentation for the analysis pipeline in Reproducible Analysis Pipeline for Data Streams (RAPIDS; www.rapids.science/1.9).

Tables 7.2 and 7.3 present hypothetical examples of how such data might be structured for call and text logs (see also, e.g., Beiwe, 2022). Importantly, these data only contain texts and calls issued from native operating system apps (called "Phone" for calls and "Messages" for texts on both iOS and Android). One limiting factor of this approach is that people may use other apps to make calls or send messages (e.g., Facebook Messenger, WhatsApp, Skype, Google Hangouts, and Facetime), which will not be captured in these logs (but rather within those apps). However, the logs allow capturing additional information about communication that would not be accessible through other apps. This, for example, enables identifying the number of communication partners characterizing ongoing communications with specific other parties (e.g., in the context of studying dyads such as romantic relationship partners) or capturing the number of characters and words in a message or the exact duration of a call. In Table 7.2 one user receives more messages than they send, while the other user sends more than they receive.

TABLE 7.2. Example of a Text Message File

User id	Device id	Type	Body word_count	Body_length	Timestamp
12345	16890253647	Inbox	26	150	06:00:01 02 12 2021 GMT+0
12345	16890253647	Inbox	22	120	07:37:12 02 12 2021 GMT+0
12345	16890253647	Sent	11	49	06:28:01 03 12 2021 GMT+0
67890	87263749726	Inbox	29	172	16:09:28 02 12 2021 GMT+1
67890	87263749726	Sent	5	28	17:13:17 03 12 2021 GMT+1
67890	87263749726	Sent	16	83	15:15:22 03 12 2021 GMT+1

TABLE 7.3. Example of a Call File

User id	Device id	Number	Type	Duration	Timestamp
12345	16890253647	A5F2J5	Incoming	9	12:03:04 02 12 2021 GMT+0
12345	16890253647	F5K8H2	Outgoing	26	16:39:21 02 12 2021 GMT+0
12345	16890253647	V2J9S5	Missed	68	07:24:14 03 12 2021 GMT+0
67890	87263749726	K9L3M2	Incoming	35	09:13:56 02 12 2021 GMT+1
67890	87263749726	K9L3M2	Outgoing	145	18:14:34 03 12 2021 GMT+1
67890	87263749726	J1B0X3	Outgoing	509	23:22:24 03 12 2021 GMT+1

User 12345 also has an early morning texting habit, while user 67890 sends most of their messages in the afternoon. Table 7.3 shows that user 67890 places calls to and receives calls from K9L3M2 (a placeholder for the unique hash that allows tracking of ongoing conversations with the same person, bot, company, or other entity without identifying them). The conversations between 67890 and K9L3M2 are also noticeably longer than the other records, suggesting the possibility of a closer relationship.

Screen Use

There are slightly varying definitions of screen use. The World Health Organization (2019), for example, refers to it as "time spent passively watching screen-based entertainment (TV, computer, mobile devices). This does not include active screen-based games where physical activity or movement is required" (p. v). The *Merriam-Webster Dictionary* defines it as "time spent watching television, playing a video game, or using an electronic device with a screen (such as a smartphone or tablet)." These definitions reveal a distinction between active and passive screen use, where the former may have beneficial implications for psychological health (Kaye, Orben, Ellis, Hunter, & Houghton, 2020). This aligns with the work by the nonprofit organization Common Sense Media, which surveys teenagers and young adults in their Common Sense Census (Common Sense, 2022). They have seen steady increases in screen time over the years, with a significant spike during the COVID-19 pandemic. Passive consumption of TV and video makes up the largest part of daily screen use, with about 3 hours of time spent by teenagers and young adults. The second largest category is gaming, with about 1.5 hours spent on this activity daily, reflecting a more active engagement with screens. While the availability of active and passive engagement options with screen media is not new, developments in phone technology have increasingly blurred the lines between TV and phones and allowed for phones to become portable TVs that users can carry in their pockets and interact with at all times (in addition to, of course, many other functionalities).

According to Reeves, Robinson, and Ram (2020), capturing screen use data may be particularly challenging, as studies have largely focused on self-reports of screen use rather than the "moment-by-moment capture of what people are doing and when" (para. 4). In past research, screen use has often been self-reported due to complexities in capturing and classifying such data. Although logging apps can help in collecting more accurate screen use data, they do not "reveal exactly what people are seeing and doing at any given moment" (Reeves et al., 2020, para. 3).

Alcott, Gentzkow, and Song (2021) conducted a study investigating screen use limits for social media use and associated effects on habit forming, self-control issues, and subjective well-being. By utilizing a program called Phone Dashboard to record screen time and establish screen use limits, 2,000 Android phone users were recruited. Participants in the experimental group had the ability to set their own screen use limits directly in Phone Dashboard. Alcott and colleagues found that screen time decreased by more than 20 minutes per day among participants in this group, suggesting a possible correlation between social media and self-control issues. This study exemplifies how a psychological study can leverage instantly capturing screen time activity rather than relying on self-report data.

Introduction of the type of objective measurement possible with smartphones is helping address difficulties in conceptualizing screen use and overcoming the limitations of self-reported data. Kaye and colleagues (2020) recommend focusing on capturing the behaviors screens are facilitating, for example, relating to social, work, or informational use, and thereby putting users' needs at the center of any investigation into the psychological and social correlates of their screen use. This may require analysis of the screen's content, however, which can be achieved through capturing and analyzing users' app usage. Another approach, as employed by the Human Screenome Project at Stanford University, takes screenshots every 5 seconds, which can allow tracking across different platforms if the software is installed on multiple devices (Ram et al., 2020). It is of note that neither of these passive approaches allows capturing whether the phone user processed the information on the screen (or, for example, was looking elsewhere) and how they perceived it (as the same content could be perceived and processed very differently depending on the person and the context they find themselves in). For example, a user might be looking up information about a medical condition that they were recently diagnosed with, or a user might be looking up the same information because they are a medical student preparing for an exam. In its most basic form (and for the purposes of this chapter), however, screen use can refer to the time the screen was on and displaying something to the user.

Table 7.4 shows a hypothetical example of a screen use file. Importantly, these data are only available on Android. Screen logs will typically capture whether the screen came on or went off (which might, for example, be caused by movement or a notification) and whether the user has unlocked or locked the screen (depending on the device, for example, via entering a PIN, or pressing a button or fingerprint reader, or via a face or eye scan).

Practical and Ethical Considerations during Study Setup

Due to the ease of collection and the availability of historic data, we suspect that there will be an increasing volume of large international datasets, studies, and collaborations as time goes on. For the sake of completeness, we therefore point out that in such cases where the data span across vastly different environments and users, systematic sources

TABLE 7.4. Example of a Screen Use File

User id	Device id	Screen status	Timestamp
12345	16890253647	Unlocked	19:03:04 02 12 2021 GMT+0
12345	16890253647	Locked	19:04:50 02 12 2021 GMT+0
12345	16890253647	On	7:35:09 02 13 2021 GMT+0
12345	16890253647	Off	7:35:12 02 13 2021 GMT+00
12345	16890253647	On	9:33:11 02 13 2021 GMT+00
12345	16890253647	Off	9:33:14 02 13 2021 GMT+00
67890	87263749726	Unlocked	09:10:45 02 12 2021 GMT+1
67890	87263749726	Locked	09:21:11 02 12 2021 GMT+1
67890	87263749726	Unlocked	11:22:16 02 12 2021 GMT+1
67890	87263749726	Locked	11:24:08 02 12 2021 GMT+1

of heterogeneity might be introduced in the data that require attention depending on the specific research questions at hand. Blunck and colleagues (2013) note that such sources might include systematic differences in user characteristics (i.e., demographics and practices), devices (i.e., properties and abilities), and environments (i.e., ecology, economy, politics, and culture). Ignoring such sources of variance can introduce systematic biases. For example, differences in phone plan cost in certain countries might influence how many calls users make and text messages they send. Additionally, the smartphone users (or those who are willing to enroll in a study) of one country might be more varied regarding age, while in another country they are predominantly of a younger age bracket.

Furthermore, ethical considerations include communicating clearly to participants which types of data will be collected (especially in the case of accessing historical data) and what will be done with them, while paying particular attention to preserving participant privacy (Tamine & Daoud, 2018). To date, we are not aware of any research showing the specific privacy risks of identifying a person from their phone log data alone, but it is likely that it would be possible to do so, given that, for example, only one spatiotemporal (i.e., latitude, longitude, and time) GPS data point can be sufficient to identify a phone user with close to 100% accuracy (Rossi, Walker, & Musolesi, 2015), or that phone users have a unique app fingerprint allowing their identification across time and even different devices (Kurtz, Gascon, Becker, Rieck, & Freiling, 2016). Phone log data should therefore be treated with the utmost caution. To ensure reproducibility by other researchers, it is advisable that such data not be shared in their raw format but, rather, only make aggregate features available publicly (for examples, see also Harari et al., 2020; Müller, Peters, Matz, Wang, & Harari, 2020).

Data Preprocessing

The particularities of log data compared to the data produced by more traditional data collection methods such as surveys or in-lab experiments are related to the data cleaning and feature computation phases as those will often be far more computationally intensive and technical than, for example, scoring a survey. However, once those steps have been completed, the resulting variables can often be dealt with and entered into statistical models in a very similar manner to how variables resulting from traditional data collection processes would be.

Data Cleaning

As with any data, it is important to inspect the files first and make sure they are in the required format for the following steps. If you are using a workflow management system such as RAPIDS (2022; see the next section), this would mean ensuring that the data format corresponds to the input requirements.

When doing manual data cleaning or if there are specific requirements, the following steps may be worth considering. First, outliers such as "failed to send" texts, "unknown" call types, NAs (i.e., missing data), duplicate, and any other atypical data points should be removed. To the best of our knowledge, this typically only affects a very small portion of users and/or records, and is less common—but certainly not impossible—in system-generated logs compared to "second-hand" logs accessed via a data collection app. Researchers should also consider validating the data entries to ensure no erroneous records are occurring when using a new data source such as a newly developed app. Second, the coding process must be conducted in a consistent way, particularly when combining different samples or data sources such as using existing data collected with different data collection apps (e.g., one data collection app might store call types as "incoming," "outgoing," and "missed," and another app might record these as "call accepted," "call made," and "call missed," respectively). Third, different time zones must be taken into account. Typically, phones will record timestamps in UTC (Coordinated Universal Time, the worldwide primary time standard) with an offset describing the difference between UTC and local time. For example, Pacific Standard Time (PST) corresponds to UTC-08:00; that is, PST is 8 hours behind UTC. Data collection apps do not necessarily follow this convention and might return the timestamp in local time (e.g., PST or GMT). However, many apps (including, e.g., the Aware framework) will provide Unix time. Unix time corresponds to the seconds that have elapsed since 00:00:00 UTC on January 1, 1970. Importantly, this does not take different time zones into account but will be, by definition, provided in UTC. Consequently, researchers working with data from participants located across different time zones will need to take this into account if they are interested in the timing of activities. For example, if the study investigates participants' daily rhythms, it would be important to adjust for different time zones so that the phone records of one participant's afternoon would not be compared with the records of another participants' night but aligned accordingly. This might get complicated further if participants travel over the course of the data collection period. If needed, Unix timestamps can be converted into local time using programming languages such as Python and R or processing tools such as RAPIDS (2022; see the section "Feature Computation" for more details). Fourth, setting a possible subset for the duration of the study (or some other period for which everyone or most participants have data) can be beneficial. Furthermore, there must be clear communication with participants to ensure institutional review board (IRB) compliance, especially for user records outside of the study period, as phone logs will allow access of historic data unless the user has emptied their memory (see the "Data Sources" section in this chapter). Ideally, computing estimates based on the same time frames is good practice and may lead to more consistent results.

Depending on the research question under investigation, one can perform any date conversions they might like, such as adding a variable for weekend days or a variable for time of the day (e.g., morning, afternoon, evening, or night). Lastly, due to the cyclical nature of such data (e.g., fewer calls/messages at night and more on Fridays; Harari et al., 2020, p. 218), one should make sure to perform due diligence prior to cleaning of time/weekly trends.

Feature Computation

Researchers processing phone log data themselves will likely find using a combination of Python and R most useful. Another option is the additional use of a data analysis system such as RAPIDS (Vega et al., 2021; for recent studies using this system, see Moshe et al., 2021; Opoku Asare et al., 2021). RAPIDS is a workflow management system for reproducible data analysis purposes and has been developed to work optimally with data captured (among others) using the AWARE (2021) framework, but it will also work on other files as long as they have the correct configuration. After installing RAPIDS on a computer, data are typically uploaded as a MySQL database or .csv file. Typically, data processing—including feature extraction—is performed at the level of the individual participant. If required for modeling, these individual variables are then merged in a following step. Time segments (frequency, periodic, or event based) are selected as well as whether data come from multiple time zones. The final configuration step is to select which features should be computed (e.g., frequency of outgoing calls, screen time), depending on which types of data are being used. Once these steps have been performed, a simple command executes use of the software for analysis.

Table 7.5 details the types of features available for the different data sources. For the first data type, calling behaviors, features are obtainable for incoming, outgoing, and missed call types. Also, the data provided by Android devices allow aggregation for specific contacts. The second data type, texting behaviors, is only available on Android, with features including type of message received and sent—again, also aggregable for specific contacts. Android features for the third data type, screen use, involves the unlock episode (i.e., the time between consecutive pairs of unlock and off events), while iOS allows consecutive pairs of unlock and lock events.

Furthermore, additional related features can be computed that rely on a combination with other data sources that lie outside of the scope of this chapter. For example, one might be interested in duration of ringing or response time to an incoming call (Stachl et al., 2020). With regards to text messages, it is possible to use data-analytical tools such as Python or R as well as additional data sources that do not get stored by the phone's OS-compute additional metrics such as time between arrival and reading of a message (Pielot, De Oliveira, Kwak, & Oliver, 2014), counts of (potentially multiple) categories of text message contents or topics (e.g., positive vs. negative words; Battestini et al., 2010), variety of simultaneous conversations (Battestini et al., 2010), keystrokes and letter deletions (Bae, Chung, Ferreira, Dey, & Suffoletto, 2018; Buschek, Bisinger, & Alt, 2018), number of words on screenshots, category of currently active applications on screen (e.g., social, games, music, and video), and indicators for screenshots in which participants generate content (e.g., typing/recording a message or social media posts; Reeves et al., 2021). Which features to compute will be guided by the research questions and potentially data availability.

Psychometric Considerations

Smartphone-based metrics such as those described in this chapter are often very skewed and might be highly variable (see, e.g., Harari et al., 2020). This needs to be considered when computing base rates and descriptive statistics and verifying any assumptions that need to be met before applying certain statistical models. Computing base rates and descriptive statistics can also be highly interesting in their own right and potentially merit the main focus of a research study. Depending on the research question at hand, it can also be helpful to explore the relationships of any computed metrics with each other and create composites; one option could be factor analysis (see, e.g., Müller et al., 2020).

Establishing reliability can be a further challenge when employing metrics that have not been previously introduced and studied with regard to their psychometric properties. Relatedly, validity issues may also arise with phone log data. Xu and colleagues (2020) note that this may be due to the choice of analytical software, as "automated algorithms

TABLE 7.5. Overview of Features Describing Calling, Texting, and Screen Use Behaviors

Data type	Possible features	References
Calling behaviors	Number of calls	Harari et al. (2020); RAPIDS (2021)
	Duration of calls	Harari et al. (2020); RAPIDS (2021)
	Android only: Number of unique hash-encoded contacts (overall or for specific call types)	RAPIDS (2021)
	Date and time for a specific call (e.g., first or last call for a specific day)	RAPIDS (2021)
Texting behaviors (Android only)	Number of texts	Harari et al. (2020); RAPIDS (2021)
	Length of texts	Harari et al. (2020); RAPIDS (2021)
	Number of unique hash-encoded contacts (overall or for specific message types)	RAPIDS (2021)
	Date and time for a specific message (e.g., first/last text for a specific day)	RAPIDS (2021)
	Count of unread SMS	Burns et al. (2011)
	Number of conversations (conversation = 2+ text messages, at least one incoming and one outgoing, with a maximum 20-minute response time)	Battestini et al. (2010)
	Number of text messages for single conversations	Battestini et al. (2010)
	Number of simultaneous conversations	Battestini et al. (2010)
	Response time	Battestini et al. (2010)
Combining calling and texting (Android only)	Similarity of calling and messaging contact lists	Stachl et al. (2020)
	Total number of call and text contacts	Stachl et al. (2020)
Screen use	Number of unlock episodes	RAPIDS (2021)
	Duration of unlock episodes	RAPIDS (2021)
	Time of first/last unlock episode for a specific day	RAPIDS (2021)
	Number and duration of lock/unlock events or screen on/off events	Abdullah et al. (2016); Wang et al. (2018)
	Overall phone (non)activity (during a specific time period, e.g., days vs. nights)	Stachl et al. (2020)

Note. Features are aggregated for a specific time period, such as a day or a week. Typically (and where possible), a range of derived statistical parameters such as mean, sum, min, max, entropy, and regularity are included for each feature.

designed to replace human coders in the information-extraction process can make mistakes" (p. 1262). In addition, validity issues could stem from the data generation process itself, as researchers have less control over system-generated data in terms of, for example, establishing the relationship between data points or variables. For instance, shifts in cultural norms about common methods of communication could change the causes of different phone use creating both validity and reliability issues. Reliability or validity issues can also arise regarding whether a certain form of communication becomes encrypted and people start using that form of communication more due to an enhanced sense of privacy, or if the phone software changes how it logs phone usage or significantly alters features (e.g., calls not being limited to voice but also offering a video option).

Visualizations

When building visualizations, key considerations are the target audience and the nature of the report in which they are included. For example, one might choose to display the data differently if individual-level visualizations are made for inclusion in feedback reports about data generated for every study participant as compared to the types of visualization one might choose to include in the write-up of a study for publication in a scientific journal. Examples of such visualizations are included in Harari and colleagues (2020) and RAPIDS as well as in Figure 7.2, which shows the duration of incoming calls for two hypothetical samples. Sample 1 consists of persons with a fairly stable calling behavior during daytime as well as across the week. Sample 2, however, seems to consist of persons who are less active in the morning but comparatively very active in the evenings and night, as well as more active during the weekend than during the week.

Another approach, frequency time charts, is illustrated in Figure 7.3 (see, e.g., Battestini et al., 2010, for additional examples). Here, the user rarely texted between midnight and 6:00 A.M., which seems to be their usual sleeping time. There is higher activity in the evening (7:00 P.M. to 11:00 P.M.) and around lunch time (10:00 A.M. to 1:00 P.M.). On Wednesdays between 3:00 P.M. and 7:00 P.M., the user seems to have some event or activity where they never text. On weekends (Friday 2:00 P.M. to Sunday 2:00 A.M.), the user seems to text more during the day and stay up longer for texting at night than during weekdays.

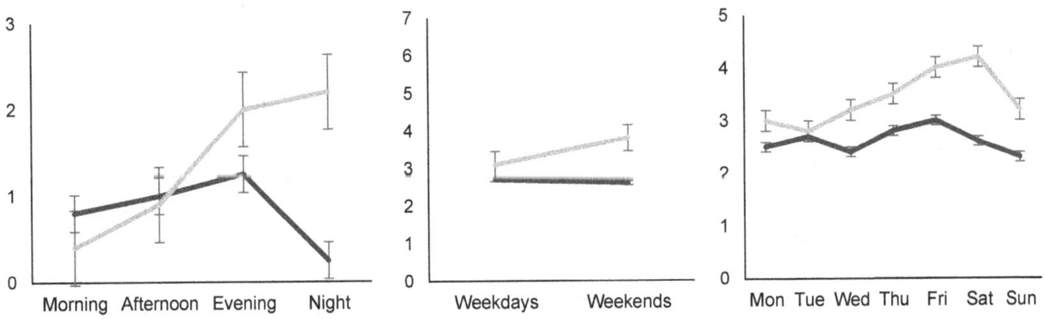

FIGURE 7.2. Example visualizations of hypothetical log data for duration of incoming calls for two different samples.

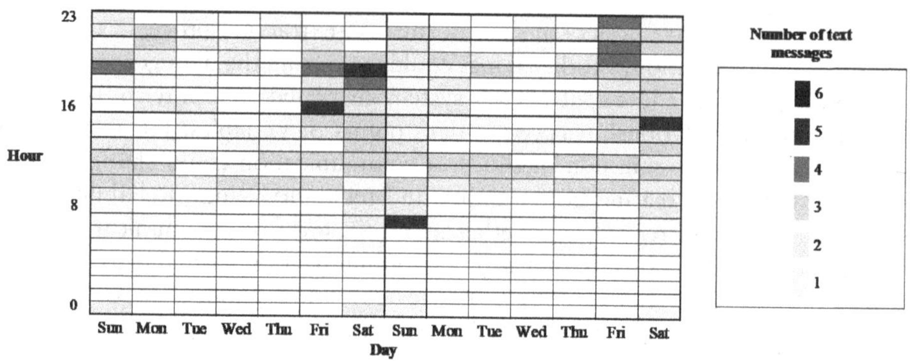

FIGURE 7.3. Time chart of text message frequency of a hypothetical user across 2 weeks.

Similar time use visualizations are also possible for screen use data (with different colors for different apps; see, e.g., the Human Screenome Project; Reeves et al., 2021). Another possibility is circular visualization, that is, displaying patterns/timelines in a circular fashion around a clock center (Reeves et al., 2021). Finally, the clustering of different (and in particular larger quantities of) variables can also be visualized with the help of heatmap colored correlation matrices (see, e.g., Stachl et al., 2020; Wang et al., 2018). Both nomothetic and idiographic approaches can be examined (or even integrated) with such data. For example, users' screen use can be ideographically assessed in their own environments, while nomothetic approaches can be employed to predict future screen use.

Limitations and Future Directions

Limitations

One main limitation of the described approach regarding phone and text logs is that people might use other apps to make calls (e.g., Skype and Facetime) and send messages (e.g., Facebook Messenger and WhatsApp). So far, the number and use of messaging apps have only been increasing over the years (Yu & Poger, 2019). In particular, more privacy-preserving options (e.g., Signal, Telegram, and Threema) have been becoming increasingly popular (Doffman, 2021; Witman, 2021). In light of this change, researchers might want to integrate multiple data sources to collect the data appropriate to their research question (e.g., integrate social media app usage behavior if social behaviors are of interest; see also Harari et al., 2020). We would consider each data source to consist of manifest variables. Researchers should consider whether these variables reflect or form latent variables. However, with the types of data described in this chapter, we imagine that in most cases these variables will be treated as manifest variables. Screen use or battery usage does not usually integrate multiple data sources because only rarely are competing (or complementary) apps for this purpose installed on people's phones. While, for example, a variety of apps and phone behaviors are related to social behaviors (e.g., phone calls, text messages, social media apps), screen usage (if enabled by the user) is usually captured only by an OS-specific app. However, validity analyses can also be performed on these variables with the help of custom-built apps (e.g., Kristensen et al., 2022) and concerted efforts to collect multiple, similar datasets for a user. In addition, there may also be opportunities for using "system" log data such as screen or battery usage for support in addition (or as opposed to) as the "main star" of the analysis. For example, Opoku Asare and colleagues (2021) investigated the percentage of battery charging and discharging to measure user activity, and Chen and colleagues (2013) predicted sleep duration from a number of data points, including the timing and duration of charge events.

Finally, the differences in available data, user behavior, and affordances between different operating systems pose a particular challenge—for both data collection and analysis. Researchers interested in collecting data across, for example, Android and iOS devices will need to use two study apps and take the different data origins into account when analyzing their data.

The mere log data also do not tell you what exactly people saw and processes—only that something was activated on the phone or used. In fact, you often probably do not even know if it was the same user operating the phone (though usually it should be). The point is that even the seemingly more objective data from logs may be devoid of psychological richness and not capture what we think or hope they might capture.

Future Directions

Future work should focus on both identifying and developing additional data sources, as well as ensuring that the currently available data are being leveraged to their maximum potential. Because what we have presented in this chapter is meant to serve as a guide or framework for analyzing phone log data, it might not fully capture the intricacies and complexities of digitally mediated behavior. Therefore, for data already at our disposal, another promising avenue is to relate log data to or combine them with other sensor data, such as calls, texts, and screen usage in different locations; co-usage or parallel activity such as navigating with help of maps app while talking on the phone; or taking a picture to send it over right away. To identify additional data sources from the smartphone in its current configuration, there are some more niche data that (1) have so far received little attention (e.g., battery status, notification settings, other system meta data), (2) have not yet been able to be turned into psychologically meaningful data (e.g., battery status and phone charging behavior), or (3) have not been able to be properly analyzed so far because more specialized and complex techniques are required (e.g., the analysis of typing patterns might require the installation of a separate keyboard and use of advanced statistical techniques such as natural language processing. Furthermore, there might be more log data in the future as phones become increasingly complex with additional sensors added, as well as the Internet of Things, virtual (and augmented) realities, and connected environmental devices and sensors. As such, it is, for example, possible that in the future log data from a smart fridge could be used to infer caloric and nutrient intake (Fujiwara et al., 2018) and for that data to be used for psychological research purposes (e.g., studying relationships between mood, self-regulation, and caloric intake).

We believe that we have only scratched the surface of what technology will enable us to do and that passively collected data will become more and more ubiquitous, informative, and powerful as we learn to leverage it. We hope that this chapter inspires more research using these types of data, as well as a rigorous approach when doing so.

Note

1. Due to conflicting information and limited information regarding Apple's data policies, one should perform their own due diligence when attempting to use iOS for phone log data.

REFERENCES

Abdullah, S., Murname, E. L., Matthews, M., Kay, M., Kientz, J. A., Gay, G., et al. (2016). Cognitive rhythms: Unobtrusive and continuous sensing of alertness using a mobile phone. *Proceedings of the 2016 ACM International Joint Conference on Pervasive and Ubiquitous Computing*, pp. 178–189.

Alcott, H., Gentzkow, M., & Song, L. (2021). *Digital addiction* (NBER Working Paper No. 28936). National Bureau of Economic Research. www.nber.org/papers/w28936

AWARE. (2021). *What Is AWARE?* https://awareframework.com/what-is-aware

Bae, S., Chung, T., Ferreira, D., Dey, A. K., & Suffoletto, B. (2018). Mobile phone sensors and supervised machine learning to identify alcohol use events in young adults: Implications for just-in-time adaptive interventions. *Addictive Behaviors, 83*, 42–47.

Battestini, A., Setlur, V., & Sohn, T. (2010). A large scale study of text-messaging use. *Proceedings of the 12th International Conference on Human Computer Interaction with Mobile Devices and Services*, pp. 229–238.

Beiwe. (2022). *Passive data.* http://wiki.beiwe.org/wiki/Passive_Data#Phone_Call_Log_Data_.28Android_Only.29

Blunck, H., Bouvin, N. O., Franke, T., Grønbæk, K., Kjaergaard, M. B., Lukowicz, P., & Wüstenberg, M. (2013). On heterogeneity in mobile sensing applications aiming at representative data collection. *Proceedings of the 2013 ACM Conference on Pervasive and Ubiquitous Computing Adjunct Publication*, pp. 1087–1098.

Bradford, A. (2021, May 11). How to view (and delete) your iPhone's call history. *Reader's Digest*. www.rd.com/article/iphone-call-history

Buschek, D., Bisinger, B., & Alt, F. (2018, April). ResearchIME: A mobile keyboard application for studying free typing behaviour in the wild. *Proceedings of the 2018 CHI Conference on Human Factors in Computing Systems*, pp. 1–14.

Chen, Z., Lin, M., Chen, F., Lane, N. D., Cardone, G., Wang, R., et al. (2013, May). Unobtrusive sleep monitoring using smartphones. In *2013 7th International Conference on Pervasive Computing Technologies for Healthcare and Workshops* (pp. 145–152). IEEE.

Common Sense. (2022). *The Common Sense Census: Media use by tweens and teens 2021.* www.commonsensemedia.org/research/the-common-sense-census-media-use-by-tweens-and-teens-2021

Doffman, Z. (2021, January 9). Do you suddenly need to stop using WhatsApp? *Forbes*. www.forbes.com/sites/zakdoffman/2021/01/09/stop-using-whatsapp-after-facebook-apple-imessage-and-signal-privacy-backlash

Fujiwara M., Moriya K., Sasaki W., Fujimoto M., Arakawa Y., & Yasumoto K. (2018). A smart fridge for efficient foodstuff management with weight sensor and voice interface. *Proceedings of the 47th International Conference on Parallel Processing Companion*, pp. 1–7.

Groves, M. R. (2011). Three eras of survey research. *Public Opinions Quarterly, 75*(5), 861–871.

Harari, G. M., Müller, S. R., Stachl, C., Wang, R., Wang, W., Bühner, M., et al. (2020). Sensing sociability: Individual differences in young adults' conversation, calling, texting, and app use behaviors in daily life. *Journal of Personality and Social Psychology, 119*(1), 204–228.

Kaye, L. K., Orben, A., Ellis, D. A., Hunter, S. C., & Houghton, S. (2020). The conceptual and methodological mayhem of "screen time." *International Journal of Environmental Research and Public Health, 17*(10), 3661.

Kristensen, P. L., Olesen, L. G., Egebæk, H. K., Pedersen, J., Rasmussen, M. G., & Grøntved, A. (2022). Criterion validity of a research-based application for tracking screen time on android and iOS smartphones and tablets. *Computers in Human Behavior Reports, 5*, 100164.

Kurtz, A., Gascon, H., Becker, T., Rieck, K., & Freiling, F. (2016). Fingerprinting mobile devices using personalized configurations. In *Proceedings on Privacy Enhancing Technologies* (pp. 4–19). DeGruyter.

Lee, S., Seo, J., & Lee, G. (2010). An adaptive speed-call list algorithm and its evaluation with ESM. In *Proceedings of the SIGCHI Conference on Human Factors in Computing Systems* (pp. 2019–2022). ACM.

Moshe, I., Terhorst, Y., Opoku Asare, K., Sander, L. B., Ferreira, D., Baumeister, H., et al. (2021). Predicting symptoms of depression and anxiety using smartphone and wearable data. *Frontiers in Psychiatry, 12*, 1–12.

Müller, S. R., Peters, H., Matz, S. C., Wang, W., & Harari, G. M. (2020). Investigating the relationships between mobility behaviours and indicators of subjective well-being using smartphone-based experience sampling and GPS tracking. *European Journal of Personality, 34*(5), 714–732.

Opoku Asare, K., Terhorst, Y., Vega, J., Peltonen, E., Lagerspetz, E., & Ferreira, D. (2021). Predicting depression from smartphone behavioral markers using machine learning methods, hyper-parameter optimization, and feature importance analysis: An exploratory study. *JMIR mHealth and uHealth, 9*(7), 1–17.

Phan, L., Modersitzki, N., Gloystein, K. K., & Müller, S. (2022, January 5). *Mobile sensing around the globe: Considerations for cross-cultural research.* https://doi.org/10.31234/osf.io/q8c7y

Pielot, M., De Oliveira, R., Kwak, H., & Oliver, N. (2014, April). Didn't you see my message?: Predicting attentiveness to mobile instant messages. In *Proceedings of the SIGCHI Conference on Human Factors in Computing Systems* (pp. 3319–3328). ACM.

Ram, N., Yang, X., Cho, M. J., Brinberg, M., Muirhead, F., Reeves, B., & Robinson, T. N. (2020). Screenomics: A new approach for observing and studying individuals' digital lives. *Journal of Adolescent Research, 35*(1), 16–50.

RAPIDS. (2022). *RAPIDS v 1.9.1.* www.rapids.science/1.9

Reeves, B., Ram, N., Robinson, T. N., Cummings, J. J., Giles, C. L., Pan, J., et al. (2021). Screenomics: A framework to capture and analyze personal life experiences and the ways that technology shapes them. *Human-Computer Interaction, 36*(2), 150–201.

Reeves, B., Robinson, T., & Ram, N. (2020). Time for the Human Screenome Project. *Nature, 577*(7790), 314–317.

Rossi, L., Walker, J., & Musolesi, M. (2015). Spatio-temporal techniques for user identification by means of GPS mobility data. *EPJ Data Science, 4*, 1–16.

Stachl, C., Au, Q., Schoedel, R., Gosling, S. D., Harari, G. M., Buschek, D., et al. (2020). Predicting personality from patterns of behavior collected with smartphones. *Proceedings of the National Academy of Sciences, 117*(30), 17680–17687.

Tamine, L., & Daoud, M. (2018). Evaluation in contextual information retrieval: Foundations and recent advances within the challenges of context dynamicity and data privacy. *ACM Computing Surveys, 51*(4), 1–36.

Vega, J., Li, M., Aguillera, K., Goel, N., Joshi, E., Durica, K. C., et al. (2021). Reproducible Analysis Pipeline for Data Streams (RAPIDS): Open source software to process data collected with mobile devices. *Frontiers in Digital Health, 3*, 1–8.

Wang, R., Wang, W., DaSilva, A., Huckins, J. F., Kelley, W. M., Heatherton, T. F., & Campbell, A. T. (2018). Tracking depression dynamics in college students using mobile phone and wearable sensing. *Proceedings of the ACM on Interactive, Mobile, Wearable and Ubiquitous Technologies, 2*(1), 1–26.

Witman, E. (2021, January 29). Is Telegram secure?: Here's what you need to know about the messaging app that rivals WhatsApp and Signa. *Business Insider.* www.businessinsider.com/is-telegram-secure

World Health Organization. (2019). *Guidelines on physical activity, sedentary behaviour and sleep for children under 5 years of age.* https://apps.who.int/iris/handle/10665/311664

Xu, H., Zhang, N., & Zhou, L. (2020). Validity concerns in research using organic data. *Journal of Management, 46*(7), 1257–1274.

Yu, S., & Poger, S. (2019). Modeling social influence in mobile messaging apps. In J. Miller, E. Stroulia, K. Lee, & L. J. Zhang (Eds.), *International Conference on Web Services 2019* (Lecture Notes in Computer Science, Vol. 11512). Springer.

CHAPTER 8

Mobile Application Usage in Psychological Research

Larissa Sust, Sanaz Talaifar, and Clemens Stachl

CHAPTER OVERVIEW

App usage data provide some of the most psychologically rich information one can collect using mobile sensing methods. Here, we discuss how data from the applications ("apps") people use to enhance the functionality of their mobile devices can advance research in all subdisciplines of psychology. First, we describe prior psychological work on app usage behavior. Next, we provide a detailed guide for researchers interested in working with app usage data. Specifically, we discuss different ways to (1) collect app usage data (e.g., usage logs, screenshots), (2) categorize individual apps and app categories, (3) analyze app usage data (e.g., considering app adoption, usage quantities, sequences, within-app behavior), and (4) enrich app usage data (e.g., using application programming interfaces [APIs], experience sampling). We conclude by discussing technical and ethical challenges posed by app usage research, as well as an outlook on the future of app usage on new kinds of mobile devices.

Virtually all user activity on a smartphone is mediated through "apps," short for "applications." Apps are defined as "self-contained software designed for a mobile device and performing specific tasks for mobile users" (Amalfitano, Fasolino, Tramontana, & Robbins, 2013, p. 002), developed with "the limitations and features of mobile devices in mind" (Clement, 2019). On a smartphone, calling, texting, surfing the Web, taking a photo, sending an email, examining a map, buying a product, listening to a song, and so on all require the user to open and interact with an application. Arguably, apps are what distinguish smartphones from regular mobile phones. After all, apps were the channel through which companies like Apple expanded the basic functionality of the phone, turning it from a device used primarily to make calls and send texts to a full-fledged computer that put the internet in people's pockets. For Apple, the competitive advantage offered by apps was so important that, in 2010, they trademarked the phrase "There's an app for that." Today, this phrase is truer than ever: There are almost 2 million apps in Apple's App Store and more than 2.5 million apps in the Google Play Store (Clement, 2020).

Given the centrality of the app to the user's experience of the smartphone, it is surprising that researchers interested in mobile sensing methods have devoted so little attention to app usage. The lack of research examining app usage is even harder to understand when one considers the kinds of psychological insights that app usage has the potential to reveal. As this chapter will show, app usage provides a rich window into people's lives and thus can be used to advance research in all subdisciplines of psychology.

This chapter provides an organizing framework for the analysis of app usage data, aiming to lower the barriers of entry for this kind of research. The first section describes prior work conducted with app usage data. After describing *what* has been done, we outline *how* researchers can go about collecting and analyzing app usage data in their own research. More specifically, in the second section, we discuss how app usage can be collected through self-reports, usage logs, and screenshots on phones running on the Android and the iPhone operating system (iOS). In the third section, we propose several ways of characterizing and analyzing the usage of individual apps and app categories, considering usage quantity, sequences, and within-app behavior. Finally, we provide an outlook on the future of app usage research.

Overview of Existing Research That Leverages App Usage

In this section, we provide a short overview of past studies that have investigated app usage for research purposes. We start by briefly reviewing research in human–computer interaction before describing app usage research in various subdisciplines of psychology. These studies serve as initial inspiration for how psychologists can leverage app usage to understand human cognition, emotion, and behavior. However, because research on app usage in psychology is still quite scarce, we provide further ideas for how it could be used in future research.

Two caveats are worth noting regarding the existing app usage research reviewed in this section. First, the vast majority of studies on mobile application usage have relied exclusively on data from Android phones because app usage data is currently almost impossible to log on iPhones. Such restrictions were implemented by Apple to protect the personal data of smartphone users, but they also impose obvious challenges to researchers. To our knowledge, only two studies have analyzed iPhone app usage by modifying the iPhone (Gordon et al., 2019; Morrison, Xiong, Higgs, Bell, & Chalmers, 2018). We return to methods for circumventing the limitations presented by iPhones (e.g., through the use of screenshots rather than app usage logs) in our section on the collection of app usage data. Second, although apps can be installed on other mobile devices like tablets, we focus specifically on smartphone app usage because this has been the focus of most research. We return to the issue of app usage on other devices in our outlook on the future of apps.

App Usage in Human–Computer Interaction Research

Most past studies on mobile app usage have been conducted by human–computer interaction (HCI) researchers interested in describing, understanding, and predicting how people use apps on their phones. (For a review of investigations of app usage in HCI, refer to Church, Ferreira, Banovic, & Lyons, 2015.) These studies examine user behavior with the goal of optimizing the usability and user experience of phones or individual apps. For example, knowing when people are likely to open an app (Hang & De Luca, 2013; Xu et al., 2013) can serve to programmatically optimize the starting routines of apps. The earliest HCI reports systematically investigating mobile application use date back to 2005 (Demumieux & Losquin, 2005; Froehlich, Chen, Consolvo, Harrison, & Landay, 2007). These early, small-scale studies were the first to keep track of app-related events that happen on early generation mobile phones through system logs. These researchers recognized logging app usage as an opportunity to objectively analyze what people do with their phones.

One of the first large-scale studies on smartphone app usage was conducted by Böhmer, Hecht, Schöning, Krüger, and Bauer (2011). Their study used a custom logging app to record app usage from 4,100 smartphone users and provided descriptive estimates on average daily app usage. Specifically, the study described app usage with regard to the time of day (e.g., less overall usage at night, news apps in the morning), the length of app usage sessions (i.e., the amount of time spent continuously using applications), and the sequence in which participants tended to use apps (e.g., "Communication–Camera–Communication"). The study also provided the first description of how apps are used differently across cultures and contexts. For example, European participants in their sample were 1.21 times more likely to use an internet browser app in comparison to participants from the United States, who seemed to rely more heavily on specific apps. Recent studies have been able to replicate most of Böhmer and colleagues' (2011) findings (Church et al., 2015; Ferreira, Goncalves, Kostakos, Barkhuus, & Dey, 2014; Gordon et al., 2019; Morrison et al., 2018; Welke, Andone, Blaszkiewicz, & Markowetz, 2016).

While research in HCI was not conducted with psychological research questions in mind, their findings and methods are very relevant to psychological science. Descriptive studies of naturalistic app usage, for example, essentially discuss what psychologists would refer to as daily behavior measured in the field. Similarly, studies in computer science aiming to predict personality traits from application usage for the purpose of personalizing smartphone services (Chittaranjan, Blom, & Gatica-Perez, 2013; De Montjoye, Quoidbach, Robic, & Pentland, 2013) can provide valuable input for research in personality and social psychology.

App Usage in Psychological Research

Compared to the breadth of empirical studies in HCI, app usage has rarely been studied in psychological science, despite the fact that the potential of smartphones for research in psychology has been highlighted repeatedly (Harari et al., 2016; Harari, Müller, Aung, & Rentfrow, 2017; Miller, 2012). The vast quantity and diversity of apps, as well as the highly idiosyncratic way they are used by each person, make app usage ideal for investigating intra- and interindividual differences in the wild. In fact, individuals' app usage data alone can successfully identify unique users (Tu et al., 2018). Perhaps unsurprisingly then, researchers in personality and differential psychology were the first to investigate how app usage maps on to individual differences in self-reported personality traits.

Initial studies in personality psychology correlated self-reported app usage and the Big Five personality traits (openness, conscientiousness, extraversion, agreeableness, and emotional stability) (Butt & Phillips, 2008; Kim, Briley, & Ocepek, 2015; Lane, 2012). These early studies did not fully capitalize on the potential of app usage for objectively capturing daily behavior since self-reports are subject to a number of limitations such as social desirability, memory-related, and response-style biases (Paulhus & Vazire, 2007; Van Vaerenbergh & Thomas, 2013). In fact, there are large discrepancies between self-reported digital media use and actual digital media use (Davidson, Shaw, & Ellis, 2022; Parry et al., 2021).

More recent and methodologically advanced studies in personality psychology have quantified app usage via direct measurement of the phone's app usage logs (Chittaranjan et al., 2013; Harari et al., 2019; Montag et al., 2015; Schoedel et al., 2019; Stachl et al., 2017, 2020). Many of these studies focused on communication and social behavior, finding that communication apps tend to be more frequently used by people with higher scores in extraversion (Harari et al., 2019; Montag et al., 2015; Stachl et al., 2017) and less frequently by people with lower scores in emotional stability (Harari et al., 2019; Stachl et al., 2020). A few studies have started to investigate apps beyond those used primarily for communication (Chittaranjan et al., 2013; Schoedel et al., 2019; Stachl et al., 2017, 2020). For example, studies show that conscientiousness is negatively associated with the use of gaming apps (Stachl et al., 2017) and positively associated with the use of weather apps (Stachl et al., 2020).

Personality traits are not the only psychological construct related to app usage data. In the area of clinical psychology, mobile app usage holds great potential for the investigation and assessment of clinically relevant constructs and psychopathology (Thomeé, 2018). Even though clinical research on app usage is scarce, one study (Gao, Li, Zhu, Liu, & Liu, 2016) showed that use of certain app categories is related to social anxiety and loneliness. For example, higher loneliness scores were associated with more frequent use of apps from the categories "health and fitness," "browser," and "social media." Findings like these might help to better explain the mechanisms perpetuating certain psychopathologies. Furthermore, if mental disorders have behavioral correlates in mobile app usage, mobile sensing could serve as a way to assess and detect these disorders earlier on.

A few pioneering studies have started to evaluate whether behavioral data from smartphones can help predict disorders such as depression, schizophrenia, and anxiety (Fukazawa et al., 2019; Saeb et al., 2016; Saeb, Lattie, Schueller, Kording, & Mohr, 2015; Wang et al., 2014). These studies have mostly relied on parameters of physical activity (e.g., accelerometer) rather than app use. However, the incorporation of app usage data could further improve the prediction of psychopathological episodes or onsets (Tuarob et al., 2017) because behaviors that are mediated by apps (e.g., music consumption, social media use) have been previously found to be related to mental disorders (Miranda & Claes, 2008; Woods & Scott, 2016). If early-stage pathologies can be predicted with sufficient accuracy, mobile apps could notify a person or health care provider about the possible onset of, for example, a depressive episode and the need to seek professional assessment and help (Ferdous, Osmani, & Mayora, 2015).

App usage data can also provide information about more specific, clinically relevant symptoms. Mood states, which are a critical aspect of the majority of mental disorders, might be reflected in mobile app usage. This is supported by preliminary results from Ferdous and colleagues (2015) who predicted stress levels from app usage logs. Although the study's very small sample (N = 28) undermines its generalizability, the study highlights the potential of longitudinal app usage data for investigating affective and other clinically relevant states. For example, sleep duration and quality, which have also been linked to psychological disorders, could be detected by considering app use throughout the night. Some sleep research shows that chronobiological daytime–nighttime behaviors can indeed be inferred from the usage of certain apps (e.g., alarm clock apps in the morning; Peng & Zhu, 2020; Schoedel et al., 2020). Again, the detection of poor mood or sleep could serve as a trigger for optimally timing clinical interventions (e.g., therapy sessions or exercises).

Because most mobile sensing studies are observational, mobile app usage can usually be considered only as a correlate of mental disorders or symptoms; its causal role in relation to such disorders remains unclear (Thomeé, 2018). The use of certain apps might very well causally contribute to psychopathology. One obvious example is smartphone addiction, which can be predicted from the increased usage of specific app categories such as social media or gaming apps (Choi et al., 2017). In contrast, mobile app usage might also have positive effects on well-being. From a health psychology perspective, there are many health and mental wellness apps (varying in quality) that aim to improve various aspects of users' well-being, ranging from apps that reduce stress to those that encourage physical exercise. Here, app usage data can help to test the negative or positive effect of the use of certain apps.

The efficacy of health apps for changing cognition or behavior has mostly been investigated in experimental designs without mobile sensing (e.g., Bostock, Crosswell, Prather, & Steptoe, 2019; Flett, Hayne, Riordan, Thompson, & Conner, 2019). However, sensing app usage could help to clarify whether health apps were regularly used. Furthermore, app usage data, including the mere presence of health apps on a person's phone, could reveal health-related behavior change goals or needs. Indeed, in 2012, one in five smartphone users in the United States had at least one health-related app installed on their phone (Krebs & Duncan, 2015).

Beyond personality and clinical psychology, the analysis of mobile app usage can also be adopted by cognitive psychologists to complement and extend rigorous laboratory studies with more objective, *in vivo* measurements of behavior. However, at this point, more exploratory research is needed to identify the cognitive correlates of mobile app usage. Aside from investigating the associations between fluid intelligence and the usage frequency of lifestyle apps (Stachl et al., 2017), these cognitive markers could, for example, be found by analyzing behavior in mobile gaming apps (Quiroga et al., 2015) or in other apps that require sensory discrimination (Melnick, Harrison, Park, Bennetto, & Tadin, 2013). Recently, researchers have analyzed app usage behaviors to identify cognitive impairments in the elderly (Rauber, Fox, & Gatys, 2019). Similarly, preliminary research has shown that app usage can discriminate between cognitively impaired and healthy adults (Gordon et al., 2019). These results provide some initial evidence that the number of apps a person uses seems to be an indicator of cognitive health. Such findings from exploratory mobile sensing research can be used for inductive theory generation and refinement. Cognitive scientists might begin to theorize about why certain patterns of app usage behavior are more indicative of cognitive functionality than others, even if the total frequency or duration of app usage is the same.

Another, more applied area of psychological research that could directly benefit from data on app usage is marketing psychology. Most obviously, many companies track the use of their branded apps to measure and enhance user engagement (Khomych, 2019). An area that has received less attention is how personality traits predicted from app usage data (Stachl et al., 2020) could improve the effectiveness of personalized advertisements within smartphone apps. A similar approach has already been tested for personality predictions based on social media usage data (Matz, Kosinski, Nave, & Stillwell, 2017).

App usage may also be relevant to researchers in industrial and organizational (I/O) psychology to the extent that apps can be used to address personnel selection and productivity in the workplace. Given the previously mentioned relationships between app usage and certain traits known to predict job performance (e.g., conscientiousness, cognitive ability; Avis, Kudisch, & Fortunato, 2002; Schmidt, 2002), app usage could be used in the future as a tool in employee selection if research shows that the predictive validity of sensed data rivals the predictive validity of data collected with more conventional assessment methods. Indeed, some companies have "gamified" their hiring practices, leveraging the assumption that skills displayed in gaming apps can be indicators of job-relevant skills (Georgiou, Gouras, & Nikolaou, 2019). It is also conceivable, though ethically questionable, to study employee productivity by tracking the amount of time spent on work-related (e.g., email apps) versus leisure apps (e.g., social media apps). Similar practices have recently produced a backlash against large companies (e.g., Lecher, 2019; Yeginsu, 2018). Therefore, we want to highlight that, especially in the realm of marketing and I/O, smartphone sensing methods generally and app usage data in particular present ethical challenges.

How to Collect App Usage Data

Now that we have highlighted existing research on mobile app usage, we describe how researchers can collect app usage data. There are different approaches to measuring app usage, which differ in both technical sophistication and the granularity of the resulting data. The approach one chooses depends in part on the operating system of the participants' devices. In recent years, the number of available mobile operating systems has shrunk from several dozen to two systems dominating the market. In 2020, Android smartphones made up about three-quarters of the worldwide smartphone market and the iOS operating system running on iPhones comprised the remaining quarter (O'Dea, 2020a). Other mobile operating systems (e.g., Windows, Blackberry) have become relatively rare and are therefore less relevant for researchers at the moment. Thus, here we focus exclusively on the Android and iOS operating systems.

Self-Reports

As previously mentioned, the very first attempts to quantify app usage behavior in psychology followed the well-beaten path of using self-reports to quantify behaviors. For example, Kim and colleagues (2015) asked participants to indicate whether they used a particular type of application, while Alkhalaf, Tekian, and Park (2018) investigated self-reported daily app usage durations. Similarly, Lane (2012) had participants rate the importance of different app types. These pioneering studies reported the first insights into app usage behavior, but their data were affected by the well-known problems inherent to self-reports (Baumeister, Vohs, & Funder, 2007; Boase & Ling, 2013; Paulhus & Vazire, 2007; Van Vaerenbergh & Thomas, 2013). In particular, given the increasing speed at which people switch between large numbers of apps, it is very difficult for participants to accurately reconstruct their app usage at fine granularities (Reeves et al., 2021). Therefore, retrospective self-reports are not a good choice for assessing app usage behavior. They are, however, useful for screening participants for different mobile operating systems or for usage of certain apps relevant to a specific research question (e.g., "Do you use apps for fishing?").

Accessing Usage Logs

The current gold-standard method for quantifying app usage involves accessing the smartphone's app usage logs. Android offers an API that lists the apps users have installed at a given point in time. This API can be incorporated into a custom sensing research app that, once installed by participants, retrieves the full list of apps on participants' devices (Frey, Xu, & Ilic, 2017; Seneviratne, Seneviratne, Mohapatra, & Mahanti, 2014a, 2014b; Xu, Frey, Fleisch, & Ilic, 2016).

To get data on the actual usage (rather than mere presence) of apps, researchers can develop more sophisticated applications that regularly retrieve system statistics for which apps are being used over a period of time. This logging approach generates a timestamp-sorted list of usage events that can be aggregated to obtain usage frequencies or durations (for more details, see the section "App Usage Quantity"). In Table 8.1, we provide an exemplary app usage log from an Android smartphone, collected with the PhoneStudy mobile sensing app (Schoedel, Kunz, et al., 2022; Stachl et al., 2020). The list contains the time and date of each event, as well as the description of the app used during the event. For example, Table 8.1 shows that the smartphone user opened the Twitter app on October 5, 2014, at 08:22:04 A.M.

Currently, there are multiple free and open-source Android research apps that read out app usage statistics (e.g., the AWARE mobile sensing framework; Ferreira, Kostakos, & Dey, 2015). In addition, a number of commercial businesses offer sensing study research services, with mobile apps capable of sensing Android app usage (e.g., EARS: Lind, Byrne, Wicks, Smidt, & Allen, 2018; the Murmuras framework: Andone et al., 2016; the Insights app: Montag et al., 2019; movisens services: Movisens GmbH, 2020). Several research groups around the world have also developed custom mobile sensing apps (e.g., the Emotion Sense app: Servia-Rodriguez et al., 2017; the StudentLife app: Wang et al., 2014), some of which allow for the logging of app use (e.g., the PhoneStudy app: Stachl et al., 2020).

For all solutions presented above, app-logging is currently possible only on the Android operating system. For iOS, it is more difficult to measure app use because Apple prohibits third-party access to app usage logs. Currently, the only option to directly access app usage logs on iPhones is to remove the software restrictions imposed by Apple with "jailbroken" devices. The jailbreak enables root access to the iOS operating system and allows for the installation of specially programmed mobile sensing applications (Gordon et al., 2019; Morrison et al., 2018). The practical implementation of the jailbreak approach for research purposes is controversial. Participants in mobile sensing studies are usually asked to use their own phones for the duration of the study. Deliberately jailbreaking participants' own iPhones is not advisable from an ethical and legal perspective since the jailbreak is not authorized and can cause warranty issues for users. One solution is to recruit iPhone users who already have jailbroken devices (Morrsion et al., 2018). However, this sample is most likely not fully representative of iOS users, as users who jailbreak their iPhones tend to be older and more technically literate (McMillan, Morrison, & Chalmers, 2013). An alternative study design was introduced by Gordon and colleagues (2019), who cooperated with Apple to provide participants with specially modified iPhones for the duration of the study period, allowing them access to phone logs. To our knowledge, Gordon and colleagues and Morrison and colleagues (2018) are the only two published studies directly measuring app usage from iPhone logs.

TABLE 8.1. App Usage and Screen Activity Logs on Android

Timestamp	Time	Date	App/activity	Android package
1,412,490,008,000.00	08:20:08	2014-10-05	ON_LOCKED	
1,412,497,210,000.00	08:20:10	2014-10-05	ON_UNLOCKED	
1,412,497,228,000.00	08:20:28	2014-10-05	Instagram	com.instagram.android
1,412,497,324,000.00	08:22:04	2014-10-05	Twitter	com.twitter.android
1,412,497,510,000.00	08:25:10	2014-10-05	Homescreen	com.android.systemui
1,412,497,516,000.00	08:25:16	2014-10-05	OFF_LOCKED	
1,412,497,523,000.00	08:25:23	2014-10-05	ON_LOCKED	
1,412,497,528,000.00	08:25:28	2014-10-05	ON_UNLOCKED	
1,412,497,531,000.00	08:25:32	2014-10-05	Weather	com.sec.android.widgetapp.ap.hero.accuweather
1,412,497,544,000.00	08:25:44	2014-10-05	Homescreen	com.android.systemui
1,412,497,572,000.00	08:26:12	2014-10-05	OFF_LOCKED	
1,412,499,304,000.00	08:55:04	2014-10-05	ON_LOCKED	
1,412,499,306,000.00	08:55:06	2014-10-05	ON_UNLOCKED	
1,412,499,306,000.00	08:55:06	2014-10-05	PopupuiReceiver	com.sec.android.app.popupuireceiver
1,412,499,336,000.00	08:55:36	2014-10-05	Push-Ups	com.runtastic.android.pushup.lite
1,412,499,397,000.00	08:56:37	2014-10-05	OFF_LOCKED	
1,412,499,921,000.00	09:05:21	2014-10-05	ON_LOCKED	
1,412,499,922,000.00	09:05:22	2014-10-05	ON_UNLOCKED	
1,412,499,927,000.00	09:05:27	2014-10-05	Wash Post	com.washingtonpost.rainbow
1,412,500,671,000.00	09:17:51	2014-10-05	SMS/MMS	com.android.mms
1,412,500,677,000.00	09:17:57	2014-10-05	Homescreen	com.android.systemui
1,412,500,680,000.00	09:18:00	2014-10-05	OFF_LOCKED	
1,412,500,756,000.00	09:19:16	2014-10-05	ON_LOCKED	

Note. The table illustrates timestamp-sorted app usage (shaded rows) and screen activity (unshaded rows) logs from an Android smartphone, collected with the PhoneStudy mobile sensing application. These logs reveal date, time, and name of a launched app, which can be used to calculate usage durations for individual apps (i.e., the time between the launch of an app and the next app launch or a screen switch off) or sessions when several apps were used. This particular user's logs reveal four active smartphone usage sessions where the apps "Instagram," "Twitter," "AccuWeather," "Runtastic Push-Ups," "Washington Post," and "SMS/MMS" were used. The phone's own system apps "Homescreen" and "PopupuiReceiver" (an app delivering pop-up notifications) were also used during these sessions.

Screenshot-Based Data Collection

Complementing the straightforward approach of accessing usage logs, researchers have developed more creative ways to measure app usage behavior with smartphone screenshots. One screenshot approach leverages the self-tracking feature included on many smartphones. Researchers can infer the daily or weekly duration of app usage from users' screenshots of the system-inherent Digital Wellbeing tool on Android (version 9 and higher) and the Screen Time application on iOS (iOS 12 and higher; Gower & Moreno., 2018; Sewall, Bear, Merranko, & Rosen, 2020). For example, participants can be instructed as part of an experience sampling protocol (Gower & Moreno, 2018; Ubochi, 2019) to take a screenshot of the Screen Time application at the end of the day. These screenshots would depict the usage duration for each app they opened that day, both on the level of individual apps and by app category (see Figure 8.1 for an exemplary screenshot). Timing is of the essence because screenshots taken too early in the day might miss important app usage behaviors. Another practical consideration is that researchers must specify whether participants should take only one screenshot of the most used

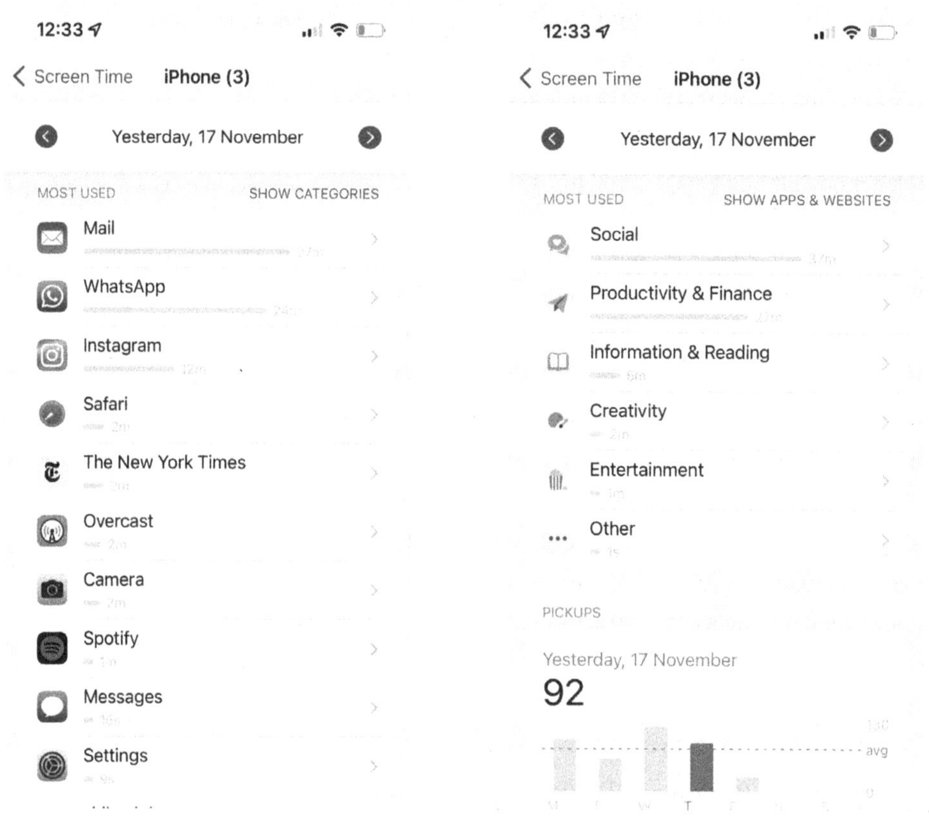

FIGURE 8.1. Manual screenshots of daily app usage durations on iOS as provided by the Apple Screen Time app. The figure on the left depicts app usage duration at the app level. The figure on the right depicts app usage duration at the category level. Screenshots can be taken for the present day or the day before. In addition to daily app usage estimates, the Apple Screen Time app also provides weekly usage estimates.

applications or several screenshots to capture all apps that have been used on a given day. Recording the most used apps may be sufficient given that smartphone users spend more than 50% of their time in one app and 97% in their top 10 apps (Comscore, 2017).

One limitation of this manual screenshot approach is that screenshots do not allow for the inference of daytime distributions or frequencies of app usage, which may be needed for certain research questions (e.g., chronotype studies). That said, given the difficulty of collecting data from iPhone app logs, this approach may be useful for researchers interested in collecting data from participants with iOS phones. Moreover, the approach might even be transferred to other, less common operating systems (e.g., Windows phones), as long as they have system-inherent or third-party apps for self-tracking app usage (e.g., the Digitox app). As a hybrid approach between screenshots and self-reports, the app usage summaries from self-tracking apps may also be assessed via questionnaires, for example, by asking participants to manually transfer their usage durations to daily (or weekly) surveys.

A second, more elaborate method for retrieving information on app usage from smartphone screenshots has recently been introduced by Reeves and colleagues (2021). They developed the Screenomics application for Android, which automatically captures screenshots of participants' visible smartphone screens at researcher-chosen intervals (e.g., every 5 seconds) whenever the screen is on (Reeves et al., 2021; Yang, Ram, Robinson, & Reeves, 2019). This method is unparalleled, as it enables researchers to capture the full app usage experience as a sequence of viewed screens, which, in turn, allows for even richer analysis. Researchers can investigate both quantitative aspects of app usage (e.g., duration or frequency) *and* qualitative aspects of the behavior performed within an app (e.g., what an individual is viewing, typing). A potential downside of this approach is that only behaviors that are visible on the screen during the sampling window (e.g., every 5 seconds) can be collected. For example, connectivity data (e.g., Bluetooth, Wifi), behaviors that occur with the screen turned off (e.g., calls, music listening, fitness tracking) or that fall outside the sampling window (e.g., some notifications), will be missed if only periodic screenshots are collected.

Researchers interested in this approach should be aware that extracting data from such a vast number of smartphone screenshots requires laborious data preprocessing efforts. To investigate app usage, screenshots have to be classified according to the specific application being used (Chiatti et al., 2019; Ram et al., 2020). The manual annotation of screenshots is very time consuming. Raters typically need an average of 2 hours to annotate 1,000 screenshots (Yang et al., 2019). Assuming average smartphone use of 3 hours per day (Wurmser, 2018), a 1-week study period would yield 15,120 screenshots (taken at 5-second intervals) and would thus require more than 30 hours of manual annotation per participant. As manual annotations can usually not be crowdsourced due to the highly sensitive nature of smartphone data, more efficient and (semi-)automated methods for information extraction are required (Chiatti et al., 2019; Reeves et al., 2021). For example, Ram and colleagues (2020) introduce a machine learning-based approach for extracting app classifications from screenshots.

Implications of Data Availability on Android versus iOS

As should be clear, the restricted accessibility of app usage data on the iOS operating system makes it difficult for psychologists to investigate the app usage of iPhone users.

Thus, it is not surprising that few studies have investigated app usage on iOS and most research has focused on Android users. This almost exclusive focus on Android users could bias the findings if systematic differences between Android versus iOS users exist. However, previous studies found no or only small differences in the demographic characteristics and personality traits of Android and iOS users (Götz, Stieger, & Reips, 2017; Shaw, Ellis, Kendrick, Ziegler, & Wiseman, 2016). The only reliable difference concerns users' budgets, as iOS users seem to be wealthier. This difference could, in turn, influence app usage behavior, as iOS users might use more premium apps and fewer free apps. Furthermore, some applications are exclusively available for either of the two systems. However, even if the availability of specific apps is not identical between both systems, it is very likely that apps of the same type and functionality are available on both systems. The potential scope of app usage behavior should therefore not be compromised for either operating system, and app usage patterns should be fairly comparable across systems.

Enriching App Usage Data

App usage data can provide detailed, quantitative information on everyday behaviors. Still, app usage data are limited with regard to the nature of behaviors. For example, use of the Spotify app does not tell us what types of music somebody likes or even if they are listening to music or a podcast (Sust, Stachl, Kudchadker, Bühner, & Schoedel, 2023). Luckily, there are multiple ways app usage data can be enriched with additional information on context, location, or subsequent behaviors. Here, we briefly introduce some suitable methods for data enrichment.

Sensor Fusion

The most obvious way to enrich app usage data is with additional data from sensors and logs on the smartphone. GPS data, for example, can be used to relate behavioral measures to different locations (Matz & Harari, 2020). In that vein, Do, Blom, and Gatica-Perez (2011) used GPS data to compare app usage frequencies at different locations (e.g., home, work, friend's house). They also leveraged Bluetooth data to create app usage durations for moments when participants were alone versus around others. Data on physical activity can also be used to better contextualize app usage. In their study, Böhmer, Hecht, Schöning, Krüger, and Bauer (2011) analyzed app usage in combination with accelerometer sensor data and found that participants in a moving state (i.e., traveling faster than 25 kilometers/hour) were 2.26 times more likely to use multimedia apps (e.g., music players). Many more traceable behaviors from smartphones can be combined with app usage data to increase the informativeness of the data with regard to different contexts and situations.

Web APIs

Another relatively easy way to enrich app usage data with additional information is through the use of standardized APIs, which enable the user to retrieve information via a standardized syntax request. In-app data on the music (i.e., songs, artists, and albums) that a participant has listened to can be used to retrieve additional information on song characteristics (Stachl et al., 2020; Sust et al., 2023). As another example, location-based

APIs (e.g., OpenStreetMaps, Google's Places, Here) can be used to enrich app usage data at different GPS positions (i.e., longitude, latitude), ground-level elevations (i.e., 1,032-m ground elevation), landmarks or places (e.g., cafés, shops), and ground types (e.g., woodland, street; see Schoedel, Kunz, et al., 2022). API calls can also be used in a sequential fashion. Once some information has been retrieved from a web API, this information can be used for further API requests.

With this approach, an initially low-dimensional dataset can quickly be enriched with additional information for much richer analyses. While most APIs offer a free limited quota for researchers, the effective labeling of app usage data can quickly exceed those quotas and inflict significant financial costs (e.g., reverse geocoding with Google's Places API [2020] currently costs $5 for 1,000 requests). Hence, it is often worthwhile to explore free alternatives, such as OpenStreetMaps (OpenStreetMap) for geodata.

Web Scraping

A cheaper, yet legally more challenging, approach to enrich app usage data is with web scraping scripts (Glez-Peña, Lourenço, López-Fernández, Reboiro-Jato, & Fdez-Riverola, 2014). The process of web scraping is similar to a human worker copying/pasting information from websites with the goal of assigning the copied information to existing data. Web scraping automates this process by using a website's underlying structure (e.g., HTML) to retrieve information from that website. While web scraping represents a more general approach to the retrieval of information from websites, it can be used specifically to enrich app usage data. Major app stores, for example, provide a range of additional information on the apps they distribute (e.g., number of downloads, popularity ratings). App stores also group apps in category systems, which can be scraped to categorize apps for research purposes (e.g., Böhmer et al., 2011; Gordon et al., 2019). In the section on analyzing app usage, we go into more detail on categorizing apps. In summary, web scraping can help to effectively enrich app usage data with additional information that is not accessible through sensors on the phone, APIs, or self-reports.

Experience Sampling

One alternative to enriching app usage data after their initial collection is to employ an event-triggered experience sampling approach during the data collection (Van Berkel, Ferreira, & Kostakos, 2017). Experience sampling items can be triggered by the launch or the prolonged usage (e.g., 20 seconds of usage) of a certain app or app category. Then, participants are prompted to answer a few short questions about their app usage. Researchers can use this approach to collect whatever information they need regarding app usage. For example, app usage data can be enriched with details about in-app behavior (e.g., What content did participants read while using a news app?), mood or cognitions related to the app use (e.g., How did participants feel after using social media apps?), or context (e.g., Were participants working or watching TV while checking their messages?). In this fashion, Ferreira and colleagues (2014) asked participants whether their app use was self-initiated or triggered by a notification and whether they were alone or in a social context while using an app.

Theoretically, the informative power of this approach seems impressive, but it is very burdensome for participants and may be problematic in terms of compliance and retention. Furthermore, the interruptions caused by the experience sampling might interfere with participants' natural app usage. Finally, experience sampling is subject to the drawbacks of self-reports mentioned earlier on.

How to Analyze App Usage

After collecting (and potentially enriching) app usage data, researchers are presented with multiple options for analyzing their data. Here, we first introduce a superordinate decision about the organization of apps as individual apps or categories, which is relevant to all analyses of app usage. Then, we present different types of information that can be extracted from app usage data and discuss their potential for informing psychology researchers about human behavior. We describe multiple approaches to analyzing each type of app usage data, summarized in Table 8.2, and illustrate each approach with examples from existing research.

Organizing App Usage

When analyzing app usage, researchers must decide how they want to characterize app usage. Next, we present the two standard options for organizing apps and discuss their advantages and limitations for the analysis of app usage. Any decisions about the following strategies should be informed by the research question at hand and should be made prior to analyzing the data.

TABLE 8.2. Summary of App Usage Data Sources and Features

			Operating system		App usage features				
Data source	**Objectivity**	**Difficulty**	**Android**	**iOS**	**Adoption**	**Quantity**	**Sequences**	**In-app behavior**	**Context**
Self-report (survey)	Low	Very Low	✓	✓	✓	✓ (gray)		✓ (gray)	✓ (gray)
Self-report (ESM)	Medium	Low	✓	✓	✓	✓ (gray)		✓	✓
App usage logs	High	High	✓		✓	✓	✓		
Screenshots (manual)	High	Medium	✓	✓	✓	✓ (gray)			
Screenshots (screenomics)	High	Very High	✓		✓	✓	✓	✓	

Note. This table reflects our interpretation of the current state of app usage data sources and features based on methods used in existing research. It is highly likely that other data sources will be developed, data from existing sources will become easier to collect, and new app usage features will be created. Data source = the method used to collect usage data on single apps or app categories; Objectivity = the degree to which the data source is free from bias; Difficulty = the difficulty of data collection and analysis for the average psychological scientist; Operating System = data source availability for participants with Android and iOS smartphones; Adoption = apps installed on participants' phones; Quantity = frequency and duration of app usage; Sequences = order in which apps or app categories are used; In-App Behavior = participants' digital behavior while using apps; Context = participants' nondigital behaviors and context during app usage. Checkmarks in gray indicate that extracting that feature from the data source is possible but not recommended.

Individual App Usage

The systematic analysis of app usage allows researchers to investigate human behavior in great detail. In particular, it allows for investigating very specific behaviors at the level of individual apps. For example, Montag and colleagues (2015) investigated whether using WhatsApp on the smartphone is related to individual differences in demographics or personality traits. Beyond its relevance in observational studies, individual app usage is also relevant to experimental studies investigating whether usage of certain apps has the desired effect. For example, clinical psychologists might be interested in analyzing whether people who regularly use a certain mindfulness app experience less stress (Bostock et al., 2019).

Analyzing the usage of one individual app is fruitful only when the app is installed by all participants (in observational studies) or at least by half of the participants (in the experimental condition). Therefore, in observational studies of individual apps, it makes sense to focus on very popular apps. Researchers interested in the use of a specific app should screen for participants who use that app (e.g., via a screening questionnaire). Another approach is to directly instruct participants to download the respective app to participate in the study. Although this reduces ecological validity in observational studies, the instructed download (and use) of a certain app can serve as a manipulation that increases internal validity in experimental settings, allowing for causal conclusions that would otherwise not be warranted.

Very often researchers are interested in the full variety of mobile app usage. In such cases, capturing app usage patterns at the single app level may be challenging because there are currently over 2 million different apps (Clement, 2020). If participants use rare apps, a large proportion of the measured data on app usage will be very sparse. Thus, one would require a very large sample to detect systematic patterns within thousands of individual apps. Instead, in cases where researchers are interested in gaining a more comprehensive portrait of participants' app usage, we recommend the use of app categories.

App Categories

It is often helpful to consider app usage behavior in terms of psychologically meaningful categories. For example, rather than examining the effect of WhatsApp use on well-being, researchers can examine the well-being effects of using communication or social media apps. This is a useful approach for a number of reasons. First, many apps serve similar functions. If a researcher is interested in the effects of digitally mediated socializing, they likely want to capture behavior on all socializing apps on an individual's phone, not just one. Second, many apps are functionally interchangeable. For example, individuals in a given sample may use Spotify *and/or* Deezer to listen to music. Researchers interested in music listening behavior would be wasting behavioral data if they considered only one of these apps. Third, analyzing app categories may be preferable to analyzing individual apps simply because the app categories capture more behavioral occurrences than the individual apps. An individual may spend only 10 minutes a day on Facebook but 1 hour a day on social media apps combined. Fourth, use of a single app is hard to interpret—one must be familiar with the respective app. In contrast, use of a meaningful app category is easier to interpret because the category is often determined by the function of the app (e.g., communication apps).

Apps can be categorized in an a priori or post-hoc manner, driven by either research questions or practical considerations. For example, some previous studies have aggregated app usage based on existing category systems suggested by app distribution platforms. Böhmer and colleagues (2011) used the category system provided by the Google Play Store (Google, 2019), and Gordon and colleagues (2019) used the categories of the App Store (Apple, 2020). However, as Stachl and associates (2017) pointed out, app categories on commercial platforms are assigned based on consumer-oriented marketing considerations rather than an optimal grouping of app content or functionality (e.g., the dating app Tinder is classified as a "Lifestyle" app, despite the existence of a more specific "Dating" app category). Because preassigned commercial categories are often too general, default categorizations should not be readily used without additional manual checks or modifications (Frey et al., 2017). For example, Stachl and colleagues (2020) manually reassigned the most frequently used apps in their sample to 70 categories. More specifically, the categories were labeled according to the app's official description available on the internet, and the results were cross-checked by three researchers. Only recently, Schoedel, Oldemeier, Bonauer, and Sust (2022) created a freely available app categorization scheme specifically for psychological research purposes. They iteratively developed and validated 26 psychologically meaningful high-level categories and manually classified over 3,000 commonly used smartphone apps reporting inter-rater agreements. However, the manual categorization of apps into semantic categories is always somewhat subjective and influenced by the cultural and temporal context, which varies over space and time. Therefore, more objective, automated approaches to the categorization of apps based on their textual descriptions or their sequential usage have been proposed (Berardi, Esuli, Fagni, & Sebastiani, 2015; Ma, Muthukrishnan, & Simpson, 2016).

Researchers can also tailor categorizations to the specific research question at hand. One way to customize app categorizations is to choose a higher or lower order to define app categories. For example, Stachl and colleagues (2020) used the higher-order category "communication and social behavior," while Harari and colleagues (2019) investigated "messaging" and "social media" as two separate categories to capture socializing behavior in greater detail. However, more narrowly defined app categories can complicate the unambiguous assignment of apps with multiple functionalities (Ma et al., 2016). For example, the Facebook app could be considered as both a "messaging" app and a "social media" app. To avoid inconsistent categorizations, researchers must very carefully define distinct categories or use a multi-label approach to assign ambiguous apps to several categories at once (e.g., Xu, Ibrahim, Zheng, & Archer, 2014). Alternatively, they might replace the app categorization by continuous ratings on category scales or percentage distributions. As an example, the Facebook app could be conceptualized as 20% "messaging" and 80% "social media." Another approach for researchers interested in app usage on a more behavioral level is abandoning app categories and describing apps in terms of their available functionalities (Xu, Dutta, Datta, & Ge, 2018). App functionalities (e.g., posting content, commenting) can either be labeled manually or extracted from app descriptions or reviews in an automated fashion (Berardi et al., 2015; Xu et al., 2018). Considering WhatsApp as an example, Xu and colleagues (2018) identified the functions "message," "address book," and "voice note," among others. Finally, it must be noted that the variety of customization approaches to app categorization introduces researcher degrees of freedom into the study of app usage. Please refer to the summary of practical recommendations on how to deal with analytical freedom in the analysis of app usage.

Extracting Information from App Usage

For both individual apps and app categories, there are multiple options for analyzing app usage data. Below, we present the most common ways to extract behavioral information from app usage data, starting with methods that are least revealing of human behavior and ending with methods that provide the most granular behavioral information. Thereby, we focus on the extraction of variables from app usage logs because, as previously mentioned, directly accessing usage logs is currently most prevalent in studies collecting app usage data in psychology.

App Adoption

Some of the first studies to investigate app usage examined which apps were installed on a given user's phone, termed *app adoption* (Seneviratne et al., 2014a, 2014b; Xu et al., 2016). The total number of installed apps is often referred to as users' app capacity (e.g., Xu et al., 2016). However, the most common measure of app adoption is the number of apps installed from different app categories (e.g., Frey et al., 2017; Gordon et al., 2019; Seneviratne et al., 2014b). For example, Xu and colleagues (2016) used the number of installations per app category to predict the Big Five personality traits. In another analysis, the researchers operationalized app adoption as a binary variable indicating whether or not participants were adopters of a certain app category. In addition, the adoption of specific apps can serve as an indicator of certain psychological characteristics. For example, the lack of apps known to collect a lot of private data could be indicative of users' privacy concerns (e.g., Gu, Xu, Xu, Zhang, & Ling, 2017; Pentina, Zhang, Bata, & Chen, 2016). Moreover, researchers can investigate changes in app adoption (e.g., the number or specific apps installed) over time. In this way, De Nadai, Cardoso, Lima, Lepri, and Oliver (2019) analyzed app adoption over a 6-month period to discover individual differences in the exploration of new apps.

Despite its many research applications, the informative power of app adoption is limited as it does not reflect actual app usage, such as how often (frequency) or for how long (duration) apps are being used (Xu et al., 2016). In other words, frequently used apps cannot be distinguished from rarely used or unused apps that users forgot about or did not bother to remove (Malmi & Weber, 2016). Preinstalled apps, in particular, are not a function of the user's individual choice (Welke et al., 2016).

App Usage Quantity

To investigate actual app usage behavior, researchers must employ measurement approaches that create continuous usage data. During preprocessing, these data can be aggregated into meaningful variables, whereby the most common metrics are usage quantities, such as frequency and duration of app usage (Böhmer et al., 2011; Gordon et al., 2019; Harari et al., 2019; Morrison et al., 2018; Stachl et al., 2017; Tu et al., 2021). While frequencies are easy to calculate by summing up usage events of a certain type (e.g., all "Homescreen" events in Table 8.1), app durations are more complicated to extract as illustrated by the following example. The app usage logs in Table 8.1 contain timestamped information on app launches but not on usage durations. Therefore, researchers have to make analytic decisions about when active app usage ends. The end of app usage may be determined by the launch of a new app so that the time interval between two app launches defines app usage duration. However, app usage can also be terminated by switching off the phone or other events such as screen activity and calls. In Table 8.1, we enriched app usage logs with information on screen use activity to calculate how long a certain app was opened before the screen was turned off or another app was opened (e.g., in line 3 of Table 8.1, Instagram was open for 1 minute and 36 seconds).

As app usage durations differ greatly between and within smartphone users, they have received special attention in research (e.g., Church et al., 2015; Ferreira et al., 2014). Ferreira and colleagues (2014) defined the concept of micro-usages as very brief interactions with an app. By clustering app usage durations, they discovered a natural break at 15 seconds, distinguishing micro-usage from more prolonged, intense app usage (see also Church et al., 2015; Gordon et al., 2019; Morrison et al., 2018). The occurrence of micro-usage depends on the different apps. For example, Ferreira and colleagues found that the majority of interactions with calendar apps are defined by micro-usage, while only 15% of browser app usages are shorter than 15 seconds.

Researchers can aggregate app usage quantities with regard to different time intervals (e.g., on an hourly, daily, or weekly level). Harari and colleagues (2019) considered the daily duration of social media and messaging app usage as relevant indicators of sociability behavior. In contrast, Böhmer and colleagues (2011) explored app usage durations and frequencies for each hour of the day. Moreover, researchers can compute usage quantities for socially defined time periods, (e.g., daytime or weekday/weekend; Stachl et al., 2020).

App Usage Sequences

The use of an app can also be considered within the context of other app usage events (Böhmer et al., 2011; Morrison et al., 2018; Peng & Zhu, 2020) by identifying "app sessions" from smartphone status logs. Continuous app usage allows researchers to organize discrete app usage into behavioral sequences, so-called app sessions (Peng & Zhu, 2020). According to their definition, app sessions include all apps that were used consecutively without the phone being shut off for a given period of time (e.g., 30 seconds; see Böhmer et al., 2011; Rauber et al., 2019). The time spent per app session is often referred to as session length (Morrison et al., 2018; Peng & Zhu, 2020). App usage sessions can either include only one app or several different apps (Peng & Zhu, 2020). So-called multi-app sessions are particularly interesting for psychologists because they reveal a variety of behavioral information. One common metric is the repertoire size calculated from the number of (unique) applications that occur during one session (e.g., Böhmer et al., 2011; Morrison et al., 2018; Peng & Zhu, 2020). For example, Gordon and colleagues (2019) used the number of different apps per session as an indicator of cognitive decline in older adults.

One measure that might reveal specific behavioral intentions is the order of apps used within one session (Peng & Zhu, 2020). Sequential patterns can be identified by pairwise sequence analysis techniques (Peng & Zhu, 2020; Rauber et al., 2019). For example, Rauber and colleagues (2019) differentiated sequences of app categories of healthy versus cognitively impaired participants. A systematic investigation of smartphone usage patterns revealed the most used app sequence to be communication apps, followed by social network apps, which might indicate a desire to socialize (Peng & Zhu, 2020). In addition, transitioning or switching between the apps within one session can be analyzed in terms of frequency, speed, or directionality (Gordon et al., 2019; Peng & Zhu, 2020).

These approaches extract typical usage sequences from empirical data in a bottom-up fashion. A complementary approach could be to predefine meaningful app usage sequences to answer specific research questions. For example, researchers could investigate whether well-being improves when people engage a mindfulness app after using a social media app. Yet another approach to app sessions is to consider them as unique characteristics of a person rather than as common behavioral patterns. Tu and colleagues (2018) were indeed able to identify participants based on the unique set of apps they used.

Expanding the scope of app sequences, Peng and Zhu (2020) suggested investigating so-called mobile trajectories. These are higher-order sequential processes in which the user may alternate between several app sessions. In this manner, Jeong, Jung, and Lee (2020) explored how people switch between work and leisure app sessions on smartphones. Considering even longer time frames, Tu and colleagues (2021) compared the weekly app usage patterns of 1,600 users over the course of 3 years, identifying long-term changes in individual app usage and relating them to the socioeconomic attributes of users.

Within-App Behavior

There is one major limitation to investigating app usage adoption, quantities, and sequences. It remains unclear what exactly participants are doing while using an application and what the intentions of their actions are (Reeves et al., 2021). Consider social media apps as an example. These apps allow users to perform diverse behaviors ranging from randomly browsing content to searching for specific content to posting their own content to commenting or communicating. These different behaviors cannot be distinguished by analyzing frequencies and durations, but they might have unique implications psychologically. In particular, active (e.g., liking or sharing content) and passive (e.g., reading comments, viewing pictures) use of social media has been shown to constitute separate behaviors with unique relations to psychological outcomes (Burke, Marlow, & Lento, 2010; Escobar-Viera et al., 2018). The ability to characterize within-app behavior would help provide answers to many more psychologically relevant questions: *While using messaging apps, who are people interacting with and what are they talking about? When browsing the internet, what are people searching for (e.g., the latest political news or movie reviews)?* These are just some examples of the very specific and diverse behavioral information that can be extracted from in-app behavior.

While some studies have started investigating these specific behaviors for certain social media platforms (e.g., Instagram; Ferwerda, Schedl, & Tkalcic, 2015), no studies have investigated the within-app behavior via mobile sensing. This is because it is currently not possible to directly collect within-app behavior on either the Android[1] or the iOS operating system due to the privacy restrictions of the respective operating systems. One of the few exceptions to such restrictions are music apps, for which custom research applications can record song listening records (Sust et al., 2023). To measure the full scope of within-app behaviors, researchers have to come up with more innovative approaches.

The Screenomics app, for example, collects high-frequent screenshot sequences of participants' app usage, which can be analyzed with regard to within-app behavior (Reeves et al., 2021). Ram and colleagues (2020) introduced different types of content-related information that can be extracted from the text and images of screenshots: active production versus passive consumption of app contents, the sentiment of the consumed media, or the presence of very specific content. For example, Reeves and colleagues (2021) searched app screenshots for keywords related to the "presidency" (e.g., "White House," "Clinton") to investigate an individual's exposure to U.S. political news. Hypothetically, app screenshots could even be analyzed with regard to the performance of specific actions, such as writing or reading text messages (Chiatti et al., 2019; Reeves et al., 2021).

Although to our knowledge there have been no systematic attempts other than the Screenomics project to analyze within-app behavior, we want to lay out some potential technical workarounds that could leverage in-app behavioral data. The most feasible option is to directly ask participants about their within-app behavior after using the respective app via event-triggered experience sampling (see our section "Enriching App Usage Data"; e.g., Randall & Rickard, 2012). A more objective, but technically more challenging, approach could build on methods for tracking keystrokes (Buschek, De Luca, & Alt, 2015) or eye movements (Paletta et al., 2014; Strobl et al., 2019) on smartphones. The position of touch or gaze while using an app could be put into context with the respective app's architecture to infer the concrete behavior performed. Furthermore, researchers could consider app usage in combination with keyboard inputs to analyze the text participants entered into the app's interface during usage (Bemmann & Buschek, 2020).

Summary of Practical Recommendations

Analysis of app usage data opens up a wide range of new possibilities for the systematic investigation of behavior in the wild. There are myriad approaches to analyzing app usage data, ranging from simple aggregations of app usage frequencies to complex model-based retrieval of within-app behavioral information. However, the diversity of analytical possibilities presented throughout this chapter also leads to a dramatic increase in the researcher's degrees of freedom (Wicherts et al., 2016). Reducing the researcher's degrees of freedom is important for restricting questionable research practices such as HARKING and p-hacking (Head, Holman, Lanfear, Kahn, & Jennions, 2015; Kerr, 1998). Thus, we highly recommend preregistering methodological decisions when analyzing app usage.

Researchers interested in conducting a study that incorporates app usage data should consider several issues during the planning and preregistration process, prior to data collection. First, researchers should decide how to collect app usage data. Even though this decision is determined in part by the researcher's technological know-how, we recommend employing objective methods for collecting continuous app usage data (e.g., data logging rather than self-report). Second, researchers should decide whether and how app usage data will be enriched. Even more importantly, researchers must think about the analysis of their collected app usage data. They must specify whether analyses will be conducted at the individual-app level (e.g., WhatsApp) or on a categorical level (e.g., communication apps), as this decision will strongly affect statistical inferences. Researchers who wish to analyze app categories must specify which categories they plan to consider (e.g., broad vs. narrow categories). Moreover, they must define how apps will be assigned to these categories (e.g., categories provided by the app store vs. manual coder labeling). For custom categorizations, ideally, the complete assignment of apps to categories should be preregistered, along with the underlying rationale (e.g., "If the app offers audio calls or texting as the primary functionality, we will assign the app category 'Communication' ").

Finally, researchers have to decide what kind of information they want to extract from the app usage data (e.g., app adoption/app usage quantities/app sessions/in-app behavior). For usage durations, in particular, they must define which smartphone events depict the end of app usage (e.g., the launch of another app and/or the next screen-lock event). Similarly, it is useful to set an upper limit for the duration of app usage because in some instances logging errors might cause implausibly long usage durations (e.g., 24 hours). Furthermore, researchers should specify for which time period app usage quantities shall be aggregated (e.g., by day or by hour).

While these are the most relevant methodological considerations, specific approaches to analyzing app usage might require even more a priori considerations. However, we recognize that with an abundance of options and few existing benchmarks in this novel field of research, creating a preregistration can be challenging. Those collecting app usage data for the first time will likely encounter issues that they did not anticipate in their preregistration and that will require ad-hoc solutions. This is a natural part of the research process, and we merely recommend that researchers report any deviations from and additions to their preregistered protocol. In addition, we would like to note that this section only covers those aspects of research transparency that are specifically relevant for analyzing app usage. For a more comprehensive discussion on the topic of researcher degrees of freedom in mobile sensing research, we refer interested readers to Chapter 3, this volume, on transparency and reproducibility.

Challenges and Future Directions for App Usage Research in Psychology

Psychological research has only just begun to scratch the surface of what is possible with app usage data. Indeed, app usage has the potential to reveal much more about people's feelings, thoughts, and behaviors than what we have mentioned thus far. Therefore, we end this chapter by providing an outlook on the future directions of mobile sensing research that incorporates app usage data. First, however, we want to discuss some of the technological, practical, and ethical challenges that researchers will need to overcome before fully realizing the full potential of app usage in psychology.

Technological Challenges

Concerning technological challenges, continuous app usage remains difficult to access as many "off-the-shelf" mobile sensing apps (e.g., Beiwe: Torous, Kiang, Lorme, & Onnela, 2016) and most research apps (e.g., Emotion Sense: Servia-Rodriguez et al., 2017) are not able to collect app usage data. In particular, it remains virtually impossible to investigate app usage on iPhones. Therefore, in samples where a majority of participants own an iPhone, a large portion of app usage behavior remains inaccessible to researchers. Perhaps the biggest technological challenge will be to develop methods to collect within-app behaviors that do not rely on self-report measures. As previously mentioned, these alternative methods are currently quite limited, and, where they do exist, they are custom-made, cumbersome, and resource-intensive for participants and researchers.

Another technological hurdle is that even when app usage is collected, processing and categorizing the respective data remain very challenging because many psychologists are not experienced in complex data analytics and computer science methodologies. In sum, technological developments that make the collection, storage, and analysis of app usage easier for the average psychological scientist would most likely increase the adoption of app usage methods in psychological research.

Of course, private corporations are already collecting iPhone app usage and within-app behavior. Therefore, one potential strategy could be accessing these existing data for use in psychological research. Public–private partnerships wherein companies provide specialized software frameworks for researchers (e.g., Apple ResearchKit) or provide them with anonymized user data in a mutually agreed upon, systematized process, have been explored in domains outside of mobile sensing (King & Persily, 2018; Stroud, Tucker, Franco, & Kiewiet de Jonge, 2020). Unfortunately, such partnerships have not always proven effective (Hegelich, 2020). Hence, a promising alternative may be legislation that guarantees public access to the public's data in a standardized form. Within such legal frameworks, several of which have already been enacted (California Consumer Privacy Act, 2018; Goodman & Flaxman, 2016), citizens can request their data from private companies and choose to donate the data to science (Christen, Domingo-Ferrer, Herrmann, & van den Hoven, 2017). However, these legal mandates will be ineffective in increasing researchers' access to app usage data unless people are educated about their data rights, know how research initiatives may benefit from their data, and are motivated to donate their data.

Ethical Challenges

We have described many ways of collecting and analyzing app usage for scientific investigations. However, the data collection methods that yield the richest, most granular, and highest quality usage data (e.g., continuous screenshots) are also the most invasive. Recruitment for mobile sensing studies will likely become more difficult the more extensive the data collection gets because participants may perceive the observation of their (in-)app usage behavior as a violation of their privacy. As the public becomes more knowledgeable about digital privacy issues, access to app usage and other sensing logs may become more restricted. Such restrictions offer significant progress for citizens' data protection rights but may impede app usage research.

Given participants' privacy concerns, compensating participants appropriately may be even more critical in mobile sensing studies collecting detailed app usage data (Keusch, Struminskaya, Antoun, Couper, & Kreuter, 2019; Kreuter, Haas, Keusch, Bähr, & Trappmann, 2020). Alternatively, nonmonetary incentives (e.g., feedback on psychological constructs) could create added value for participants who participate in app usage studies (Servia-Rodriguez et al., 2017). Another solution may be to use more sophisticated, technical approaches to better protect users' privacy. For example, recent technologically sophisticated techniques like federated learning, distributed computing, differential privacy, and on-device data aggregation techniques allow researchers to minimize the collection of personal data by training predictive models directly on the user's smartphone, avoiding downloading user data to centralized servers, and performing parts of the analysis on different machines (McMahan, Moore, Ramage, Hampson, & Aguera y Arcas, 2016; Wang et al., 2019). These techniques, however, are very complex and will require psychologists to cooperate with computer scientists and software engineers to execute effectively.

The Future of App Usage on Other Smart Devices

Smartphones are currently the most popular mobile device. Half of the world population owns a smartphone (O'Dea, 2020b), so it is unsurprising that smartphones have been the focus of most mobile app research. Yet, apps can also be installed on other mobile devices that are increasing in popularity, such as tablet computers or smartwatches (Musil, 2016; Zickuhr & Rainie, 2019). App usage on these devices can be collected and analyzed similarly to app usage on smartphones. However, there are differences in methodological considerations across the different devices that need to be better understood to advance the analysis of app usage beyond smartphones. Some differences that are already apparent relate to the types of apps and their usage frequencies on various devices, such as smartwatches versus smartphones.

Regarding the types of apps available, a systematic analysis of 14,000 smartwatch apps found that many smartwatch apps fall into categories similar to smartphone app categories (e.g., games, music/audio). However, one of the most popular smartwatch app categories was personalization (i.e., apps that change the interface of the watch; Chauhan, Seneviratne, Kaafar, Mahanti, & Seneviratne, 2016), which is an uncommon smartphone app category in the current literature. In contrast, only 9% of smartwatch apps fall in the communication category (Visuri et al., 2017), which is a crucial app category for smartphones, whose original purpose is to facilitate communication (Bröhl et al., 2018). Therefore, different app categorizations might be needed for different devices, depending on the device's central functionalities and the age of the respective technology (e.g., novel technologies usually offer increased personalization functionalities).

The nature of app usage also differs on different types of devices. Similar to smartphone users (Ferreira et al., 2014), smartwatch users tend to engage in micro-usage of apps; however, the average session length is even shorter on smartwatches (Visuri et al., 2017). Smartphone and smartwatch app usage behaviors also differ in that smartwatch users rarely launch the apps directly (Liu et al., 2017). Instead, smartwatch apps send frequent push notifications and remain active in the background. Thus, Liu and colleagues (2017) distinguish between two components of smartwatch app usage: app activity (wherein the app is visibly present on the interface) and app service (wherein the app operates in the background without being visibly present on the interface), with app activity being less common than app service. App activity is less frequent in part because the user interface of smartwatches is so small and visually impoverished, precluding many behaviors that people can perform on smartphone and tablet apps (Chun, Dey, Lee, & Kim, 2018).

In contrast to the increasing popularity of research on smartwatch app usage, only a few studies have investigated app usage on tablet computers, even though 75% of tablet users have downloaded an app to their device, and 38% use six or more tablet apps every week (Purcell, 2011). Studies that have examined app use on tablets have focused on rather narrow applied settings like classrooms and hospitals (Amelink, Scales, & Tront, 2012; Diliberto-Macaluso & Hughes, 2016; Rick, 2012; Zhao, Tai-Seale, Longhurst, & Clay, 2019). Given the greater similarity between the tablet and smartphone user interface, the smartphone app data collection and analysis methods described in this chapter are likely to be more generalizable to tablets than smartwatches. However, future work should more systematically document which devices people use for different app-mediated behaviors so that researchers interested in a given behavior can collect data from the most relevant device.

An even more promising direction that future mobile sensing research could take is to combine sensor log streams from different devices. While the smartphone plays a central role in many people's lives, app usage logged on multiple devices should provide a more complete picture of a person's daily behaviors than app usage logged on their smartphone alone. Consumers tend to increasingly own additional smart devices that could provide complementary sensing and logging capabilities (Westcott et al., 2019). This is particularly important since many apps are now synchronized across multiple devices that a person may own (Årsand, Muzny, Bradway, Muzik, & Hartvigsen, 2015; Liu et al., 2017) and people sometimes use multiple devices simultaneously (Jokela, Ojala, & Olsson, 2015). That said, integrating data from multiple devices is a topic that all mobile sensing research (not just app usage research) will need to tackle. For a more in-depth discussion on mobile sensing beyond the smartphone, see Chapter 12, this volume.

Toward More Experimental App Usage Studies

Many have called for more experimental and confirmatory studies in mobile sensing research to add the benefit of high internal validity (i.e., establishing causality) to the benefits of high ecological validity already inherent to mobile sensing studies (Gordon et al., 2019; Rachuri et al., 2010). However, like other mobile sensing studies, research with a focus on app usage tends to be purely observational and exploratory. We believe that app usage research, in particular, is uniquely suitable for experimental manipulations and confirmatory research (even if, by definition, mobile sensing offers less control over experimental conditions).

One interesting avenue for future research is to randomly assign participants to use different versions of a researcher-developed app, with each version hypothesized to have diverging effects according to a priori theorizing. To provide a more concrete example, different behavioral feedback mechanisms within a health app could be tested for their effects on adherence to an exercise protocol, measured via the smartphone's sensors. Or the same app could be installed for all participants but with random assignment of how the app is framed psychologically (e.g., goal-oriented or leisure-oriented; Stieger et al., 2020). Alternatively, participants could be randomly assigned to either continue their app usage as usual or to remove certain apps from their phones, allowing researchers to examine the psychological effects of removing various features of digital media from daily life. For example, researchers randomly assigned participants to deactivate their Facebook account and found that well-being increased and political polarization decreased (Allcott, Braghieri, Eichmeyer, & Gentzkow, 2020). A similar study could be conducted with app usage by having participants delete all social media or news-related apps from their phone.

As a closing remark, we want to emphasize that app usage research, in general, is not only suitable for nomothetic investigations. The richness of app usage data also allows for an increased focus on idiographic processes in the modeling of the individuals. Highlighted by recent research (Ram et al., 2020) and in contrast to traditional analytic approaches emphasizing between-subjects and group-level analyses, app usage, and mobile sensing data, in general, can provide detailed reflections of a given individual's unique daily behavioral trajectories (Harari et al., 2016).

Conclusion

The quantitative analysis of app usage offers a uniquely comprehensive view of *in vivo* human activities. Obviously, the analysis of app usage data depends on the continued existence of apps. Recent technological trends suggest that apps may not always maintain their supremacy in the user experience. We are witnessing the rise of speech- and camera-based devices (e.g., Amazon's Alexa or Auctify's glasses) that fulfill voice requests ("Alexa, play music") and mediate what people see. Even though these devices access apps in the background, the user's experience is no longer dependent on interaction with clearly recognizable, self-contained apps. In other words, the user may ask the device to play music rather than to open the Spotify app. Therefore, in the future, analyzing app usage at the level of the individual app may be less meaningful. This may be even more true if devices are replaced by technologies that are integrated more seamlessly into the human body (i.e., brain–computer interfaces) that do not require the user to consciously interact with apps in the ways they do currently on their devices.

However, currently and for the foreseeable future, apps are the organizing principle that allows users to both navigate and expand the functionalities of their smartphones. Until there is a radical shift in how the smartphone user's experience is organized, we anticipate that mobile apps will continue to dominate people's digital life. Thus, mobile app usage data is a valuable and largely untapped source of information about people's thoughts, feelings, and behaviors. We believe that psychological scientists who leverage this new source of information in their research will uncover important new insights about human life in the 21st century.

Note

1. It is possible but not advisable to retrieve within-app behavior by exploiting accessibility services on Android phones.

REFERENCES

Alkhalaf, A. M., Tekian, A., & Park, Y. S. (2018). The impact of WhatsApp use on academic achievement among Saudi medical students. *Medical Teacher, 40*(1), 10–14.

Allcott, H., Braghieri, L., Eichmeyer, S., & Gentzkow, M. (2020). The welfare effects of social media. *American Economic Review, 110*(3), 629–676.

Amalfitano, D., Fasolino, A. R., Tramontana, P., & Robbins, B. (2013). Testing android mobile applications: Challenges, strategies, and approaches. *Advances in Computers, 89*, 1–52.

Amelink, C. T., Scales, G., & Tront, J. G. (2012). Student use of the Tablet PC: Impact on student learning behaviors. *Advances in Engineering Education, 3*(1), 1–17.

Anderson, I., Gil, S., Gibson, C., Wolf, S., Shapiro, W., Semerci, O., & Greenberg, D. M. (2020). "Just the way you are": Linking music listening on Spotify and personality. *Social Psychological and Personality Science, 12*(4), 561–571.

Andone, I., Błaszkiewicz, K., Eibes, M., Trendafilov, B., Montag, C., & Markowetz, A. (2016). Menthal: A framework for mobile data collection and analysis. *Proceedings of the 2016 ACM International Joint Conference on Pervasive and Ubiquitous Computing: Adjunct*, pp. 624–629.

Apple. (2020). *App Store*. www.apple.com/ios/app-store.

Årsand, E., Muzny, M., Bradway, M., Muzik, J., & Hartvigsen, G. (2015). Performance of the first combined smartwatch and smartphone diabetes diary application study. *Journal of Diabetes Science and Technology, 9*(3), 556–563.

Avis, J. M., Kudisch, J. D., & Fortunato, V. J. (2002). Examining the incremental validity and adverse impact of cognitive ability and conscientiousness on job performance. *Journal of Business and Psychology, 17*(1), 87–105.

Baumeister, R. F., Vohs, K. D., & Funder, D. C. (2007). Psychology as the science of self-reports and finger movements: Whatever happened to actual behavior? *Perspectives on Psychological Science, 2*(4), 396–403.

Bemmann, F., & Buschek, D. (2020). LanguageLogger: A mobile keyboard application for studying language use in everyday text communication in the wild. *Proceedings of the ACM on Human-Computer Interaction, 4*(EICS), 1–24.

Berardi, G., Esuli, A., Fagni, T., & Sebastiani, F. (2015, April). Multi-store metadata-based supervised mobile app classification. *Proceedings of the 30th Annual ACM Symposium on Applied Computing*, pp. 585–588.

Boase, J., & Ling, R. (2013). Measuring mobile phone use: Self-report versus log data. *Journal of Computer-Mediated Communication, 18*(4), 508–519.

Böhmer, M., Hecht, B., Schöning, J., Krüger, A., & Bauer, G. (2011). Falling asleep with Angry Birds, Facebook and Kindle: A large-scale study on mobile application usage. *Proceedings of the 13th International Conference on Human Computer Interaction with Mobile Devices and Services*, pp. 47–56.

Bostock, S., Crosswell, A. D., Prather, A. A., & Steptoe, A. (2019). Mindfulness on-the-go: Effects of a mindfulness meditation app on work stress and well-being. *Journal of Occupational Health Psychology, 24*(1), 127.

Bröhl, C., Rasche, P., Jablonski, J., Theis, S., Wille, M., & Mertens, A. (2018). Desktop PC, tablet PC, or smartphone? An analysis of use preferences in daily activities for different technology generations of a worldwide sample. In *International Conference on Human Aspects of IT for the Aged Population* (pp. 3–20). Springer.

Burke, M., Marlow, C., & Lento, T. (2010). Social network activity and social well-being. *Proceedings of the SIGCHI Conference on Human Factors in Computing Systems*, pp. 1909–1912.

Buschek, D., De Luca, A., & Alt, F. (2015). Improving accuracy, applicability and usability of keystroke biometrics on mobile touchscreen devices. *Proceedings of the 33rd Annual ACM Conference on Human Factors in Computing Systems*, pp. 1393–1402.

Butt, S., & Phillips, J. G. (2008). Personality and self reported mobile phone use. *Computers in Human Behavior, 24*(2), 346–360.

California Consumer Privacy Act (CCPA). (2018). https://oag.ca.gov/privacy/ccpa

Chauhan, J., Seneviratne, S., Kaafar, M. A., Mahanti, A., & Seneviratne, A. (2016). Characterization of early smartwatch apps. *2016 IEEE International Conference on Pervasive Computing and Communication Workshops (PerCom Workshops)*, pp. 1–6.

Chiatti, A., Davaasuren, D., Ram, N., Mitra, P., Reeves, B., & Robinson, T. (2019). *Guess what's on my screen?: Clustering smartphone screenshots with active learning*. https://arxiv.org/abs/1901.02701.

Chittaranjan, G., Blom, J., & Gatica-Perez, D. (2013). Mining large-scale smartphone data for personality studies. *Personal and Ubiquitous Computing, 17*(3), 433–450.

Choi, J., Rho, M. J., Kim, Y., Yook, I. H., Yu, H., Kim, D. J., et al. (2017). Smartphone dependence classification using tensor factorization. *PloS One, 12*(6), e0177629.

Christen, M., Domingo-Ferrer, J., Herrmann, D., & van den Hoven, J. (2017). Beyond informed consent—Investigating ethical justifications for disclosing, donating or sharing personal data in research. In T. M. Powers (Ed.), *Philosophy and computing* (pp. 193–207). Springer.

Chun, J., Dey, A., Lee, K., & Kim, S. (2018). A qualitative study of smartwatch usage and its usability. *Human Factors and Ergonomics in Manufacturing and Service Industries, 28*(4), 186–199.

Church, K., Ferreira, D., Banovic, N., & Lyons,

K. (2015). Understanding the challenges of mobile phone usage data. *Proceedings of the 17th International Conference on Human-Computer Interaction with Mobile Devices and Services*, pp. 504–514.

Clement, J. (2019, August 1). *Topic: Mobile app usage*. Statista. www.statista.com/topics/1002/mobile-app-usage

Clement, J. (2020, September 1). *Number of apps available in leading app stores as of 1st quarter 2020*. Statista. www.statista.com/statistics/276623/number-of-apps-available-in-leading-app-stores.

Comscore. (2017). *The 2017 U.S. mobile app report*. www.comscore.com/Insights/Presentations-and-Whitepapers/2017/The-2017-US-Mobile-App-Report

Davidson, B., Shaw, H., & Ellis, D. A. (2022). Fuzzy constructs in technology usage scales. *Computers in Human Behavior, 133*, 107206.

De Montjoye, Y. A., Quoidbach, J., Robic, F., & Pentland, A. (2013). Predicting personality using novel mobile phone-based metrics. *Proceedings of the 6th International Conference on Social Computing, Behavioral-Cultural Modeling, and Prediction*, pp. 48–55.

De Nadai, M., Cardoso, A., Lima, A., Lepri, B., & Oliver, N. (2019). Strategies and limitations in app usage and human mobility. *Scientific Reports, 9*(1), 1–9.

Demumieux, R., & Losquin, P. (2005). Gather customer's real usage on mobile phones. *Proceedings of the 7th International Conference on Human Computer Interaction with Mobile Devices and Services*, pp. 267–270.

Diliberto-Macaluso, K., & Hughes, A. (2016). The use of mobile apps to enhance student learning in introduction to psychology. *Teaching of Psychology, 43*(1), 48–52.

Do, T. M. T., Blom, J., & Gatica-Perez, D. (2011). Smartphone usage in the wild: A large-scale analysis of applications and context. *Proceedings of the 13th International Conference on Multimodal Interfaces*, pp. 353–360.

Escobar-Viera, C. G., Shensa, A., Bowman, N. D., Sidani, J. E., Knight, J., James, A. E., et al. (2018). Passive and active social media use and depressive symptoms among United States adults. *Cyberpsychology, Behavior, and Social Networking, 21*(7), 437–443.

Ferdous, R., Osmani, V., & Mayora, O. (2015). Smartphone app usage as a predictor of perceived stress levels at the workplace. *Proceedings of the 2015 9th International Conference on Pervasive Computing Technologies for Healthcare, Pervasive Health*, pp. 225–228.

Ferreira, D., Goncalves, J., Kostakos, V., Barkhuus, L., & Dey, A. K. (2014). Contextual experience sampling of mobile application micro-usage. *Proceedings of the 16th International Conference on Human-Computer Interaction with Mobile Devices and Services*, pp. 91–100.

Ferreira, D., Kostakos, V., & Dey, A. K. (2015). AWARE: Mobile context instrumentation framework. *Frontiers in ICT, 2*, 6.

Ferwerda, B., Schedl, M., & Tkalcic, M. (2015, September). Predicting personality traits with instagram pictures. *Proceedings of the 3rd Workshop on Emotions and Personality in Personalized Systems 2015*, pp. 7–10.

Flett, J. A., Hayne, H., Riordan, B. C., Thompson, L. M., & Conner, T. S. (2019). Mobile mindfulness meditation: A randomised controlled trial of the effect of two popular apps on mental health. *Mindfulness, 10*(5), 863–876.

Frey, R. M., Xu, R., & Ilic, A. (2017). Mobile app adoption in different life stages: An empirical analysis. *Pervasive and Mobile Computing, 40*, 512–527.

Froehlich, J., Chen, M. Y., Consolvo, S., Harrison, B., & Landay, J. A. (2007). MyExperience: A system for in situ tracing and capturing of user feedback on mobile phones. *MobiSys'07: Proceedings of the 5th International Conference on Mobile Systems, Applications and Services*, pp. 57–70.

Fukazawa, Y., Ito, T., Okimura, T., Yamashita, Y., Maeda, T., & Ota, J. (2019). Predicting anxiety state using smartphone-based passive sensing. *Journal of Biomedical Informatics, 93*, 103151.

Gao, Y., Li, A., Zhu, T., Liu, X., & Liu, X. (2016). How smartphone usage correlates with social anxiety and loneliness. *PeerJ, 4*, e2197.

Georgiou, K., Gouras, A., & Nikolaou, I. (2019). Gamification in employee selection: The development of a gamified assessment. *International Journal of Selection and Assessment, 27*(2), 91–103.

Glez-Peña, D., Lourenço, A., López-Fernández, H., Reboiro-Jato, M., & Fdez-Riverola, F. (2014). Web scraping technologies in an API world. *Briefings in Bioinformatics, 15*(5), 788–797.

Goodman, B., & Flaxman, S. (2016). *European Union regulations on algorithmic decision-making and a "right to explanation."* http://arxiv.org/abs/1606.08813

Google. (2019). *Android Apps on Google Play.* https://play.google.com/store/apps

Google. (2020). *Places API.* https://developers.google.com/places/web-service/overview

Gordon, M. L., Gatys, L., Guestrin, C., Bigham, J. P., Trister, A., & Patel, K. (2019). App usage predicts cognitive ability in older adults. *Proceedings of the 2019 CHI Conference on Human Factors in Computing Systems*, pp. 1–12.

Götz, F. M., Stieger, S., & Reips, U. D. (2017). Users of the main smartphone operating systems (iOS, Android) differ only little in personality. *PloS One, 12*(5), e0176921.

Gower, A. D., & Moreno, M. A. (2018). A novel approach to evaluating mobile smartphone screen time for iPhones: Feasibility and preliminary findings. *JMIR mHealth and uHealth, 6*(11), e11012.

Gu, J., Xu, Y. C., Xu, H., Zhang, C., & Ling, H. (2017). Privacy concerns for mobile app download: An elaboration likelihood model perspective. *Decision Support Systems, 94*, 19–28.

Hang, A., & De Luca, A. (2013). Oh app, where art thou?: On app launching habits of smartphone users. *Proceedings of the 15th International Conference on Human-Computer Interaction with Mobile Devices and Services*, pp. 392–395.

Harari, G. M., Lane, N. D., Wang, R., Crosier, B. S., Campbell, A. T., & Gosling, S. D. (2016). Using smartphones to collect behavioral data in psychological science: Opportunities, practical considerations, and challenges. *Perspectives on Psychological Science, 11*(6), 838–854.

Harari, G. M., Müller, S. R., Aung, M. S., & Rentfrow, P. J. (2017). Smartphone sensing methods for studying behavior in everyday life. *Current Opinion in Behavioral Sciences, 18*, 83–90.

Harari, G. M., Müller, S. R., Stachl, C., Wang, R., Wang, W., Bühner, M., et al. (2019). Sensing sociability: Individual differences in young adults' conversation, calling, texting, and app use behaviors in daily life. *Journal of Personality and Social Psychology, 19*(1), 204–228.

Head, M. L., Holman, L., Lanfear, R., Kahn, A. T., & Jennions, M. D. (2015). The extent and consequences of p-hacking in science. *PLOS Biology, 13*(3), e1002106.

Hegelich, S. (2020). Facebook needs to share more with researchers. *Nature, 579*(7800), 473–473.

Jeong, Y., Jung, H., & Lee, J. (2020). Cyberslacking or smart work: Smartphone usage log-analysis focused on app-switching behavior in work and leisure conditions. *International Journal of Human–Computer Interaction, 36*(1), 15–30.

Jokela, T., Ojala, J., & Olsson, T. (2015). A diary study on combining multiple information devices in everyday activities and tasks. In *Proceedings of the 33rd Annual ACM Conference on Human Factors in Computing Systems* (pp. 3903–3912).

Kerr, N. L. (1998). HARKing: Hypothesizing after the results are known. *Personality and Social Psychology Review, 2*(3), 196–217.

Keusch, F., Struminskaya, B., Antoun, C., Couper, M. P., & Kreuter, F. (2019). Willingness to participate in passive mobile data collection. *Public Opinion Quarterly, 83*(S1), 210–235.

Khomych, A. (2019, November 25). *How to measure user engagement in mobile apps: Key metrics and strategies.* https://appfollow.io/blog/metrics-to-measure-user-engagement-in-mobile-apps

Kim, Y., Briley, D. A., & Ocepek, M. G. (2015). Differential innovation of smartphone and application use by sociodemographics and personality. *Computers in Human Behavior, 44*, 141–147.

King, G., & Persily, N. (2018). A new model for industry–academic partnerships. *PS: Political Science and Politics*, 1–7.

Krebs, P., & Duncan, D. T. (2015). Health app use among US mobile phone owners: A national survey. *JMIR mHealth and uHealth, 3*(4), e101.

Kreuter, F., Haas, G.-C., Keusch, F., Bähr, S., & Trappmann, M. (2020). Collecting survey and smartphone sensor data with an app: Opportunities and challenges around privacy and informed consent. *Social Science Computer Review, 38*(5), 533–549.

Lane, W. (2012). The influence of personality traits on mobile phone application preferences. *Journal of Economics and Behavioral Studies, 4*(5), 252–260.

Lecher, C. (2019, April 25). *How Amazon automatically tracks and fires warehouse workers for "productivity."* www.theverge.com/2019/4/25/18516004/amazon-warehouse-fulfillment-centers-productivity-firing-terminations

Lind, M. N., Byrne, M. L., Wicks, G., Smidt, A. M., & Allen, N. B. (2018). The effortless assessment of risk states (EARS) tool: An interpersonal approach to mobile sensing. *JMIR Mental Health, 5*(3), e10334.

Liu, X., Chen, T., Qian, F., Guo, Z., Lin, F. X., Wang, X., et al. (2017). Characterizing smartwatch usage in the wild. *Proceedings of the 15th Annual International Conference on Mobile Systems, Applications, and Services*, pp. 385–398.

Ma, Q., Muthukrishnan, S., & Simpson, W. (2016). App2vec: Vector modeling of mobile apps and applications. *2016 IEEE/ACM International Conference on Advances in Social Networks Analysis and Mining (ASONAM)*, pp. 599–606.

Malmi, E., & Weber, I. (2016). *You are what apps you use: Demographic prediction based on user's apps.* http://arxiv.org/abs/1603.00059

Matz, S. C., & Harari, G. M. (2020). Personality–place transactions: Mapping the relationships between big five personality traits, states, and daily places. *Journal of Personality and Social Psychology, 120*(5), 1367–1385.

Matz, S. C., Kosinski, M., Nave, G., & Stillwell, D. J. (2017). Psychological targeting as an effective approach to digital mass persuasion. *Proceedings of the National Academy of Sciences, 114*(48), 12714–12719.

McMahan, H. B., Moore, E., Ramage, D., Hampson, S., & Aguera y Arcas, B. (2016). Communication-efficient learning of deep networks from decentralized data. *Proceedings of the 20th International Conference on Artificial Intelligence and Statistics (AISTATS).* http://arxiv.org/abs/1602.05629

McMillan, D., Morrison, A., & Chalmers, M. (2013). A comparison of distribution channels for large-scale deployments of iOS applications. In *Developments in technologies for human-centric mobile computing and applications* (pp. 222–239). IGI Global.

Melnick, M. D., Harrison, B. R., Park, S., Bennetto, L., & Tadin, D. (2013). A strong interactive link between sensory discriminations and intelligence. *Current Biology, 23*(11), 1013–1017.

Miller, G. (2012). The smartphone psychology manifesto. *Perspectives on Psychological Science, 7*(3), 221–237.

Miranda, D., & Claes, M. (2008). Personality traits, music preferences and depression in adolescence. *International Journal of Adolescence and Youth, 14*(3), 277–298.

Montag, C., Baumeister, H., Kannen, C., Sariyska, R., Meßner, E. M., & Brand, M. (2019). Concept, possibilities and pilot-testing of a new smartphone application for the social and life sciences to study human behavior including validation data from personality psychology. *J—Multidisciplinary Scientific Journal, 2*(2), 102–115.

Montag, C., Błaszkiewicz, K., Sariyska, R., Lachmann, B., Andone, I., Trendafilov, B., et al. (2015). Smartphone usage in the 21st century: Who is active on WhatsApp? *BMC Research Notes, 8*(1), 331.

Morrison, A., Xiong, X., Higgs, M., Bell, M., & Chalmers, M. (2018). A large-scale study of iPhone app launch behaviour. *Proceedings of the 2018 CHI Conference on Human Factors in Computing Systems*, pp. 1–13.

Movisens GmbH. (2020). *movisensXS*. Author.

Musil, S. (2016, February 19). *Smartwatches now more popular than Swiss watches, thanks to Apple.* www.cnet.com/news/smartwatches-now-more-popular-than-swiss-watches-thanks-largely-to-apple

O'Dea, S. (2020a, August 17). *Market share of mobile operating systems worldwide 2012–2020.* Statista. https://www.statista.com/statistics/272698/global-market-share-held-by-mobile-operating-systems-since-2009

O'Dea, S. (2020b, August 20). *Number of smartphone users worldwide from 2016 to 2021.* Statista. https://www.statista.com/statistics/330695/number-of-smartphoneusers-worldwide

OpenStreetMap. (n.d.). https://www.openstreetmap.org/#map=17/48.10862/11.81247

Paletta, L., Neuschmied, H., Schwarz, M., Lodron, G., Pszeida, M., Ladstätter, S., et al. (2014). Smartphone eye tracking toolbox: Accurate gaze recovery on mobile displays.

Proceedings of the Symposium on Eye Tracking Research and Applications, pp. 367–368.

Parry, D. A., Davidson, B. I., Sewall, C. J., Fisher, J. T., Mieczkowski, H., & Quintana, D. S. (2021). A systematic review and meta-analysis of discrepancies between logged and self-reported digital media use. *Nature Human Behaviour*, 1–13.

Paulhus, D. L., & Vazire, S. (2007). The self-report method. In R. W. Robins, R. C. Fraley, & R. F. Krueger (Eds.), *Handbook of research methods in personality psychology* (pp. 224–239). Guilford Press.

Peng, T. Q., & Zhu, J. J. (2020). Mobile phone use as sequential processes: From discrete behaviors to sessions of behaviors and trajectories of sessions. *Journal of Computer-Mediated Communication, 25*(2), 129–146.

Pentina, I., Zhang, L., Bata, H., & Chen, Y. (2016). Exploring privacy paradox in information-sensitive mobile app adoption: A cross-cultural comparison. *Computers in Human Behavior, 65*, 409–419.

Purcell, K. (2011, November 2). *Half of adult cell phone owners have apps on their phones.* Pew Research. https://www.pewresearch.org/internet/2011/11/02/half-of-adult-cell-phone-owners-have-apps-on-their-phones

Quiroga, M. Á., Escorial, S., Román, F. J., Morillo, D., Jarabo, A., Privado, J., et al. (2015). Can we reliably measure the general factor of intelligence (g) through commercial video games?: Yes, we can! *Intelligence, 53*, 1–7.

Rachuri, K. K., Musolesi, M., Mascolo, C., Rentfrow, P. J., Longworth, C., & Aucinas, A. (2010). EmotionSense: A mobile phones based adaptive platform for experimental social psychology research. *Proceedings of the 12th ACM International Conference on Ubiquitous Computing*, pp. 281–290.

Ram, N., Yang, X., Cho, M. J., Brinberg, M., Muirhead, F., Reeves, B., et al. (2020). Screenomics: A new approach for observing and studying individuals' digital lives. *Journal of Adolescent Research, 35*(1), 16–50.

Randall, W. M., & Rickard, N. S. (2012). Development and trial of a mobile experience sampling method (m-ESM) for personal music listening. *Music Perception: An Interdisciplinary Journal, 31*(2), 157–170.

Rauber, J., Fox, E. B., & Gatys, L. A. (2019). *Modeling patterns of smartphone usage and their relationship to cognitive health.* https://arxiv.org/abs/1911.05683

Reeves, B., Ram, N., Robinson, T. N., Cummings, J. J., Giles, C. L., Pan, J., et al. (2021). Screenomics: A framework to capture and analyze personal life experiences and the ways that technology shapes them. *Human–Computer Interaction, 36*(2), 150–201.

Rick, J. (2012). Proportion: A tablet app for collaborative learning. In *Proceedings of the 11th international conference on interaction design and children* (pp. 316–319).

Saeb, S., Lattie, E. G., Schueller, S. M., Kording, K. P., & Mohr, D. C. (2016). The relationship between mobile phone location sensor data and depressive symptom severity. *PeerJ, 4*, e2537.

Saeb, S., Zhang, M., Karr, C. J., Schueller, S. M., Corden, M. E., Kording, K. P., et al. (2015). Mobile phone sensor correlates of depressive symptom severity in daily-life behavior: An exploratory study. *Journal of Medical Internet Research, 17*(7), e175.

Schmidt, F. L. (2002). The role of general cognitive ability and job performance: Why there cannot be a debate. *Human Performance, 15*(1–2), 187–210.

Schoedel, R., Au, Q., Völkel, S. T., Lehmann, F., Becker, D., Bühner, M., et al. (2019). Digital footprints of sensation seeking. *Zeitschrift für Psychologie, 226*(4), 232–245.

Schoedel, R., Kunz, F., Bergmann, M., Bemmann, F., Bühner, M., & Sust, L. (2022). Snapshots of Daily Life: Situations Investigated Through the Lens of Smartphone Sensing. *PsyArXiv.*

Schoedel, R., Oldemeier, M., Bonauer, L., & Sust, L. (2022). Systematic categorisation of 3091 smartphone applications from a large-scale smartphone sensing dataset. *Journal of Open Psychology Data, 10*(1), 7.

Schoedel, R., Pargent, F., Au, Q., Völkel, S. T., Schuwerk, T., Bühner, M., et al. (2020). To challenge the morning lark and the night owl: Using smartphone sensing data to investigate day–night behaviour patterns. *European Journal of Personality, 34*(5), 733–752.

Seneviratne, S., Seneviratne, A., Mohapatra, P., & Mahanti, A. (2014a). Predicting user traits from a snapshot of apps installed on a smartphone. *ACM SIGMOBILE Mobile Computing and Communications Review, 18*(2), 1–8.

Seneviratne, S., Seneviratne, A., Mohapatra, P.,

& Mahanti, A. (2014b). Your installed apps reveal your gender and more! *SPME 2014—Proceedings of the ACM MobiCom Workshop on Security and Privacy in Mobile Environments*, pp. 1–5.

Servia-Rodríguez, S., Rachuri, K. K., Mascolo, C., Rentfrow, P. J., Lathia, N., & Sandstrom, G. M. (2017). Mobile sensing at the service of mental well-being: A large-scale longitudinal study. *Proceedings of the 26th International Conference on World Wide Web*, pp. 103–112.

Sewall, C. J. R., Bear, T. M., Merranko, J., & Rosen, D. (2020). How psychological well-being and usage amount predict inaccuracies in retrospective estimates of digital technology use. *Mobile Media & Communication, 8*(3), 379–399.

Shaw, H., Ellis, D. A., Kendrick, L. R., Ziegler, F., & Wiseman, R. (2016). Predicting smartphone operating system from personality and individual differences. *Cyberpsychology, Behavior, and Social Networking, 19*(12), 727–732.

Stachl, C., Au, Q., Schoedel, R., Gosling, S. D., Harari, G. M., Buschek, D., et al. (2020). Predicting personality from patterns of behavior collected with smartphones. *Proceedings of the National Academy of Sciences, 117*(30), 17680–17687.

Stachl, C., Hilbert, S., Au, J. Q., Buschek, D., De Luca, A., Bischl, B., et al. (2017). Personality traits predict smartphone usage. *European Journal of Personality, 31*(6), 701–722.

Stieger, M., Wepfer, S., Rüegger, D., Kowatsch, T., Roberts, B. W., & Allemand, M. (2020). Becoming more conscientious or more open to experience?: Effects of a two-week smartphone-based intervention for Personality change. *European Journal of Personality, 34*(3), 345–366.

Strobl, M. A., Lipsmeier, F., Demenescu, L. R., Gossens, C., Lindemann, M., & De Vos, M. (2019). Look me in the eye: Evaluating the accuracy of smartphone-based eye tracking for potential application in autism spectrum disorder research. *Biomedical Engineering Online, 18*(1), 1–12.

Stroud, N. J., Tucker, J. A., Franco, A., & Kiewiet de Jonge, C. P. (2020, August 31). *A proposal for understanding social media's impact on elections: Peer-reviewed scientific research.* https://medium.com/@2020_election_research_project/a-proposal-for-understanding-social-medias-impact-on-elections-4ca5b7aae10

Sust, L., Stachl, C., Kudchadker, G., Bühner, M., & Schoedel, R. (2023). Personality computing with naturalistic music listening behavior: Comparing audio and lyrics preferences. *Collabra: Psychology, 9*(1), 75214.

Thomée, S. (2018). Mobile phone use and mental health. A review of the research that takes a psychological perspective on exposure. *International Journal of Environmental Research and Public Health, 15*(12), 2692.

Torous, J., Kiang, M. V., Lorme, J., & Onnela, J. P. (2016). New tools for new research in psychiatry: A scalable and customizable platform to empower data driven smartphone research. *JMIR Mental Health, 3*(2), e16.

Tu, Z., Cao, H., Lagerspetz, E., Fan, Y., Flores, H., Tarkoma, S., et al. (2021). Demographics of mobile app usage: Long-term analysis of mobile app usage. *CCF Transactions on Pervasive Computing and Interaction, 3*(3), 235–252.

Tu, Z., Li, R., Li, Y., Wang, G., Wu, D., Hui, P., et al. (2018). Your apps give you away. *Proceedings of the ACM on Interactive, Mobile, Wearable and Ubiquitous Technologies, 2*(3), 1–23.

Tuarob, S., Tucker, C. S., Kumara, S., Giles, C. L., Pincus, A. L., Conroy, D. E., et al. (2017). How are you feeling?: A personalized methodology for predicting mental states from temporally observable physical and behavioral information. *Journal of Biomedical Informatics, 68*, 1–19.

Ubochi, E. O. A. (2019). *Apple's screen time: The utility of digital wellness software in curbing smartphone dependency.* Unpublished doctoral dissertation, Florida Institute of Technology.

Van Berkel, N., Ferreira, D., & Kostakos, V. (2017). The experience sampling method on mobile devices. *ACM Computing Surveys (CSUR), 50*(6), 1–40.

Van Vaerenbergh, Y., & Thomas, T. D. (2013). Response styles in survey research: A literature review of antecedents, consequences, and remedies. *International Journal of Public Opinion Research, 25*(2), 195–217.

Visuri, A., Sarsenbayeva, Z., van Berkel, N., Goncalves, J., Rawassizadeh, R., Kostakos, V., et al. (2017). Quantifying sources and types of smartwatch usage sessions. *Proceedings of the 2017 CHI Conference on Human Factors in Computing Systems*, pp. 3569–3581.

Wang, R., Chen, F., Chen, Z., Li, T., Harari, G., Tignor, S., et al. (2014). StudentLife: Assessing mental health, academic performance and behavioral trends of college students using smartphones. *Proceedings of the 2014 ACM International Joint Conference on Pervasive and Ubiquitous Computing*, pp. 3–14.

Wang, K., Mathews, R., Kiddon, C., Eichner, H., Beaufays, F., & Ramage, D. (2019). *Federated evaluation of on-device personalization.* http://arxiv.org/abs/1910.10252

Westcott, K., Loucks, J., Littmann, D., Wilson, P., Srivastava, S., & Ciamp, D. (2019). *Connectivity and mobile trends survey.* https://www2.deloitte.com/us/en/insights/industry/telecommunications/connectivity-mobile-trends-survey.html

Welke, P., Andone, I., Blaszkiewicz, K., & Markowetz, A. (2016). Differentiating smartphone users by app usage. *Proceedings of the 2016 ACM International Joint Conference on Pervasive and Ubiquitous Computing*, pp. 519–523.

Wicherts, J. M., Veldkamp, C. L. S., Augusteijn, H. E. M., Bakker, M., van Aert, R. C. M., & van Assen, M. A. L. M. (2016). Degrees of freedom in planning, running, analyzing, and reporting psychological studies: A checklist to avoid p-hacking. *Frontiers in Psychology, 7*, 1832.

Woods, H. C., & Scott, H. (2016). # Sleepyteens: Social media use in adolescence is associated with poor sleep quality, anxiety, depression and low self-esteem. *Journal of Adolescence, 51*, 41–49.

Wurmser, Y. (2018, June 18). *Mobile time spent 2018.* www.emarketer.com/content/mobile-time-spent-2018

Xu, Q., Ibrahim, G., Zheng, R., & Archer, N. (2014). Toward automated categorization of mobile health and fitness applications. *Proceedings of the 4th ACM MobiHoc Workshop on Pervasive Wireless Healthcare*, pp. 49–54.

Xu, R., Frey, R. M., Fleisch, E., & Ilic, A. (2016). Understanding the impact of personality traits on mobile app adoption—Insights from a large-scale field study. *Computers in Human Behavior, 62*, 244–256.

Xu, X., Dutta, K., Datta, A., & Ge, C. (2018). Identifying functional aspects from user reviews for functionality-based mobile app recommendation. *Journal of the Association for Information Science and Technology, 69*(2), 242–255.

Xu, Y., Lin, M., Lu, H., Cardone, G., Lane, N., Chen, Z., et al. (2013). Preference, context and communities: A multi-faceted approach to predicting smartphone app usage patterns. *Proceedings of the 2013 International Symposium on Wearable Computers*, pp. 69–76.

Yang, X., Ram, N., Robinson, T., & Reeves, B. (2019). Using screenshots to predict task switching on smartphones. *Extended Abstracts of the 2019 CHI Conference on Human Factors in Computing Systems*, pp. 1–6.

Yeginsu, C. (2018, February 1). If workers slack off, the wristband will know. (And Amazon has a patent for it.) *New York Times.* www.nytimes.com/2018/02/01/technology/amazon-wristband-tracking-privacy.html

Zhao, B., Tai-Seale, M., Longhurst, C., & Clay, B. (2019). Utilization of hospital room hospitality features on patient-controlled tablet computers: Cohort study. *JMIR mHealth and uHealth, 7*(6), e13964.

Zickuhr, K., & Rainie, L. (2019, December 31). *Tablet and e-reader ownership.* Pew Research. www.pewresearch.org/internet/2014/01/16/tablet-and-e-reader-ownership

CHAPTER 9

Examining Well-Being in Situated Contexts with Computational Modeling of Social Media Data

Koustuv Saha and Munmun De Choudhury

CHAPTER OVERVIEW

A core aspect of our lives is often embedded in the communities where we live. The interconnectedness of our interactions and experiences impinges on our well-being. A better understanding of well-being will help us devise proactive support strategies. However, the existing methodologies used to assess well-being are limited in both scale and timeliness. These limitations are being surmounted by our ubiquitous technologies. Given their ubiquity and wide use, social media can be considered a "passive sensor" that can provide a complementary source of unobtrusive and naturalistic data regarding well-being. This chapter showcases research on well-being in two situated communities (which are geographically co-located, diverse, and close-knit communities where individuals share distinctive social ties), college campuses, and workplaces, based on methods from machine learning, time-series, natural language, and causal inference analysis of social media data. In this chapter, first, we leverage social media data on online communities on Reddit to study the evolution of stress following gun violence events on college campuses, and second, we leverage LinkedIn data to measure the role of ambiguity and its relationship to workplace productivity and well-being. These studies have theoretical, practical, and methodological implications for various stakeholders, including researchers, practitioners, and policymakers. This research can provide building tools and applications through these digital and sensing data-driven methodologies to support well-being.

Introduction

The past few years have seen an increasing interest in the research and development of passive sensing approaches to improve our understanding of our well-being. Simultaneously, research reveals that social media technologies provide unique advantages as a passive sensing modality (Saha et al., 2019f). Social media platforms, such as Facebook, Twitter, Instagram, Reddit, Snapchat, and LinkedIn, are pervasive and widely used by large populations (Greenwood, Perrin, & Duggan, 2016), enabling individuals to share thoughts and connect with others. The social media provide a low-cost, large-scale, nonintrusive means of data collection, which not only focuses on the linguistic and social behaviors of individuals but also may reveal naturalistic patterns of mood, behavior, cognition, psychological states, and social milieu, both in real time and across longitudinal time (Golder & Macy, 2011). Simultaneously, research has utilized social media platforms as a "passive sensor" (Saha, Chan, de Barbaro, Abowd, & De Choudury, 2017) and an unobtrusive source of behavioral data self-recorded and self-initiated by individuals in their natural settings. Considerable research highlights the potential and feasibility of the ability of social media data-driven approaches to (semi-)automatically assess the health and well-being of both individuals and communities (Chancellor & De Choudhury, 2020; Culotta, 2014; De Choudhury & Counts, 2013; Guntuku, Buffone, Jaidka, Eichtaedt, & Ungar, 2019; Saha et al., 2019f).

Language can help us understand the individual's psychological state (Pennebaker & Chung, 2007). In recent years, several studies have demonstrated that social media data can help us to understand the psychological and mental health states of individuals and communities (Spiro, 2016). Researchers have leveraged social media data at scale to quantitatively identify conditions and symptoms related to diseases (Paul & Dredze, 2011), disease contagion (Sadilek, Kautz, & Silenzio, 2012), mood and depressive disorders (De Choudhury & Counts, 2013), mental health (Birnbaum, Ernala, Rizvi, De Choudhury, & Kane, 2017; Coppersmith, Dredze, Harman, & Holingshead, 2015; Saha et al., 2019f), posttraumatic stress disorder (Coppersmith, Harman, & Dredze, 2014), eating disorders (Chancellor, Lin, Goodman, Zerwas, & De Choudhury, 2016), suicidal ideation (De Choudhury, Kiciman, Dredze, Coppersmith, & Kumar, 2016), psychotic symptoms (Ernala, Rizvi, Birnbaum, Kane, & De Choudhury, 2017), addictive behaviors (Moreno, Christakis, Egan, Brockman, & Becker, 2011), grief (Brubaker, Kivran-Swaine, Taber, & Hayes, 2012; Glasgow, Fink, & Boyd-Graber, 2014), and substance use (Chancellor, Nitzburg, Hu, Zampieri, & De Choudhury, 2019; Saha et al., 2019f). From the standpoint of collective well-being, Culotta (2014) inferred county-level mental health using Twitter data.

Relatedly, the social media have facilitated analysis of personality traits and their relationship to psychological and psychosocial well-being, through machine learning and linguistic analysis (Quercia, Kosinski, Stillwell, & Crowcroft, 2011; Kosinski, Stillwell, & Graepel, 2013; Schwartz et al., 2013). In addition, crisis literature has found promising evidence supporting the potential of social media language to better understand the psychological impacts of external events and crisis (De Choudhury et al., 2014; Mark et al., 2012; Palen, 2008; Starbird, Palen, Hughes, & Vieweg, 2010). This body of work highlights that online platforms have become a safe haven for people, enabling them to interact and express themselves during their times of upheavals (Al-Ani, Mark, & Semaan, 2010; Fitzhugh, Gibson, Spiro, & Butts, 2016; Mark et al., 2012; Starbird et al., 2010). Notably, Cohn, Mehl, and Pennebaker (2004) studied psychological markers using social media language following 9/11.

Social Media and Well-Being in Situated Communities

According to Murphey (1999), communities are grounded in locally meaningful realities. Consequently, situated communities are typically defined as groups of people in geographic spaces where they share some form of physical co-location (workplaces, residential compounds, neighborhoods, and localities, school and college campuses), or even physically co-located interests and demography. Here, individuals share social interactions and bear common and distinctive social ties and interests, including third places (i.e., places where people spend time between home ["first" place] and work ["second" place]; Oldenburg, 1999). Individuals belonging to the same situated communities often access common resources and institutions dedicated to the well-being and prosperity of these individuals (Poland & Maré, 2005).

The social ecological model implies the interdependence of behavior and well-being among individuals and the community in which they are situated (Sallis & Owen, 1998; Walcott-McQuigg, Zerwic, Dan, & Kelley, 2001). Therefore, through the interconnectedness and interdependencies that derive from human interactions, experiences, and concerns, individual and collective well-being become interlinked in situated communities. For example, crime or violence in a neighborhood will cause alertness and anxiety among all or most neighborhood residents. The absence of appropriate and proactive support strategies may exacerbate the neighborhood's overall well-being manifold owing to these interdependencies and interconnectedness in situated communities. For instance, the lack of timely supportive interventions following an external crisis can proliferate community-cascading acute stress experiences, leading to several negative consequences. The overwhelming amount of stress that usually follows crisis can lead to long-term negative mental health outcomes, including posttraumatic stress disorder, acute stress disorder, borderline personality disorder, or adjustment disorder (Wood, Foy, Layne, Pynoos, & Boyd James, 2002). A better understanding of psychosocial dynamics can help devise strategies to address well-being concerns in situated communities.

However, capturing the subjective aspects of individual lives in their situated contexts is a challenging undertaking (Atkinson, Bagnall, Corcoran, South, & Curtis, 2020). Traditional and most existing approaches to understanding behavior and well-being in these communities are limited and are typically reactive (Tourangeau, Rips, & Rasinski, 2000). These approaches are based largely on discrete occurrences of events, and there is no way to continually and comprehensively assess well-being dynamics in situated communities. Studies of human behavior and well-being have typically relied on self-reported survey data from individuals. In the last few decades, these approaches have been found to have a variety of limitations. For instance, self-reported data suffer from subjective assessments, recall, and hindsight biases. These surveys are often retrospective. That is, information is gathered after an event has occurred or after an individual has experienced a specific change (Tourangeau et al., 2000). Recent research has recognized the value of in-the-moment data recording and acquisition approaches. One prominent example centers on using active logging approaches, such as ecological momentary assessments (EMAs) capturing an individual's momentary state (Wang et al., 2014). However, active sensing involves the challenges of scale, access, and cost (Scollon, Prieto, & Diener, 2009). EMAs are often disseminated through prompts to impose a response burden on participants through disruptions (Suh, Shahriaree, Hekler, & Kientz, 2016). This leads to a tradeoff between balancing the construct validity of participant responses and their compliance (Chan et al., 2018). Subsequently, researchers have employed various forms of passive sensing (Wang et al., 2014), such as logging an individual's phone usage or tracking physical activity via wearable sensors, and these sensing technologies have been significantly successful in studying human behavior, well-being, and psychosocial dynamics (Wang et al., 2014).

Social media represent one such passive sensing platform, whose promise is situated in the notion that many human behaviors and attributes have social underpinnings when viewed through the lens of the social-ecological model (Catalano, 1979). This chapter seeks to overcome the gap in studying well-being in situated communities by using social media data. In particular, we focus on two situated communities: *college campuses* and *workplaces*. These communities are unique in age, demographics, and socioeconomic characteristics, as well as day-to-day activities, goals, and concerns.

Social Media and Well-Being in College Campuses

College campuses are close-knit, largely geographically co-located communities, where students typically experience mental well-being concerns (Eisenberg, Golberstein, & Gollust, 2007). Colleges are valued institutions that help build upon a society's foundations and serve as an arena where the growth and stability of future generations begin. With regard to the population of college students, Ellison, Steinfield, and Lampe (2007) found a positive relationship between social media usage and maintenance of social capital, and Manago, Taylor, and Greenfield (2012) found that social media help college students satisfy their psychosocial needs. Given the near-universal use of social media among youth (Pew Research Center, 2021) and because social media platforms enable individuals to share and disclose mental health issues (Eisenberg, Hunt, & Speer, 2012), researchers have begun to leverage social media as an unobtrusive and passive source of data to infer and understand the mental health and well-being of college students (Liu, Zhu, & Young, 2018; Mark, Wang, Niiya, & Reich, 2016; Moreno, Jelenchick, et al., 2011). Of particular relevance is the work of Bagroy, Kumaraguru, and De Choudhury (2017), who built a collective mental health index of colleges employing social media (Reddit) data. Manago and colleagues (2012) found that social networking helps satisfy the psychosocial needs of college students, and Moreno, Jelenchick, and colleagues (2011) studied mental health disclosures by college students on social media. Prior research has also inferred other behavioral and psychological attributes of college students, using social media (Mark et al., 2016; Valkenburg, Peter, & Schouten, 2006). Recent research has revealed the construct validity of social media-based mental health assessments of college students in predicting on-campus mental health consultations (Saha, Yousuf, Boyd, Pennebaker, & De Choudhury, 2022).

Social Media and Well-Being in Workplaces

In the last decade, researchers have used social media technologies to study employee behavior in the workplace (De Choudhury & Counts, 2013). For example, IBM researchers (Ehrlich & Shami, 2010) compared employees' use of social media platforms, particularly their motivations for using these platforms (Twitter). They reported that, both at home and at work, social media made workers, especially mobile workers, feel more connected to other employees and helped boost their position in the workplace. Studies found that social media use is positively correlated with workplace well-being (Shami, Nichols, & Chen, 2014). Increased social media interactions within the workplace, through platforms such as IBM's Beehive, were found to improve both personal and professional networking, career advancements, and innovation (DiMicco et al., 2008; Farzan et al., 2008; Geyer et al., 2008). Other works have also found that social media technologies have promoted positive relationships between workplace and employee behavior (De Choudhury & Counts, 2013; Erez, Misangyi, Johnson, LePine, & Halverson, 2008; Fowler & Christakis, 2008; Guillory et al., 2011). In an early work, Skeels and Grudin (2009) conducted a longitudinal study of employee motivations and use of social media platforms. Taken together, social media use, both within and outside of the workplace, contribute to the worker's well-being and professional stature through increased connectivity, reputation building, and networking opportunities. Social media and online engagement platforms have facilitated efforts to study employee behavior and satisfaction (Archambault & Grudin, 2012; De Choudhury & Counts, 2013; Mitra, Muller, Sadt Shami, Golestani, & Masli., 2017; Shami, Yang, et al., 2014; Skeels & Grudin, 2009). Analytical and computational approaches on language and network dynamics have gleaned correlates of employee job satisfaction and well-being, such as engagement (Hickman, Saha, De Choudhury, & Tay, 2019; Mitra et al., 2017; Shami, Muller, Pal, Masli, & Geyer, 2015), employee affect (De Choudhury & Counts, 2013; Saha et al., 2019c), social pulse (Shami, Nichols, et al., 2014), reputation (Jacovi, Guy, Kremer-Davidson, Porat, & Aizenbud-Reshef, 2014), organizational relationships (Brzozowski, 2009; Gilbert, 2012; Mitra & Gilbert, 2012), and workplace behavior (Mark, Iqbal, Czerwinski, & Johns, 2014). Anonymized platforms such as Glassdoor provide "safe spaces" for employees to share and assess their workplace experience (Boyd & Ellison, 2007; Kollock, 1999) and to measure organizational culture (Das Swain et al., 2020). These studies indicate the value of unobtrusive data sources in understanding workplace experiences.

This chapter highlights research that examines problems applicable to and critical for situated communities and leverages social media data that reflect the online analog of offline (physically co-located) situated communities. For example, we leverage college subreddit data for college campuses where college students express and share topics and interests about their day-to-day academic, personal, and college lives (Saha & De Choudhury, 2017; Saha, Weber, & De Choudhury, 2018). Similarly, we leverage LinkedIn data for employees in workplace communities in order to show how employees' job roles relate to their workplace performance and experiences (Saha et al., 2019e). These datasets uniquely allow us to capture the social and environmental context required for a better understanding of well-being. Thus, the contributions highlighted in this chapter are threefold: (1) using social media data that particularly and uniquely capture the behavior of situated communities, (2) adopting theory-driven computational and causal methods to make conclusive research claims on well-being dynamics, and (3) discussing the challenges given the limitations of social media data and how methods combining social media and other behavioral data can circumvent these challenges toward reaching a comprehensive understanding of human behavior.

Employing an interdisciplinary context that includes psychology and the social sciences and considering theoretical, practical, design, methodological, and ethical perspectives has implications for a variety of stakeholders, including researchers, practitioners, administrators, and policymakers. A major implication of these studies concerns building tools and applications that leverage these data-driven methodologies to improve well-being in practice. The following two sections review our research conducted in two situated communities: college campuses and workplaces. Particularly showcased is the role of social media in a variety of dimensions concerning mental and psychological well-being.

Measuring Stress Associated with Gun Violence on College Campuses

In this section, we discuss our prior research on the use of computational methods to infer mental well-being (stress) in crisis situations (e.g., gun violence incidents; Saha & De Choudhury, 2017). College students undergo stress throughout the year due to academic, personal relationships, environmental, and social factors (Ross, Niebling, & Heckert, 1999). Mental health concerns are pervasive in the college student population (Hirsch & Ellis, 1996). Crises on college campuses can cause acute stress and have long-term negative consequences, including posttraumatic stress, acute stress, borderline personality, or adjustment disorders (Wood et al., 2002). Violent incidents on college campuses ranging from mass shootings to acts of terrorism have proliferated in the recent past. A survey from Everytown for Gun Safety Support Research[1] reports that between 2013 and 2016, 76 incidents of gun violence occurred on U.S. college campuses, resulting in more than 100 casualties. Many of these incidents not only affect those involved in the incidents directly, but also leave profound negative psychological impacts on the general campus community (Zajacova, Lynch, & Espenshade, 2005). It is vital to understand the potential impacts of violent incidents on the college student's psyche.

Two complementary research directions guided our work. First, studies in psycholinguistics and crisis informatics presented promising evidence that the language shared on social media could help us determine the psychological states of individuals and collectives (De Choudhury, Monroy-Hernandez, & Mark, 2014; Mark et al., 2012; Starbird et al., 2010). Second, over 90% of young adults or individuals of college age use social media.[2] This facilitated our ability to study college students' mental well-being unobtrusively and passively (Bagroy et al., 2017). Our three research aims were as follows:

- Aim 1: Infer stress expressions in social media posts.
- Aim 2: Quantify *temporal* changes in stress expressions following gun violence incidents on campuses.
- Aim 3: Quantify *linguistic* changes in stress expressions following gun violence incidents on campuses.

We studied gun violence incidents reported between 2012 and 2016 on 12 U.S. college campuses. For each campus, we obtained data from corresponding college subreddits. For the first aim, we developed an inductive transfer learning approach to infer stress expressed in Reddit posts, which achieved a mean accuracy of 82%. Using this classifier, we identified high-stress posts shared in the 12 college subreddits. Then, targeting the second and third aims, we developed techniques drawing from the time-series and natural language analysis. Complete details of the study are available in Saha and De Choudhury (2017); here we summarize our approach to collecting and analyzing the social media data and the main findings to illustrate how social media data can help us understand and predict mental well-being on college campuses.

Data

Gathering Campus-Specific Gun Violence Data

For our study (Saha & De Choudhury, 2017), we adopted the definition of gun violence on college campuses, as published by Everytown for Gun Safety Support Research[3]: "a shooting involving discharge of a firearm inside a college building or on campus grounds and not in self-defense." Everytown for Gun Safety is an American nonprofit organization that conducts gun violence research in the United States. However, since there is no single database for gun violence incidents on college campuses, we adopted a snowball approach to curate our dataset (Ayers, Althouse, Leas, Alcorn, & Dredze, 2016; Pavlick & Callison-Burch, 2016): (1) We collected a seed list of gun violence incidents on U.S. college campuses from Everytown for Gun Safety Research; we also used this list in prior work (Ayers et al., 2016); (2) we augmented this seed list with additional incidents that satisfy the same definition we cited above (we consulted credible online sources in an iterative fashion).[4] Our curated list consisted of gun-related incidents of violence that took place both on and in close proximity to the college campus between 2012 and 2017.

Finding a Campus-Specific Social Media Data Source

The social media data source of our study is Reddit, particularly college subreddits. In colleges with subreddits, we filtered at least 500 subscribers on the day of the campus incident, guided by prior work (see Bagroy, Kumaraguru, & De Choudhury, 2017). Twelve such colleges met the criteria, and there were between 969 (r/NAU) and 8,936 (r/OSU) subscribers in these subreddits.

Compiling Treatment and Control Data from Social Media

Because our study examined statistical differences in the expression of stress around gun violence incidents, we ensured that the measured differences in stress were indeed attributable to the incidents rather than to other unobserved or latent variables. In the statistics literature, these concerns regarding quantification of an "outcome" (stress) are typically mitigated by adopting randomized experiments, where, given a "treatment" (gun violence incident) in the target population, an equivalent population is assigned to a "control" (gun violence free) condition to rule out the effects that might be attributable to confounding or omitted variables (Holland, 1986; Petticrew et al., 2005). Since an experimental approach was inappropriate for our study, we adopted matching to compile our data, drawing from the causal inference literature (Rosenbaum & Rubin, 1985). Specifically, for each of the 12 incidents, we identified two separate time periods of campus subreddit data collection: a treatment period and a control period.

1. *Treatment period.* We identified a period of 2 months before and 2 months after the gun violence incident on each campus. Our rationale for marking this as our period of analysis was based on prior work published by Kumar, Dredze, Coppersmith, and De Choudhury (2015), which observed that the effects of societal upheaval persisted for only a limited period of time. Because we focused on college campuses that tended to follow a 4-month semester or a 2.5-month quarterly academic system, we deduced that a 4-month period around each incident that closely followed the academic system would help us detect meaningful stress changes attributable to the incident.

2. *Control period.* For the combined period of 2 months before and 2 months after the gun-related violence incident on each campus, we identified an equivalent period of 4 months from the previous year. Gathering data from the same period in the past year (when no gun violence was reported) is likely to rule out confounding effects in the measuring temporal or linguistic differences in stress attributable to academic calendar factors, or seasonal and periodic events that impact students' experiences, lifestyle, and activities. Because we identified this period specific to each campus, we ruled out the possibility of incorporating confounding effects attributable to campus characteristics or the nature of student population and their demographics.

We used Google BigQuery to collect data from each college subreddit during the *Treatment* and *Control* periods. This dataset consisted of 113,337 posts[5] (Table 9.1). We further demarcated each *Treatment* and *Control* dataset into before and after samples based on whether the date of a post in the *Treatment* (or *Control*) dataset was prior to or followed the reported incident at the corresponding campus (or the same date in the previous year).

TABLE 9.1. Gun Violence in U.S. College Campuses during 2012-2016 Used in Our Work

College	Incident	#n	Subreddit	Users	#Posts
University of Southern California	2012-10-31	4	r/USC	1,143	2,676
University of Maryland	2013-02-12	3	r/UMD	2,201	9,578
University of Central Florida	2013-03-18	1	r/ucf	2,886	13,708
Massachusetts Institute of Technology	2013-04-18	3	r/mit	1,568	1,682
Purdue University	2014-01-21	1	r/Purdue	3,605	11,172
University of California Santa Barbara	2014-05-23	21	r/UCSantaBarbara	3,278	17,682
Florida State University	2014-11-20	4	r/fsu	3,859	8,150
University of South Carolina	2015-02-05	2	r/Gamecocks	1,903	1,661
University of North Carolina at Chapel Hill	2015-02-10	3	r/chapelhill	2,025	1,177
North Arizona University	2015-10-09	4	r/NAU	969	1,025
University of California, Los Angeles	2016-06-01	2	r/ucla	6,301	9,454
Ohio State University	2016-11-28	14	r/OSU	8,936	35,372

Note. We also include the date, number of casualties (#*n*), and descriptive statistics of the corresponding sub-Reddit communities

Aim 1: Infer Stress Expressions in Social Media Posts

It is hard to obtain large-scale ground-truth stress expressions data on social media. To overcome this challenge, we adopted a transfer learning approach through which we built a supervised machine learning model to classify stress expressions in posts into the binary labels *High Stress* and *Low Stress*. We used this classifier to machine label posts in the college subreddits.

Our stress class definition is based on the established psychometric measure of stress as per the Perceived Stress Scale (PSS; Cohen, Kamarck, & Mermelstein, 1983). The widely used 10-item version of PSS identifies three categories: (1) Scores ranging from 0 to 13, minimal stress; (2) 14–26, moderate stress; and (3) 27–40, extreme stress. Typically, factor analysis (Hewitt et al., 1992) reveals two factors, based on this scoring. This motivates our choice of two classes: *Low Stress* and *High Stress*.

We collected all 1,402 posts from the subreddit *r/stress* from December 2010 to January 2017. The *r/stress* community allows individuals to self-report and disclose stressful experiences and is a support community. For example, two (paraphrased) post excerpts say: "*Feel like I am burning out (again . . .) Help: what do I do?*"; and "*How do I calm down when I get triggered?*." The community is heavily moderated, so we considered these 1,402 posts as ground-truth data for *High Stress* posts. Next, we obtained a second dataset of over 100,000 random posts from subreddits listed on Reddit's landing page. We randomly sampled 2,000 posts from this dataset and considered it as ground-truth data for *Low Stress* posts.

On the above training dataset, we obtained features for the stress classifier: We used Stanford CoreNLP's sentiment analysis model to retrieve the sentiment class of the posts and the top 500 n-grams ($n = 3$). We developed a binary support vector machine (SVM) classifier (with a linear kernel) for detecting *High Stress* and *Low Stress* in posts. We used this classifier to machine label all *Before* and *After* posts shared in the *Control* and *Treatment* datasets associated with the 12 campuses.

Corresponding to our first aim, we present the results of the machine learning classifier of stress. Our binary SVM classifier uses 5,000 n-gram features and three boolean sentiment features, Positive, Negative, and Neutral; the number of n-gram features was determined based on systematic parameter sweep. We used a k-fold ($k = 5$) cross-validation technique to evaluate our model and achieved a mean accuracy of 0.82. This accuracy beats the baseline accuracy (based on a chance model) of 0.68 on this dataset. Table 9.2 reports the performance metrics of the stress classifier, and Figure 9.1 shows the receiver operating characteristic (ROC) curve of the same. We find that our classifier yields a low number of false positives (average precision 0.82), as well as low false negatives (average recall 0.82), indicating robust performance on test data. Table 9.3 reports the top 30 features of our stress classifier.

To understand the temporal and linguistic dynamics of *High Stress*, we applied the stress classifier to machine label the posts. With the help of three human raters, who were expert in social media analytics and affect dynamics, we validated a random sample of 151 of the classifier labeled posts (79 *High Stress* and 72 *Low Stress* posts). Our experts adopted the Perceived Stress Scale (Cohen et al., 1983) to examine how stressful experiences from the scale (e.g., feelings of nervousness, anger, lack of control) are expressed in each post. Our raters reached a high agreement (Fleiss's kappa = 0.84), and we found an accuracy of 82% for the stress classification.

TABLE 9.2. Performance Metrics of Stress Classification per *k*-Fold Cross-Validation (*k* = 5)

Metric	Mean	Stdev.	Median	Max.
Accuracy	0.82	0.11	0.78	0.90
Precision	0.83	0.14	0.77	0.92
Recall	0.82	0.09	0.78	0.88
F1-score	0.82	0.11	0.79	0.89
ROC-AUC	0.90	0.08	0.78	0.95

Aim 2: Quantify Temporal Changes in Stress Expressions around Campus Gun Violence

We examined the temporal variability of *High Stress* expressed in subreddit posts around each campus gun violence (*Treatment* data) and a similar period in the previous year (*Control* data). We aggregated posts shared per day, and then we normalized the number of posts labeled as *High Stress* on each day. In order to assign weightage to the number of *High Stress* posts on a day as well as its proportion in this normalization, we employed a variant of the TF-IDF (term frequency-inverse document frequency) estimation technique: We multiplied the proportion of *High Stress* posts in a day with the squared root of their count on the same day. We obtained the temporal variability in stress for both *Control* and *Treatment* datasets, spanning the *Before* and *After* periods. Then, we used 0–lag cross correlation to assess how the manifestations of *High Stress* around incidents differ from the same in a comparable time frame in the past.

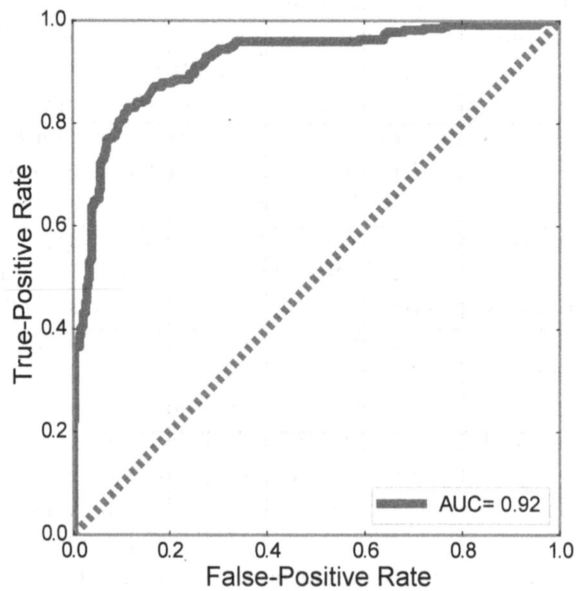

FIGURE 9.1. ROC curve for the stress classifier.

TABLE 9.3. Top 30 Features in Stress Classifier

Feature	p	log(score)	Feature	p	log(score)	Feature	p	log(score)	Feature	p	log(score)
stress	***	9.63	thank	***	6.20	breathing	***	6.44	health	***	5.87
try	***	7.46	meet	***	6.17	techniques	***	6.33	week	***	5.86
work	***	7.20	life	***	6.07	feel	***	6.30	minutes	***	5.83
anxiety	***	7.05	sleep	***	6.03	exercise	***	6.30	doctor	***	5.83
meditation	***	6.88	problems	***	5.98	time	***	6.25	mental	***	5.83
help	***	6.81	control	***	5.95	play	***	6.23	relax	***	5.72
focus	***	6.62	job	***	5.89	body	***	6.21	stressful	***	5.67
luck	***	6.62	good	***	5.87						

Note. Statistical significance reported after Bonferroni correction.
***$p < .001$.

We quantified changes in stress expressions by estimating the trend of *High Stress* before and after the incidents. We computed z-scores of *High Stress* posts on each day for the *Before* and *After* samples in the *Treatment* dataset. We also measured an average change in z-scores between *Before* and *After* samples.

Time Domain Analysis of High-Stress Posts

Figure 9.2 shows the normalized volume of *High Stress* content in the *Treatment* and *Control* datasets. We find that *High Stress* posts are shared in the college subreddits throughout the period spanning across the *Treatment* and *Control* datasets, in varying degrees. These posts consist of content ranging across varieties of academic and college-life-specific topics including, admission, examinations, and assignments. This observation aligns with prior literature that situates various college-life-specific factors that are attributable to student stress (Ross et al., 1999); that stress is a persistent psychological observation among college students (Bayram & Bilgel, 2008). When we examine the day of the gun violence incident and its vicinity, we observe a peak in the normalized volume of *High Stress* posts in a majority of the subreddits that is considerably distinct in r/ucf, r/Purdue, r/UCSantaBarbara, r/NAU, r/OSU. The peak in stress in the *Treatment* year, as compared to the *Control* year, suggests that campus gun violence contributes to increased stress immediately following the incident. We find that the mean normalized stress in the *Treatment* year is higher than the same for *Control* across all campuses (1.35 vs. 1.19). A cross-correlation analysis of the temporal occurrences of *High Stress* posts in *Control* and *Treatment* datasets shows statistical significance.

How does the expression of *High Stress* in the college subreddits change in the aftermath of the gun violence incidents compared to the incident before? To answer this question, we report the findings of our proposed before–after analysis. A 0-lag cross-correlation for *Before* and *After* samples within the *Treatment* dataset shows statistical significance. Next, we computed the z-scores of *High Stress* expressed on each day. The mean change in z-score between *Before* and *After* samples ranged from −0.30 (r/NAU) to 0.83 (r/Purdue), with 9 out of 12 subreddits exhibiting a positive change in expression of *High Stress*. We conducted Mann-Whitney U tests of *Before* and *After* day-wise z-scores,

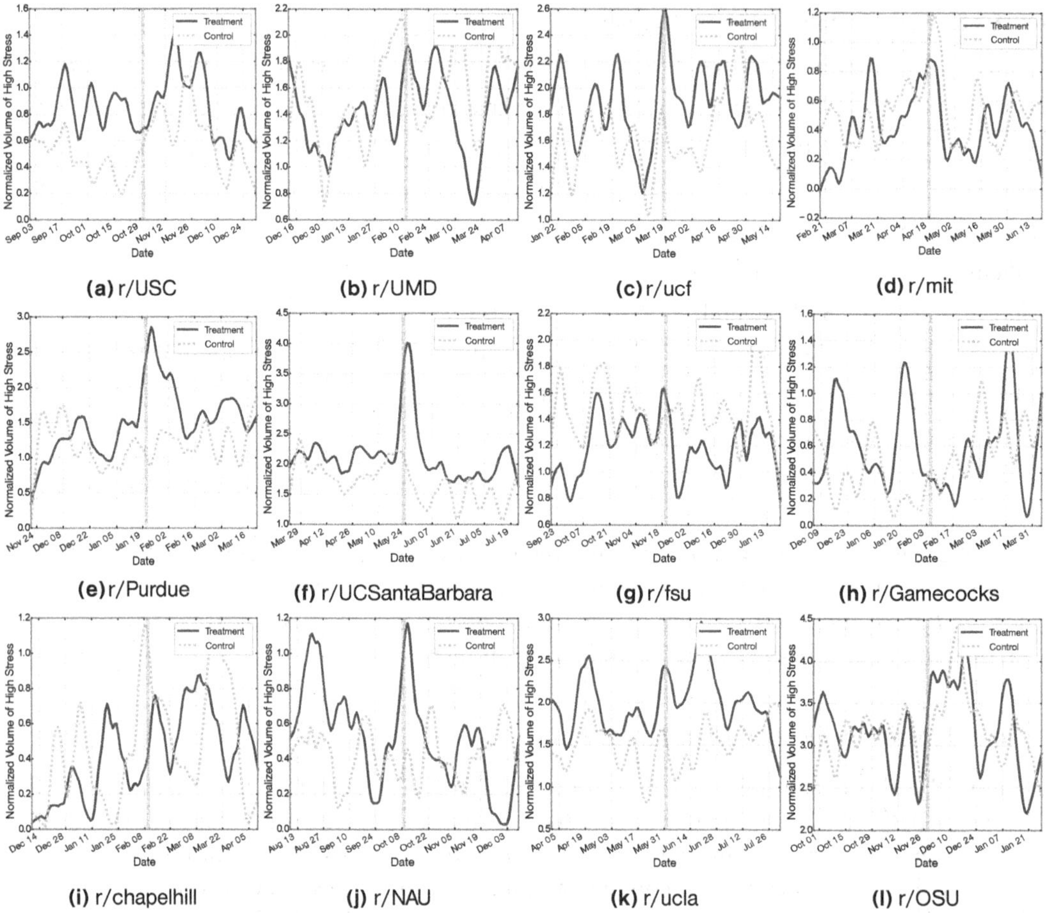

FIGURE 9.2. Temporal variation in the expression of *High Stress*. The reference line represents the date of gun violence incident.

revealing the statistical significance for each subreddit. More careful examination indicates that the *z*-scores of *High Stress* in the days following the incident in most of the subreddits have a trend line (based on fitting a linear model) yielding a negative slope. Specifically, we observe the most negative slopes in the cases of r/Purdue (–0.03) and r/OSU (–0.03). However, the trend line fits for *High Stress* *z*-scores in the *Before* period do not show such a trend—the mean slope during the period preceding the gun violence incidents is 0.001, revealing approximately a stable pattern.

Overall, our results suggest that the expression of *High Stress* in the aftermath of gun violence shows an abrupt shift in temporal pattern, peaking significantly around the day of the incidents, and thereafter showing a downward trend.

Frequency Domain Analysis of High-Stress Posts

Our final analysis for the second aim centers around understanding how the various gun violence incidents on campuses disrupt the periodicity of sharing *High Stress* posts. Working within the frequency domain, we apply Fast-Fourier Transform (FFT) on the distribution of *High Stress* posts in *Treatment* data. For each college subreddit, Figure 9.3 shows the distribution of frequencies *F(t)* during *Before* and *After* periods as heatmaps. The color intensity of a cell in a specific heatmap indicates the probability of a certain frequency, *P(F(t))* (measured in terms of days). Discussing our main observations from the heatmaps, in case of r/USC (Figure 9.3(a)), we find that *High Stress* posts in the *Before* period show high periodicity (i.e., exhibit peaks in expression) around every 4 and 13 days, whereas the same in the *After* period occurred every 5, 7, and 11 days.

We note that for r/Gamecocks, which we found to show an aberrant pattern compared to other subreddits in the time domain analysis, according to its frequency domain analysis distribution heatmap (Figure 9.3h), there was a significant change in the periodicity of expression of high stress following the gun violence incident at the University of Southern Carolina (14% change in spectral density and a SMAP difference of 17).

Aim 3: Quantify Linguistic Changes in Stress Expressions around Campus Gun Violence

For this aim, we adopted two language analyses: (1) psycholinguistic characterization and (2) open-vocabulary linguistic analysis.

Psycholinguistic Characterization

We characterized the psycholinguistics of *High Stress* posts in *Treatment* data using Linguistic Inquiry and Word Count (LIWC; Pennebaker, Mehl, & Niederhoffer, 2003). We compared *High Stress Treatment* posts from the *Before* and *After* samples across (1) *affective attributes* (anger, anxiety, negative, and positive affect, sadness, swear), (2) *cognitive attributes* (causation, inhibition, cognitive mechanics, discrepancies, negation, tentativeness, certainty), (3) *perception* (feeling, hearing, insight, seeing, perception),

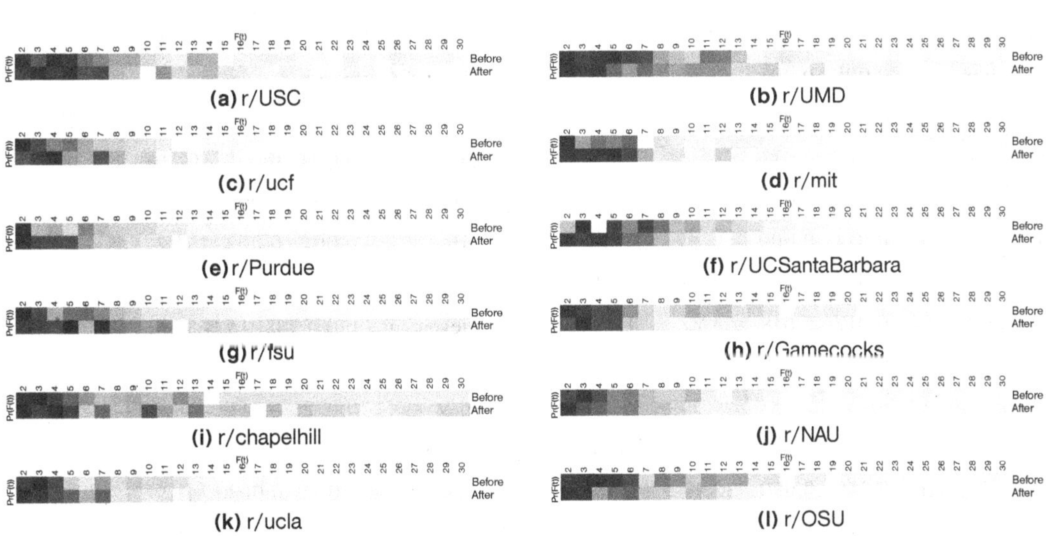

FIGURE 9.3. Frequency distribution heatmaps of stress in the *Treatment* dataset. The *x*-axis, *F(t)*, represents frequency, where *t* is in terms of days; the density of color, *Pr(F(t))*, represents the probability of *High Stress* at *F(t)*.

(4) *interpersonal focus* (categories: first person singular and plural, second person, third person, indefinite pronoun), (5) *temporal references* (future tense, past tense, present tense), (6) *lexical density and awareness* (adverbs, verbs, article, exclusive, inclusive, preposition, quantifier, auxiliary verbs, relative, conjunction), (7) *biological concerns* (bio, body, death, health, sexual), (8) *personal concerns* (achievement, home, money, religion), and (9) *social concerns* (family, friends, humans, social, work). We conducted Welch's *t*-test, followed by Benjamini-Hochberg-Yekutieli False Discovery Rate (FDR) correction (Table 9.4).

AFFECT

Starting with *Affective Attributes*, we observe that *High Stress* posts in the *After* dataset show higher occurrences of *anger*, *negative affect*, and *swear* words. Some example post

TABLE 9.4. Welch's *t*-Test Comparing the Psycholinguistic Attributes of High-Stress Treatment Posts Shared before and after Gun Violence Incidents

Category	*Before*	*After*	Δ%	*t*-stat.	*p*	Category	*Before*	*After*	Δ%	*t*-stat.	*p*
Affective Attributes						***Temporal References***					
Anger	0.008	0.010	23.34	3.558	***	Future Tense	0.037	0.035	−6.15	−2.15	*
Anxiety	0.007	0.003	−61.81	−11.499	***	Past Tense	0.056	0.061	8.58	3.79	***
Negative Affect	0.007	0.009	20.55	3.376	***	Present Tense	0.116	0.113	−2.20	−1.79	*
Positive Affect	0.072	0.036	−50.56	−27.978	***	***Lexical Density and Awareness***					
Sadness	0.002	0.002	14.42	1.554	*	Article	0.117	0.144	22.93	16.72	***
Swear	0.006	0.007	12.46	1.5765	*	Exclusive	0.032	0.064	99.31	33.66	***
Cognitive Attributes						Preposition	0.219	0.181	−17.38	−21.99	***
Causation	0.027	0.013	−51.95	−23.312	***	Quantifier	0.023	0.043	86.01	25.47	***
Inhibition	0.008	0.005	−36.48	−7.824	***	***Biological Concerns***					
Negation	0.029	0.041	41.90	13.334	***	Bio	0.012	0.014	10.62	2.48	**
Perception						Body	0.004	0.005	16.30	2.07	***
Feel	0.004	0.006	34.59	3.225	**	Health	0.003	0.007	97.39	8.84	***
Hear	0.014	0.009	−35.49	−7.518	***	Death	0.001	0.003	155.22	6.41	***
Insight	0.041	0.020	−50.24	−26.544	***	***Personal and Social Concerns***					
Percept	0.017	0.018	4.22	1.137	*	Achievement	0.037	0.016	−55.66	−25.51	***
See	0.019	0.018	−7.11	−1.896	*	Home	0.005	0.009	93.94	10.15	***
Interpersonal Focus						Money	0.022	0.011	−48.75	−16.66	***
1st P. Plural	0.013	0.010	−24.94	−5.011	***	Religion	0.003	0.004	43.82	2.87	**
1st P. Singular	0.061	0.080	32.47	15.864	***	Family	0.002	0.003	41.67	2.61	**
3rd P.	0.015	0.012	−18.78	−3.740	**	Friends	0.004	0.006	65.55	5.35	***

Note. Statistical significance reported after Benjamini–Hochberg–Yekutieli False Discovery Rate Correction.
***$p < .001$; **$.001 < p < .01$; *$01 < p < .05$.

snippets include, "*why the hell do they have a giant assault rifle?*" and "*I guess since campus is a gun free zone we're all fucked.*" At the same time, *High Stress* posts in the *After* period show significantly lowered levels of *positive affect* words. This indicates that the students may be engaging over Reddit to express their relatively higher negative perceptions, reactions, and thoughts apropos the gun violence incidents.

Cognition and Perception

For *Cognition* and *Perception*, we observe that words related to *causation*, *inhibition*, and *insight* are used significantly less often in the *After* period. Prior work has attributed this psycholinguistic expression to lowered cognitive functioning (Bagroy et al., 2017), which is a symptom of high stress. However, *negation* words occur more frequently in the *After* period, and so do the words related to *feel*. Per prior work (Pennebaker et al., 2003), this kind of greater perceptual expressiveness is associated with language that depicts personal and first-hand accounts of events and experiences. Likewise, in our case, they indicate that the subreddit users are more expressive of their feelings in the aftermath of the campus gun violence incidents.

Linguistic Style

Corresponding to linguistic style attributes, *Before* and *After High Stress* posts show distinctive *Interpersonal Focus*. We find that the use of *first person singular* pronouns increases by 32% after gun violence, but that of *first person plural* and *third person* pronoun words decreases. We conjecture that users posting in the college subreddits may be resorting to social media to share their personal experiences and opinions about the incident. In the case of *Temporal References*, we find reduced use of *future* and *present* tense, and increased use of *past* tense in the *After* period. Higher use of the past tense indicates tendency to recollect prior experiences and events (Tausczik & Pennebaker, 2010), which in our case, might be an orientation toward discussing the gun violence incident on the campus.

Biological Concerns

Our results show that words referring to *bio*, *body*, *health*, and *death* increase in the *After* period. We conjecture that the *High Stress* posts shared following the gun violence incidents tend to relate to the after-effects, casualties, and implications of the incident for students' safety, well-being, and life.

Personal and Social Concerns

We observe revealing patterns for *Personal* and *Social Concerns*. First, words related to *achievement* occur significantly less (55%) in the period *After* the gun violence incidents. The lower usage of *achievement* words indicates a decline in engagements in career and academic topic-related discussions in the aftermath of the campus gun-related violence. Next, we find that the usage of words relating to social life and relationships, notably, *family*, *friends*, and *home*, increase *After* the incidents. Through these social orientation words, we ask the subreddit users to share social well-being impressions and perceptions of solidarity in the context of the incidents. In addition, some of these incidents, such as the UNC Chapel Hill or the OSU attack were violence attributed to religious radicalism or religious hate crime, which we conjecture contribute to the higher occurrence of *religion* words in the *After* period.

Open-Vocabulary Lexical Analysis

We examined the lexical cues shared in *High Stress* posts in *Treatment* data around the gun violence incidents. We analyzed linguistic markers as manifested in the subreddits immediately after gun violence on a college campus. Within the *High Stress Treatment* posts, we first extracted the 30 most frequently occurring *n*-grams (n = 1,2,3) on the day of the incident. Figure 9.4 shows the 30-day *Before* and *After* temporal trends of usage of *n*-grams. We find that "class" occurs consistently in *High Stress* posts until the incident dates, but its usage declines considerably in the following week. In contrast, keywords such as "people," "friend," "hope," and "feel" showed increased occurrence in the immediate aftermath of the event—aligning with the observations from the psycholinguistic analysis and involving the emergence of a social orientation and greater perceptual expression following the incidents. The *n*-grams describing the nature, manifestation, and implications of the specific campus incidents (e.g., "police," "shooting," "safe," and "gun") had dense and increased concentration of usage following the day of the incident.

We drilled down further for each of the 12 colleges and, employing the Log Likelihood Ratio (LLR) measure, we extracted the top 50 *n*-grams (n = 3) from the *High Stress* posts within 7 days following the day of gun violence, and then we compared the occurrences in *High Stress* posts in the 7 days preceding the day of the incident. Table 9.5 reports the *n*-grams, for which we obtained an LLR of over 0.75. We find keywords specific to the gun violence incidents such as the geographical sites (e.g., "*campus center*" in r/USC, "*tower 1*" in r/ucf, "*isla vista*" in r/UCSantaBarbara, "*library*" in r/fsu, "*public health*" in r/Gamecocks, and "*parking*" in r/OSU). Additionally, we find the presence

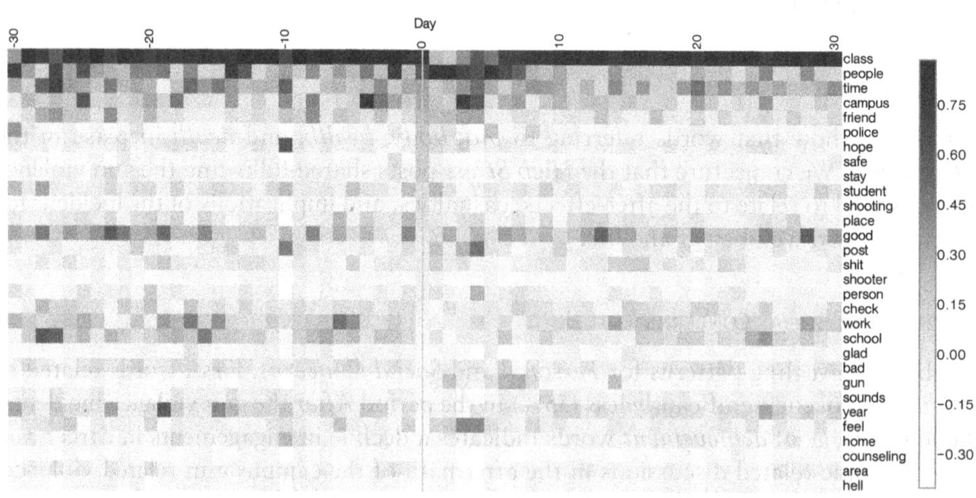

FIGURE 9.4. Top 30 keywords used in *High Stress* posts around the day of gun violence incident (day = 0).

of "*muslims*" in r/chapelhill and r/OSU, where the incidents were attributed to religious hate crimes or radicalism. We find keywords relating to the victim or the perpetrator's name and occupations. Summarily, this analysis shows that the high stress expressed in the posts of the college subreddits in the immediate aftermath of the gun-related violence may be a consequence of the incidents in the respective campuses.

Implications

We employed a causal inference-based analytical approach, in conjunction with computational techniques, to examine the evolution stress following gun violence events on college campuses. Compared to a control (gun violence-free) time period on each campus, our methods revealed a change in the volume of posts expressing high stress following the violent incidents, including a considerable change in the patterns of stress expressed in the immediate aftermath of the incidents. Psycholinguistic characterization of the high stress posts indicates that campus populations exhibited reduced cognitive processing and greater self-attention and social orientation, and that they participated

TABLE 9.5. Lexicon of Selected *n*-Grams ($n = 1, 2, 3$) Occurring Considerably Higher in Posts Shared 7 Days after the Day of Gun-Related Violence, as Compared to 7 Days before the Day of Gun-Related Violence

Subreddit	*After > Before* (*LLR* ≥ (0.75))
r/USC	problems, night, security, shooting, party, events, fingerprint, entrances, email, dps, campus center, event, trojan, defense, safe
r/UMD	athletics, gun, supercar, cars, shoot, department, school, fire, community, sports, college, park
r/ucf	assault, assault rifle, weapon, tower 1, rifle, gun, police
r/mit	state, lincoln, stay safe, watertown, officer, officers, police, scanner, second, shots, shots fired, house, bpd, unknown, clear, confirmed, custody, dexter, fired, fuck, spruce, suspect, black, boston
r/Purdue	shooter, police, shooting, news, place, building, ee, campus, guy, heard, day, gt, know, student, people, today
r/UCSanta-Barbara	videos, victims, gun, mental, isla vista, guy, news, community, post, police, person, help, feel, love, iv, life, point, friends
r/fsu	mental, safe, shooting, strozier, ok, news, library, shooter, friends, victims, hope, stay, post, time, people, information, good
r/Gamecocks	alert, murder/suicide, public health, public health research, research center, shooter, shooting, students, support, lockdown, faculty staff, counseling center, building, health research center, cancelled
r/chapelhill	pretty, muslims, writing, religion, high, hicks, help, pound, students, execution style, execution, universal, world, abusalha, 30 serv, support, parking, unc
r/NAU	astronomy, jones, kill, kill people, meth, problem, harder, professors, self, self defense, shooter, shot, tour, guns kill people, year, guns, fight, class, defense, gun, asu, shooting
r/ucla	safe, confirmed, police, klug, shooter, gun, guns, health, mental, saying, professor, situation
r/OSU	safe, police, muslims, gun, removed, parking, post, stay, wrong

more in death-related conversations. Additionally, a lexical analysis of high stress posts shows distinctive temporal trends in the use of incident-specific words, providing further evidence of the impact of the incidents on the stress responses of campus populations.

Theoretical Implications

We presented our findings in the context of psychological theories surrounding trauma and crisis and made two major observations: (1) Psychological stress may be automatically inferred from social media content by employing supervised learning approaches and (2) inferred stress levels on a college campus may indicate the responses of individuals exposed to the reported gun-related violence incident. To arrive at these findings, we made a methodological contribution in our study as to how stress changes, both temporal and linguistic, can be measured following a violent incident on campus, drawing from machine learning and time-series analysis techniques. Therefore, our work has implications for researchers' study of the sociopsychological responses of a population exposed to a crisis. We discuss these implications below.

Freud (2003) argued that external reality (e.g., traumatic events) can have profound effects on an individual's pysche and can be the cause of emotional upheaval, stress, and traumatic neurosis. He suggested that the personal impact of the trauma, the inability to find conscious expressions for it, and the unpreparedness of the individual can cause a breach to the stimulus barrier and overwhelm the defense mechanisms (Freud, 1977). Our study examined these theoretical constructs in a data-driven manner. For instance, the linguistic analytical methods suggest that distinctive psycholinguistic cues in high-stress posts are shared after a gun violence incident compared to before the incident. As an example, language related to biological concerns increases remarkably following the incident. In contrast, more general topics closely related to stress in a college population, such as financial and career-related concerns, are significantly reduced following the incident.

Furthermore, a notable finding of our study comes from the incident-specific lexical analysis: The content shared on social media immediately following the violent incidents appears to be largely topically related to the events themselves. McCann and Pearlman (1990), working within the framework of cognitive theory, proposed seven fundamental psychological need areas that arise following a crisis event: frame of reference, safety, dependency/trust of self and others, power, esteem, intimacy, and independence. Words such as "stay safe," "support," "hope," "help," and "self," whose usage increases in high-stress social media posts following violent incidents, are some of the expressions that many need at such times.

Our methods also help reveal the nuances in acute stress responses on college campuses following violent incidents, which tend to offset more persistent chronic stress expressions. For instance, although students experience stress throughout the year for both academic and personal reasons (Ross et al., 1999), a college campus's stress expression changes considerably after gun violence. In essence, as campus social media posts reveal, stress as a construct is prevalent (possibly chronic in nature) across time; yet the nature of this construct changes drastically (possibly becoming more acute) around a critical crisis incident. This also reveals the temporal and linguistic "signatures" of expression of such acute stress, such as altered periodicities or increase/decrease in specific psycholinguistic words which can be gleaned with our proposed machine learning and time-series analysis approaches. These findings support similar observations that have been made regarding the manifestation of psychological states in response to chronic violence (De Choudhury et al., 2014), war (Mark et al., 2012), and terrorist attacks (Lin & Margolin, 2014). Moreover, in close alignment with prior work (Al-Ani et al., 2010), we also observe that postviolence acute stress levels subside within days to follow and approach the baseline levels of generally persistent chronic stress. This interpretation is consistent with prior work on crisis informatics (Mark et al., 2012) and with Foa, Steketee, and Rothbaum's (1989) emotional processing theory.

Practical Implications

Our proposed techniques provide a mechanism for quantifying the impacts and severity of a crisis, as well as the corresponding community responses. Our techniques can be used as unobtrusive sensors of stress and the linguistic and temporal changes it brings during crises. These methodologies may be leveraged in future situations where causes of stress may not be so apparent or known, as was the case in our study assessing stress and associated student responses in everyday—crisis free—contexts, where a variety of day-to-day but unanticipated academic, personal, or social concerns may contribute to stress.

For instance, since sudden bursts of stress can be detrimental in the long term, McFarlane (2010), with our work, population-centric stress tracking tools can be built. These tools can significantly advance current practices in terms of how college authorities engage with the student community following crisis incidents. Typically, these practices include broad campus-wide communication of the context and outcomes of the incident, followed by specialized programs to direct psychological counseling and rehabilitation support to students who may need help. Our work can complement existing techniques and tools for assessing stress among individuals (Þórarinsdóttir, Kessing, & Faurholt-Jepsen, 2017). Using tools that leverage our methods, college authorities can learn about the pervasiveness of stress following a crisis event and the extent to which its normal pattern has been disrupted. This can enable them to make more informed decisions about the nature of crisis communication that should take place on campus, such as balancing informational alerts with adequately sensitive and focused assurance. Additionally, administrators will be able to reach a better understanding of students' counseling or rehabilitation resource needs. They will also be able to identify specific stress-induced temporal or linguistic responses that negatively impact specific student groups. This can allow them to take adequate action in a timely manner (e.g., conducting campus-wide awareness and mitigation campaigns on mental well-being, or making tailored provisions to improve the student body's mental resilience and morale.

Furthermore, since we leverage social media of the specific affected communities (college campuses), they can help identify their unique "signatures" or idiosyncratic patterns in stress expressions. Our approaches may also help discover the presence of protective factors surrounding stress in specific communities/campuses, including how a campus's stress expression deviates from an expected pattern of stress on any campus affected by a similar crisis. This information can be valuable to crisis rehabilitation efforts, including how specific campuses may adopt policies or strategies to enhance the idiosyncratic aspects relating to the community, that exacerbate or protect against stress.

Finally, we note that the impact of a violent incident transcends observed casualties, and its perception can be very subjective at an individual level. Our work provides a way to account for the "invisible wounds" (Holdeman, 2009) or "hidden casualties" (Prothrow-Stith & Quaday, 1995) in a crisis, which tend not to get reported or measured adequately. In essence, we observe that in the aftermath of campus gun-related violence, campus-specific social media like Reddit acts as a unique platform, allowing campus populations to express their emotions and stress their circumstances, (semi)anonymously, amid feelings of fear and trauma. These techniques enable the capturing of a "quantitative narrative" of these self-disclosed stress experiences of campus populations exposed to crisis events, which, we believe, can eventually inform historical accounts about campus life – insights critical to ensuring the well-being of situated communities.

Using LinkedIn Data to Measure Role Ambiguity in the Workplace

In this section, we discuss social-media-based modeling approaches to assessing well-being in another form of situated community—the workplace (Saha et al., 2019e). Employee satisfaction and well-being are of prime interest to both individuals and organizations. Researchers have concluded that employee-subjective well-being is one of the prime determinants of important outcomes that range across (1) health and longevity, (2) income, productivity, and organizational behavior, and (3) individual and social behavior (De Neve, Diener, Tay, & Xuereb, 2013). We present a research study that is motivated to help fill the gaps in state-of-the-art assessments of workplace well-being metrics. The study has implications for designing individual- and organization-facing tools designed to improve organizational functioning and well-being.

The complexities related to an individual's job role, or the *expectations applied to an individual within and beyond an organization's boundaries*, can impact their job satisfaction (Van Sell, Brief, & Schuler, 1981). In fact, any sort of discrepancy between *what* an employer expects and *what* an employee does at the workplace can impact well-being and performance, as employees can find themselves pulled in various directions as they try to respond to the many statuses they hold. According to role theory, role conflict, role ambiguity, and role overload are three aspects of the job role that contribute to workplace stress (Kahn, Wolfe, Quinn, Snoek, & Rosenthal, 1964; Pearce, 1981). Among the role constructs, role ambiguity has been considered to be the most significant one, and it is also the focus of the current study (Kahn et al., 1964).

Role ambiguity broadly includes uncertainties about role definition, expectations, responsibilities, tasks, and behaviors involved in one or more facets of the task environment (Jackson & Schuler, 1985; Kahn et al., 1964; Schmidt, Roesler, Kusserow, & Rau, 2014). Role ambiguity has both objective and subjective components. Objective role ambiguity refers to external conditions in the individual's workplace environment, whereas subjective role ambiguity relates to the amount of ambiguity that the individual perceives in their workplace owing to the information gap they face (Kahn et al., 1964). Furthermore, role ambiguity leads to dissatisfaction, distrust, lack of loyalty, turnover, absenteeism, low performance, anxiety-stress, and increased heart rate (Van Sell et al., 1981). There is sufficient evidence demonstrating how role ambiguity negatively affects one's organizational life in terms of their physiological, behavioral, psychological, and performance-related measures (Kahn, Byosiere, & Dunnette, 1992; Schmidt et al., 2014).

Traditionally, role ambiguity is measured using survey instruments that record employee responses to their perceived clarity of assigned tasks, expectations on the job, expectations of peers, and if these peers explicitly mention their expectations from the focal employee (Rizzo, House, & Lirtzman, 1970). In particular, these methods not only suffer from subjective biases (Smith, Tisak, & Schmieder, 1993), but also are only able to capture the "perceived" component of role ambiguity. Individuals may or may not be aware that they are working on things beyond their job requirements, such as when there is an information gap, or if they are investing their effort to gain knowledge and experience (Fried, Ben-David, Tiegs, Avital, & Yeverechyahu, 1998; King & King, 1990). Thus, it is unclear how useful these measures are (Ritter, Matthews, Ford, & Henderson, 2016). Researchers have argued that the lack of an instrument capable of measuring objective and perceived facets of ambiguity may impede both theory development and application of research results (Breaugh & Colihan, 1994).

Furthermore, as a result of the technology adopted in the workplace, the landscape of work is evolving at an unprecedented speed. This changed landscape demands continuous development of skills (Chancellor & Counts, 2018; Jhaver, Cranshaw, & Counts, 2019). A recent study by McKinsey Global Institute has predicted enormous workforce transitions in the years ahead. By 2030, it is estimated that as many as 375 million workers globally will likely need to transition to new occupational categories and learn new skills (Manyika et al., 2017). However, no approach has been defined to proactively gauge individuals' fit with their assigned roles, nor has any guidance been provided regarding interventions that will help overcome role ambiguity. An organization that can proactively deal with role ambiguity will benefit from employees with increased satisfaction, well-being, and productivity.

Our study has contributed to the research gap and advances the theory by introducing a novel way of measuring role ambiguity. Juxtaposing traditional surveys with modern sensor-derived measures of well-being, we combine methods adopted from natural language analysis and statistical modeling to examine the relationship of LinkedIn-based Role Ambiguity (LibRA) with the well-being and job performance of individuals. Specifically, we focus on three objectives:

- To measure role ambiguity using unobtrusively obtained LinkedIn data.
- To examine the relationship of LibRA with individual well-being and job performance.
- To investigate what factors may contribute to one's LibRA, relating to their intrinsic traits, LinkedIn's platform-specific characteristics, preferences, and goals of use of professional social networking service.

Data

Study Background

The dataset in this study (Saha et al., 2019e) originated primarily from a large-scale multisensor study of workplace behaviors called the Tesserae Project (Mattingly et al., 2019; Mirjafari et al., 2019; Saha et al., 2019a). This study, approved by the Institutional Review Board (IRB), recruited 757 participants, all of whom were information workers in cognitively demanding fields (e.g., engineering, consultancies, management) across the United States. These participants were recruited from January 2018 through July 2018 and completed an initial set of questionnaires related to demographics, job performance, personality, intelligence, affect, anxiety, alcohol and tobacco use, exercise, sleep, and stress, personal attributes, and well-being, administrated via psychometrically validated survey instruments. They also received daily surveys on a set of these attributes and three sensors: location-tracking Bluetooth beacons; a wearable device (smartwatch); and a phone agent—a smartphone application (Wang et al., 2014). In addition, some participants authorized collection of their historical social media data. As compensation, they either received a series of staggered stipends totaling up to $750 or participated in a set of weekly lottery drawings (multiples of $250 drawings), depending on their employer restrictions. Because the participants were enrolled over a 6-month period (January–July 2018) in a staggered fashion, data collection varied, with a range of time between 59 and 97 days (or an average of 68 days).

Social Media Data: LinkedIn

Social media was deployed as a passive sensing modality of behaviors and well-being in Tesserae (Mattingly et al., 2019; Saha et al., 2019a). The study asked the participants to provide their Facebook and LinkedIn data (unless they did not consent to do so or did not have either account); consent was sought only from those participants who had existing Facebook or LinkedIn accounts prior to entering the study.

Of the 757 participants in the study, 529 provided their LinkedIn data. Our work accounts for those with self-described portfolios and their passively sensed and self-reported well-being and job performance data. Therefore, we filtered out "blinded" participants and those without any self-description in their LinkedIn profile, particularly in their profile and job summary. This led us to a LinkedIn dataset of 257 individuals. All the ensuing analyses in this study were limited to these 257 individuals' data. For every participant, we obtained their self-presented profile and job summary, which included current and previous jobs.

Self-Reported Data

During enrollment, participants responded to a set of initial survey questionnaires related to demographics (age, sex, education, type of occupation, role in the company, and income). They additionally answered an initial survey questionnaires of personality traits and executive function. We also collected self-reported data on job performance. These are described below.

For the 257 participants with *complete* LinkedIn data, we obtained their big-five personality traits, as assessed by the Big Five Inventory (BFI-2) scale (Soto & John, 2017; Tett, Jackson, & Rothstein, 1991), and executive function, especially their fluid and crystallized intelligence, as assessed by the Shipley scale (Cattell, 1987; Schneider & McGrew, 2012; Shipley, 2009).

For job performance, we obtained two kinds of measures: Task Performance and Organizational Citizenship. To assess task performance, we used two scales, IRB (In-Role Behavior; Williams & Anderson, 1991) and ITP (Individual Task Proficiency; Griffin, Neal, & Parker, 2007). The IRB scale contains seven items, including questions such as *adequately performed assigned duties, failed to perform essential duties, and performed expected tasks*, each of which can be rated on a scale of 1 (strongly disagree) to 7 (strongly agree). The ITP scale contains three items: *carried out core parts of the job well, completed core tasks well using standard procedures, and ensured that the tasks were completed properly*. Each of these items can be rated on a scale of 1 (very little) to 5 (a great deal). For organizational citizenship, we administered the Organizational Citizenship Behavior scale (Fox, Spector, Goh, Bruursema, & Kessler, 2012). Organizational citizenship characterizes an individual's activities that are not typically or formally rewarded by the management or voluntary activities that are outside one's core responsibilities but that promote the welfare and effectiveness of the organization and its members (Cortina & Luchman, 2012; Organ, 1988).

Passively Sensed Behavior and Well-Being Data

To passively sense participants' behavior and the well-being measures of participants, the study deployed three modalities of sensing technologies (Bin Morshed et al., 2019; Mattingly et al., 2019): (1) Bluetooth beacons were provided to the participants (two static and two portable Gimbal beacons; API, 2018) to essentially sense their presence at work and home locations, and consequently to help assess their commute and desk time as well; (2) a wearable (Garmin Vivosmart (API); Garmin, n.d.) was provided to each participant to continually track their health measures, such as heart rate, arousal, and physical activity in the form of sleep, footsteps, and calories lost; and (3) a smartphone application was installed on the participants' smartphones to leverage their smartphone-based mobile sensors to track their mobility and physical activity (Wang et al., 2014).

Objective 1. Measuring Role Ambiguity from LinkedIn (LibRA)

Defining and Assessing LibRA: LinkedIn-Based Role Ambiguity

Drawing on the theoretical definition of role ambiguity, we operationalized LinkedIn-based Role Ambiguity (LibRA) as the *quantified differences in the self-explained roles and responsibilities of the individual against that posted by the company for the same role in the organization*. We obtained the self-explained job summary from an individual's LinkedIn profile, and for each specific role of individuals, the company provided a job description. These job descriptions are typically posted on job posting websites, such as *Glassdoor, LinkedIn, Indeed*, and the *Google job search portal*—where the Google job search portal collates both exact and nearest matching job descriptions from multiple websites, including the company's own website (LinkedIn, Glassdoor, Indeed, etc.) and sorts them relative to the search query. Figure 9.5 shows an example LinkedIn role description and company-published role description for the same role of Software Development Engineer at the same location of the company.

We first mapped the above self-reported LinkedIn job descriptions, and the company described job descriptions in a multidimensional space of job aspects, for which we leveraged O*NET. O*NET[6] is an online database and job ontology that contains a comprehensive list of jobs and their descriptions, elaborating on eight notable aspects of the job role: *abilities*, *interests*, *knowledge*, *skills*, *work activities*, *work context*, *work styles*, and *work values*. These aspects are grounded in the literature and have been used in prior work to study employee behavior (Tambe & Hitt, 2012).

We used word-embeddings, particularly pretrained GloVe vectors (Pennington et al., 2014; Saha et al., 2019f), to project the role descriptions of individuals and companies in a 50-dimensional word-vector space to obtain rich lexico-semantic context surrounding

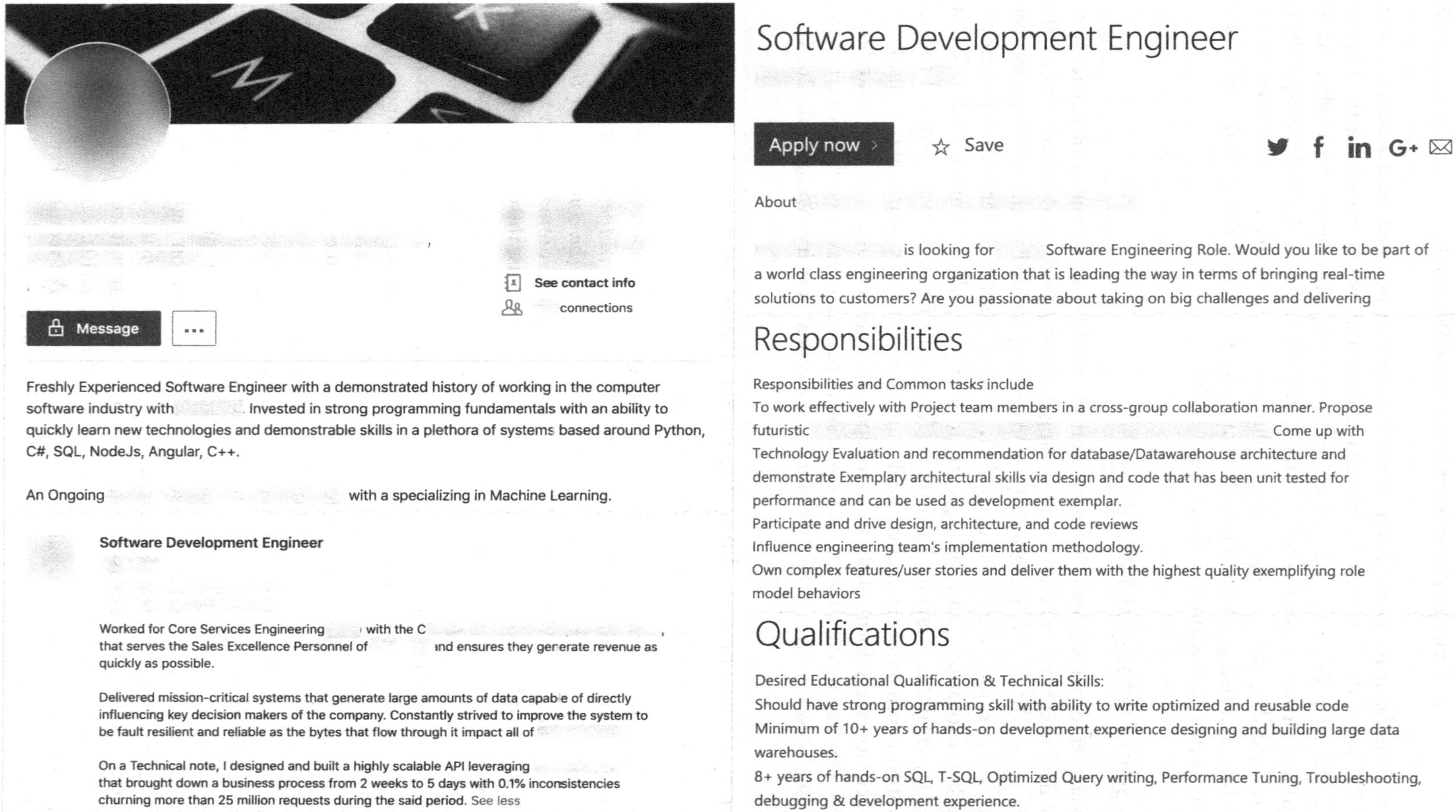

FIGURE 9.5. Left: Role summary of a Software Development Engineer as described on LinkedIn. Right: Job description of a Software Development Engineer as posted on the company webpage.

the hand-curated job descriptors above (Saha et al., 2019d). We used cosine similarities to obtain two vector projections in the eight-dimensional job aspect space per individual i: (1) one that is obtained from their LinkedIn summary (v_1^i) and (2) one that is obtained from the same role's company description (v_2^i). Then, the overall LibRA is measured as the euclidean distance between v_1^i and v_2^i. We obtained the aspect-wise LibRA of an individual as the absolute difference per dimension of v_1^i and v_2^i.

Evaluating the Validity of LibRA against the Gold Standard

We draw on modern validity theory (Crocker & Algina, 1986) to compare the LibRA of the individuals against a gold-standard validated survey on measuring role ambiguity. The Michigan Assessment of Organization survey instrument measures an individual's role ambiguity, role conflict, and role overload (Nadler, Jenkins, Cammann, & Lawler, 1975). We randomly sampled a subset of 77 participants from our entire participant pool to answer the Michigan Assessment of Organization survey (Nadler et al., 1975). Correlating the survey-based role ambiguity with LibRA, we found Spearman's correlation coefficient to be 0.22 ($p < .05$). Consequently, a statistically significant correlation does imply criterion validity and hints at construct validity in our claim that LibRA does contain information that is also captured by gold-standard, validated survey instruments on role ambiguity.

Objective 2. Examining the Relationship of LibRA with Well-Being and Performance

Theoretical Underpinnings and Hypotheses

Role Ambiguity and Well-Being

While there is no single conceptualization of well-being, the broad categories that well-being encompasses are physiological, psychological, and behavioral aspects (Kahn et al., 1992; Schmidt et al., 2014). Within the scope of our dataset, we study the relationship of LibRA with one's physiological measures (heart rate and sleep: Caplan & Jones, 1975; Chang & Hancock, 2003), psychological measures (stressful arousal: Sullivan & Bhagat, 1992), and behavior at the workplace (time spent at the desk and time spent at the workplace: Zenger & Lazzarini, 2004). Specifically, we test for the following hypotheses in the relationship of LibRA with well-being attributes.

- H1. Greater role ambiguity is associated with increased heart rate.
- H2. Greater role ambiguity is associated with increased arousal.
- H3. Greater role ambiguity is associated with decreased sleep.
- H4. Greater role ambiguity is associated with reduced work hours.

Role Ambiguity and Job Performance

Role ambiguity refers to the uncertainty regarding tasks that an employee needs to perform as part of their job role in the company. An employee with greater clarity will be able to better perform the required tasks. Lower role ambiguity makes it easier to meet expectations, helps the employee to become more motivated, and encourages such intrinsically motivated employees to perform more efficiently (Frey & Osterloh, 2001; Furnham, Eracleous, & Chamorro-Premuzic, 2009). We studied the relationship of LibRA with two dimensions of job performance (Rotundo & Sackett, 2002; Viswesvaran & Ones, 2000; Williams & Anderson, 1991): (1) task performance and (2) organizational citizenship behavior. We tested the following hypotheses:

- H5. Greater role ambiguity is associated with decreased task performance.
- H6. Greater role ambiguity is associated with decreased organizational citizenship.

Testing Hypotheses and the Convergent Validity of LibRA

To establish the convergent validity of LibRA, we adopted a theory-driven approach to outline hypotheses on the relationship of LibRA with job performance and well-being. We studied the relationship of LibRA with passively sensed well-being and job performance measures. For every well-being or performance measure *M*, we built linear regression models with *M* as the dependent variable, and LibRA as an independent variable and controlled for demographic, personality, and executive function measures per individual. For all the regression models, we used the variance inflation factor (VIF) to eliminate multicollinearity of covariates (if any) (O'Brien, 2007).

Testing Hypothesis 1. Greater Role Ambiguity Is Associated with Increased Heart Rate

High heart rate is associated with an increase in stress (Benetos, Rudnichi, Thomas, Safar, & Guize, 1999; Hellhammer & Schubert, 2012). Greater role ambiguity is associated with increased heart rate, which is identified as a major predictor of coronary heart rate (Benetos et al., 1999; Caplan & Jones, 1975). We obtained the participants' heart rate measures through the wearable sensor and fit a linear regression model with the average heart rate in the study period per individual. Given that physical activities are associated with heart rate (Goodie, Larkin, & Schauss, 2000), we controlled for each participant's physical activity. The regression model reveals a positive standardized coefficient (0.10) with statistical significance for LibRA (Table 9.6). This supports our Hypothesis 1.

Testing Hypothesis 2. Greater Role Ambiguity Is Associated with Increased Arousal

Arousal is a physiological response that is related to one's heart rate variability and is associated with stress, fatigue, and anxiety (Dienstbier, 1989; Hellhammer & Schubert, 2012). These well-being measures are known to become exacerbated in the presence of role ambiguity (Abramis, 1994; Caplan & Jones, 1975). In our project, the wearable sensor allows us to obtain participant arousal, particularly their sympathetic nervous system (SNS) arousal measures in a continuous fashion. In particular, for every individual, it scores the arousal level from restful to stressful on a scale of 1–100 at every 3-minute granularity. Here, the restful duration is when an individual relaxes or recovers from stress (API). We build two separate regression models, one with median duration of high

TABLE 9.6. Summary of Standardized Coefficients of Regression Models of Well-Being

Covariates	Std. Coeff.	Covariates	Std. Coeff.	Covariates	Std. Coeff.
H_1 (Heart Rate)		H_2 (Arousal)			
$\mathcal{M}$ = Heart Rate, $R^2 = 0.16^*$		$\mathcal{M}$ = Stressful Duration, $R^2 = 0.65^*$		$\mathcal{M}$ = Restful Duration, $R^2 = 0.47^{**}$	
Exercise Duration	0.53**	Age	0.69**	Job: Non-IT	0.31*
Shipley: Abs.	-0.81*	Edu: Grad. School	-0.24*	**LibRA**	-0.22***
Agreeableness	0.91*	Tenure: 4	-1.59*		
Conscientiousness	-0.78*	**LibRA**	0.42***		
LibRA	0.10*				
H_3 (Sleep)		H_4 (Work-Hours)			
$\mathcal{M}$ = Sleep Duration, $R^2 = 0.19^{***}$		$\mathcal{M}$ = Duration at Work		$\mathcal{M}$ = Duration at Desk	
Income: $50K-75K	0.21*	Edu.: College	0.23***	Duration at Work	0.18*
Agreeableness	-0.14*	Edu.: Grad. School	0.21***	Edu: College	-0.09
Tenure: 7 Yrs.	-1.74*	Income: $50K-75K	0.14***	Edu: Grad.	-0.04
Job: Non-IT	0.15**	Income: $100K-125K	-0.18***	Edu: Master's	0.04
LibRA	-0.16***	Shipley: Abs.	0.01***	Income: $100K-125K	0.09*
		Extraversion	0.09***	Income: $125K-150K	0.08*
		Conscientiousness	0.05***	Tenure: <1 Yr.	-0.18***
		Neuroticism	0.12**	Tenure: 2 Yrs.	0.18***
		Tenure: 6 Yrs.	-0.16***	Tenure: 3 Yrs.	0.26***
		Tenure: 7 Yrs.	-0.15***	Tenure: 4 Yrs.	0.09***
		Tenure: 8 Yrs.	-0.31***	Tenure: 8 Yrs.	0.15***
		Job: Non-IT	0.20***	Job: Non-IT	-0.03*
		LibRA	-0.41***	**LibRA**	-0.12**

stressful arousal (75–100), and one with median duration of restful arousal (1–25) per individual. We find that LibRA shows a positive standardized coefficient (0.42) in the former model and a negative standardized coefficient (–0.22) in the latter model (Table 9.6). This suggests that individuals with high LibRA are more likely to show higher stressful arousal and lower restful arousal. Therefore, our observations support Hypothesis 2.

Testing Hypothesis 3. Greater Role Ambiguity Is Associated with Decreased Sleep

Sleep is important to an individual's well-being; it reduces the negative impact of stress as well as improving overall health (Blaxton, Bergeman, Whitehead, Braum, & Payne, 2017). Given that stress reduces sleep, and sleep reduces stress, a stressed person is likely to sleep less (Van Reeth et al., 2000). If role ambiguity is stressful, we hypothesize that high role ambiguity will correspond with reduced sleep duration. The wearable sensor collected participant sleep durations. We build a linear regression model with median duration of sleep per individual. We find that LibRA shows a negative standardized coefficient (–0.16) with statistical significance (Table 9.6). Therefore, Hypothesis 3 is supported in our dataset.

Testing Hypothesis 4. Greater Role Ambiguity Is Associated with Decreased Work-Hours

Role ambiguity is known to affect an individual's workplace behavior (Pearce, 1981). The Bluetooth beacons sense if a participant is at work, at home, or commuting; it additionally captures how long the participant is at and away from the desk. We built two regression models, one with the duration at work and the other with the duration at desk when at work (this model additionally controlled for duration at work). For these distributions,

χ^2 tests could not reject the null hypotheses that they were significantly different from a Poisson distribution ($p > 0.05$). Therefore, instead of using purely linear regression models, we built negative binomial regression models (Hilbe, 2011) that essentially regress the logarithm of the dependent variables with the independent variables (Hilbe, 2011). We found that LibRA shows a negative standardized coefficient in both models (–0.41 for duration at work and –0.12 for duration at desk; see Table 9.6). This suggests that individuals with high LibRA are not only less likely to spend time at work, but also less likely to spend time at desk when at work. These observations support Hypothesis 4.

Testing Hypothesis 5. Greater Role Ambiguity Is Associated with Decreased Task Performance

For the measures of In-Role Behavior (IRB) and Individual Task Performance (ITP), we built two linear regression models each—one that uses an aggregated (median) value of task performance and one that uses a change in task performance over the duration of the study. We found that LibRA shows a negative association with both *aggregated ITP* (–0.33) and *change in ITP* (–0.20) per individual. Similarly, LibRA also shows a negative association with both *aggregated IRB* (–0.29) and *change in IRB* (–0.20) per individual (Table 9.7). Our observations suggest that individuals with higher LibRA not only have a greater likelihood of performing badly at work, but also their performance worsens over time. Therefore, our observations support Hypothesis 5.

Testing Hypothesis 6. Greater Role Ambiguity Is Associated with Decreased Organizational Citizenship

Like the above, we built two linear regression models—one that uses an aggregated (median) value of Organizational Citizenship Behavior (OCB) and one that uses a change in OCB over the duration of the study. We found that LibRA shows a negative association with both aggregated OCB and change in OCB per individual (Table 9.7). These observations suggest that individuals with higher LibRA show a greater likelihood of poorer OCB, which also worsens over time — a tendency associated with being disinclined to be

TABLE 9.7. Summary of Standardized Coefficients of Regression Models of Task Performance

Covariates	Std. Coeff.	Covariates	Std. Coeff.	Covariates	Std. Coeff.
H_5 (Task Performance)				H_6 (Org. Citizenship Behavior)	
$\mathcal{M}$ = ITP, $R^2 = 0.29^{***}$		$\mathcal{M}$ = IRB, $R^2 = 0.29^{***}$		$\mathcal{M}$ = OCB, $R^2 = 0.24^{***}$	
Income: L	-0.38*	Openness	0.13**	Supervisor: Yes	0.24***
Income: Q	0.40**	Consc.	1.13*	Extraversion	0.34***
Openness	1.07*	Tenure: 8	0.17*	Tenure: 6	-0.14*
Consc.	1.30***	LibRA	-0.29*	Tenure: 7	-0.20**
Tenure: 6	-0.15*			LibRA	-0.10**
LibRA	-0.33***				
$\mathcal{M}$ = Δ ITP, $R^2 = 0.13^{*}$		$\mathcal{M}$ = Δ IRB, $R^2 = 0.17^{***}$		$\mathcal{M}$ = Δ OCB, $R^2 = 0.22^{*}$	
Extraversion	0.69*	Openness	0.91**	Supervisor: Yes	-0.26*
Consc.	-1.37***	Consc.	-0.84*	Agreeableness	-1.80*
LibRA	-0.20*	Tenure: 7	-0.19*	Tenure: 5	0.21*
		Tenure: 8	-0.26**	LibRA	-0.25***
		Tenure: 9	-0.18**		
		LibRA	-0.20**		

altruistic or help colleagues at workplace. Therefore, our observations support Hypothesis 6.

Objective 3. Investigating the Factors Affecting LibRA

Finally, we studied the factors that contribute to LibRA assessment. We investigated the extent to which appropriating data shared online may bring forth new dimensions to consider while employing LibRA for practical use. We delved deeper using a qualitative examination of a sample of our dataset described below. We separately matched those pairs of individuals who belonged to IT roles and those who belonged to non-IT roles. Figure 9.6 plots the pair-wise Mahalanobis distances and the absolute differences in their role ambiguities. We focus on those individuals (the shaded region in Figure 9.6) who are similar in individual attributes but show high differences in LibRA.

Next, among the individuals in the above sample, we manually looked at their LinkedIn job descriptions. While these individuals were very similar in personality, demographic traits, and roles in the company (because of matching), we found differences in their style of writing and LinkedIn self-presentation (also highlighted in the Figure 9.6 examples). Given the affordances and the uniqueness of LinkedIn as a professional social networking platform, we deduced a few plausible reasons that could potentially influence the virtual self-presentation of the individuals, and in turn, lead to varied inferred role ambiguity. We now discuss these factors, which are not disjointed and could be interrelated.

Individuals' Organizational Behavior

Individuals who are looking for new jobs or endeavors may write a more detailed portfolio on LinkedIn profiles, whereas individuals who are generally "settled" are not as likely to provide detailed descriptions (Skeels & Grudin, 2009). This could also be a *different type* of job than what they are currently involved in altogether as well. An alternative conjecture could also be that only a few individuals write and "highlight" *work experiences*, rather than describing responsibilities and tasks at work. We also found individuals who described their role with people skills beyond their tasks. These could be individuals who exhibit proactive behaviors in the organizations (Crant, 2000): they show anticipatory, change-oriented, and self-initiated behavior and tend to act in advance of a future situation rather than react later. Although these individuals have high role ambiguity, they may show desirable individual characteristics (proactive behavior and leadership traits) in organizations (Bateman & Crant, 1993; Crant, 2000).

Individual-Intrinsic Factors

Prior research has shown that people may self-promote and appear honest and less deceptive on their professional social networking profiles (Guillory & Hancock, 2012; Van Dijck, 2013). However, the degree and the way in which they self-present themselves can vary. We can look at it from the perspective of growth versus fixed mindset (Dweck, 2009). Those with a "fixed mindset" believe their abilities are innate, whereas those with a "growth mindset" believe that abilities can be acquired through effort and study. Complementary research has also coined the expressions benefit mindset, global

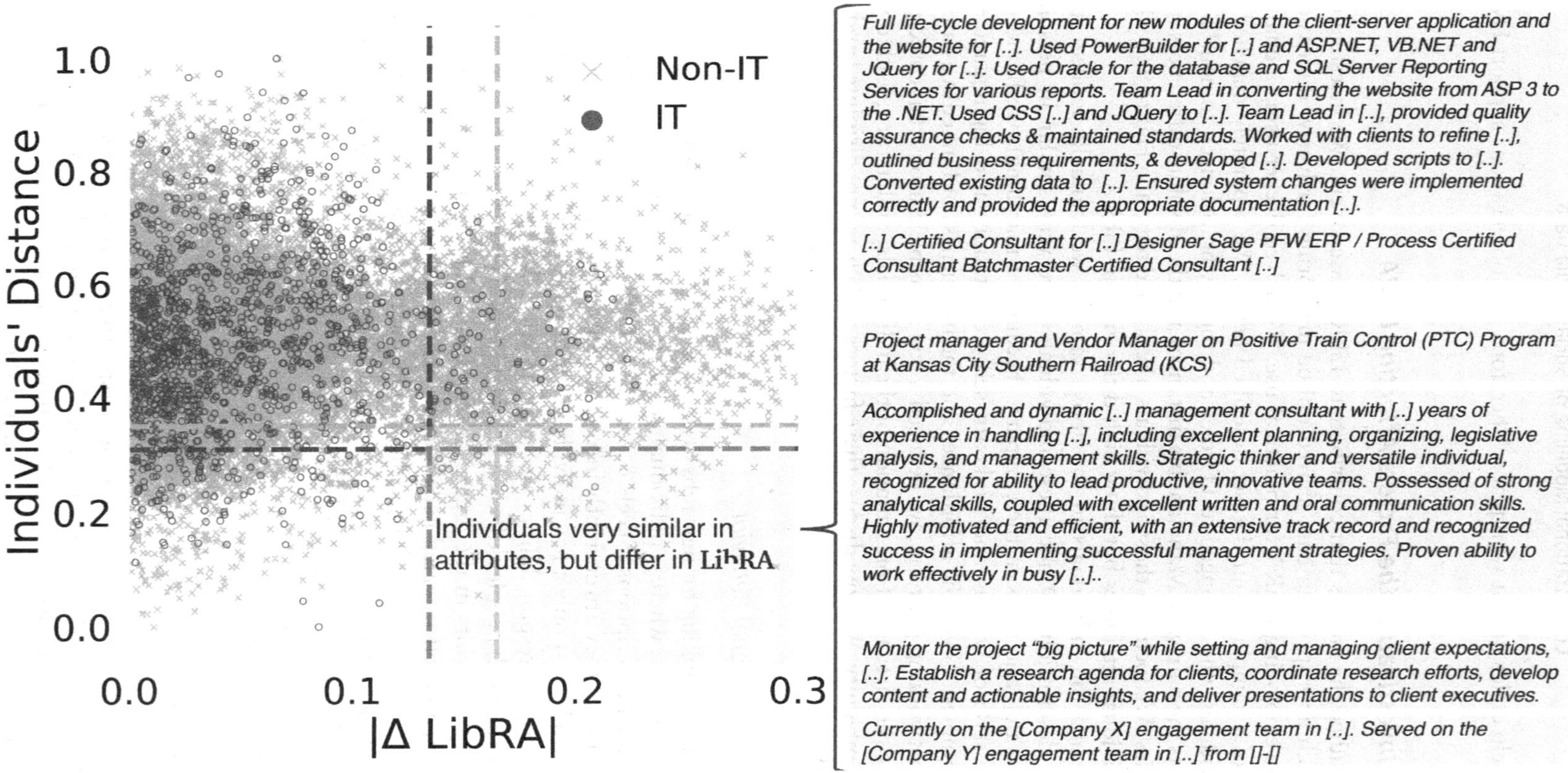

FIGURE 9.6. Pairwise differences in individual attributes and corresponding differences in LibRA. Example excerpts show differences in LinkedIn descriptions of pairs of individuals with very similar individual attributes (low differences) but large differences in LibRA.

mindset, productive mindset, and defensive mindset, all of which illustrate the intrinsic behaviors of individuals who contribute to their skill development, proficiency, and self-presentation in organizations (Buchanan & Kern, 2017; Gupta & Govindarajan, 2002). We conjecture that similar traits permeate online self-promotion practices on LinkedIn.

Job-Related Factors

Ambiguity in job titles adds ambiguity to the job role. We find pairs of individuals where one is an Associate, while the other is a Specialist. Both of these titles are generic and do not convey much information to the employees. In contrast, the fact that recently companies have been coming up with "cool" job titles (e.g., *ninja*) to gain visibility and distinctiveness can add other complexities to role ambiguity (Sapone, 2019). Additionally, some individuals may work on confidential projects, and they are bound by nondisclosure agreements. Furthermore, the size of a company can influence the self-description behaviors (Zide, Elman, & Shahani-Denning, 2014).

Audience, Privacy, and Platform Factors

Finally, use of the LinkedIn platform varies across individuals. Two participants in our sample described what their company does, rather than their roles. LinkedIn also functions as a marketplace for job seekers, and individuals tend to share credible information because they have a conceptualization of an "invisible audience" (Bernstein et al., 2013), and they do not want to appear as dishonest (Guillory & Hancock, 2012). At the same time, employee surveillance and subjective expectation of privacy shares a competing relationship, and the perception of being "surveilled" can influence one's self-disclosure on the platform (Ghoshray, 2013; Jacobson & Tufts, 2013; Tufekci, 2008). Furthermore, the employee's own mental models about LinkedIn privacy might be a factor behind what they share (Caramujo & da Silva, 2015).

Implications

Our findings align with the propositions put forth by role theory, that greater LibRA measure is associated with factors related to depleted well-being such as increased heart rate, increased arousal, decreased sleep, and decreased work hours, and is associated with lower job performance such as decreased task performance and decreased organizational citizenship behavior. Our work has theoretical and practical implications surrounding this new measure of role ambiguity assessed from people's professional social networking data from the perspective of employees, organizations, and social computing platforms.

Theoretical Implications

Traditionally, registries and census organizations have served as an analogous source of data for people's professional portfolios. Our study revealed the feasibility of measuring a role-related construct (here LibRA) at scale via a previously unexplored, low-cost, and unobtrusive source of data. Research is advancing in ways that these data can be used to operationalize and derive existing measures in novel ways. Thereby, this study revisits old questions in labor economics where existing efforts have been limited to statistical numbers such as salary distribution and unemployment rates. This study can potentially complement these numbers with richer information on satisfaction and well-being at scale.

Our work lays the foundation for studying employee well-being through unobtrusive online data sources that set up marketplaces for employees. These data sources include other professional networking websites such as Meetup, Xing, and Jobcase. Being platform-agnostic (i.e., demonstrating interoperability across operating platforms), methods in this study can be easily replicated in other platforms or other contexts.

This work shows a means to objectively assess the differences in "what the individual considers and self-describes themselves to be doing," "what the company hired them for, or what their job description states." That is, the individual may only be showing normative and socially influenced behavior at work, or they may show there is an information gap, or reveal that they intend to invest more effort in learning and gathering experience themselves. These behaviors are oblivious to the presence of role ambiguity. It is challenging to capture such "unaware role ambiguities" using traditional approaches, as they are tuned to measure the "perceived role ambiguity." Language can reflect differences in personal as well as situational traits (Goffman, 1981). This additionally makes our measure less subjectively biased than traditional methods of measuring role ambiguity.

Practical Implications

Presently, job and skillset training at organizations is not streamlined (Noe, Hollenbeck, Gerhart, & Wright, 2017). Either organizations train a lot of employees in a batch, or they mentor them individually. However, with more information regarding how employees perceive their role, employers can identify the area of training required that will reduce role ambiguity and enhance the productivity of employees. This method can help reduce the time to identify such role ambiguity gaps, reducing training and employee well-being costs. This, in turn, can improve employee retention for companies by identifying turnover intentions.

Aligning with and confirming the literature (Ladany & Friedlander, 1995), our findings suggest that LibRA is not dependent on individual differences such as personality, gender, supervisory role, and executive function. This can inform organizations how these roles or titles can be transformed to match the skill-level, task-assignment level, and incentive-level restructuring. The interest in human resource management is still nascent, but it is promising in the research literature. Cross-disciplinary literature pertaining to workplaces and online technologies provide potential use-cases attracting the attention of designers (Shami, Yang, et al., 2014). Our work has a number of implications for designing and developing organization-centric technologies, as follows:

1. First, tools can be built that suggest carefully chosen, fine-tuned job titles for companies, based on LibRA (Baron & Bielby, 1986; Grant et al., 2014). This implication is particularly important because younger organizations sometimes offer (higher-ranking or impressive-sounding) titles to employees in lieu of higher salaries, but this strategy has been reported to backfire due to increased role ambiguity, which affects employee productivity and well-being (Sapone, 2019). Adopting tools that inform organizations about existing ambiguities in specific job roles, therefore, may help protect against workplace stress (Lazarus, 1995). Moreover, job agencies and resume-matching

consultancies already are making heavy use of professional social networking platforms such as LinkedIn (Koch, Gerber, & de Klerk, 2018). Such agencies can use the insights gained from our approach to match and recommend suitable jobs to prospective employees.

2. Second, this study can help design workplace tools and dashboards to enhance organizational "health" or functioning. Such dashboards can unobtrusively and proactively assess employee role ambiguities at scale, taking employees' privacy considerations into account. In fact, many companies already provide their employees with internal social media platforms (DiMicco et al., 2008), online engagement forums, or even email profile description spaces, where they can regularly update their self-explained expertise and role descriptions, along with manager- or peer-appraised testimonials. By leveraging such internal datasets, companies can potentially adopt these dashboards to gauge role ambiguity to make informed role matching for open positions in internal hiring. Companies can restructure and reassign current employees with appropriate incentivization and compensation on their task and workload.

Conclusion

As noted above, spatial and contextual attributes influence the well-being of individuals and collectives within situated communities (Galster, 1998). Therefore, ensuring that the members cope with psychological and cognitive demands is essential for both individual and collective well-being. This requires identifying and understanding psychological changes in the circumstances of both normalcy and crisis.

This chapter highlighted the computational techniques and frameworks used to measure well-being in situated communities employing social media data and advocated building rigorous but ethical approaches by critically reflecting about practical and real-world consequences. We situated the findings in an interdisciplinary context, including psychology and social science, and we discussed theoretical, practical, and methodological implications catering to a variety of stakeholders, including researchers, practitioners, administrators, and policymakers.

Nonetheless, the computational use of social media data for understanding the well-being of situated communities does raise some unavoidable ethical considerations. In recent years, data-driven behavioral inferences, like the kind discussed in this chapter, have come under scrutiny due to privacy breaches such as the Cambridge Analytica scandal (Cadwalladr & Graham-Harrison, 2018). This work renews attention to the challenges that may arise when college student or employee data are appropriated for surveillance purposes in a situated community; as Van Dijck (2013) noted, "LinkedIn's functionality goes beyond its self-claimed ambition as a professional matchmaker, and ventures into behavioral monitoring." With research like this, use of people's online self-presentation to infer their offline behavior (with high-risk outcomes such as one's mental health or profession) heightens several complexities related to one's perception of ethics and privacy, and consequently their behavior on social media.

More elaborately, as per Goffman's theory of self-presentation Goffman (1959), individuals may present two kinds of information: one that they intend to "give off" and one that "leaks through" without any intention (Goffman, 1959; Miller, 1995). This implies that both of the intentions may be present in the data used for this research. Socially connecting with peers online may provide social support as well as support the bridging and bonding of social capital and publishing role descriptions. Online portfolios on social media may benefit the individuals in many ways, including professional development and support of career growth. However, we recognize that studies such as the ones presented in this chapter may appropriate these data without the awareness of the individuals themselves. College campus administrators may use these data to identify which students are likely to succeed academically, while employers may make inferences about role ambiguity and subsequent job satisfaction to make decisions on rewarding, promotions, or even retention and layoffs. To regulate such practices through the use of social media data, student and employee rights protection agencies and lawmaking bodies should consider issuing guidelines on how organizations engage in data-driven decision making for their student bodies, workforces, and broadly situated communities.

In addition, individuals may also start gaming the system and describe themselves in language that is more attuned with positive mental health or their role descriptions at work to gain academic, professional, or social advantages (Van Dijck, 2013). Such deceptive behavior calls for action for stakeholders with diverse interests ranging from academia and industry, as this adds complexities, and they may even impact the social computing ecosystem of use on Reddit or LinkedIn in contrast to how it is used currently. This may, in turn, bring into question the potential efficacy of using social media data prospectively to design interventions or support policy and decision making for improved well-being outcomes, via what is known as the "observer effect" (de Bianchi, 2013). Future research that involves stakeholders in situated communities and participatory approaches will be needed to unpack and overcome these challenges, as well as build trust in how social media-based computational inferences may support broader societal good.

Finally, we acknowledge limitations in the use of campus-specific social media data in modeling stress to identify the after-effects of violent incidents. First and importantly, we recognize that, although college students or information workers in various companies constitute a demographic in which social media penetration is among the highest (Greenwood et al., 2016), possibly because not every student or employee uses them. Our approach therefore cannot account for social media nonuse or for those who use platforms whose data cannot be collected for research purposes in an ethical manner. Augmenting our data with other social media sources (e.g., Twitter), including individuals' self-reported (qualitative and quantitative) data or other forms of passively sensed signals (e.g., smartphone or wearable use) can circumvent some of these limitations. They constitute promising directions for future work that employs computational approaches for assessing well-being.

Notes

1. everytownresearch.org.
2. pewinternet.org.
3. www.everytown.org.
4. These sources include gunviolencearchive.org, time.com, motherjones.com, huffingtonpost.com, and en.wikipedia.org.

5. We refer to *posts* within college sub-Reddits as a unified term for both posts and comments.

6. O*Net (*onetonline.org*) is developed under the sponsorship of the U.S. Department of Labor/Employment and Training Administration (USDOL/ETA).

REFERENCES

Abramis, D. J. (1994). Work role ambiguity, job satisfaction, and job performance: Meta-analyses and review. *Psychological Reports, 75*(3; Pt. 2), 1411–1433.

Al-Ani, B., Mark, G., & Semaan, B. (2010). Blogging in a region of conflict: Supporting transition to recovery. In *CHI '10: Proceedings of the SIGCHI Conference on Human Factors in Computing Systems* (pp. 1069–1078). ACM.

API. (2018). *Employer access to employee social media: Applicant screening, "friend" requests and workplace investigations, 2018.*

Archambault, A., & Grudin, J. (2012). A longitudinal study of Facebook, LinkedIn, and Twitter use. In *CHI '12: Proceedings of the SIGCHI Conference on Human Factors in Computing Systems* (pp. 2741–2750). ACM.

Atkinson, S., Bagnall, A.-M., Corcoran, R., South, J., & Curtis, S. (2020). Being well together: Individual subjective and community wellbeing. *Journal of Happiness Studies, 21*, 1903–1921.

Ayers, J. W., Althouse, B. M., Leas, E. C., Alcorn, T. M., & Dredze, M. (2016). *Can big media data revolutionarize gun violence prevention?* arXiv preprint arXiv:1611.01148.

Bagroy, S., Kumaraguru, P., & De Choudhury, M. (2017). A social media based index of mental well-being in college campuses. *Proceedings of the 2017 CHI Conference on Human Factors in Computing Systems.*

Baron, J. N., & Bielby, W. T. (1986) The proliferation of job titles in organizations. *Administrative Science Quarterly, 31*(1), 561–586.

Bateman, T. S., & Crant, J. M. (1993). The proactive component of organizational behavior: A measure and correlates. *Journal of Organizational Behavior, 14*(2), 103–118.

Bayram, N., & Bilgel, N. (2008). The prevalence and socio-demographic correlations of depression, anxiety and stress among a group of university students. *Social Psychiatry and Psychiatric Epidemiology, 43*(8), 667–672.

Benetos, A., Rudnichi, A., Thomas, F., Safar, N., & Guize, L. (1999). Influence of heart rate on mortality in a French population: Role of age, gender, and blood pressure. *Hypertension, 33*(1), 44–52.

Bernstein, M. S., Bakshy, E., Burke, M., & Karrer, B. (2013). Quantifying the invisible audience in social networks. In *Proceedings of the SIGCHI Conference on Human Factors in Computing Systems* (pp. 21–30). ACM.

Bin Morshed, M. B., Liu, R., D'Mello, S. K., De Choudhury, M., Abowd, G. D., & Plotz, T. (2019). Prediction of mood instability with passive sensing. *Proceedings of the ACM on Interactive, Mobile, Wearable and Ubiquitous Technologies, 3*(3).

Birnbaum, M. L., Ernala, S. K., Rizvi, A. F., De Choudhury, M., & Kane, J. K. (2017). A collaborative approach to identifying social media markers of schizophrenia by employing machine learning and clinical appraisals. *Journal of Medical Internet Research, 19*(8).

Blaxton, J. M., Bergeman, C. S., Whitehead, B. R., Braun, M. E., & Payne, J. D. (2017). Relationships among nightly sleep quality, daily stress, and daily affect. *Journals of Gerontology: Series B, 72*(3), 363–372.

Boyd, D. M., & Ellison, N. B. (2007). Social network sites: Definition, history, and scholarship. *Journal of Computer-Mediated Communication, 13*(1), 210–230.

Breaugh, J. A., & Colihan, J. P. (1994). Measuring facets of job ambiguity: Construct validity evidence. *Journal of Applied Psychology, 79*(2), 191.

Brubaker, J. R., Kivran-Swaine, F., Taber, L., & Hayes, G. R. (2012). Grief-stricken in a crowd: The language of bereavement and distress in social media. *Sixth International AAAI Conference on Weblogs and Social Media, 6*(1), 42–49.

Brzozowski, M. J. (2009). Watercooler: Exploring an organization through enterprise social media. *Proceedings of the ACM 2009 Inter-*

national Conference on Supporting Group Work, pp. 219–228.

Buchanan, A., & Kern, M. L. (2017). The benefit mindset: The psychology of contribution and everyday leadership. *International Journal of Wellbeing, 7*(1), 1–11.

Cadwalladr, C., & Graham-Harrison, E. (2018). Revealed: 50 million Facebook profiles harvested for Cambridge Analytica in major data breach. *The Guardian*, p. 17.

Caplan, R. D., Jones, K. W. (1975). Effects of work load, role ambiguity, and Type A personality on anxiety, depression, and heart rate. *Journal of Applied Psychology, 60*(6), 713–719.

Caramujo, J., & Rodrigues da Silva, A. M. (2015). *Analyzing privacy policies based on a privacy-aware profile: The Facebook and Linkedin case studies.* 2015 IEEE 17th Conference on Business Informatics.

Catalano, R. (1979). *Health, behavior and the community: An ecological perspective.* Pergamon Press.

Cattell, R. B. (Ed.). (1987). *Intelligence: Its structure, growth and action.* North-Holland.

Chan, L., Das Swain, V., Kelley, C., de Barbaro, K., Abowd, G. D., & Wilcox, L. (2018). Students' experiences with ecological momentary assessment tools to report on emotional well-being. *Proceedings of the ACM on Interactive, Mobile, Wearable and Ubiquitous Technologies, 2*(1), 1–29.

Chancellor, S., & Counts, S. (2018). Measuring employment demand using internet search data. *CHI '18: Proceedings of the 2018 CHI Conference on Human Factors in Computing Systems, 122*, 1–14.

Chancellor, S., & De Choudhury, M. (2020). Methods in predictive techniques for mental health status on social media: A critical review. *NPJ Digital Medicine, 3*(1), 1–11.

Chancellor, S., Lin, Z., Goodman, E., Zerwas, S., & De Choudhury, M. (2016, February). Quantifying and predicting mental illness severity in online pro-eating disorder communities. *CSCW '16 Proceedings of the 19th ACM Conference on Computer Supported Cooperative Work and Social Computing*, pp. 1171–1184.

Chancellor, S., Nitzburg, G., Hu, A., Zampieri, F., & De Choudhury, M. (2019). Discovering alternative treatments for opioid use recovery using social media. *CHI '19: Proceedings of the 2019 CHI Conference on Human Factors in Computing Systems, 124*, 1–15.

Chang, E., & Hancock, K. (2003). Role stress and role ambiguity in new nursing graduates in Australia. *Nursing and Health Sciences, 5*(2), 155–163.

Cohen, S., Kamarck, T., & Mermelstein, R. (1983). A global measure of perceived stress. *Journal of Health and Social Behavior, 24*(1), 385–396.

Cohn, M. A., Mehl, M. R., & Pennebaker, J. W. (2004). Linguistic markers of psychological change surrounding September 11, 2001. *Psychological Science, 15*(10), 687–693.

Coppersmith, G., Dredze, M., Harman, C., & Hollingshead, K. (2015). From ADHD to SAD: Analyzing the language of mental health on Twitter through self-reported diagnoses. *Proceedings of the 2nd Workshop on Computational Linguistics and Clinical Psychology: From Linguistic Signal to Clinical Reality*, pp. 1–10.

Coppersmith, G., Harman, C., & Dredze, M. (2014). Measuring post traumatic stress disorder in Twitter. *Eighth International AAAI Conference on Weblogs and Social Media, 8*(1), 579–582.

Cortina, J. M., & Luchman, J. N. (2012). Personnel selection and employee performance. In I. B. Weiner, N. W. Schmitt, & S. Highhouse (Eds.), *Handbook of psychology: Vol. 12. Industrial and organizational psychology* (pp. 143–183). Wiley.

Crant, J. M. (2000). Proactive behavior in organizations. *Journal of Management, 26*(3), 435–462.

Crocker, L., & Algina, J. (1986). *Introduction to classical and modern test theory.* Cengage.

Culotta, A. (2014). Estimating county health statistics with Twitter. *Proceedings of the SIGCHI Conference on Human Factors in Computing Systems*, pp. 1335–1344.

Das Swain, V., Saha, K., Reddy, M. D., Rajvanshy, H., Abowd, G. D., & De Choudhury, M. (2020, April). Modeling organizational culture with workplace experiences shared on glassdoor. *CHI '20: Proceedings of the 2020 CHI Conference on Human Factors in Computing Systems*, pp. 1–15.

de Bianchi, M. S. (2013). The observer effect. *Foundations of Science, 18*(2), 213–243.

De Choudhury, M., & Counts, S. (2013). Understanding affect in the workplace via social media. *CSCW '13: Proceedings of the 2013 Conference on Computer Supported Cooperative Work*, pp. 303–316.

De Choudhury, M., Counts, S., & Gamon, M. (2012). Not all moods are created equal!: Exploring human emotional states in social media. In J. G. Breslin, N. B. Ellison, J. G. Shanahan & Z. Tufekci (Eds.), *ICWSM*. AAAI Press.

De Choudhury, M., Kiciman, E., Dredze, M., Coppersmith, G., & Kumar, M. (2016, May). Discovering shifts to suicidal ideation from mental health content in social media. *Proceedings of the SIGCHI Conference on Human Factors in Computing Systems*, pp. 2098–2110.

De Choudhury, M., Monroy-Hernandez, A., & Mark, G. (2014, April). Narco emotions: Affect and desensitization in social media during the Mexican drug war. *CHI '14: Proceedings of the SIGCHI Conference on Human Factors in Computing Systems*, pp. 3563–3572.

De Neve, J.-E., Diener, E., Tay, L., & Xuereb, C. (2013). The objective benefits of subjective well-being. In J. Helliwell, R. Layard, & J. Sachs (Eds.), *World Happiness Report 2013*. UN Sustainable Development Solutions Network.

Dienstbier, R. A. (1989). Arousal and physiological toughness: Implications for mental and physical health. *Psychological Review, 96*(1), 84.

DiMicco, J., Geyer, W., Millen, D. R., Dugan, C., & Brownholtz, B. (2009, January 5–8). *People sensemaking and relationship building on an enterprise social network site*. 42st Hawaii International Conference on Systems Science (HICSS-42 2009).

DiMicco, J., Millen, D. R., Geyer, W., Dugan, C., Brownholtz, B., & Muller, M. (2008, November 8–12). Motivations for social networking at work. *Proceedings of the 2008 ACM Conference on Computer Supported Cooperative Work, CSCW 2008*.

Dweck, C. S. (2009). Mindsets: Developing talent through a growth mindset. *Olympic Coach, 21*(1), 4–7.

Ehrlich, K., & Shami, N. S. (2010, May 23–26). Microblogging inside and outside the workplace. *Proceedings of the Fourth International Conference on Weblogs and Social Media, ICWSM 2010*.

Eisenberg, D., Golberstein, E., & Gollust, S. E. (2007). Help-seeking and access to mental health care in a university student population. *Medical Care, 45*(7), 594–601.

Eisenberg, D., Hunt, J., & Speer, N. (2012). Help seeking for mental health on college campuses: Review of evidence and next steps for research and practice. *Harvard Review of Psychiatry, 20*(4), 222–232.

Ellison, N. B., Steinfield, C., & Lampe, C. (2007). The benefits of Facebook "friends": Social capital and college students' use of online social network sites. *Journal of Computer-Mediated Communication, 12*(4), 1143–1168.

Erez, A., Misangyi, V. F., Johnson, D. E., LePine, M. A., & Halverson, K. C. (2008). Stirring the hearts of followers: Charismatic leadership as the transferal of affect. *Journal of Applied Psychology, 93*(3), 602.

Ernala, S. K., Rizvi, A. F., Birnbaum, M. L., Kane, J. M., & De Choudhury, M. (2017). Linguistic markers indicating therapeutic outcomes of social media disclosures of schizophrenia. *Proceedings of the ACM on Human-Computer Interaction, 1*(43), 1–2.

Farzan, R., DiMicco, J. M., Millen, D. R., Dugan, C., Geyer, W., & Brownholtz, E. A. (2008, April 5–10). Results from deploying a participation incentive mechanism within the enterprise. *Proceedings of the 2008 Conference on Human Factors in Computing Systems, CHI 2008*.

Fitzhugh, S. M., Gibson, C. B., Spiro, E. S., & Butts, C. T. (2016). Spatio-temporal filtering techniques for the detection of disaster-related communication. *Social Science Research, 59*, 137–154.

Foa, E. B., Steketee, G., & Olasov Rothbaum, B. (1989). Behavioral/cognitive conceptualizations of post-traumatic stress disorder. *Behavior Therapy, 20*(2), 155–176.

Fowler, J. H., Christakis, N. A. (2008). Dynamic spread of happiness in a large social network: Longitudinal analysis over 20 years in the Framingham Heart Study. *British Medical Journal, 337*, 1–9.

Fox, S., Spector, P. E., Goh, A., Bruursema, K., & Kessler, S. R. (2012). The deviant citizen: Measuring potential positive relations between counterproductive work behaviour and organizational citizenship behaviour. *Journal of Occupational and Organizational Psychology, 85*(1). 199–220.

Freud, S. (1977). *Inhibitions, symptoms and anxiety.* Norton.

Freud, S. (2003). *Beyond the pleasure principle.* Penguin.

Frey, B. S., & Osterloh, M. (2001). *Successful management by motivation: Balancing intrinsic and extrinsic incentives.* Springer Science + Business Media.

Fried, Y., Ben-David, H. A., Tiegs, R. B., Avital, N., & Yeverechyahu, U. (1998). The interactive effect of role conflict and role ambiguity on job performance. *Journal of Occupational and Organizational Psychology, 71*(1), 19–27.

Furnham, A., Eracleous, A., & Chamorro-Premuzic, T. (2009). Personality, motivation and job satisfaction: Hertzberg meets the big five. *Journal of Managerial Psychology, 24*(8), 765–779.

Galster, G. (1998). A stock/flow model of defining racially integrated neighborhoods. *Journal of Urban Affairs, 20*(1), 43–51.

Garmin Connet Developer Program. (n.d.). *Health API.* http://developer.garmin.com/gc-developer-program/health-api

Geyer, W., Dugan, C., DiMicco, J., Millen, D. R., Brownholtz, B., & Muller, M. (2008, April). Use and reuse of shared lists as a social content type. *CHI '08: Proceedings of the SIGCHI Conference on Human Factors in Computing Systems*, pp. 1545–1554.

Ghoshray, S. (2013). Employer surveillance versus employee privacy: The new reality of social media and workplace privacy. *Northern Kentucky Law Review, 40*, 593.

Gilbert, E. (2012, February). Phrases that signal workplace hierarchy. *CSCW '12: Proceedings of the ACM 2012 Conference on Computer Supported Cooperative Work*, pp. 1037–1046.

Glasgow, K., Fink, C., & Boyd-Graber, J. L. (2014). "Our grief is unspeakable": Automatically measuring the community impact of a tragedy. *Eighth International AAAI Conference on Weblogs and Social Media, 8*(1), 161–179.

Goffman, E. (1981). *Forms of talk.* University of Pennsylvania Press.

Goffman, E. (1959). *The presentation of self in everyday life.* Doubleday.

Golder, S. A., & Macy, M. W. (2011). Diurnal and seasonal mood vary with work, sleep, and daylength across diverse cultures. *Science, 333*(6051), 1878–1881.

Goodie, J. L., Larkin, K. T., & Schauss, S. (2000). Validation of polar heart rate monitor for assessing heart rate during physical and mental stress. *Journal of Psychophysiology, 14*(3), 1591.

Grant, A. M., Berg, J. M., & Cable, D. M. (2014). Job titles as identity badges: How self-reflective titles can reduce emotional exhaustion. *Academy of Management Journal, 57*(4), 1201–1225.

Greenwood, S., Perrin, A., & Duggan, M. (2016). *Demographics of social media users in 2016.* Pew Research Center.

Griffin, M. A., Neal, A., & Parker, S. K. (2007). A new model of work role performance: Positive behavior in uncertain and interdependent contexts. *Academy of Management Journal, 50*(2), 327–347.

Guillory, J., & Hancock, J. T. (2012). The effect of Linkedin on deception in resumes. *Cyberpsychology, Behavior, and Social Networking, 15*(3), 135–140.

Guillory, J., Spiegel, J., Drislane, M., Weiss, B., Donner, W., & Hancock, J. (2011, May). Upset now?: Emotion contagion in distributed groups. *CHI '11: Proceedings of the SIGCHI Conference on Human Factors in Computing Systems*, pp. 745–748.

Guntuku, S. C., Buffone, A., Jaidka, K., Eichstaedt, J. C., & Ungar, L. H. (2019). Understanding and measuring psychological stress using social media. *arXiv:* 1811.07430

Gupta, A. K., & Govindarajan, V. (2002). Cultivating a global mindset. *Academy of Management Perspectives, 16*(1), 116–126.

Hellhammer, J., & Schubert, M. (2012). The physiological response to trier social stress test relates to subjective measures of stress during but not before or after the test. *Psychoneuroendocrinology, 37*(1), 119–124.

Hewitt, P. L., Flett, G. L., & Mosher, S. W. (1992). The perceived stress scale: Factor structure and relation to depression symptoms in a psychiatric sample. *Journal of Psychopathology and Behavioral Assessment, 14*(3), 247–257.

Hickman, L., Saha, K., De Choudhury, M., & Tay, L. (2019). *Automated tracking of components of job satisfaction via text mining of Twitter data.* ML Symposium, SIOP.

Hilbe, J. M. (2011). *Negative binomial regression.* Cambridge University Press.

Hirsch, J. K., & Ellis, J. B. (1996). Differences

in life stress and reasons for living among college suicide ideators and non-ideators. *College Student Journal, 30*(3), 377–386.

Holdeman, T. C. (2009). Invisible wounds of war: Psychological and cognitive injuries, their consequences, and services to assist recovery. *Psychiatric Services, 60*(2), 273.

Holland, P. W. (1986). Statistics and causal inference. *Journal of the American Statistical Association, 81*(396), 945–960.

Jackson, S. E., & Schuler, R. S. (1985). A meta-analysis and conceptual critique of research on role ambiguity and role conflict in work settings. *Organizational Behavior and Human Decision Processes, 36*(1), 16–78.

Jacobson, W. S., & Tufts, S. (2013). To post or not to post: Employee rights and social media. *Review of Public Personnel Administration, 33*(1), 84–107.

Jacovi, M., Guy, I., Kremer-Davidson, S., Porat, S., & Aizenbud-Reshef, N. (2014). The perception of others: Inferring reputation from social media in the enterprise. *Proceedings of the 17th ACM Conference on Computer Supported Cooperative Work and Social Computing*, pp. 756–766.

Jhaver, S., Cranshaw, J., & Counts, S. (2019). Measuring professional skill development in U.S. cities using Internet search queries. *Proceedings of the International AAAI Conference on Web and Social Media, 13*(1), 267–277.

Kahn, R. L., Byosiere, P., & Dunnette, M. D. (1992). Stress in organizations. In L. M. Hough (Ed.), *Handbook of industrial and organizational psychology* (Vol. 3, pp. 571–650). Consulting Psychologists Press.

Kahn, R. L., Wolfe, D. M., Quinn, R. P., Snoek, J. D., & Rosenthal, R. A. (1964). *Organizational stress: Studies in role conflict and ambiguity.* Wiley.

King, L. A., & King, D. W. (1990). Role conflict and role ambiguity: A critical assessment of construct validity. *Psychological Bulletin, 107*(1), 48.

Koch, T., Gerber, C., & de Klerk, J. J. (2018). The impact of social media on recruitment: Are you linked in? *SA Journal of Human Resource Management, 16*(1), 1–14.

Kollock, P. (1999). The economies of online cooperation. *Communities in Cyberspace, 220.*

Kosinski, M., Stillwell, D., & Graepel, T. (2013). Private traits and attributes are predictable from digital records of human behavior. *Proceedings of the National Academy of Sciences, 110*(15), 5802–5805.

Kumar, M., Dredze, M., Coppersmith, G., & De Choudhury, M. (2015). Detecting changes in suicide content manifested in social media following celebrity suicides. *Proceedings of the 26th ACM Conference on Hypertext and Social Media Association for Computing Machinery*, pp. 85–94.

Ladany, N., & Friedlander, M. L. (1995). The relationship between the supervisory working alliance and trainees' experience of role conflict and role ambiguity. *Counselor Education and Supervision, 34*(3), 220–231.

Lazarus, R. S. (1995). Psychological stress in the workplace. In R. Crandall & P. L. Perrewe (Eds.), *Occupational stress: A handbook* (2nd ed., Vol. 1, pp. 3–14). Routledge.

Lin, Y. R., & Margolin, D. (2014). The ripple of fear, sympathy and solidarity during the Boston bombings. *EPJ Data Science, 3*(1), 31.

Liu, S., Zhu, M., & Young, S. D. (2018). Monitoring freshman college experience through content analysis of tweets: Observational study. *JMIR Public Health and Surveillance, 4*(1), e5.

Manago, A. M., Taylor, T., & Greenfield, P. M. (2012). Me and my 400 friends: The anatomy of college students' Facebook networks, their communication patterns, and well-being. *Developmental Psychology, 48*(2), 369–380.

Manyika, J., Lund, S., Chui, M., Bughin, J., Woetzel, J., Batra, P., Ko, R., & Sanghvi, S. (2017). *Jobs lost, jobs gained: Workforce transitions in a time of automation.* McKinsey Global Institute.

Mark, G., Bagdouri, M., Palen, L., Martin, J., Al-Ani, B., & Anderson, K. (2012). Blogs as a collective war diary. *CSCW '12: Proceedings of the ACM 2012 Conference on Computer Supported Cooperative Work*, pp. 37–46.

Mark, G., Iqbal, S. T., Czerwinski, M., & Johns, P. (2014). Bored Mondays and focused afternoons: The rhythm of attention and online activity in the workplace. *Proceedings of the SIGCHI Conference on Human Factors in Computing Systems* (pp. 3025–3034). ACM.

Mark, G., Wang, Y., Niiya, M., & Reich, S. (2016). Sleep debt in student life: Online attention focus, Facebook, and mood. *Proceedings of the 2016 CHI Conference on Human Factors in Computing Systems*, pp. 5517–5528.

Mattingly, S. M., Gregg, J. M., Audia, P., Bayraktaroglu, A. E., Campbell, A. T., Chawla, N. V., et al. (2019, May). The Tesserae project: Large-scale, longitudinal, *in situ*, multimodal sensing of information workers. (2019, May). The tesserae project: Large-scale, longitudinal, *in situ*, multimodal sensing of information workers. *Extended Abstracts of the 2019 CHI Conference on Human Factors in Computing Systems*, pp. 1–8.

McCann, I. L., & Pearlman, L. A. (1990). *Psychological trauma and the adult survivor: Theory, therapy, and transformation*. Brunner-Routledge.

McFarlane, A. C. (2010). The long-term costs of traumatic stress: Intertwined physical and psychological consequences. *World Psychiatry, 9*(1), 3–10.

Miller, H. (1995). *The presentation of self in electronic life: Goffman on the internet*. Embodied Knowledge and Virtual Space Conference (Vol. 9).

Mirjafari, S., Masaba, K., Grover, T., Wang, W., Audia, P., Campbell, A. T., et al. (2019). Differentiating higher and lower job performers in the workplace using mobile sensing. *Proceedings of the ACM on Interactive, Mobile, Wearable and Ubiquitous Technologies, 2*(1), 1–23.

Mitra, T., & Gilbert, E. (2012). Have you heard?: How gossip flows through workplace email. *Proceedings of the International AAAI Conference on Web and Social Media, 6*(1), 242–249.

Mitra, T., Muller, M., Sadat Shami, N., Golestani, A., & Masli, M. (2017). Spread of employee engagement in a large organizational network: A longitudinal analysis. *Proceedings of the ACM on Human-Computer Interaction, 1*, 1–20.

Moreno, M. A., Christakis, D. A., Egan, K. G., Brockman, L. N., & Becker, T. (2011). Associations between displayed alcohol references on Facebook and problem drinking among college students. *Archives of Pediatrics and Adolescent Medicine, 166*(2), 157–163.

Moreno, M. A., Jelenchick, L. A., Egan, K. G., Cox, E., Young, H., Gannon, K. E., et al. (2011). Feeling bad on Facebook: Depression disclosures by college students on a social networking site. *Depression and Anxiety, 28*(6), 447–455.

Murphey, D. A. (1999). Presenting community-level data in an "outcomes and indicators" framework: Lessons from Vermont's experience. *Public Administration Review, 59*(1), 76–82.

Nadler, D. A., Jenkins, G. D., Cammann, C., & Lawler, E. E. (1975). *The Michigan Organizational Assessment Package: Progress Report II*. Institute for Social Research, University of Michigan.

Noe, R. A., Hollenbeck, J. R., Gerhart, B., & Wright, P. M. (2017). *Human resource management: Gaining a competitive advantage*. McGraw-Hill Education.

O'Brien, R. M. (2007). A caution regarding rules of thumb for variance inflation factors. *Quality and Quantity, 41*(5), 673–690.

Oldenburg, R. (1999). *The great good place: Cafes, coffee shops, bookstores, bars, hair salons, and other hangouts at the heart of a community*. Da Capo Press.

Organ, D. W. (1988). *Organizational citizenship behavior: The good soldier syndrome*. Lexington Books/DC Heath.

Palen, L. (2008). Online social media in crisis events. *Educause Quarterly, 31*(3), 76–78.

Paul, M. J., & Dredze, M. (2011). You are what you Tweet: Analyzing Twitter for public health. *Proceedings of the International AAAI Conference on Web and Social Media, 5*(1), 265–272.

Pavlick, E., & Callison-Burch, C. (2016). The gun violence database. *arXiv preprint arXiv:1610.01670*.

Pearce, J. L. (1981), Bringing some clarity to role ambiguity research. *Academy of Management Review, 6*(4), 665–674.

Pennebaker, J. W., & Chung, C. K. (2007). Expressive writing, emotional upheavals, and health. In T. A. Revenson & R. A. R. Gurung (Eds.), *Handbook of health psychology* (pp. 263–284). Routledge.

Pennebaker, J. W., Mehl, M. R., & Niederhoffer, K. G. (2003). Psychological aspects of natural language use: Our words, our selves. *Annual Review of Psychology, 54*(1), 547–577.

Pennington, J., Socher, R., & Manning, C. D. (2014). GloVe: Global vectors for word representation. *EMNLP, 14*, 1532–1543.

Petticrew, M., Cummins, S., Ferrell, C., Findlay, A., Higgins, C., Hoy, C., Kearns, A., & Sparks, L. (2005). Natural experiments: An underused tool for public health? *Public Health, 119*(9), 751–757.

Pew Research Center. (2021). *Social media fact sheet.* Retrieved from pewinternet.org/fact-sheet/social-media

Poland, M., & Maré, D. C. (2005). *Defining geographic communities* (Motu Working Paper 05-09). Motu Economic and Public Policy Research Trust.

Þórarinsdóttir, H., Kessing, L. V., & Faurholt-Jepsen, M. (2017). Smartphone-based self-assessment of stress in healthy adult individuals: A systematic review. *Journal of Medical Internet Research, 19*(2), e41.

Prothrow-Stith, D., & Quaday, S. (1995). *Hidden casualties: The relationship between violence and learning.* National Association of Elementary School Principals.

Quercia, D., Kosinski, M., Stillwell, D., & Crowcroft, J. (2011). Our Twitter profiles, our selves: Predicting personality with Twitter. *2011 IEEE Third International Conference on Privacy, Security, Risk and Trust and 2011 IEEE Third International Conference on Social Computing*, pp. 180–185.

Ritter, K.-J., Matthews, R. A., Ford, M. T., & Henderson, A. A. (2016). Understanding role stressors and job satisfaction over time using adaptation theory. *Journal of Applied Psychology, 101*(12), 1655.

Rizzo, J. R., House, R. J., & Lirtzman, S. I. (1970). Role conflict and ambiguity in complex organizations. *Administrative Science Quarterly*, pp. 150–163.

Rosenbaum, P. R., & Rubin, D. B. (1985). Constructing a control group using multivariate matched sampling methods that incorporate the propensity score. *The American Statistician, 39*(1), 33–38.

Ross, S. E., Niebling, B. C., & Heckert, T. M. (1999). Sources of stress among college students. *Social Psychology, 61*(5), 841–846.

Rotundo, M., & Sackett, P. R. (2002). The relative importance of task, citizenship, and counterproductive performance to global ratings of job performance: A policy-capturing approach. *Journal of Applied Psychology, 87*(1), 66.

Sadilek, A., Kautz, H. A., & Silenzio, V. (2012). Modeling spread of disease from social interactions. *Proceedings of the International AAAI Conference on Web and Social Media (ICWSM), 5*(1), 322–329.

Saha, K., Bayraktaraglu, A. E., Campbell, A., Chawla, N. V., De Choudhury, M., et al. (2019a). Social media as a passive sensor in longitudinal studies of human behavior and wellbeing. *Conference on Human Factors in Computing Systems, Paper No. CS12*, pp. 1–8.

Saha, K., Chan, L., de Barbaro, K., Abowd, G. D., & De Choudhury, M. (2017). Inferring mood instability on social media by leveraging ecological momentary assessments. *Proceedings of the ACM on Interactive, Mobile, Wearable, and Ubiquitous Technologies, 1*(3), 1–27.

Saha, K., Chandrasekharan, E., & De Choudhury, M. (2019b). Prevalence and psychological effects of hateful speech in online college communities. *Proceedings of the 10th ACM Conference on Web Science*, pp. 255–264.

Saha, K., & De Choudhury, M. (2017). Modeling stress with social media around incidents of gun violence on college campuses. *Proceedings of the ACM on Human-Computer Interaction, 1*(CSCW), Article No. 92, 1–27.

Saha, K., Reddy, M. D., Das Swain, V., Gregg, J. M., Grover, T., Lin, S., Martinez, G. J., Mattingly, S. M., et al. (2019c). Imputing missing social media data stream in multisensor studies of human behavior. *Proceedings of International Conference on Affective Computing and Intelligent Interaction (ACII 2019).*

Saha, K., Reddy, M. D., & De Choudhury, M. (2019d). Joblex: A lexico-semantic knowledgebase of occupational information descriptors. *11th International Conference on Social Informatics (SocInfo).*

Saha, K., Reddy, M. D., Mattingly, S. M., Moskal, E., Sirigiri, A., & De Choudhury, M. (2019e). Libra: On linkedin based role ambiguity and its relationship with wellbeing and job performance. *Proceedings of the ACM on Human-Computer Interaction, 3, Issue CSCW*, pp. 1–30.

Saha, K., Sugar, B., Torous, J., Abrahao, B., Kıcıman, E., & De Choudhury, M. (2019f). A social media study on the effects of psychiatric medication use. *Proceedings of the International AAAI Conference on Web and Social Media, 13*(1), 440–451.

Saha, K., Weber, I., & De Choudhury, M. (2018). A social media based examination of the effects of counseling recommendations after student deaths on college campuses. In *Proceedings of the International AAAI Conference on Web and Social Media, 12*(1).

Saha, K., Yousuf, A., Boyd, R. L., Pennebaker, J. W., & De Choudhury, M. (2022). Social media discussions predict mental health consultations on college campuses. *Nature Scientific Reports, 12*(1), 1–11.

Sallis, J. F., & Owen, N. (1998). *Behavioral medicine and health psychology; Vol. 3. Physical activity and behavioral medicine.* SAGE.

Sapone, Marcela. medium.com/@MsSapone/why-titles-will-kill-your-startup-58402c5b6954, 2019.

Schmidt, S., Roesler, U., Kusserow, T., & Rau, R. (2014). Uncertainty in the workplace: Examining role ambiguity and role conflict, and their link to depression–a meta-analysis. *European Journal of Work and Organizational Psychology, 23*(1), 91–106.

Schneider, W. J., & McGrew, K. S. (2012). The Cattell–Horn–Carroll model of intelligence. In D. P. Flanagan & P. L. Harrison (Eds.), *Contemporary intellectual assessment: Theories, texts, and issues* (pp. 99–144). Guilford Press.

Schwartz, H. A., Eichstaedt, J. C., Kern, M. L., et al. (2013). Personality, gender, and age in the language of social media: The open-vocabulary approach. *PLOS ONE, 8*(9), e73791.

Scollon, C. N., Prieto, C.-K., & Diener, E. (2009). Experience sampling: Promises and pitfalls, strength and weaknesses. In *Assessing well-being* (pp. 157–180). Springer.

Shami, N. S., Muller, M., Pal, A., Masli, M., & Geyer, W. (2015). Inferring employee engagement from social media. *Proceedings of 33rd Annual ACM Conference on Human Factors in Computing System*, pp. 3999–4008.

Shami, N. S., Nichols, J., & Chen, J. (2014). Social media participation and performance at work: A longitudinal study. In *Proceedings of the SIGCHI Conference on Human Factors in Computing Systems* (pp. 115–118). ACM.

Shami, N. S., Yang, J., Panc, L., Dugan, C., Ratchford, T., Rasmussen, J. C., et al. (2014). Understanding employee social media chatter with enterprise social pulse. *Proceedings of the 17th ACM Conference on Computer Supported Cooperation Work and Social Computing*, pp. 379–392.

Shipley, W. C. (2009). *Shipley-2: Manual.* WPS.

Skeels, M. M., & Grudin, J. (2009). When social networks cross boundaries: A case study of workplace use of Facebook and Linkedin. *Proceedings of the 2009 ACM International Conference on Supporting Group Work*, pp. 95–104.

Smith, C. S., Tisak, J., & Schmieder, R. A. (1993). The measurement properties of the role conflict and role ambiguity scales: A review and extension of the empirical research. *Journal of Organizational Behavior, 14*(1), 37–48.

Soto, C. J., & John, O. P. (2017). The next Big Five Inventory (BFI-2): Developing and assessing a hierarchical model with 15 facets to enhance bandwidth, fidelity, and predictive power. *Journal of Personality and Social Psychology, 113*(1), 117.

Spiro, E. S. (2016). Research opportunities at the intersection of social media and survey data. *Current Opinion in Psychology, 9*, 67–71.

Starbird, K., Palen, L., Hughes, A. L., & Vieweg, S. (2010). Chatter on the red: What hazards threat reveals about the social life of microblogged information. *Proceedings of the 2010 ACM Conference on Computer Supported Cooprative Work, CSCW 2010*, pp. 241–250.

Suh, H., Shahriaree, N., Hekler, E. B., & Kientz, J. A. (2016). Developing and validating the user burden scale: A tool for assessing user burden in computing systems. In *Proceedings of the 2016 CHI Conference on Human Factors in Computing Systems* (pp. 3988–3999). ACM.

Sullivan, S. E., & Bhagat, R. S. (1992). Organizational stress, job satisfaction and job performance: Where do we go from here? *Journal of Management, 18*(2), 353–374.

Tambe, P., & Hitt, L. M. (2012). Now it's personal: Offshoring and the shifting skill composition of the US information technology workforce. *Management Science, 58*(4), 678–695.

Tausczik, Y. R., & Pennebaker, J. W. (2010). The psychological meaning of words: LIWC and computerized text analysis methods. *Journal of Language and Social Psychology, 29*(1), 24–54.

Tett, R. P., Jackson, D. N., & Rothstein, M. (2000). Personality measures as predictors of job performance: A meta-analytic review. *Personnel Psychology, 44*(4), 703–742.

Tourangeau, R., Rips, L. J., & Rasinski, K. (2000). *The psychology of survey response.* Cambridge University Press.

Tufekci, Z. (2008). Can you see me now?: Audience and disclosure regulation in online social network sites. *Bulletin of Science, Technology and Society, 28*(1), 20–36.

Valkenburg, P. M., Peter, J., & Schouten, A. P. (2006). Friend networking sites and their relationship to adolescents' well-being and social self-esteem. *CyberPsychology and Behavior, 9*(5), 584–590.

van Dijck, J. (2013). *The culture of connectivity: A critical history of social media.* Oxford University Press.

Van Reeth, O., Weibel, L., Spiegel, K., Leproult, R., Dugovic, C., & Maccari, S. (2000). Physiology of sleep (Review)–interactions between stress and sleep: From basic research to clinical situations. *Sleep Medicine Reviews, 4*(2), 201–219.

Van Sell, M., Brief, A. P., & Schuler, R. S. (1981). Role conflict and role ambiguity: Integration of the literature and directions for future research. *Human Relations, 34*(1), 43–71.

Viswesvaran, C., & Ones, D. S. (2000). Perspectives on models of job performance. *International Journal of Selection and Assessment, 8*(4), 216–226.

Walcott-McQuigg, J. A., Zerwic, J. J., Dan, A., & Kelley, M. A. (2001). An ecological approach to physical activity in African American women. *Medscape Women's Health, 6*(6), 3.

Wang, R., Chen, F., Chen, Z., Li, T., Harari, G., Tignor, S., Zhou, X., et al. (2014, September). Studentlife: Assessing mental health, academic performance and behavioral trends of college students using smartphones. *UbiComp '14: Proceedings of the 2014 ACM International Joint Conference on Pervasive and Ubiquitous Computing*, pp. 3–14.

Williams, L. J., & Anderson, S. E. (1991). Job satisfaction and organizational commitment as predictors of organizational citizenship and in-role behaviors. *Journal of Management, 17*(3), 601–617.

Wood, J., Foy, D. W., Layne, C., Pynoos, R., & Boyd James, C. (2002). An examination of the relationships between violence exposure, posttraumatic stress symptomatology, and delinquent activity: An "ecopathological" model of delinquent behavior among incarcerated adolescents. *Journal of Aggression, Maltreatment and Trauma, 6*(1), 127–147.

Zajacova, A., Lynch, S. M., & Espenshade, T. J. (2005). Self-efficacy, stress, and academic success in college. *Research in Higher Education, 46*(6), 677–706.

Zenger, T. R., & Lazzarini, S. G. (2004). Compensating for innovation: Do small firms offer high-powered incentives that lure talent and motivate effort? *Managerial and Decision Economics, 25*(6–7), 329–345.

Zide, J., Elman, B., & Shahani-Denning, C. (2014). Linkedin and recruitment: How profiles differ across occupations. *Employee Relations, 36*(5), 583–604.

CHAPTER 10

Behavioral Audio Signal Processing in Mobile Sensing Research

Rajat Hebbar, Arindam Jati, Tiantian Feng, Ramon Reyes, Alexander F. Danvers, Matthias R. Mehl, and Shrikanth S. Narayanan

CHAPTER OVERVIEW

Convergent advances in on-device computing and machine learning are creating possibilities for the ubiquitous use of wearable devices in a variety of health-related applications. Audio is an essential stream of information that can be measured via such devices. Audio sensing in naturalistic settings can provide insight into a person's day-to-day life and hence infer meaningful patterns in their lifestyle from an acoustic perspective. Egocentric audio recordings can provide important cues about a person's mental state and well-being (e.g., stress, social interaction patterns, as well as the ambient context of a person's surroundings). In this chapter, we provide an overview of mobile audio acquisition methods and fundamental audio processing techniques, showcasing some of the state-of-the-art methodologies in this domain. We discuss example studies that highlight the utility of audio-derived cues for a variety of applications in psychology research and practice.

Acquiring Audio in Mobile Settings

Investigating audio signals in natural environments can help researchers model and understand social activity in everyday life (Narayanan & Georgiou, 2013; Pantic, Pentland, Nijholt, & Huang, 2006). Traditional audio sensing systems, such as handheld microphones and lapel mics, are cumbersome, hard to use, expensive, and not scalable. They also present risks to privacy by recording and storing raw audio. Driven by the recent advances in microelectronics technology, many modern wearable sensors and mobile devices today can capture important audio information (e.g., egocentric audio, environmental audio) about an individual over a prolonged period in real-world settings.

Additionally, these wearable and mobile sensors can now gather audio data for human behavior analysis without relying on sensors installed in physical infrastructure. The audio data captured from these modern sensing systems have opened new possibilities for understanding human behavior (Jiang et al., 2018; Sashima & Kawamoto, 2019; S. Yang et al., 2018).

Audio Sensing Overview

In this section, we introduce two broad types of audio sensing: environmental audio sensing and egocentric audio sensing. Then, we will go over the challenges of utilizing mobile technologies to sense and sample audio information. Finally, we will introduce some state-of-the-art systems in sensing audio information in the natural environment.

Environmental Audio Sensing

It has been well established that environmental audio is a rich source of information that can be used to make inferences about our surroundings, such as event detection and location classification. Two research fields associated with audio analysis are audio event detection (Gemmeke et al., 2017) and acoustic scene classification (Stowell, Giannoulis, Benetos, Lagrange, & Plumbley, 2015). The infrastructure used for such tasks include the installation of microphones.

The traditional method of recording audio is to connect several low-cost microphones to a single computer and run audio analysis on that computer. However, this infrastructure requires the installation of long wires between the personal computers and the microphones, and may not be achievable for the study running in a natural environment. Some recent researchers have prototyped audio sensing devices using mobile sensing devices. One example is the iSENSE platform (Buschmann & Pfisterer, 2007), which consists of compact data-logging devices called PINPoint, which can periodically sense environmental audio. The Mobile Sensing Platform (Choudhury et al., 2008) is another such sensing system, and EnviroMic is another recently designed low-cost experimental prototype of a distributed acoustic monitoring system working in the outdoor environment (Luo et al., 2007). This system aims to monitor acoustic information among animal populations. The system can coordinate audio sampling tasks among different sensors deployed in the environment.

Egocentric Audio Sensing

With the availability of multisensor wearable devices (e.g., GoPro), egocentric (centered around a certain person) audio recordings have become popular in many areas such as extreme sports, health monitoring, and lifelogging. In egocentric audio, the world is recorded from the user's perspective, capturing the context of the user's activities. (Figure 10.1 shows a generic egocentric audio processing framework). Audio information from the egocentric view allows researchers to track human behaviors automatically and objectively. Such audio data also have important elements in the field of activity recognition (Stork, Spinello, Silva, & Arras, 2012), emotion classification (Busso et al., 2004), and context inference (Cai, Lu, Hanjalic, Zhang, & Cai, 2006).

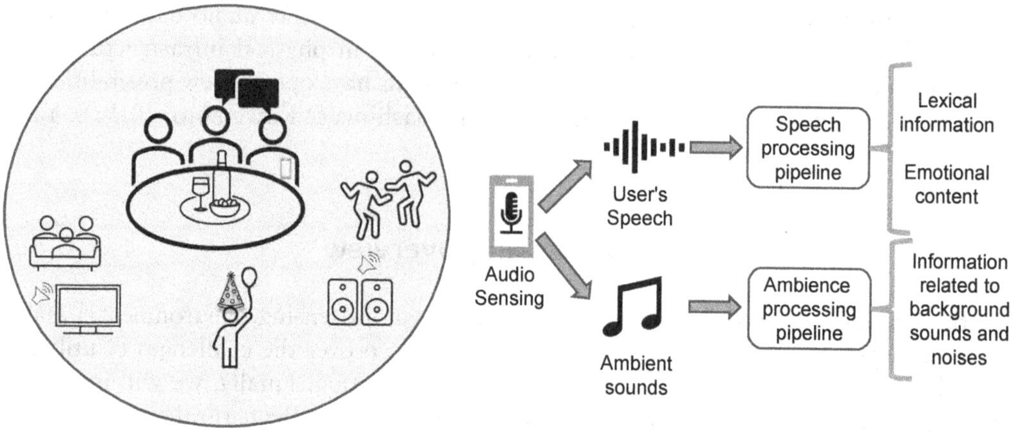

FIGURE 10.1. Egocentric audio sensing and processing.

The early developed solutions for sensing egocentric audio, such as EAR (Mehl, Pennebaker, Crow, Dabbs, & Price, 2001), can record small fractions of audio from an egocentric perspective at regular intervals. However, these sensing systems pose privacy concerns by recording and saving the raw audio. Some recent egocentric audio sensing systems, like SoundSense (H. Lu et al., 2009), are capable of running machine learning techniques on resource-limited mobile devices to classify and record the activities users are performing. Similar mobile platforms, like EmotionSense (Rachuri et al., 2010), can detect emotion as well as activities and surroundings from the audio. These devices perform on-device training and classification for privacy protection.

Challenges

In this section, we discuss the challenges in acquiring audio (both environmental and egocentric audio) in mobile settings for human behavior research.

Background Noise

The signal-to-noise ratio (SNR) is typically low in an audio signal collected in the natural environment, making postprocessing a challenging task. This is particularly problematic in environmental audio sensing systems when the recording microphone is far from the acoustic sources. Researchers have proposed installing multiple audio recording modules in the surroundings to resolve this problem. Similar to environmental audio sensing systems, the egocentric audio recording solutions, like SoundSense and EAR (electronically activated recorder), usually suffer from poor recording quality because people commonly carry phones in their pockets or handbags. Hip-worn device holsters, commonly used in EAR studies, are also far from the wearer's mouth. To improve the quality of audio recordings in an egocentric sensing setup, researchers have designed recording solutions, such as TAR (TILES Audio Recorder) (Feng, Nadarajan, Vaz, Booth, & Narayanan, 2018), that can be easily placed close to the wearer's mouth.

Privacy

Privacy protection has already been recognized as an important issue in the design of audio sensing applications. Audio recordings from both the environment or egocentric view can contain sensitive information about an individual. Thus, it would be problematic to record, store, and transmit raw audio during the data collection process. A possible solution to this problem is to store task-specific features instead of raw audio recordings, such that neither verbal speech nor lexical content can be reconstructed (Langheinrich, 2001). These features are referred to as privacy-sensitive features that preserve information about conversation style and dynamics. For example, StudentLife (R. Wang et al., 2014) is a recent study that implements applications on smartphone devices to process audio on the fly and record features. TILES is another large-scale human behavior study in the hospital environment that implemented a wearable audio recording system to record audio features from health care providers. Some other systems choose to directly infer and save high-level descriptors from the audio data to preserve user privacy. These high-level descriptors include emotions, audio events, and surrounding context.

Ease of Use

Ease of use is a critical factor in the development of audio sensing solutions. Human behavior study typically takes place in a naturalistic environment. Thus, the installation of audio data collection sensors needs to require minimum effort. Researchers are recommended to deploy wireless sensor nodes for sensing environmental audio. Additionally, wearable and mobile data logging hardware are ideal tools to collect egocentric audio data. Some customization on the hardware may be considered as presented in TAR and EAR (Feng et al., 2018; Mehl et al., 2001) to increase the comfort of participants in wearing the sensors.

Scalability

A big hurdle in designing audio sensing systems presented in the human behavior study is the solution's scalability. Here, scalability is associated with the ability to deploy an increasing number of systems and the ability to adopt modifications from different contributors. For example, many notable efforts in developing wearable audio recorders include devices like the Sociometer (Choudhury & Pentland, 2003), which are not commercially available, making large-scale deployment prohibitive. Implementing the audio sensing solutions using commercially available hardware and open-source software can improve scalability. For example, commercially available smartwatches and smartphones are good options in the design of audio sensing systems. Open hardware like Arduino (www.arduino.cc) can be considered as candidates for customized design audio sensing applications. Open-source software tools, such as openSMILE (Eyben, Wöllmer, & Schuller, 2010) and Kaldi (Povey et al., 2011), can be configured to run on many hardware devices.

Sampling and Battery Life

One common challenge for designing audio sensing systems for human behavior study is the mobile device's limited battery capacity. The sampling process in mobile devices is a major source of power consumption. For instance, empirical results in TAR show that the mobile devices can run for 10 hours with low sampling frequency, but the battery would be drained entirely within 6 hours if the device sampled half of the time. Hence, excessive energy consumption may become a major obstacle to broader acceptance of mobile audio sensing services in human behavioral studies. To achieve energy efficiency in mobile sensing applications, researchers proposed periodic sensing and sleeping techniques (Y. Wang, Krishnamachari, Zhao, & Annavaram, 2010) instead of continuous sampling. Machine learning approaches such as the Markov Decision Process have been integrated into mobile sensing devices to obtain the "optimal" data sampling policy (Y. Wang, Krishnamachari, & Annavaram, 2012). Applying these sampling approaches can also reduce redundant information since environmental audio events or conversations do not happen continuously by nature.

Audio Features

As discussed in the last section, extracting audio features plays an important role in preserving privacy in audio sensing applications. Additionally, audio features provide discriminative information useful for classification tasks while neglecting background noise and other confounding factors. Over the last several decades, a plethora of audio features have been designed in the field of audio analysis. (Refer to Alías, Socoró, & Sevillano, 2016, for details on various features.) Many of these features were developed for specific tasks such as speech recognition, speaker recognition, and audio context classification. Thus, the selection of robust audio features plays a critical role in different audio sensing applications for human behavior study. The audio feature extraction approach is typically based on frame-based processing. During this process, the audio signals are first divided into frames, often using a Hamming or Hanning window (Prabhu, 2014). Subsequently, features are extracted from each frame, and this sequence of feature vectors is used to represent an audio signal. Here, we focus on presenting five types of audio features commonly used in audio analysis: time-domain, frequency-domain, cepstrum, energy, and perceptually driven features.

Time-Domain Features

Frequently used time-domain audio features include zero crossing rate and waveform extrema. Zero crossing rate is the number of times the sign of the signal changes in a given window. It measures the abnormality of an audio segment. The waveform extrema features state the maximum and minimum values in the signal (Swain, Routray, & Kabisatpathy, 2018).

Frequency-Domain Features

Frequency-domain features such as harmonicity, spectral centroid, spectral flatness, spectral roll-off, spectral moment, band energy, bandwidth, fundamental frequency, and spectral flux are frequently included with other developed sets of features. Most of these features provide measures about spectrum shape (Chu, Narayanan, & Kuo, 2009).

Cepstrum Features

Cepstral features are typically computed on the cepstrum, which is the inverse Fourier transform of the log-magnitude of the signal power spectrum. The most widely used features in this category are Mel-frequency cepstral coefficients (MFCCs). This feature set has wide applications such as speaker recognition, emotion detection, and audio event detection (Lu & Zhang, 2002).

Energy Features

Frequently used energy features include signal energy, log energy derivatives, and energy entropy. Signal energy is the total signal energy over a frame, and log energy derivatives are derivatives of logarithm power in adjacent data frames. Energy entropy is calculated over the energies extracted from a set of audio frames. These features have applications in audio event detection, emotion recognition, and so on (Swain et al., 2018).

Perceptually Driven Features

Perceptually driven features are time-domain, frequency-domain, or cepstral features that consider the human auditory and vocal structure. For example, the Mel-scale in MFCCs is used to mimic the nonlinear perception of the human ear to different frequencies. Two other feature sets of this kind are prosodic and voice quality features (Friedland, Vinyals, Huang, & Muller, 2009). Commonly used prosodic features are pitch and intensity. Voice quality features include jitter (pitch modulation), shimmer (amplitude modulation), unvoiced rate (proportion of unvoiced frames in a sequence), and harmonic-to-noise ratio (proportion of periodic vs. nonperiodic signal).

Speech Processing Pipeline

The field of speech processing has seen rapid advancements over recent decades. Speech processing has found applications in people's daily lives in the form of virtual assistants, mobile applications, and teleconferences, to name a few. With significant advances in computational power over the last decade, real-time speech processing is now a reality that lends itself to on-device applications such as mobile phones, smart devices, and egocentric recorders. In this section, we discuss a few speech processing modules that are salient to many such applications.

Voice Activity Detection

The primary module in any speech processing pipeline is invariably a voice activity detection (VAD) system. The role of this module is to detect the absence/presence of human voices in an audio recording. Such a system requires a high resolution of operation (typically 10 ms) to detect pauses between words and account for variable rate of speech across people and conversational settings (Ramirez, Górriz, & Segura, 2007).

Early efforts in VAD explored statistical methods, particularly using likelihood ratio tests to determine VAD decisions (Sohn, Kim, & Sung, 1999). The Gaussian statistical models were replaced by Laplacian and Gamma distributions (Chang, Kim, & Mitra, 2006), shown to result in robust parametric representation of noisy speech. Other approaches include energy-based methods (Renevey & Drygajlo, 2001). While such methods work for clean audio conditions, they often degrade in regions of low-SNR and nonstationary noise types such as babble (Ramirez, Segura, Benıtez, De La Torre, & Rubio, 2004). Deep-learning-based methods have been effective in modeling large amounts of data augmented with a variety of noise types. Recurrent neural networks were shown to be able to effectively capture context to outperform traditional methods (Hughes & Mierle, 2013), and convolutional neural networks have also been shown to be powerful lightweight counterparts in many applications (Sehgal & Kehtarnavaz, 2018).

Variability in acoustic conditions and a large number of background noise types pose challenges to most VAD systems. For example, VAD systems developed for meeting domains have been shown to perform poorly in conditions with atypical background audio conditions such as music and nonstationary noise (Sahidullah & Saha, 2012). Since VAD is used as a preprocessing module for subsequent speech systems such as speech recognition, speaker recognition and/or diarization, gender identification, and the like, its use comprises most speech processing applications, including virtual assistants such as Alexa and Siri, teleconferencing systems, and hearing aids. Consequently, a VAD system is required to have low computational latency for any real-time application. Furthermore, since errors in a VAD system propagate through subsequent systems, such errors would adversely affect the end-application.

Features

Early approaches used relatively simple audio features such as pitch, energy, and zero-crossing rate (Graf, Herbig, Buck, & Schmidt, 2015). Due to differences in the nature of frequency distributions in speech and nonspeech regions, spectral features such as linear predictive coefficients and MFCCs have also become popular features. With increases in computational resources and the evolution of deep-learning methods, spectrograms have become increasingly popular, since they contain uncompressed spectral information, providing more detailed input representation compared to MFCCs.

Online VAD

With the increased use of real-time voice assistants and teleconferencing applications, online VAD systems are a crucial element to processing speech in real time. A direct application for online VAD in psychology is in wearable devices like TAR, providing richer information and reducing the load on coders. A key necessity for an online VAD system is low computational latency. Consequently, features that are lightweight and easy to extract are favored for real-time applications. The International Telecommunication Union has specified a standard for VAD (*ITU-T Recommendation database*, n.d.), which is widely used for Voice over Internet Protocol applications. This VAD uses full band energy, low band energy, zero crossing rate, and line spectral frequencies as features. VAD solutions have been proposed for embedded systems, including smart-technology devices such as phones, watches, and earphones (Lezzoum, Gagnon, & Voix, 2014; Sehgal & Kehtarnavaz, 2018).

Speaker Diarization

Speaker diarization is the task of classifying speech segments into different speaker identities, answering the question "who spoke and when?" (Park et al., 2021). Traditional diarization systems comprise multiple sequential modules, commonly, voice activity detection, speaker-homogeneous segmentation, speaker clustering, and speaker labeling of clusters, as depicted in Figure 10.2. Additionally, modules for the purposes of resegmentation, cluster recombination, and overlap detection have also been developed to improve the performance of diarization systems over time.

The bulk of effort in advancing diarization systems over the years has focused on three aspects of the pipeline (Park et al., 2021): (1) developing speaker-discriminative features for clustering, (2) similarity metric for computing affinity matrix, and (3) the clustering algorithm. Cosine similarity and probabilistic linear discriminant analysis (Sell & Garcia-Romero, 2014), a supervised similarity metric, are commonly used similarity metrics. Agglomerative hierarchical clustering and spectral clustering are the most popular clustering techniques (Park et al., 2021), with hierarchical clustering being favored for long-form data due to its ability to cluster without knowing the number of speakers a priori. Speaker diarization tends to perform poorly in audio conditions with diverse acoustic backgrounds (e.g., models developed on controlled audio domains such as telephonic speech and meetings deployed on in-the-wild audio; Park et al., 2021). This problem has been largely alleviated with the procurement of large-scale "in-the-wild" labeled datasets (Chung, Nagrani, & Zisserman, 2018; Ryant et al., 2019). Challenges remain in nonconventional domains, however, such as egocentric audio. Dealing with a variable and unknown number of speakers also remains an open challenge.

Speaker diarization finds applications in many audio domains that involve multiparty interactions such as telephone conversations, meetings, broadcast news, counseling sessions, and multimedia. For many of these applications, detecting speaker identities can also be an intermediary step toward further analysis such as role recognition, audio indexing, and retrieval. In psychology, diarization is useful in separating speech from the speaker of interest from those in their surroundings. Diarization can also be used to develop speaker-specific models to enhance other systems such as speech and emotion recognition.

Features

A key necessity for features used for speaker diarization is high interspeaker variability and low intraspeaker variability for improved speaker discriminability. Ideally, such

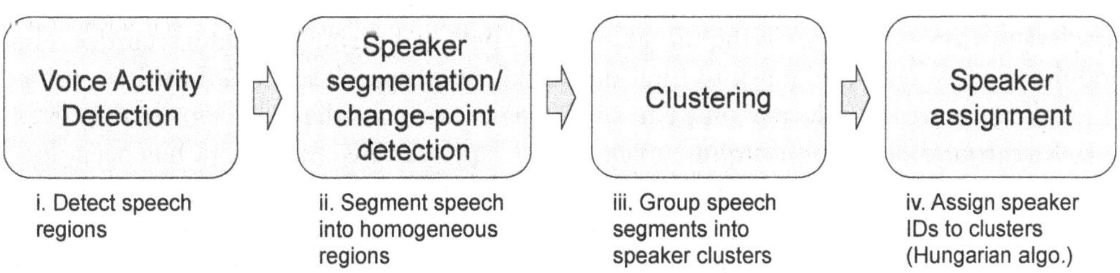

FIGURE 10.2. Speaker diarization pipeline.

features must also be disentangled from sources of audio variability such as channel information and background music/noise.

Due to the compressed yet robust nature of MFCCs, they are the most commonly used audio features in several applications, including speaker diarization. Typically, 13–23 MFCC coefficients, along with their first and/or second derivatives, are used. Other audio features include pitch, line spectrum pairs (Lu & Zhang, 2002), perceptual linear prediction (PLP) coefficients, and prosodic features (Friedland et al., 2009). Total variability modeling was used to decompose speech features into speaker and channel-dependent factors (Dehak, Kenny, Dehak, Dumouchel, & Ouellet, 2010). The resulting representation of speaker-specific characteristics, called the i-vector, can be estimated using expectation maximization. First developed for the task of speaker verification, i-vectors have since been used for speaker diarization (Park et al., 2021; Sell & Garcia-Romero, 2014). More recently, neural-network-based features developed on speaker-labeled datasets have outperformed i-vector-based methods for most applications. Some of the popular embeddings include x-vectors (Snyder, Garcia-Romero, Sell, Povey, & Khudanpur, 2018) and d-vectors (Wan, Wang, Papir, & Moreno, 2018). In addition to leveraging large amounts of data, these representations impose fewer constraints on the distribution of features as compared to i-vectors.

Online Diarization

In online diarization systems, the framework is quite different, since decisions can be made only using speech data up to a given time. There are two key differences from offline systems: (1) homogeneous speech segmentation is replaced by a speaker change point detection, and (2) speaker clustering is replaced by open-set speaker tracking (Kwon & Narayanan, 2003b). Because the number of speakers is not known a priori, speaker tracking is done in an online fashion, with new speakers being enrolled on the fly. Since the amount of data for new speakers is often not enough to build robust speaker models, generic speaker models on a predetermined training set were developed as a way of initializing speaker models (Kwon & Narayanan, 2003b). Several modeling techniques have been explored for these generic models, including Universal Background Models and Gender Background Models (Kwon & Narayanan, 2003a, 2005). Recently, neural-network-based approaches have been explored. One prominent method uses recurrent neural networks as a generative method of updating speakers (Zhang et al., 2019).

Foreground Speech Detection

In the context of egocentric audio, a special application of speaker diarization is foreground speech detection, that is, detecting speech from the person wearing the audio recorder. This module acts as a temporal mask to filter out background speech sources. In this scenario, all speakers, apart from the person wearing the device, are considered background sources. Since foreground detection is unique to egocentric applications, little work has been done in literature exploring methods for this task. A recent work explored using existing meeting databases with stationary microphone setups to develop methods that can be used for egocentric devices (Nadarajan, Somandepalli, & Narayanan, 2019). Another work showed that features obtained from VAD tasks can be transfer-learned for foreground detection in a coarsely labeled setup on audio collected using EAR (Hebbar et al., 2021).

Automatic Speech Recognition

Automatic speech recognition (ASR) is the task of transcribing a segment of recorded audio by decoding the sequence of words spoken. ASR is one of the most widely used speech processing modules that bridges the gap to natural language processing, which is the field of study of human language, for example, English, in the form of words, sentences and documents. As such, ASR systems find use in applications such as sentiment analysis, machine translation, and text classification (Junqua & Haton, 2012).

Typical ASR systems comprise three submodules: (1) feature extraction module, (2) acoustic model (AM), and (3) language model (LM) (Yu & Deng, 2016), as shown in Figure 10.3. AM is used to model a predefined set of acoustic phonemes. Phonemes, typically monosyllabic sound-forms, form the building blocks for words in a language. A typical set for English consists of 44 phonemes, which in combination can be used to pronounce every word in a given lexicon (dictionary), even accounting for multiple pronunciations. The task of the AM is to produce a set of probabilities for each phoneme through time. These probabilities are then decoded to find the phoneme sequence that maximizes the probability of a given word being spoken.

Traditionally, Gaussian mixture models (GMM) based on Hidden Markov models (HMM) systems have been widely used for AMs (Benzeghiba et al., 2007). Here, GMMs are used to model individual phonemes based on audio features. HMMs, parametrized by an initial probability vector and transition probability matrix, model the transition between different GMM states. More recently, deep neural-networks have replaced GMMs in the AM, giving rise to hybrid DNN-HMM systems (Yu & Deng, 2016).

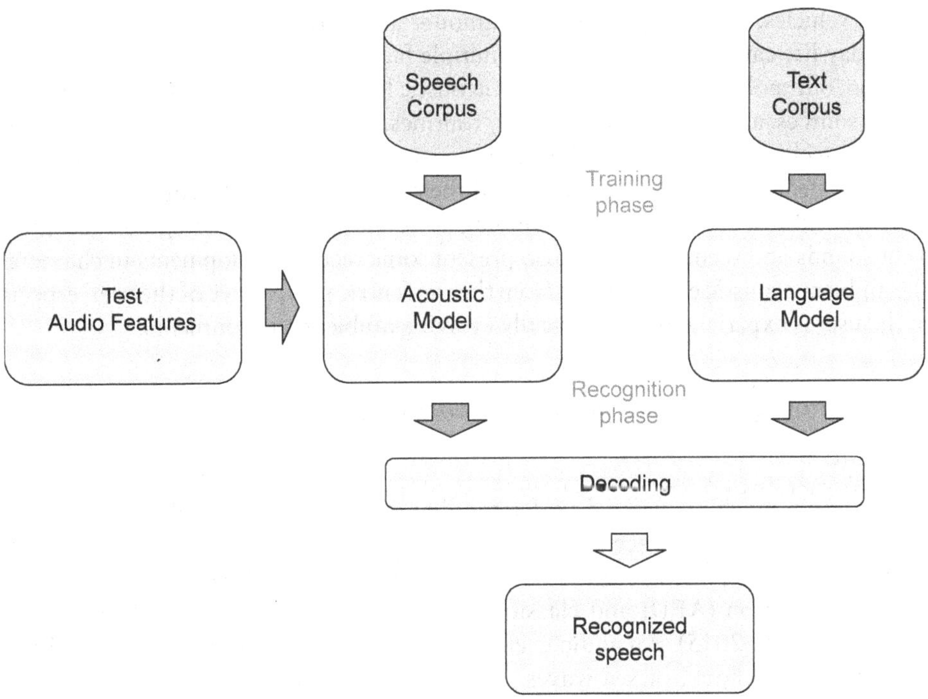

FIGURE 10.3. Automatic speech recognition schematic.

LM is used to detect the most probable sequence of words, using the knowledge of most commonly co-occurring words. The typical LM is an n-gram, which models the probability of n words occurring in sequence. More recently, neural network models have replaced n-grams to develop more powerful LM using large amounts of data.

In the context of on-device processing for egocentric applications, end-to-end systems have been proposed, including connectionist-temporal-classification, recurrent-neural-network transducer, and attention-based models (Kim et al., 2020). These are not only low latency but also have been shown to outperform traditional methods.

Apart from the typical challenges of channel variability and background noise, there are a few challenges that are unique to ASR (Benzeghiba et al., 2007). ASR tends to degrade in cases of spontaneous speech, as opposed to read-speech. Incomplete pronunciation, merging together of words, and colloquial speech pose challenges to AM. Non-native speakers of a language (e.g., English) develop different dialects of the language, which leads to increased acoustic variability, posing additional challenges to the AM. Similarly, the frequency of words in the spoken language is different from those in the written language, and also changes between different cultures, adversely affecting the LM. Child speech also poses challenges to ASR, especially during the development stage of a child's speech production.

Ambient Acoustic Events and Scenes

The human auditory system experiences a multitude of different sounds in the environment – from natural sources like chirping birds and waterfalls, or artificial sources like machines, vehicles, or music players. The amount and variety of sounds we encounter in our everyday life can vary depending on multiple factors—for example, the nature of our occupation, our mobility between different acoustic locales, duration of exposure to different sound sources, and even habits and daily routines. With the rapid advancement of wearable sensing technology, it is becoming easier to capture and sense acoustic cues from both the user (the person wearing the sensor) and their ambient environment. In the following section, we will discuss automated technologies developed for detecting and recognizing ambient sounds and scenes. We will also present some recent developments in characterizing the ambient acoustic environment from the egocentric perspective of the user, especially when the user is experiencing dynamically evolving ambient environments.

Detection and Classification of Audio Events and Acoustic Scenes

Audio Events

The first step in machine-assisted understanding of the effects of ambient acoustics on our life is to detect the presence and type of a particular sound, and identify its duration of activity. This has spawned a broad area of research in "machine hearing," known as audio event detection (AED) and classification (Gemmeke et al., 2017; Hershey et al., 2017; Stowell et al., 2015). An audio event is defined as a specific type of sound, like the alarm clock, door knock, or sea waves. Audio event detection refers to the human-like ability of machines to understand and recognize a particular sound and its onset and offset times. Classification refers to categorizing the detected sound into a predefined semantic audio class labels such as door knock. The semantic class labels are generally annotated by humans following a predefined ontology such as the audio set ontology defined in Gemmeke and colleagues (2017).

Acoustic Scenes

While audio event detection can give us useful information about the sound and noise sources in the surrounding environment, we are also interested in the overall acoustic ambience popularly known as the acoustic scene (Barchiesi, Giannoulis, Stowell, & Plumbley, 2015; Mesaros et al., 2017; Stowell et al., 2015). Typical examples of acoustic scenes are park, office, kitchen, and restaurant. An acoustic scene is generally composed of several audio events. Acoustic scene classification (ASC) can be defined as predicting the semantic label of an ambient environment from an audio stream recorded in that environment. Detecting the acoustic scene might be helpful to an AED system as well, since the acoustic scene can provide prior information about which audio events might be present. For example, a typical office acoustic scene might consist of audio from human speech, keyboards, phones, and air conditioner vents.

Machine Learning Pipeline

While AED and ASC are related, most of the prior literature tackles the two problems separately. Although there are numerous different methods for each of those tasks (good survey articles are Barchiesi et al., 2015; Mesaros et al., 2017; Stowell et al., 2015, and some examples provided at the end of this section), the basic principle is learning a supervised audio classifier. The only differences between these methods are the semantic labels used for classification. Figure 10.4 shows a typical machine learning pipeline for learning an audio classifier.

The preprocessing module represents all the (optional) audio signal-level preprocessing steps such as resampling, normalization, and removing silence regions. The acoustic feature extraction module extracts some time-frequency representation of the audio signal such as spectrogram, mel-spectrogram, or MFCC features. The learning model is a classifier that is being trained to predict the semantic class of the audio signal. Recently, deep neural networks (Goodfellow, Bengio, & Courville, 2016) have become the most widely employed approach to classification due to their impressive learning capabilities (Hershey et al., 2017).

Examples of the "Learning Model"

Here we briefly describe the different learning models (see Figure 10.4) proposed for audio event detection and classification and acoustic scene classification.

Audio Event Detection and Classification

Classical methods (Mesaros, Heittola, Eronen, & Virtanen, 2010) include the usage of GMM, non-negative matrix factorization, and support vector machines. Recently, neural networks have replaced classical techniques. Convolutional neural networks trained on

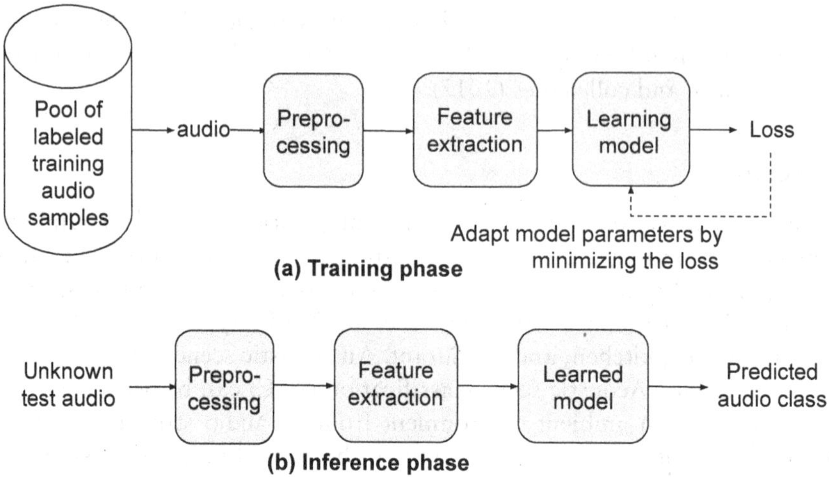

FIGURE 10.4. Typical machine learning pipeline for audio classification (audio event or acoustic scene).

~70 million YouTube recordings with "weak labels" (Hershey et al., 2017) set a new standard in this field. Another approach proposed models trained on weakly labeled audio, which can be transferred to other tasks (Kumar, Khadkevich, & Fugen, 2018).

Acoustic Scene Classification

There are two main approaches to learning a model for ASC (Stowell et al., 2015). The first one can be thought of as a "bag-of-frames" approach. It computes a long-term statistical distribution of low-level audio features, and tries to map it to the semantic label of the acoustic scenes. MFCC features were found to be effective in this approach. A classical bag-of-frames approach used GMMs for each class to model their distributions (Aucouturier, Defreville, & Pachet, 2007). Recently, convolutional networks were used to learn appropriate filters and the feature-to-class mapping during training (Hershey et al., 2017). Recurrent networks, effective in capturing context, have also been used for several sound event recognition tasks (Phan et al., 2017).

The second approach for ASC exploits the relationship between AED and ASC, based on the idea of an acoustic scene as a "dictionary of acoustic atoms." They generally try to learn intermediate representations (or atoms) that indicate a set of high-level features. The atoms generally represent audio events that constitute the final acoustic scene. Matching pursuits (Chu et al., 2009) is one such technique.

Egocentric Perspective

To investigate the effect of ambient sounds on physiological and psychological health, acoustic scenes and events a person experiences must be analyzed from their egocentric perspective. It is further useful if the person encounters dynamically evolving acoustic scenes. For example, nurses in a hospital might encounter diverse acoustic environments in their work shift, as they move from one location to another—for example, from nursing station to patient room, to lounge, and to medication center. Each one of these locales has unique acoustic characteristics. For example, nursing stations might have more human speech compared to the medication centers, and thus, they can represent different acoustic scenes. To continuously track acoustic scenes as the nurse moves, we need two important tools discussed so far in this chapter: (1) wearable sensing that can capture audio from the user's surroundings and (2) an algorithm that can predict the background acoustic scene at a particular point of time. Limited research efforts have been made in the egocentric domain. A recent work explored dynamically varying acoustic scenes that the staff, wearing TAR devices, encounter in a large critical care hospital (Jati et al., 2021). Significant correlations were found between different behavioral and psychological attributes of the employees and the dynamics of their movement between different acoustic scenes in the workplace.

Applications in Psychology

In this section, we discuss the role of human speech and ambient audio in psychology, and how the audio processing systems described in this chapter can be useful for psychologists.

Several acoustic measures have been associated with increased symptoms of clinical depression, using severity on the Hamilton Depression Rating Scale (HDRS) scale as a proxy. It was found that speaking rate and pitch variations were highly negatively correlated with HDRS scores (higher score ⇒ greater severity; Cannizzaro, Harel, Reilly, Chappell, & Snyder, 2004). Another study showed that pause time between utterances decreased as symptom severity decreased in patients (Yang, Fairbairn, & Cohn, 2012). Speaking rate has been shown to increase at the onset of Parkinson's disease, due to reduced articulator movement, at the cost of articulation clarity (Cannizzaro et al., 2004). However, later stages of the disease are characterized by reduced speech rates.

A study based on self-reported assessments showed that social well-being is closely associated with both the quantity and quality of interactions (Sun, Harris, & Vazire, 2019). Life satisfaction is also associated with the amount of alone time, conversation time, and substantive conversations (Milek et al., 2018). Additionally, personality traits have been associated with speech patterns (Tackman et al., 2020). Research has also characterized the psychologically meaningful aspects of nonverbal audio content. For example, acoustic characteristics could be used to distinguish between affiliative, reward-based, and dominant laughter (Wood, Martin, & Niedenthal, 2017).

Certain natural sounds tend to have positive effects on our mind, for example, in recovering from a stressful situation (Alvarsson, Wiens, & Nilsson, 2010). On the contrary, certain ambient sounds and noises can be harmful to our physiological and psychological health as well. For example, exposure to ambient noise was found to cause change in heart rate variability (Kraus et al., 2013), elicit annoyance (Clark & Stansfeld, 2007), disturb sleep patterns (Muzet, 2007; Stansfeld & Matheson, 2003), and even act as a stressor (Westman & Walters, 1981). The effect of noisy acoustic environments on job performance is well known and has been extensively studied. Depending on the subjective noise sensitivity, workplace sounds and noises can cause increased annoyance (Clark & Stansfeld, 2007) and decreased concentration (Banbury & Berry, 2005), which eventually leads to decreased productivity and job performance (Mak & Lui, 2012). This motivates the need to understand the type, intensity, and duration of exposure to different sounds and noises to analyze their effects on our physiological and psychological health.

Conducting studies like those we have described can be laborious and time consuming, and are usually only performed at a small scale, in terms of number of participants and number of days recorded. In the context of egocentric devices, state-of-the-art audio processing modules described in the prior sections can be used to reduce the processing time and largely automate the feature-extraction process. Foreground detection can be used to isolate the foreground speaker of interest, following which vocal prosodic features of interest can be extracted and analyzed as was done in the studies shown. In certain cases, it may be of interest to analyze speech from the participants' partner, or other social environments (such as friends and colleagues). In this case, a more complex speaker diarization system can be used to segregate speakers. Qualitative studies demand the need for content-based analysis. Nature of conversation, sentiment, and quality of interaction can be estimated from the text transcription, which is the product of an ASR system. Finally, ASC can be used to detect ambient scenes, which provide cues to a person's daily routines.

Conclusions and Future Directions

Mobile audio sensing is a relatively recent phenomenon that has been made possible due to recent advances in hardware infrastructure, software tools, as well as cutting-edge research in audio technology. In this chapter, we provide a window into the array of commonly used speech processing and ambient sensing techniques, and how they can be adapted to the egocentric setting. Several studies discussed in this chapter show the relevance of audio analysis to psychological health and monitoring, and how incorporating such tools into egocentric devices can help scale and automate the monitoring. The field of egocentric audio processing is still young and provides scope for several threads of research directions. While these are promising signs, it is important to keep in mind the challenges that such applications face, such as privacy, resource constraints and scalability hurdles in hardware.

REFERENCES

Alías, F., Socoró, J. C., & Sevillano, X. (2016). A review of physical and perceptual feature extraction techniques for speech, music and environmental sounds. *Applied Sciences, 6*(5), 143

Alvarsson, J. J., Wiens, S., & Nilsson, M. E. (2010). Stress recovery during exposure to natural sound and environmental noise. *International Journal of Environmental Research and Public Health, 7*(3), 1036–1046.

Aucouturier, J. J., Defreville, B., & Pachet, F. (2007). The bag-of-frames approach to audio pattern recognition: A sufficient model for urban soundscapes but not for polyphonic music. *Journal of Acoustical Society of America, 122*(2), 881–891.

Banbury, S. P., & Berry, D. C. (2005). Office noise and employee concentration: Identifying causes of disruption and potential improvements. *Ergonomics, 48*(1), 25–37.

Barchiesi, D., Giannoulis, D., Stowell, D., & Plumbley, M. D. (2015). Acoustic scene classification: Classifying environments from the sounds they produce. *IEEE Signal Processing Magazine, 32*(3), 16–34.

Benzeghiba, M., De Mori, R., Deroo, O., Dupont, S., Erbes, T., Jouvet, D., et al. (2007). Automatic speech recognition and speech variability: A review. *Speech Communication, 49*(10–11), 763–786.

Buschmann, C., & Pfisterer, D. (2007). isense: A modular hardware and software platform for wireless sensor networks. *6. Fachgespräch Sensornetzwerke*, 15.

Busso, C., Deng, Z., Yildirim, S., Bulut, M., Lee, C. M., Kazemzadeh, A., et al. (2004). Analysis of emotion recognition using facial expressions, speech and multimodal information. *Proceedings of the 6th International Conference on Multimodal Interfaces*, pp. 205–211.

Cai, R., Lu, L., Hanjalic, A., Zhang, H.-J., & Cai, L.-H. (2006). A flexible framework for key audio effects detection and auditory context inference. *IEEE Transactions on Audio, Speech, and Language Processing, 14*(3), 1026–1039.

Cannizzaro, M., Harel, B., Reilly, N., Chappell, P., & Snyder, P. J. (2004). Voice acoustical measurement of the severity of major depression. *Brain and Cognition, 56*(1), 30–35.

Chang, J.-H., Kim, N. S., & Mitra, S. K. (2006). Voice activity detection based on multiple statistical models. *IEEE Transactions on Signal Processing, 54*(6), 1965–1976.

Choudhury, T., Borriello, G., Consolvo, S., Haehnel, D., Harrison, B., Hemingway, B., et al. (2008). The mobile sensing platform: An embedded activity recognition system. *IEEE Pervasive Computing, 7*(2), 32–41.

Choudhury, T., & Pentland, A. (2003). Sensing and modeling human networks using the sociometer. *Proceedings of the Seventh IEEE International Symposium on Wearable Computers*, pp. 216–222.

Chu, S., Narayanan, S., & Kuo, C.-C. J. (2009). Environmental sound recognition with time frequency audio features. *IEEE Transactions on Audio, Speech, and Language Processing, 17*(6), 1142–1158.

Chung, J. S., Nagrani, A., & Zisserman, A. (2018). *Voxceleb2: Deep speaker recognition.* https://arxiv.org/abs/1806.05622v2

Clark, C., & Stansfeld, S. A. (2007). The effect of transportation noise on health and cognitive development: A review of recent evidence. *International Journal of Comparative Psychology, 20*(2), 145–158.

Dehak, N., Kenny, P. J., Dehak, R., Dumouchel, P., & Ouellet, P. (2010). Front-end factor analysis for speaker verification. *IEEE Transactions on Audio, Speech, and Language Processing, 19*(4), 788–798.

Eyben, F., Wöllmer, M., & Schuller, B. (2010). Opensmile: The Munich versatile and fast open-source audio feature extractor. *Proceedings of the 18th ACM International Conference on Multimedia*, pp. 1459–1462.

Feng, T., Nadarajan, A., Vaz, C., Booth, B., & Narayanan, S. (2018). Tiles audio recorder: An unobtrusive wearable solution to track audio activity. *Proceedings of the 4th ACM Workshop on Wearable Systems*, pp. 33–38.

Friedland, G., Vinyals, O., Huang, Y., & Muller, C. (2009). Prosodic and other long-term features for speaker diarization. *IEEE Transactions on Audio, Speech, and Language Processing, 17*(5), 985–993.

Gemmeke, J. F., Ellis, D. P., Freedman, D., Jansen, A., Lawrence, W., Moore, R. C., et al. (2017). Audio set: An ontology and human-labeled dataset for audio events. *2017 IEEE International Conference on Acoustics, Speech and Signal Processing (ICASSP)*, pp. 776– 780.

Goodfellow, I., Bengio, Y., & Courville, A. (2016). *Deep learning.* MIT press.

Graf, S., Herbig, T., Buck, M., & Schmidt, G. (2015). Features for voice activity detection: A comparative analysis. *EURASIP Journal on Advances in Signal Processing, 2015*(1), 91.

Hebbar, R., Papadopoulos, P., Reyes, R., Danvers, A. F., Polsinelli, A. J., Moseley, S. A., et al. (2021). Deep multiple instance learning for foreground speech localization in ambient audio from wearable devices. *EURASIP Journal on Audio, Speech, and Music Processing, 2021*(1), 1–8.

Hershey, S., Chaudhuri, S., Ellis, D. P., Gemmeke, J. F., Jansen, A., Moore, R. C., et al. (2017). CNN architectures for large-scale audio classification. *2017 IEEE International Conference on Acoustics, Speech and Signal Processing (ICASSP)*, pp. 131–135.

Hughes, T., & Mierle, K. (2013). Recurrent neural networks for voice activity detection. *2013 IEEE International Conference on Acoustics, Speech and Signal Processing*, pp. 7378–7382.

Itu-t Recommendation Database. (n.d.). https://

www.itu.int/ITU-T/recommendations/rec.aspx?rec=4415&lang=en.

Jati, A., Nadarajan, A., Peri, R., Mundnich, K., Feng, T., Girault, B., et al. (2021). Temporal dynamics of workplace acoustic scenes: Egocentric analysis and prediction. *IEEE/ACM Transactions on Audio, Speech, and Language Processing, 29*, 756–769.

Jiang, L., Gao, B., Gu, J., Chen, Y., Gao, Z., Ma, X., et al. (2018). Wearable long-term social sensing for mental wellbeing. *IEEE Sensors Journal, 19*(19), 8532–8542.

Junqua, J. C., & Haton, J. P. (2012). *Robustness in automatic speech recognition: Fundamentals and applications* (Vol. 341). Springer Science & Business Media.

Kim, C., Gowda, D., Lee, D., Kim, J., Kumar, A., Kim, S., et al. (2020). *A review of on-device fully neural end-to-end automatic speech recognition algorithms*. https://arxiv.org/abs/2012.07974

Kraus, U., Schneider, A., Breitner, S., Hampel, R., Ruckel, R., Pitz, M., et al. (2013). Individual daytime noise exposure during routine activities and heart rate variability in adults: a repeated measures study. *Environmental Health Perspectives, 121*(5), 607–612.

Kumar, A., Khadkevich, M., & Fugen, C. (2018). Knowledge transfer from weakly labeled audio using convolutional neural networks for sound events and scenes. *2018 IEEE International Conference on Acoustics, Speech and Signal Processing (ICASSP)*, pp. 326–330.

Kwon, S., & Narayanan, S. (2003a). *A method for on-line speaker indexing using generic reference models*. Eighth European Conference on Speech Communication and Technology.

Kwon, S., & Narayanan, S. (2003b). A study of generic models for unsupervised on-line speaker indexing. *2003 IEEE Workshop on Automatic Speech Recognition and Understanding*, pp. 423– 428.

Kwon, S., & Narayanan, S. (2005). Unsupervised speaker indexing using generic models. *IEEE Transactions on Speech and Audio Processing, 13*(5), 1004–1013.

Langheinrich, M. (2001). Privacy by design—principles of privacy-aware ubiquitous systems. *International Conference on Ubiquitous Computing*, pp. 273–291.

Lezzoum, N., Gagnon, G., & Voix, J. (2014). Voice activity detection system for smart earphones. *IEEE Transactions on Consumer Electronics, 60*(4), 737–744.

Lu, H., Pan, W., Lane, N. D., Choudhury, T., & Campbell, A. T. (2009). Soundsense: Scalable sound sensing for people-centric applications on mobile phones. *Proceedings of the 7th International Conference on Mobile Systems, Applications, and Services*, pp. 165–178.

Lu, L., & Zhang, H.-J. (2002). Speaker change detection and tracking in real-time news broadcasting analysis. *Proceedings of the Tenth ACM International Conference on Multimedia*, pp. 602–610.

Luo, L., Cao, Q., Huang, C., Abdelzaher, T., Stankovic, J. A., & Ward, M. (2007). Enviromic: Towards cooperative storage and retrieval in audio sensor networks. *27th International Conference on Distributed Computing Systems (ICDCS'07)*, pp. 34–34.

Mak, C. M., & Lui, Y. (2012). The effect of sound on office productivity. *Building Services Engineering Research and Technology, 33*(3), 339–345.

Mehl, M. R., Pennebaker, J. W., Crow, D. M., Dabbs, J., & Price, J. H. (2001). The electronically activated recorder (ear): A device for sampling naturalistic daily activities and conversations. *Behavior Research Methods, Instruments, and Computers, 33*(4), 517–523.

Mesaros, A., Heittola, T., Benetos, E., Foster, P., Lagrange, M., Virtanen, T., et al. (2017). Detection and classification of acoustic scenes and events: Outcome of the dcase 2016 challenge. *IEEE/ACM Transactions on Audio, Speech, and Language Processing, 26*(2), 379–393.

Mesaros, A., Heittola, T., Eronen, A., & Virtanen, T. (2010). Acoustic event detection in real life recordings. *2010 18th European Signal Processing Conference*, pp. 1267–1271.

Milek, A., Butler, E. A., Tackman, A. M., Kaplan, D. M., Raison, C. L., Sbarra, D. A. et al. (2018). "Eavesdropping on happiness" Revisited: A pooled, multisample replication of the association between life satisfaction and observed daily conversation quantity and quality. *Psychological Science, 29*(9), 1451–1462.

Muzet, A. (2007). Environmental noise, sleep and health. *Sleep Medicine Reviews, 11*(2), 135–142.

Nadarajan, A., Somandepalli, K., & Narayanan,

S. S. (2019). Speaker agnostic foreground speech detection from audio recordings in workplace settings from wearable recorders. *ICASSP 2019–2019 IEEE International Conference on Acoustics, Speech and Signal Processing (ICASSP)*, pp. 6765–6769.

Narayanan, S., & Georgiou, P. G. (2013). Behavioral signal processing: Deriving human behavioral informatics from speech and language. *Proceedings of the IEEE, 101*(5), 1203–1233.

Pantic, M., Pentland, A., Nijholt, A., & Huang, T. S. (2006). Human computing and machine understanding of human behavior: A survey. *Proceedings of the 8th International Conference on Multimodal Interfaces (ICMI)*, pp. 239–248.

Park, T. J., Kanda, N., Dimitriadis, D., Han, K. J., Watanabe, S., & Narayanan, S. (2021). *A review of speaker diarization: Recent advances with deep learning.* https://arxiv.org/abs/2101.09624

Phan, H., Koch, P., Katzberg, F., Maass, M., Mazur, R., & Mertins, A. (2017). *Audio scene classification with deep recurrent neural networks.* https://arxiv.org/abs/1703.04770

Povey, D., Ghoshal, A., Boulianne, G., Burget, L., Glembek, O., Goel, N., et al. (2011). *The kaldi speech recognition toolkit.* IEEE 2011 Workshop on Automatic Speech Recognition and Understanding.

Prabhu, K. M. (2014). *Window functions and their applications in signal processing.* Taylor & Francis.

Rachuri, K. K., Musolesi, M., Mascolo, C., Rentfrow, P. J., Longworth, C., & Aucinas, A. (2010). Emotionsense: A mobile phones based adaptive platform for experimental social psychology research. *Proceedings of the 12th ACM International Conference on Ubiquitous Computing*, pp. 281–290.

Ramirez, J., Górriz, J. M., & Segura, J. C. (2007). Voice activity detection. fundamentals and speech recognition system robustness. *Robust Speech Recognition and Understanding, 6*(9), 1–22.

Ramirez, J., Segura, J. C., Benıtez, C., De La Torre, A., & Rubio, A. (2004). Efficient voice activity detection algorithms using long-term speech information. *Speech Communication, 42*(3–4), 271–287.

Renevey, P., & Drygajlo, A. (2001). *Entropy based voice activity detection in very noisy conditions.* Seventh European Conference on Speech Communication and Technology.

Ryant, N., Church, K., Cieri, C., Cristia, A., Du, J., Ganapathy, S., et al. (2019). *The second DIHARD diarization challenge: Dataset, task, and baselines.* https://arxiv.org/abs/1906.07839

Sahidullah, M., & Saha, G. (2012). *Comparison of speech activity detection techniques for speaker recognition.* https://arxiv.org/abs/1210.0297.

Sashima, A., & Kawamoto, M. (2019). Towards sensing and sharing auditory context information using wearable devices. *Joint European Conference on Machine Learning and Knowledge Discovery in Databases*, pp. 54–59.

Sehgal, A., & Kehtarnavaz, N. (2018). A convolutional neural network smartphone app for real-time voice activity detection. *IEEE Access, 6*, 9017–9026.

Sell, G., & Garcia-Romero, D. (2014). Speaker diarization with PLDA i-vector scoring and unsupervised calibration. *2014 IEEE Spoken Language Technology Workshop (SLT)*, pp. 413–417.

Snyder, D., Garcia-Romero, D., Sell, G., Povey, D., & Khudanpur, S. (2018). X-vectors: Robust dnn embeddings for speaker recognition. *2018 IEEE International Conference on Acoustics, Speech and Signal Processing (ICASSP)*, pp. 5329–5333.

Sohn, J., Kim, N. S., & Sung, W. (1999). A statistical model-based voice activity detection. *IEEE Signal Processing Letters, 6*(1), 1–3.

Stansfeld, S. A., & Matheson, M. P. (2003). Noise pollution: non-auditory effects on health. *British Medical Bulletin, 68*(1), 243–257.

Stork, J. A., Spinello, L., Silva, J., & Arras, K. O. (2012). Audio-based human activity recognition using non-Markovian ensemble voting. *2012 IEEE RO-MAN: The 21st IEEE International Symposium on Robot and Human Interactive Communication*, pp. 509–514.

Stowell, D., Giannoulis, D., Benetos, E., Lagrange, M., & Plumbley, M. D. (2015). Detection and classification of acoustic scenes and events. *IEEE Transactions on Multimedia, 17*(10), 1733–1746.

Sun, J., Harris, K., & Vazire, S. (2019). Is well-being associated with the quantity and quality of social interactions? *Journal of Personality and Social Psychology, 119*(6), 1478.

Swain, M., Routray, A., & Kabisatpathy, P. (2018). Databases, features and classifiers for speech emotion recognition: A review. *International Journal of Speech Technology, 21*(1), 93–120.

Tackman, A. M., Baranski, E. N., Danvers, A. F., Sbarra, D. A., Raison, C. L., Moseley, S. A., et al. (2020). 'Personality in its natural habitat revisited: A pooled, multi-sample examination of the relationships between the big five personality traits and daily behaviour and language use. *European Journal of Personality, 34*(5), 753–776.

Wan, L., Wang, Q., Papir, A., & Moreno, I. L. (2018). Generalized end-to end loss for speaker verification. *2018 IEEE International Conference on Acoustics, Speech and Signal Processing (ICASSP)*, pp. 4879–4883.

Wang, R., Chen, F., Chen, Z., Li, T., Harari, G., Tignor, S., et al. (2014). Studentlife: assessing mental health, academic performance and behavioral trends of college students using smartphones. *Proceedings of the 2014 ACM International Joint Conference on Pervasive and Ubiquitous Computing*, pp. 3–14.

Wang, Y., Krishnamachari, B., & Annavaram, M. (2012). Semi-Markov state estimation and policy optimization for energy efficient mobile sensing. *2012 9th Annual Communications Society Conference on Sensor, Mesh and Ad Hoc Communications and Networks (SECON)*, pp. 533–541.

Wang, Y., Krishnamachari, B., Zhao, Q., & Annavaram, M. (2010). Markov optimal sensing policy for user state estimation in mobile devices. *Proceedings of the 9th ACM/IEEE International Conference on Information Processing in Sensor Networks*, pp. 268–278.

Westman, J. C., & Walters, J. R. (1981). Noise and stress: a comprehensive approach. *Environmental Health Perspectives, 41*, 291–309.

Wood, A., Martin, J., & Niedenthal, P. (2017). Towards a social functional account of laughter: Acoustic features convey reward, affiliation, and dominance. *PloS One, 12*(8), e0183811.

Yang, S., Gao, B., Jiang, L., Jin, J., Gao, Z., Ma, X., et al. (2018). IoT structured long-term wearable social sensing for mental wellbeing. *IEEE Internet of Things Journal*, 6(2), 3652–3662.

Yang, Y., Fairbairn, C., & Cohn, J. F. (2012). Detecting depression severity from vocal prosody. *IEEE Transactions on Affective Computing, 4* (2), 142–150.

Yu, D., & Deng, L. (2016). *Automatic speech recognition*. Springer.

Zhang, A., Wang, Q., Zhu, Z., Paisley, J., & Wang, C. (2019). Fully supervised speaker diarization. *ICASSP 2019–2019 IEEE International Conference on Acoustics, Speech and Signal Processing (ICASSP*), pp. 6301–6305.

CHAPTER 11

Acquisition and Analysis of Camera Sensor Data (Lifelogging)

Edison Thomaz and Mariella Dimiccoli

CHAPTER OVERVIEW

In this chapter, we discuss wearable imaging in the context of human lifestyle and behavior sensing. We consider imaging as both context information to derive labels for other sensor data and as a measure of daily situations to study people's lives. We begin with a brief historical perspective and discuss how the capture of everyday situations and activities can be used as an alternative to direct observation in field studies; our focus is on the acquisition of ground-truth labels to train activity recognition systems. Next, we describe the practical challenges associated with wearable cameras, such as placement and positioning, and we contrast these challenges against those of other popular sensing modalities. Several lifelogging application scenarios are presented, including event segmentation, localization, dietary monitoring, action recognition, and social interaction analysis. The chapter concludes with lifelogging privacy considerations, future opportunities, and best practices and recommendations for how to best leverage wearable cameras in research.

Introduction

Over the last two decades, advances in camera technologies and computer vision algorithms have greatly expanded the role of wearable imaging in mobile sensing. Hardware advances are largely attributed to the skyrocketing adoption of the smartphone in the last 10 years, which has been driving innovations in mobile technologies at a fast pace. Because camera performance has become increasingly important to smartphone users, today's high-end handsets contain not one but multiple specialized cameras (e.g., wide, ultra-wide, telephoto). Consequently, small, lightweight, powerful camera systems designed for mobile phones have become widely available and have made their way into embedded devices and wearable computing platforms. On the software side, deep-learning algorithms and the increasing computing capability of today's systems has fueled breakthroughs in computer vision. These developments have contributed to new performance heights in tasks such as object detection, motion tracking, action recognition, pose estimation, and semantic segmentation. This chapter focuses on wearable imaging and how these developments have created new opportunities in mobile lifelogging. We consider imaging as both context information to derive labels for other sensor data and as a measure of daily situations to study people's lives.

Personal Capture of Everyday Situations and Activities

Fundamentally, wearable imaging involves capturing photos and videos with an outward-facing camera mounted on the body. Early work in wearable imaging, which is also referred to as *egocentric vision*, stretches back more than two decades, with pioneering work in human-centered wearable computing by Mann (1997) and Starner (1999).

Years later, and inspired by early visions of pervasive life capture (Bush, 1945), research in the field gave rise to lifelogging, the practice of recording one's own everyday situations and activities through the lens of digital technologies. While the granularity of capture and the digital tools employed in lifelogging vary, the richness in detail and unique perspective afforded by wearable cameras made these devices popular with early lifeloggers. Designed to be worn around the neck on a lanyard, the SenseCam enabled early work in visual lifelogging (Gemmell, Bell, Lueder, Drucker, & Wong, 2002; Hodges et al., 2006). In addition to having a camera capable of passively capturing a photograph every 20 seconds, it also contained motion, temperature, light, and passive infrared sensors. SenseCam proved useful in health research, validating the use of egocentric imaging for many applications such as rehabilitation of individuals with cognitive impairment and brain injuries (Hodges, Berry, & Wood, 2011), diet behavior monitoring (Castro et al., 2015; Hossain, Imtiaz, Ghosh, Bhaskar, & Sazonov, 2020; Thomaz, Parnami, Essa, & Abowd, 2013), and physical activity tracking (Ekelund et al., 2020). While the SenseCam was created exclusively as a research tool and is no longer supported, it inspired many commercial products focused on mobile situations and activity capture such as the GoPro camera and movisensXS.[1]

Lifelogging Camera Recordings as an Interpretable Proxy for Direct Observation

Mobile sensing is motivated by the opportunity to leverage sensors in smartphones and wearable devices to make inferences about people in their lives; people's physiological health, emotional state, social interactions, daily activities, the environment in which they live, and much more. To translate low-level sensor data (e.g., accelerometer data, sounds) into high-level predictions about complex behaviors such as dancing, supervised machine learning methods are typically used, and *annotated examples* must be obtained as part of model training. An annotated example consists of the raw sensor data collected during a target activity and a label that uniquely describes the activity (e.g., cooking, writing).

In laboratory experiments, where participants perform tasks while being continuously monitored by researchers, it is often possible to acquire sensor data and annotate it accurately. Annotation labels are often created by the researchers themselves upon reviewing recorded videos of the activities. However, in real-world and free-living settings, when individuals perform activities in a naturalistic way, often spontaneously and unobserved, obtaining labels is a significant challenge. As noted by Bao and Intille (2004), the most realistic training and test data for mobile sensing is real-world data acquired from subjects as they go about their day, performing their everyday tasks.

Traditionally, three approaches have been utilized to address the challenges of data annotation: direct observation, retrospective self-report of activities, and self-reports obtained through experience sampling method (Larson & Csikszentmihalyi, 2014). Direct observation requires a researcher to monitor individuals throughout the day; it is highly intrusive in natural environments, does not scale well to large numbers of participants, and can be costly. Crucially, it is not a good fit for activities and situations that are inherently private such as personal grooming and bathroom activities. With self-report surveys, individuals fill out a form indicating what they did and when after events occurred. This method addresses the key limitations of direct observation, but it also suffers from important shortcomings. Most critically, retrospective self-report instruments are prone to recall errors and biases (Napa Scollon, Prieto, & Diener, 2009) and do not offer the temporal precision required to be accurately associated with the underlying sensor data. Lastly, self-reports obtained through the experience sampling method (ESM) deliver prompts to individuals throughout the day, requiring them to input what they are doing *in situ*. While recall errors are eliminated with this approach, biases can still influence what is ultimately reported. Additionally, ESM is usually highly burdensome and disruptive since they force individuals to constantly interrupt their activities. Consequently, experience sampling compliance tends to drop over time as individuals get fatigued and progressively ignore prompts. Despite these factors, ESM has been extensively adopted, and various platforms have been implemented in support of experience sampling in the Ubicomp community (Froehlich, Chen, Consolvo, Harrison, & Landay, 2007; Xiong, Huang, Barnes, & Gerber, 2016).

Recently, the availability of wearable imaging has opened up new possibilities in data annotation. Wearable cameras that were originally designed to capture everyday situations and activities have been successfully appropriated for data labeling. The same richness in detail that made wearable cameras appealing to lifeloggers also proved to be highly useful in data annotation. While methodological limitations and weaknesses remain, a wearable camera recording egocentric photos and videos on a regular basis is effectively a proxied version of a scalable, less intrusive, and more private form of direct observation.

High Data Volume: The Need for Segmentation and Summarization

Whether to capture personal situations and activities or to support annotation for human behavior analysis, one of the most significant challenges in passive wearable imaging is handling large amounts of rich visual data. A system designed to capture photos every 30 seconds can generate over 2,000 images per day, or approximately 700,000 images every year. This magnitude of data demands efficient methods for summarization with minimum semantic loss. Systems designed for data aggregation and basic visualization have been implemented (Thomaz, 2020), but deeper transformations of long, untrimmed, and continuous egocentric streams into meaningful temporal segments are critical. These segments share semantic attributes such as backgrounds and sounds characterizing the same event. Semantic attributes are typically modeled by appearance-based features, such as objects, scenes, and people.

Because of the limited amount of annotated data for this task, temporal segmentation cannot be efficiently addressed by using supervised learning. Recently, Dias and Dimiccoli (2018) proposed a neural network-based model and a long short-term memory network (LSTM)-based model performing a self-supervised pretext task consisting of predicting the concept vectors of temporal neighbor frames, given the concept vector of the current frame. For example, since one frame contains concepts such as *dishes, glasses, knife*, and *tap*, the pretext task is to guess what concepts are present in temporally neighboring frames, that is, in a time interval before and just after the given frame. The ground truth for this pretext task can be obtained without manual annotations by just applying an object detector (or whatever feature extractor) to each frame. As a by-product of this pretext task, the model will modify feature frames to make them more similar to those of frames having the same temporal context, and therefore likely to belong to the same event. In this way, the single-image sequence itself is used to learn new features, without need for an annotated training dataset. This approach has shown interesting results and has been revisited (Garcia del Molino, Lim, & Tan, 2018). More recently, Dimiccoli and Wendt (2020) proposed a joint feature learning and clustering approach that learns a low-dimensional representation that reflects a temporal and semantic structure of events. Once the image sequence (e.g., over 2 hours) has been partitioned into semantically homogeneous segments (e.g., five episodes), a visual summary is typically obtained by extracting one or more key frames for each segment.

Automated Recognition of Human Activities and Context

Over the last decade, advances in machine learning and computer vision algorithms have amplified the capabilities of wearable imaging. While first-person photos were only used as a basis for data annotation in the past, they can now take the place of other forms of sensor data as input into classifiers of human behaviors and context. In particular, the rapid development of supervised deep-learning-based approaches in recent years has made it possible to partially cope with the technical challenges imposed by wearable devices by leveraging large training datasets. The first and most characteristic challenge for activity recognition from egocentric visual data is that only the camera wearer's hands are sometimes visible throughout the images, and hence the recognition methods can rely only on scene context such as manipulated objects, other people, and the environment. Much of the research on first-person action recognition from videos has been focused on exploiting different egocentric features: the camera wearer's visible hands (Cartas, Dimiccoli, & Radeva, 2017a), the objects with which the wearer interacts (McCandless & Grauman, 2013), head motion (also called ego-motion; Poleg, Arora, & Peleg, 2014), gaze (Li, Liu, & Rehg, 2018) and, their temporal structure (Cartas, Radeva, & Dimiccoli,

2021), or a combination of them (Cartas, Luque, Radeva, Segura, & Dimiccoli, 2019). A deeper overview of these methods and their applicability to real-world scenarios can be found in Dimiccoli, Cartas, and Radeva (2019). This section provides more details on activity recognition from visual lifelogging that is captured by lifelog cameras over a long period of time (from one to several weeks), since they are more suited to daily activity monitoring and lifestyle characterization.

Early approaches to daily activity monitoring via wearable photo cameras have focused on a single user or a few users and have leveraged contextual information to deal with the ambiguity of pictorial information. In particular, focusing on a single user, Castro and colleagues (2015) exploited the fact that typically the same activity takes place in the same room or at the same time of the day, and they used color and time metadata in a random forest fusion strategy to improve activity classification obtained with a convolutional neural network (CNN). A generalization of this approach to multiple users has used the output of different layers of a CNN as contextual information (Cartas, Marín, Radeva, & Dimiccoli, 2017). While these approaches have modeled each image as independent of all the others, more recently long short-term memory network-based approaches have modeled the temporal coherence at the object/context level of temporally adjacent images to improve classification performance.

Since visual lifelogs are typically very long, Cartas, Dimicoli, and Radeva (2017b) proposed different training strategies for a CNN + LSTM architecture that use overlapping batches of consecutive frames instead of a single long sequence. Recently, all these algorithms have been tested on a new large-scale dataset, the ADLEgodataset (Cartas, Radeva, & Dimiccoli, 2020), acquired by 15 people wearing a Narrative Clip camera in an unconstrained setting. It includes 35 activities of daily life acquired during 12.7 days on average for each person, for a total of 191. For people seen during training, the CNN + LSTM trained in a sliding window fashion achieved 80.12% accuracy for the 35 activities. Conversely, for unseen people, best performance was achieved at 79.87% without previous event segmentation.

Given a new egocentric dataset representing activities of daily living, a recommended strategy for analysis would be to apply a standard action recognition algorithm such as those described by Cartas and colleagues (2017a), with a domain adaptation strategy by Cartas and associates (2020). Using a small amount of labeled data of this new dataset will ensure better predictions (Cartas et al., 2020).

Wearable Camera Placement and Orientation

An important consideration when using and deploying wearable cameras is determining where the camera should be placed on the body and what its orientation should be. Both of these parameters directly affect what can be captured and should be picked according to the envisioned application or data collection goal. Following SenseCam, which pioneered the use of wearable cameras in lifelogging, wearable cameras have been traditionally worn on the chest (see Figure 11.1). Facing directly forward, the camera records a frontal view of activities, capturing the wearer's hands, overall context, items in the environment, and objects manipulated. Head-mounted cameras produce images with these characteristics as well, but at eye level, which allows for a larger and more dynamic field-of-view since the camera follows head movements. However, both of these

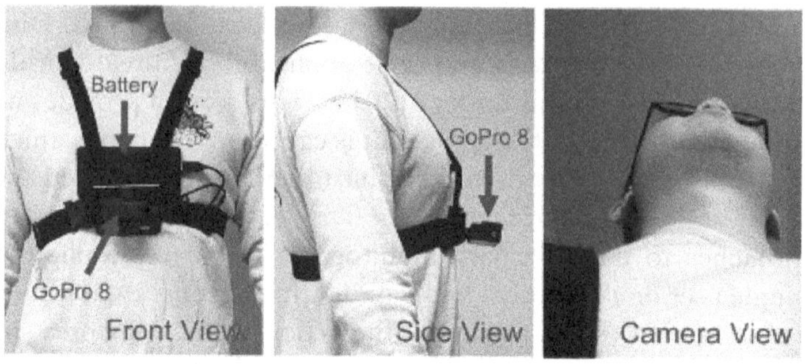

FIGURE 11.1. Setup showing a chest-mounted wearable camera pointing upwards.

camera positions pose privacy challenges and, since they can easily capture bystanders without their consent, we discuss the privacy considerations of wearable cameras in more detail in the "Mitigating Privacy Concerns" section. When chest-mounted cameras are pointed upward, these privacy concerns are minimized since the field of view includes the wearer's head and usually a ceiling as background. This orientation is useful to track personal health behaviors involving head or facial activities such as eating, drinking, and brushing teeth. On the other hand, the amount of contextual detail provided is limited since the camera does not capture the individual's surroundings.

A promising placement for wearable cameras is on the head but pointing downward instead of forward (see Figure 11.2). In this orientation, the privacy of bystanders is preserved, as is the case with the upward-facing chest camera, but with the advantage of capturing much more contextual information. The first to experiment with this camera position was Starner, Weaver, and Pentland (1998) more than two decades ago while implementing an American Sign Language (ASL) recognizer; a baseball cap-mounted camera captured video of the user's hands, which were tracked for gestures.

Researchers have explored other placements for wearable cameras as well. Alharbi and colleagues (2018) examined two alternative camera locations: shoulder and wrist. In

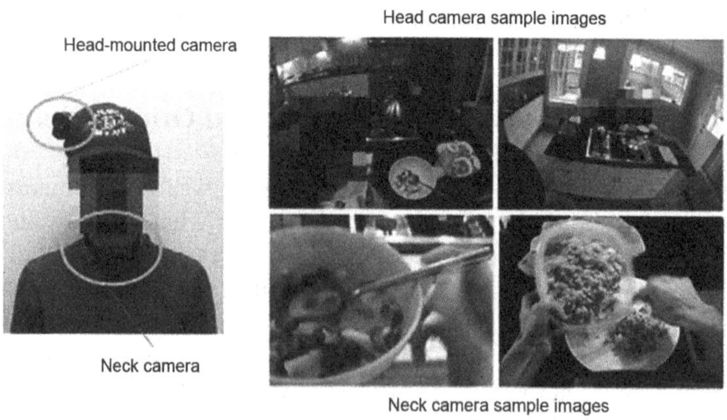

FIGURE 11.2. Camera placement and orientation provide different perspectives, with implications for the size of the field of view, what activities get captured, and privacy exposure.

a study with 24 participants, the shoulder camera was deemed very similar to the chest camera in terms of its visibility on the body, but it was less recognizable as a camera. Not surprisingly, the wrist camera was considered the least obtrusive and least noticeable of the options considered. Additionally, participants reported more control and flexibility on the recording functionality; one participant reported that it is easy to cover the camera when going to the bathroom, for example. On the other hand, due to motion artifacts, the quality of imaging recorded on the wrist is usually of lower quality than what is captured with a head or chest-mounted camera.

Health Applications

Situation and activity capture from a first-person perspective permits the objective recording and observation of activities in real-world settings that are highly relevant to health and clinical applications, such as dietary intake and sedentary behaviors (Doherty et al., 2013). Monitoring and quantifying lifestyle behaviors *in situ* is highly useful as it guides policy and serves as the starting point for interventions. In this section, we provide examples of how wearable imaging has been applied toward measuring activities of daily living, dietary behaviors, and social interactions.

Physical Activity and Sedentary Behaviors

Numerous studies have shown the link between health outcomes and physical activity. More recently, measures quantifying *lack of physical activity* have gained attention. Sedentary behaviors are extremely relevant even for individuals who might be considered active (Ekelund et al., 2020). However, sedentary behaviors and physical activities have been traditionally recorded using accelerometers, and they have relied on questionnaires for ground truth. However, as previously discussed, self-report methods are prone to errors, biases, and inaccuracies. Using a wearable camera as a proxy for direct observation, Kerr and colleagues (2013) compared sedentary behavior estimates between wearable imaging and accelerometry, showing a 30-minute per day difference between the two. In addition to being more temporally accurate, the wearable camera provided much greater insight into the sedentary activities themselves. More specifically, accelerometers are unable to identify detailed type and context behavioral information. Not surprisingly, TV watching is strongly correlated with sedentarism and obesity in adults and children. Zhang and Rehg (2018) used head-mounted wearable cameras to detect moments of screen-watching during daily life activities. In their work, they show that wearable cameras do not provide a measure of visual attention, but attention to screens can be reliably inferred by detecting and tracking the location of screens within the camera's field of view.

Automated Dietary Monitoring

Recording in a truly objective manner when, what, and how much individuals eat is one of the most challenging behavior-tracking problems health researchers face today. The variability in the types of food people eat and how they eat it make this effort particularly difficult. The ability to reveal what people consume in a visual way, whether at home or not, that is, without instrumenting the environment, has motivated researchers to explore wearable imaging for many years. For instance, Sun and colleagues (2015) developed a complete custom wearable system aimed at dietary monitoring a decade ago. But as previously discussed, one hurdle with passive sensing is that significant amounts of sensor data are typically collected and must be later reviewed for patterns of interest. With wearable imaging, this means examining thousands of images every day for every single person, which is an extremely large undertaking. Thomaz, Parnami, Bidwell, and colleagues (2013) investigated the feasibility of scaling the annotation task by outsourcing it to crowdworkers. In a study that included 17,575 egocentric images captured in real-world settings, detecting eating moments was possible with 89.68% accuracy. However, the recall measure was only 63.26%, underscoring the difficulty of spotting every eating moment.

Short eating episodes such as eating snacks on the go were particularly difficult to detect using a passive, time-lapsed photographic approach. To record such eating moments, the photo capture had to be perfectly timed with intake gestures, which can be sparse. An example of this scenario is shown in Figure 11.3; out of many first-person photos taken while the participant was driving to work, only one photo provided evidence that an eating event occurred. To make matters even more challenging, the lighting conditions when the photos were taken makes recognition of objects particularly difficult.

While determining *when* someone eats is important and a keystone to automated dietary monitoring, the central question that drives most researchers in the field is *what* a person consumes and *how much*.

Many efforts have been made to automatically recognize foods in photographs that have been manually, and thus explicitly, captured, such as Platemate (Noronha, Hysen, Zhang, & Gajos, 2011). However, fewer implementations have been studied from the context of lifelogging. Bettadapura, Thomaz, Parnami, Abowd, and Essa (2015) showed how to automatically determine food when eating in restaurants. In this work, they leveraged the location of where the picture was taken to infer the restaurant. With additional information about the restaurant obtained using online resources, coupled with state-of-the-art computer vision techniques, the researchers showed they could recognize the food being consumed. More recently, Fitbyte captures visuals of the food through instrumented eyeglasses as a person eats; the capture is triggered by motion sensors that detect food intake (Bedri, Li, Khurana, Bhuwalka, & Goel, 2020). Lastly, researchers have also

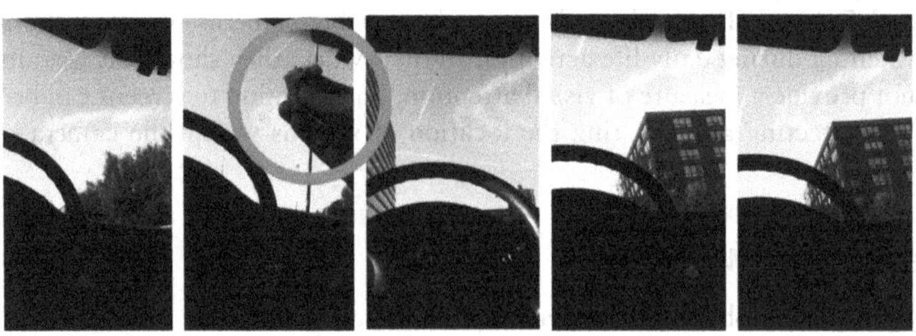

FIGURE 11.3. Consecutive first-person photos in which only one shows evidence of an eating activity, with the food circled. Short eating episodes such as eating snacks on the go can be difficult to detect using a time-lapsed wearable camera.

attempted to use egocentric imaging to estimate *how much* people eat, by capturing photos during the course of a meal (Liu et al., 2012).

Social Interactions Analysis

Social interactions are a fundamental and integral part of human life. It is well known that being *socially* connected promotes a person's overall and psychological *health* (Umberson & Karas Montez, 2010). Advances in sensing technology and wearable cameras have offered the opportunity to observe and objectively analyze human social interactions in a naturalistic setting and over a long period of time. However, detecting social interaction beyond the mere presence of other people, from an unconstrained stream of images, by relying solely on nonverbal features, is a challenging task.

Most prior work focused on detecting social interactions from egocentric images or photostreams (Aghaei, Dimiccoli, & Radeva, 2015, 2016b) have exploited the theory of F-formations proposed by Kendon (1976). When humans get involved in social interactions, they tend to stand in determined close positions to other interacting people to avoid occlusions, and they organize orientations in order to naturally place the focus on the subjects of interest. F-formation is hence defined as a geometric pattern that people instinctively tend to form when interacting. More specifically, the *o*-space within an F-formation is a convex empty space surrounded by the people involved in a social interaction, where every participant looks inward into it and no external people are allowed in this region (see Figure 11.4). A typical approach to detect such patterns from videos is to extract a bird's view model of the scene, where mutual distances between people and their head orientations are visualized as if the scene was recorded from the top, as shown in Figure 11.4.

Research based on this approach first localizes the appearance of each person in the scene along the video or photo-stream (see Figure 11.5). Afterward, head pose and 3D location for each person along the sequence are estimated to build the set of features for the analysis. To estimate the distance of each individual from the camera, typically a regression model that learns the depth relationships on a two-dimensional surface is trained. The analysis of temporal change in these features is crucial for detecting and understanding social interactions. Toward this goal, several strategies have been

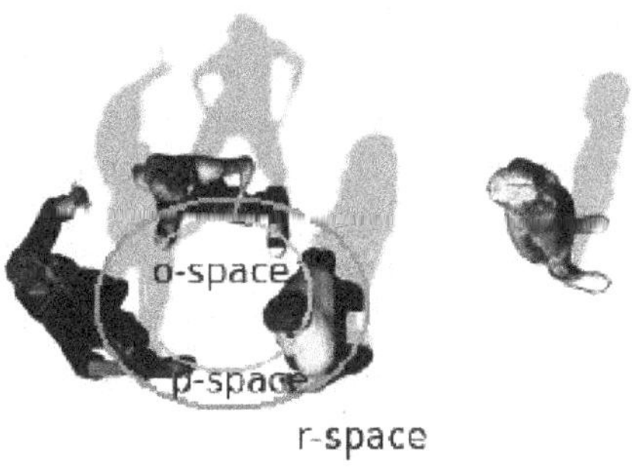

FIGURE 11.4. Example of F-formation, a geometrical pattern formed by interacting people. The o-space is shared by interacting people, the p-space is the space where interacting people stand, and people in the r-space are not interacting.

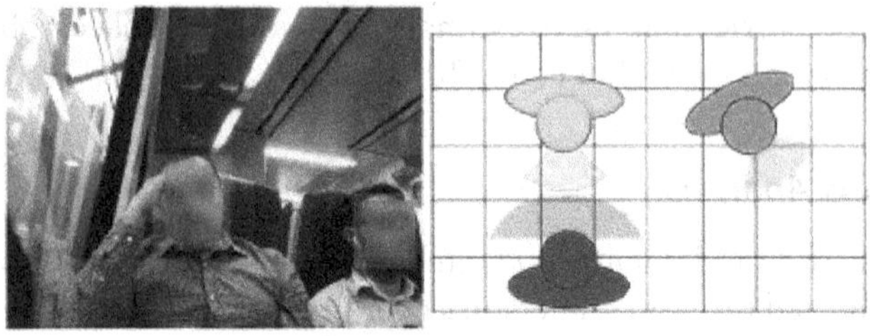

FIGURE 11.5. Example of a bird's view model extracted from an egocentric image. The bottom person on the right image corresponds to the camera wearer. Image from Aghaei et al. (2015).

proposed. While Aghaei and colleagues (2015) adopt a voting strategy, the more recent approach by Aghaei and colleagues (2016b) models F-formation detection as a binary classification problem (interacting/noninteracting). A sequence is represented by a multi-dimensional time series, where at each time step, a feature vector represents a frame, and the time series is classified using an LSTM (Aghaei et al., 2016b).

Only a few works have gone beyond the detection task in the egocentric domain (Aghaei, Dimiccoli, Ferrer, & Radeva, 2018; Aghaei, Dimiccoli, & Radeva, 2017; Aimar, Radeva, & Dimiccoli, 2019). Aghaei and colleagues (2018) introduced a pipeline for automatically characterizing the social patterns of a person from the analysis of egocentric photostreams of a user over a long period of time, and showed its effectiveness on a test user. To discover people with whom the camera wearer interacts more often, Aghaei and colleagues (2017) used a fully unsupervised approach for face clustering from egocentric photo-streams collected over a long period of time. Since a person's appearance may change drastically on different days or even at different times of the day, this problem is very challenging. To cope with the extreme intraclass variability of faces, first the appearance of multiple faces into a same event is tracked (Aghaei, Dimiccoli, & Radeva, 2016a), and then considering a set of constraints (for instance, faces in a same image correspond to different individuals), similar faces across the events are clustered into an unknown number of groups.

Aghaei and colleagues (2018) classifies social interactions into formal and informal meetings. A formal meeting is defined as a preplanned event where two or more people come together at a preplanned place at a particular time to discuss specific matters for the purposes of achieving a specific goal. Meanwhile, an informal meeting is more casual, requires less planning, and usually can take place at any casual space ranging from a park to a hall. Classification is achieved by leveraging several features, including global image features extracted from a pretrained CNN that characterize the surrounding environment, and facial expression (emotion) features.

The proposed pipeline was validated on a test set acquired by one user who wore the camera under free-living conditions over a 1-month period. It is worth noting that the test user did not participate in acquiring the training set used for training the model. An example of a social interaction temporal map that can be obtained using this approach is shown in Figure 11.6.

A more detailed classification of people's social life in visual lifelogs, based on Bugental's domain-based social theory (Bugental, 2000), has been recently proposed by Aimar and colleagues (2019). Bugental's theory includes specific domains with examples

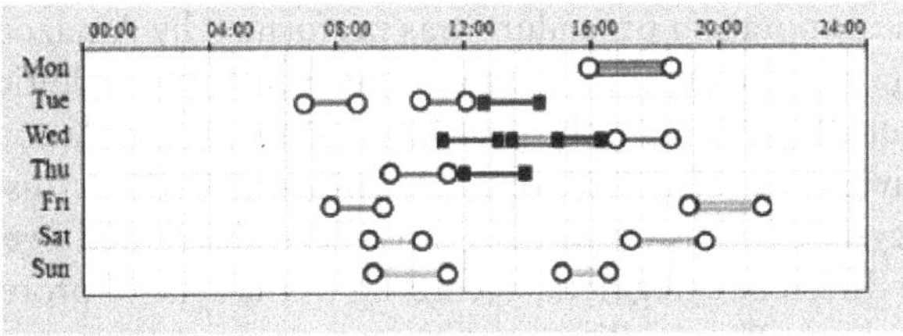

FIGURE 11.6. Example of social interaction temporal map of a user during 1 week. Different colors correspond to different people the user was interacting with. Multiple lines are indicative of a social interaction with multiple persons. Circles and squares indicate informal and formal meetings respectively. Image from Aghaei et al. (2018).

of common relations, characterized by specific attributes and behaviors. Specifically, it includes 5 domains (coalitional group, attachment, reciprocity, hierarchical power, mating) and 16 related subcategories.

A psychology study aimed at detecting social interactions from pictures collected by a wearable lifelogging camera should rely on Aghaei and colleagues (2016b). If instead the goal is to understand the type of social interactions, in Bugental's spirit, the individual is having, then Aimar and colleagues (2019) should be the reference work. For a more detailed characterization of the person's social style in terms of frequency, diversity, and duration, the work by Aghaei and associates (2018) proposes a complete pipeline.

Mitigating Privacy Concerns

As we have shown, photos and videos captured with wearable cameras can provide accurate depictions of an individual's activities and context *in situ*, enabling a large number of applications. However, this power and capability comes with a significant tradeoff: privacy concerns. Passive egocentric vision often records sensitive or undesirable information on the person wearing the camera, whether at home, at work, around family, or in public spaces. As a result, conducting human-subject studies that involve wearable imaging demands special attention. In particular, institutional review boards (IRBs) often impose strict requirements on the collection, manipulation, and annotation of egocentric photos and videos. Specific concerns include whether individuals can be identified in the photos and how they will be annotated, if necessary. For example, in the context of an automated dietary monitoring application, Thomaz and colleagues (2013) employed a two-stage review procedure to meet the demands of the IRB office at their institution and get approval to conduct their study. In the first step, all participants who wore the wearable camera were required to review all captured images and delete any photos they were not comfortable sharing with the research team. In the second phase, the researchers gained access to the photos and reviewed them for any other evidence that could pose a threat to participants. Additionally, researchers were required to discard any first-person photo that depicted an individual, whether fully or partially. As individuals went on about their day while wearing the camera (e.g., meeting friends, having meals, taking public transportation), it was common for the images to record other people, that is, bystanders, or the camera wearer (e.g., when facing a mirror). All of these photos had to be deleted. In this specific case, the annotation procedure was performed by Amazon Mechanical Turk workers, that is, nontrustworthy third parties, which called for additional precautionary steps to reduce or, ideally, eliminate the possibility of privacy violations.

To address privacy concerns in wearable imaging without discarding photos, a vast array of privacy-mitigating techniques have been developed over the years. These approaches fall into different categories, according to the type of protection they attempt to provide and for whom. Wearability permits unconstrained movement; therefore, it is valuable to have mechanisms that support capture in certain locations and not others. This was the impetus behind PlaceAvoider, which applies image analysis to identify and blacklist rooms where photos should not be taken (Templeman, Korayem, Crandall, & Kapadia, 2014). The approach required individuals to take photographs of sensitive areas such as bathrooms and bedrooms, which were then used to build visual models of these spaces. As researchers pointed out, this approach is complementary to GPS, which can locate the device within a geographical area but is not reliable enough indoors. Additionally, it does not require special instrumentation in every room such as beacons or custom-built imaging disablers (Hightower & Borriello, 2001; Truong, Patel, Summet, & Abowd, 2005).

Perhaps counterintuitively, even everyday situations and activities that might seem low-risk from a privacy standpoint can still pose acute threats to privacy. A particularly relevant scenario is the capture of computer and phone screens. For example, an office worker whose job involves performing tasks on a computer might have username, passwords, and sensitive documents revealed by egocentric photos. In fact, recent studies indicate that computer screens represent the most significant privacy concern for those wearing cameras since so much time is often spent in front of devices that display sensitive information (Hoyle et al., 2014). To address this concern, Korayem, Templeman, Chen, Crandall, and Kapadia (2016) explored how computer vision approaches could be used to automatically detect screens in egocentric photos. This proved challenging as object detection with first-person imaging requires examining photos that are often blurry and hard to interpret. Using CNNs and models pretrained with ImageNet (Krizhevsky, Sutskever, & Hinton, 2012), the researchers obtained around 90% accuracy in screen detection when testing with 1,842 first-person photos captured in naturalistic settings by 36 participants.

Beyond those wearing the camera, egocentric vision can also be highly concerning to others who might end up photographed or video-recorded. In other words, wearable imaging has the potential to greatly enhance the vulnerability of bystanders (Ferdous, Chowdhury, & Jose, 2017). Egocentric photos might catch bystanders in embarrassing situations or undesirable poses, or they may reveal information they would rather not have on record. Denning, Dehlawi, and Kohno (2014) examined how bystanders respond to the presence of augmented reality (AR) glasses with built-in cameras. In this work, the researchers wore a mock AR device in cafés around a city over the course of 12 field sessions and conducted semistructured interviews with 31 individuals on their reactions to the device. They found that bystanders assumed these devices were used for recording and "were predominantly split between having indifferent and negative reactions to the device." In a different study, lifeloggers stated that bystanders should be informed about lifelogging devices (Hoyle et al., 2014).

When it comes to protecting the privacy of bystanders in egocentric photos, the obvious approach is to employ face detection and simply delete photos that uniquely identify a person in front of the camera. This approach is suboptimal, however. Photos that pose privacy concerns might also contain evidence of behaviors or any other information relevant to a given relevant task. Representations such as the privacy-saliency matrix were developed to make this balance explicit (Thomaz, Parnami, Bidwell, Essa, & Abowd, 2013). Instead of deleting photos with faces, a common approach is to obfuscate them through selecting filtering (Vishwamitra, Knijnenburg, Hu, & Caine, 2017). Similarly, an interesting solution is to anonymize the photos instead of blurring or blocking them. Ren, Lee, and Ryoo (2018) showed promising results using generative adversarial networks (GANs). An *anonymizer* modifies the original video to remove privacy-sensitive information while attempting to maximize spatial action detection performance, and a *discriminator* extracts privacy-sensitive information from the anonymized videos.

Before faces can be blurred, blocked, or anonymized, they must first be *reliably* detected. Over the last decade, deep-learning algorithms have greatly improved the performance of computer vision tasks, enabling higher performance accuracies in object detection and identification (Krizhevsky et al., 2012), but further progress is needed for facial recognition. In particular, while face detection algorithms are very accurate today, they are not immune to false negatives in unconstrained environments (Masi, Wu, Hassner, & Natarajan, 2018). Even a single lapse in facial recognition could result in a considerable privacy threat. One way to avoid missing faces in first-person images is to blur the entire photo, regardless of whether it contains faces. This approach guarantees that if there are faces, they are not clearly visible and thereby do not pose a privacy concern. Additionally, any other piece of information in view that could be sensitive information (e.g., a bank account number) is also protected. The downside of this method is that all images are affected, which comes at the expense of lower inference accuracy. Examining a dataset of 84,078 egocentric images, Dimiccoli, Marín, and Thomaz (2018) studied the trade-off between image quality and inference performance. Their research demonstrated a statistically significant positive relationship between the amount of image degradation and participants' willingness to be captured by wearable cameras.

Future Outlook and Opportunities

As discussed in this chapter, wearable cameras have been successfully explored in numerous applications over the past two decades. During this time, much has changed in the technology landscape, and new opportunities have emerged. Camera systems have advanced significantly due in large part to the introduction and rapid adoption of smartphones and portable action cameras. The pace of smartphone development in particular has demanded increasingly more sophisticated imaging sensing hardware, driving down costs and making these components available to myriad devices such as indoor cameras and aerial drones. Compact and powerful image sensors, sometimes referred to as *imagers*, are now liberating wearable cameras from their traditional form factor (e.g., worn on a lanyard) to a much wider range of placements such as mounted on eyeglasses. Additionally, factors that previously limited the use of imagers are no longer as critical as they used to be. For example, power consumption has always been a concern with imaging systems, but recent imagers can capture grayscale images at 30 frames per second (FPS), using less than 1 mW.[2] Processing photo and video streams in real time is now also possible thanks to optimization in CNNs and the introduction of frameworks such as MobileNet, which offer competitive performance in computer vision tasks (Howard et al., 2017). Real-time inference of human activities under low-power conditions is a critical capability because it greatly enhances privacy protection. This feature eliminates the need for photos and videos to be saved and transferred to another device for analysis. Fully self-contained imagers that output inferences without providing access to the raw data, and thus mitigating privacy concerns, could become widely acceptable as sensors of human-centered activities.

Thanks to enhancements in power, computational inference, and onboard data processing, we foresee an increase in usage of imagers in the future. In the context of wearables, we expect the development of new lifelogging and behavior sensing systems that make use of multiple imagers, each capturing a different perspective depending on placement and orientation. This is important because existing wearable cameras are constrained in what they can capture by their single-lens field of view. A multi-imager system could embed all cameras into one device such as a smartwatch (Tong, Tailor, & Lane, 2020) or consist of several imagers that can be individually placed on different parts of the body as needed to suit a specific type of capture or application. New directions in imaging technology (e.g., 360-degree cameras) provide new alternatives for expanding the reach of lifelogging as well.

From a human-centered perspective, privacy and social discomfort have been important factors limiting wider adoption of passive wearable imaging technology. Most people are not comfortable in the presence of others who could be recording movements and behaviors passively; the sight of an exposed camera lens is often cause for concern. However, social media has greatly increased the prominence of photos and videos in popular culture and the public discourse. As a result, perceptions around camera-based devices, being captured on camera, and the utility and applications of photos in general are rapidly evolving. Cameras are all around us; police officers wear them as body cameras, doorbell cameras record us as we stroll by homes in our neighborhoods, and emerging camera-based augmented reality systems promise breakthrough new applications that will change the way we learn, work, and play. While we do not anticipate that individuals will be comfortable with wearable cameras in the short term, societal changes will likely increase acceptance of wearable imaging in the future.

Best Practices for Using Lifelogging in Research

Consider a scenario in which a psychologist is interested in exploring the extent to which people's social behaviors change depending on who they are with. As an example, an individual might be reserved and timid with family but highly extroverted with friends. Traditionally, researchers have had to depend on self-reported instruments such as surveys filled out by the study participants themselves to answer these types of research questions. However, these instruments are known to suffer from numerous limitations and biases. As discussed, lifelogging offers a rich and compelling alternative to capturing situations, settings, and individual behaviors in a passive and unbiased way. In this section, we provide practical guidance for how to employ lifelogging in a research study in key areas while taking into account considerations that have been discussed in this chapter.

Selecting a Device

The GoPro and other cameras similar to it have been extensively used in lifelogging research for many years. When meeting capture requirements, these cameras continue to be a reliable option. An alternative approach to using a traditional camera is to program a smartphone to record video and audio and have participants wear the phone on a lanyard around the neck. We have had success with this approach since it offers a large degree of flexibility; for example, capture intervals are not restricted to presets (e.g., recording a photo every 30 seconds and 60 seconds only), and additional data can be captured alongside video clips and photos (e.g., audio, inertial measurements from the device's sensors, location). Moreover, smartphones can be configured to process audio, videos and photos as they are captured in order to perform additional tasks (e.g., classify foreground versus background speech) or minimize privacy risks (e.g., blur faces that are captured in the first-person photos). Lastly, the communication capabilities of phones can also be useful, such as to log data capture metrics in a remote server and allow researchers to verify that data collection in the field is taking place as expected. We should note that despite the popularity of chest-mounted cameras, the use of head-mounted cameras has increased substantially in the last few years thanks to the availability of new devices such as the Vuzix Blade, Pupil Labs, ZShades, ORDRO EP6, iVue Rincon 1080, and Weeview. Looking forward, this trend will likely continue as augmented reality (AR) technologies mature. Devices such as Spectacles and Ray-Ban Stories, designed specifically for the consumer market, have the potential to become socially acceptable, which is an essential requirement for lifelogging systems aiming to capture natural behaviors.

Setting a Sampling Frequency

Determining how often to take a snapshot or record a video clip is usually one of the first steps when setting up and configuring a lifelogging system. Data collection frequency tends to be application specific, and collecting more data than necessary imposes an extra strain on battery power, a scarce resource in a mobile setting. It is often useful to conduct a pilot study to determine what the sampling frequency should be, with the goal of optimizing activity capture fidelity. In the event that power consumption is an issue, contextual triggers can be considered. With triggers, data capture is not continuous; instead, it is initiated only when a contextual criterion is met, such as when the individual is in a specific location, a certain amount of physical activity is detected, or an auditory signal is present (e.g., speech). Once a capture pipeline has been established, capturing data is straightforward and thousands of images or hours of videos can be easily recorded. However, the more data that are collected, the more effort and time must be allocated to annotation—and the higher the privacy risk that participants are exposed to.

Obtaining IRB Approval

The process of obtaining IRB approval to run a lifelogging study varies greatly depending on the institution and expertise of the IRB officers assigned to review the study protocol. Capturing audio, video, and photos in real time will understandably be cause for concern. To protect the privacy of bystanders, a basic first step is to clearly communicate that face detection algorithms will be applied to the data and identified faces will be blurred. However, face detection alone might not be enough. In one of our experiences, we were required to agree to eliminate photos that contained any body part based on the argument that any part of the body could uniquely identify an individual (e.g., a ring on a finger, a tattoo on a leg). The implications of this decision were significant; we could neither automate nor outsource this body part identification task and so we had to review all photos manually, greatly increasing our workload. Also, it forced us to discard many photos that contained evidence of activities and context that we were interested in. Other measures that have proved successful in demonstrating sensitivity to privacy concerns include (1) requiring participants to review their own photos and videos and delete any data they would rather not share with researchers, (2) instructing participants to temporarily remove the lifelogging device or turn it off in certain settings and events (e.g., bathroom, religious activity), and (3) processing data onboard the lifelogging device if at all possible, thus eliminating the need to save the photos and video after capture.

Lifelogging is usually associated with capture of photos and videos, but special attention must be dedicated to audio as well. For privacy protection, it is possible to apply filters to the data in order to make speech and other relevant sounds unintelligible to a human while preserving the underlying characteristics of the signal for machine analysis. Overall, given the nuances of these various techniques and potential for misinterpretation, we have found it productive and time-saving to review the procedures and methods of a lifelogging study with the IRB officer in person. Lastly, and beyond institutional approach, it is important to be aware of and follow regulations regarding privacy protection and security of communications. For example, in the United States, many states require that all parties consent to recordings. In these states, an individual who is lifelogging should let others in their vicinity know that a recording is taking place. In practice, this has been achieved by researchers having lifelogging study participants wear a badge communicating that a recording is in progress.

Visualizing, Annotating, and Processing Images and Videos

Researchers have often employed custom solutions to visualize, annotate, and analyze lifelogging data. It is not uncommon for companies that make wearable cameras to provide tools that can be used to retrieve and browse media captured by the cameras, but these packages do not include support for data annotation and processing. One of the difficulties of working with lifelogging data is that it might be combined with data from other sensors (e.g., smartwatch inertial measurements), and thus a data synchronization step is required. However, while not specialized for lifelogging, general-purpose tools for audio and video recordings exist. One of the most popular packages is ELAN, which has been successfully adapted to lifelogging data (Wittenburg, Brugman, Russel, Klassmann, & Sloetjes, 2006).

Notes

1. www.movisens.com/de/produkte/movisensxs
2. www.himax.com.tw.

REFERENCES

Aghaei, M., Dimiccoli, M., & Radeva, P. (2015, December). Towards social interaction detection in egocentric photo-streams. In *Eighth International Conference on Machine Vision (ICMV 2015)* (Vol. 9875, pp. 218–222). SPIE.

Aghaei, M., Dimiccoli, M., & Radeva, P. (2016a). Multi-face tracking by extended bag-of-tracklets in egocentric photo-streams. *Computer Vision and Image Understanding, 149*, 146–156.

Aghaei, M., Dimiccoli, M., & Radeva, P. (2016b, December). With whom do I interact?: Detecting social interactions in egocentric photo-streams. In *2016 23rd International Conference on Pattern Recognition (ICPR)* (pp. 2959–2964). IEEE.

Aghaei, M., Dimiccoli, M., & Radeva, P. (2017, September). All the people around me: Face discovery in egocentric photo-streams. In *2017 IEEE International Conference on Image Processing (ICIP)* (pp. 1342–1346). IEEE.

Aghaei, M., Dimiccoli, M., Ferrer, C. C., & Radeva, P. (2018). Towards social pattern characterization in egocentric photo-streams. *Computer Vision and Image Understanding, 171*, 104–117.

Aimar, E. S., Radeva, P., & Dimiccoli, M. (2019, September). Social relation recognition in egocentric photostreams. In *2019 IEEE International Conference on Image Processing (ICIP)* (pp. 3227–3231). IEEE.

Alharbi, R., Stump, T., Vafaie, N., Pfammatter, A., Spring, B., & Alshurafa, N. (2018). I can't be myself: Effects of wearable cameras on the capture of authentic behavior in the wild. *Proceedings of the ACM on Interactive, Mobile, Wearable and Ubiquitous Technologies, 2*(3), 1–40.

Bao, L., & Intille, S. S. (2004, April). Activity recognition from user-annotated acceleration data. In *International Conference on Pervasive Computing* (pp. 1–17). Springer.

Bedri, A., Li, D., Khurana, R., Bhuwalka, K., & Goel, M. (2020, April). Fitbyte: Automatic diet monitoring in unconstrained situations using multimodal sensing on eyeglasses. *Proceedings of the 2020 CHI Conference on Human Factors in Computing Systems*, pp. 1–12.

Bettadapura, V., Thomaz, E., Parnami, A., Abowd, G. D., & Essa, I. (2015, January). Leveraging context to support automated food recognition in restaurants. In *2015 IEEE Winter Conference on Applications of Computer Vision* (pp. 580–587). IEEE.

Bugental, D. B. (2000). Acquisition of the algorithms of social life: A domain-based approach. *Psychological Bulletin, 126*(2), 187.

Bush, V. (1945). As we may think. *Atlantic Monthly, 176*(1), 101–108.

Cartas, A., Dimiccoli, M., & Radeva, P. (2017a). Batch-based activity recognition from egocentric photo-streams. In *Proceedings of the IEEE International Conference on Computer Vision Workshops*, pp. 2347–2354.

Cartas, A., Dimiccoli, M., & Radeva, P. (2017b, February). Detecting hands in egocentric videos: Towards action recognition. In *International Conference on Computer Aided Systems Theory* (pp. 330–338). Springer.

Cartas, A., Luque, J., Radeva, P., Segura, C., & Dimiccoli, M. (2019). Seeing and hearing egocentric actions: How much can we learn? *Proceedings of the IEEE/CVF International Conference on Computer Vision Workshops.*

Cartas, A., Marín, J., Radeva, P., & Dimiccoli, M. (2017, June). Recognizing activities of daily living from egocentric images. In *Iberian Conference on Pattern Recognition and Image Analysis* (pp. 87–95). Springer.

Cartas, A., Radeva, P., & Dimiccoli, M. (2020). Activities of daily living monitoring via a wearable camera: Toward real-world applications. *IEEE Access, 8*, 77344–77363.

Cartas, A., Radeva, P., & Dimiccoli, M. (2021, January). Modeling long-term interactions to enhance action recognition. In *2020 25th International Conference on Pattern Recognition (ICPR)* (pp. 10351–10358). IEEE.

Castro, D., Hickson, S., Bettadapura, V., Thomaz, E., Abowd, G., Christensen, H., et al. (2015, September). Predicting daily activities from egocentric images using deep learning. *Proceedings of the 2015 ACM International Symposium on Wearable Computers*, pp. 75–82.

Denning, T., Dehlawi, Z., & Kohno, T. (2014, April). In situ with bystanders of augmented reality glasses: Perspectives on recording and privacy-mediating technologies. *Proceedings of the SIGCHI Conference on Human Factors in Computing Systems*, pp. 2377–2386.

Dias, C., & Dimiccoli, M. (2018). Learning event representations by encoding the temporal context. *Proceedings of the European Conference on Computer Vision (ECCV) Workshops.*

Dimiccoli, M., Bolanos, M., Talavera, E., Aghaei, M., Nikolov, S. G., & Radeva, P. (2017). Sr-clustering: Semantic regularized clustering for egocentric photo streams segmentation. *Computer Vision and Image Understanding, 155*, 55–69.

Dimiccoli, M., Cartas, A., & Radeva, P. (2019). Activity recognition from visual lifelogs: State of the art and future challenges. In X. Alameda-Pineda, E. Ricci, & N. Sebe (Eds.), *Multimodal behavior analysis in the wild* (pp. 121–134). Elsevier.

Dimiccoli, M., Marín, J., & Thomaz, E. (2018). Mitigating bystander privacy concerns in egocentric activity recognition with deep learning and intentional image degradation. *Proceedings of the ACM on Interactive, Mobile, Wearable and Ubiquitous Technologies, 1*(4), 1–18.

Dimiccoli, M., & Wendt, H. (2020). Learning event representations for temporal segmentation of image sequences by dynamic graph embedding. *IEEE Transactions on Image Processing, 30*, 1476–1486.

Doherty, A. R., Hodges, S. E., King, A. C., Smeaton, A. F., Berry, E., Moulin, C. J., et al. (2013). Wearable cameras in health: The state of the art and future possibilities. *American Journal of Preventive Medicine, 44*(3), 320–323.

Ekelund, U., Tarp, J., Fagerland, M. W., Johannessen, J. S., Hansen, B. H., Jefferis, B. J., et al. (2020). Joint associations of accelero-meter measured physical activity and sedentary time with all-cause mortality: A harmonised meta-analysis in more than 44 000 middle-aged and older individuals. *British Journal of Sports Medicine, 54*(24), 1499–1506.

Ferdous, M. S., Chowdhury, S., & Jose, J. M. (2017). Analysing privacy in visual lifelogging. *Pervasive and Mobile Computing, 40*, 430–449.

Froehlich, J., Chen, M. Y., Consolvo, S., Harrison, B., & Landay, J. A. (2007, June). MyExperience: A system for *in situ* tracing and capturing of user feedback on mobile phones. *Proceedings of the 5th International Conference on Mobile Systems, Applications and Services*, pp. 57–70.

Garcia del Molino, A., Lim, J. H., & Tan, A. H. (2018, October). Predicting visual context for unsupervised event segmentation in continuous photo-streams. *Proceedings of the 26th ACM International Conference on Multimedia*, pp. 10–17.

Gemmell, J., Bell, G., Lueder, R., Drucker, S., & Wong, C. (2002, December). MyLifeBits: fulfilling the Memex vision. *Proceedings of the Tenth ACM International Conference on Multimedia*, pp. 235–238.

Hightower, J., & Borriello, G. (2001). Location systems for ubiquitous computing. *Computer, 34*(8), 57–66.

Hodges, S., Berry, E., & Wood, K. (2011). SenseCam: A wearable camera that stimulates and rehabilitates autobiographical memory. *Memory, 19*(7), 685–696.

Hodges, S., Williams, L., Berry, E., Izadi, S., Srinivasan, J., Butler, A. et al. (2006, September). SenseCam: A retrospective memory aid. In *International Conference on Ubiquitous Computing* (pp. 177–193). Springer.

Hossain, D., Imtiaz, M. H., Ghosh, T., Bhaskar, V., & Sazonov, E. (2020, July). Real-time food intake monitoring using wearable egocnetric camera. In *2020 42nd Annual International Conference of the IEEE Engineering in Medicine and Biology Society (EMBC)* (pp. 4191–4195). IEEE.

Howard, A. G., Zhu, M., Chen, B., Kalenichenko, D., Wang, W., Weyand, T. et al. (2017). *Mobilenets: Efficient convolutional neural networks for mobile vision applications.* https://arxiv.org/abs/1704.04861

Hoyle, R., Templeman, R., Armes, S., Anthony, D., Crandall, D., & Kapadia, A. (2014, September). Privacy behaviors of lifeloggers using wearable cameras. *Proceedings of the 2014 ACM International Joint Conference on Pervasive and Ubiquitous Computing*, pp. 571–582.

Kendon, A. (1976). Spatial organization in social encounters: The F-formation system. *Man–Environment Systems, 6*, 291–296.

Kerr, J., Marshall, S. J., Godbole, S., Chen, J., Legge, A., Doherty, A. R.,et al. (2013). Using the SenseCam to improve classifications of sedentary behavior in free-living settings. *American Journal of Preventive Medicine, 44*(3), 290–296.

Korayem, M., Templeman, R., Chen, D., Crandall, D., & Kapadia, A. (2016, May). Enhancing lifelogging privacy by detecting screens. *Proceedings of the 2016 CHI Conference on Human Factors in Computing Systems*, pp. 4309–4314.

Krizhevsky, A., Sutskever, I., & Hinton, G. E. (2012). Imagenet classification with deep convolutional neural networks. *Advances in Neural Information Processing Systems, 25*, 1097–1105.

Larson, R., & Csikszentmihalyi, M. (2014). The experience sampling method. In *Flow and the foundations of positive psychology* (pp. 21–34). Springer.

Li, Y., Liu, M., & Rehg, J. M. (2018). In the eye of beholder: Joint learning of gaze and actions in first person video. *Proceedings of the European Conference on Computer Vision (ECCV)*, pp. 619–635.

Liu, J., Johns, E., Atallah, L., Pettitt, C., Lo, B., Frost, G. et al. (2012, May). An intelligent food-intake monitoring system using wearable sensors. In *2012 Ninth International Conference on Wearable and Implantable Body Sensor Networks* (pp. 154–160). IEEE.

Mann, S. (1997). Wearable computing: A first step toward personal imaging. *Computer, 30*(2), 25–32.

Masi, I., Wu, Y., Hassner, T., & Natarajan, P. (2018, October). Deep face recognition: A survey. In *2018 31st SIBGRAPI Conference on Graphics, Patterns and Images (SIBGRAPI)* (pp. 471–478). IEEE.

McCandless, T., & Grauman, K. (2013, May). Object-centric spatio-temporal pyramids for egocentric activity recognition. *British Machine Vision Conference, 2*, 3.

Napa Scollon, C., Prieto, C. K., & Diener, E. (2009). Experience sampling: Promises and pitfalls, strength and weaknesses. In E. Diener (Ed.), *Assessing well-being* (pp. 157–180). Springer.

Noronha, J., Hysen, E., Zhang, H., & Gajos, K. Z. (2011, October). Platemate: crowdsourcing nutritional analysis from food photographs. *Proceedings of the 24th Annual ACM Symposium on User Interface Software and Technology*, pp. 1–12.

Poleg, Y., Arora, C., & Peleg, S. (2014). Temporal segmentation of egocentric videos. *Proceedings of the IEEE Conference on Computer Vision and Pattern Recognition*, pp. 2537–2544.

Ren, Z., Lee, Y. J., & Ryoo, M. S. (2018). Learning to anonymize faces for privacy preserving action detection. *Proceedings of the European Conference on Computer Vision (ECCV)*, pp. 620–636.

Starner, T. (1999). *Wearable computing and contextual awareness*. Unpublished doctoral dissertation, Massachusetts Institute of Technology.

Starner, T., Weaver, J., & Pentland, A. (1998). Real-time American sign language recognition using desk and wearable computer based video. *IEEE Transactions on Pattern Analysis and Machine Intelligence, 20*(12), 1371–1375.

Sun, M., Burke, L. E., Baranowski, T., Fernstrom, J. D., Zhang, H., Chen, H. C., et al. (2015). An exploratory study on a chest-worn computer for evaluation of diet, physical activity and lifestyle. *Journal of Healthcare Engineering, 6*(1), 1–22.

Templeman, R., Korayem, M., Crandall, D. J., & Kapadia, A. (2014). PlaceAvoider: Steering first-person cameras away from sensitive spaces. *Network and Distributed System Security(NDSS) Symposium, 14*, 23–26.

Thomaz, E. (2020, March). Activiome: A system for annotating first-person photos and multimodal activity sensor data. In *2020 IEEE International Conference on Pervasive Computing and Communications Workshops (PerCom Workshops)* (pp. 1–6). IEEE.

Thomaz, E., Parnami, A., Bidwell, J., Essa, I., & Abowd, G. D. (2013, September). Technological approaches for addressing privacy concerns when recognizing eating behaviors with wearable cameras. *Proceedings of the 2013 ACM International Joint Conference on Pervasive and Ubiquitous Computing*, pp. 739–748.

Thomaz, E., Parnami, A., Essa, I., & Abowd, G. D. (2013, November). Feasibility of identifying eating moments from first-person images leveraging human computation. *Proceedings of the 4th International SenseCam and Pervasive Imaging Conference*, pp. 26–33.

Tong, C., Tailor, S. A., & Lane, N. D. (2020,

March). Are accelerometers for activity recognition a dead-end? *Proceedings of the 21st International Workshop on Mobile Computing Systems and Applications*, pp. 39–44.

Truong, K. N., Patel, S. N., Summet, J. W., & Abowd, G. D. (2005, September). Preventing camera recording by designing a capture-resistant environment. In *International Conference on Ubiquitous Computing* (pp. 73–86). Springer.

Umberson, D. & Karas Montez, J. (2010). Social relationships and health: A flashpoint for health policy. *Journal of Health and Social Behavior, 51*(1, Suppl.), S54–S66.

Vishwamitra, N., Knijnenburg, B., Hu, H., & Kelly Caine, Y. P. (2017). Blur vs. block: Investigating the effectiveness of privacy-enhancing obfuscation for images. *Proceedings of the IEEE Conference on Computer Vision and Pattern Recognition Workshops*, pp. 39–47.

Wittenburg, P., Brugman, H., Russel, A., Klassmann, A., & Sloetjes, H. (2006). ELAN: A professional framework for multimodality research. *5th International Conference on Language Resources and Evaluation (LREC 2006)*, pp. 1556–1559.

Xiong, H., Huang, Y., Barnes, L. E., & Gerber, M. S. (2016, September). Sensus: a cross-platform, general-purpose system for mobile crowdsensing in human-subject studies. *Proceedings of the 2016 ACM International Joint Conference on Pervasive and Ubiquitous Computing*, pp. 415–426.

Zhang, Y. C., & Rehg, J. M. (2018). Watching the TV watchers. *Proceedings of the ACM on Interactive, Mobile, Wearable and Ubiquitous Technologies, 2*(2), 1–27.

CHAPTER 12

Beyond the Smartphone

The Future of Wearables as Mobile Sensors

Kristof Van Laerhoven

CHAPTER OVERVIEW

Wearable sensors hold multiple advantages: Having sensors that are closer, *on the skin*, to the human user allows for more information and, when those sensors are worn throughout the day (and, in many cases, even night and day), the data these sensors produce tend to cover many aspects of the user's life. This chapter attempts to predict what type of wearable sensors—for there are many—and to what extent wearables will be particularly attractive as mobile sensors in psychology. As is the case with predictions, this only makes sense when looking at the prevailing and current trends in research in the area of wearable sensing, in order to be able to extrapolate what might become feasible in the coming years and decades. Technology-wise, this does not only depend on the sensors themselves: Other key components that have become common in wearables, such as wireless communication and energy demands, are equally important in this picture. Furthermore, the concept of wearable sensing does not depend only on the used hardware components: The information that is generated from the sensor signals, and where and how this information is analyzed, abstracted, and interpreted, are equally important. From these analyses of what will become technically possible in wearable sensing, a set of promising applications is extracted and presented in the final section of this chapter.

Introduction

Wearable computing as a scientific discipline has been around since 1997, when there was barely a commercial market for wearables—certainly not the vast market we see today (Martin, Starner, Siewiorek, Kunze, & Van Laerhoven, 2021). Wearable sensors in psychology and medical research predate this field, with wearable actigraphs, pedometers, and similar devices already in use for decades in psychological experiments and studies before that (Benoit, Royant-Parola, Borbely, Tobler, & Widlöcher, 1985; Brown, Smolensky, D'Alonzo, & Redman, 1990). This chapter gives an overview of what we can expect to emerge in terms of new modalities and information that can be gathered from human study participants, and how these new technologies can be expected to impact psychology in the near and far future. The focus will be mostly on sensor technologies that have become mature or are nearly ready to be integrated in wearables. What this chapter avoids is a prediction on which devices will appear on the market and become available as wearable mass-deployment tools for psychology, in a similar way that smartphones have now become ubiquitous and mobile sensors, simply because this entails many other factors such as marketing and social acceptance.

A first goal of this chapter is thus to provide an overview of what wearable sensors are coming up for use in psychology research. What is already certain is that several technological breakthroughs that are happening as we write or read this will lead to novel ways to extract more, more reliable, and more fine-grained information from humans. Wearable devices will not only become increasingly smaller and more comfortable to wear, but will also deliver more useful information over longer time spans. It is important to keep in mind, though, that the information these new sensor devices deliver will not always be as crisp and clear to interpret from the start. Actigraphs initially recorded with so-called counts of a person's amount of physical activity over time, but they were then found to be hard to translate across different devices that used different mechanical constructs to generate these counts. Similarly, many newer sensors might initially deliver data that will be hard to reproduce or translate in future studies.

A second goal of this chapter is to stress that future wearables are about to increasingly produce estimates of much higher-level information than the absolute measurements that we are used to today. Instead of collecting the raw inertial data of a smartwatch or counting steps, for instance, these wearables will increasingly be able to directly deliver what physical activities the user performs—"playing the piano for 2.5 hours," "cooking dinner for 20 minutes," or "rock climbing in the afternoon"—or what affective states the wearer might be in. This is much more attractive, both from a technological perspective as there is less information to store and communicate at a relatively low processing cost, and from an information perspective as well, for these data are easier to interpret. But it also holds dangers and pitfalls: These predictions will never work with 100% accuracy for every use, and the methods—algorithms running on the wearable, basically—that perform these predictions will be susceptible to certain biases. An outstanding question is whether dealing with such inaccuracies will be a small price to pay for avoiding having to spend a lot of the wearable's energy in collecting large amounts of "raw" sensor data that require large efforts in retrospective "big data" analysis.

In the next sections, this chapter first describes the large variety of wearable devices and then details in a nonexhaustive list how sensors offer great potential to impact psychology in terms of the information they can objectively measure over long periods of time, before putting them into perspective in terms of what values they really capture. After that, some research trends are described that detail how wearables will be able to capture large amounts of data, whose analysis and extraction of essential information can be useful for psychology, especially in "in the wild" experiments where participants are observed through the wearable sensors over longitudinal recording sessions and in their natural habitats.

Types of Wearables

Wearable devices come in a surprisingly large variety, depending on the scenario in which they are deployed and where on the body they are worn. Beyond the classical activity trackers that are typically worn on the hip or wrist (Kim, He, Lyons, & Starner, 2007), other form factors include glasses and rings (Colley, Inget, Lappalainen, & Häkkilä, 2017) embedded in shoes, textile garments, tattoos applied on the skin (Vega et al., 2017), and so-called earables that are worn in the ears (Kawsar et al., 2018). Research methods have been devised that quantify the wearing comfort of these devices (Knight, Baber, Schwirtz, & Bristow, 2002), and best practices have emerged in the past decades that link, for particular sensors, the optimal placement to increase the measurement reliability.

Guidelines on human factors surrounding wearability were first introduced in Gemperle, Kasabach, Stivoric, Bauer, and Martin (1998) and have since then been updated regularly for newer technologies and application considerations. The work of Zeagler (2017) has contributed a web-based set of body maps with references and design considerations, detailing for all areas on the body where a designer should most likely place a wearable device. These maps also show that the most likely locations for wearable technology to be successful in general are the hands, wrists, forearms, upper arms, upper chest area above the breast, forehead, ears, and mid-thighs. Keep in mind the ongoing miniaturization of sensors as well as the drive for producing system-on-chips that not only led to smaller and more energy-efficient, but also more reusable designs (Saleh et al., 2006).

Sensors to Look Out for in Wearables

Certain sensing technologies have in past years been rapidly miniaturized and integrated in wearable prototypes. As we will show, some of the most prolific ones are introduced to give a sense of what type of sensors might experience a widespread breakthrough in commercial wearables to come out in the future. These are roughly listed here in order of certainty of appearance in future wearables, with the first one already present in most people.

Inertial Sensors

Inertial sensors cover a family of sensors that can measure orientation and changes in orientation, so that they are optimal for characterizing movements of the body they are attached to (Randell & Muller, 2000). They have been used to measure the amount of motion, as well as to detect particular gestures, ranging from step counting to counting and analyzing training exercises in sports. In terms of advances in miniaturization and integration, inertial sensors have experienced one of the most remarkable transitions in the past decades. These sensors are nowadays referred to as inertial measurement units (IMUs), which is appropriate as these are not single sensors but rather a grouping of about a dozen sensors (accelerometers, gyroscope, and magnetometers, all sensing in three dimensions) integrated in the same package (Ayazi, 2011). They can be regarded as successors of the old actigraphy devices and accelerometers, since they basically sense motion, while delivering much more accurate data in terms of movement and sensor orientation over time (Fong, Ong, & Nee, 2008). Current sensors have been so minimized through MEMS technology advances, that they occupy only a tiny footprint on any device, and they are mass-produced in such high batches that their cost has dropped to an all-time low. As a result, IMUs are integrated into almost every wearable device, smart watches, smart glasses, or wireless earbuds. Their low-energy footprint has enabled large studies in which participants are monitored over longer periods of time through such wearables, for instance (Purta et al., 2016).

Meanwhile, the miniaturization of mechanical and electrical sensor designs for IMUs has stabilized; both research and industry have now predominantly focused on digitally processing the sensor signals, locally on the sensor chip. Off-the-shelf sensor devices come with their own processing capabilities, which meanwhile can be reprogrammed as well, and they deliver many functions, including sensor fusion and detection of patterns of interest within the sensor signals. Wearable developers "just" need to glue the IMU to a processor, which then can digitally speak to each other and where much of the information extraction is done on the IMU, freeing up capabilities on the wearable's main processor. IMU sensors offer a blueprint for many sensors that, due to their popularity, might follow a similar evolution in becoming tiny, low-cost, and requiring little energy.

Electrocardiography, Electrodermal Activity, Electrooculography, Electromyography, and Photoplethysmography

The following set of sensors, which detects a person's vital signs, has been used in a medical context for decades. In all these sensor types, their proper attachment to the human body is critical for their readings. The electrode design or the mechanical attachment design that keeps the sensor placed firmly on the skin so that motion and skin condition will not change the readings is just as important as how their signals are amplified and filtered. For standard three-point electrocardiography (or ECG), three electrodes are placed on the wearer's torso, measuring the depolarization and repolarization of the heart muscle during each heartbeat. For clinical purposes, 12-lead ECG is typically used, whereas wearable devices have recently been introduced that perform one-lead ECG, such as the Apple Watch Series 4 and above (Strik et al., 2020). ECG samples are collected with frequencies up to 1,024 samples per second. When collected at such high frequency, the signal is capable of downsampling to 256 readings per second without loss of information (Soleymani, Lichtenauer, Pun, & Pantic, 2011). This results in a signal that allows capture of the heart rate, heart rate variability, and other parameters related to the cardiac cycle. For additional details on physiological recordings in daily life, see also Chapter 6, this volume.

Electrodermal activity (EDA) records skin resistance or skin conductance by measuring resistance between two electrodes that are placed on the skin, usually where the wearer tends to sweat (Dawson, Schell, & Filion, 2000). This sensor is particularly susceptible to the wearer's skin type, as well as external influences such as changing humidity, temperature, or physical activity. Relative changes in the signal have been shown to be useful, however, and wearables such as the Empatica E4 (*https://www.empatica.com/research/e4/*) have integrated this sensor and provide measurements at rates of several readings per second (Milstein & Gordon, 2020).

Electromyogram (EMG) sensors have not yet been widely incorporated in wearables but nevertheless show much promise for use in analyses of human movement (Kleissen, Buurke, Harlaar, & Zilvold, 1998). In EMG, electrodes are attached to the skin above a muscle; the difference in electrical potential generated when the muscle cells are activated is then recorded by the surface electrodes. Measurements are typically recorded from 30 to 1,000 samples per second (van Boxtel, 2001). Depending on how the electrodes are attached to the skin, noise from movement or nearby muscles tends to enter the signal, often requiring substantial filtering of the signal. The muscles around the eyes can be monitored using a similar principle with the help of electrooculography (EOG) electrodes that can be built in the nose pad and bridge of glasses to detect the wearer's eye movement and events such as blinking. An early wearable product that integrated such sensors is the JINS MEME glasses (Uema & Inoue, 2017).

The overall measurement principle of photoplethysmography (PPG) is straightforward: The sensor is placed on the skin of the user and uses a light source (typically a light-emitting diode [LED]) to illuminate the skin, as well as a light sensor to measure over time how much light is reflected back from (or through, for the fingertip or earlobe for example) the skin (Tamura, Maeda, Sekine, & Yoshida, 2014). Blood flow through the skin tissue is in this way picked up, allowing several interesting measures to be extracted from the resulting signal, such as the person's pulse or heart rate variability, but also other information such as breathing rate or the blood's oxygen levels. Wearables have seen a proliferation of PPG as these sensors do not need electrodes to be placed on the skin, though other problems, such as motion artifacts when the pressure on the skin changes or when ambient light interferes with the photodiodes, do remain. Furthermore, where the sensor is placed has a significant effect on the signal quality (Hartmann et al., 2019).

Location, Microphones, Cameras, and Depth Sensors

Until now, the sensors we have mentioned in this section have been introspective; they are placed on and are directed to the wearer's skin and directly provide information about the wearer. What is happening in the wearer's environment may be equally interesting: The information used ever since mobile phones obtained integrated GPS and wireless locationing capabilities is location tracking over time. The modules that allow a device to sense its location are only slowly moving toward some wearable devices, however. Sensor types that are equally lacking a pervasive presence in current wearables constitute some of the more interesting modalities in terms of producing data straightforward enough to interpret: sounds (Franke, Lukowicz, Kunze, & Bannach, 2009), images, and video clips from a wearable device can provide valuable data for use in psychological trials in multiple ways. Early prototypes in this area include the Microsoft SenseCam (Chowdhury, Ferdous, & Jose, 2016), which has the formfactor of a large pendant or clip that can be attached to clothing. With miniaturized (three-dimensional) cameras, which include depth data of the scenes they observe, slowly finding their way in mobile smartphones, these can also be expected to appear in wearable devices. Because of the energy they need to conduct the sensing, though, as well as the amount of data generated (sound requires thousands of samples per second, images or video frames are represented by large matrices of color [and depth] data), they will not likely be introduced in the near future for small wearables that need to operate over longer periods of time.

The above categories have been listed as some of the more interesting wearable-specific sensors for psychology research. This is also just a subset of sensors that will be integrated in wearables, as many other, nonwearable, computing devices such as smartphones already contain valuable sensors (as discussed in Chapter 13, this volume). Excellent examples here are the array of sensors that can be used to localize a user from their smartphone, or the log which other users (through Bluetooth communication) were close by. Further developments for these sensors can and likely will eventually lead to their integration into wearable devices that the user carries more often, and is especially promising for obtaining a more complete coverage over time (Van Laerhoven, Borazio, & Burdinski, 2015). The following section will cover a subsequent challenge that follows after the physical sensor packages are obtained in hardware: the analysis and processing of their output data.

Making Sense of the Sensor Data

Many of the sensors discussed in the previous section have become available as miniature, energy-efficient packages that can be directly integrated into wearables. This does not mean, however, that all of them will definitely find their way into every commercial wearable device in the future or that their data can reliably be used across multi-user psychological studies. Some key differences in the way they operate and in the signals that these sensor chips deliver are as follows.

- *Sensors' output data can be delivered in absolute units or relative values.* Inertial sensors tend to come with calibration routines and to deliver values that come in well-defined units such as milli-g/s (for the amount of acceleration) or representations such as quaternions (for full IMU sensors, giving the sensor a three-dimensional orientation within a specified orientation frame; see Grützmacher, Kempfle, Van Laerhoven, & Haubelt, 2021). When attaching the sensor to another person on another day, but being exposed to the same acceleration or orientation, the resulting values will be comparable across these different persons. This is not the case for the raw data collected by EDA sensors or PPG sensors, for instance: Integrated sensors that measure reflected light for a particular setup, or charge or voltage differences between particular electrodes, provide a raw signal that will differ significantly between users, skin types, sensor properties, or situations. If any of these parameters are changed—a PPG sensor using a different light intensity, the user moving their limbs, the environment being warmer or more humid—the resulting measurements will likely be completely different.

- *Filters almost always impact the sensor data.* All sensors described in the previous section can provide users or researchers with the measurements as they were picked up, but this "raw" signal in this case can be highly variable. Every sensor is prone to noise, drift, or other sources of error that result in a sensor signal that rarely matches the aimed-for information. To remedy this problem, sensors therefore contain multiple analog or digital constructs that modify the original physical signal, making it smoother and in the process losing some information about the measurement process (Wolling, Heimes, & Van Laerhoven, 2019). Reconstructing or reproducing the exact settings in which data are collected as a result becomes much harder as physical sensor chips are phased out and replaced by others. For some of the sensor types discussed earlier in this chapter, these changes can be bounded within a small margin of error, so that the recorded information can be considered to be reliable and reusable. For other sensor types, however, there exists an inherent danger that the recorded data are nearly impossible to compare to similar data at a later stage.

- *Sensors' estimates often obfuscate accuracy.* An increasing number of sensor packages comes with embedded processing capabilities to provide an early abstraction of the raw signal or deliver the output data in absolute units, for instance, as heartbeats per minute or step count. (The LIS2DS12 accelerometer, for instance, has an internal step counter and step detection in the chip package.[1]) Among the dangers of locally processing such estimates and aggregated metrics are that (1) they tend to be sensor-specific and (2) they often lack clear accuracy measures for these estimates: The algorithms that do the translation between the raw data and the estimates are rarely documented well and might have been written for one particular application, for example a step counter for noncritical fitness applications. Such algorithms might produce data that seem to have a clear unit (e.g., steps or heartbeats per minute), but since these embedded algorithms differ between sensors, the accuracy of these measurements might differ significantly: Data from one study with one sensor series can thus become difficult to compare to other data from another study with a different sensor manufacturer, version, or firmware.

- *The importance of the energy footprint.* Why are the above differences important to wearable sensors in particular? For most of the previously discussed sensors, processing the data within a wearable module is significantly more energy efficient than storing or forwarding the data via a wireless communication link, with wireless communication being orders of magnitude more energy demanding than sampling and processing sensor data (Razzaque & Dobson, 2014). Since the wearable form-factor favors small, comfortable to wear, and energy-efficient components, designers of these wearable sensors are facing a tradeoff: Either the sensor produces a large amount of data that contain all details but also cost a lot of energy to be stored or transferred, or the data are abstracted within the sensor chip to lead to an energy-efficient component but with a loss of generalization. Having a wearable unit that is able to hold longer on one battery charge is in view of this tradeoff often seen as more attractive than providing data that allow a more thorough analysis at a later time.

The foregoing discussion is worth keeping in mind when selecting wearable devices; the type and make of the integrated sensors often have a large impact and applicability for psychological studies. In the next section, we describe several research trends that take the abstraction of sensor data one step further by fusing information over time and from multiple sensors into higher-level concepts, such as user activity or affective state. Currently, most of these trends assume that data are collected and that analysis takes place on computing equipment with sufficient memory and processing resources. For some of these research trends, first steps have already been taken to embed these systems into the wearable devices themselves.

Wearable Sensor Information

The physical sensor devices that are integrated in wearable form represent one interesting aspect; what is eventually done with their data is an equally interesting one. The previous section has shown that many sensors provide so much data that their storage locally on the wearable, or transferring these data wirelessly elsewhere, is expensive in terms of energy. An alternative to abstracting the sensor signals that we can see in current sensors is the compression of sensor data: Similar to how images or movies that are taken with a camera are heavily compressed, usually only a fraction of the original data is retained, and other sensors routinely use compression to keep the amount of data down to a sustainable amount. The processing power needed to perform the compression typically outweighs the fact that only a fraction of the data needs to be stored or sent wirelessly. A second set of methods (and those we will focus on in this section), go beyond compression by extracting only the essential information needed for later applications from the sensor data. The advantage of this is a significantly lower-energy footprint (making the wearable smaller and requiring less recharging interruptions), which makes the resulting dataset smaller and less prone to contain private data from the study participants that is "hidden" in the large quantities of recorded sensor streams. With the aforementioned techniques and processing methods in mind, the next subsections will describe types of information that could impact future psychology research tremendously. The eventual aim is the wearable device's automatic and *in vivo* recognition of a person's activity, affect, and attention (Van Laerhoven, 2021).

Wearable Activity Recognition

The first activity recognition papers using wearable sensors, such as Van Laerhoven and Cakmakci (2000), demonstrated the feasibility of using data from body-worn accelerometers to detect physical activities such as sitting, standing, walking, running, climbing stairs, or riding a bicycle. This research was followed by varying the location where these sensors were being placed (from more data-friendly locations such as the knee to more comfortable and easier to wear locations such as the wrist, or by having multiple sensors) and by improving the accelerometers by combining them with gyroscopes and magnetometers to be able to track orientation of the sensor more reliably (as an IMU, see also the section "Sensors to Look Out for in Wearables"). Activity recognition has meanwhile grown into its own research area in which many sensors and algorithms have been evaluated on a growing number of benchmark datasets that hold the sensor recordings of volunteers performing several target activities that are to be detected. Important to note here is that activity recognition with wearable sensors has witnessed several waves in the way these research projects were set up and validated over the past decades. (For additional details, see also Chapter 5, this volume.)

Early research efforts focused on hardware prototypes that integrated and combined new sensors, such as capacitive sensing around the neck (Lukowicz, Amft, Roggen, & Cheng, 2010), sensing pressure changes in a house (Patel, Reynolds, & Abowd, 2008), or detection of activities with minute motions such as the EOG reading (Troester, Bulling, & Roggen, 2011). The main goal of these studies was to demonstrate that such modalities could in principle, often in well-controlled lab studies, be used as an interesting sensor modality to discern certain activities. These research contributions were less focused on the maximization of the detection accuracy of such systems or the demonstration that such systems could work in any environment.

Following these first explorations, more research in sensor data analysis and classifiers in activity recognition has led to focus on the accuracy of the systems. Best practices emerged that were combined into a common evaluation pipeline, in which researchers pressed for more realistic sensor data and reproducibility (Blanke, Larlus, Van Laerhoven, & Schiele, 2010), as well as demonstrated the need for proper evaluation procedures (Hammerla & Plötz, 2015). These studies had less focus on the perfect usability or durability of the sensor systems under consideration.

Activity recognition has now arrived in a third phase where researchers use wearable sensors that tend to target deployments with actual users, over longer stretches of time, in real-world settings. More focus is currently also being placed on the system's usability, durability, and applicability. As current machine learning approaches have moved to deep-learning models that allow so-called end-to-end learning, typical models now concentrate on convolutional neural networks (CNNs) and long short-term memory (LSTM) models, but also other alternatives are under consideration, for example, Murahari and Plötz (2018). The interesting concept of transfer learning promises to be able to learn models for activity classification from large datasets and to transfer—not learn from scratch—the learned model to new data or activities. Transfer learning has proven to be especially useful in computer vision research, where large image databases have already been collected. With regard to activity recognition from wearable data, this concept is still very much in its infancy (Hoelzemann & Van Laerhoven, 2020).

Wearable Affect Recognition

Current research has expanded from image-based affect recognition to the wearable approach, as image-based systems can only perform a temporal- and spatial-limited assessment of a person's affect state, for instance while driving (Affectiva, www.affectiva.com) or when triggered by the person (Abadi et al., 2015). Affect recognition systems that are wearable can detect the user's affective state continuously, 24 hours per day, 7 days a week, and ubiquitously, throughout the person's day-to-day routines. Initial research on these approaches such as Gjoreski, Luštrek, Gams, and Gjoreski (2017) or Budner, Eirich, and Gloor (2017) have shown that large amounts of long-term data can be used for a more comprehensive analysis that might even point to overall behavioral patterns of the wearer. These publications also regularly use correlations between affective states and environmental conditions, such as outdoor temperature, weather conditions, location, short audio analysis (such as detection of laughter), sleep quality information, calendar metadata, and nearby persons, to map this information to situations where the person tends to be stressed. Essential for such a correlation analysis is contextual information to make the analysis understandable and insightful.

In a recent and comprehensive survey on wearable affect recognition, Schmidt, Reiss, Dürichen, and Van Laerhoven (2019) pointed out four other challenges besides long-term reasoning that remain to be tackled in this field: valence detection, hardware, datasets, and algorithmic challenges. For *valence* detection, physiological changes and the arousal axis of the circumplex model (Valenza, Citi, Lanatá, Scilingo, & Barbieri, 2014) have been linked in many previous studies. It is therefore not that surprising that approaches of stress detection and arousal assessment (Valenza, Lanata, & Scilingo, 2012) report accuracies of such methods that are high and encouraging. Valence-related changes in human physiology are subtler, though, and more difficult to detect automatically and consequently show poorer results, such as in Schmidt, Reiss, Dürichen, and Van Laerhoven (2018). *Hardware* to record physiological data in affect recognition studies is mostly limited to smartwatch-like devices such as the Empatica E4 or chest-worn belts such as AutoSense (Ertin et al., 2011). Smart patches have to date found little application in affect recognition studies, but sensors and processing hardware can be integrated into the fabric (Reiss, Amft, & Barfield, 2015). Typical information such as ECG, EDA, and inertial data is bound to be supplemented by blood pressure (Vrijkotte, Van Doornen, & De Geus, 2000) information such as pulse wave transit time (Gesche, Grosskurth, Küchler, & Patzak, 2012), body microphones on the chest or abdomen (Pandia, Ravindran, Cole, Kovacs, & Giovangrandi, 2010), and chemical-electrophysiological sensors (Imani et al., 2016). More *datasets* to test affect recognition approaches are constantly being introduced; robust affect recognition systems are ideally benchmarked on redundant data streams and different affective states (stress, amusement, neutral), such as the WESAD (WEarable Stress and Affect Data set; Schmidt et al., 2018) benchmark. *Algorithmic challenges* are continually being solved in recent research as well: With end-to-end approaches such as deep neural networks like CNNs, methods to preprocess the sensor signals (called features) to allow classification is no longer such a big design problem. These methods are more challenging to implement on smaller wearable devices, however (Bhattacharya & Lane, 2016).

Wearable Attention Recognition

For decades, attention has been focused on wearable interfaces, for wearable devices can be used anywhere and anytime. Thad Starner's prediction still holds: that is, that the issue of attention, especially divided attention that focuses on the ability to allocate attention to simultaneous tasks, in wearable interfaces "will be key to developing compelling wearable products in the future" (2002, p. 91). With the advent of smart glasses, which incorporate miniature cameras that point inward at the wearer's pupils (Morimoto, Koons, Amir, & Flickner, 2000), enabling the user's gaze tracking, attention recognition has become a third type of application with a large spectrum of sensing applications for psychology. Although cameras are still relatively large and power hungry, several such systems have become cost-effective for shorter or laboratory-bound studies. At the same time, generic methods to analyze the camera data and fuse this with other sensors, such as inertial sensing data, have emerged (Kassner, Patera, & Bulling, 2014).

Added to eye-tracking modules, which use cameras worn near the eyes, have come newer types of sensing devices. One modality that has seen first integrations into commercial products is the earlier-mentioned EOG electrodes embedded in smart glasses (Kunze, Utsumi, Shiga, Kise, & Bulling, 2013); these electrodes can coarsely detect eye movements and blinking, allowing one to distinguish what type of document the wearer is reading. Small on-skin patches have proven feasible in capacitive sensing of the wearer's eye blinking in first studies (Luo, Fu, Chu, Vega, & Kao, 2020). New techniques for ongoing attention detection and eye-tracker calibration (Murauer, Haslgrübler, & Ferscha, 2018) also are used for researching aspects of attention, during both strenuous tasks and everyday activities, such as face-to-face conversations (Gupta, Strivens, Tag, Kunze, & Ward, 2019) and moments of eye contact between adults and children (Ye et al., 2012). Wearable attention research has thus expanded from ever accurate tracking of coordinates where the user's gaze is focusing at, to a more diverse set of data involving attention information.

Conclusions

This chapter presents an overview of current trends in wearable sensing systems. The ultimate aim was to predict what types of wearable sensors might become available in the future and in particular how these might impact future psychological studies.

What information can be collected from people in future studies through wearable sensors? We have seen that presently robust and detailed *movement and activity* of the wearer through IMUs can already be captured in current wearable devices. The near future will see mostly improvements in how these data can be analyzed and interpreted on the sensor devices themselves. Other pieces of information entail *vital signs* of the user. Most of these are of course already known in psychology, but wearables allow this information to be captured in a person's daily routines, in their day-to-day lives, and over much longer 24/7 periods of time. *Video and depth* data offer visual information that researchers can easily interpret afterward, with a multitude of applications in validating other sensor data.

Which challenges do wearable sensor technologies pose? Usage of wearable sensors should always take the reproducibility and accuracy of the information they deliver into consideration. Many sensor technologies have become mature enough to deliver data that can be compared and interpreted, even when the devices are no longer available, but plenty of systems have been introduced in which this is more difficult. The rapid developments in the area of sensor chips is one reason, but another reason is the drive especially in wearables for a quick abstraction of sensor data to keep systems small and energy efficient.

Three types of information that can be extracted and abstracted from the wearable sensors' data streams were proposed as especially promising, which in the future could be delivered by a wearable device: (physical) activities, affect, and attention. Although we are still far from having commercial systems that can deliver any type of activity, affective state, or attention model, some systems have started to emerge that can reliably deliver *some* basic concepts in this direction. For activity recognition systems, some wearable systems are capable of counting steps, identifying fitness workouts, or detecting basic activities such as sleeping or sitting still over prolonged stretches of time. For affect detection systems, binary stress detection approaches have shown good performance results in selected, controlled settings. For attention, coarse eye motions and eye blinks can be detected.

The final, more technical message of this chapter is that opportunistic, Big Data-driven approaches (all that can be sensed is recorded, leaving it to after-the-fact analysis on high-performance clusters of computing power to extract the more important information) are not likely to become widely adopted in wearable sensing in the near future. Wearables need to remain comfortable, primarily (apart from other factors such as having appealing designs and being socially acceptable), and current battery technologies do not allow wearables to store or send more than the most essential data only. This bottleneck often leads wearable device developers to favor abstracting the sensor data as soon as possible to keep the system small and low power, as a tradeoff. Approaches that aim at recording the original, more precise, and large amounts of data do remain harder to implement.

Note

1. www.st.com/en/mems-and-sensors/lis2ds12.html.

REFERENCES

Abadi, M. K., Subramanian, R., Kia, S. M., Avesani, P., Patras, I., & Sebe, N. (2015). DECAF: MEG-based multimodal database for decoding affective physiological responses. *IEEE Transactions on Affective Computing, 6*(3), 209–222.

Ayazi, F. (2011, June). Multi-DOF inertial MEMS: From gaming to dead reckoning.

2011 16th International Solid-State Sensors, Actuators and Microsystems Conference, pp. 2805–2808.

Benoit, O., Royant-Parola, S., Borbely, A. A., Tobler, I., & Widlöcher, D. (1985). Circadian aspects of motor activity in depressed patients. *Acta Psychiatrica Belgica, 85*(5), 582–592.

Bhattacharya, S., & Lane, N. D. (2016, March). From smart to deep: Robust activity recognition on smartwatches using deep learning. *2016 IEEE International Conference on Pervasive Computing and Communication Workshops (PerCom Workshops)*, pp. 1–6.

Blanke, U., Larlus, D., Van Laerhoven, K., & Schiele, B. (2010). *Standing on the shoulders of other researchers: A position statement.* www.researchgate.net/profile/Kristof-Van-Laerhoven/publication/216439945_Standing_on_the_Shoulders_of_Other_Researchers_-_A_Position_Statement/links/0fcfd50b35b5dd607e000000/Standing-on-the-Shoulders-of-Other-Researchers-A-Position-Statement.pdf

Brown, A. C., Smolensky, M. H., D'Alonzo, G. E., & Redman, D. P. (1990). Actigraphy: A means of assessing circadian patterns in human activity. *Chronobiology International, 7*(2), 125–133.

Budner, P., Eirich, J., & Gloor, P. A. (2017). *"Making you happy makes me happy": Measuring individual mood with smartwatches.* https://arxiv.org/abs/1711.06134

Chowdhury, S., Ferdous, M. S., & Jose, J. M. (2016, September). Exploring lifelong sharing and privacy. *Proceedings of the 2016 ACM International Joint Conference on Pervasive and Ubiquitous Computing: Adjunct*, pp. 553–558.

Colley, A., Inget, V., Lappalainen, T., & Häkkilä, J. (2017, September). Ring form factor: A design space for interaction. *Proceedings of the 2017 ACM International Symposium on Wearable Computers*, pp. 178–179.

Dawson, M., Schell, A., & Filion, D. (2000). The electrodermal system. In J. T. Cacioppo, L. G. Tassinary, & G. Berntson (Eds.), *Handbook of psychophysiology* (2nd ed., pp. 200–223). Cambridge University Press.

Ertin, E., Stohs, N., Kumar, S., Raij, A., Al'Absi, M., & Shah, S. (2011, November). AutoSense: unobtrusively wearable sensor suite for inferring the onset, causality, and consequences of stress in the field. *Proceedings of the 9th ACM Conference on Embedded Networked Sensor Systems*, pp. 274–287.

Fong, W. T., Ong, S. K., & Nee, A. Y. C. (2008). Methods for in-field user calibration of an inertial measurement unit without external equipment. *Measurement Science and technology, 19*(8).

Franke, T., Lukowicz, P., Kunze, K., & Bannach, D. (2009, September). Can a mobile phone in a pocket reliably recognize ambient sounds? *2009 International Symposium on Wearable Computers*, pp. 161–162.

Gemperle, F., Kasabach, C., Stivoric, J., Bauer, M., & Martin, R. (1998, October). Design for wearability. *Second International Symposium on Wearable Computers*, pp. 116–122.

Gesche, H., Grosskurth, D., Küchler, G., & Patzak, A. (2012). Continuous blood pressure measurement by using the pulse transit time: comparison to a cuff-based method. *European Journal of Applied Physiology, 112*(1), 309–315.

Gjoreski, M., Luštrek, M., Gams, M., & Gjoreski, H. (2017). Monitoring stress with a wrist device using context. *Journal of Biomedical Informatics, 73*, 159–170.

Grützmacher, F., Kempfle, J., Van Laerhoven, K., & Haubelt, C. (2021). fastSW: Efficient piecewise linear approximation of quaternion-based orientation sensor signals for motion capturing with wearable IMUs. *Sensors, 21*(15), 5180.

Gupta, A., Strivens, F. L., Tag, B., Kunze, K., & Ward, J. A. (2019, September). Blink as you sync: Uncovering eye and nod synchrony in conversation using wearable sensing. *Proceedings of the 23rd International Symposium on Wearable Computers*, pp. 66–71.

Hammerla, N. Y., & Plötz, T. (2015, September). Let's (not) stick together: pairwise similarity biases cross-validation in activity recognition. *Proceedings of the 2015 ACM International Joint Conference on Pervasive and Ubiquitous Computing*, pp. 1041–1051.

Hartmann, V., Liu, H., Chen, F., Hong, W., Hughes, S., & Zheng, D. (2019). Toward accurate extraction of respiratory frequency from the photoplethysmogram: Effect of measurement site. *Frontiers in Physiology, 10*, 732.

Hoelzemann, A., & Van Laerhoven, K. (2020, September). Digging deeper: towards a better understanding of transfer learning for human activity recognition. *Proceedings of the 2020 International Symposium on Wearable Computers*, pp. 50–54.

Imani, S., Bandodkar, A. J., Mohan, A. M., Kumar, R., Yu, S., Wang, J., et al. (2016). A wearable chemical–electrophysiological hybrid biosensing system for real-time health and fitness monitoring. *Nature Communications, 7*(1), 1–7.

Kassner, M., Patera, W., & Bulling, A. (2014, September). Pupil: An open source platform for pervasive eye tracking and mobile gaze-based interaction. *Proceedings of the 2014 ACM International Joint Conference on Pervasive and Ubiquitous Computing: Adjunct Publication*, pp. 1151–1160.

Kawsar, F., Min, C., Mathur, A., Montanari, A., Acer, U. G., & Van den Broeck, M. (2018, November). esense: Open earable platform for human sensing. *Proceedings of the 16th ACM Conference on Embedded Networked Sensor Systems*, pp. 371–372.

Kim, J., He, J., Lyons, K., & Starner, T. (2007, October). The gesture watch: A wireless contact-free gesture based wrist interface. *2007 11th IEEE International Symposium on Wearable Computers*, pp. 15–22.

Kleissen, R. F. M., Buurke, J. H., Harlaar, J., & Zilvold, G. (1998). Electromyography in the biomechanical analysis of human movement and its clinical application. *Gait and Posture, 8*(2), 143–158.

Knight, J. F., Baber, C., Schwirtz, A., & Bristow, H. W. (2002, October). The comfort assessment of wearable computers. *Proceedings. Sixth International Symposium on Wearable Computers*, pp. 65–72.

Kunze, K., Utsumi, Y., Shiga, Y., Kise, K., & Bulling, A. (2013, September). I know what you are reading: Recognition of document types using mobile eye tracking. *Proceedings of the 2013 International Symposium on Wearable Computers*, pp. 113–116.

Lukowicz, P., Amft, O., Roggen, D., & Cheng, J. (2010). On-body sensing: From gesture-based input to activity-driven interaction. *Computer, 43*(10), 92–96.

Luo, E., Fu, R., Chu, A., Vega, K., & Kao, H. L. (2020, September). Eslucent: an eyelid interface for detecting eye blinking. *Proceedings of the 2020 International Symposium on Wearable Computers*. pp. 58–62.

Martin, T., Starner, T., Siewiorek, D., Kunze, K., & Van Laerhoven, K. (2021). 25 years of ISWC. Time flies when you're having fun. *IEEE Pervasive Computing, 20*(3), 72–78.

Milstein, N., & Gordon, I. (2020). Validating measures of electrodermal activity and heart rate variability derived from the empatica e4 utilized in research settings that involve interactive dyadic states. *Frontiers in Behavioral Neuroscience 14*, 148.

Morimoto, C. H., Koons, D., Amir, A., & Flickner, M. (2000). Pupil detection and tracking using multiple light sources, *Image and Vision Computing, 18*(4), 331–335.

Murahari, V. S., & Plötz, T. (2018, October). On attention models for human activity recognition. *Proceedings of the 2018 ACM International Symposium on Wearable Computers*, pp. 100–103.

Murauer, M., Haslgrübler, M., & Ferscha, A. (2018, September). Natural pursuits for eye tracker calibration. *Proceedings of the 5th International Workshop on Sensor-based Activity Recognition and Interaction*, pp. 1–10.

Pandia, K., Ravindran, S., Cole, R., Kovacs, G., & Giovangrandi, L. (2010, March). Motion artifact cancellation to obtain heart sounds from a single chest-worn accelerometer. *2010 IEEE International Conference on Acoustics, Speech and Signal Processing*, pp. 590–593.

Patel, S. N., Reynolds, M. S., & Abowd, G. D. (2008, May). Detecting human movement by differential air pressure sensing in HVAC system ductwork: An exploration in infrastructure mediated sensing. In *International Conference on Pervasive Computing* (pp. 1–18). Springer.

Purta, R., Mattingly, S., Song, L., Lizardo, O., Hachen, D., Poellabauer, C., et al. (2016, September). Experiences measuring sleep and physical activity patterns across a large college cohort with fitbits. *Proceedings of the 2016 ACM International Symposium on Wearable Computers*, pp. 28–35.

Randell, C., & Muller, H. (2000, October). Context awareness by analysing accelerometer data. *Fourth International Symposium on Wearable Computers*, pp. 175–176.

Razzaque, M. A., & Dobson, S. (2014). Energy-efficient sensing in wireless sensor networks using compressed sensing. *Sensors, 14*(2), 2822–2859.

Reiss, A., Amft, O., & Barfield, W. (2015).

Design challenges of real wearable computers. In *Fundamentals of wearable computers and augmented reality* (pp. 583–618). CRC Press.

Saleh, R., Wilton, S., Mirabbasi, S., Hu, A., Greenstreet, M., Lemieux, G., et al. (2006). System-on-chip: Reuse and integration. *Proceedings of the IEEE, 94*(6), 1050–1069.

Schmidt, P., Reiss, A., Dürichen, R., & Van Laerhoven, K. (2018, October). Labelling affective states "in the wild": Practical guidelines and lessons learned. *Proceedings of the 2018 ACM International Joint Conference and 2018 International Symposium on Pervasive and Ubiquitous Computing and Wearable Computers*, pp. 654–659.

Schmidt, P., Reiss, A., Dürichen, R., & Van Laerhoven, K. (2019). Wearable-based affect recognition—A review. *Sensors, 19*(19), 4079.

Soleymani, M., Lichtenauer, J., Pun, T., & Pantic, M. (2011). A multimodal database for affect recognition and implicit tagging. *IEEE Transactions on Affective Computing, 3*(1), 42–55.

Starner, T. E. (2002). Attention, memory, and wearable interfaces. *IEEE Pervasive Computing, 1*(4), 88–91.

Strik, M., Caillol, T., Ramirez, F. D., Abu-Alrub, S., Marchand, H., Welte, N., et al. (2020). Validating QT-interval measurement using the Apple Watch ECG to enable remote monitoring during the COVID-19 pandemic. *Circulation, 142*(4), 416–418.

Tamura, T., Maeda, Y., Sekine, M., & Yoshida, M. (2014). Wearable photoplethysmographic sensors—past and present. *Electronics, 3*(2), 282–302.

Troester, G., Bulling, A., & Roggen, D. (2011) What's in the eyes for context-awareness? *IEEE Pervasive Computing, 10*(2), 48–57.

Uema, Y., & Inoue, K. (2017, September). JINS MEME algorithm for estimation and tracking of concentration of users. *Proceedings of the 2017 ACM International Joint Conference on Pervasive and Ubiquitous Computing and Proceedings of the 2017 ACM International Symposium on Wearable Computers*, pp. 297–300.

Valenza, G., Citi, L., Lanatá, A., Scilingo, E. P., & Barbieri, R. (2014). Revealing real-time emotional responses: A personalized assessment based on heartbeat dynamics. *Scientific Reports, 4*(1), 1–13.

Valenza, G., Lanata, A., & Scilingo, E. P. (2012). The role of nonlinear dynamics in affective valence and arousal recognition. *IEEE Transactions on Affective Computing, 3*(2), 237–249.

van Boxtel, A. (2001). Optimal signal bandwidth for the recording of surface EMG activity of facial, jaw, oral, and neck muscles. *Psychophysiology, 38*(1), 22–34.

Van Laerhoven, K. (2021). The three A's of wearable and ubiquitous computing: activity, affect, and attention. *Frontiers in Computer Science, 3.*

Van Laerhoven, K., Borazio, M., & Burdinski, J. H. (2015). Wear is your mobile? Investigating phone carrying and use habits with a wearable device. *Frontiers in ICT, 2*, 10.

Van Laerhoven, K., & Cakmakci, O. (2000). What shall we teach our pants? *Fourth International Symposium on Wearable Computers (ISWC 2000).*

Vega, K., Jiang, N., Liu, X., Kan, V., Barry, N., Maes, P., et al. (2017, September). The dermal abyss: Interfacing with the skin by tattooing biosensors. *Proceedings of the 2017 ACM International Symposium on Wearable Computers*, pp. 138–145.

Vrijkotte, T. G., Van Doornen, L. J., & De Geus, E. J. (2000). Effects of work stress on ambulatory blood pressure, heart rate, and heart rate variability. *Hypertension, 35*(4), 880–886.

Wolling, F., Heimes, S., & Van Laerhoven, K. (2019). Unity in Diversity: Sampling Strategies in Wearable Photoplethysmography. *IEEE Pervasive Computing, 18*(3), 63–69.

Ye, Z., Li, Y., Fathi, A., Han, Y., Rozga, A., Abowd, G. D., et al. (2012, September). Detecting eye contact using wearable eye-tracking glasses. *Proceedings of the 2012 ACM Conference on Ubiquitous Computing*, pp. 699–704.

Zeagler, C. (2017, September). Where to wear it: functional, technical, and social considerations in on-body location for wearable technology 20 years of designing for wearability. *Proceedings of the 2017 ACM International Symposium on Wearable Computers*, pp. 150–157.

CHAPTER 13

Viva Experience Sampling

Combining Passive Mobile Sensing with Active Momentary Assessments

Ulrich W. Ebner-Priemer and Philip Santangelo

CHAPTER OVERVIEW

Combining passive mobile sensing with active assessments is a silver bullet in psychological everyday life research, as both approaches can highly benefit from each other. Enriching e-diaries with continuous mobile sensing allows triggering the right question at the right time point. Conversely, enriching mobile sensing with momentary assessments enables us to understand the psychological content of mobile sensing parameters. After a short introduction to e-diary research, two main themes structure this chapter. In the first part, we will highlight conceptual and design issues of sensor-triggered e-diaries and add practical examples from research using activity-triggered, GPS-triggered, physiology-triggered, and audio- or video-triggered e-diaries. In the second part, we will explain how e-diary assessments enable uncovering the psychological content of pure sensing parameters. We close our chapter by presenting the ambulatory assessment toolbox as well as highlighting conclusions, limitations, and prospects.

E-Diaries as an Active Assessment Tool in Psychology

During the last decade, e-diaries became more and more used in psychological research, driven by technological progress in the area of digital mobile tools (e.g., smartphones), the general population's increasing acceptance of those tools, as well as advances in statistical approaches to analyze the resulting longitudinal data. Multiple terms have been used to describe e-diary methods in psychology, including the experience sampling method (ESM; Csikszentmihalyi & Larson, 1987), ecological momentary assessment

(EMA; Stone & Shiffman, 1994), or ambulatory assessment (Fahrenberg & Myrtek, 1996). These terms are often used interchangeably, although their historical antecedents and original aims differ (Wilhelm, Perrez, & Pawlik, 2012). Usually, we adopt the term *ambulatory assessment* (Trull & Ebner-Priemer, 2013) in accordance with the name of the primary organization that brings together investigators of daily-life research methods, the Society for Ambulatory Assessment (www.ambulatory-assessment.org). However, for the present chapter, our focus is on how to combine passive mobile sensing with active e-diary assessments and, therefore, to avoid confusion, we refrain from using higher-ranking terms such as ambulatory assessment or ecological momentary assessment. To gain more basic information on conventional diary approaches, see Mehl and Conner (2012).

Although terms and their meaning are subject to debate, these methods are distinctly characterized by a set of specific features or advantages, namely, (1) the assessment in real-life environments, therewith limiting lab-based biases and increasing the ecological validity of findings (Reis, 2012); (2) the assessment in real time, or close to real time, therewith limiting retrospective distortions (Schwarz, 2012); and (3) the focus on investigating within-subject mechanisms, processes, and dynamics, therewith enabling an idiographic focus (Hamaker, 2012). Above all, these methods are sought to provide a representative and (nearly) unbiased sample of an individual's emotions, thoughts, and behaviors as they unfold in daily life.

In comparison with classical retrospective questionnaire-based research in psychology, e-diary research involves additional methodological decisions, most importantly the time-based design. As mentioned earlier, e-diaries are best suited to catch emotions, thoughts, and behaviors as they occur dynamically in daily life. As those parameters (e.g. emotions) cannot be assessed continuously, specific sampling strategies have to be designed to catch those dynamics. Sampling strategies can be very heterogeneous and span from high-frequency sampling such as having e-diary assessments every 15 minutes (Ebner-Priemer, Kuo, et al., 2007) to once-daily end-of-day diaries over a total assessment period of one year or more (Ebner-Priemer et al., 2020). When defining a time-based design, the first question is about the goal of the assessment itself. Shiffman (2007), and quite similarly Fahrenberg, Myrtek, Pawlik, and Perrez (2007), differentiate specific strategies, such as getting complete coverage of the phenomena of interest over time (e.g., having the exact number of smoked cigarettes), drawing representative samples of moments or events in everyday life (having, e.g., hourly ratings of the current mood) or mapping the dynamics of specific processes. Although higher-order strategies or rules on how to design these sampling strategies are rarely at hand, one common understanding is that the sampling frequency must fit the dynamics of interest (Bolger, Davis, & Rafaeli, 2003; Ebner-Priemer & Sawitzki, 2007). Thus, faster changing psychological processes (i.e., processes with a higher dynamic) should be assessed with a higher sampling frequency, that is, more assessments within a given time frame. However, when designing the sampling scheme, the researcher has to carefully balance the sampling time interval, the number of items at each assessment, and the length of the assessment period to ensure high acceptance, good compliance, and low reactivity (Santangelo, Bohus, & Ebner-Priemer, 2014; Wrzus & Neubauer, 2021). This balance can be achieved by trying to keep the number of repeated inquiries and the assessment period as short as possible and only as long and as frequent as necessary (Dejonckheere & Erbas, 2021).

Enhancing E-Diary Assessments with Passive Mobile Sensing and Real-Time Analysis: The Case of Sensor-Triggered Diaries

Even with elaborated time-based designs, one major obstacle in e-diary research is still the ability to deliver the right question at the right time point. This endeavor may sound trivial, but it can be most complex, especially when the events of interest are rare. A practical example may be helpful to clarify this point. In one of our studies, we were interested in the effects of a green environment on mood (Tost et al., 2019). How can we ensure that during the rare moments of visiting parks or walking through the woods, e-diary assessments are posed? Context-triggered e-diary assessments can do the trick, with passive sensing on environmental data, screening continuously how green the environment is, real-time analyses to identify moments of interest (e.g., parks), and context-triggered assessments to obtain mood assessments in those specific situations and moments of interest. Those sensor-triggered assessments are not yet included in mainstream psychological research, partly because of hard- and software constraints, but multiple empirical studies have been conducted, mainly in the following four areas: (1) activity-triggered e-diaries, (2) physiology-triggered e-diaries, (3) GPS-triggered e-diaries, and (4) audio- or video-triggered assessments.

Sensor-Triggered E-Diaries: The Rationale

We begin our explanation of the rationale of sensor-triggered e-diaries using the example of activity-triggered e-diaries, as this is, in our view, the most easily explained sensor-triggered diary (Ebner-Priemer, Koudela, Mutz, & Kanning, 2013; Kanning, Ebner-Priemer, & Schlicht, 2013). The encompassing research question in several papers on this topic was to examine the relationship between physical activity and mood with the hypothesis that physical activity can improve momentary mood. In a paper from 2013, Ebner-Priemer, Koudela, Mutz, and Kanning nicely visualized the underlying idea of triggered assessments as pictured in Figure 13.1.

Figure 13.1A depicts physical activity assessed via a wearable fixed on the hip over a 24-hour time course in a single subject (three-dimensional accelerometer varioport-E; rectified AC-values were smoothed by a moving average over 10 minutes). The 24-hour time course is characterized by low physical activity during nighttime (22.00 through 06.00) and several peaks of high physical activity during daytime (e.g., at around 07.00, 15.00, and 17.00 on day 1 and at around 08.00 on day 2). What would happen if we were to combine this passive mobile sensing with fixed e-diary assessments like assessments every 60 minutes? E-diary assessments would temporarily coincide with some peaks of physical activity, as illustrated in Figure 13.1B, but other peaks would be missed; that is, those peaks would not be accompanied with e-diary ratings, and no information about these rather rare events would be gathered. To address the relationship between physical activity and momentary mood via e-diary ratings, the maximization of the variance is key. In the example at hand, this would mean obtaining e-diary assessments during all episodes of high physical activity as well as during episodes of low physical activity, as depicted in Figure 13.1C. This results in the maximization of assessed variance, or, in other words, an intentional oversampling of episodes of interest, which in our example are the rare events of high physical activity. (Of course, there are caveats to consider, such as ensuring that data from the entire spectrum is represented; we will attend to these

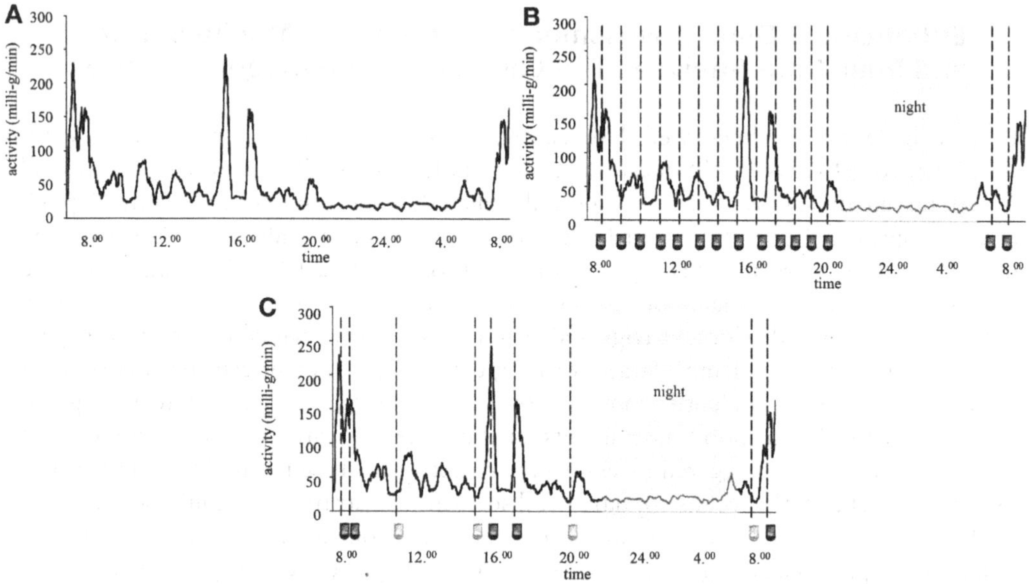

FIGURE 13.1. (A) Time course over 24 hours of physical activity (10-minute moving average) in a single subject; (B) combined with a fixed e-diary assessment in 1-hour intervals; or (C) combined with an interactive e-diary assessment. From Ebner-Priemer et al. (2013).

caveats in detail later in this chapter.) Such an approach might be best understood when compared to classical laboratory research. One indisputable advantage of laboratory research is the possibility of experimental manipulation. The experimenter defines which stimuli will be presented to the participant. To achieve meaningful findings, significant stimuli are usually presented. To study in a laboratory context how physical activity influences mood states, an experimenter would try to cover the full range of physical activity. Just letting participants walk at 2.3, 2.4, and 2.5 miles per hour (mph) might not be sufficient to reveal the existing effects. Adding experimental conditions with 2.0, 4.0, and 6.0 miles per hour, therewith including the full natural spectrum, would maximize the variance of the independent variable. This very same idea, namely, getting the full spectrum of possible experiences, constitutes the basis of sensor-triggered diaries, with the additional advantages of heightened ecological validity.

Whereas in hindsight it is evident when to trigger assessments (e.g., around 07.00, 15.00, and 17.00 at day 1 in our example), it is unfortunately much more complex in real time. Related to Figure 13.1B, it seems evident that in order to investigate the relationship between physical activity and mood, the peak of physical activity at 17.00 should be accompanied by an e-diary mood assessment. Under the assumption that the relationship between both parameters is linear, a huge effect on mood should be expected at this time point. However, from a real-life perspective, it is unclear, at this very moment, if this peak will still increase from 150 to 250 milli-g, as the peak before at around 16:00, or if the current 150 milli-g will stay the maximum. In other words, we are searching for significant events without knowing the width of these events, which vary between and within participants. Some participants are rather active, whereas others are true couch potatoes. In addition, physical activity does also differ within-subjects, with weekends showing different patterns compared to weekdays. We have used adaptive thresholds in our studies to cover this issue. In the following, we will report our real-time algorithm to detect episodes of physical activity in more detail. However, this is again just an illustrative example, as the other sensor-triggered diaries work in a quite similar fashion.

Setting Up a Sensor-Triggered E-Diary: Conceptual Decisions

Incredible, yet not much noticed, pioneer work on sensor-triggered assessments was already done in the last century by Michael Myrtek (summarized in Myrtek, 2004). Most of our conceptual decisions are based on his valuable work, which will be described in more detail in the next section on physiology-triggered e-diaries. From a conceptual point of view, several basic decisions have to be made when setting up an algorithm for sensor-triggered assessments: (1) defining events, (2) considering the dynamical relations between the parameters of interest, (3) defining the number of intended events, (4) deciding about the adaptive threshold, and (5) defining how to determine thresholds (see also Ebner-Priemer et al., 2013, for further details). We provide insights into the theoretical and empirical basis for these five decisions in the given example for activity-triggered e-diaries as reported in Ebner-Priemer and colleagues (2013):

1. Following the work of Myrtek (2004), we defined three events as triggers for the e-diary: an activity event, an inactivity event, and a time-limited event. Assessing both, the event of interest and the opposite event (i.e., instances of activity and inactivity in this example), might sound trivial, but we have seen empirical studies in which researchers forgot to assess their control condition, thereby making analyses nearly impossible. Time-limit events are interspersed when no activity or inactivity events are detected over a longer period of time. To have time-limit events, that is, having assessments at least every 2 hours, provides assessments during normal/medium values of the parameter of interest (which might be useful in case of nonlinear relations) and enables statistical control of autocorrelation processes. Moreover, these time-limit events may provide the participant with the information that the system is still running properly.

2. Considering the expected dynamical relation between the parameters of interest, in our case physical activity and mood, is also of great importance. Based on the prior e-diary-based work of Schwerdtfeger, Eberhardt, and Chmitorz (2008) in which they showed that the temporal relation between affective states and physical activity was most pronounced in short periods, and also based on the guidelines (Haskell et al., 2007) that postulate that being physically active for a minimum of 10 minutes leads to health benefits, we assumed that relatively short time frames would be most suitable. Accordingly, we have set the length of an event at 10 minutes.

3. As the number of events per day, we chose 10, as this comes with reasonable participant burden, still enables us to consider autocorrelations, and permits every event type several times a day.

4. Thresholds were defined to be adaptive: When physical activity, measured in milli-g, was low throughout the data collection period (i.e., a very inactive subject), both the activity and the inactivity thresholds decreased from one e-diary assessment to the next. In this way, e-diary assessments during the most active and least active episodes were

determined for each subject regardless of the absolute amount of activity. This approach also works fine for very active individuals: When too many activity episodes are detected (which is the same as too few inactivity episodes), the thresholds for both the activity and the inactivity episodes are increased to obtain less e-diary ratings during their individual most active and more e-diary scores during individual least active episodes. To achieve a similar number of events, we set the aspired ratio for activity/inactivity episodes to 1:1. Technically, we stored the number of detected (and triggered) events and simultaneously calculated the ratio between inactivity and activity episode-based triggers. After at least six triggers (settling phase), adapting the thresholds was activated. If the (activity/inactivity)–trigger ratio was above 2.05, both thresholds were increased by 5%, and if the ratio was below 0.95, both thresholds were decreased by 5%. In addition, the occurrence of time-limit triggers (i.e., no activity or inactivity event could be detected), the threshold for activity episodes was decreased by 5% and the threshold for inactivity episodes was increased by 5% (i.e., increasing the chance for both events). See also Meschtscherjakov, Reitberger, and Tscheligi (2010) on adaptive thresholds for user behavior-driven and context-triggered experience sampling.

5. We defined the thresholds using a combination of theoretical, empirical, and time-based design considerations. Again, details can be found in the paper by Ebner-Priemer and colleagues (2013). There we also validated our activity-triggered approach showing that the assessment of rare events (mood assessment during physically active episodes) was quadrupled compared to a random e-diary sampling. However, it must be noted as a limitation that the ability to improve the number of assessed events of interest is constricted by the actual frequency of those events. For example, assessing a bedridden patient, no algorithm will be able to find an actual active episode. Although our algorithm uses adaptive thresholds, which are not fixed to absolute values but we look for the most active episodes in each participant, the algorithm fails in subjects with no variability regarding their activity. Good feasibility and compliance of activity-triggered assessments have been reported in the literature (e.g., Dunton, Dzubur, & Intille, 2016).

Beyond Activity-Triggered E-Diaries: Methodological Considerations and Studies

A subtheme of activity-triggered e-diaries is sedentariness-triggered e-diaries, as they also use acceleration data from wearables. However, sedentariness is more than missing activity, from both an empirical and a conceptual perspective. There is growing evidence that sedentariness is a risk factor for human health over and above low physical activity (World Health Organization [WHO], 2020). In particular, longer sedentary bouts, such as more than 30 minutes of uninterrupted sitting, may lead to detrimental health effects (WHO, 2020). Importantly, definitions of sedentariness have two components: body posture and movement intensity or energy expenditure. The Sedentary Behavior Research Network (Tremblay et al., 2017, p. 9) defined sedentariness as "any waking behavior characterized by an energy expenditure ≤ 1.5 metabolic equivalents (METs), while in a sitting, reclining, or lying posture." Accordingly, it is of great importance to reveal body posture from the acceleration device to estimate sedentariness.

In a methodological paper, Giurgiu, Niermann, Ebner-Priemer, and Kanning (2020) described their approach for sedentariness-triggered assessments, combining an accelerometer with real-time analyses capabilities (move 4; www.movisens.com) via Bluetooth Low Energy to an e-diary (movisensXS; www.movisens.com) for real-time feedback. In detail, a thigh-worn sensor analyzes data on body position (differentiating between a sitting or lying position, and an upright position; for details on how to get body position data from accelerative signals, see Chapter 5, this volume) and sends this information in real time to the smartphone. Each time a specific, uninterrupted amount of time was spent in a sedentary posture (e.g., 20 or 30 minutes), the e-diary was triggered.

Giurgiu, Niermann, and colleagues (2020) could show in multiple datasets that the sedentariness-triggered algorithm captured about 83% of all sedentary bouts, which was superior to simulations of randomly triggered prompts. These authors even argued that not using a sedentariness-triggered design poses the risk of an incomplete picture of sedentariness since rare events (such as sedentary bouts while on public transport) might be missed. Convincingly, the authors argued that their real-time feedback algorithm might be the prospective basis for just-in-time adaptive interventions (JITAIs; Nahum-Shani et al., 2018) to reduce sedentariness and its negative health outcomes.

As JITAIs are handled by Nahum-Shani in Chapter 30, this volume, we just want to emphasize that tailored suggestions for physical activity based on context (Klasnja et al., 2019) or on past activity (Mayer et al., 2018) are promising, as is the possibility of detecting eating behavior via accelerometry. Goldstein, Hoover, Evans, and Thomas (2021) report on an accelerative-device-driven algorithm that tracks eating lapses in obese participants, demonstrating discrepancies of reports (and their distributions) that compare device-based detection to time-based e-diary assessments. Expanding on such a setup, Mondol and colleagues (2020) report a system that combines smart wearables, smartphones, Bluetooth beacons, and an eating gesture detection algorithm to monitor family eating dynamics in all members of a family simultaneously.

Activity-Triggered E-Diaries: Empirical Findings

The activity-triggered approach has been successfully used in a series of studies to tackle the real-life relationship between physical activity and mood in healthy populations (Reichert et al., 2016, 2017) and patient samples (Reichert, Schlegel, et al., 2020), in students (Kanning, Ebner-Priemer, & Brand, 2012), and the elderly (Kanning, Ebner-Priemer, & Schlicht, 2015), showing that both constructs are associated across time. Using activity-triggered e-diaries, Reichert and colleagues (2016) revealed that mood is an antecedent driving spontaneous nonexercise activity (such as climbing stairs or catching the train) within a person's everyday life (replicated by Koch et al., 2018, in adolescents). Reichert and colleagues (2017) also found that structured exercise activities (such as jogging and playing soccer) versus spontaneous nonexercise activities (such as climbing stairs, catching the train) do show distinct within-subject effects on mood (replicated for incidental activities by Koch et al., 2020, in adolescents).

Similar to activity-triggered approaches, the sedentariness-triggered e-diaries not only revealed superiority in methodological studies over and above pure random sampling but could also contribute substantial findings to the existing literature (Kanning, Niermann, Ebner-Priemer, & Giurgiu, 2021). To reduce sedentary time, for example, with JITAIs, it is important to understand its antecedents and consequences, as well as its social and environmental contexts, such as where, when, and with whom it takes place, and what people are doing while being sedentary. Giurgiu and colleagues (2019; Giurgiu,

Plotnikoff, et al., 2020) investigated the relationship between sedentary behavior and mood in everyday life and found evidence of a reciprocal relationship between both constructs. Put simply, being more sedentary in daily life led to lower levels of well-being and energy (Giurgiu et al., 2019), whereas higher momentary ratings of valence and energetic arousal predicted lower amounts of subsequent sedentary behavior, moderated by context (home vs. work; Giurgiu, Plotnikoff, et al., 2020). In addition, the article by Giurgiu, Koch, and colleagues (2020) was one of the first studies indicating that in everyday life on a within-subject level, breaking up sedentary behavior may indeed enhance one's mood.

GPS-Triggered Diaries: Empirical Findings

Contextual factors have a critical impact on human behavior, emotions, thoughts, and symptomatology. Examples from a clinical perspective include the influence of interpersonal interactions at work on depressive symptomatology, the occurrence of anxiety and panic in an elevator, and substance use depending on the social setting or persons present. Thus, when assessing human behavior, emotions, thoughts, and symptomatology, knowledge of context is of great importance. Fortunately, aspects of context can be estimated via geolocation (e.g., via GPS tracking). Froehlich and colleagues (2006) had 15 years before already assessed the geolocation and investigated its relationship to personal experience, combining e-diaries with GPS tracking. Again using geolocation tracking, Epstein and colleagues (2014) showed a decreased craving in polydrug users when being located in more disordered neighborhoods. In a similar vein, Gustafson and colleagues (2014) implemented real-time feedback based on GPS data into a smartphone application, aiming to provide mental support for patients with alcohol use disorder when approaching their favorite bar.

Real-time analyses of GPS data during patients' daily lives allow detection of situations/contexts of interest and obtaining additional parameters and information via GPS-triggered assessments. The goal here again is to be able to obtain detailed information in very specific situations. One of the first examples of GPS-triggered diaries is the landmark study from Froehlich, Chen, Smith, and Potter (2006) with the intriguing title "Voting with Your Feet: An Investigative Study of the Relationship between Place Visit Behaviour and Preference." They triggered new e-diary assessments, when the analyzed GPS signal shifted from "mobile" to "stationary" and remained in that state for at least 10 minutes, revealing a new place visit.

In a more recent study, we investigated how inner-city green spaces relate to affective well-being and its neurobiological underpinnings (Tost et al., 2019). Prior work suggested that urbanicity had negative effects on the prevalence of mental disorders and also on neural social stress processing. However, the underlying factors of these negative effects (such as air pollution and light or noise exposure) remained unknown. To shed light on these questions, Tost and colleagues (2019) monitored whereabouts continuously over 1 week using GPS tracking in two separate samples (33 participants and 52 participants, respectively). A combined assessment strategy was implemented so that mood ratings were collected via GPS-triggered e-diaries as well as via time-based samplings, that is, the assessments were randomly prompted during the daytime within a range of 40 to 100 minutes. The GPS-trigger algorithm monitored the distance between the current and the previous locations of the participants in real time and triggered additional e-diary assessments, whenever distances larger than 500 meters were covered. The sampling strategy was implemented in movisensXS (movisens GmbH, https://xs.movisens.com).

The algorithm was based on two methodological studies showing the superiority of GPS-triggered e-diary assessment when searching for rare environmental contexts, such as parks and other areas with high green density (Dorn et al., 2015; Törnros et al., 2016). In detail, Dorn and colleagues (2015) added a spatial component incorporating the land use associated with the participant's location, resulting in more unique trigger positions and an increase of triggers at less frequently visited land uses, helping to obtain a spatial spreading of the e-diary assessed locations. Törnros and colleagues (2016) simulated four different sampling schemes: two location-based sampling schemes incorporating the environmental characteristics (land use and population density), a pure time-based sampling scheme triggering reports every hour as well as an activity-triggered design. Their location-based sampling obtained more unique trigger positions, more triggers during rarely visited types of land use, and a greater spatial spread compared to the sampling strategies based on time or distance.

However, the GPS-triggered e-diaries not only were interesting from a methodological perspective but also delivered meaningful findings concerning content (Tost et al., 2019). Urban greenery (lawns, shrubs, trees) were mapped via high-resolution (20 × 20 cm) aerial photographs of the region to momentary mood ratings. Both samples of Tost and colleagues (2019) showed a positive relationship between urban greenery and mood. Multilevel analyses revealed a green space-induced mood enhancement. In addition, interindividual differences of this intraindividual relationship suggest that individuals with higher psychological risk especially benefited from this momentary mechanism, as well as participants who showed less activation in the dorsolateral prefrontal cortex (a structure associated with emotion regulation) during negative emotion processing. In further analyses on this dataset with GPS-triggered e-diaries, Reichert, Braun, and colleagues (2020) were able to show a specific association of everyday life activity with momentary mood ratings mediated by the subgenual part of the anterior cingulate cortex, a key emotion regulatory site.

In an ongoing multisite addiction research consortium (Heinz et al., 2020), we are assessing trajectories of losing and regaining control over drug intake. From a methodological perspective, this is challenging as multiple time frames might be of importance at the same time. Losing control might happen subtly over many months, but also on an hourly basis. Accordingly, we set up a sophisticated time-based design with various real-time algorithms to catch meaningful variance across different time frames, with a 12-month assessment period per participant. Specifically, we implemented geofence-triggered e-diaries. Drinking spots in the study region were subjected to a digital map. An interactive algorithm triggers participants to fill out e-diary assessments when they approach such a spot.

Physiology-Triggered E-Diaries: Empirical Findings

The godfather of triggered diaries is, without doubt, Michael Myrtek. He started a research program developing physiology-triggered e-diaries in the 1990s (summarized in Myrtek, 2004) as a member of the Psychophysiological Research Group at the University of Freiburg (Germany). Being interested in psychophysiological covariation in daily life, he developed a real-time algorithm to separate emotional and physical influences on physiological processes, the so-called additional heart rate. As extensively explicated by de Geus and Gevonden in Chapter 6, this volume, on physiological measures in daily life, physiological processes heavily depend on physical behavior, such as physical activity and posture (see also Brouwer, van Dam, van Erp, Spangler, & Brooks, 2018). In detail, physiological processes are more dependent on posture (more explained variance) than on psychological processes (less explained variance). Accordingly, it is inevitable to control for these confounds, if we are interested in the psychological influences such as emotions or stress on these physiological processes. Myrtek (2004) called the heart rate part, which was partly corrected for activity influences, "additional heart rate." As pronounced affective episodes are quite rare in daily life (i.e., they do not happen several times a day in regular intervals; for an excellent illustration of such a rare occasion, see Wilhelm & Grossman, 2010), Myrtek monitored heart rate and physical activity in daily life and separated in real time heart rate increases, which were not caused by physical activity, the so-called additional heart rate. This additional heart rate was taken as a physiological indicator of momentary emotional activation or mental stress (for a critical view and alternative possibilities to explore real-life estimates of emotion based on heart rate, see Brouwer et al., 2018). When the recorder–analyzer system detected that the additional heart rate exceeded a certain threshold, a handheld PC was triggered, which in turn signaled the participant to self-report momentary affective states. Our earlier reported activity-triggered diary methods were strongly influenced by Myrtek's work, as he already integrated currently used components such as adaptive thresholds and time-limit events. His real-time additional-heart-rate-triggered algorithm has been used and validated in many studies measuring a total of 1,300 participants over a 24-hour period each (Myrtek, 2004); these studies investigated psychological phenomena such as interoception, perceptions of emotions, as well as stress at work and during leisure time. Unfortunately, applications of physiology-triggered diaries in everyday life are still extremely rare, which can be partly explained by the fact that most physiological recorder systems do not provide real-time analyses and interfaces for e-diaries. However, the progress in mobile digital technology in the last decade has made such approaches much easier to implement, and, although still far from being a mainstream method, we see new studies with physiology-triggered e-diaries popping up occasionally. We will report those studies in the next section of this chapter.

More recent studies that used the original algorithm by Myrtek (2004) did investigate, for example, the relation between affect, memory, and physiological processes in daily life. Loeffler, Myrtek, and Peper (2013) could demonstrate that psychophysiological arousal (additional heart rate) at the time of encoding word lists in daily life, enhanced the recall of negative words in negative emotional conditions, whereas low psychophysiological arousal did facilitate the recall of positive words, therewith evidencing the ecological validity of traditional laboratory findings. In a follow-up paper, Loeffler and Peper (2014) broadened their findings to include psychophysiological instability. Ebner-Priemer and colleagues (2008; Ebner-Priemer, Welch, et al., 2007) also used Myrtek's original algorithm to investigate psychophysiological covariation in patients with borderline personality disorder. Although they could show, as expected, heightened additional heart rate in the patient sample (Ebner-Priemer, Welch, et al., 2007) as well as significant relations between affective reports and physiological parameters in daily life (Ebner-Priemer et al., 2008), investigating physiological parameters in mental health samples comes with limitations as some mental health medications are known for their effects on cardiovascular processes (Ebner-Priemer, Welch, et al., 2007).

In a more recent paper, Hoemann and colleagues (2020) used a physiology-triggered e-diary approach, which they label "context-aware experience sampling." They used real-time analyses to trigger e-diaries during heart rate increases, which were not accompanied by physical activity. Due to technical reasons, they only used 8-hour recordings and manually adjusted thresholds. As a novel and promising approach, they used machine learning to better understand the huge variability within and between participants as well as within and across emotion categories (see also Hoemann et al., 2021).

Van Halem, Van Roekel, Kroencke, Kuper, and Denissen (2020) reported a very rare example of an electrodermal-activity-triggered e-diary. Electrodermal activity (EDA) is a very interesting signal, as it is purely driven by sympathetic activity. This is in contrast to heart rate, which is driven by sympathetic and parasympathetic branches of the heart (for details, see the contribution of de Geus and Gevonden in Chapter 6, this volume). EDA is less robust and not so easy to assess in daily life. However, van Halem and colleagues (2020) provided participants with gelled electrodes attached to the palmar surface and added kinesiology tape and special gloves to ensure proper fit in daily life situations. Triggers were both random and based on momentary increases in the skin conductance level (SCL) controlled for physical activity (steps). The algorithm was implemented in movisensXS in combination with an EdaMove3 sensor (both from www.movisens.com). As an adaptive algorithm was not at hand, van Halem and colleagues based their thresholds at the beginning of each recording on a previously acquired distribution of SCL values. During the ongoing recording, they increasingly complemented the group threshold by personal cutoffs based on the person's own SCL distribution. As hypothesized, the authors could show a meaningful relation between sympathetic activation (SCL) and subjective ratings of arousal and positive energy. Even more worth reading is their methodological considerations on how to define future SCL-triggered e-diaries, taking the dependency of level and slope of these signals into account (law of initial values). The groundwork for heart rate variability-triggered e-diaries has been set by Verkuil, Brosschot, Tollenaar, Lane, and Thayer (2016).

Audio- or Video-Triggered E-Diaries: Empirical Findings

Wu and colleagues (2021) reported a fascinating approach using hearing aids to trigger e-diaries to shed light on compliance and missing data in e-diary assessments. In detail, they recruited hearing aid users and provided specific study hearing aids capable of logging and transmitting environmental sound information in real time to a connected smartphone which in turn triggered e-diary assessments. Logging data on unanswered e-diary prompts revealed that missing data occurred systematically in situations that were less quiet and contained more speech, noise, and machine sounds, pointing to more challenging environments. Regarding the advantages of using real-time analyses and feature extraction of highly sensitive data on privacy, see also the section "Conclusions, Limitations, and Future Prospects" on future prospects in this chapter. Regarding video data, real-time analysis and logging using Google glasses have been described (e.g., by Ye, Moynagh, Albatal, & Gurrin, 2014).

Enhancing Passive Mobile Sensing with E-Diary Assessments

Although up to now we have highlighted just the advantages of adding mobile sensing to classical e-diary research, especially promoting the possibilities of continuous real-time analyses and sensor-triggered diaries, the opposite method, enhancing mobile sensing with e-diary assessments, is, of course, also very promising. Whereas mobile sensing data can be assessed over prolonged periods of time with a high sampling frequency and low participant burden, those parameters (like smartphone on/off, number of phone calls, physical activity estimated by GPS, and acceleration data of the smartphone) are mostly not the psychological parameters of interest but rather are just approximations of psychologically relevant parameters. This becomes evident when we look at physical activity. Physical activity has been successfully used to predict the course of Parkinson's disease, depressive symptomatology, the success of hip replacement, cancer-related fatigue, fitness level, epileptic seizure, personality traits, pain, cardiovascular processes, manic episodes, and so on. But what do we know if we detect decreased physical activity over the past week in a given participant? Is this evidence for increased pain, for an upcoming depressive episode, for influenza, or for COVID? Considering classical psychometric concepts, the reliability in assessing physical activity via accelerometers is usually high, but the validity clearly depends on the construct of interest. Frankly, many digital phenotyping parameters are unspecific (data upload, incoming calls, battery power) and are not very closely related to the psychological phenomena of interest. E-diary assessments can help to better understand mobile sensing parameters.

The automated real-time prediction of upcoming affective episodes in patients with bipolar disorder may serve as an example to further elaborate this issue. In this scenario, mobile sensing or digital phenotyping is a prime candidate (Ebner-Priemer & Santangelo, 2020; Ebner-Priemer et al., 2020), as mobile sensing parameters are closely related to the psychopathology of interest (e.g., altered sleep, altered activity, altered communicativeness) and prevention of new episodes is a major treatment goal. The basic idea of these approaches is quite simple. Namely, those mobile sensing parameters that are closely related to psychopathological features are monitored and analyzed in real time, and if an algorithm detects that a critical number of parameters exceed certain thresholds, the patient or the treating psychiatrist is alarmed (Mühlbauer et al., 2018). However, how do we train such an algorithm? We need high-resolution ground truth labels to learn what critical thresholds and parameters are.

The golden standard in digital phenotyping in bipolar patients was for a long time to have diagnostic interviews each month (Ebner-Priemer & Santangelo, 2020). However, such assessments do not deliver dimensional fluctuating values of real-time psychopathology continuously over prolonged periods of time. In other words, with such infrequent assessments a precise determination of a beginning new episode is impossible. However, this would be exactly the information we need for training our algorithms. Thus, a more promising approach is to statistically combine retrospective dimensional and categorical interviews (covering the last weeks) with daily e-diary self-ratings, resulting in a latent psychopathology variable dimensionally fluctuating from day to day (see Ebner-Priemer et al., 2020). In other words, mobile sensing can profit from e-diaries to fully leverage its potential.

Conclusions, Limitations, and Future Prospects

As stated several times in this chapter, we see great potential in combining passive mobile sensing with more active e-diary assessments, leveraging benefits for both approaches. Or stated in other words, we do not understand what we consider an artificial differentiation between mobile sensing and e-diary assessments. Both share the same advantages and goals, like getting ecological valid data in real time to model within-subject dynamics, predicting upcoming events, and delivering personalized interventions at the right moments. Accordingly, our technological setup, the Ambulatory Assessment toolbox (see

Figure 13.2), intertwines both approaches inseparably (see also Kubiak & Smyth, 2019, for such a mobile sensing framework).

The Ambulatory Assessment toolbox expanded significantly during the last decade. Meanwhile, location tracking and sensing smartphone parameters (digital phenotypes) complement the more classical parameters such as e-diaries and physiological assessments. Real-time onboard analyses, in addition, enable all kinds of triggered diaries, real-time predictions, and just-in-time interventions. They all support our ambition to understand, predict, and change human behavior and experience in daily life.

After praising the advantages of combining mobile sensing with e-diary assessments, we have to describe some practical and a few more specific limitations. First, not all wearables and e-diary systems can conduct real-time analyses and provide interfaces to work together properly. Accordingly, we emphasize that if real-time interactions between sensor and smartphone are of interest, a careful selection of devices and extensive testing are indispensable. Second, technological possibilities for sensor-triggered assessments increase steadily. To infer social interactions, Bluetooth and Radio-Frequency Identification tracking of nearby devices can be used; to track physical activity and traveling, Magnetometer and Geolocation are useful; weather conditions assessed by barometers and microphone, camera, and touch sensors offer additional possibilities for potential sensor-triggered assessments. However, for psychological phenomena for which no continuously accessible objective data exist, real-time monitoring and analyses to trigger e-diary assessments are an option. In such cases, proxies for psychological assessments are used, sometimes with limited validity. Accordingly, heart rate variability is a common proxy for relaxation, stress, rumination, and cognitive demands, just to name a few.

Third, another related limitation concerns the frequency of the phenomena of interest. Triggered e-diaries will only be able to prompt participants if the expected behavior occurs. For example, if researchers are interested in drinking episodes in bars, but the participant does not visit these spots, there will be no drinking-spot-triggered assessments. Thus, to actually profit from the sensor-triggered assessments to increase insights into the variable of interest over and above a time-triggered assessment scheme, one has to choose the triggers with great care

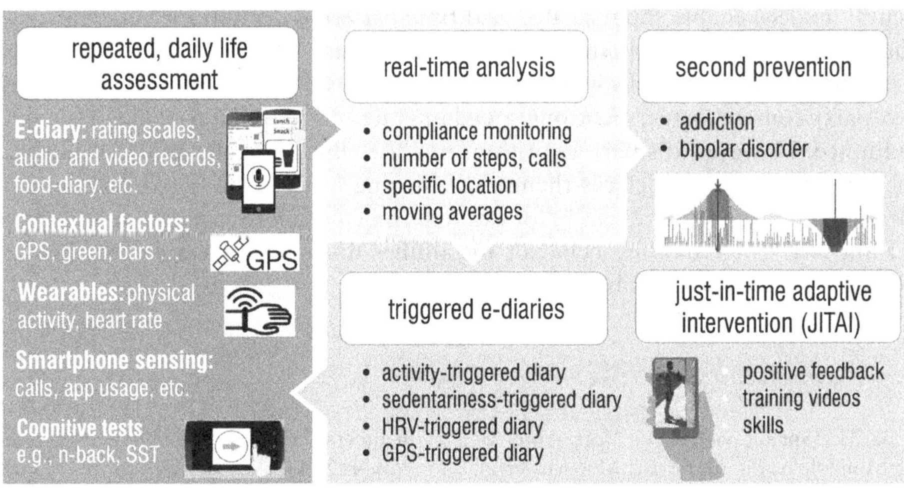

FIGURE 13.2. Ambulatory Assessment toolbox.

Fourth, algorithms cannot foresee the duration of events. If we aim to understand the psychological effects of strolling, it remains difficult to initiate an e-diary assessment directly after such an event, as we do not know its total duration in advance. In other words, triggering an assessment after 30 minutes of strolling might come too early, as the participant would show this behavior for a whole hour (for a discussion on timing, see also op den Akker, Moualed, Jones, & Hermens, 2011). Even more convincing examples can be made for sedentariness. To investigate the activity–affect relation, we triggered e-diaries after a defined period of activity. However, another promising approach might be to search for 5 minutes of rest terminating a physical activity episode. This would answer questions regarding how participants feel after episodes of physical activity and not during such episodes. Unfortunately, the dynamic processes and relations of psychological phenomena are still rarely investigated (Trull, Lane, Koval, & Ebner-Priemer, 2015). Combining different sampling procedures (such as sensor-triggered prompts, time-out prompts [when the searched phenomenon is not at hand for a given period], and pure random prompts) might help to enlarge the amount of variance captured.

Fifth, when investigating the advantages of sensor-triggered e-diaries, the most convincing evidence would be to show increased correlations between both parameters of interests (such as physical activity and mood) when using sensor-triggered e-diaries compared to time-based assessments in a single dataset. Unfortunately, there are no datasets at hand that simultaneously used sensor-triggered and time-based assessment of the same participant during the same time frame. More sophisticated designs should be implemented in future studies.

As the last limitation, we mention that sensor-triggered e-diaries with interventional feedback (which might overlap conceptually with just-in-time adaptive interventions by a large degree) might fall under specific regulation by respective authorities, such as the FDA (U.S. Food and Drug Administration) or the EMA (European Medicines Agency), which might come with tremendous restrictions regarding both hard- and software.

Quite briefly, we want to report on future prospects. All the current developments in technology, such as making devices mobile, smart, connected, and miniaturized (Ponnada et al., 2022), will push these methods, as well as their widespread use in the general population. In addition, recent advances in artificial intelligence (AI; such as deep-learning or all-neural models) enable sophisticated real-time pattern detection for personalized psychology (Koppe, Guloksuz, Reininghaus, & Durstewitz, 2019). The next major step, at least in our view, might be AI solving current data protection problems in mobile sensing. In two-party consent states, recording social interactions via speech or video is currently quite limited. However, if smart algorithms might enable real-time analyses and feature extraction on the mobile devices themselves, storing just the extracted pseudonymized features might push future research, for example, on emotion recognition in speech (Salekin et al., 2017) or on eating behavior in families documented via videos (Bell et al., 2019), just to name two possibilities.

REFERENCES

Bell, B. M., Spruijt-Metz, D., Vega Yon, G. G., Mondol, A. S., Alam, R., Ma, M., et al. (2019). Sensing eating mimicry among family members. *Translational Behavioral Medicine, 9*(3), 422–430.

Bolger, N., Davis, A., & Rafaeli, E. (2003).

Diary methods: Capturing life as it is lived. *Annual Review of Psychology, 54*, 579–616.

Brouwer, A. M., van Dam, E., Van Erp, J. B., Spangler, D. P., & Brooks, J. R. (2018). Improving real-life estimates of emotion based on heart rate: A perspective on taking metabolic heart rate into account. *Frontiers in Human Neuroscience, 12*, Article 284.

Csikszentmihalyi, M., & Larson, R. (1987). Validity and reliability of the experience-sampling method. *Journal of Nervous and Mental Disease, 175*(9), 526–536.

Dejonckheere, E., & Erbas, Y. (2021). Designing an experience sampling study. In I. Myin-Germeys & P. Kuppens (Eds.), *The open handbook of experience sampling methodology: A step-by-step guide to designing, conducting, and analyzing ESM studies* (pp. 33–70). Center for Research on Experience Sampling and Ambulatory Methods.

Dorn, H., Törnros, T., Reichert, M., Salize, H-J., Tost, H., Ebner-Priemer, U., et al. (2015). Incorporating land use in a spatiotemporal trigger for ecological momentary assessments. *GI_Forum—Journal for Geographic Information Science*, 1–2015, 113–116.

Dunton, G. F., Dzubur, E., & Intille, S. (2016). Feasibility and performance test of a real-time sensor-informed context-sensitive ecological momentary assessment to capture physical activity. *Journal of Medical Internet Research, 18*(6), Article No. e106.

Ebner-Priemer, U. W., Koudela, S., Mutz, G., & Kanning, M. (2013). Interactive multimodal ambulatory monitoring to investigate the association between physical activity and mood. *Frontiers in Psychology, 3*, Article No. 596.

Ebner-Priemer, U. W., Kuo, J., Kleindienst, N., Welch, S. S., Reisch, T., Reinhard, I., et al. (2007). State affective instability in borderline personality disorder assessed by ambulatory monitoring. *Psychological Medicine, 37*(7), 961 970.

Ebner-Priemer, U. W., Kuo, J., Schlotz, W., Kleindienst, N., Rosenthal, Z., Detterer, L., et al. (2008). Distress and affective dysregulation in patients with Borderline Personality Disorder: A psychophysiological ambulatory monitoring study. *Journal of Nervous and Mental Disease, 196*(4), 314–320.

Ebner-Priemer, U. W., Mühlbauer, E., Neubauer, A. B., Hill, H., Beier, F., Santangelo, P., et al. (2020). Digital phenotyping—Towards replicable findings with comprehensive assessments and integrative models in bipolar disorders. *International Journal of Bipolar Disorders, 8*, Article No. 35.

Ebner-Priemer, U., & Santangelo, P. (2020). Digital phenotyping: Hype or hope? *Lancet Psychiatry, 7*(4), 297–299.

Ebner-Priemer, U. W. & Sawitzki, G. (2007). Ambulatory assessment of affective instability in Borderline Personality Disorder—The effect of the sampling frequency. *European Journal of Psychological Assessment, 23*(4), 238–247.

Ebner-Priemer, U. W., Welch, S. S., Grossman, P., Reisch, T., Linehan, M. M., & Bohus, M. (2007). Psychophysiological ambulatory assessment of affective dysregulation in Borderline Personality Disorder. *Psychiatry Research, 150*(3), 265–275.

Epstein, D. H., Tyburski, M., Craig, I. M., Phillips, K. A., Jobes, M. L., Vahabzadeh, M., et al. (2014). Real-time tracking of neighborhood surroundings and mood in urban drug misusers: Application of a new method to study behavior in its geographical context. *Drug and Alcohol Dependence, 134*, 22–29.

Fahrenberg, J., & Myrtek, M. (Eds.). (1996). *Ambulatory assessment. Computer-assisted psychological and psychophysiological methods in monitoring and field studies*. Hogrefe.

Fahrenberg, J., Myrtek, M., Pawlik, K., & Perrez, M. (2007). Ambulatory assessment-monitoring behavior in daily life settings. *European Journal of Psychological Assessment, 23*(4), 206–213.

Froehlich, J., Chen, M. Y., Smith, I. E., & Potter, F. (2006, September). Voting with your feet: An investigative study of the relationship between place visit behavior and preference. In P. Dourish & A. Friday (Eds.), *UbiComp 2006: Ubiquitous Computing. 8th International Conference* (pp. 333–350). Springer.

Giurgiu, M., Koch, E. D., Ottenbacher, J., Plotnikoff, R. C., Ebner-Priemer, U. W., & Reichert, M. (2019). Sedentary behavior in everyday life relates negatively to mood: An ambulatory assessment study. *Scandinavian Journal of Medicine and Science in Sports, 29*(9), 1340–1351.

Giurgiu, M., Koch, E. D., Plotnikoff, R. C., Ebner-Priemer, U. W., & Reichert, M. (2020). Breaking up sedentary behavior optimally to enhance mood. *Medicine and Science in Sports and Exercise, 52*(2), 457–465.

Giurgiu, M., Niermann, C., Ebner-Priemer, U., & Kanning, M. (2020). Accuracy of sedentary behavior–triggered ecological momentary assessment for collecting contextual information: Development and feasibility study. *JMIR Mhealth and Uhealth, 9*, Article No. e17852.

Giurgiu, M., Plotnikoff, R. C., Nigg, C. R., Koch, E. D., Ebner-Priemer, U. W., & Reichert, M. (2020). Momentary mood predicts upcoming real-life sedentary behavior. *Scandinavian Journal of Medicine and Science in Sports, 30*(7), 1276–1286.

Goldstein, S. P., Hoover, A., Evans, E. W., & Thomas, J. G. (2021). Combining ecological momentary assessment, wrist-based eating detection, and dietary assessment to characterize dietary lapse: A multi-method study protocol. *Digital Health, 7*, Article No. 2055207620988212.

Gustafson, D. H., McTavish, F. M., Chih, M.-Y., Atwood, A. K., Johnson, R. A., Boyle, M. G., et al. (2014). A smartphone application to support recovery from alcoholism: A randomized clinical trial. *JAMA Psychiatry 71*(5), 566–572.

Hamaker, E. L. (2012). Why researchers should think "within-person": A paradigmatic rationale. In M. Mehl & T. Connor (Eds.), *Handbook of research methods for studying daily life* (pp. 43–61). Guilford Press.

Haskell, W. L., Lee, I. M., Pate, R. R., Powell, K. E., Blair, S. N., Franklin, et al. (2007). Physical activity and public health: Updated recommendation for adults from the American College of Sports Medicine and the American Heart Association. *Circulation, 116*(9), 1081–1093.

Heinz, A., Kiefer, F., Smolka, M., Endrass, T., Beste, C., Beck, A., et al. (2020). Losing and regaining control over drug intake—from trajectories to mechanisms and interventions. *Addiction Biology, 25*, Article No. e12866.

Hoemann, K., Khan, Z., Feldman, M. J., Nielson, C., Devlin, M., Dy, J., et al. (2020). Context-aware experience sampling reveals the scale of variation in affective experience. *Scientific Reports, 10*(1), 1–16.

Hoemann, K., Khan, Z., Kamona, N., Dy, J., Barrett, L. F., & Quigley, K. S. (2021). Investigating the relationship between emotional granularity and cardiorespiratory physiological activity in daily life. *Psychophysiology, 58*(6), Article No. e13818.

Kanning, M., Ebner-Priemer, U. W., & Brand, R. (2012). Autonomous regulation mode moderates the effect of actual physical activity on affective states: An ambulant assessment approach on the role of self-determination. *Journal of Sport and Exercise Psychology, 34*(2), 260–269.

Kanning, M., Ebner-Priemer, U. W., & Schlicht, W. (2013). How to investigate within-subject associations between physical activity and momentary affective states in everyday life: A position statement based on a literature overview. *Frontiers in Psychology, 4*, Article No. 187.

Kanning, M., Ebner-Priemer, U. W., & Schlicht, W. (2015). Using activity triggered e-diaries to reveal the associations between physical activity and affective states in elderly's daily living. *International Journal of Behavioral Nutrition and Physical Activity, 12*, Article 111.

Kanning, M., Niermann, C., Ebner-Priemer, U. W., & Giurgiu, M. (2021). The context matters—not all prolonged sitting bouts are equally related to momentary affective states: An ambulatory assessment with sedentary-triggered E-diaries. *International Journal of Behavioral Nutrition and Physical Activity, 18*, Article 106.

Klasnja, P., Smith, S., Seewald, N. J., Lee, A., Hall, K., Luers, B., et al. (2019). Efficacy of contextually tailored suggestions for physical activity: A micro-randomized optimization trial of HeartSteps. *Annals of Behavioral Medicine, 53*(6), 573–582.

Koch, E. D., Tost, H., Braun, U., Gan, G., Giurgiu, M., Reinhard, I., et al. (2018). Mood and physical activity in adolescents: Ambulatory assessment data reveals distinct within-subject associations between mood dimensions and non-exercise activity. *Frontiers in Psychology, 9*, Article No. 268.

Koch, E. D., Tost, H., Braun, U., Gan, G., Giurgiu, M., Reinhard, I., et al. (2020). Relationships between incidental physical activity, exercise, and sports with subsequent mood in adolescents. *Scandinavian Journal of Medicine and Science in Sports, 30*(11), 2234–2250.

Koppe, G., Guloksuz, S., Reininghaus, U., & Durstewitz, D. (2019). Recurrent neural networks in mobile sampling and intervention. *Schizophrenia Bulletin, 45*(2), 272–276.

Kubiak, T., & Smyth, J. M. (2019). Connecting domains—ecological momentary assessment in a mobile sensing framework. In H. Baumeister & C. Montag (Eds.), *Digital phenotyping and mobile sensing* (pp. 201–207). Springer.

Loeffler, S. N., Myrtek, M., & Peper, M. (2013). Mood-congruent memory in daily life: Evidence from interactive ambulatory monitoring. *Biological Psychology, 93*(2), 308–315.

Loeffler, S. N., & Peper, M. (2014). Affect and memory in real life: Evaluating the utility of interactive ambulatory assessment. *Zeitschrift für Neuropsychologie, 25*(4), 267–278.

Mayer, J. S., Hees, K., Medda, J., Grimm, O., Asherson, P., Bellina, M., et al. (2018). Bright light therapy versus physical exercise to prevent co-morbid depression and obesity in adolescents and young adults with attention-deficit/hyperactivity disorder: Study protocol for a randomized controlled trial. *Trials, 19*, Article No. 140.

Mehl, M. R., & Conner, T. S. (Eds.). (2012). *Handbook of research methods for studying daily life.* Guilford Press.

Meschtscherjakov, A., Reitberger, W., & Tscheligi, M. (2010, August). MAESTRO: Orchestrating user behavior driven and context triggered experience sampling. In E. Barakova, B. de Ruyter, & A. Spink (Eds.), *MB '10: Proceedings of the 7th International Conference on Methods and Techniques in Behavioral Research* (pp. 1–4). Association for Computing Machinery.

Mondol, M. A. S., Bell, B., Ma, M., Alam, R., Emi, I., Preum, S. M., et al. (2020). *MFED: A system for monitoring family eating dynamics.* https://arxiv.org/abs/2007.05831

Mühlbauer, E., Bauer, M., Ebner-Priemer, U. W., Ritter, P., Hill, H., Beier, F., et al. (2018). Effectiveness of smartphone-based ambulatory assessment (SBAA-BD) including a predicting system for upcoming episodes in the long-term treatment of patients with bipolar disorders: Study protocol for a randomized controlled single-blind trial. *BMC Psychiatry, 18*, Article 349.

Myrtek, M. (2004). *Heart and emotion: Ambulatory monitoring studies in everyday life.* Hogrefe & Huber.

Nahum-Shani, I., Smith, S. N., Spring, B. J., Collins, L. M., Witkiewitz, K., Tewari, A., et al. (2018). Just-in-time adaptive interventions (JITAIs) in mobile health: Key components and design principles for ongoing health behavior support. *Annals of Behavioral Medicine, 52*(6), 446–462.

op den Akker, H., Moualed, L. S., Jones, V. M., & Hermens, H. J. (2011). A self-learning personalized feedback agent for motivating physical activity. In S. Frattasi & N. Marchetti (Eds.), *ISABEL '11: Proceedings of the 4th international symposium on applied sciences in biomedical and communication technologies* (pp. 1–5). Association for Computing Machinery.

Ponnada, A., Wang, S., Chu, D., Do, B., Dunton, G., & Intille, S. (2022). Intensive longitudinal data collection using microinteraction ecological momentary assessment: Pilot and preliminary results. *JMIR Formative Research, 6*(2), e32772.

Reichert, M., Braun, U., Gan, G., Reinhard, I., Giurgiu, M., Ma, R., et al. (2020). A neural mechanism for affective well-being: Subgenual cingulate cortex mediates real-life effects of non-exercise activity on energy. *Science Advances, 6*, Article No. eaaz8934.

Reichert, M., Schlegel, S., Jagau, F., Ebner-Priemer, U. W., Hartmann, A., & Zeeck, A. (2020). Mood and dysfunctional cognitions constitute within-subject antecedents and consequences of exercise in eating disorders. *Psychotherapy and Psychosomatics, 89*(2), 119–121.

Reichert, M., Tost, H.; Reinhard, I., Schlotz, W., Zipf, A., Salize, H.-J., et al. (2017). Exercise vs. non-exercise activity: e-diaries unravel distinct effects on mood. *Medicine and Science in Sports and Exercise, 49*(6), 763–773.

Reichert, M., Tost, H., Reinhard, I., Zipf, A., Salize, H.-J., Meyer-Lindenberg, A., et al. (2016). Within-subject associations between mood dimensions and non-exercise activity: An ambulatory assessment approach using repeated real-time and objective data. *Frontiers in Psychology, 7*, Article No. 918.

Reis, H. T. (2012). Why researchers should think "real-world": A conceptual rationale. In M. Mehl & T. Connor (Eds.), *Handbook of research methods for studying daily life* (pp. 3–21). Guilford Press.

Salekin, A., Chen, Z., Ahmed, M. Y., Lach, J., Metz, D., De La Haye, K., et al. (2017). Distant emotion recognition. *Proceedings of the*

ACM on Interactive, Mobile, Wearable and Ubiquitous Technologies, 1(3), 1–25.

Santangelo, P., Bohus, M., & Ebner-Priemer, U. W. (2014). Ecological momentary assessment in borderline personality disorder: A review on recent findings and methodological challenges. *Journal of Personality Disorders, 28*(4), 555–576.

Schwarz, N. (2012). Why researchers should think "real-time": A cognitive rationale. In M. Mehl & T Connor (Eds.), *Handbook of research methods for studying daily life* (pp. 22–42). Guilford Press.

Schwerdtfeger, A., Eberhardt, R., & Chmitorz, A. (2008). Is there an association between everyday-life physical activity and psychological wellbeing?—A methodological study using ambulatory monitoring. *Zeitschrift für Gesundheitspsychologie, 16*(1), 2–11.

Shiffman, S. (2007). Designing protocols for ecological momentary assessment. In A. A. Stone, S. Shiffman, A. A. Atienza, & L. Nebeling (Eds.), *The science of real-time data capture: self-reports in health research* (pp. 27–53). Oxford University Press.

Stone A. A., Shiffman S. (1994). Ecological momentary assessment (EMA) in behavioral medicine. *Annals of Behavioral Medicine, 16*(3), 199–202.

Törnros, T., Dorn, H., Reichert, M., Ebner-Priemer, U. W., Salize, H.-J., Tost, H., et al. (2016). A comparison of temporal and location-based sampling strategies for GPS-triggered electronic diaries. *Geospatial Health, 11*(3), 335–341.

Tost, H., Reichert, M., Braun, U., Reinhard, I., Peters, R., Lautenbach, S., et al. (2019). Neural correlates of individual differences in affective benefit of real-life urban green space exposure. *Nature Neuroscience, 22*(9), 1389–1393.

Tremblay, M. S., Aubert, S., Barnes, J. D., Saunders, T. J., Carson, V., Latimer-Cheung, A. E., et al. (2017). Sedentary behavior research network (SBRN)–terminology consensus project process and outcome. *International Journal of Behavioral Nutrition and Physical Activity, 14*(1), 1–17.

Trull, T. J. & Ebner-Priemer, U. W. (2013). Ambulatory assessment. *Annual Review of Clinical Psychology, 9*, 151–176.

Trull, T. J., Lane, S. P., Koval, P., & Ebner-Priemer, U. W. (2015). Affective dynamics in psychopathology. *Emotion Review, 7*(4), 355–361.

van Halem, S., Van Roekel, E., Kroencke, L., Kuper, N., & Denissen, J. (2020). Moments that matter?: On the complexity of using triggers based on skin conductance to sample arousing events within an experience sampling framework. *European Journal of Personality, 34*(5), 794–807.

Verkuil, B., Brosschot, J. F., Tollenaar, M. S., Lane, R. D., & Thayer, J. F. (2016). Prolonged non-metabolic heart rate variability reduction as a physiological marker of psychological stress in daily life. *Annals of Behavioral Medicine, 50*(5), 704–714.

Wilhelm, F. H., & Grossman, P. (2010). Emotions beyond the laboratory: Theoretical fundaments, study design, and analytic strategies for advanced ambulatory assessment. *Biological Psychology, 84*(3), 552–569.

Wilhelm, P., Perrez, M., & Pawlik, K. (2012). Conducting research in daily life: A historical overview. In M. Mehl & T. Connor (Eds.), *Handbook of research methods for studying daily life* (pp. 62–86). Guilford Press.

World Health Organization. (2020). *WHO guidelines on physical activity and sedentary behaviour.* Author.

Wrzus, C., & Neubauer, A. B. (2021). Ecological momentary assessment: A meta-analysis on designs, samples, and compliance across research fields. *Assessment*, Article No. 10731911211067538.

Wu, Y. H., Xu, J., Stangl, E., Pentony, S., Vyas, D., Chipara, O., et al. (2021). Why ecological momentary assessment surveys go incomplete: When it happens and how it impacts data. *Journal of the American Academy of Audiology, 32*(1), 16–26.

Ye, T., Moynagh, B., Albatal, R., & Gurrin, C. (2014, August 27–29). *Real-time behavioural analysis using Google Glass.* Paper presented at the 9th International Conference on Methods and Techniques in Behavioral Research, Wageningen, the Netherlands.

PART III

Analysis of Mobile Sensing Data

CHAPTER 14

A Psychometric Perspective on Mobile Sensing Data

Michael Eid and Jana Holtmann

CHAPTER OVERVIEW

This chapter discusses how the three major psychometric criteria of objectivity, reliability, and validity can be applied to determine the quality of mobile sensing data. In particular, modern statistical approaches for analyzing interindividual and intraindividual measurement precision and reliability, and a combination of both, are described and illustrated. Based on a layered, hierarchical model for personal sensing data, several aspects of validity are discussed. In order to assess the validity of mobile sensing data, recommendations with respect to unit and value calibration are formulated. Several approaches for estimating the agreement of mobile sensing data with gold-standard measures (mean squared deviation, concordance correlation coefficient, limits of agreement, total deviation index, latent variable approaches) are presented and illustrated. Moreover, issues concerning construct, convergent, criterion-related, and ecological validity are examined. Finally, recommendations of the German Data Forum concerning data collection, reliability, and validity are presented.

Introduction

In recent years, wearable sensors have become an innovative measurement tool that has been increasingly applied in quite different areas of psychology (see Chapters 20 to 32, this volume). Like all other measurement tools of the empirical sciences, they have to meet certain quality standards to ensure that the data gathered in empirical studies can be trusted and that conclusions drawn from the results of these studies are valid. In this chapter, we discuss specific challenges of mobile sensing that are related to the three major psychometric quality criteria of objectivity, reliability, and validity. We will treat each quality criterion separately, and present psychometric approaches to analyze these quality criteria for mobile sensing data. We will focus on wearable sensors such as activity trackers but will discuss psychometric issues with respect to other types of sensor data (e.g., communication behavior) in the discussion section.

Data Collection and Objectivity

The first important step in the construction of a psychological measurement such as an ability test or a questionnaire is the process of item construction and item selection. The meaning of the psychological measurement strongly depends on the items and the way the item responses are integrated into a single (or multiple) measurement(s). This process has to be well documented, transparent, and traceable. Wearables do not consist of different items, but modern wearables assess a variety of different signals that are typically integrated into a single measurement. For example, accelerometers are widely used to assess physical activity (e.g., Henriksen, Johansson, Hartvigsen, Grimsgaard, & Hopstock, 2020; von Haaren-Mack, Bussmann, & Ebner-Priemer, 2020). Accelerometers differ not only in the sensors being used, but also in the way raw signals are filtered and processed (Chen, Janz, Zhu, & Brychta, 2012). Often, not the raw signals per se are stored but only the processed data (Chen et al., 2012). In order to understand the final measurement provided by a wearable, the data processing steps have to be well documented. However, in particular for consumer-wearable activity trackers, the data processing methods are typically not provided by sensor manufacturers but kept secret (Evenson, Goto, & Furberg, 2015). In particular, if the data stemming from different sensors are combined (e.g., using GPS data in combination with accelerometer and physiological measurement) to get a measure (e.g., indicating activity), the algorithm of combining the data is often not documented (Düking, Fuss, Holmberg, & Sperlich, 2018). Moreover, the data processing methods applied can change between hardware and software updates made by the same manufacturer, which complicates the comparison of measurements over time (Rat für Sozial, & Wirtschaftsdaten [RatSWD; German Data Forum], 2020). Therefore, the version of the sensors and software used should be well documented (Düking et al., 2018), and the benefits and drawbacks of using consumer products for scientific research should be seriously weighed against the use of scientific products (RatSWD, 2020).

Also, the correct placement of the wearable is important. For example, not all parts of the body are equally suited for the placement of wearable activity sensors, and there are areas that are preferable for specific purposes (Yang & Hsu, 2010). Moreover, placing sensors at multiple areas simultaneously is often necessary to get accurate measurements (Komukai & Ohmura, 2019). Therefore, the correct placement is important and concerns the quality standard of *objectivity* (e.g., Price, 2017), in particular *implementation objectivity* (Schermelleh-Engel, Kelava, & Moosbrugger, 2006). In this context, objectivity means that the result of the measurement does not depend on the person who has fixed the wearable at the body parts prescribed. In order to make an appropriate replication study possible, the documentation of the placement of the wearables is necessary (Düking et al., 2018).

As wearables can produce implausible data, it is recommended to check the data quality directly after the data collection (von Haaren-Mack et al., 2020) and remove implausible values. Depending on the researcher being responsible for data checking, the results could differ between researchers. This concerns the *statistical evaluation objectivity* (Schermelleh-Engel et al., 2006). All preprocessing steps conducted by a researcher before the creation of the final dataset have to be considered for judging statistical evaluation objectivity. Therefore, in order to make replication studies possible and to check the quality criterion of statistical evaluation objectivity, the datasets belonging to different steps of data preprocessing should be stored separately and every step of data preprocessing should be documented. Moreover, statistical evaluation objectivity also refers to all statistical analyses that are done using the data provided by wearables. If, for example, statistical learning methods are used for activity recognition (e.g., Balli & Sağbas, 2017), these analyses have to be documented (e.g., by providing the program codes along with the datasets).

Measurement Precision and Reliability

A second major quality criterion for psychological measurements is high measurement precision. The measurement of a psychological construct should not be distorted by measurement error. We use the term *construct* in a broad sense as a latent variable underlying an observable behavior, feeling, or thought. That means that behaviors such as bodily activity are also considered as constructs as they can typically not be assessed without measurement error. If one was able to measure a psychological construct under the same conditions repeatedly, the obtained measurement values should not differ from each other. However, measurement error cannot be completely avoided in empirical studies. Therefore, it is important to assess the degree of measurement precision. In measurement error theory, also called classical psychometric test theory (e.g., Lord & Novick, 1968; Steyer, 2015), an observed variable Y is decomposed into a latent true score variable T and a measurement error variable E:

$$Y = T + E \tag{14.1}$$

Moreover, the variance of the observed variable Y can be decomposed into the variance of the true score variable T and the variance of the measurement error variable E (Lord & Novick, 1968):

$$\sigma_Y^2 = \sigma_T^2 + \sigma_E^2 \tag{14.2}$$

The error variance σ_E^2 and the standard deviation of the error variable σ_E, the standard error of measurement (*SEM*), are measures of measurement precision. If the values of the observed variable stem from different individuals, the *SEM* indicates the degree of *inter*individual differences that are due to measurement error. If the values of the observed variable stem from the same individual (measured repeatedly), the *SEM* indicates the degree of *intra*individual differences that are due to measurement error. The smaller the *SEM*, the higher is the precision of measurement.

Because the value of the *SEM* depends on the metric of the observed variable, it is difficult to use the *SEM* to compare the precision of measurement across different measurements. In order to make the values comparable, the error variance can be divided by the variance of the observed variable. This *unreliability* coefficient

$$Unrel(Y) = \frac{\sigma_E^2}{\sigma_Y^2} \tag{14.3}$$

can take on values between 0 (perfect precision) and 1 (perfect imprecision). The counterpart of the unreliability coefficient is the *reliability* coefficient

$$Rel(Y) = \frac{\sigma_T^2}{\sigma_Y^2} \tag{14.4}$$

indicating the precision of measurement in a standardized form, taking on values from 0 (perfect imprecision) to 1 (perfect precision). If the values of the observed variable indicate interindividual differences, we call the reliability coefficient *interindividual reliability* (sometimes also called *between-person reliability*; Schuurman & Hamaker, 2019). If the values of the observed variables are repeatedly obtained from the same individual, we call it *intraindividual reliability* (sometimes also called *within-person reliability*; Schuurman & Hamaker, 2019). If multiple measurements are available from multiple individuals, interindividual differences in intraindividual reliability can be considered (see Holtmann, Eid, & Kanning, Chapter 15, this volume; Schuurman & Hamaker, 2019). All three aspects offer interesting insights into the measurement quality of wearables and will be shortly discussed.

Interindividual Precision and Reliability

High interindividual reliability is important if one is interested in interindividual differences. If a researcher wants to analyze interindividual differences in activity, it is important that interindividual differences in the observed activity scores mainly represent interindividual differences in true activity scores. High reliability values indicate that observed activity differences are mainly due to true activity differences. A reliability coefficient of 0 indicates that there are no true interindividual differences and that analyzing interindividual differences is not reasonable in a study.

Because the variance of an observed variable is decomposed into two parts (true score variance, error variance), it is not possible to estimate the true score and error variance based on one observed variable. In measurement error theory, measurement models have been developed that allow the estimation of the true score and error variances as well as the reliability coefficients. These models require that the construct of interest (e.g., activity) is assessed by multiple wearables (e.g., activity trackers, accelerometers) at the same time (see, e.g., Kubala et al., 2020). There are, in general, two approaches to obtain multiple measurements (e.g., Evenson et al., 2015; RatSWD, 2020): *Interdevice reliability* requires that the multiple wearables under study are the same products, that is, that they stem from the same production series of the same manufacturer and therefore do not differ in their general characteristics (parallel-form method; e.g., Eid & Schmidt, 2014). *Intradevice reliability* refers to the repeated measurement with the exact same device (retest method; e.g., Eid & Schmidt, 2014). Interindividual differences in fluctuations over time, however, only indicate measurement error influences if the construct under consideration is stable over time. If this is not the case, fluctuations are also due to true situational influences. Separating situational influences from measurement error in the case of only one measurement (with one device) on each occasion of measurement, however, requires the application of rather complex psychometric methods to disentangle unsystematic measurement error from systematic situational influences (RatSWD, 2020).

Therefore, application of the intradevice method for analysis of interindividual reliability is limited, and it is typically not applied (Evenson et al., 2015).

Classical unidimensional models of measurement error theory (classical test theory), which can be applied to estimate the reliability based on multiple measurements, assume that the different wearables measure the same construct C (e.g., activity). In the most general model, the model of τ-congeneric variables (Jöreskog, 1971), it is assumed that the true score variables T_i belonging to the different wearables ($i = 1, \ldots, k$) are linear functions of the common construct to be assessed:

$$T_i = \alpha_i + \lambda_i \cdot C \quad (14.5)$$

where α_i denotes an intercept term, λ_i a (factor) loading, and C the factor capturing the common construct measured by the true score variables T_i. Consequently, the observed variables can be decomposed in the following way:

$$Y_i = T_i + E_i = \alpha_i + \lambda_i \cdot C + E_i \quad (14.6)$$

For the variance of an observed variable, the following decomposition holds:

$$\sigma^2_{Y_i} = \sigma^2_{T_i} + \sigma^2_{E_i} = \lambda_i^2 \cdot \sigma^2_C + \sigma^2_{E_i} \quad (14.7)$$

Because the mean values of the error variables are $0(\mu_{E_i} = 0)$, the mean values of the observed variables are decomposed in the following way:

$$\mu_{Y_i} = \mu_{T_i} + \mu_{E_i} = \alpha_i + \lambda_i \cdot \mu_C \quad (14.8)$$

The intercepts α_i and the loading parameters λ_i indicate that the wearables can differ in the metric in which they assess the construct. For example, if body temperature is measured by one wearable in degrees Celsius and by another wearable in degrees Fahrenheit, the intercepts and loading parameters will differ, as Celsius and Fahrenheit measurements are linear functions of each other. Because the construct can be measured by methods that differ in their metrics—like Celsius and Fahrenheit—it is necessary to give the construct a metric in order to be able to give the scores of the construct C a meaning. This is also necessary for estimating the model parameters that depend on the metric of the construct chosen. There are different ways to give the factor a metric. For this chapter, we define the metric of a factor by fixing one intercept α_i to 0 and one factor loading λ_i to 1. For reasons of simplicity, these restrictions can be put on the first observed variable: $\alpha_1 = 0$ and $\lambda_1 = 1$. As a consequence, the construct equals the true score variable of the first observed variable: $C = T_1$

The model of τ-congeneric variables is a one-factor model of factor analysis. The parameters of the model—the intercepts α_i and loading parameters λ_i as well as the variances σ^2_C and $\sigma^2_{E_i}$—can be estimated if there are at least three observed variables (i.e., wearables applied). The assumptions of the models can be tested if there are at least four observed variables (wearables applied; e.g., Steyer, 2015). If the model fits the data, the error variances and the *SEM* of the wearables can be interpreted as the degree of interindividual imprecision, and the reliability coefficients can be estimated and interpreted as a measure of interindividual reliability. In order to estimate the parameters and test the model assumptions, software for confirmatory factor analysis (CFA), such as the freely available R package lavaan (Rosseel, 2012), can be used. Many textbooks are available showing how such models can be specified and tested (e.g., Gana & Broc, 2019, for lavaan; Brown, 2015, for other software packages such as LISREL, Mplus, EQS, and SAS/CALIS).

The requirement of at least four observed wearables for testing the model is demanding because wearing four wearables might not always be possible. However, several special cases of the model of τ-congeneric variables can be applied with fewer observed variables. For example, if the wearables (e.g., activity monitors) stem from the same production series and are placed at parts of the body that ensure the same construct is measured (see, e.g., Picard, Fedor, & Ayzenberg, 2016), they can be considered to be interchangeable. In this case, it is reasonable to assume that the single wearables do not differ in the intercepts, loadings, and error variances. These assumptions that define the model of τ-parallel variables can be tested, and the model parameters can be estimated with only two observed variables (e.g., two activity watches from the same product series). The model of τ-parallel variables implies that the observed variables do not differ in their means and variances. In this case, the reliability coefficient equals the intraclass correlation coefficient (ICC; McGraw & Wong, 1996). For example, according to the analyses by Kubala and colleagues (2020), the assumptions of equal means and equal variances seem to be reasonable for analyzing the reliability of activity monitors stemming from the same production series. These researchers found relatively large reliability coefficients for assessing sleep time by commercial activity monitors (ICC between .86 and .99).

BOX 14.1. Empirical Application: Measurement of Total Sleep Time with Activity Monitors

We will illustrate some statistical methods with a dataset that was simulated and based on results reported by Kubala and colleagues (2020). In their study, several commercial activity monitors were compared with a gold-standard accelerometer (Actiwatch). To estimate interdevice reliability, a subsample of participants had to wear two wearables of the same product line at the same time. We denote with CW the consumer wearable and GSW the gold-standard wearable. Data were simulated for 100 individuals. We use the simulated data only to describe the general proceeding and how results could be interpreted. In order to estimate the interdevice reliability, a model of τ-parallel variables was specified separately for each device. (As we show later in this chapter, the analyses of the different devices could also be combined in one model.) Such a model fits well for both CW ($\chi^2_2 = 2.357$, $df = 2$, $p = 0.308$) and GSW ($\chi^2_2 = 1.263$, $df = 2$, $p = 0.532$). Because the intercepts and error variances are equal within the model, three parameters were estimated for each model. The factor mean (mean sleeping time in minutes) is 464.375 for CW and 417.213 for GSW. The error variance for CW is 2,846.755 and 111.473 for GSW. Therefore, the *SEMs* are 53.355 (CW) and 10.558 (GSW). Because both wearables are measuring sleeping time with the same metric (minutes), the *SEMs* can be compared, showing that the measurement precision is higher for GSW than for CW. The factor variances are 17,185.086 (CW) and 5,970.908 (GSW). Therefore, the reliabilities are .858 (CW) and .982 (GSW). The results show that the measurement precision is very high for GSW but lower for CW.

Other special cases of the model of τ-congeneric variables are less restrictive than the model of τ-parallel variables (see, e.g., Bandalos, 2018; Eid & Schmidt, 2014; Steyer, 2015). All these models can be analyzed with computer programs for CFA, and they can be tested against each other to find the most parsimonious, well-fitting model. They can also be applied to test specific hypotheses about the measurement quality of different wearables.

Intraindividual Precision and Reliability

Intraindividual precision and reliability refer to the situation when the different scores of an observed variable stem from a single individual. Mobile sensing studies are often longitudinal studies in which individuals are repeatedly measured over many occasions of measurement. In such a design, the true score of an individual can vary across time, indicating variability in true states (e.g., momentary activity). Intraindividual reliability indicates to which degree the observed variability is due to true state variability (e.g., Hu et al., 2016). In fact, all the requirements that have been discussed for interindividual reliability are also true for intraindividual reliability by replacing individuals with occasions of measurement. In particular, multiple observed variables and a measurement model are required. However, traditional models of CFA can usually not simply be applied by just replacing individuals with occasions of measurement. Traditional unidimensional models of CFA assume that the units of measurement (e.g., individuals) are independent from each other. This assumption might not be reasonable for time-series data, in which a serial dependency of the scores across time is common (e.g., autocorrelation). In order to take care of this serial dependency, models of CFA for single-case data have been developed. For example, dynamic factor analysis (Browne & Zhang, 2007; Molenaar, 1985) allows the CFA of single-case data by taking the serial dependency into account. The freely available software DyFa2.03 (Browne & Zhang, 2005), and also the commercial program Mplus (Muthén & Muthén, 1998–2017), allow the estimation of a dynamic factor model. The assessment of individual *SEM* is necessary if one wants to use mobile sensing for individual assessment and calculate confidence intervals for person parameters (factor scores, true scores) under the assumption of individual differences in *SEM*.

Interindividual Differences in Intraindividual Precision and Reliability

If individuals differ in measurement precision, the analysis of such differences might be important for mobile sensing research in order to understand the conditions for measurement precision. The analysis of interindividual differences in intraindividual precision is possible if multivariate time-series data are available from many individuals (e.g., Schuurman & Hamaker, 2019). Recent developments in psychometric modeling such as dynamic structural equation modeling (DSEM; see Asparouhov, Hamaker, & Muthén, 2018; also see Holtmann et al., Chapter 15, this volume) allow the estimation of interindividual differences in intraindividual error variances (typically quantified with respect to the logarithm of the error variance).

Multivariate time series from multiple individuals also make it possible to analyze characteristics of the dynamic process. For example, interindividual differences in intraindividual variability (true systematic state fluctuations; e.g., Nesselroade & Ram, 2004) have gained interest in many different areas such as affect (e.g., Eid & Diener, 1999) or clinical psychology (e.g., Ebner-Priemer et al., 2007). Intraindividual variability and instability are typically assessed by the intraindividual standard deviation or the mean square successive difference (e.g., Ebner-Priemer, Eid, Kleindienst, Stabenow, & Trull, 2009). Interindividual reliability can also be estimated for dynamic features such as intraindividual variability (Du & Wang, 2018; Eid & Diener, 1999).

Validity

Validity is the most important quality criterion of empirical research. According to Messick (1989, p. 13), "validity is an integrated evaluative judgment of the degree to which empirical evidence and theoretical rationales support the *adequacy* and *appropriateness* of *inferences* and *actions* based on test scores and other modes of assessment." Hence, validity in mobile sensing research refers to all inferences based on mobile sensing data. These inferences can be quite complex and can refer to different levels of human behavior and experiences. Mohr, Zhang, and Schueller (2017) have proposed a layered, hierarchical model for personal sensing data that they consider a "sensemaking framework" (p. 25) and that could be used as a framework for validity studies. This model consists of four levels, ranging from different raw sensor data (lowest level) to different clinical constructs (highest level). In order to illustrate how this framework can be used for validity studies, the layers for three single-sensor types (location, movement, ambient light) are extracted from the more comprehensive figure in Mohr and colleagues (2017, Figure 1) and presented here in Table 14.1 along with respective validity issues. From a psychometric perspective, construct validity is the most important validity concept. It refers to the question of whether the inferences from the measurements to the underlying construct are adequate and appropriate (Messick, 1995). All other validity facets mentioned in Table 14.1—with the exception of ecological validity—are facets of construct validity and refer to specific inferences and strategies to analyze construct validity.

Level 1: Single Sensors

The different sensors are considered on Level 1 of Mohr and colleagues' (2017) framework. There exist, for example, many different accelerometers and activity trackers (e.g., Henriksen et al., 2020). They are applied for quite different purposes, for example, the monitoring of activity (e.g., duration, intensity), energy expenditure, or sleep (e.g., Henriksen et al., 2020; Kubala et al., 2020). Different sensors also differ in the way the raw signal is processed. Accelerometers, for example, can differ in their outcome measures (e.g., counts per unit time) because of "different transducers, amplifiers, sampling frequencies, and signal filters" (Chen et al., 2012, p. 15). There can be strong differences in the measurement quality between sensors, in particular, if consumer-based wearables are also applied (Peake, Kerr, & Sullivan, 2018). Therefore, a basic important question is to which degree these sensors measure what they intend to measure and to which degree inferences with respect to the intended purpose are valid. Two aspects have to be considered. The first aspect refers to the basic signals that are obtained (e.g., the number of steps counted) and whether these signals are the same (or very similar) when obtained by different sensors and—in the best case—by a gold-standard method. In order to analyze this question, different sensors have to be worn at the same time (e.g., Kubala et al.,

TABLE 14.1. Part of the Layered, Hierarchical Sensemaking Framework of Mohr et al. (2017) for Location and Movement Sensors

Layer	Relevant variables	Validity issues
Clinical state	Depression Anxiety Other clinical constructs	*Construct validity* Separating trait from state and dynamic aspects *Criterion-related validity* Prediction and separation of clinical constructs and groups by integration of different behavioral markers *Ecological validity* Representativeness of situations, contexts, time points?
High-level behavioral markers	Hedonic activity Psychomotor activity Fatigue Stress Social avoidance	*Construct validity* Appropriate integration of low-level features *Convergent validity* Convergence with nonsensor-based assessment of constructs (e.g., self-report, observer data)
Low-level features	Activity type (e.g., walk, run, or drive) Movement intensity Bedtime/waketime	*Construct validity* Assessment of context, annotations *Convergent validity* Convergence with nonsensor-based assessment of constructs (e.g., ambulatory self-report assessment, day reconstruction method)
Sensors	Location (e.g., GPS or Wi-Fi) Movement (e.g., gyroscope or accelerometer) Ambient light	*Construct/convergent validity* Gold-standard validation

Note. The first two columns are extracted from Figure 1 in Mohr et al. (2017, p. 26).

2020). High agreement across sensors indicates high convergent validity. The second aspect refers to the validity of the conclusions drawn with respect to the intended purpose. Because the data obtained by a sensor can be used for different purposes, validity with respect to each purpose has to be analyzed, and the validity of the conclusions obtained by the same sensor can differ between purposes (Bassett, Rowlands, & Trost, 2012). One way to analyze this type of validity is to compare the sensor measures with gold-standard methods for different purposes. For example, a gold-standard method for the measurement of sleep is polysomnography (Kubala et al., 2020), and a gold-standard method for the assessment of energy expenditure is the doubly labeled water technique (Plasqui & Westerterp, 2007).

Calibration

A first important aspect for analyzing the quality of a sensor and a basis for validity studies is *calibration* (Bassett et al., 2012). Bassett and colleagues (2012) distinguish between two types of calibration: unit calibration and value calibration. *Unit calibration* refers to the question of whether a sensor correctly measures the direct signal. It can be analyzed by gold-standard physical calibration checks (see Bassett et al., 2012). *Value calibration* refers to the transformation of a direct signal into other measurement units that are needed for the intended purpose (Bassett et al., 2012). For example, for measuring energy expenditure or activity intensity by accelerometers, different value calibrations are necessary (Bassett et al., 2012). Value calibration of accelerometers, for example, requires that data from (1) multiple individuals being representative for the intended population who (2) perform different activities (covering an appropriate range of intensity and being representative for the intended purpose), (3) obtained by different wearables, and (4) simultaneously assessed criterion variables are collected (Bassett et al., 2012; Welk, 2005). Based on these data, value calibration can be done by applying statistical methods such as regression analysis or pattern recognition methods (Bassett et al., 2012; see Chapters 17 and 18, this volume, on machine learning and neural networks, respectively). Bassett and colleagues discuss the strengths and weaknesses of different value calibration methods. After calibration has been done, the validity of conclusions that are drawn based on these derived values has to be assessed in validation studies by analyzing the convergence and agreement with gold-standard methods.

Agreement

Agreement indicates the similarity of two measures. Choudhary and Nagaraja (2017, p. 6) define perfect agreement by $P(Y_1 = Y_2) = 1$, where Y_1 and Y_2 are two different measurements and P denotes the probability. Considering the difference $D = Y_2 - Y_1$, perfect agreement means that the probability that the difference for a randomly selected individual from the population equals 0 is 1: $P(D = 0) = 1$. This definition of perfect agreement requires that the two measurements obtained by the two different methods (e.g., gold standard and sensor) do not differ in their metric. If, for example, activity duration is measured by one method in seconds and by the other measure in milliseconds, perfect agreement would not be possible. However, if the two metrics can be transformed into each other (e.g., multiplying seconds by 1,000), the difference values can be considered for the values transformed into the same metric. Defining perfect agreement in this way is reasonable for analyzing the convergent validity of measurements obtained in the unit calibration step, but it might be questionable for validating measurements obtained in the value calibration step because such calibrated values of accelerometers might differ in their metric from gold-standard methods, such as polysomnography or the doubly labeled water technique. In these cases, regression-based methods might be more appropriate (see the section "Latent Agreement").

Disagreement is represented by the difference, D, between the two measurements, for example, the sensor measurement and the gold-standard measurement. This difference is sometimes divided by the value of the gold-standard measurement to get a more comparable measure of disagreement (Shcherbina et al., 2017). Carstensen (2010) and Choudhary and Nagaraja (2017) give a comprehensive overview of different biometric approaches for measuring agreement, statistical models, and graphical approaches for various research designs (e.g., multiple methods, longitudinal designs) and different data situations (e.g., continuous data, categorical data), the planning of agreement studies, and sample size determination. They also discuss in detail how special data situations such as non-normal distributions and heteroscedasticity can be dealt with. Given the space limitations, we will only present some basic concepts and selected measures of agreement and illustrate them with our simulated datasets that stem from a multivariate normal distribution.

Mean Squared Deviation

The mean squared deviation (*MSD*) is the mean value of the squared difference variable D^2 (Lin, 2000):

$$MSD = \mu_{D^2} \tag{14.9}$$

Perfect agreement will be present if *MSD* equals 0. The larger the *MSD*, the larger is the amount of disagreement. The value of the *MSD* depends on the difference of the means ($\mu_{Y_2} - \mu_{Y_1}$), the variances ($\sigma^2_{Y_1}$, $\sigma^2_{Y_2}$), the standard deviations (σ_{Y_1}, σ_{Y_2}), and the correlation $\rho_{Y_1Y_2}$ of the two variables Y_1 and Y_2 in the following way (Choudhary & Nagaraja, 2017, p. 54):

$$MSD = \left(\mu_{Y_2} - \mu_{Y_1}\right)^2 + \sigma^2_{Y_1} + \sigma^2_{Y_2} - 2 \cdot \rho_{Y_1Y_2} \cdot \sigma_{Y_1} \cdot \sigma_{Y_2} \tag{14.10}$$

If the first method is, for example, the gold-standard method, the mean difference ($\mu_{Y_2} - \mu_{Y_1}$) can be interpreted as a mean bias. It is important to note that a perfect correlation ($\rho_{Y_1Y_2} = 1$) is not sufficient to get a perfect agreement (*MSD* = 0). Perfect agreement additionally requires that the mean bias ($\mu_{Y_2} - \mu_{Y_1}$) is 0 and that the variances are equal. This shows that the assumption of agreement is much stronger than that of a perfect correlation.

Concordance Correlation Coefficient

The values of the *MSD* have a lower but no upper limit. In order to obtain a measure of agreement whose values are bounded by –1 and 1 (like the correlation coefficient), the *MSD* is rescaled in the following way (Choudhary & Nagaraja, 2017; Lin, 1989) that defines the concordance correlation coefficient (CCC):

$$\text{CCC} = 1 - \frac{MSD}{MSD_0} = \rho_{Y_1Y_2} \cdot \text{C}_\text{b}, \text{ with } \text{C}_\text{b} = \frac{2 \cdot \sigma_{Y_1} \cdot \sigma_{Y_2}}{\left(\mu_{Y_1} - \mu_{Y_2}\right)^2 + \sigma^2_{Y_1} + \sigma^2_{Y_2}} \tag{14.11}$$

MSD_0 is the *MSD* value that one obtains by assuming that the two measures are uncorrelated ($\rho_{Y_1Y_2} = 0$):

$$MSD_0 = \left(\mu_{Y_1} - \mu_{Y_2}\right)^2 + \sigma^2_{Y_1} + \sigma^2_{Y_2}$$

The CCC equals 0 if the two measures are uncorrelated. It reaches its maximum in the case of perfect agreement (*MSD* = 0). The CCC equals –1 if the two measures are perfectly negatively correlated ($\rho_{Y_1Y_2} = -1$) and do not differ in their means and variances. Lin (1989) has shown that the CCC equals the Pearson correlation

BOX 14.2. Empirical Application: *MSD* and *CCC*

We illustrate the coefficients of agreement by estimating their value for the measurement of total sleep time by the first GSW and the first CW. The *MSD* is relatively large: *MSD* = 15,903.905, even if one takes into consideration that the metric is squared minutes. The *CCC* was estimated with the CCC function of the R package DescTools (Signorell et al., 2021). This function estimates the *CCC* according to Lin's (1989) equation using the empirical variances (sum of squares divided by the sample size n, not by $n - 1$). The estimated *CCC* value and its two-sided 95% confidence interval are

$$\widehat{CCC} = .414,\ CI_{95\%} = [.280; .532]$$

This value is significantly different from 0 and indicates a moderate agreement between the two activity monitors. The estimated *CCC* is smaller than the correlation coefficient of $r = .525$ because (1) the mean difference is 48.815, indicating that the CW overestimates the total sleep time by 48.815 minutes compared to the GSW (which indicates a rather strong bias), and (2) the standard deviation of the CW is larger (136.339) compared to the GSW (78.489). The estimated scale shift equals 1.737 and indicates strong differences in the standard deviations. Also, the estimated location shift of 0.472 indicates a substantive bias. The estimated bias constant of 0.789 indicates a diminution of the correlation factor that is due to differences in the location and scale of the two methods.

multiplied by a bias correction factor C_b that indicates to which degree the regression line for the two variables deviates from the 45-degree line passing through the origin. Hence, the *CCC* is the product of a coefficient indicating precision ($\rho_{Y_1Y_2}$) and a coefficient indicating accuracy (C_b) (Lin, 2000). According to Lin (2000, p. 255), precision indicates "how closely observations fall on the fitted linear line," whereas accuracy indicates "how closely the fitted line agrees with the identity line." The difference in the standard deviations can be expressed as a standardized effect-size measure that is called *scale shift* (Lin, 1989, p. 258): $v = \sigma_1/\sigma_2$. A standardized effect size for the mean difference is the *location shift* relative to the scale (Lin, 1989, p. 258): $u = (\mu_1 - \mu_2)/\sqrt{\sigma_1 \cdot \sigma_2}$.

Other Measures of Agreement

There are two other measures of agreement that are used for special purposes and that we will describe shortly.

Limits of Agreement

Another approach to measure agreement based on the difference variable D is the *limits of agreement* (LoA) approach (Bland & Altman, 1999; Choudhary & Nagaraja, 2017). It assumes that the difference variable D is normally distributed with the mean value μ_D and the standard deviation σ_D. A measure of agreement is the interval around μ_D that covers the middle $100 \cdot (1 - p)$% of the population distribution of D (Choudhary &

Nagaraja, 2017, p. 60). This can be estimated by the sample mean $\overline{x}_D$ and sample standard deviation $\hat{\sigma}_D$. The $100 \cdot (1 - p)\%$ limits of agreement are defined by the lower limit $\overline{x}_D - z_{(1-p)/2} \cdot \hat{\sigma}_D$ and the upper limit $\overline{x}_D + z_{(1-p)/2} \cdot \hat{\sigma}_D$ of this interval.

Total Deviation Index

A further measure of agreement is the *total deviation index* [$TDI(1-p)$; Lin, 2000], which is defined as follows (Choudhary & Nagaraja, 2017):

$$TDI(1 - p) = 100(1 - p)\text{th percentile of } |D| \tag{14.12}$$

The smaller the value of $TDI(1 - p)$, the larger is the agreement. For a fixed p value and a fixed criterion δ of sufficient agreement, the hypotheses H_0: $TDI(1 - p) \geq \delta$ and H_1: $TDI(1 - p) < \delta$ can be tested by calculating an upper $100 \cdot (1 - \alpha)\%$ confidence limit ul for $TDI(1 - p)$ and comparing it with δ (Choudhary & Nagaraja, 2017; Lin, 2000). If $ul < \delta$, a sufficient limit of agreement is obtained.

Latent Agreement

The agreement measures presented so far are calculated for two different devices (e.g., wearable, gold-standard measure). The disagreement can be due to different reasons. First, the disagreement might only be due to the imprecision with which each device measures the construct under consideration. Second, the disagreement might be due to structural differences between the devices, for example, differences in the mean values (mean bias), in the discrimination ability (bias with respect to the variances), or in the way that individuals interact with the measurement such that the amount of disagreement depends on the individual. This source of disagreement would imply that the true scores underlying the two measurements are generally not the same. Third, disagreement can be due to both sources. In order to separate the two sources of disagreement, it is important to obtain at least two measures of the same method at the same time. For measurements obtained by a wearable, this can be managed by wearing two devices of the same model. For example, in the validity study of Kubala and colleagues (2020), a subsample of participants wore two commercial activity monitors of the same model type of the same manufacturer on the same (nondominant) wrist. For the gold-standard measure, it is also necessary to obtain two measures by wearing two devices of the same type. If gold-standard measures refer to physical measurements like the doubly labeled water method, one can use, for example, duplicate measurements (e.g., Trabulsi et al., 2003).

Having two indicators (observed variables) i for each device, a two-factor CFA model can be applied (see Figure 14.1a). In this model there is one factor for each method k (e.g., gold-standard method, wearable) on which the two observed variables (belonging to the same method) load. Because the two measurements were obtained by applying the same type of device two times, it is reasonable to assume that the two measurements obtained for each device are exchangeable and that a model of τ-parallel variables is appropriate. This model assumes equal intercepts, loadings, and error variances for the two indicators, implying equal means and variances for the observed variable:

$$Y_{ik} = T_{ik} + E_{ik} = C_k + E_{ik} \tag{14.13}$$

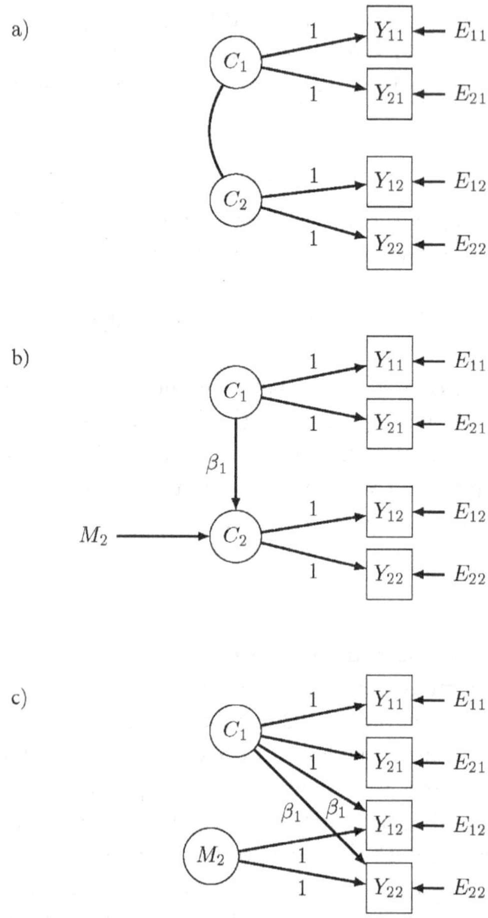

FIGURE 14.1. Latent variable models for analyzing agreement. (a) Correlated factor model, (b) latent regression model, (c) two-method measurement model. Y_{ik}, observed variable; C_k, latent construct (factor); M_2, latent method residual variable; E_{ik}, residual error variable; β_1, regression coefficient; i, indicator; k, method.

This model assumes that there is perfect *latent intra-device agreement* on the level of true scores for the two measurements and that observed intra-device disagreement is only due to unsystematic measurement error.

Latent Inter-Device Agreement and CCC: The Two-Factor Model

The *latent inter-device agreement* can be scrutinized by analyzing the associations between the two factors. The latent factor means μ_{C_1} and μ_{C_2}, variances $\sigma^2_{C_1}$ and $\sigma^2_{C_2}$, covariance $\sigma_{C_1C_2}$, and correlation $\rho_{C_1C_2}$ can be taken into consideration. Moreover, the CCC can be estimated by entering the estimated latent parameters into Equation 14.11. CFA allows us to test several hypotheses that are important for evaluating latent agreement measured by the CCC: (1) equality of factor means: $\mu_{C_1} = \mu_{C_2}$, (2) equality of factor variances: $\sigma^2_{C_1} = \sigma^2_{C_2}$, and (3) perfect correlation: $\rho_{C_1C_2} = 1$.

BOX 14.3. Empirical Application: Latent *CCC*

In our empirical application with two CW and two GSW, the correlated two-factor model with a τ-parallel measurement model for each factor fits the data very well (χ^2_7 = 4.730, df = 7, p = .693). Assuming equal factor means, factor variances, and a perfect correlation results in models not fitting the data. The latent CCC and 95% bootstrap confidence interval were estimated with the computer program Mplus (Muthén & Muthén, 1998–2017) using 1,000 bootstrap samples and model constraints to define the latent CCC. The estimated latent CCC value and its two-sided 95% confidence interval are

$$\widehat{CCC} = .470,\ CI_{95\%} = [.346; .587]$$

The value of the latent CCC is higher than the observed one because of the correction for measurement error. The estimated latent CCC is smaller than the latent correlation of .589 because the factor means (μ_{C_1} = 417.213, μ_{C_2} = 464.375) and variances ($\sigma^2_{C_1}$ = 5970.909, $\sigma^2_{C_2}$ = 17184.869) differ.

Perfect latent inter-device agreement requires that all three assumptions hold; that means that all true score variables are equal, but the observed variables belonging to different devices can differ in the error variances (and the reliabilities):

$$Y_{ik} = T_{ik} + E_{ik} = C + E_{ik} \tag{14.14}$$

If the error variances are also the same, a model of τ-parallel variables holds.

Analyzing Bias: Two-Method Measurement Model

The two-factor model can be reformulated by regressing the factor of the method that has to be validated on the factor of the gold-standard method (see Figure 14.1b). The latent regression is defined by

$$C_2 = \beta_0 + \beta_1 \cdot C_1 + M_2 \tag{14.15}$$

As a consequence, the expected value and the variance of C_2 (assessed by the method to be validated) depend on the expected value and variance of C_1 (assessed by the gold-standard method) in the following way:

$$\mu_{C_2} = \beta_0 + \beta_1 \cdot \mu_{C_1} \tag{14.16}$$

$$\sigma^2_{C_2} = \beta^2_1 \cdot \sigma^2_{C_1} + \sigma^2_{M_2} \tag{14.17}$$

The intercept β_0 is called *fixed bias*, and the regression slope β_1 is called *proportional bias* or *level-dependent bias* by Choudhary and Nagaraja (2017, p. 13). The values of the latent regression residual variable M_2 indicate the deviation of an individual score on C_2 from its expectation given C_1: $M_2 = C_2 - \mu_{C_2|C_1}$, where $\mu_{C_2|C_1} = E(C_2|C_1)$. A positive value, for example, indicates that the individual score on the method to be validated is higher than expected given the value obtained by the gold-standard method. The values on M_2 represent the *individual method bias* (Geiser, Eid, West, Lischetzke, & Nussbeck, 2012). If the variance of $M_2 = 0$, then there is no individual bias at all.

The expected difference $C_2 - C_1$ for a given value of C_1 is called *conditional method bias* and can be calculated by (see Geiser et al., 2012, for a proof):

$$\mu_{(C_2-C_1)|C_1} = \beta_0 + (\beta_1 - 1) \cdot C_1 \tag{14.18}$$

If $\beta_1 = 1$ the conditional bias does not depend on the value obtained by the gold-standard method, but it only depends on β_0. If in addition $\beta_0 > 0$, there is a positive fixed bias, and the values obtained by the method to be validated are higher than the values obtained by the gold-standard method by the fixed value β_0. This explains why the intercept β_0 is called *fixed bias*. If $\beta_0 < 0$, there is a negative fixed bias. If $\beta_1 = 1$ and $\beta_0 = 0$, the conditional method bias is 0.

If $\beta_1 > 1$, the conditional bias increases with the values obtained by the gold-standard method. If $\beta_1 < 1$, the conditional bias decreases with the values obtained by the gold-standard method. This shows that, if $\beta_1 \neq 1$, the bias depends on and is proportional to the values obtained by the gold-standard method, explaining its name *proportional bias* or *level-dependent bias*.

The unconditional expected value $\mu_{(C_2-C_1)}$ is called *general method bias* and can be calculated by (see Geiser et al., 2012, for a proof):

$$\mu_{(C_2-C_1)} = \beta_0 + (\beta_1 - 1) \cdot \mu_{C_1} \tag{14.19}$$

The general bias is 0 if $\beta_1 = 1$ and $\beta_0 = 0$. That means that, on average, there is no bias. However, there could still be individual biases.

Perfect agreement refers to the situation that $\beta_0 = 0$, $\beta_1 = 1$, and $\sigma^2_{M_2} = 0$. That means there is no bias at all. *Perfect consistency*, on the other hand, requires only that $\sigma^2_{M_2} = 0$. In this case, the latent correlation is 1, and the rankings of the individuals on both variables are identical. This could be the case, for example, if the two methods differ in their metric (like temperatures measured in degrees Celsius and Fahrenheit). In this case, perfect agreement can be obtained by rescaling the values of the non-gold-standard method so that they are equivalent to the gold-standard method. The degree of consistency can be measured by the *consistency coefficient* (Eid, Lischetzke, Nussbeck, & Trierweiler, 2003):

$$Con(C_2) = \frac{\beta_1^2 \cdot \sigma^2_{C_1}}{\sigma^2_{C_2}} = \frac{\beta_1^2 \cdot \sigma^2_{C_1}}{\beta_1^2 \cdot \sigma^2_{C_1} + \sigma^2_{M_2}} \tag{14.20}$$

The consistency coefficient corresponds to the coefficient of determination in regression analysis; that is, it is a squared (latent) correlation. It is a measure of convergent validity that only considers the degree of linear relationship and not the agreement per se. It is particularly reasonable as a measure of convergent validity if the methods differ in their metrics. Its counterpart, the method specificity coefficient, represents that part of the variance of the second factor that is due to method effects, that is, individual biases (Eid et al., 2003):

$$MSpe(C_2) = \frac{\sigma^2_{M_2}}{\sigma^2_{C_2}} = \frac{\sigma^2_{M_2}}{\beta_1^2 \cdot \sigma^2_{C_1} + \sigma^2_{M_2}} \tag{14.21}$$

The model depicted in Figure 14.1b is equivalent to the model depicted in Figure 14.1c. The model in Figure 14.1c is called the *two-method measurement model* (Graham, 2012; Lawes, Schultze, & Eid, 2020). It can be applied to analyze the same bias questions as we have discussed for the model in Figure 14.1b. In this reformulated model, the method-specific residual variable M_2 is a factor that can be related to other variables. This is important, for example, for analyzing individual method effects (Koch, Holtmann, Bohn, & Eid, 2018). If one wants to understand why a measurement obtained by a wearable (e.g., accelerometer) differs from the expected value given the gold-standard measure (e.g., the doubly labeled water method), the two-method model would be the appropriate measurement model to analyze this research question. If method effects can be explained by covariates, these covariates can then be used to correct the nonstandard measurements in order to get measures that are closer to the gold-standard method.

The two-method measurement model is used in planned missing data designs to optimize the statistical power for predicting a criterion variable, given a fixed research budget. For example, if a researcher wants to predict physical or mental health (criterion variable) by energy expenditure, energy expenditure can be measured by the expensive gold-standard doubly labeled water method or by a less expensive but less valid activity

BOX 14.4. Empirical Application: Two-Method Measurement Model

The two-method measurement model is a reformulation of the correlated two-factor model and shows, therefore, the same fit. The estimated regression coefficient is close to 1 ($\hat{\beta}_1 = 0.998$). A model in which this parameter is fixed to 1 fits the data very well ($\chi^2_8 = 4.730$, $df = 8$, $p = 0.786$) and is not significantly worse than the model with a free regression slope (the χ^2 difference equals 0). This shows that there is no *proportional* or *level-dependent bias*. In this model, the estimated intercept is $\hat{\beta}_0 = 47.213$, which is significantly different from 0 ($p < .001$). Hence, there is a strong *fixed bias* of 47.213. Because the regression slope equals 1, the fixed bias equals the estimated factor mean difference of 47.213 minutes of sleep time. Because the slope equals 1, the *conditional method bias* (Equation 14.18) equals the fixed bias, which means that the conditional bias is independent from the value of the gold-standard method. That means that one expects the same conditional mean difference of the two methods for each value of the gold-standard method. Because the two factors are not perfectly correlated, there is a certain amount of *individual method bias*. The method specificity coefficient and its 95% bootstrap confidence interval (1,000 bootstrap samples) are

$$MSpe(C_2) = \frac{\hat{\sigma}^2_{M_2}}{\beta_1^2 \, \hat{\sigma}^2_{C_1} + \hat{\sigma}^2_{M_2}} = \frac{11{,}232.438}{1 \cdot 5{,}970.826 + 11{,}232.438} = .693, \; CI_{95\%} = [.595; .769]$$

This shows that 69.3% of the true CW variance is not predicted by the GSW factor and that there is a strong amount of individual bias. The consistency coefficient, on the other hand, shows that 30.7 % of the variance is predictable by the gold-standard method ($Con(C_2) = .307$, $CI_{95\%} = [.230; .404]$).

tracker. The researcher has a fixed research budget and wants to optimize the prediction by obtaining the lowest standard error of the regression coefficient predicting health by the gold-standard method, given this fixed research budget. It can be shown that this aim can be achieved by a planned missing data design in which all participants provide data for the health measures and the activity tracker measures, but only a randomly selected subsample is additionally assessed by the expensive gold-standard method. The optimal sample sizes of the whole sample and the subsample can be determined if the research budget, the costs of the two methods, and the expected model parameters are known. Lawes and colleagues (2020) provide a program that can be used to determine the optimal sample size.

Assessing Low-Level Features: Combination of Different Sensors

Whereas Level 1 of Mohr and colleagues' (2017) framework refers to the quality of single sensors, Level 2 considers the assessment of low-level features by the combination of different sensors. According to Mohr and associates, "features are constructs measured by, and proximal to, the sensor data" (p. 25). Feature examples are *location type* (e.g., home, work) that are inferred from location sensors like GPS or *activity type* (e.g., walk, drive) that are measured using several sensors (e.g., location and movement sensors). There are different methods to infer features from sensor data. Features can be defined by researchers based on their expertise but also by statistical methods such as machine learning. The inference of features from sensor data has to be validated. Often the measurement of context information (such as the situations in which individuals are) and the integration of other information obtained by nonsensor methods are necessary. This information can be obtained by self-reports or other reports. In order to get this information, the collection of sensor data can be combined with ambulatory assessment procedures that allow the assessment of activities, feelings, situations, contexts, and locations in real time and *in situ*, for instance, via self-reports. For example, von Haaren-Mack and colleagues (2020) recommend combining accelerometry with electronic diaries. They emphasize that activity-triggered e-diaries (interactive multimodal ambulatory monitoring) are a promising method to assess self-reports triggered by and linked to specific activities. These self-reports can also be used to validate inferences from sensor data to features obtained by statistical methods. Context information can also be assessed retrospectively by the day reconstruction method (Kahneman, Krueger, Schkade, Schwarz, & Stone, 2004). Day reconstruction means that participants retrospectively split the day into different episodes and describe what they were doing, feeling, and so on. This method can be adapted to specific purposes. The information obtained can be compared with the sensor data collected in specific episodes. Compared to ambulatory assessment procedures, however, this method has the disadvantage that it depends on retrospective assessments. Because the collection of additional data such as context information is often necessary to understand the psychological meaning of sensor data and their combinations, it has to be an integral part of the research and validation process.

Assessing High-Level Behavioral Markers: Integration of Low-Level Features

According to Mohr and colleagues (2017, p. 26), "behavioral markers are higher-level features, reflecting behaviors, cognitions, and emotions, that are measured using low-level features and sensor data." As examples they present behavioral markers such as hedonic activity, fatigue, depressed mood, or stress. They emphasize that most often, machine learning and data-mining methods are used to infer high-level behavior markers from low-level features and sensor data. These methods are presented in several chapters in this volume. The validity of these inferences has to be analyzed. Several validation methods have been developed for machine learning methods (see Brandmaier, Chapter 17, this volume) that can be applied. Moreover, for many constructs it might be necessary to analyze how measures obtained by these methods converge with measures stemming from other methods, for example, the self-report of behavioral markers such as depressed mood, stress, and social avoidance. For example, if fatigue is inferred from location type, activity type, and movement intensity (Mohr et al., 2017), this inferred indicator of fatigue can be correlated with self-report measures of fatigue and should show a certain degree of convergent validity.

Analyzing More Global Psychological Constructs

The highest level of Mohr and colleagues' (2017) framework is called *clinical state* and comprises more global constructs such as depression or anxiety. The term *clinical state* is certainly due to the fact that Mohr and associates' work was published in a journal of clinical psychology. In a broader sense, this highest level refers to all types of psychological constructs that are defined based on high-level behavioral markers. In order to measure constructs such as depression, behavioral markers have to be assessed repeatedly over time, and inferences based on these longitudinal data have to be validated. For example, depressed mood has to be measured repeatedly in daily lives, and its stability or persistence across time has to be considered. This also holds true for behavioral markers such as hedonic activity or social avoidance. Many statistical models for longitudinal data analysis have been developed in recent years that can be applied to separate stable components from variable components varying systematically due to situational influences as well as unsystematic measurement errors (e.g., Cole, Martin, & Steiger, 2005; Eid, Holtmann, Santangelo, & Ebner-Priemer, 2017; Hamaker, Kuiper, & Grasman, 2015; Steyer, Mayer, Geiser, & Cole, 2015). These models also have been extended to intensive longitudinal data with many occasions of measurements. DSEM (Asparouhov et al., 2018), for example, integrates models of time series and multilevel analysis with models of CFA and allows the analysis of interindividual differences in longitudinal processes in a sophisticated way. For example, it is possible to scrutinize interindividual differences in different components of a dynamic process, such as interindividual differences in intraindividual variability, inertia, and measurement error variances (see Holtmann et al., Chapter 15, this volume).

Validity issues, however, do not only refer to data analytic methods but also to design issues. Inferences about more global constructs based on repeatedly measured sensor data, such as depression, require that the situations in which the data are collected are randomly selected or at least representative of a person's life. If the selection of situations is biased, the ecological validity, a facet of external validity, is threatened (RatSWD, 2020). It is likely that individuals do not wear wearables in all situations of their life, and for ethical, in particular privacy reasons, they are allowed to interrupt and stop the data collection process. Moreover, some sensors like location sensors (e.g., GPS) are not able to collect data everywhere (e.g., in a subway). This can challenge the validity of conclusions about habitual behaviors and feelings, the distribution of states, and dynamic aspects of behaviors and feelings. Therefore, assessment of situational information, information about the use of wearables, and individual deviations from the intended data collection plan is recommended.

Another aspect of external validity is the sampling of individuals (RatSWD, 2020). If individuals are not randomly sampled from an underlying population, the results of a study might not be generalizable to the whole population. From a psychometric point of view, this might be a problem when statistical norms (comparable with norms for psychometric tests and questionnaires) are developed. This is not yet the case. However, given the strong influence of mobile sensing on psychological assessment, the development of statistical norms might be an important future endeavor. Therefore, the sampling process should be well documented in each mobile sensing study (RatSWD, 2020).

Summary and Recommendations

Traditional psychometric quality criteria that are widely used in psychology can be applied to mobile sensing data. They have to take the peculiarities of the assessment and data production process into account. This chapter has shown how psychometric methods can be used to analyze facets of objectivity, reliability, and validity. The analysis of these quality criteria typically requires basic psychometric research projects because many requirements (such as wearing multiple sensors and availability of gold-standard measures) are usually not and do not have to be fulfilled in every research project. However, researchers applying special mobile sensing methods should make sure that these quality criteria have been analyzed in previous research projects focusing on the measurement quality of these sensing methods. Construction of an intelligence test requires extensive basic psychometric research; it is also necessary that basic psychometric research programs are established for mobile sensing research. If the results of such basic psychometric studies are not available, researchers should exploit all available data in terms of validity analyses. For example, they can split the total length of their study into different periods, analyze the stability of their measures, and check whether these stability coefficients are plausible. They can look at the correlation structure of their measures and check if they are in line with theoretical expectations. Even if they are not able to conduct a comprehensive psychometric study, they can think about how to integrate some of the aspects presented in this chapter to enhance the possibility of checking their data quality (e.g., by administering two instead of one wearable and collecting multimethod data such as additional situational data or questionnaire data).

This chapter focused on wearable mobile sensing. The methods for analyzing reliability and agreement, for example, are based on the concept of measurement error of physics (which is also the basic concept of measurement error theory in psychometrics) and the availability of gold-standard methods. Psychometrically speaking, they typically refer to so-called reflective indicators that can be considered observed variables of an underlying latent variable (such as the models depicted in Figure 14.1). At first glance, they do not refer to composite (formative) indicators. Composite indicators are linearly weighted to represent the psychological characteristic of interest (Bollen & Bauldry, 2011). They are the independent variables for defining a dependent formative variable (construct) and are not dependent manifest variables of an underlying independent variable (construct). For example, a researcher might be interested in combining different behavioral measures of social activity (e.g., log-file behavior, frequency of outgoing calls, posting behavior) for optimally predicting satisfaction with social relationships. In this case, there is no underlying construct. Even in this case, however, concepts and ideas presented in this chapter can be used to analyze the quality of such composite scores. For example, the day can be divided into 30-minute periods, each of which is randomly assigned to two time sets. Based on the behavioral indicators assessed in the two time sets, a composite can be calculated for each of them, and the strength of the two composites' correlation can be checked.

The German Data Forum has developed recommendations for data collection using new information technology (RatSWD, 2020). The recommendations on data collection, reliability, and validity are depicted in Figures 14.2–14.4, with the permission of the German Data Forum. They also summarize the major recommendations given in this chapter.

1. Data collection requires comprehensive **documentation of the data collection process.** Documentation of data collection using new information technology should contain information on the following aspects:
   - All **sensors and software used** (manufacturer, type, production year, software version)
   - **Raw data** that were collected and stored
   - All the **data processing steps** leading to the derived data
   - **Contextual information** (e.g., the situation in which the data were collected)
2. Researchers should **weigh the benefits of consumer products against more expensive, scientific products.** Measuring attributes of interest without access to raw data or knowledge of the product's signal processing is hard to justify in a scientific context.
3. Sensor data should be recorded as **raw data in a standard format** and in their original (native) resolution. The use of lossless types of compression is advisable.
4. If the device already processes sensor data into higher-quality information, it is important to know the way it does so. If **data analytics procedures** such as machine learning are employed for such processes, training data and the respective model should be documented, and program codes and program versions should be provided.
5. Manufacturers should **archive the documentation of all their sensors and data processing algorithms for all versions of the sensors.** However, this is unlikely with common consumer products. It is therefore advisable to archive the data sheets when buying a product. Researchers should also try to document hard- and software updates.

FIGURE 14.2. Recommendations of the German Data Forum: Data collection. From RatSWD (2020, p. 14).

1. Information on the **measurement precision of sensors** should be made transparent by manufacturers and documented in scientific publications that rely on sensor data.
2. Empirical research projects should make transparent the **methods used to determine measurement precision.** This can be done using a range of methods (e.g., parallel-forms method, testing-retesting method).
3. When reducing complex data (e.g., audio, video, text data) using coding procedures, the **quality of the reduction techniques** should be **documented** (e.g., through assessing intercoder reliability, that is, the level of agreement between different coders).

FIGURE 14.3. Recommendations of the German Data Forum: Reliability. From RatSWD (2020, p. 15).

Construct Validity

1. For sensors used in scientific studies, validation studies should demonstrate the **convergence with gold-standard methods.**

2. The validity of results based on sensors should be examined in **theory-driven validation studies** (including the use of other data sources, e.g., behavioral observations and questionnaires).

3. In the case of ambiguous signals, the **validity of inferences** should be verified—to the extent that this is consistent with standards of data protection and research ethics—by including additional methods as well as by documenting the data collection context. This is particularly important when collecting data on physiological processes in everyday life situations.

4. Whenever data are generated or evaluated using algorithms, technical validation studies should be used to assess the **correctness of algorithms**. Moreover, these data should be matched with real-world data ("ground truth"). To the extent possible, this comparison should be performed and documented in every data collection process (using subsamples). Pilot studies should at least be used where this is not possible in real-life applications.

External Validity

5. It must be documented when **selective samples of situations lead to missing data** and—if possible and reasonable—it must be reconstructed and corrected using appropriate methods. These can include the following:

   a. **Subsequent interviewing of participants** (e.g., using appropriately implemented questions on a smartphone); this can give some indication of reasons for missing data and possibly facilitate the reconstruction of missing data. However, such subsequent questioning can be viewed negatively by the respondents.

   b. Assessing selectivity in the recorded situations can be made possible by **comparing** the frequency of occurrence of such situations in datasets collected **through different methods** (mobile sensing, experience sampling, field observations, questionnaires). Studies that do this systematically are extremely rare, however, there are some examples are to be found in research on illegal drugs (Linas et al., 2016).

   c. If viable (depending on the burden on the participants and existing resources), the **data collection period or data collection frequency can be increased.** Data can be collected every 60, 30, or 15 minutes, for a brief duration in certain situations. It is also possible to survey levels of acceptance, or annoyance, and to estimate the influence on survey compliance. Generally, such procedures may lead to higher compliance (Trull & Ebner-Priemer, 2013). Yet, systematic studies on this issue are also still very rare (Stone et al., 2003).

   d. To estimate the amount of missing data, it can help to document how often participants resorted to **editing and censoring** their data.

   e. Providing **incentives** for participation (e.g., financial compensation) can increase compliance (Göritz, 2014).

(continued)

FIGURE 14.4. Recommendations of the German Data Forum: Validity. From RatSWD (2020, pp. 19 and 20).

6. **Missing data** through **selective sampling of individuals** must be documented and—if possible and reasonable—**reconstructed and corrected** using appropriate methods. Researchers can rely, for this purpose, on established methods from survey research (Kreuter, Haas, Keusch, Bähr, & Trappmann, 2018; Schupp & Wolf, 2015):
   a. In order to be able to analyze the selectivity of participants and to adjust for it (using statistical techniques such as weighting), it will be useful to **randomly select participants from data sources** that contain relevant information on participants and nonparticipants. These can be administrative data, such as population registers or existing representative surveys. The advantage of sampling from surveys (Kreuter et al., 2018) is that researchers can bring in questions that measure important target variables of the following technology-based survey, e.g., their usage intensity or survey equivalents of the variables later to be measured using new technology. Models can then show whether a study's participants differ from nonparticipants regarding the study's key measures.
   b. Data from participants (and, if applicable, the control group) can be **compared with external data sources and statistics.**
   c. Data from participants and nonparticipants can be **linked with commercial microgeographic data** (e.g., infas 360) (for the survey context, see Sinibaldi, Trappmann, & Kreuter, 2014).
   d. Nonparticipants can be interviewed about **reasons for nonparticipation.**
   e. If the researchers themselves oversee recruiting, they can have recruiters **observe or estimate information on participants and nonparticipants** (West, 2013).
   f. It must be documented whether and to what extent devices (e.g., smartphones, fitness trackers) are shared with other individuals. This can be done by:
      - depending on the aim of the analysis, explicitly **excluding the sharing of wearables** used for the study in the **informed consent** form for the scientific study,
      - interviewing participants, if sensible, whether and to what extent devices were shared or used by others. **Devices used by several individuals can be excluded** or—depending on the aim of the analysis—be given special consideration,
      - using machine-learning-based algorithms to identify variations in user behavior and to assign the collected data to various users (Ochoa, Bort, & Porcar, 2018). This must take data protection regulations into account.

FIGURE 14.4. *(continued)*

REFERENCES

Asparouhov, T., Hamaker, E. L., & Muthén, B. (2018). Dynamic structural equation models. *Structural Equation Modeling: A Multidisciplinary Journal, 25*(3), 359–388.

Balli, S., & Sağbas, E. A. (2017). The usage of statistical learning methods on wearable devices and a case study: Activity recognition on Smartwatches. In T. Hokimoto (Ed.), *Advances in statistical methodologies and their application to real problems* (pp. 259–277). IntechOpenScience.

Bandalos, D. L. (2018). *Measurement theory and applications for the social sciences.* Guilford Press.

Bassett, D. R., Jr., Rowlands A. V., & Trost, S. G. (2012). Calibration and validation of wearable monitors. *Medicine and Science in Sports and Exercise, 44*(1, Suppl. 1), S32–S38.

Bland, J. M., & Altman, D. G. (1999). Measuring agreement in method comparison studies. *Statistical Methods in Medical Research, 8*(2), 135–160.

Bollen, K. A., & Bauldry, S. (2011). Three Cs in measurement models: Causal indicators, composite indicators, and covariates. *Psychological Methods, 16*(3), 265–284.

Brown, T. A. (2015). *Confirmatory factor analysis for applied research* (2nd ed.). Guilford Press.

Browne, M. W., & Zhang, G. (2005). *User's guide: DyFa: Dynamic factor analysis of lagged correlation matrices, version 2.03*

[Computer software and manual]. https://psychology.osu.edu/dr-browne-software

Browne, M. W., & Zhang, G. (2007). Developments in the factor analysis of individual time series. In R. Cudeck & R. C. MacCallum (Eds.), *Factor analysis at 100: Historical developments and future directions* (pp. 265–291). Erlbaum.

Carstensen, B. (2010). *Comparing clinical measurement methods: A practical guide*. Wiley.

Chen, K. Y., Janz, K., Zhu, W. & Brychta, R. J. (2012). Redefining the roles of sensors in objective physical activity monitoring. *Medicine and Science in Sports and Exercise, 44*(1, Suppl. 1), S13–S23.

Choudhary, P. K., & Nagaraja, H. N. (2017). *Measuring agreement: Models, methods, and applications*. Wiley.

Cole, D. A., Martin, N. C., & Steiger, J. H. (2005). Empirical and conceptual problems with longitudinal trait-state models: Introducing a trait-state-occasion model. *Psychological Methods, 10*(1), 3–20.

Du, H., & Wang L. (2018). Reliabilities of intraindividual variability indicators with autocorrelated longitudinal data: Implications for longitudinal study designs. *Multivariate Behavioral Research, 53*(4), 502–520.

Düking, P., Fuss, F. K., Holmberg, H.-C., & Sperlich, B. (2018). Recommendations for assessment of the reliability, sensitivity, and validity of data provided by wearable sensors designed for monitoring physical activity. *JMIR mHealth and uHealth*, 6(4),e102.

Ebner-Priemer, U. W., Eid, M., Kleindienst, N., Stabenow, S., & Trull, T. J. (2009). Analytic strategies for understanding affective (in)stability and other dynamic processes in psychopathology. *Journal of Abnormal Psychology, 118*(1), 195–202.

Ebner-Priemer, U. W., Kuo, J., Kleindienst, N., Welch, S. S., Reisch, T., Reinhard, I., et al. (2007). State affective instability in borderline personality disorder assessed by ambulatory monitoring. *Psychological Medicine, 37*(7), 961–970.

Eid, M. & Diener, E. (1999). Intraindividual variability in affect: Reliability, validity, and personality correlates. *Journal of Personality and Social Psychology, 76*(4), 662–676.

Eid, M., Holtmann, J., Santangelo, P. & Ebner-Priemer, U. (2017). On the definition of latent-state-trait models with autoregressive effects: Insights from LST-R theory. *European Journal of Psychological Assessment, 33*(4), 285–295.

Eid, M., Lischetzke, T., Nussbeck, F. W., & Trierweiler, L. I. (2003). Separating trait effects from trait-specific method effects in multitrait-multimethod models: A multiple indicator CT-C(M-1) model. *Psychological Methods, 8*(1), 38–60.

Eid, M., & Schmidt, K. (2014). *Testtheorie und Testkonstruktion* [*Test theory and test construction*]. Hogrefe.

Evenson, K. R., Goto, M. M., & Furberg, R. D. (2015): Systematic review of the validity and reliability of consumer-wearable activity trackers. *International Journal of Behavioral Nutrition and Physical Activity, 12*, 159.

Gana, K., & Broc, G. (2019). *Structural equation modeling with lavaan*. Iste.

Geiser, C., Eid, M., West, S. G., Lischetzke, T. & Nussbeck, F. W. (2012). A comparison of method effects in two confirmatory factor models for structurally different methods. *Structural Equation Modeling: A Multidisciplinary Journal, 19*(3), 409–436.

Göritz, A. S. (2014). Incentive effects. In U. Engel, B. Jann, P. Lynn, A. Scherpenzeel, & P. Sturgis (Eds.), *Improving survey methods: Lessons from recent research* (pp. 339–350). Routledge.

Graham, J. W. (2012). *Missing data*. Springer.

Hamaker, E. L., Kuiper, R. M., & Grasman, R. P. P. P. (2015). A critique of the cross-lagged panel model. *Psychological Methods, 20*(1), 102–116.

Henriksen, A., Johansson, J., Hartvigsen, G., Grimsgaard, S., & Hopstock, L. (2020). Measuring physical activity using triaxial wrist worn polar activity trackers: A systematic review. *International Journal of Exercise Science, 13*(4), 438–454.

Hu, Y., Nesselroade, J. R., Erbacher, M. K., Boker, S. M., Burt, S. A., Keel, P. K., et al. (2016). Test reliability at the individual level. *Structural Equation Modeling: A Multidisciplinary Journal, 23*(4), 532–543.

Jöreskog, K. G. (1971). Statistical analysis of sets of congeneric tests. *Psychometrika, 36*(2), 109–133.

Kahneman, D., Krueger, A. B., Schkade, D. A., Schwarz, N., & Stone, A. A. (2004). A survey method for characterizing daily life experience: The day reconstruction method. *Science, 306*(5702), 1776–1780.

Koch, T., Holtmann, J., Bohn, J., & Eid, M. (2018). Explaining general and specific factors in longitudinal, multimethod, and bifactor models: Some caveats and recommendations. *Psychological Methods, 23*(3), 505–523.

Komukai, K., & Ohmura, R. (2019). Optimizing of the number and placements of wearable IMUs for automatic rehabilitation recording. In N. Kawaguchi, N. Nishio, D. Roggen, S. Inoue, S. Pirttikangas, & K. van Laerhoven (Eds.), *Human activity sensing: Corpus and applications* (pp. 3–15). Springer Nature.

Kreuter, F., Haas, G.-C., Keusch, F., Bähr, S., & Trappmann, M. (2018). Collecting survey and smartphone sensor data with an app: Opportunities and challenges around privacy and informed consent. *Social Science Computer Review, 38*(5), 533–549.

Kubala, A. G., Gibbs, B. B., Buysse, D. J., Patel, S. R., Hall, M. H., & Kline, C. E. (2020). Field-based measurement of sleep: Agreement between six commercial activity monitors and a validated accelerometer. *Behavioral Sleep Medicine, 18*(5), 637–652.

Lawes, M., Schultze, M., & Eid, M. (2020). Making the most of your research budget: efficiency of a three-method measurement design with planned missing data. *Assessment, 27*(5), 903–920.

Lin, L. I.-K. (1989). A concordance correlation coefficient to evaluate reproducibility. *Biometrics, 45*(1), 255–268.

Lin, L. I.-K. (2000). Total deviation index for measuring individual agreement with applications in laboratory performance and bioequivalence. *Statistics in Medicine, 19*(2), 255–270.

Linas, B. S.; Genz, A., Westergaard, R. P., Chang, L. W., Bollinger, R. C., Latkin, C., et al. (2016). Ecological momentary assessment of illicit drug use compared to biological and self-reported methods. *Journal of Medical Internet Research mHealth and uHealth, 4*(1), e27.

Lord, F. M., & Novick, M. R. (1968). *Statistical theories of mental test scores.* Addison-Wesley.

McGraw, K. O., & Wong, S. P. (1996). Forming inferences about some intraclass correlation coefficients. *Psychological Methods, 1*(1), 30–46.

Messick, S. (1989). Validity. In R. L. Linn (Ed.), *Educational measurement* (3rd ed., pp. 13–103). Macmillan.

Messick, S. (1995). Validity of psychological assessment: Validation of inferences from persons' responses and performances as scientific inquiry into score meaning. *American Psychologist, 50*(9), 741–749.

Mohr, D. C., Zhang, M., & Schueller, S. M. (2017). Personal sensing: Understanding mental health using ubiquitous sensors and machine learning. *Annual Review of Clinical Psychology, 13*, 23–47.

Molenaar, P. C. M. (1985). A dynamic factor model for the analysis of multivariate time series. *Psychometrika, 50*, 181–202.

Muthén, L. K., & Muthén, B. O. (1998–2017). *Mplus user's guide* (8th ed.). Muthén & Muthén.

Nesselroade, J. R., & Ram, N. (2004). Studying intraindividual variability: What we have learned that will help us understand lives in context. *Research in Human Development, 1*(1–2), 9–29.

Ochoa, C., Bort, C., & Porcar, J. M. (2018): Who is who with behavioural data. An algorithm to attribute the device's navigation to users sharing the same device. *Frontiers of Marketing Data Science Journal, 1*, 43–62.

Peake, J. M., Kerr, G., & Sullivan, J. P. (2018). A critical review of consumer wearables, mobile applications, and equipment for providing biofeedback, monitoring stress, and sleep in physically active populations. *Frontiers in Physiology, 9*, 743.

Picard, R. W., Fedor, S., & Ayzenberg, Y. (2016). Multiple arousal theory and daily-life electrodermal activity asymmetry. *Emotion Review, 8*(1), 62–75.

Plasqui, G., & Westerterp, K. R. (2007). Physical activity assessment with accelerometers: An evaluation against doubly labeled water. *Obesity, 15*(10), 2371–2379.

Price, L. R. (2017). *Psychometric methods: Theory into practice.* Guilford Press.

Rat für Sozial & Wirtschaftsdaten [German Data Forum] (2020): *Data collection using new information technology: Recommendations on data quality, data management, research ethics, and data protection.* https://www.konsortswd.de/wp-content/uploads/RatSWD_Output6.6_Data-collection-newIT_EN.pdf

Rosseel, Y. (2012). lavaan: An R package for structural equation modeling. *Journal of Statistical Software, 48*(2), 1–36.

Schermelleh-Engel, K., Kelava, A., & Moosbrugger, H. (2006). Gütekriterien [Quality standards for tests]. In F. Petermann & M. Eid (Eds.), *Handbuch der psychologischen diagnostik* [*Handbook of psychological assessment*] (pp. 420–433). Hogrefe.

Schupp, J., & Wolf, C. (Eds.). (2015). *Nonresponse bias. Qualitätssicherung sozialwissenschaftlicher umfragen* [*Nonresponse bias. Quality assurance of social science surveys*]. Springer.

Schuurman, N. K., & Hamaker, E. L. (2019). Measurement error and person-specific reliability in multilevel autoregressive modeling. *Psychological Methods, 24*(1), 70–91.

Shcherbina, A., Mattsson, C. M., Waggott, D., Salisbury, H., Christle, J. W., Hastie, T., et al. (2017). Accuracy in wrist-worn, sensor-based measurements of heart rate and energy expenditure in a diverse cohort. *Journal of Personalized Medicine, 7*(2), 3.

Signorell, A., Aho, K., Alfons, A., Anderegg, N., Aragon, T., Arachchige, C., et al. (2021). *Package 'DescTools'* [Reference manual]. https://cran.r-project.org/web/packages/DescTools/index.html

Sinibaldi, J., Trappmann, M., & Kreuter, F. (2014). Which is the better investment for nonresponse adjustment: Purchasing commercial auxiliary data or collecting interviewer observations? *Public Opinion Quarterly, 78*(2), 440–473.

Steyer, R. (2015). Classical (psychometric) test theory. In J. D. Wright (Ed.), *International encyclopedia of the social and behavioral sciences* (2nd ed., pp. 785–791). Elsevier.

Steyer, R., Mayer, A., Geiser, C. & Cole, D. A. (2015). A theory of states and traits—revised. *Annual Review of Clinical Psychology, 11*, 71–98.

Stone, A., Broderick, J., Schwartz, J., Shiffman, S., Litcher-Kelly, L., & Calvanese, P. (2003). Intensive momentary reporting of pain with an electronic diary: Reactivity, compliance, and patient satisfaction. *Pain, 104*(1–2), 343–351.

Trabulsi, J., Troiano, R. P., Subar, A. F., Sharbaugh, C., Kipnis, V., Schatzkin, A., et al. (2003). Precision of the doubly labeled water method in a large-scale application: Evaluation of a streamlined-dosing protocol in the Observing Protein and Energy Nutrition (OPEN) study. *European Journal of Clinical Nutrition, 57*, 1370–1377.

Trull, T. J., & Ebner-Priemer, U. (2013). Ambulatory assessment. *Annual Review of Clinical Psychology, 9*(1), 151–176.

von Haaren-Mack, B., Bussmann, J. B. J., & Ebner-Priemer, U. W. (2020). Physical activity monitoring. In L. M. Cohen, K. Sweeny, & M. L. Robbins (Eds.), *The Wiley encyclopedia of health psychology: Vol. 2: The social bases of health behavior* (pp. 447–458). Wiley.

Welk, G. J. (2005). Principles of design and analyses for the calibration of accelerometry-based activity monitors. *Medicine and Science in Sports and Exercise, 37*(11, Suppl.), S501–S511.

West, B. T. (2013): An examination of the quality and utility of interviewer observations in the National Survey of Family Growth. *Journal of the Royal Statistical Society: Series A. Statistics in Society, 176*(1), 211–225.

Yang, C.-C., & Hsu, Y.-L. (2010). A review of accelerometry-based wearable motion detectors for physical activity monitoring. *Sensors, 10*(8), 7772–7788.

CHAPTER 15

Dynamic Structural Equation Modeling for the Analysis of Mobile Sensing Data

Jana Holtmann, Michael Eid, and Martina Kanning

CHAPTER OVERVIEW

This chapter describes modeling strategies for the analysis of mobile sensing data by dynamic structural equation modeling (DSEM; Asparouhov, Hamaker, & Muthén, 2018). DSEM combines time-series modeling, multilevel modeling, structural equation modeling, and time-varying effects modeling within one modeling framework. Thereby, DSEM covers a large variety of powerful modeling strategies suited for the analysis of intensive longitudinal data. The described models separate stable between-person differences from within-person temporal dynamics and measurement error components. On the within-person level, reciprocal dependencies between latent variables across time are modeled. On the between-person level, individual differences in the within-person dynamics or average levels, as well as associations with external covariates, can be modeled. Several extensions of the model (e.g., random measurement error, inclusion of time-varying covariates) are discussed. We illustrate the models with an application for the joint analysis of physical activity (accelerometer; wearable sensor data) and self-reported energetic arousal (electronic diary data).

Introduction

Recent technological advances have initiated an increase in the use of different ambulant data collection methods, with longitudinal data being collected more intensively and at the same time less invasively (Mehl & Conner, 2012; Trull & Ebner-Priemer, 2014). A shift in data collection methods toward mobile sensing thereby proliferates intensive longitudinal data (ILD) in the psychological sciences. These new ILD typically consist of a large number of repeated measurements (from one or more individuals), which are closely spaced in time. ILD with many measurements that are taken within short time intervals are usually gathered to investigate stable processes (as opposed to developmental processes; see, e.g., Jongerling, Laurenceau, & Hamaker, 2015; McNeish & Hamaker, 2020; Ram & Gerstorf, 2009). In stable processes, dynamics across time are assumed to consist mainly of short-term variability around a stable mean, as no systematic changes or long-lasting developments are expected within a short assessment period (e.g., several days). Research questions thereby often focus on time-dependent (co-)variation between different variables that occur within the individual, calling for an idiographic approach to studying longitudinal data (Molenaar, 2004). This within-person variability across time is the main focus when analyzing stable process data (Ram & Gerstorf, 2009) and when investigating questions regarding within-person dynamic interactions between several variables across time, interindividual differences in these dynamics, or the effect of covariates on the presence of peaks and valleys in the dynamic process. A researcher might, for instance, investigate how physical activity (PA) and energetic arousal (EA) reciprocally influence each other across time within the same person. Is there a reciprocal cross-lagged association between PA and experienced energy level? Does high PA lead to a directly following increase or a decrease in energy level, and does a high-energy level predict an increase in PA? Why do some people show larger variability in their experienced energy level? And which external covariates explain why energy level is higher than expected at certain time points or why the effect of PA on subsequent energy levels is higher for some persons than for others? These questions refer to dynamics that occur on the within-person level; that is, they tackle reciprocal relationships between PA and EA within a person across time. Furthermore, we are interested in interindividual differences in these dynamics, as, for instance, PA may lead to a burst of energy in some individuals, while others who do not regularly exercise may rather feel exhausted while doing it.

The aforementioned technical developments and the increased availability of ILD stimulated advances in statistical models to analyze ILD (e.g., Asparouhov et al., 2018; Hedeker, Mermelstein, & Demirtas, 2008; Lane, Gates, Pike, Beltz, & Wright, 2019; Oravecz, Tuerlinckx, & Vandekerckhove, 2009). Models that are suited to answer the aforementioned questions are, among others, multilevel time-series models, which separate stable between-person differences from within-person temporal dynamics (Asparouhov et al., 2018; Jongerling et al., 2015, Schuurman, Ferrer, de Boer-Sonnenschein, & Hamaker, 2016; Song & Ferrer, 2012). On the within-person level, individual time series capture within-person dynamics across time. On the between-person level, individual differences in within-person dynamics and associations with external covariates can be modeled. Furthermore, by fitting a model for an entire (random) sample of individuals, group effects capturing average effects across individuals are estimated, thereby facilitating the generalization of results to a larger population of individuals.

One disadvantage of classical (multilevel) autoregressive time-series models is that they do not consider potential measurement error in the variables. However, many constructs of interest in psychological research are not directly observable, and measurements are not perfectly reliable (see Eid & Holtmann, Chapter 14, this volume). It has been shown that if measurements are affected by measurement error, disregarding this measurement error in autoregressive models may result in bias of the autoregressive parameters (Schuurman & Hamaker, 2019; Schuurman, Houtveen, & Hamaker, 2015; Staudenmayer & Buonaccorsi, 2005). In latent variable models (e.g., confirmatory factor analysis [*CFA*], structural equation modeling [*SEM*]), measurement error is accounted for by using multiple (parallel) indicators to measure the latent construct of interest.

The DSEM approach introduced by Asparouhov and colleagues (2018) combines multivariate time-series modeling with multilevel modeling, as well as structural equation modeling. To this date, DSEM has been applied to the analysis of mobile sensing data in only a few instances, such as the joint modeling of smartphone use and procrastination (Aalbers, vanden Abeele, Hendrickson, de Marez, & Keijsers, 2021) or of physical activity and sleep time in schoolchildren (Armstrong et al., 2021).

In this chapter, we introduce the basic ideas of DSEM, illustrate its use for the joint analysis of sensor and self-report ambulatory assessment (AA) data, and discuss several model extensions for extended research questions.

DSEM for Wearable Sensor and Self-Report AA Data

In the following, we will shortly introduce both single- and multiple-indicator models and discuss differences between the two model variants.[1] In most applications, signals obtained from wearable devices will be measured using one measurement device, thereby providing only one measured indicator variable. In this case, single-indicator models need to be used. In contrast, in AA studies collecting self-report data, it is common that participants are asked to rate several items intended to measure a common underlying psychological construct. The availability of several items per construct provides the possibility of applying multiple-indicator models. Hence, in applications investigating the joint dynamics between signals obtained from wearable devices and self-reported ambulatory assessments, hybrid models combining both a single-indicator measurement model (for the wearable device data) and a multiple-indicator measurement model (for the self-reported data obtained with more than one item per construct) will be common. This last case is illustrated in the data application section, in which the joint dynamics of PA and self-reported EA across time are analyzed. We present the example of PA and EA for a wearable device measure and a self-report measure, respectively, in the following model descriptions.

Measurement Models

Suppose EA is assessed by self-reports using two items, $Y_{E1,it}$ and $Y_{E2,it}$, which are repeatedly administered to participants ($i = 1, \ldots, N$) across several measurement time points ($t = 1, \ldots, T$). As a special case of a multilevel structural equation model, DSEM allows for a decomposition of the observed variables $Y_{E1,it}$ and $Y_{E2,it}$ into several latent between- and within-level components (see Figure 15.1A). The latent variables $\mu_{E1,i}$ and $\mu_{E2,i}$ denote the person-specific and indicator-specific latent means of $Y_{E1,it}$ and $Y_{E2,it}$ across time, respectively:

$$Y_{E1,it} = \mu_{E1,i} + Y_{E1,it}^{(w)} \tag{15.1}$$

$$Y_{E2,it} = \mu_{E2,i} + Y_{E2,it}^{(w)} \tag{15.2}$$

These person-specific mean variables $\mu_{E1,i}$ and $\mu_{E2,i}$ can be considered as latent trait variables that are stable across the observed time period. Between-person differences in these trait scores thereby reflect systematic trait-like differences between persons; for instance, some persons may generally feel a higher level of EA as compared to other

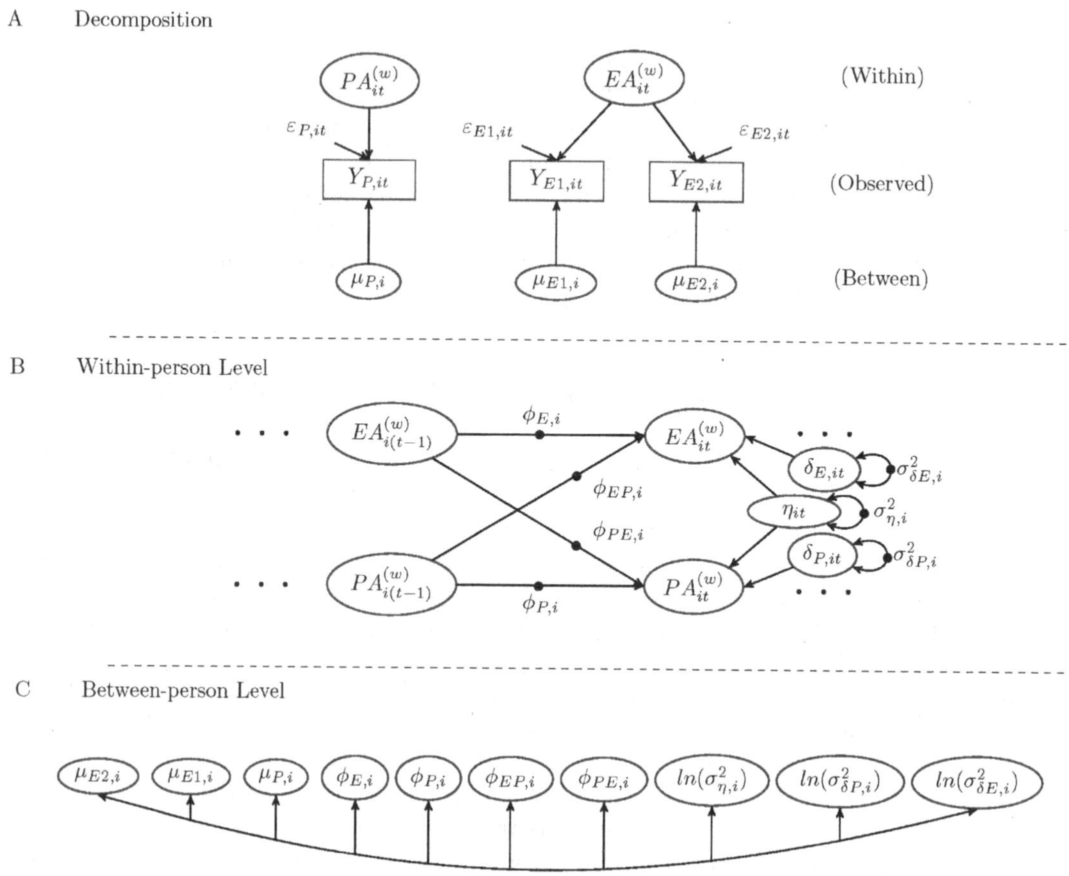

FIGURE 15.1. Measurement model (A; decomposition), latent between-person (B), and latent within-person (C) model for the dynamic structural equation model of physical activity (PA) and energetic arousal (EA). Following Curran and Bauer (2007) and Hamaker et al. (2018), circles indicate that the parameter of the respective path is estimated as a latent variable with a mean and variance at the between-person level. *i*: individual; *t*: time point; $Y_{E1,it}$/$Y_{E2,it}$/$Y_{P,it}$: Observed variables of EA, indicator 1 and 2, and PA; $EA^{(w)}_{it}$/$PA^{(w)}_{it}$: latent within-person variables of EA and PA; $\mu_{E1,i}$/$\mu_{E2,i}$/$\mu_{P,i}$: random, person-specific mean of the respective construct and indicator; $\varepsilon_{E1,it}$/$\varepsilon_{E2,it}$/$\varepsilon_{P,it}$: measurement error variables; $\phi_{E,i}$/$\phi_{P,i}$: random, person-specific autoregressive effects; $\phi_{EP,i}$: person-specific slope of the latent cross-lagged regression of $EA^{(w)}_{it}$ at time *t* on $PA^{(w)}_{i(t-1)}$ at time $(t-1)$; $\phi_{EP,i}$: person-specific slope of the latent cross-lagged regression of $PA^{(w)}_{it}$ at time point *t* on $EA^{(w)}_{i(t-1)}$ at time point $(t-1)$; η_{it}: common factor for the innovations; $\delta_{E,it}$/$\delta_{P,it}$: residual innovations not shared with the respective other construct at time *t*; $ln(\sigma^2_{\eta,i})$ / $ln(\sigma^2_{\delta E,i})$ / $ln(\sigma^2_{\delta P,i})$: logarithm of the random, person-specific common and residual innovation variances for person *i*.

persons on average. By modeling separate latent trait variables for each indicator, the model accounts for potential time-invariant item heterogeneity (Eid, Holtmann, Santangelo, & Ebner-Priemer, 2017). The variables $Y^{(w)}_{E1,it}$ and $Y^{(w)}_{E2,it}$ capture the time-specific deviations of the observed variables from this stable person mean. The superscript (w) indicates that these are within-level variables that capture the within-person fluctuation of the scores around the person-specific stable trait across time. A person might for instance show a high habitual level of EA (e.g., trait $\mu_{E1,i}$) but a reduced level as compared to their habitual level at a specific time point (e.g., negative value of $Y^{(w)}_{E1,it}$).

In multiple-indicator models, it is assumed that the two indicators measure a common within-level factor. That is, the two variables $Y^{(w)}_{E1,it}$ and $Y^{(w)}_{E2,it}$ are assumed to measure a common within-level latent factor of energetic arousal, $EA^{(w)}_{it}$ (see Figures 15.1A and 15.2). That part of $Y^{(w)}_{E1,it}$ and $Y^{(w)}_{E2,it}$ that is not shared across the two indicators and thereby is not captured by $EA^{(w)}_{it}$ is represented in the measurement error variables $\varepsilon_{E1,it}$ and $\varepsilon_{E2,it}$:

$$Y^{(w)}_{E1,it} = EA^{(w)}_{it} + \varepsilon_{E1,it} \quad (15.3)$$

$$Y^{(w)}_{E2,it} = EA^{(w)}_{it} + \varepsilon_{E2,it} \quad (15.4)$$

That is, residual variance (variation due to $\varepsilon_{E1,it}$ or $\varepsilon_{E2,it}$) and true within-person fluctuations (variation in $E^{(w)}_{it}$) across time are separated by factorizing two parallel indicators.[2] The measurement error variables are assumed to be independently and identically normally distributed with $\varepsilon_{E1,it} \sim N(0,\sigma^2_{\varepsilon E1})$, $\varepsilon_{E2,it} \sim N(0,\sigma^2_{\varepsilon E2})$ and $cov(\varepsilon_{E1,it}, \varepsilon_{E2}) = 0$.

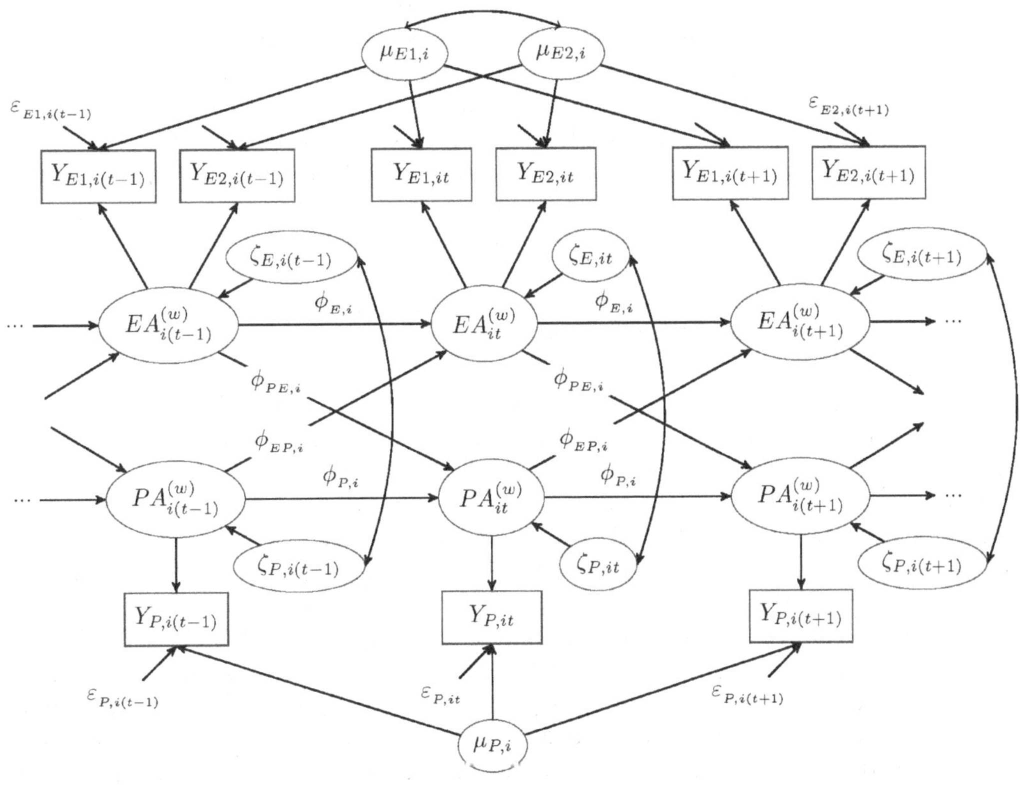

FIGURE 15.2. Alternative representation of the measurement and latent within-person model for the dynamic structural equation model of physical activity (PA) and energetic arousal (EA). i: individual; t: time point; $Y_{E1,it}/Y_{E2,it}/Y_{P,it}$: Observed variables of EA, indicator 1 and 2, and PA; $EA^{(w)}_{it}/PA^{(w)}_{it}$: latent within-person state variables of EA and PA; $\mu_{E1,i}/\mu_{E2,i}/\mu_{P,i}$: random, person-specific mean of the respective construct and indicator; $\varepsilon_{E1,it}/\varepsilon_{E2,it}/\varepsilon_{P,it}$: measurement error variables; $\phi_{E,i}/\phi_{P,i}$: random, person-specific autoregressive effects; $\phi_{EP,i}$: person-specific slope of the latent cross-lagged regression of $EA^{(w)}_{it}$ at time t on $PA^{(w)}_{i(t-1)}$ at time $(t-1)$; $\phi_{PE,i}$: person-specific slope of the latent cross-lagged regression of $PA^{(w)}_{it}$ at time point t on $EA^{(w)}_{i(t-1)}$ at time point $(t-1)$; $\zeta_{E,it}/\zeta_{P,it}$: latent innovations of EA and PA.

Suppose physical activity was measured by one accelerometer and actual PA was averaged across predefined time periods, for instance, by splitting the timeline into consecutive 10-minute intervals or by averaging PA across a specified time interval preceding an electronic diary prompt. Consequently, one observed indicator is available for modeling PA, calling for a single-indicator model. In this model, the observed variable $Y_{P,it}$ for person *i*'s PA at time point *t* is decomposed into three parts:

$$Y_{P,it} = \mu_{P,i} + PA_{it}^{(w)} + \varepsilon_{P,it} \tag{15.5}$$

where $\mu_{P,i}$ is the latent person-specific average PA level across the observed time period, $PA_{it}^{(w)}$ denotes the latent within-person deviation of the true PA at time *t* from the person-specific mean level $\mu_{P,i}$, and $\varepsilon_{P,it}$ denotes a residual variable. Note that in case of a single-indicator model, residual variance and true within-person fluctuations across time are not separated by factorizing two parallel indicators. The separation of both components is possible only if the dynamic process across time is modeled. As elaborated in the next section, it is assumed that the dynamics on the within-person level show a systematic pattern in that true within-person fluctuations are serially dependent across time, for instance, following an autoregressive (AR) process of order 1 (AR[1] or potentially higher). That is, true levels of $PA_{it}^{(w)}$ at time *t* are assumed to show carryover effects to subsequent time points. In contrast, the residual variables $\varepsilon_{P,it}$ are assumed to be serially uncorrelated (independently and identically normally distributed with mean zero across all time points *t*). That is, the residual variable $\varepsilon_{P,it}$ in the single-indicator measurement model captures all within-person fluctuations that are not carried forward in time—that is, deviations from the stable person mean $\mu_{P,i}$ that do not affect subsequent levels of $Y_{P,it}$. The residual variable $\varepsilon_{P,it}$ might therefore capture any time-specific components that are unsystematic, such as measurement error, but also other fluctuations due to time-specific situational effects that are of short duration and have no impact on future states of the measured construct. Whether external effects on the process are captured by $PA_{it}^{(w)}$ or $\varepsilon_{P,it}$ (referred to as measurement error in the following) therefore depends in part on the frequency of measurements taken and the time interval between adjacent observations (Schuurman et al., 2015). This single-indicator model variant is referred to as the (two-level) measurement error AR(1) [MEAR(1)] model in the univariate case in Asparouhov and colleagues (2018) and as the measurement error vector AR(1) (MEVAR(1)) model in the multivariate case in Schuurman and Hamaker (2019). It has to be stressed that estimation of this model requires large sample sizes on the within-person level (see Asparouhov et al., 2018). That is, in order to separate $PA_{it}^{(w)}$ and $\varepsilon_{P,it}$ in empirical applications, a large number of measurement time points per person (e.g., ≥200) is required. It is therefore recommended to reduce model complexity in smaller samples by reducing the number of random effects in the model (e.g., by holding measurement error variance, innovation variance, or both equal across persons). In order to separate the two error components more appropriately, multiple indicators of the same construct are recommended. In some applications using questionnaire data, multiple indicators can be obtained by grouping the items into different parcels.

Within-Person Processes

On the within-person level, the dynamic interplay of occasion-specific state variables across time is modeled. DSEMs can accommodate a large variety of modeling strategies, including autoregressive and moving average effects of flexible order (see Asparouhov et al., 2018, and Asparouhov & Muthén, 2020, for a detailed description of different models covered by the DSEM framework).

BOX 15.1. Autocorrelation, Autoregressive Effects, and Moving Average Effects

Autocorrelation refers to the correlation of a variable with itself at previous time points, with the lag of the autocorrelation quantifying the temporal distance between the correlated time series. For instance, a lag-1 autocorrelation is simply the correlation of each observation with the directly preceding observation of the same variable. Analogously, a lag-k autocorrelation is the correlation of a variable with its observations k time points earlier. Autocorrelated series can be modeled by *autoregressive (AR) effects* of order k, regressing a variable on its past k values. An AR(*1*) process is, for instance, given by

$$Y_t = c + \phi Y_{(t-1)} + \varepsilon_t \tag{15.6}$$

The autoregressive parameter ϕ in Equation 15.6 should assume values in the interval (–1; 1) only, as $|\phi| \leq 1$ implies a nonstationary time series (Hamilton, 1994). A series is called (weakly) stationary if its mean, variance, and autocovariance are constant across time (the autocorrelation only depends on the time lag between the correlated series; Hamilton, 1994). The stationarity of the series should be ensured before estimating a time-series model (see Box 15.6).

As an alternative to AR effects, serial dependency might be explained by a *moving average (MA) process*, in which the current value of a variable is regressed on previous random shocks, with a respective time lag q. An MA(q) process is, for instance, given by

$$Y_t = \mu + \theta_1 \varepsilon_{(t-1)} + \theta_2 \varepsilon_{(t-2)} + \ldots + \theta_q \varepsilon_{(t-q)} + \varepsilon_t \tag{15.7}$$

with independent and identically distributed ε_t (with mean 0 and variance σ^2). Both AR and MA components might be combined within one model (so-called ARMA(p, q) models). AR and MA components result in different autocorrelated series, and the decision on the respective model and order p and q of the AR and MA components can, for instance, be based on visual inspections of plots of the autocorrelation function and partial autocorrelation functions (Jebb, Tay, Wang, & Huang, 2015). In practice, AR models might be preferred due to ease of interpretation of the model parameters. As shown by Granger and Morris (1976), an AR(p) model with an additional random measurement error term (White Noise; WN), which is not carried forward in time, can be equivalently modeled by an ARMA(p, p) model without this random measurement error. However, Schuurman and colleagues (2015) found that the AR(p) + WN model performed better with respect to parameter recovery. We refer the interested reader to Jebb and colleagues (2015) for an introduction to time-series analysis for psychological research.

In the following, we focus on the simplest and most common case of autoregressive and cross-lagged effects of order 1. The respective within-level latent dynamics are depicted in Figure 15.1B. An alternative representation of the decomposition and within-level dynamics is given in Figure 15.2. In this model, it is assumed that the time-specific within-level occasion-specific variables $EA_{it}^{(w)}$ and $PA_{it}^{(w)}$ show serial dependency across time. The serial dependency within a variable is modeled by an autoregressive process of order 1, regressing the latent occasion-specific variable at time point t on the latent occasion-specific variable at the previous time point $t - 1$. Additionally, it is assumed that EA and PA reciprocally affect each other across time:

$$EA_{it}^{(w)} = \phi_{E,i}\, EA_{i(t-1)}^{(w)} + \phi_{EP,i}\, PA_{i(t-1)}^{(w)} + \zeta_{E,it} \tag{15.8}$$

$$PA_{it}^{(w)} = \phi_{P,i}\, PA_{i(t-1)}^{(w)} + \phi_{PE,i}\, EA_{i(t-1)}^{(w)} + \zeta_{P,it} \tag{15.9}$$

The autoregressive parameters $\phi_{E,i}$ and $\phi_{P,i}$ quantify the carryover effect of EA and PA, respectively, across subsequent measurement time points. The strength of the AR parameter indicates how each variable affects itself across time. A positive AR effect indicates that scores of subsequent measurement occasions are positively correlated and are thereby similar (e.g., a relatively high value is followed by a relatively high value). AR effects are sometimes termed inertia, and positive values are interpreted as a sign for resistance to change across time (Suls, Green, & Hillis, 1998). AR effects close to zero indicate that future values cannot be well predicted by past values and that the return from elevated or reduced levels to baseline levels is relatively fast. A negative AR effect, in contrast, indicates that relatively elevated levels are typically followed by relatively low levels and vice versa (a pattern that is rather uncommon for psychological constructs).

The cross-lagged parameters $\phi_{EP,i}$ and $\phi_{PE,i}$ capture the effect of PA on subsequent EA and vice versa (controlled for autoregressive effects). A positive cross-lagged effect $\phi_{PE,i}$ would, for instance, indicate that a high level of EA is associated with a subsequent elevated level of PA (controlled for previous PA). That is, the cross-lagged effects capture potential reciprocal effects between PA and EA over time, that is, predictive relationships. Note that these are within-person associations, which are to be interpreted relative to the person-mean. That is, the cross-lagged effects capture whether an elevated activity score relative to the respective person's average activity predicts an increase or decrease in the person's energetic arousal level (relative to the person's average energy level), and vice versa.

All autoregressive and cross-lagged parameters in Equations 15.8 and 15.9 are assumed to be constant across time points t, but have an index i, indicating that they are estimated as person-specific parameters. That is, subjects may vary with respect to the degree of autoregressive as well as reciprocal effects between psychological and physical states. While it is possible to reduce model complexity by fixing the respective parameters to equality across persons, the possibility of modeling interindividual differences in latent within-person dynamics is an attractive feature for the analysis of sensor data with DSEM and mirrors the observation that intraindividual dynamics are likely to vary across persons. Note that sample-size requirements increase with model complexity. See, for instance, Schultzberg and Muthén (2018) for required sample sizes for different model variants.

The variables $\zeta_{E,it}$ and $\zeta_{P,it}$ capture components in $EA_{it}^{(w)}$ and $PA_{it}^{(w)}$ that remain unexplained by previous within-level states (fluctuations around the predicted trajectory). These autoregressive residuals are termed innovations or dynamic errors and capture the effect of perturbations on the system at time t by anything not accounted for in the model (e.g., unobserved events). The term *dynamic error* mirrors the idea that the innovations are carried forward to future time points through the autoregressive effects and thereby affect future values of the system. This characteristic distinguishes dynamic errors from measurement errors, which are specific to a single time point. Note that in order for measurement error and innovations to be distinguishable in the single-indicator case, the series has to contain a substantive amount of time dependency. If the AR and cross-lagged effects equal zero, these two sources of variance cannot be separated and the model is not identified. For small dynamic effects (close to zero), empirical identification might become difficult (Schuurman et al., 2015). In this case, it is recommended that measurement error variances be fixed to zero.

The variances of these innovations are measures of unexplained true-score variability across time. Within-level variance (innovation as well as measurement error variance) is typically estimated as a fixed parameter across clusters (here: persons) in multilevel analyses. Restricting within-level innovation variances to equality implies that unexplained variation in the time series, and thereby the predictability of upcoming values, is equally high for all persons. However, persons may potentially vary with respect to the quantity and quality in which external events are experienced as well as to their sensitivity and reactivity with respect to these events and thereby with respect to their unexplained variation (peaks and valleys) in their temporal dynamics. Recent developments allow for the estimation of person-specific innovation variances and thereby for investigating interindividual differences in intraindividual variability across time as well as correlates of such interindividual differences (multilevel location scale model; Hedeker, Mermelstein, & Demirtas, 2008; Jongerling et al., 2015). As shown by Jongerling and colleagues (2015), ignoring interindividual differences in innovation variances can result in biased estimates of the autoregressive effects (see also Asparouhov et al., 2018). Considering interindividual differences in innovation variances, the innovations are assumed to be multivariate normally distributed with mean zero and subject-specific variances, $\sigma^2_{\zeta E,i}$ and $\sigma^2_{\zeta P,i}$, and covariance $\sigma_{\zeta EP,i}$, that is,

$$\begin{pmatrix} \zeta_{E,it} \\ \zeta_{P,it} \end{pmatrix} \sim MVN\left(\begin{bmatrix} 0 \\ 0 \end{bmatrix}, \begin{bmatrix} \sigma^2_{\zeta E,i} & \sigma_{\zeta EP,i} \\ \sigma_{\zeta EP,i} & \sigma^2_{\zeta P,i} \end{bmatrix} \right) \tag{15.10}$$

The person-specific innovation covariances capture the temporal coupling between the innovations of PA and EA. That is, the covariance reflects the amount to which external and internal unobserved factors simultaneously affect PA and EA at the same time point and thereby models the temporal coupling of time-specific components in both constructs (i.e., in the deviations from values predicted based on past observations). Following Hamaker, Asparouhov, Brose, Schmiedek, and Muthén (2018), these person-specific covariances are modeled by a common factor η_{it}:

$$\zeta_{E,it} = \eta_{it} + \delta_{E,it} \tag{15.11}$$

$$\zeta_{P,it} = \eta_{it} + \delta_{P,it} \tag{15.12}$$

where η_{it} captures the commonalities between the innovations, and $\delta_{E,it}$ and $\delta_{P,it}$ are construct-specific, unique components of the innovations, which are uncorrelated across constructs (see Figure 15.1B). The common factor and the residual (unique) innovations are assumed to be independently and identically normally distributed for each person i, with $\eta_{it} \sim N(0,\sigma^2_{\eta,i})$, $\delta_{E,it} \sim N(0,\sigma^2_{\delta E,i})$, and $\delta_{P,it} \sim N(0,\sigma^2_{\delta P,i})$. This approach is taken as it ensures that the covariance matrix of the innovations is positive definite for each individual (Hamaker et al., 2018). A disadvantage of this approach is that innovation covariances have to be a priori specified to be either positive or negative for all individuals. A negative correlation is obtained by setting the factor loading of η_{it} in either Equation 15.11 or Equation 15.12 to –1. Based on the decomposition in Equations 15.11 and 15.12, the innovation variances $\sigma^2_{\zeta E,i}$ and $\sigma^2_{\zeta P,i}$ are only indirect model parameters given by the sum of the innovation covariance and the respective residual innovation variance:

$$\sigma_{\zeta EP,i} = \sigma^2_{\eta,i} \tag{15.13}$$

$$\sigma^2_{\zeta E,i} = \sigma^2_{\eta,i} + \sigma^2_{\delta E,i} \tag{15.14}$$

$$\sigma^2_{\zeta P,i} = \sigma^2_{\eta,i} + \sigma^2_{\delta P,i} \tag{15.15}$$

BOX 15.2. Unequal Time Intervals between Observations

Unequal time intervals between adjacent observations pose a challenge for the analysis of intensive longitudinal data. Unequally spaced observations might not be prevalent in signals obtained with wearable sensors if these are measured continuously. However, nonequidistant observations (across time and/or individuals) are frequent in experience sampling data, in which participants might be prompted at random time points, participants might miss to answer a prompt, or nighttime interrupts measurements taken in intervals of 1 to 2 hours during day time over several days.

The models presented above are discrete time models, in which the strengths of the lagged effects (autoregressive and cross-lagged) are specific to the respective time interval between the observations. Furthermore, the models assume that the lagged effects are constant across time. There are different ways to account for varying distances between adjacent observations. For instance, in Mplus (Muthén & Muthén, 1998–2017), researchers can make use of the `tinterval` option provided for DSEM analyses. A dataset with equally spaced observations is approximated by inserting missing values between subsequent observed values according to the desired time interval specified by the user. That is, a time grid with fixed time increments is imposed on the supposedly continuous time dimension, creating segments of the specified length. Mplus appends the data by inserting missing values to each grid not containing an observation. The inserted missing values can be easily estimated and updated in each Markov chain Monte Carlo sampling step (see Box 15.3), along with the remaining model parameters and latent variables. Thereby, lagged effects obtain a constant interpretation with respect to the requested time interval.

The choice of an appropriate time grid is crucial, as the quality of the estimation depends on the accuracy with which the time intervals between the observations are approximated, as well as on the amount of missing data that are inserted. With respect to the specified time scale, larger requested (transformed) time intervals were found to lead to more bias in parameter estimates (Asparouhov et al., 2018). In contrast, smaller requested time intervals lead to more accurate approximations of the original observed time scale, while inserting larger amounts of missing data, which might lead to convergence problems. Asparouhov and colleagues (2018) recommend inserting between 80 and 95% of missing data, depending on model complexity, while choosing a time interval that is interpretable from a substantial point of view (with respect to the time metric of the observations).

Note that this is an approximate solution in which observed values falling into a specific segment of the imposed time grid may have been observed at any time within this segment and might be slightly shifted forward or backward in time by the algorithm. See, for instance, Voelkle and Oud (2013) or Oravecz and colleagues (2009) for an alternative, continuous time-modeling approach.

Alternative Model for Within-Person Processes: Simultaneous/Concurrent Regression

In the dataset analyzed in the present illustrative application, each participant's PA was averaged across the 10 minutes preceding a person's self-reported EA during preprocessing. That is, the dataset contains one measure of PA, indicating average actual PA in the 10 minutes directly preceding reported EA (both located in the same line of the datafile). Time intervals between self-reports of EA varied across persons and between measurement occasions, with a median of 45 minutes and a mean of 108 minutes. That is, the measurements of EA at occasion $(t - 1)$ were, on average, observed 108 minutes before the observation at occasion t, while PA was observed for the 10 minutes preceding each EA measurement. We accounted for the variation in the time intervals between adjacent EA measurements, such that model parameters are estimated for a time interval of approximately 30 minutes between two measurement occasions t and $(t - 1)$ (see Box 15.2 for further information). Additionally, to account for the large differences between the time lag between previous PA and subsequent EA and the time lag between previous EA and subsequent PA in the present dataset, we used a different variant of the within-level model structure described above. That is, we chose to model the effect of PA on EA as a simultaneous regression effect, where the most recent observation of PA to predict EA is that of the same measurement occasion:

$$EA_{it}^{(w)} = \phi_{E,i}\, EA_{i(t-1)}^{(w)} + \beta_{EP,i}\, PA_{it}^{(w)} + \phi_{EP,i}\, PA_{i(t-1)}^{(w)} + \zeta_{E,it} \tag{15.16}$$

where $\phi_{E,i}$ is the autoregressive effect of EA, $\beta_{EP,i}$ captures the effect of PA on the level of EA directly following the PA measure (simultaneous regression), and $\phi_{EP,i}$ captures the effect of PA on EA with a time lag of approximately 30–40 minutes. In contrast, for predicting PA by EA, the most recent observation of EA is that obtained at the foregoing measurement occasion:

$$PA_{it}^{(w)} = \phi_{P,i}\, PA_{i(t-1)}^{(w)} + \phi_{PE,i}\, EA_{i(t-1)}^{(w)} + \zeta_{P,it} \tag{15.17}$$

As a result of the simultaneous regression of $EA_{it}^{(w)}$ on $PA_{it}^{(w)}$ of the same measurement occasion, the innovation of EA, $\zeta_{E,it}$, is a residual with respect to $PA_{it}^{(w)}$, such that the innovations between EA and PA are modeled to be uncorrelated, with

$$\zeta_{E,it} \sim N\left(0, \sigma^2_{\zeta E,i}\right) \tag{15.18}$$

$$\zeta_{P,it} \sim N\left(0, \sigma^2_{\zeta P,i}\right) \tag{15.19}$$

See Figure 15.3 for a visual representation of the within-level dynamics in the model including a simultaneous regression.

Between-Level Structure

On the between-person level, interindividual differences in the stable trait variables and in the within-person dynamics, as well as associations between these person-specific parameters, are modeled (see Figure 15.1C). As in standard multilevel models, the individual parameters from the within-person level are assumed to come from a distribution with a mean corresponding to the average effect across persons (fixed effect) and a variance of person-specific deviations from this average effect (random effect). That is, the person-specific variables and parameters are decomposed into average, fixed effects γ and person-specific deviations from the respective fixed effect, u_i. For the model with a simultaneous regression effect (see Equations 15.16–15.19), this decomposition is given by

$$\begin{bmatrix} \mu_{E1,i} \\ \mu_{E2,i} \\ \mu_{P,i} \\ \phi_{E,i} \\ \phi_{P,i} \\ \phi_{EP,i} \\ \phi_{PE,i} \\ \beta_{EP,i} \\ ln\left(\sigma^2_{\zeta E,1}\right) \\ ln\left(\sigma^2_{\zeta P,1}\right) \end{bmatrix} = \begin{bmatrix} \gamma_{\mu E1} \\ \gamma_{\mu E2} \\ \gamma_{\mu P} \\ \gamma_{\phi E} \\ \gamma_{\phi P} \\ \gamma_{\phi EP} \\ \gamma_{\phi PE} \\ \gamma_{\beta EP} \\ \gamma_{\sigma\zeta E} \\ \gamma_{\sigma\zeta P} \end{bmatrix} + \begin{bmatrix} u_{\mu E1,i} \\ u_{\mu E2,i} \\ u_{\mu P,i} \\ u_{\phi E,i} \\ u_{\phi P,i} \\ u_{\phi EP,i} \\ u_{\phi PE,i} \\ u_{\beta EP,i} \\ u_{\sigma\zeta E,i} \\ u_{\sigma\zeta P,i} \end{bmatrix} \tag{15.20}$$

The fixed effects $\gamma_{\mu E1}$, $\gamma_{\mu E2}$, and $\gamma_{\mu P}$ are the average trait levels of EA and PA across all persons (expectations of the latent trait variables); the fixed effects $\gamma_{\phi E}$, $\gamma_{\phi P}$, $\gamma_{\phi EP}$, $\gamma_{\phi PE}$, and $\gamma_{\beta EP}$ reflect the average AR, cross-lagged, and simultaneous regression effects across all individuals; and $\gamma_{\sigma\zeta E}$ and $\gamma_{\sigma\zeta P}$ denote the average individual log-innovation variances of EA and PA, respectively. The individual deviations u_i are assumed to come from a multivariate normal distribution, that is, $\boldsymbol{u}_i \sim MVN(0, \boldsymbol{\Psi})$, where $\boldsymbol{\Psi}$ is the covariance matrix of the random effects (in this case with dimension 10×10). The variances in $\boldsymbol{\Psi}$ quantify the variation in the individual parameters across individuals, for instance, the amount of interindividual differences in trait scores of EA and PA or in cross-lagged effects between the latent states of EA and PA. The covariances capture the associations between the person-specific parameters; for instance, a positive correlation between $u_{\mu E1,i}$ / $u_{\mu E2,i}$ and $u_{\mu P,i}$ would indicate that persons with high trait levels of EA tend to also have high trait levels of PA, and vice versa.

On the between-person level, random effects are modeled as latent variables, such that the between-person level model can also contain measurement equations (e.g., a common between-person factor for the two trait factors of EA) or structural equations. That is, factor models or path models can be specified on the between-person level, with the possibility of including additional (latent or observed) time-invariant variables as predictors or outcomes of the random effects. We could, for instance, use external variables such as age, body mass index, or athleticism to explain interindividual differences in persons' average levels of or unexplained variability in PA and EA. Interindividual differences in the parameters describing average levels and dynamics of PA across time might be used to predict differences in indices of health or well-being.

Note that the logs of the person-specific variances ($ln(\sigma^2_{\zeta E,i})$ and $ln(\sigma^2_{\zeta P,i})$) are modeled on the between-person level; that is, $\gamma_{\sigma\zeta E}$ and $\gamma_{\sigma\zeta P}$ refer to the average log of the innovation variances, and $u_{\sigma\zeta E,i}$ and $u_{\sigma\zeta P,i}$ refer to the individual deviations of the individual log innovation variances from the average log innovation variances. The respective variance in $\boldsymbol{\Psi}$ is the variance (across persons) of the log of the individual innovation variances. Individual innovation variances are thereby assumed to follow a log-normal distribution on the between-person level (Asparouhov et al., 2018), ensuring that estimates of innovation variances will be positive for each individual (Hamaker et al., 2018). Additionally, the log of the variances can be easily modeled within a multivariate normal distribution alongside the remaining random effects to investigate potential correlations between person-specific innovation variances and stable trait levels or dynamic (lagged) parameters. This log transformation should be kept in mind when interpreting coefficients regarding innovation variances on the between-person level (e.g., when including predictor variables for individual innovation variances on the between-person level; see, e.g., McNeish & Hamaker, 2020, for an illustrative interpretation of such regression coefficients).

In theory, any of the random effects could be excluded from the model, or between-level covariances could be set to zero for parsimony. In case of low variation across participants (i.e., very small random effect variances), it might be advisable to reduce model complexity by fixing the respective parameter across individuals. Furthermore, we recommend adjusting model complexity to the available between- and within-level sample sizes (see Schultzberg & Muthén, 2018, and Asparouhov et al., 2018, for simulation studies).

BOX 15.3. Bayesian Estimation and Markov Chain Monte Carlo Sampling

Dynamic *SEMs* in Mplus are estimated in a Bayesian framework using Markov chain Monte Carlo (MCMC) sampling techniques. We will not provide a detailed coverage of Bayesian statistics or MCMC sampling here, but we will provide a very short introduction of the basic idea and terminology. Note that MCMC sampling can be used as a computational tool to facilitate estimation of complex models, without necessarily relying on the philosophical underpinnings of Bayesian methods (Asparouhov et al., 2018). For detailed information on Bayesian statistics and MCMC estimation, we refer the reader to Kruschke (2015), McElreath (2020), or Gelman and colleagues (2014), and for short introductions, we refer the reader to Kruschke, Aguinis, and Joo (2012), van de Schoot and colleagues (2014), or Song and Lee (2012).

In Bayesian statistics, parameters are considered random variables, and the uncertainty about a parameter's value is reflected in the parameter's probability distribution. Prior beliefs about a parameter's distribution are updated with information from observed data to obtain a posterior probability distribution of the respective parameter (Song & Lee, 2012). That is, while classical estimation procedures such as maximum likelihood (ML) estimation provide a point estimate for each parameter, Bayesian statistics provides a (posterior) distribution for each model parameter. Prior beliefs regarding a parameter's location may, for instance, stem from previous research results. This prior belief, as well as the uncertainty associated with it, are quantified in terms of a prior distribution. Disregarding philosophical differences, Bayesian and ML approaches are asymptotically equivalent (Song & Lee, 2012), with the effect of the prior distribution decreasing with increasing sample sizes. Furthermore, if researchers do not wish to incorporate prior beliefs into the analysis, they can make use of uninformative prior distributions (also called flat or diffuse priors, which contain no or little information on the parameter's location within the admissible parameter space). Per default, Mplus uses uninformative prior distributions; for details, see Asparouhov and Muthén (2010) and Asparouhov and colleagues (2018). Recently, McNeish (2019) has proposed the use of weakly informative, so-called admissible-range-restricted priors to improve the performance of DSEMs in small sample sizes.

For many complex models, the joint posterior distribution of the model parameters cannot be derived analytically, such that sampling methods are needed. That is, posterior distributions are approximated by use of MCMC methods. MCMC is an iterative sampling process that generates a Markov chain of draws from the posterior distribution, generating a large representative sample of parameter values from the posterior (see Kruschke, 2015, or McElreath, 2020, for an introduction). A parameter's posterior distribution can then be described by summarizing the MCMC samples drawn from the posterior, for example, by use of a measure of central tendency (e.g., mean or median), the standard deviation, as well as percentiles of the posterior distribution. For instance, the 2.5 and 97.5 percentiles serve as boundaries of a 95% credible interval (CI; as an analog of a confidence interval). Different from classical frequentist confidence intervals, the interpretation of a 95% credible interval is that, given the observed data, there is a 95% probability that the true parameter lies within the interval. CIs may be consulted to decide whether a parameter estimate can be considered to be different from a previously specified value (e.g., zero). Note that relying on CIs to test deviations from zero is not advisable for variance parameters, as these are often precluded from assuming negative values by use of corresponding priors (see below for alternative decision rules regarding variance parameters). Typically, at least two parallel MCMC chains are sampled, with a large number of iterations (determining the sample size of draws from the posterior), where a certain percentage of draws at the beginning of the chain is discarded (burn-in; since the chain may not yet have converged to the target distribution). Researchers may decide to use only every *k*th sampled value to avoid high autocorrelation between the samples.

An advantage of MCMC procedures is that (nonlinear) transformations of the estimated model parameters can be easily sampled, along with their respective CIs, even if these parameters follow unknown or possibly skewed distributions. Furthermore, missing data are sampled, along with the remaining model parameters in each MCMC iteration, from its respective conditional posterior distribution, taking the within-person dynamics (serial dependency) into account. Thereby, data that are missing at random can be easily handled within MCMC estimation, without further required modeling steps or loss of information.

Estimation via MCMC sampling requires careful checks of convergence diagnostics to ensure that the sampler has converged to the target distribution. To this end, convergence statistics such as the Potential Scale Reduction (PSR; Gelman-Rubin convergence diagnostic; Gelman & Rubin, 1992) should be combined with visual diagnostics of trace plots, autocorrelation plots, and posterior density plots. The PSR is a convergence criterion for parallel MCMC chains, which is based on comparing within-chain and between-chain variance, with a value of 1 indicating that the chains have converged to a common distribution (see Asparouhov & Muthén, 2010, for details). For guidelines on convergence checking and the interpretation of MCMC plots, see, for example, Kruschke (2015, Ch. 7.5) or McElreath (2020, Ch. 9). For a checklist of steps in the practical implementation of Bayesian estimation, see Depaoli and van de Schoot (2017).

For the purpose of model comparisons of DSEMs estimated by MCMC methods, Mplus (version 8.4, Muthén & Muthén, 1998–2017) currently provides the deviance information criterion (DIC) as well as Bayes factors (BF). The DIC (Asparouhov et al., 2018; Spiegelhalter, Best, Carlin, & van der Linde, 2002) can be used as an index of relative model fit for nested or non-nested models, given that the models have the same latent variables (with relatively lower DIC values indicating better model fit). That is, the DIC should be implemented with caution, as it cannot be naively applied for comparisons of any two possible models, and DIC estimation tends to be unstable in complex time-series models including latent variables (Asparouhov et al., 2018; Asparouhov & Muthén, 2020). The Bayes factor is a likelihood ratio quantifying the relative evidence in the data for an hypothesis over a competing hypothesis (for details see, e.g., Hoijtink, Mulder, van Lissa, & Gu, 2019). For details on how to request BFs for variance parameters in Mplus, see Muthén and Asparouhov (2012). To decide on the necessity to include random effects in the model, Asparouhov and Muthén (personal communication, July 2, 2021) recommend a different approach, using a cutoff value of $z > 3$, with z = parameter estimate / standard error.

Illustrative Application to Physical Activity and Energetic Arousal Data

We applied the dynamic *SEM* described above to data on physical activity (accelerometer) and energetic arousal (self-report) obtained in a convenience sample of undergraduate students and citizens of a city in the southern part of Germany in 2009. Self-report ratings of EA were assessed via electronic diaries (e-diaries, smartphones), which prompted participants randomly about every 45 minutes during a predefined 14-hour daytime period (8:00 A.M. to 10:00 P.M.) across 1 to 3 days. EA was assessed with two items of the short mood scale (Wilhelm & Schoebi, 2007), which has been explicitly developed and evaluated for AA studies. It is a bipolar scale (tired vs. wake; energetic vs. nonenergetic). Participants answered to the prompt "At this moment, I feel . . . " by moving a slider from the left end (e.g., tired) to the right end (e.g., wake). We changed the original 7-point rating scale to a 6-point scale to force participants to decide between the two poles. Inverse items were recoded such that high values reflect high levels of EA.

PA was assessed continuously and objectively with hip-worn accelerometers (varioport-e, Becker, Meditech, Karlsruhe). Accelerometers are used to measure the intensity, rate of occurrence, and duration of a physically active episode. To analyze associations between PA and EA, the activity values during the 10 minutes preceding each entry into the e-diary were averaged. For further information on the conducted data preprocessing steps see Kanning (2013). To reduce the skewness of the PA measure, actual PA was rescaled by taking its natural logarithm, resulting in a measure of actual PA measured in log-milli-g, with observed values in the range between –7.07 and 7.18 (with mean = 3.86, 25% quantile = 2.94, median = 4.08, and 75% quantile = 4.84). Note that on this scale, pure sitting episodes would elicit values of around 2.3, walking episodes of around 5.9, and jogging episodes of around 6.9.

The dataset comprised observations from 166 participants, of which 84 were female, with an average age of 40.5 years (min = 18, max = 74, *SD* = 17.8, median = 30.5). Note that only participants who provided at least 10 valid self-reports were included in the present analyses. On average, the resulting dataset includes observations on 19.2 time points per person (min = 10, max = 42, median = 19), with a median time interval between adjacent observations of 45 minutes (min = 3 minutes, 25% quantile = 39 minutes, 75% quantile = 68 minutes, max = 26 hours). To account for nonequidistant observations, we made use of the `tinterval` option in Mplus, which was set to produce approximately equal time intervals of 30 minutes. An interval of 30 minutes was chosen because it should sufficiently well approximate the observed time intervals reported

BOX 15.4. Standardization in Multilevel Time-Series Models

In the analysis of ILD, we are typically interested in comparing the relative strengths of different predictor variables in the dynamics of psychological processes that occur on the within-person level. That is, between-person differences in average trait levels are not of primary interest when we are judging the relative strengths of cross-lagged effects on the within-person level. As proposed by Schuurman and colleagues (2016), to compare the relative strengths of different predictors in the within-person dynamics, the parameters should be standardized on the within-person level. By standardizing on the within-person level, standardized cross-lagged effects quantify the proportion of uniquely explained variance in the within-person dynamics, considering each individual's unique variability in the covariate and outcome across time (i.e., some individuals may have larger/smaller variances for the same psychological construct). To obtain within-person standardized estimates, regression coefficients are standardized for each individual separately (similar to standardization in $n = 1$ time-series models) and then are averaged across individuals to obtain an average standardized effect estimate (Schuurman et al., 2016). Furthermore, the proportion of variance explained by the within-person dynamics is calculated on the within-person level and is subsequently averaged to obtain an average R^2 estimate for within-level (latent) variables. Within-person standardized autoregressive and cross-lagged effects can be interpreted as the person-specific standard deviations that the outcome variable increases when the predictor variable increases by one person-specific standard deviation (Schuurman et al., 2016), controlling for the autoregressive dependency. In contrast, between-level parameters are standardized based on the between-person variances.

above (using time intervals of 15 minutes did produce convergence problems). Using a time interval of 30 minutes, approximately 70% missings were inserted into the dataset.

With no prior hypotheses on the parameter locations, we used the uninformative prior distributions provided as default priors in Mplus (see Asparouhov & Muthén, 2010, as well as Asparouhov et al., 2018, for details). MCMC estimation was conducted using two MCMC chains, which ran with a minimum of 600,000 iterations per chain with a thinning factor of 40. That is, only every 40th iteration per chain was used as a sample for constructing the posterior distribution. The first half of each chain was discarded as a burn-in period. That is, posterior distributions comprised at least 15,000 samples. MCMC sampling was stopped when the PSR fell below a threshold of 1.01 for the first time after the minimum number of iterations was sampled. Mixing of the MCMC chains was further checked by visual inspection of trace plots.

Due to the described preprocessing steps, an average PA measure was available for the 10 minutes directly preceding each EA self-report. Therefore, we applied the model that includes a simultaneous regression effect of PA on EA, as described above and depicted in Figure 15.3. For comparisons and interpretation of within-person dynamics, we make use of average within-person standardized estimates (Schuurman et al., 2016).

Within-Person Dynamics

The results in Table 15.1 show that both PA and EA exhibit positive autocorrelation across time, with average within-person standardized AR effects of 0.711 for EA (95% CI [0.653; 0.757]) and 0.498 for PA (95% CI [0.421; 0.591]). This implies that persons who feel energetic at one occasion tend to feel similarly energetic at the next one (30 minutes later), with high carryover effects. If the level of EA is perturbed by an external

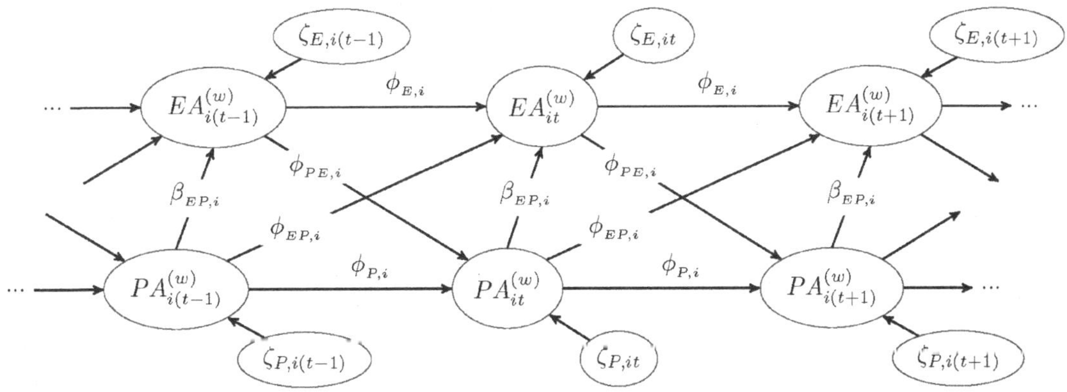

FIGURE 15.3. Latent within-person dynamics in the dynamic structural equation model with a simultaneous effect of physical activity (PA) on energetic arousal (EA). *i*: individual; *t*: time point; $EA^{(w)}_{it}/PA^{(w)}_{it}$: latent within-person variables of EA and PA; $\beta_{EP,i}$: person-specific slope of the latent simultaneous regression of $EA^{(w)}_{it}$ at time *t* on $PA^{(w)}_{it}$ at time *t*; $\phi_{E,i}/\phi_{P,i}$: random, person-specific autoregressive effects; $\phi_{EP,i}$: person-specific slope of the latent cross-lagged regression of $EA^{(w)}_{it}$ at time *t* on $PA^{(w)}_{i(t-1)}$ at time $(t-1)$; $\phi_{PE,i}$: person-specific slope of the latent cross-lagged regression of $PA^{(w)}_{it}$ at time point *t* on $EA^{(w)}_{i(t-1)}$ at time point $(t-1)$; $\zeta_{E,it}/\zeta_{P,it}$: latent innovations of EA and PA.

TABLE 15.1. Parameter Estimates of the DSEM of Energetic Arousal and Physical Activity

	Energetic arousal		Physical activity	
	Estimate	95% CI	Estimate	95% CI
Unstandardized parameter estimates				
$Var(\varepsilon_{E1}) / Var(\varepsilon_P)$	0.713	[0.661; 0.767]	0.254	[0.131; 0.363]
$Var(\varepsilon_{E2})$	0.454	[0.413; 0.497]		
Fixed effects				
$\gamma_{\mu E1} / \gamma_{\mu P}$	3.228	[3.096; 3.377]	3.859	[3.774; 3.941]
$\gamma_{\mu E2}$	3.035	[2.916; 3.153]		
$\gamma_{\phi E} / \gamma_{\phi P}$	0.712	[0.665; 0.765]	0.511	[0.424; 0.597]
$\gamma_{\beta EP}$	0.368	[0.266; 0.504]		
$\gamma_{\phi EP} / \gamma_{\phi PE}$	−0.260	[−0.394; −0.161]	0.115	[0.048; 0.188]
$\gamma_{\sigma\zeta P} / \gamma_{\sigma\zeta P}$	−1.383	[−1.670; −1.147]	−0.462	[−0.758; −0.197]
Random effect variances				
μ_{E1} / μ_P	0.551	[0.401; 0.764]	0.102	[0.056; 0.171]
μ_{E2}	0.330	[0.221; 0.480]		
ϕ_E / ϕ_P	0.023	[0.013; 0.040]	0.048	[0.029; 0.079]
β_{EP}	0.062	[0.029; 0.127]		
ϕ_{EP} / ϕ_{PE}	0.047	[0.020; 0.101]	0.028	[0.011; 0.062]
$ln(\sigma^2_{\zeta E}) / ln(\sigma^2_{\zeta P})$	1.179	[0.786; 1.811]	0.709	[0.419; 1.161]
Standardized parameter estimates				
Within-person standardization (averaged across clusters)				
ϕ_E / ϕ_P	0.711	[0.653; 0.757]	0.498	[0.421; 0.591]
β_{EP}	0.364	[0.288; 0.479]		
ϕ_{EP} / ϕ_{PE}	−0.256	[−0.378; −0.168]	0.120	[0.062; 0.174]
$\sigma^2_{\zeta E} / \sigma^2_{\zeta P}$	0.334	[0.278; 0.386]	0.616	[0.539; 0.677]
R-squared				
Within-level (averaged across clusters)				
Y_{E1} / Y_P	.570	[.537; .601]	.815	[.716; .919]
Y_{E2}	.666	[.634; .697]		
$EA^{(w)} / PA^{(w)}$	.666	[.614; .720]	.384	[.323; .461]

Note. Estimated parameters denote posterior medians and 95% CIs denote Bayesian credibility intervals. Within-person standardized parameters are within-person-level standardized estimates averaged across clusters. R^2 measures for $EA^{(w)}/PA^{(w)}$ denote averaged within-person explained variance with respect to the measurement-error-free latent construct on the within-person level, and those for Y_{E1}, Y_{E2}, and Y_P refer to explained variance in the observed variables on the within-person level. *E/EA*: energetic arousal; *P/PA*: physical activity; *E1*: first item of energetic arousal (awake); *E2*: second item of energetic arousal (energetic); β_{EP}: person-specific simultaneous regression coefficient of $EA^{(w)}_{it}$ on $PA^{(w)}_{it}$; $\varepsilon_{E1}/\varepsilon_{E2}/\varepsilon_P$: measurement error variables; $\gamma_{\phi E}/\gamma_{\phi P}$: average autoregressive effect of $EA^{(w)}/PA^{(w)}$; $\gamma_{\beta EP}$: average effect of the simultaneous regression of $EA^{(w)}_{it}$ on $PA^{(w)}_{it}$; $\gamma_{\phi EP}$: average effect of the cross-lagged regression of $EA^{(w)}_{it}$ on $PA^{(w)}_{i(t-1)}$; $\gamma_{\phi PE}$: average effect of the cross-lagged regression of $PA^{(w)}_{it}$ on $EA^{(w)}_{i(t-1)}$; $\gamma_{\sigma\zeta E}/\gamma_{\sigma\zeta P}$: average log innovation variance of latent construct $EA^{(w)}/PA^{(w)}$; $ln(\sigma^2_{\zeta E})/ln(\sigma^2_{\zeta P})$: logarithm of the random, person-specific innovation variances; $\mu_{E1}/\mu_{E2}/\mu_P$: random, person-specific mean of the respective construct and indicator; ϕ_E/ϕ_P: random, person-specific autoregressive effects; ϕ_{EP}: person-specific slope of the latent regression of $EA^{(w)}_{it}$ at time point t on $PA^{(w)}_{i(t-1)}$ at time point $(t-1)$; ϕ_{PE}: person-specific slope of the latent regression of $PA^{(w)}_{it}$ at time point t on $EA^{(w)}_{i(t-1)}$ at time point $(t-1)$; $Y_{E1}/Y_{E2}/Y_P$: observed variables of EA, indicator 1 and 2, and PA; $EA^{(w)}/PA^{(w)}$: latent within-person state variables of EA and PA.

event (e.g., lack of sleep, a strong coffee), EA is expected to only slowly return to the person's respective baseline level. Although there is a positive carryover from PA levels at one occasion to PA at the next occasion, this effect is smaller for PA as compared to EA.

With respect to the simultaneous effect, we observe that PA in the temporally preceding 10 minutes affects EA such that higher PA is associated with higher levels of EA (average within-person standardized effect: β_{EP} = 0.364, 95% CI [0.288; 0.479]). In contrast, higher levels of PA lead to lower levels of EA 30 to 40 minutes later (ϕ_{EP} = −0.256, 95% CI [−0.378; −0.168]). That is, on average, higher PA is followed by a direct/simultaneous increase in EA, with a subsequent decrease in EA half an hour later. EA at time $t-1$ affects the level of PA at time t, with higher levels of *EA* predicting higher levels of PA 20 to 30 minutes later (ϕ_{PE} = 0.120, 95% CI [0.062; 0.174]).

Autoregressive, simultaneous and cross-lagged regression effects vary substantially across individuals, with random effect variances ranging from 0.023 to 0.062 (see Table 15.1). Note that, although the reported variances may seem small, autoregressive parameters are restricted to the interval [−1; 1], such that small variances may indicate substantial between-person variance. For instance, under the assumption of normality, an average autoregressive effect of $\gamma_{\phi P}$ = 0.511 (fixed effect of PA) with a random effect variance of 0.048 implies that 95% of the individuals' person-specific autoregressive effects lie between [.082; .940]. That is, there seem to be substantial interindividual differences in the dynamic processes within persons. As estimates of variance parameters are prevented from dropping below zero by the Mplus default prior distributions, the respective credibility intervals are less informative with respect to a deviation of random effect variances from zero (unless the lower bound is far above zero). We requested the Bayes factors for the hypotheses that the random effect variances are smaller than 0.001. In this case, a BF of x suggests that a model in which the respective variance is < 0.001 is x times more likely than a model with a variance deviating from zero. Often, a BF > 3 is used as a cutoff for positive evidence against the comparison hypothesis (here: nonzero random-effect variance; Kass & Raftery, 1995). For the present model, the values of the requested BFs suggest keeping all random effects in the model (BFs < 3 in all cases). Using the rule of thumb that variances with $z < 3$ (with z = parameter estimate / standard error) can be dropped from the model, we could consider excluding the random effects for the cross-lagged and the simultaneous regression effects (see Table 15.1). Note that there is no harm in including a random effect if the true parameter is nonrandom, given the required sample sizes for the respective model complexity are met. Otherwise, it is recommended that nonessential random effects be excluded from the model. In the case of substantial random effect variances, considering the fixed effects only might be misleading, and fixed effects close to zero do not necessarily indicate that the respective parameter (e.g., cross-lagged effect) could be excluded from the model.

The average innovation variances for latent state EA and PA are exp(−1.383) = 0.251 and exp(−0.462) = 0.630, respectively. Within-person standardized innovation variances averaged across persons are 0.334 (CI = [0.278; 0.386]) for EA and 0.616 (CI = [0.539; 0.677]) for PA, indicating that, on average, there is a larger amount of unexplained variability in PA as compared to EA. Innovation variances of both EA and PA vary across persons, with random effect variances on the log-scale of 1.179 and 0.709. These log-scale random effects can be interpreted such that, for instance, under the assumption of normality, 95% of the individuals' innovation variances of EA fall in the interval between $\exp(-1.383 - 1.960 \cdot \sqrt{1.179}) = 0.030$ and $\exp(-1.383 + 1.960 \cdot \sqrt{1.179}) = 2.107$.

Extension: Random Measurement Error Variances and Covariance

The presented DSEMs can be extended by including person-specific measurement error variances and covariances. Assume PA and EA were measured by one indicator variable, respectively. In this case, the measurement models are single-indicator models for both variables, with the respective measurement error variables $\varepsilon_{E,it}$ and $\varepsilon_{P,it}$ capturing all effects on the within-level constructs that are not carried forward to the next measurement occasion. That is, they capture any perturbations that are truly time-point specific in that they do not affect future states of the process. Thereby, when jointly modeling multiple constructs across time, measurement error variables might correlate across constructs within persons and measurement time points. A positive correlation would indicate that an unobserved external event resulted in a simultaneous increase or decrease of both variables at the same time, while being so spurious that the effect does not last to the next measurement occasion. Assume, for instance, that energetic arousal and tense arousal are modeled jointly in a bivariate DSEM across time. An unexpected loud noise occurring nearby might lead to a sudden increase in a person's tense arousal and energetic arousal levels at that moment in time, while the effect dissipates immediately after the person has made out the (harmless) source of the experienced noise. The increases in both energetic and tense arousal subside quickly and are not carried forward to the next

BOX 15.5. Within-Person Reliabilities

Multilevel time-series models offer the possibility of estimating different types of reliability for the observed variables: reliability with respect to trait scores and reliability with respect to within-person fluctuations across time (Schuurman & Hamaker, 2019). The first type of reliability is the relevant entity for inferences regarding interindividual trait differences, which Schuurman and Hamaker (2019) call between-person reliability. The second type of reliability is relevant for inferences regarding intraindividual variations across time. Within-person reliability refers to the proportion of within-person true-score variance relative to the total within-person variance across time, a measure that may vary across individuals. Between-person differences in within-person variability may therefore originate from interindividual differences in autoregressive and cross-lagged effects as well as innovation variances on the one hand and, in case measurement error variances are modeled as random parameters, differences in measurement error variability on the other hand. Average within-person reliability as well as the variance of within-person reliabilities across individuals can be inspected. In the model with random measurement error variances, the estimated average within-person reliabilities are .623 (CI [.594; .652]) and .693 (CI [.665; .720]) for the two indicators of EA and .692 (CI [.539; 0.819]) for PA. Note that for single-indicator measurement models (used for PA in the present example), the error variable may partly contain reliable, time-specific components (see the section "Measurement Models"), which might lower the reliability estimates. Within-person reliabilities varied across persons with a central 95% interval of [.30; .90] for the item awake, a central 95% interval of [.25; .93] for the item energetic, and a central 95% interval of [.28; .92] for physical activity.

measurements taken 1 or 2 hours later. A substantive correlation between concurrent residual variables of the two constructs thereby indicates that these do not only capture random measurement error, but also partly contain systematic effects caused by unobserved external factors. In a DSEM model with correlated error variables, the residual variables $\varepsilon_{E,it}$ and $\varepsilon_{P,it}$ are assumed to be multivariate normally distributed with person-specific error variances and covariance:

$$\begin{pmatrix} \varepsilon_{E,it} \\ \varepsilon_{P,it} \end{pmatrix} \sim MVN\left(\begin{bmatrix} 0 \\ 0 \end{bmatrix}, \begin{bmatrix} \sigma^2_{\varepsilon E,i} & \sigma_{\varepsilon EP,i} \\ \sigma_{\varepsilon EP,i} & \sigma^2_{\varepsilon P,i} \end{bmatrix} \right) \quad (15.21)$$

We extended the model in the current data application to incorporate random, person-specific residual variances for both PA and EA. Note that in case of multiple-indicator models, in which measurement error variance is identified by use of two parallel indicators, it is not reasonable to model correlations between random measurement error variables of different constructs (e.g., PA and EA in the present data application), as measurement error variables are theoretically expected to only consist of random noise. That is, we did not include simultaneous correlations between the error variable of PA and the measurement error variables of EA. Parameter estimates are presented in Table 15.2. In comparison to the model with fixed error variances (assuming the error variances are the same for all individuals), average (measurement) error variance for PA has increased (average within-level standardized variance of 0.308 as compared to 0.185), with a respective decrease of the average within-person reliability of PA (see Box 15.5).[3] The transition from fixed to random error variances changed the parameters of the within-level dynamics. Specifically, with respect to the average within-person standardized effects, the simultaneous effect of PA on EA increased to 0.457 (stronger positive effect), the cross-lagged effect of PA on EA half an hour later decreased to −0.350 (stronger negative effect), and the cross-lagged effect of EA on PA half an hour later decreased to 0.097 (slightly smaller positive effect). On average, autoregressive and cross-lagged effects could explain 68.8% and 47.3% of the within-person latent occasion-specific variance in EA and PA, respectively. Random effect variances as well as further parameter estimates along with their credibility intervals are given in Table 15.2.

Between-Person Associations

For parsimony, between-level random effect correlations are presented for the model without random measurement error and if substantially differing from zero only. As expected, we observe a strong positive correlation between the stable trait levels of the two indicators of *EA* ($r(\mu_{E2}, \mu_{E1})$ = .721; *CI* = [.586; .815]), indicating that the stable trait measured by the item awake is positively correlated with the stable trait measured by the item energetic. Stable trait levels of PA substantially correlate with stable levels of EA ($r(\mu_P, \mu_{E1})$ =.305 and $r(\mu_P, \mu_{E2})$ = .425 with CIs [.009; .555] and [.112; .666], respectively), indicating that there is systematic between-person association between persons' average amount of PA and EA. Furthermore, individuals with high average levels of EA tend to show less unexplained (occasion-specific) variability in their dynamics of EA across time ($r(\mu_{E1}, ln(\sigma^2_{\zeta E}))$ = −.334 and $r(\mu_{E2}, ln(\sigma^2_{\zeta E}))$ = −.343 with CIs [−.553; −.086] and [−.589; −.063]), while individuals with higher average levels of PA tend to show less

TABLE 15.2. Parameter Estimates of the DSEM of Energetic Arousal and Physical Activity with Random Measurement Error Variances

	Energetic arousal		Physical activity	
	Estimate	95% CI	Estimate	95% CI
Unstandardized parameter estimates				
Fixed effects				
$\gamma_{\mu E1}/\gamma_{\mu P}$	3.240	[3.097; 3.380]	3.861	[3.773; 3.944]
$\gamma_{\mu E2}$	3.023	[2.900; 3.145]		
$\gamma_{\phi E}/\gamma_{\phi P}$	0.709	[0.641; 0.769]	0.587	[0.483; 0.686]
$\gamma_{\beta EP}$	0.469	[0.301; 0.713]		
$\gamma_{\phi EP}/\gamma_{\phi PE}$	−0.351	[−0.579; −0.195]	0.088	[0.017; 0.162]
$\gamma_{\sigma\zeta E}/\gamma_{\sigma\zeta P}$	−1.449	[−1.760; −1.193]	−0.909	[−1.374; −0.471]
$\gamma_{\sigma\varepsilon E1}/\gamma_{\sigma\varepsilon P}$	−0.694	[−0.876; −0.523]	−1.194	[−2.036; −0.723]
$\gamma_{\sigma\varepsilon E2}$	−1.194	[−1.287; −0.891]		
Random effect variances				
μ_{E1}/μ_P	0.566	[0.419; 0.772]	0.112	[0.065; 0.180]
μ_{E2}	0.376	[0.267; 0.529]		
ϕ_E/ϕ_P	0.028	[0.014; 0.049]	0.045	[0.026; 0.078]
β_{EP}	0.099	[0.041; 0.248]		
ϕ_{EP}/ϕ_{PE}	0.075	[0.028; 0.196]	0.034	[0.014; 0.071]
$ln(\sigma^2_{\zeta E})/ln(\sigma^2_{\zeta P})$	1.198	[0.781; 1.806]	0.930	[0.407; 1.806]
$ln(\sigma^2_{\varepsilon E1})/ln(\sigma^2_{\varepsilon P})$	0.909	[0.631; 1.304]	1.227	[0.595; 2.756]
$ln(\sigma^2_{\varepsilon E2})$	0.982	[0.696; 1.400]		
Standardized parameter estimates				
Within-person standardization (averaged across clusters)				
ϕ_E/ϕ_P	0.707	[0.650; 0.770]	0.591	[0.492; 0.694]
β_{EP}	0.457	[0.317; 0.653]		
ϕ_{EP}/ϕ_{PE}	−0.350	[−0.552; −0.206]	0.097	[0.037; 0.162]
$\sigma^2_{\zeta E}/\sigma^2_{\zeta P}$	0.312	[0.242; 0.372]	0.527	[0.417; 0.611]
$\sigma^2_{\varepsilon E1}/\sigma^2_{\varepsilon P}$	0.377	[0.348; 0.406]	0.308	[0.181; 0.461]
$\sigma^2_{\varepsilon E2}$	0.307	[0.280; 0.335]		

(continued)

TABLE 15.2. *(continued)*

	Energetic arousal		Physical activity	
	Estimate	95% CI	Estimate	95% CI
R-squared				
Within-level (averaged across clusters)				
Y_{E1}/Y_P	.623	[.594; .652]	.692	[.539; 0.819]
Y_{E2}	.693	[.665; .720]		
$EA^{(w)}/PA^{(w)}$	.688	[.628; .758]	.473	[.389; .583]

Note. Estimated parameters denote posterior medians and 95% CIs denote Bayesian credibility intervals. Within-person standardized parameters are within-person-level standardized estimates averaged across clusters. R^2 measures for $EA^{(w)}/PA^{(w)}$ denote averaged within-person explained variance with respect to the measurement-error-free latent construct on the within-person level, and those for Y_{E1}, Y_{E2}, and Y_P refer to explained variance in the observed variables on the within-person level. E/EA: energetic arousal; P/PA: physical activity; $E1$: first item of energetic arousal (awake); $E2$: second item of energetic arousal (energetic); β_{EP}: person-specific simultaneous regression coefficient of $EA_{it}^{(w)}$ on $PA_{it}^{(w)}$; $\gamma_{\phi E}/\gamma_{\phi P}$: average autoregressive effect of $EA^{(w)}/PA^{(w)}$; $\gamma_{\beta EP}$: average effect of the simultaneous regression of $EA_{it}^{(w)}$ on $PA_{it}^{(w)}$; $\gamma_{\phi EP}$: average effect of the cross-lagged regression of $EA_{it}^{(w)}$ on $PA_{i(t-1)}^{(w)}$; $\gamma_{\phi PE}$: average effect of the cross-lagged regression of $PA_{it}^{(w)}$ on $EA_{i(t-1)}^{(w)}$; $\gamma_{\sigma\zeta E}/\gamma_{\sigma\zeta P}$: average log innovation variance of latent construct $EA^{(w)}/PA^{(w)}$; $\gamma_{\sigma\varepsilon E1}/\gamma_{\sigma\varepsilon E2}/\gamma_{\sigma\varepsilon P}$: average (fixed effect) of the logarithm of the random measurement error variance for indicator 1 and 2 for EA/PA; $ln(\sigma_{\zeta E}^2)/ln(\sigma_{\zeta P}^2)$: logarithm of the random, person-specific innovation variances; $\sigma_{\varepsilon E1}^2 / \sigma_{\varepsilon E2}^2 / \sigma_{\varepsilon P}^2$: random, person-specific error variances; $\mu_{E1}/\mu_{E2}/\mu_P$: random, person-specific mean of the respective construct and indicator; ϕ_E/ϕ_P: random, person-specific autoregreesive effects; ϕ_{EP}: person-specific slope of the latent regression of $EA_{it}^{(w)}$ at time point t on $PA_{i(t-1)}^{(w)}$ at time point $(t-1)$; ϕ_{PE}: person-specific slope of the latent regression of $PA_{it}^{(w)}$ at time point t on $EA_{i(t-1)}^{(w)}$ at time point $(t-1)$; $Y_{E1}/Y_{E2}/Y_P$: Observed variables of EA, indicator 1 and 2, and PA; $EA^{(w)}/PA^{(w)}$: latent within-person state variables of EA and PA.

unexplained (occasion-specific) variability in PA across time ($r(\mu_P, ln(\sigma_{\zeta P}^2))$ = –.545; *CI* = [–.796; –.215]). Higher carryover in PA is associated with less unexplained variability in PA across time ($r(\phi_P, ln(\sigma_{\zeta P}^2))$ = –.363; CI = [–.636; –.021]). The same holds for EA ($r(\phi_E, ln(\sigma_{\zeta E}^2))$ = –.709; CI = [–.873; –.455]). Individuals who experience a weaker positive simultaneous effect of PA on EA tend to also have a weaker negative effect of PA on EA half an hour later ($r(\phi_{EP}, \beta_{EP})$ = –.788; CI = [–.931; –.468]). That is, individuals tend to vary with respect to the strength of the effect that PA exerts on EA in general. Additionally, individuals with comparatively large degrees of unexplained variability in PA (innovation variance) tend to exhibit weaker positive simultaneous effects of PA on EA ($r(ln(\sigma_{\zeta P}^2), \beta_{EP})$ = –.533; CI = [–.781; –.177]) and weaker negative (i.e., negative values closer to zero) cross-lagged effects of PA on EA ($r(ln(\sigma_{\zeta P}^2), \phi_{EP})$ = .450; CI = [.024; .753]).

In conclusion, the results suggest that high PA is associated with a simultaneous increase in experienced EA and a decrease in EA half an hour later. The results are in line with previous research. For instance, AA studies observed that EA and momentary volume of PA were positively associated, whereas this association subsided over time (Kanning & Schoebi, 2016; Reichert et al., 2016).

Further Model Extensions

Besides including covariates as predictors or outcomes on the between-person level (see the section "Between-Level Structure"), we may be interested in including time-varying covariates in our model. We might for instance ask why EA shows variability across time and which covariates (e.g., quality and length of the last night's sleep or contextual effects of work and leisure time; Kanning, 2013) might explain observed drops and increases in EA. Time-varying (observed or latent) covariates can be easily incorporated into the DSEM, while researchers have to decide whether the effects of time-varying covariates are assumed to carry forward in time or are truly time-specific. For instance, if a time-varying (observed or latent) covariate X_{it} is added as a predictor variable in Equation 15.8, X_{it} affects $EA_{it}^{(w)}$ at time t but also at later time points, as the effect is carried forward in time by an indirect effect of X_{it} on future EA by the autoregressive effect of EA. (This type of model is called an *indirect model* by Asparouhov et al., 2018). Alternatively, in the model termed *direct model* in Asparouhov and colleagues (2018), X_{it} only affects concurrent $EA_{it}^{(w)}$, and there is no accumulated effect of X_{it} across time. This is achieved by separating the structural and autoregressive parts of the model, with X_{it} being part of the structural model. For instance, in the direct model, autoregression for within-level EA is modeled for the residuals f_{it} of EA after controlling for X_{it}:

$$EA_{it}^{(w)} = \theta_i X_{it} + f_{it} \tag{15.22}$$

$$f_{it} = \phi_{E,i} f_{i(t-1)} + \zeta_{E,it} \tag{15.23}$$

Equation 15.22 specifies the structural part of the model which includes the contemporaneous regressions between the variables (nondynamic), and Equation 15.23 specifies the residual part (dynamic part of $EA_{it}^{(w)}$). Note that the meaning and interpretation of the regression parameters differ between the two modeling strategies, with parameters in the direct model sometimes being easier to interpret (e.g., when X_{it} represents time in a growth curve model). Asparouhov and Muthén (2020) propose selecting a modeling approach (direct or indirect) by the focus of the research question (i.e., focus on contemporaneous relations vs. dynamic structural relations) or by determining the appropriate model for a covariate by estimation of a full model (both indirect and direct effects) and inspection of the respective regression coefficients. The modeling framework to model autoregressive processes on the structural regression residuals (direct model) is termed residual DSEM (RDSEM), which is discussed in detail in Asparouhov and Muthén. They present several alternative modeling strategies for the inclusion of covariates and address further issues such as identification, the exogeneity of covariates, or the effect of missing data to adjust for unequally spaced observations. They conclude that (1) it is advisable to treat the covariate as an endogenous variable and account for its autocorrelation across time instead of treating it as exogenous and that (2) the estimation of the structural regression coefficients is more robust with respect to how unequally spaced time intervals are treated when using the direct (RDSEM) as compared to the indirect modeling approach.

BOX 15.6. Trends, Cyclical Effects, and Growth Curve Models

The models described in this chapter are suited to analyze stable process data. That is, the outcome variables are assumed to not systematically change across the observed time period, and fluctuations center around a stable mean value across time. Time-series models require the series to be stationary, which implies (among other assumptions; see Box 15.1) that the expected value of the series is constant across time. If the assumption of stationarity is violated by a trend in the data, the series has to be detrended before model estimation, or the trend can be directly modeled within the model by including time as a time-varying covariate (Jebb et al., 2015). In the same vein, seasonal or cyclical effects (e.g., weekly cycles) have to be addressed as they violate the stationarity assumption by introducing a recurring pattern of change in the series' mean.

To model subject-specific linear trends in EA, time can be included as a predictor of EA on the within-person level, resulting in the estimation of a linear growth curve model:

$$EA_{it}^{(w)} = \theta_i t + f_{it} \tag{15.24}$$

$$f_{it} = \phi_{E,i} f_{i(t-1)} + \zeta_{E,it} \tag{15.25}$$

where t denotes time and θ_i captures the linear growth of individual i across time. Note that in Equations 15.24 and 15.25, we chose a direct modeling approach; that is, the autoregressive part is modeled separately from the trend/growth curve component, such that the conditional expectation of EA depends only on its trait value as well as on t_i, facilitating the interpretation of the model parameters (see Asparouhov et al., 2018). This model can be easily specified by use of RDSEM. Analogously, cyclical components could, for instance, be specified by use of sine or cosine functions of time in Equation 15.24 (see, e.g., Liu & West, 2016; Zhou, Wang, & Zhang, 2019). Another approach to model growth in DSEM is to use a cross-classified DSEM (see the following section).

Cross-Classified DSEM

Another form of nonstationarity that might occur in intensive longitudinal data arises from changes in the dynamic parameters across time. The models covered in this chapter assume that the dynamic effects are constant across time; for instance, autocorrelation does not change over the observation period, and the effect of time-varying covariates is the same across all measurement occasions. This assumption is relaxed in time-varying effects models, which allow for time-specific effects in the intercepts, autoregressive parameters, or within-level relationships between variables (e.g., Bringmann, Ferrer, Hamaker, Borsboom, & Tuerlinckx, 2018; Tan, Shiyko, Li, Li, & Dierker, 2012). Besides the aforementioned modeling techniques that are unified in the DSEM framework (i.e., multilevel, time series, and structural equation modeling), DSEM also comprises time-varying effects modeling by modeling time-varying effects as random effects across time within a cross-classified modeling approach. That is, cross-classified DSEM incorporates both person-specific and time-specific random effects. By modeling changes in intercepts and slopes across time by means of time-specific random effects, it is not necessary to specify a functional form of the effects over time. However, a prerequisite for estimating time-specific effects by a cross-classified DSEM is that the time scale is aligned across all individuals (Asparouhov et al., 2018). A requirement that is not met in many intensive longitudinal datasets (for instance, when participants are prompted to respond to an e-diary question at random times during the day, as is the case in the presented application) might, however, be quite often met when data are obtained continuously across time by wearable sensors and are potentially split into equivalent time intervals for every participant by the researcher.

Summary

The flexibility of the DSEM framework allows extensive modeling strategies, and myriad different models can be specified under the umbrella of DSEM, the presentation of which is beyond the scope of this chapter. Besides the manifold advantages and possibilities offered by DSEM, a small note of caution has to be added with respect to the sample size requirements of the models. That is, modeling person-specific dynamics on the within-person level, including random effects for many or even all relevant model parameters, requires a large number of repeated measurements per person. When combining data from wearable sensors with e-diaries, the required number of observed time points (e.g., more than 50, 100, or even 200, depending on model complexity; see Asparouhov et al., 2018; Schultzberg & Muthén, 2018) might exceed the actual number of available observations in many datasets. In this case, it might be necessary to reduce model complexity by reducing the number of random effects in the model. However, if continuously measured signals from wearable sensors are analyzed without additional data from e-diaries, the amount of available time points should easily surmount the required sample sizes, with many potential areas of application. One such application of the DSEM model described in this chapter is the analysis of dyadic data obtained with wearable sensors. For instance, research on emotional synchrony investigated the temporal coupling between behavior, emotional experiences, and their underlying physiology in parent–child dyads or romantic couples (e.g., Amole, Cyranowski, Wright, & Swartz, 2017; Woody, Feuer, Sosoo, Hastings, & Gibb, 2016). That is, when focusing, for instance, on the synchrony of heart rate variability, heart rate variability could be measured in parallel for each member of the dyad across an extended time period. The resulting time series from each dyad can be analyzed by treating each member of the dyad as a different variable in a bivariate DSEM. In this example, cross-lagged effects and innovation correlations would provide dyad-specific indices of the temporal coupling of heart rate variability between the two members of a dyad (also see Laurenceau & Bolger, 2012).

Another possible area of application is for the purpose of validating measurements obtained with wearable sensors (see Eid & Holtmann, Chapter 14, this volume). To assess construct validity, the latent agreement between measurements obtained by two devices of the same type or by devices of different types (e.g., a gold-standard method and a comparison method) can be investigated. That is, several devices designed to measure the same variable are worn simultaneously, and the latent agreement between the devices can be investigated with respect to the average signal as well as the temporal fluctuations captured by each device.

For the purpose of this chapter, we focused on one modeling approach within the extensive DSEM framework that might be the most commonly applied model for the analysis of e-diary and wearable sensor data. We discussed several model extensions, such as random measurement error or the inclusion of time-invariant and time-varying covariates. However, only a fraction of the DSEM modeling capabilities fits into one single chapter. We therefore encourage interested readers to dive into the extensive literature covering advanced DSEM models and further modeling alternatives and model extensions.

Notes

1. In the following, the terms *single* and *multiple indicator* refer to the number of observed variables per latent construct (measurement model). In contrast, the terms *univariate* and *multivariate* refer to the number of constructs included in one model.

2. Note that in longitudinal models with two or more indicators per latent construct, a tau-congeneric measurement structure (see Eid & Holtmann, Chapter 14, in this volume) with time-invariant but freely estimated factor loadings per indicator could be specified (intercepts on the within-level are set to zero by definition). For ease of model presentation, we focus on the more parsimonious model variant with loading parameters fixed to one in the following example.

3. Note, however, that judging by the Bayes factor as well as the $z > 3$ rule of thumb, the random measurement error for PA could be excluded from the model in the present data. Furthermore, the present data do not comprise the number of within-level observations per person required for accurate parameter estimation for a model of this complexity, and results are presented for illustrative purposes only.

REFERENCES

Aalbers, G., vanden Abeele, M. M. P., Hendrickson, A. T., de Marez, L., & Keijsers, L. (2021). Caught in the moment: Are there person-specific associations between momentary procrastination and passively measured smartphone use? *Mobile Media and Communication, 10*(1), 115–135.

Amole, M. C., Cyranowski, J. M., Wright, A. G. C., & Swartz, H. A. (2017). Depression impacts the physiological responsiveness of mother–daughter dyads during social interaction. *Depression and Anxiety, 34*, 118–126.

Armstrong, B., Beets, M. W., Starrett, A., Brazendale, K., Turner-McGrievy, G., Saelens, B. E., et al. (2021). Dynamics of sleep, sedentary behavior, and moderate-to-vigorous physical activity on school versus nonschool days, *Sleep, 44*(2), zsaa174.

Asparouhov, T., Hamaker, E. L., & Muthén, B. (2018). Dynamic structural equation models. *Structural Equation Modeling: A Multidisciplinary Journal, 25*(3), 359–388.

Asparouhov, T., & Muthén, B. (2010). *Bayesian analysis in Mplus: Technical implementation* (Mplus technical report, Version 3). www.statmodel.com/download/Bayes3.pdf

Asparouhov, T., & Muthén, B. (2020). Comparison of models for the analysis of intensive longitudinal data. *Structural Equation Modeling: A Multidisiplinary Journal, 27*(2), 275–297.

Bringmann, L. F., Ferrer, E., Hamaker, E. L., Borsboom, D., & Tuerlinckx, F. (2018). Modeling nonstationary emotion dynamics in dyads using a time-varying vector-autoregressive model. *Multivariate Behavioral Research, 53*(3), 293–314.

Curran, P. J., & Bauer, D. J. (2007). Building path diagrams for multilevel models. *Psychological Methods, 12*, 283–297.

Depaoli, S., & van de Schoot, R. (2017). Improving transparency and replication in Bayesian statistics: The WAMBS-Checklist. *Psychological Methods, 22*(2); 240–261.

Eid, M., Holtmann, J., Santangelo, P., & Ebner-Priemer, U. (2017). On the definition of latent-state-trait models with autoregressive effects. *European Journal of Psychological Assessment, 33*(4), 285–295.

Gelman, A., Carlin, J. B., Stern, H. S., Dunson, D. B., Vehtari, A., & Rubin, D. B. (2014). *Bayesian data analysis* (3rd ed.). Chapman & Hall/CRC.

Gelman, A., & Rubin, D. B. (1992). Inference

from iterative simulation using multiple sequences. *Statistical Science, 7,* 457–472.

Granger, C. W. J., & Morris, M. J. (1976). Time series modelling and interpretation. *Journal of the Royal Statistical Society, Series A, 139,* 246–257.

Hamaker, E. L., Asparouhov, T., Brose, A., Schmiedek, F. & Muthén, B. (2018). At the frontiers of modeling intensive longitudinal data: dynamic structural equation models for the affective measurements from the COGITO study. *Multivariate Behavioral Research, 53*(6), 820–841.

Hamilton, J. D. (1994). *Time series analysis.* Princeton University Press.

Hedeker, D., Mermelstein, R. J., & Demirtas, H. (2008). An application of a mixed-effects location scale model for analysis of Ecological Momentary Assessment (EMA) data. *Biometrics, 64,* 627–634.

Hoijtink, H., Mulder, C., van Lissa, C., & Gu, X. (2019). A tutorial on testing hypotheses using the Bayes Factor. *Psychological Methods, 24,* 539–556.

Jebb, A. T., Tay, L., Wang, W. & Huang, Q. (2015). Time series analysis for psychological research: Examining and forecasting change. *Frontiers in Psychology, 6,* 727.

Jongerling, J., Laurenceau, J.-P., & Hamaker, E. L. (2015). A multilevel AR(1) model: Allowing for inter-individual differences in trait-scores, inertia, and innovation variance. *Multivariate Behavioral Research, 50,* 334–349.

Kanning, M. (2013). Using objective, real-time measures to investigate the effect of actual physical activity on affective states in everyday life differentiating the contexts of working and leisure time in a sample with students. *Frontiers in Psychology, 3,* 602.

Kanning, M., & Schoebi, D. (2016). Momentary affective states are associated with momentary volume, prospective trends, and fluctuations of daily physical activity. *Frontiers in Psychology Movement Science and Sport Psychology, 7,* 744.

Kass, R. E., & Raftery, A. E. (1995). Bayes factors. *Journal of the American Statistical Association, 90,* 773–795.

Kruschke, J. K. (2015). *Doing Bayesian data analysis: A tutorial with R, JAGS, and Stan* (2nd ed.). Elsevier.

Kruschke, J. K., Aguinis, H., & Joo, H. (2012). The time has come: Bayesian methods for data analysis in the organizational sciences. *Organizational Research Methods, 15*(4), 722–752.

Lane, S. T., Gates, K. M., Pike, H. K., Beltz, A. M., & Wright, A. G. (2019). Uncovering general, shared, and unique temporal patterns in ambulatory assessment data. *Psychological Methods, 24*(1), 54.

Laurenceau, J., & Bolger, N. (2012). Analyzing diary and intensive longitudinal data from dyads. In M. Mehl & T. S. Conner (Eds.), *Handbook of research methods for studying daily life* (pp. 407–422). Guilford Press.

Liu, Y., & West, S. G. (2016). Weekly cycles in daily report data: An overlooked issue. *Journal of Personality, 84,* 560–579.

McElreath, R. (2020). *Statistical rethinking. A Bayesian course with examples in R and Stan* (2nd ed.). CRC Press.

McNeish, D. (2019). Two-level dynamic structural equation models with small samples. *Structural Equation Modeling: A Multidisciplinary Journal, 26*(6), 948–966.

McNeish, D., & Hamaker, E. L. (2020). A primer on two-level dynamic structural equation models for intensive longitudinal data in M*plus*. *Psychological Methods, 25*(5), 610–635.

Mehl, M. R., & Conner, T. S. (Eds.). (2012). *Handbook of research methods for studying daily life.* Guilford Press.

Molenaar, P. C. M. (2004). A manifesto on psychology as idiographic science: Bringing the person back into scientific psychology, this time forever. *Measurement, 2*(4), 201–218.

Muthén, L. K., & Asparouhov, T. (2012). *New developments in Mplus Version 7: Part 2.* www.statmodel.com/download/handouts/V7Part2.pdf

Muthén, L. K., & Muthén, B. O. (1998–2017). *Mplus user's guide* (8th ed.). Muthén & Muthén.

Oravecz, Z., Tuerlinckx, F., & Vandekerckhove, J. (2009). A hierarchical Ornstein–Uhlenbeck model for continuous repeated measurement data. *Psychometrika, 74*(3), 395–418.

Ram, N., & Gerstorf, D. (2009). Time-structured and net intraindividual variability: Tools for examining the development of dynamic characteristics and processes. *Psychology and Aging, 24,* 778–791.

Reichert, M., Tost, H., Reinhard, I., Zipf, A., Salize, H.-J., Meyer-Lindenberg, A., et al. (2016). Within-subject associations between mood dimensions and non-exercise activity: An ambulatory assessment approach using repeated real-time and objective data. *Frontiers of Psychology, 7*, 918.

Schultzberg, M., & Muthén, B. (2018). Number of subjects and time points needed for multilevel time-series analysis: A simulation study of dynamic structural equation modeling. *Structural Equation Modeling: A Multidisciplinary Journal, 25*, 495–515.

Schuurman, N. K., Ferrer, E., de Boer-Sonnenschein, M., & Hamaker, E. L. (2016). How to compare cross-lagged associations in a multilevel autoregressive model. *Psychological Methods, 21*(2), 206–221.

Schuurman, N. K., Houtveen, J. H., & Hamaker, E. L. (2015). Incorporating measurement error in $n = 1$ psychological autoregressive modeling. *Frontiers in Psychology, 6*, 1038.

Schuurman, N. K., & Hamaker, E. L. (2019). Measurement error and person-specific reliability in multilevel autoregressive modeling. *Psychological Methods, 24*(1), 70–91.

Song, H., & Ferrer, E. (2012). Bayesian estimation of random coefficient dynamic factor models. *Multivariate Behavioral Research, 47*(1), 26–60.

Song, X.-Y., & Lee, S.-Y. (2012). A tutorial on the Bayesian approach for analyzing structural equation models. *Journal of Mathematical Psychology, 56*, 135–148.

Spiegelhalter, D. J., Best, N. G., Carlin, B. P., & van der Linde, A. (2002). Bayesian measures of model complexity and fit. *Journal of the Royal Statistical Society, Series B. 64*, 583–639.

Staudenmayer, J., & Buonaccorsi, J. P. (2005). Measurement error in linear autoregressive models. *Journal of the American Statistical Association, 100*, 841–852.

Suls, J., Green, P., & Hillis, S. (1998). Emotional reactivity to everyday problems, affective inertia, and neuroticism. *Personality and Social Psychology Bulletin, 24*, 127–136.

Tan, X., Shiyko, M. P., Li, R., Li, Y., & Dierker, L. (2012). A time-varying effect model for intensive longitudinal data. *Psychological Methods, 17*(1), 61–77.

Trull, T. J., & Ebner-Priemer, U. (2014). The role of ambulatory assessment in psychological science. *Current Directions in Psychological Science, 23*, 466–470.

van de Schoot, R., Kaplan, D., Denissen, J., Asendorpf, J. B., Neyer, F. J., & van Aken, M. A. G. (2014). A gentle introduction to Bayesian analysis: Applications to developmental research. *Child Development, 85*, 842–860.

Voelkle, M. C., & Oud, J. H. L. (2013). Continuous time modelling with individually varying time intervals for oscillating and non-oscillating processes. *British Journal of Mathematical and Statistical Psychology, 66*, 103–126.

Wilhelm, P., & Schoebi, D. (2007). Assessing mood in daily life: Structural validity, sensitivity to change, and reliability of a short-scale to measure three basic dimensions of mood. *European Journal of Psychological Assessment, 23*, 258–267.

Woody, M. L., Feurer, C., Sosoo, E. E., Hastings, P. D., & Gibb, B. E. (2016). Synchrony of physiological activity during mother–child interaction: Moderation by maternal history of major depressive disorder. *Journal of Child Psychology and Psychiatry, 57*(7), 843–850.

Zhou, L., Wang, M., & Zhang, Z. (2019). Intensive longitudinal data analyses with dynamic structural equation modeling. *Organizational Research Methods, 24*(2), 219–250.

CHAPTER 16

Dynamic Network Analysis

Emorie D. Beck and Stuti Thapa

CHAPTER OVERVIEW

Psychological dynamics are central to psychological theories. However, the methods for capturing psychological dynamics have lagged far behind the theories, leaving researchers to rely on nondynamic methods for theory testing and building. Such a mismatch between theories and methods creates a gap that can threaten the psychological process. From the perspective of a longtime theory–method gap in personality psychology, this chapter illustrates how dynamic methods can help to close this gap. We review four statistical methods for estimating dynamic networks from time series of data of active and passive sensing: association networks, graphical vector autoregressive models, unified structural equational models, and dynamic exploratory graph analysis. Using a focal participant, we demonstrate the shared and unique features of each of these methods, make recommendations for when to use each of these models, and highlight core challenges these and other dynamic methods will have to tackle moving forward.

Dynamic Systems Analysis

Since the rise of empirical psychology in the 19th century, psychologists have attempted to specify theories of psychological processes and phenomena, including consciousness (Wundt, 1911), attitudes (G. W. Allport, 1954), personality (e.g., G. W. Allport, 1960; Baumert et al., 2017; Beck & Jackson, 2020b, 2020d), work performance (Campbell & Wiernik, 2015; Dalal, Bhave, & Fiset, 2014), intergroup processes (F. H. Allport, 1920), and more. A common feature of these theories is that they specify how one or more psychological processes and/or phenomena unfold over short and long time spans. In other words, psychological theories are dynamic. For example, theories of personality suggest that personality should drive the types of situations individuals select to participate in (e.g., Emmons & Diener, 1986), that individuals should modify the situations they encounter (e.g., Funder & Colvin, 1991), and that situations should impact personality as both a stable entity (e.g., Wrzus, Wagner, & Riediger, 2016) and as its expression (e.g., Sherman, Rauthmann, Brown, Serfass, & Jones, 2015). These theories also suggest that how individuals navigate these patterns between personality and situations reflects personality itself (e.g., Mischel & Shoda, 1995). Despite this, personality is typically studied by looking at how broad, aggregated, and often decontextualized personality traits (1) predict the life events people experience (e.g., Beck & Jackson, 2021b), (2) change over time (e.g., Graham et al., 2020), and (3) are predicted by events or experiences individuals have (e.g., Bleidorn, 2012; Bleidorn et al., 2013). Thus, the dynamic nature of the theory is not reflected in either the measurement or the modeling of personality specifically and psychology more broadly. This has led to a widening gap between theories of psychology and the methods applied to test them, but such gaps between theory and method in psychology can have great consequences for theory building and testing.

In this chapter, we address the theory–method gap in psychology from the perspective of the study of personality. We summarize broad classes of dynamic psychological theories in personality, how challenges to collecting dynamic data have widened the theory–method gap, how active and passive mobile sensing data have the opportunity to close this gap, and how dynamic networks can aid analyzing and interpreting such data in alignment with dynamic psychological theories. We specifically highlight four network models: graphical vector autoregressive models (graphical VAR), unified structural equation models (uSEM), dynamic exploratory graph analysis (dynEGA), and how dynamic theory can guide associated analytical decisions. Finally, we close by connecting these back to psychology more broadly.

Personality Dynamics

Allport and the Rise of Personality Theory

The role of dynamics in the study of personality goes back to its earliest days of personality psychology. Gordon Allport, one of the "fathers" of personality as an empirical discipline (e.g., 1937), wrote about personality as a dynamic phenomenon. As he defined it, personality was "the dynamic organization within the individual of those psychophysical systems that determine his unique adjustments to his environment" (Allport, 1937, p. 48). Each piece of this definition deserves consideration and underscores dynamic elements of personality theory. First, the definition explicitly uses the word "dynamic," implying that personality is not simply a static factor over time. Second, personality is an organization, or structure, albeit a dynamic one. Third, personality exists within the individual or is idiographic or person-specific. Fourth, what makes up the structure of personality is (psychophysical) systems, meaning that the structure (or the organization of features that are relevant) within an individual may dynamically shift over time and across situations. Finally, personality is explicitly about unique adjustments to the environment, which are likely to be unique to them. In other words, transactions with the environment are also best considered idiographically.

Despite this dynamic core of one of the earliest theories of personality by a founder of the field who remains heavily cited to this day, the personality literature over the past century largely concerns studies of population-level (i.e., variable-centered, nomothetic approaches) personality traits and their relationship to outcomes (e.g., Beck & Jackson, 2021b), how they change (e.g., Graham et al., 2020), and what they are associated with more broadly. This is a strong contrast to the person-level (i.e., person-centered, idiographic approach) that Allport advocated for in his definition of personality. Some have labeled this contrast the two sciences of personality—one whose goal was to describe how people differed from one another on shared attributes (a nomothetic approach) and another whose goal was to describe and explain individuals holistically (an idiographic approach), with a focus on why people behaved similarly or differently across time and contexts (see Beck & Jackson, 2021d; Winter & Barenbaum, 1999).

According to Allport (1937, 1968), what these nomothetic approaches captured were not the dynamic structures alluded to in his definition. Instead, these "common" traits captured measurable aspects of psychological experience and behavior that are often experienced or exhibited by many people in a similar manner. In other words, common traits reflected similar idiographic traits (and variability in those traits) across people, but, as they reflect idiographic traits, such common traits have no true (i.e., causal) reality of their own. Instead, Allport (1960) saw personality as an open system made up of a number of other psychophysical systems. Indeed, he laid out theoretical evidence of ways in which personality theory and research adhered to the main criteria of open systems: (1) input and output of both energy and matter; (2) homeostasis (i.e., equilibria), both achieved and maintained even across great disruption; (3) an increase in the order of the system over time; and (4) transactional relationships with the environment (Allport, 1960). Allport also argued that nomothetic conceptualizations of personality were a closed system that were a consequence of the open-system nature of the idiographic personality.

Cattell and the Data Box

Despite his theoretical contributions to personality, Allport did much less to test those theoretical propositions. For example, how we could measure and model personality idiographically and link that with nomothetic personality traits was largely not addressed. Instead, studies by Raymond Cattell largely structured work toward measuring and modeling personality at different levels of aggregation. In introducing the *data box*, Cattell (1946a) argued that persons could be conceptualized into three dimensions that indexed people (P_1 to P_N), variables (X_1 to X_p), and occasions or time (T_1 to T_t). Different ways of "slicing" or aggregating across dimensions of the data box reflected the wide array of questions psychologists could ask and answer. For example, typical nomothetic questions focus on the person (P) and variable (X) dimensions and aggregate across the occasion (T) dimension, thereby addressing the question of the structure of individual differences within a population of people, which he termed the *R-technique* (see Figure 16.1).

Cattell's work on the data box and factor-analytic approaches moved forward both the science of between-person differences and the study of idiographic personality dynamics. Indeed, he formalized methods for estimating idiographic personality structure by slicing the data box into variable (X) and occasion (T) dimensions and fixing the person dimension (see Figure 16.1). He termed this slicing of the data box the *P-technique*, in

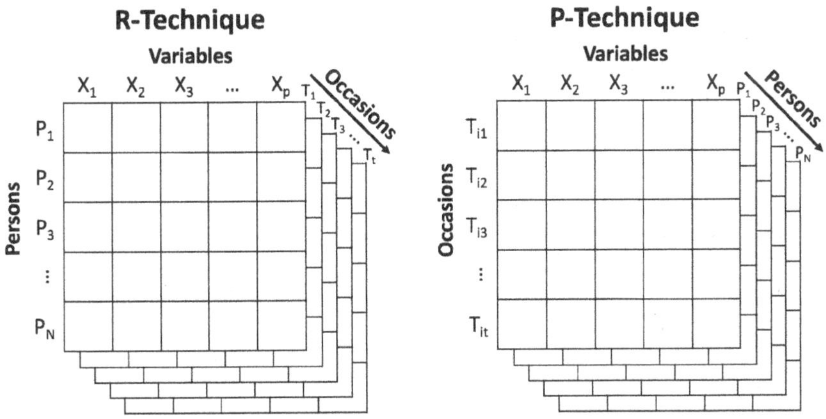

FIGURE 16.1. Two ways to "slice" Cattell's (1946b) data box to produce *R*-technique (nomothetic) and P-technique (idiographic) factor-analytic structures. In the *R*-technique, one collapses across or slices across the occasions dimension (*T*) to get the common structure of variables across people, perhaps solely applicable to a particular time or population. In the *P*-technique, one slices across individuals to find the unique structure of variables within a particular person across time.

which factor-analytic models were applied to $X \times T$ matrices for individual people (Cattell, 1943). However, the goal of *P-technique* was to reduce the data to smaller clusters that could be subsumed under a single label rather than to understand the dynamic complexities of how the underlying indicators unfolded within and across people. Such methods would emerge later and will be the focus of later sections of this chapter.

Challenges in Dynamic Data Collection

One major factor in the theory–method gap in the study of personality has been that the available means for and methods of collecting dynamic data have been quite limited. Empirically understanding how personality unfolds over time often requires time-series data, and most statistical techniques require rather large sets of data in order to be able to capture and uncover dynamic features well. But the rise of smartphones has created new opportunities for psychological researchers to collect dynamic data in everyday life. First, the experience sampling method (ESM; Csikszentmihalyi & Larson, 1987), which we will refer to as "active sensor data" because it requires participants to actively provide responses, allowed researchers to collect repeated samples of sets of variables from an individual multiple times within or across days or weeks. Second, smartphones are also constantly collecting so-called passive sensor data, including audio data (from microphones), accelerometer data, location data, and social media posts, among others. Finally, smartphones and computers can be linked to other passive sensor devices, such as physiological monitors of heart rate, blood pressure, skin conductance, sleep quality, and movement.

Together, these new sources of data provide a unique opportunity to capture times-series data that can be used to better understand personality—and other psychological, social, and biological phenomena—more dynamically. The collection of such data opens up new opportunities for assessing all the dimensions of Cattell's data box by making it easier to collect multiple observations (*T*) from different individuals (*P*) across sets of variables (*X*). In other words, researchers could tackle large-dimension person (*P*) × observation (*T*) questions, fixing the variable (*X*), among others.

Recent Work on Within-Person Personality Processes

Although Allport and Cattell, among others, advocated for the consideration of dynamic and dispositional approaches to understanding personality, the latter half of the 20th century saw personality largely diverge on two tracks—one interested in how personality unfolds over time and another examining personality as broad, aggregated traits. Fueled by the rise of the experience sampling method in particular, an emphasis on within-person variability began to work its way back into personality near the turn of the century. In the 1970s and 1980s, both Zuckerman (1979) and Buss and Craik (1980) had contended that personality traits were aggregates of personality states. At the turn of the 21st century, Fleeson (2001) updated this proposition and demonstrated its empirical validity using ESM data. This and later empirical work became the basis of whole trait theory (Conner, Tennen, Fleeson, & Barrett, 2009; Fleeson, 2004; Fleeson & Jayawickreme, 2015). Means, standard deviations, and other density distribution parameters of personality states captured the descriptive properties of personality, while leaving the explanatory properties of personality largely open.

In addition, increased computing power made regression-based techniques for dealing with dynamic, time-series data in which participants have multiple observations more available. Statistically, such data are considered nested, with observations nested within person. Nested data violate assumptions of independence of errors in basic linear regression and require specialized methods, such as multilevel modeling (MLM). Unlike basic regression, MLM allows one to estimate different error terms for observations and units/groups (i.e., persons), thus, explicitly modeling within-person variability (Holtmann, Eid, & Kanning, Chapter 15, this volume; Snijders & Bosker, 2011). Moreover, it allows researchers to condition such variability on broader, person-level phenomena as well as momentary factors. As such, some have argued that MLM is "idiothetic" and helps to bridge the gap between nomothetic assessments of personality that focus on between-person differences and idiographic assessments of personality that focus on within-person variability (e.g., Conner et al., 2009).

Personality: Descriptive, Predictive, and Explanatory

Despite its promise, MLM is a statistical model, that is, a tool to test theories, not create them. Stated simply, a statistical method alone cannot dissolve idiographic-nomothetic tensions (see Fried, 2020) without having a clear and precise link with theories of personality. Many personality theorists have clearly argued that personality states vary over time and should be connected to personality traits (e.g., Baumert et al., 2017; Fleeson, 2001; Fleeson & Jayawickreme, 2015), but the links these theories offer for why states are linked to traits do not align with the theories. Indeed, the data-generating process, such as the open system Allport (1960) advocated, of the unfolding of complex psychological phenomena is unlikely to be captured with MLM. Several researchers have laid out evidence suggesting that using between-person models, like factor analysis and MLM, to investigate "within-person processes," which are often thought be the data-generating entities, is often misleading and does not allow for strong (causal) conclusions (Borsboom, Mellenbergh, & van Heerden, 2003; Fisher, Medaglia, & Jeronimus, 2018; Molenaar, 2004). Such an observation should not be taken lightly, as it suggests that inferences based on between-person models may be misleading at best and wholly incorrect at worst, which could lead to a new kind of credibility crisis in psychology (Moeller, 2021).

Dynamic Methods for Mobile Sensing

In the first sections, we argued that psychology is facing a gap between theory and methods. Then, we briefly introduced challenges to collecting data for answering dynamic questions as well as a small subset of methods often applied to dynamic data. Using personality as an example, we detailed work on the dynamic nature of personality theories as well as how factor analysis and latent traits are not good candidate data-generating (i.e., explanatory) models for personality, as well as most psychological constructs. In this section, we next detail a different class of methods that rely on dynamic systems theories and network analysis that show promise for closing the theory–method gap when integrated with mobile sensing data. Before beginning, we want to note that although the methods detailed below draw upon machine learning methods in some cases, we will be focusing on time-series and dynamic systems model approaches, leaving the details of machine learning methods to other chapters in this volume (e.g., Chapter 17, this volume) and elsewhere (e.g., Renner et al., 2020).

First, network approaches provide a framework for thinking about psychological measurement that extends across levels of multiple dimensions of Cattell's data box. Based on dynamic systems theory, a network approach asserts that latent traits are emergent properties of interactions among a set of indicators, rather than simply showing how levels of a variable tend to discriminate among individuals (e.g., Cramer et al., 2012). In other words, such models assume that indicators, not latent traits, are causal and that the processes through which latent traits emerge as measurable phenomena emerge from reliable patterning among indicators that have diverse causal underpinnings.

Network approaches have seen an explosion (e.g., Robinaugh, Hoekstra, Toner, & Borsboom, 2020), with some touting the great advantages these models offer (Beck & Jackson, 2021c; Borsboom & Cramer, 2013; Cramer et al., 2012), and others reflecting some of the downfalls (e.g., Forbes, Wright, Markon, & Krueger, 2019, 2021; although see Jones, Williams, & McNally, 2021, for a rejoinder), particularly in cross-sectional research that does not utilize time-series designs. Such cross-sectional work can, in some cases, merely reify the methods and findings of existing structural theory–method gaps in the guise of using models used in the study of dynamics. Networks highlight and summarize relationships among indicators, visually and quantitatively representing relationships between indicators that reveal both direct (i.e., relationships between two indicators) and indirect (i.e., relationships between two indicators separated by one or more intermediate indicators) relationships between them. However, only a few studies have used network approaches to examine personality (e.g., Beck & Jackson, 2020a, 2021c; Christensen, Cotter, & Silvia, 2019; Costantini et al., 2019; A. G. C. Wright et al., 2019). Despite the promise of these studies, the dearth of research on this topic makes it unclear to what extent network approaches apply to the time series of passive and active mobile sensing data.

Importantly, a network approach is not a single model; there are a growing number of instantiations and parameterizations of network-based models, four of which we will focus on in the present chapter: correlations, graphical vector autoregressive models (graphical VAR), unified structural equation models (uSEM), and dynamic exploratory graph analysis (dynEGA). Rather, network approaches, much like other structural methods such as factor analysis, are a set of statistical tools that can be applied to the pairwise relationships among a number of indicators, typically structured as matrices. And the models that underlie them are those that result in such matrix-structured estimates. Broadly, the rows and columns indicate the nodes (or variables) under investigation, while the cells of the matrices represent the edges (or relationships) among the nodes. Below, we will demonstrate each of these four methods using an example participant from Beck and Jackson (2020a). In that paper, Beck and Jackson demonstrated each of these methods except dynEGA. The present chapter additionally extends this to dynEGA and includes a more detailed comparison of each. The data come from a longitudinal experience sampling study of personality that collected nine indicators of four of the Big Five (Extraversion [2], Agreeableness [2], Conscientiousness [2], and Neuroticism [3]) four times per day (approximately 4 hours apart) for 2 weeks. This resulted in a multivariate time series for each participant with $p = 9$ indicators and $t = \sim 56$ time points. Although this example uses active sensor data, passive sensor data can also be readily incorporated into each of these models.

Concerns and Considerations in Node Selection

Before considering each of the methods, we first want to highlight that a critical part of matching theory and methods is also the design and measures of a study. Indeed, theory–method gaps can also arise when the indicators or variables used are not in alignment with theoretical propositions. Thus, perhaps the most important question when considering whether to represent and understand data or models from a network perspective concerns the definitions of the nodes and edges (Beck & Jackson, 2021c; Piccirillo, Beck, & Rodebaugh, 2019)—that is, what are the indicators (nodes) and the relationships among them (edges)? For example, should the lowest-level measurement unit be raw mobile sensing data, or should the data be composited into higher-order constructs (e.g., to reduce multicollinearity a priori)? Just as important as the definition of the nodes is the definition of the edges, which can represent adjacency (or co-occurrences), correlations, partial correlations, frequencies, individual differences, and more (see Beck & Jackson, 2021e; Wood, Spain, & Harms, 2017). Moreover, the edges can represent different time scales. Contemporaneous (also known as lag 0; *while* relationships) relationships estimate probabilistic within-person same time point relationships—that is, the tendency for two manifestations of personality to occur at the same time (i.e., co-occur)—and can be thought of as "while" relationships. In contrast, lagged and cross-lagged relationships (also known as lag 1 or simply "lagged"; *if–then* contingent relationships) estimate probabilistic within-person, cross-time point and cross-indicator (or cross-lagged) relationships—that is, the tendency for two manifestations of personality to follow the other across measurement occasions—and can be thought of as *if–then* relationships, partialing out associations with other features (e.g., J. C. Wright & Mischel, 1987). Below, we integrate these relationships within the discussion of each method, beginning with introducing the basics of networks in the association networks before linking them to personality theory.

Association Networks

The simplest time-series procedure for constructing a "dynamic" network is zero-order correlations among the variables (X) dimension across the time (T) dimension for each person individually (see Figure 16.2). Called "association networks," these are the correlation matrices that P-technique factor analysis (or any other form of factor analysis or principal components analysis) attempts to reduce. Figure 16.2 shows a visual representation of the steps from raw data to representing person-specific correlations as a network.

These association networks traditionally focus on concurrent associations among psychological, behavioral, or other states, which results in a symmetric matrix. But the data can also be lagged in order to look at bidirectional associations among the indicators (i.e., a nonsymmetric matrix). Relative to zero-order association networks, cross-lagged networks have some advantages. They are more dynamic by considering how levels of states are associated across time rather than at the same time. Because most psychological theories concern the changes in states, cross-lagged models come closer to aligning with theories.

Moreover, they offer a method for testing complex sets of relationships that are a hallmark of many key models of personality (G. W. Allport, 1937; Cervone, 2005; Mischel & Shoda, 1995), thus providing initial inroads for closing the theory–method gap in personality. Such relationships are complex not only in that they can include a large number of predictors but also in what those predictors are. For example, within such a framework, one can include different forms of active and passive sensor data, such as ESM, location data, heart rate, and more.

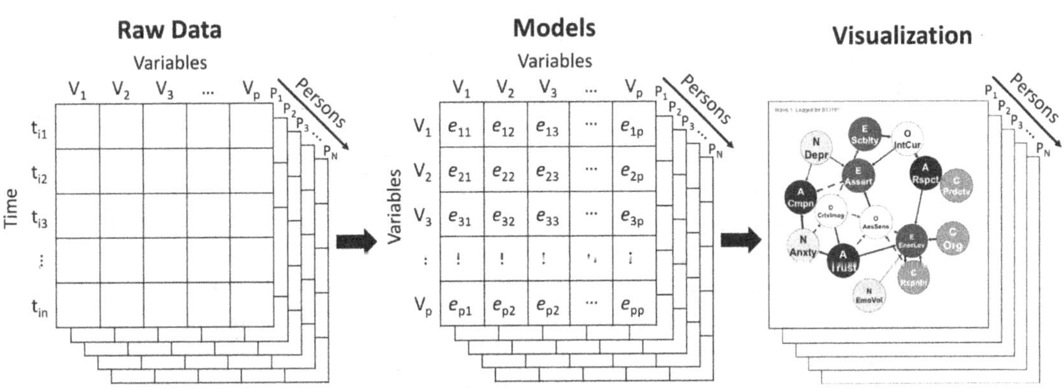

FIGURE 16.2. A simplified analytic procedure for using network tools on idiographic time-series data from raw data (left) to modeling relationships among variables (V_1 to V_P) and formatting them as a matrix (middle) to visually displaying them as a network.

How do such models help close the theory–method gap? To illustrate, we will consider a dynamic theory of personality and how these methods can be applied. Conditional frameworks of personality (J. C. Wright & Mischel, 1987) propose that personality can be conceived of as *if–then* relationships between behaviors and contexts. *If– thens* are also reflective of an open systems perspective (i.e., external influences impact the system, but it retains its coherence; G. W. Allport, 1960). When conceptualizing cross-lagged VAR models in these frameworks, we see how these models, coupled with sensor data, close the theory–method gap. Lagged relationships can capture *if–then* contingent relationships, while contemporaneous associations capture *while* relationships. In other words, cross-lagged VAR models allow personality researchers to test for conditional associations that characterize the study of how personality unfolds in the context of individuals' daily lives.

For example, the first row of Figure 16.3 shows the contemporaneous and lagged association network of one participant. Because association networks allow all pathways to be estimated (i.e., there is no feature selection procedure), all edges are plotted. To help ease understanding of the visualization, stronger associations have darker and thicker lines, positive associations have solid lines, and negative associations have dashed lines. There is, for example, a dark, thick, and dashed edge between two indicators of Conscientiousness, reliable and lazy, which indicates that *while* this participant felt they were not reliable, they also felt lazy and vice versa. The dark, thick, and solid edge between reliable (Conscientiousness) and outgoing (Extraversion), in contrast, indicates that *while* this participant felt outgoing (E), they also felt reliable (C) and vice versa. Of all the nodes, the reliable (C) node has the darkest, thickest edges between it and other nodes, which indicates that many of this participant's other experiences tended to covary with how reliable they felt.

In the lagged networks, there are also arrows on the edges, indicating the temporal direction of the effect. As can be seen in the figure, the worried (Neuroticism) node has dark, thick dashed lines from it to lazy (Conscientiousness), rude (Agreeableness), relaxed (N), and kind (A). In other words, *if* someone was worried (N) at present, *then* they would be likely to be less lazy (C), rude (A), relaxed (N), and kind (A) at the next time point. Other nodes, like outgoing (E), have thin pale lines extending from it, suggesting that it does not strongly predict experiences at the next time point. It also suggests that there were a number of strong reciprocal effects, including the strong positive one between rude (A) and relaxed (N), suggesting that *if* . . . this participant was more relaxed (N) now, *then* they were rude (A) later and vice versa. Finally, there were a number of self-feedback loops, which are often thought of as inertia in the emotion literature. When positive, like the one for lazy (C), this indicates that laziness was a self-perpetuating cycle (Ong & Ram, 2017). *If* they acted lazy, *then* this participant was likely to continue to do so. Negative feedback loops, like the small one for quiet (E), are thought to represent negative reinforcement cycles (Hamaker, Grasman, & Kamphuis, 2016). In this case, it could indicate that being quiet had negative consequences such that the participant was likely to change their behavior.

Association networks, which are based on zero-order correlations, have some disadvantages, particularly when there is overlapping variance among the indicators. Thus, some have argued for the importance of examining the unique relationships among the indicators using partial correlations or regression (e.g., Epskamp & Fried, 2018). In such cases, the possibility of overcontrolling or overfitting the model increases (assuming the

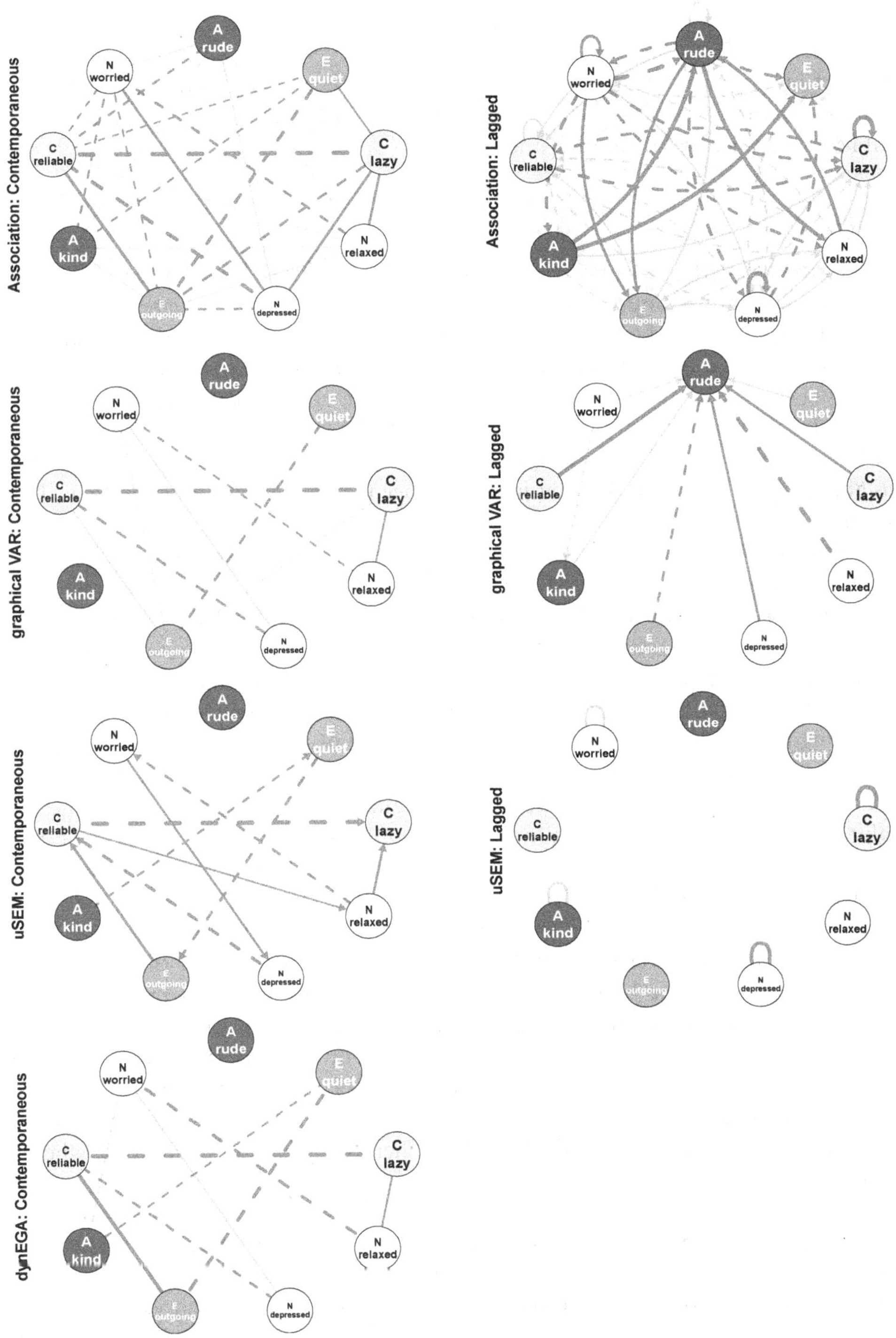

FIGURE 16.3. Sample network visualizations of four different network models: association networks (top row), graphical vector autoregressive (graphical VAR) models (second row), unified structural equation models (uSEM; third row), and dynamic exploratory graph analysis (dynEGA) using generalized linear local approximation of derivatives (GLLA; bottom row). For each, the right column indicates contemporaneous (lag 0, *while*) relationships among indicators, while the left column indicates lagged (lag 1, *if–then*) relationships among indicators.

number of observations remains constant). Recently, there have been a number of proposed models for examining such complex models without overfitting, which we will detail now: graphical VAR, uSEM, and dynEGA.

Graphical VAR

New techniques for the basic lagged, or vector autoregressive (VAR) model (e.g., Bringmann et al., 2016; Epskamp, Waldorp, Mõttus, & Borsboom, 2018; Gates & Molenaar, 2012; Wild et al., 2010), have been proposed and implemented (in a limited manner) to account for dynamic relationships among predictors. Typically, these use some method for pruning model pathways to prevent or reduce the effects of multicollinearity (e.g., graphical LASSO; Friedman, Hastie, & Tibshirani, 2008). These methods produce partial correlations or multiple regression coefficients, which capture the unique relationships among diverse phenomena that may influence manifestations of psychological phenomena.

Graphical VAR uses a two-stage procedure to estimate two networks: a within-time, contemporaneous network (i.e., a symmetrical matrix) and an across-time, cross-lagged network (i.e., a nonsymmetrical matrix; Epskamp & Fried, 2018; Wild et al., 2010). The lagged and contemporaneous networks are estimated sequentially, such that lagged networks are estimated by regressing each indicator on all other indicators (including the focal indicator itself) at the previous time point. Contemporaneous networks are estimated using the concentration matrix (i.e., the inverse) of the residual covariance matrix of the lagged networks to detrend participants' responses (e.g., Flury & Levri, 1999).

To prevent overfitting, these models are regularized using a variant of the *least absolute shrinkage and selection operator* (LASSO; Tibshirani, 1996), graphical LASSO (glasso; Friedman et al., 2008). Essentially, regularization uses a constraint to prevent overfitting. Edges that fall below the constraint are set to 0, which effectively reduces the dimensionality of the network by eliminating the estimation of these pathways. glasso includes a tuning parameter that can be set to control the sparsity of the network (the dimensions set to 0). The best-fitting network is found by testing a range of penalty parameters (lambda) for both the contemporaneous and lagged networks and using an information criterion to compare the models at different values of the tuning parameter. Different values of the hyperparameter gamma can be chosen to optimize prediction accuracy in order to minimize an information criterion, such as the Bayesian information criterion (BIC) or the extended BIC (eBIC; Chen & Chen, 2008). Notably, when the hyperparameter gamma is set to 0, the information criterion is simply BIC.

Graphical VAR produces two sets of $p \times p$ matrices of partial correlations, symmetric partial contemporaneous correlations (PCCs), and asymmetric partial directed correlations (PDCs), which are derived from the regression coefficients. First, the PDCs are calculated by rescaling the regression coefficients using the residual variances on the diagonal of the residual covariance matrix. Next, the PCCs are estimated by taking the inverse of the residual covariance matrix (see Wild et al., 2010).

The resulting networks from the graphical VAR procedure can be understood to be similar to the association networks presented in the previous section. However, there are three key differences. First, rather than zero-order correlations, these networks represent the partial correlations between each indicator after partialing out overlapping with variance with all other indicators. Second, because graphical VAR uses regularization to constrain the edges, not all edges are present. Third, the contemporaneous network is based on the residuals of the lagged network. As a result, the contemporaneous network in Figure 16.3 can be interpreted as *while* relationships. For example, *while* this participant felt lazy, they tended to not feel lazy or depressed. However, how reliable they felt had no association to how worried they felt, but *while* they felt worried, they felt more depressed and less outgoing.

The lagged network suggests a different, more interpretable pattern than the association network. As is clear in Figure 16.3, almost all of the edges point toward the rude (A) node. In other words, *if* this participant felt quiet (E), reliable (C), depressed (N), lazy (C), or kind (A) now, *then* they tended to be ruder (A) later. In contrast, *if* they were more outgoing (E), worried (N), and relaxed (N) now, *then* they tended to be less rude (A) later. There were only two small self-feedback-loops for the lazy (C) and depressed (N) nodes. Both of these were the strongest self-feedback-loops in the lagged association network as well and indicate that feeling lazy (C) or depressed (N) had strong inertia—that is, *if* the participant felt this way, *then* they were likely feeling similar at the next time point.

uSEM

uSEM is another method for estimating partial contemporaneous and lagged relationships between indicators (Gates, Molenaar, Hillary, Ram, & Rovine, 2010; Kim, Zhu, Chang, Bentler, & Ernst, 2007). Although its overall goal to estimate these contemporaneous and lagged associations is similar to graphical VAR, it differs in a few key ways. First, rather than sequentially estimating a lagged and contemporaneous network, respectively, uSEM estimates these contemporaneous and lagged estimates simultaneously. As a result, uSEM does not result in two $p \times p$ networks, one symmetric and one asymmetric. Instead, it results in a $p \times 2{*}p$ asymmetric matrix, which has been split up and visualized separately in Figure 16.3, for comparison with other methods. Second, rather than using regularization to penalize the regression coefficients, uSEM uses an iterative, automatic search procedure for retaining pathways in the model using Lagrange multiplier tests. Starting with an empty model, the procedure adds each indicator and tests the overall improvement in model fit according to the Lagrange multiplier tests. The variable that results in the largest jump in the test is included. Then the procedure is repeated with the remaining variables until there is no longer a significant jump in the Lagrange multiplier tests.

uSEM allows researchers to answer similar questions as graphical VAR and association networks. However, its implementation within the group iterative multiple model estimation (GIMME) procedure also provides a unique opportunity for merging idiographic and group-level approaches and easy implementation in R using the gimme package (Lane et al., 2021). The GIMME procedure is a data driven procedure for estimating both group-level and idiographic patterns of pathways in time-series data (Lane, Gates, Pike, Beltz, & Wright, 2019). As currently implemented in the gimme package (Lane, Gates, Molenaar, Hallquist, & Pike, 2016) in R, the procedure estimates a series of uSEMs for each person and constructs a group-level structure based on the individual-level models. It does not estimate a group-level matrix of point estimates. Instead, it produces a group-level matrix of pathways that will be estimated for all individuals. uSEM uses an iterative procedure for retaining pathways in the individual models using Lagrange multiplier tests. The GIMME procedure begins by estimating the pathways to be retained at the group-level (i.e., in all individual-level models) by estimating individual-level models and retaining group-level pathways for those paths that were shared by 75% of the participants. Starting with a null model, pathways are iteratively added to the group-level structure (i.e., in all participants' final unique models) when the largest proportion of individuals (above a chosen threshold, 75% by default) show a better model fit according to the Lagrange multiplier tests. This procedure is continued until no additional pathways improve fit above the threshold. Idiographic models are then built using the uSEM procedure described earlier.

The difference between the glasso regularization used by graphical VAR and the stepwise Lagrange multiplier tests is important. Regularization retains or eliminates all pathways simultaneously by optimizing a fit criterion like eBIC or BIC (among others) and choosing the best-fitting model. In contrast, uSEM iteratively adds paths to the model that optimizes Lagrange multiplier tests. Although these can produce almost identical results to regularized graphical VAR models, some longitudinal evidence suggests that graphical VAR models demonstrate somewhat better test–retest consistency than GIMME models in shorter time series (e.g., $N \sim 50$ assessments/person; Beck & Jackson, 2020a, 2021b). However, recent promising work has aimed to integrate regularization into the GIMME procedure in so-called hybrid GIMME (Luo et al., 2023). This procedure can now be readily implemented using the gimme package in R.

The uSEM models can be interpreted similarly to the graphical VAR models with two main exceptions. Although both the uSEM and graphical VAR models represent partial associations between indicators, uSEM coefficients are not correlations unless they are provided standardized data or unless the coefficients themselves were standardized based on the residual covariance matrix. In addition, the contemporaneous associations are directed and simultaneously estimated with lagged associations, which results in directed contemporaneous associations. Although these are still interpreted as the same time-point associations, the goal is to better understand how changes in one may precede changes in the other. For example, the strong, negative association between reliable (C) and lazy (C) evidenced by the dark, thick dashed line between the two nodes, was evidence across each method. However, in uSEM, this association is directed, such that feeling reliable (C) precedes feeling less lazy (C). Similarly, uSEM suggests that the positive association between worried (N) and depressed (N) is directional, such that feeling worried (N) precedes feeling depressed (N).

Using uSEM as part of the GIMME procedure, this participant's lagged network only contains self-feedback-loops. Each of the nine nodes has a self-feedback loop. Of these, five are positive, suggesting self-perpetuating cycles. *If* the participant felt worried (N), depressed (N), kind (A), reliable (C), or lazy (C) now, *then* they were likely to feel similarly later. They also had four negative self-feedback loops, suggesting negative reinforcement patterns. *If* they felt relaxed (N), quiet (E), outgoing (E), or rude (A) now, *then* they were likely to feel less so later.

dynEGA

Finally, dynEGA is a network-based approach that merges network science with dynamic systems theory through derivatives (Golino, Christensen, Moulder, Kim, & Boker, 2022). Rather than examining levels of indicators that co-occur (contemporaneous) or covary across fixed intervals (lagged), dynEGA examines the extent to which changes in levels of indicators covary over time. From a theoretical perspective, this has the advantage of more closely capturing how psychological phenomena change over time rather than just whether they tend to have similar levels at observed moments. More pragmatically, by using derivatives, they also overcome issues introduced by missing assessments when using fixed interval lags as in the previously described methods (see the section "Choosing a Network Model" below for a more thorough discussion).

In order to estimate these networks, the first step is to take the raw time-series data of levels of indicators across time and transform them into derivatives using the generalized local linear approximation (GLLA; Boker, Deboeck, Edler, & Keel, 2010; Deboeck, Montpetit, Bergeman, & Boker, 2009). Using time-delay embedding, first- (velocity) and second- (acceleration or changes in velocity) order derivatives are estimated using GLLA. Then, patterns of associations of derivatives among the derivatives are evaluated using exploratory graph analysis (Golino et al., 2020; Golino & Epskamp, 2017).

Like graphical VAR, dynEGA uses glasso regularization using eBIC for tuning parameter selection for purposes of feature selection and to help prevent overfitting. But unlike both graphical VAR and uSEM, dynEGA also specifically focuses on understanding network topology as part of the model fitting procedure. dynEGA specifically uses community detection algorithms in order to understand how nodes cluster together, similar to how factor-analytic approaches can be applied for dimension reduction of psychometric data (e.g., Golino et al., 2020). Although multiple community detection algorithms are available, both in general and as implemented in the EGAnet package in R, in the example participant in the bottom row of Figure 16.3, we opted for the Louvain community detection algorithm (Blondel, Guillaume, Lambiotte, & Lefebvre, 2008). It has several advantages relative to other community detection algorithms, including its speed, its multilevel structure, and its overall performance (Gates, Henry, Steinley, & Fair, 2016).

Unlike association networks, graphical VAR, and GIMME, dynEGA does not produce both lagged and contemporaneous matrices of associations among indicators. Rather, both level and change are incorporated into a single matrix that captures partial correlations of change or the degree to which different indicators have similar velocity across the time series. As shown in the bottom row of Figure 16.3, the resulting symmetric matrix of associations can be visually represented similar to contemporaneous networks. The network shares many of the same edges as graphical VAR and uSEM, with many of the main differences being smaller (i.e., thinner and lighter) edges. As is clear in the figure, *if* reliability (C) was decreasing, *then* laziness (C) also tended to be increasing and vice versa. In addition, *if* laziness (C) was increasing, *then* relaxation (N) was also often increasing and rudeness (A) was sometimes decreasing. Indeed, one major difference between the graphical VAR network and the dynEGA network is the greater number of associations between changes in rudeness (A) with changes in other nodes. In graphical VAR, rudeness (A) was strongly predicted by previous time-point levels of other indicators in the lagged network but was not associated with any indicators in the contemporaneous network. In contrast, in the dynEGA network, increases in rudeness (A) were weakly associated with increases in how outgoing (E) the participant was as well as how reliable (C) they felt as well as with decreases in laziness (C), as noted previously. This may be because dynEGA is incorporating both level and change into the associations, while graphical VAR attempts to separate these out by sequentially estimating lagged and contemporaneous associations, respectively.

dynEGA additionally emphasizes how the nodes cluster via community detection, in this case using Louvain. The Louvain algorithm identified three communities in this participant's experiences, with (1) rude (A), lazy (C), reliable (C), and depressed (N); (2) quiet (E), outgoing (E), and kind (A); and (3) relaxed (N) and worried (N) all falling into communities. This is notable because it suggests that the participant's experiences did not fall neatly into their putative Big Five domains. Instead, we learn that this participant's experiences of depression (N) and how rude (A) they are linked to how lazy (C) and reliable (C) they feel, while how kind (A) they are is more related to how quiet (E) and outgoing (E) they feel. In other words, the participant's more affiliative behaviors appear to be linked to how social they feel, while some emotions and behavioral responses are linked more to productivity.

Choosing a Network Model

In the previous section, we described four different network models that can be applied to time-series data, such as those collected via active (e.g., EMA) or passive sensing (e.g., mobile sensing). None of these models is the "correct" choice under all conditions. Rather, each model has unique features and advantages under different conditions. Briefly, in this section, we will make a small number of recommendations to help guide the choice of a model on the basis of research questions, temporal properties of the data, and design considerations.

First, an important consideration when choosing a model is the structure of the data. Lagged methods, such as those used in lagged association networks, graphical VAR, and uSEM assume fixed intervals between assessments. If the intervals are not fixed, either due to a different sampling schedule (e.g., pseudo random, event contingent, etc.), late responses, missing responses, or overnight periods, the lags are agnostic to the different intervals between assessments. Such gaps can have two consequences:

1. The most common recommendation to deal with missing assessments is to add empty rows to the time series. Then, because lags are created by shifting the rows of the time series, missing values can multiply. Thus, even with relatively high adherence to sampling protocols, researchers could be left with less than 50% of usable observations when using lags. When missing periods are due to overnight periods and there are multiple assessments per day, another alternative is to use multilevel models in which observations can be nested within days to parse day variance from observation variance. However, this does not fully solve the issue when using lagged estimates without adding empty rows for overnight periods. Moreover, their application to the models described above can require more data due to the need to estimate parameters at both the observation and day level.

2. To the extent that the observed interval is critical in capturing contingent relationships, unequal intervals could greatly reduce both the sensitivity and specificity of the lagged model. Some more recently developed models, like continuous time VAR models (CT-VAR; de Haan-Rietdijk, Voelkle, Keijsers, & Hamaker, 2017; Ryan, Kuiper, & Hamaker, 2018), aim to deal with the limitations of assumptions of fixed interval lags, but the necessary data requirements (upward of 100 assessments of each indicator) can sometimes be prohibitive, particularly when coupling less frequent active sensing with more frequent passive sensing. But dynEGA performs well even under these conditions,

with time-delayed GLLA showing good performance on short time series and regularization increasing the sparsity of the network as a whole (Golino et al., 2020; Hardt, Boker, & Bergeman, 2020).

Second, the choice of model also depends on which aspects of a network are of interest. For example, in some cases, contemporaneous, concurrent associations alone may be of interest, making the estimation of lagged networks seem unnecessary. However, it is not possible to estimate only contemporaneous associations using either graphical VAR or uSEM. Rather, in both cases, both lagged and contemporaneous associations will always be estimated. In such cases, simply examining an association network of contemporaneous correlations may seem sufficient, coupled with follow-up examinations of the network topology via techniques like the Louvain community detection algorithm. However, examining contemporaneous associations alone ignores the autocorrelative structure of multivariate time series, which can confound and introduce bias into estimates of contemporaneous associations (McCleary, Hay, Meidinger, & McDowall, 1980). Thus, many recommend detrending the time series through differencing or residual-based regression approaches (Wang & Maxwell, 2015), which is similar to the residual-based approach used by graphical VAR's sequential estimation of lagged and contemporaneous associations (Wild et al., 2010). uSEM does so indirectly at best, which may not fully account for the trends in the data, so detrending preprocessing is recommended prior to analysis. Finally, dynEGA directly captures the autocorrelative structure of the data using time-delay embedding and by examining associations of change (i.e., GLLA derivatives).

Given each of these, how do you choose a model? Our general recommendation is that no model should be taken as ground truth. Each should be examined across a range of tuning parameters, data cleaning choices, and modeling choices in order to better understand the robustness of the results. Similar to multiverse (Steegen, Tuerlinckx, Gelman, & Vanpaemel, 2016) and specification curve analyses (Simonsohn, Simmons, & Nelson, 2020), this recommendation suggests considering how differences across methods can bias our inferences when selecting a single model or specification of a model. Instead, by examining the impact of a range of choices, we can better understand the robustness and boundary conditions of the observed patterns, associations, and more. For example, the models presented in Figure 16.1 suggest that while the contemporaneous associations were quite consistently recovered across methods, the lagged associations differed greatly. This suggests that the lagged associations are likely unstable and should be interpreted with caution at best and disregarded completely at worst. These comparisons are also in line with the test–retest consistency of these models across 1 year (Beck & Jackson, 2020a) and the COVID-19 pandemic (Beck & Jackson, 2021a), which suggest much better consistency for contemporaneous associations than lagged associations.

Considering all of this together, we want to highlight that the goal of using these methods is to most aptly and accurately represent the research question at hand and the data available to test it. There will never be one "correct" model to apply to a set of data or to answer a research question, so researchers are left with the challenge of addressing the theory–method match in each research endeavor and at each stage of each endeavor. Above we have aimed to demonstrate a series of models that can be used to estimate dynamic associations in multivariate time-series data from active and passive mobile sensing. Furthermore, we linked these conditional and open systems frameworks of personality to demonstrate how interpreting the models in line with these helps to close the theory–method gap (G. W. Allport, 1960; Beck & Jackson, 2020a, 2020b; Wright & Mischel, 1987).

Personality as a Dynamic System

As demonstrated above, using network tools can help to close the theory–method gap by examining associations among features dynamically in ways that address questions raised by Allport, Cattell, and others. Below, we outline a few final considerations and possible additions to the dynamic network models reviewed in the previous section, most of which take advantage of a key passive sensor datapoint collected in almost all studies: date and time stamps. More broadly, in our view, mobile sensing data are ideal to expand and answer these questions because of the possibility of more frequent assessment.

Formal and Verbal Theories of Personality Dynamics

In 1957, Cattell noted the importance of incorporating time effects into models of personality. In addition to discussing periodicity and cycles in psychological states, he argued that accounting for different time effects is important for creating reliable models from which conclusions can be drawn, writing that "the task of research is first to establish statistically and experimentally the nature of the rhythms and then to trace them to internal physiological or external environmental sources, or both" (Cattell, 1957, p. 610).

More colloquially, timing is an important dimension in understanding personality. When we consider the theories we have about the personalities of others, the frequency of, duration of, and change in experiences all play an important role in the ways we understand them. Colloquial phrases such as "[They] are so often tired" (frequency), "[They] can get stuck in an anxious state for days" (duration), and "[They] can turn on a dime" (change), all highlight how time is an explicit part of how we understand and describe the personalities of others.

Thus, the methods appropriate for building personality theory require that the way that manifestations unfold over time, not just their momentary or aggregated levels, are incorporated. Although autocorrelations can help to capture persistence and dynEGA can help to capture rates of change, none of the previously reviewed methods is, at face value, able to deal with cyclical processes, time of day effects, and diurnal cycles. Below, however, we close our discussion of these methods by briefly reviewing evidence on such cycles in psychological phenomena and how they can be incorporated into dynamic network models.

Cycles in Psychological Processes

When describing the personality of others, another frequent description includes time of day effects. You might hear, for example, "Don't talk to [them] in the morning. [They]'ll chew your head off!" or "I tend to fade after lunch." Such descriptors signal possible diurnal cycles in psychological processes and phenomena. Indeed, accumulating evidence suggests not only that some psychological processes demonstrate reliable diurnal pattern (e.g., Broughton, 1975; Stone, Smyth, Pickering, & Schwartz, 1996) across people but also that there are individual differences in such diurnal patterns that partially underlie broader individual differences. Some studies have tested how such cycles relate to broader between-person traits, such as higher circadian rhythm values (i.e., more pronounced 24-hour cycles) of phone usage being associated with Extraversion (Wang et al., 2018). Other studies have tested how passive mobile sensing indicators are associated with active mobile sensing indicators, such as personality states. One such study found that time of day was associated with Extraversion across people using both linear regression and machine learning prediction models (Rüegger et al., 2020).

Although such studies examining diurnal cycles and time of day effects of mobile sensing data are great steps forward, most such studies still search for group-level patterns or attempt to link the patterns to between-person personality traits. Many of these studies do not report the variability of mobile sensing indicators either within or across people. Thus, there are many theoretically relevant open questions about how diurnal cycle and time of day effects can be used to better understand personality and other psychological phenomena, such as whether we can detect behavioral descriptors such as "I tend to fade after lunch," how such patterns cluster together within and across people, and so on.

Quite simply, these diurnal and time of day effects can be included as nodes in the dynamic network methods reviewed in the previous sections (see Beck & Jackson, 2021b; e.g., code on calculating each of the terms below). First, for example, a time of day node that is dummy coded as "morning," "midday," "afternoon," "evening," and "night" could help address differences in each of the other nodes across the day. In other words, particularly when coupled with feature selection techniques, like glasso, any edges between these nodes and nodes from active or passive sensing indicate a time of day effect, partialing out all other relationships between other nodes—that is, a robust time of day effect for that indicator. Second, cosinor terms can be included, particularly when denser, passive sensing data are utilized. The most commonly used terms are both one- and two-period sine and cosine functions of decimal time (since midnight). Because these represent a more continuous but more complex method for addressing time of day effects, we recommend using them with careful planning and attention. Finally, trends can be included, such as linear, quadratic, and cubic trends across the time series. These are particularly important when the act of completing active or passive sensing is thought to potentially impact participants' behaviors and experiences. By including such trends across time, researchers can directly address questions about changes in the levels of the indicators across time as well as interpret associations among them adjusting for such trends.

Conclusion

Psychology is a dynamic science, yet much of the study of psychology relies on aggregating across dynamics of psychological phenomena and looking at individual differences or group-level differences of such aggregates. This creates a gap between psychological theories and the methods used to test them. In this chapter, we discussed how dynamic passive and active mobile sensing data can be used to help close the gap. Using theoretical and empirical findings from the domain of personality psychology, we argued for both the importance of dynamics for studying and testing personality theory and for its utility in everyday life.

Our representation of both personality theory and dynamic methods was far from exhaustive. Rather, we hoped to demonstrate how theoretical propositions, both simple and complex, both narrow and sweeping, could be linked to dynamic methods better suited to testing the proposition than methods that rely on aggregates. In the simplest case, we argued that propositions that personality is a readiness for response (Allport, 1937) could be captured by looking at personality as rates of change of personality states. In a broader, more complex case, we highlighted how Allport's (1960) proposition that personality is an open system could be tested using dynamic systems approaches that build structural and mathematical models of dynamic features.

We believe that by bringing the theory–method gap in personality specifically and psychology more broadly to the fore, psychologists can make more active and informed choices in their model selection in ways that will better align theory and methods. By demonstrating a small number of dynamic models, we hope that readers of this chapter will consider how they may relate to theories in all disciplines of psychology. Moreover, we hope that much as we endeavored to start with a theory and then make the case for why different models test its proposition, readers of this chapter will walk similar avenues and test old dynamic questions with new dynamic methods.

ACKNOWLEDGMENTS

Emorie D. Beck was supported by National Institute on Aging Grant Nos. T32 AG00030-3, R01-AG067622, and R01-AG018436. Stuti Thapa was supported by the Gratitude to God Grant from John Templeton Foundation.

REFERENCES

Allport, F. H. (1920). The influence of the group upon association and thought. *Journal of Experimental Psychology, 3*(3), 159–182.

Allport, G. W. (1937). *Personality: A psychological interpretation.* Holt.

Allport, G. W. (1954). *The nature of prejudice.* Addison-Wesley.

Allport, G. W. (1960). The open system in personality theory. *The Journal of Abnormal and Social Psychology, 61*(3), 301–310.

Allport, G. W. (1968). *The person in psychology: Selected essays.* Beacon Press.

Baumert, A., Schmitt, M., Perugini, M., Johnson, W., Blum, G., Borkenau, P., et al. (2017). Integrating personality structure, personality process, and personality development. *European Journal of Personality, 31*(5), 503–528.

Beck, E. D., & Jackson, J. J. (2020a). Consistency and change in idiographic personality: A longitudinal ESM network study. *Journal of Personality and Social Psychology, 118*(5), 1080–1100.

Beck, E. D., & Jackson, J. J. (2020b). Idiographic traits: A return to Allportian approaches to personality. *Current Directions in Psychological Science, 29*(3), 301–308.

Beck, E. D., & Jackson, J. J. (2021a). Idiographic personality coherence: A quasi experimental longitudinal ESM study. *European Journal of Personality, 36*(3), 391–412.

Beck, E. D., & Jackson, J. J. (2021b). A mega-analysis of personality prediction: Robustness and boundary conditions. *Journal of Personality and Social Psychology.*

Beck, E. D., & Jackson, J. J. (2021c). Network approaches to representing and understanding personality dynamics. In D. Wood, S. J. Read, P. D. Harms, & A. Slaughter (Eds.), *Measuring and modeling persons and situations* (pp. 465–497). Academic Press.

Beck, E. D., & Jackson, J. J. (2021d). *Personalized behavior prediction: An idiographic person–situation test.* PsyArXiv.

Beck, E. D., & Jackson, J. J. (2021e). Within-person variability. In J. F. Rauthmann (Ed.), *The handbook of personality dynamics and processes* (pp. 75–100). Academic Press.

Bleidorn, W. (2012). Hitting the road to adulthood: Short-term personality development during a major life transition. *Personality and Social Psychology Bulletin, 38*(12), 1594–1608.

Bleidorn, W., Klimstra, T. A., Denissen, J. J. A., Rentfrow, P. J., Potter, J., & Gosling, S. D. (2013). Personality maturation around the world: A cross-cultural examination of social-investment theory. *Psychological Science, 24*(12), 2530–2540.

Blondel, V., Guillaume, J.-L., Lambiotte, R., & Lefebvre, E. (2008). Identification multi-échelle de la structure communautaire de très grands graphes (D. Simplot-Ryl & S. Tixeuil, Trans.). In *10ème Rencontres Francophones sur les Aspects Algorithmiques des Télécommunications (AlgoTel'08)* (pp. 61–64). https://hal.inria.fr/inria-00374457

Boker, S. M., Deboeck, P. R., Edler, C., & Keel, P. K. (2010). Generalized local linear approximation of derivatives from time series. In S. M. Chow, E. Ferrer, & F. Hsieh (Eds.), *Statistical methods for modeling human dynamics: An interdisciplinary dialogue.* (pp. 161–178). Routledge/Taylor & Francis Group.

Borsboom, D., & Cramer, A. O. J. (2013). Network analysis: An integrative approach to the structure of psychopathology. *Annual Review of Clinical Psychology, 9*(1), 91–121.

Borsboom, D., Mellenbergh, G. J., & van Heerden, J. (2003). The theoretical status of latent variables. *Psychological Review, 110*(2), 203–219.

Bringmann, L. F., Pe, M. L., Vissers, N., Ceulemans, E., Borsboom, D., Vanpaemel, W., et al. (2016). Assessing temporal emotion dynamics using networks. *Assessment, 23*(4), 425–435.

Broughton, R. (1975). Biorhythmic variations in consciousness and psychological functions. *Canadian Psychological Review/Psychologie Canadienne, 16*(4), 217–239.

Buss, D. M., & Craik, K. H. (1980). The frequency concept of disposition: Dominance and prototypically dominant acts. *Journal of Personality, 48*(3), 379–392.

Campbell, J. P., & Wiernik, B. M. (2015). The modeling and assessment of work performance. *Annual Review of Organizational Psychology and Organizational Behavior, 2*, 47–74.

Cattell, R. B. (1943). The description of personality: Basic traits resolved into clusters. *The Journal of Abnormal and Social Psychology, 38*(4), 476–506.

Cattell, R. B. (1946a). *Description and measurement of personality.* World Book.

Cattell, R. B. (1946b). Personality structure and measurement. I. The operational determination of trait unities. *British Journal of Psychology, 36*, 88–103.

Cattell, R. B. (1957). *Personality and motivation structure and measurement.* World Book.

Cervone, D. (2005). Personality architecture: Within-person structures and processes. *Annual Review of Psychology, 56*(1), 423–452.

Chen, J., & Chen, Z. (2008). Extended Bayesian information criteria for model selection with large model spaces. *Biometrika, 95*(3), 759–771.

Christensen, A. P., Cotter, K. N., & Silvia, P. J. (2019). Reopening openness to experience: A network analysis of four openness to experience inventories. *Journal of Personality Assessment, 101*(6), 574–588.

Conner, T. S., Tennen, H., Fleeson, W., & Barrett, L. F. (2009). Experience sampling methods: A modern idiographic approach to personality research. *Social and Personality Psychology Compass, 3*(3), 292–313.

Costantini, G., Richetin, J., Preti, E., Casini, E., Epskamp, S., & Perugini, M. (2019). Stability and variability of personality networks: A tutorial on recent developments in network psychometrics. *Dynamic Personality Psychology, 136*, 68–78.

Cramer, A. O. J., van der Sluis, S., Noordhof, A., Wichers, M., Geschwind, N., Aggen, S. H., et al. (2012). Dimensions of normal personality as networks in search of equilibrium: You can't like parties if you don't like people. *European Journal of Personality, 26*(4), 414–431.

Csikszentmihalyi, M., & Larson, R. (1987). Validity and reliability of the experience-sampling method. *Journal of Nervous and Mental Disease, 175*(9), 526–536.

Dalal, R. S., Bhave, D. P., & Fiset, J. (2014). Within-person variability in job performance: A theoretical review and research agenda. *Journal of Management, 40*(5), 1396–1436.

Deboeck, P. R., Montpetit, M. A., Bergeman, C. S., & Boker, S. M. (2009). Using derivative estimates to describe intraindividual variability at multiple time scales. *Psychological Methods, 14*(4), 367–386.

de Haan-Rietdijk, S., Voelkle, M. C., Keijsers, L., & Hamaker, E. L. (2017). Discrete- vs. continuous-time modeling of unequally spaced experience sampling method data. *Frontiers in Psychology, 8*. https://www.frontiersin.org/article/10.3389/fpsyg.2017.01849

Emmons, R. A., & Diener, E. (1986). Situation selection as a moderator of response consistency and stability. *Journal of Personality and Social Psychology, 51*(5), 1013–1019.

Epskamp, S., & Fried, E. I. (2018). A tutorial on regularized partial correlation networks. *Psychological Methods, 23*(4), 617–634.

Epskamp, S., Waldorp, L. J., Mõttus, R., & Borsboom, D. (2018). The Gaussian graphical model in cross-sectional and time-series data. *Multivariate Behavioral Research, 53*(4), 453–480.

Fisher, A. J., Medaglia, J. D., & Jeronimus, B. F. (2018). Lack of group-to-individual generalizability is a threat to human subjects research. *Proceedings of the National Academy of Sciences, 115*(27), E6106.

Fleeson, W. (2001). Toward a structure- and process-integrated view of personality: Traits as density distributions of states. *Journal of Personality and Social Psychology, 80*(6), 1011–1027.

Fleeson, W. (2004). Moving personality beyond the person-situation debate: The challenge and the opportunity of within-person variability. *Current Directions in Psychological Science, 13*(2), 83–87.

Fleeson, W., & Jayawickreme, E. (2015). Whole trait theory. *Integrative Theories of Personality, 56*, 82–92.

Flury, B. D., & Levri, E. P. (1999). Periodic logistic regression. *Ecology, 80*(7), 2254–2260.

Forbes, M. K., Wright, A. G. C., Markon, K. E., & Krueger, R. F. (2019). The network approach to psychopathology: Promise versus reality. *World Psychiatry, 18*(3), 272–273.

Forbes, M. K., Wright, A. G. C., Markon, K. E., & Krueger, R. F. (2021). Quantifying the reliability and replicability of psychopathology network characteristics. *Multivariate Behavioral Research, 56*(2), 224–242.

Fried, E. I. (2020). Theories and models: What they are, what they are for, and what they are about. *Psychological Inquiry, 31*(4), 336–344.

Friedman, J., Hastie, T., & Tibshirani, R. (2008). Sparse inverse covariance estimation with the graphical lasso. *Biostatistics, 9*(3), 432–441.

Funder, D. C., & Colvin, C. R. (1991). Explorations in behavioral consistency: Properties of persons, situations, and behaviors. *Journal of Personality and Social Psychology, 60*(5), 773–794.

Gates, K. M., Henry, T., Steinley, D., & Fair, D. A. (2016). A Monte Carlo evaluation of weighted community detection algorithms. *Frontiers in Neuroinformatics, 10*. www.frontiersin.org/article/10.3389/fninf.2016.00045

Gates, K. M., & Molenaar, P. C. M. (2012). Group search algorithm recovers effective connectivity maps for individuals in homogeneous and heterogeneous samples. *NeuroImage, 63*(1), 310–319.

Gates, K. M., Molenaar, P. C. M., Hillary, F. G., Ram, N., & Rovine, M. J. (2010). Automatic search for fMRI connectivity mapping: An alternative to Granger causality testing using formal equivalences among SEM path modeling, VAR, and unified SEM. *NeuroImage, 50*(3), 1118–1125.

Golino, H. F., Christensen, A. P., Moulder, R., Kim, S., & Boker, S. M. (2022). Modeling latent topics in social media using dynamic exploratory graph analysis: The case of the right-wing and left-wing trolls in the 2016 US elections. *Psychometrika, 87*(1), 156–187.

Golino, H. F., & Epskamp, S. (2017). Exploratory graph analysis: A new approach for estimating the number of dimensions in psychological research. *PLoS One, 12*(6), e0174035.

Golino, H. F., Shi, D., Christensen, A. P., Garrido, L. E., Nieto, M. D., Sadana, R., et al. (2020). Investigating the performance of exploratory graph analysis and traditional techniques to identify the number of latent factors: A simulation and tutorial. *Psychological Methods, 25*(3), 292–320.

Graham, E. K., Weston, S. J., Gerstorf, D., Yoneda, T. B., Booth, T., Beam, C. R., et al. (2020). Trajectories of Big Five personality traits: A coordinated analysis of 16 longitudinal samples. *European Journal of Personality, 34*(3), 301–321.

Hamaker, E. L., Grasman, R. P. P. P., & Kamphuis, J. H. (2016). Modeling BAS dysregulation in bipolar disorder: Illustrating the potential of time series analysis. *Assessment, 23*(4), 436–446.

Hardt, K., Boker, S. M., & Bergeman, C. S. (2020). A note on the usefulness of constrained fourth-order latent differential equation models in the case of small t. *Psychometrika, 85*(4), 1016–1027.

Jones, P. J., Williams, D. R., & McNally, R. J. (2021). Sampling variability Is not nonreplication: A Bayesian reanalysis of Forbes, Wright, Markon, and Krueger. *Multivariate Behavioral Research, 56*(2), 249–255.

Kim, J., Zhu, W., Chang, L., Bentler, P. M., & Ernst, T. (2007). Unified structural equation modeling approach for the analysis of multisubject, multivariate functional MRI data. *Human Brain Mapping, 28*(2), 85–93.

Lane, S. T., Gates, K., Fisher, Z., Arizmendi, C., Molenaar, P., Hallquist, M., et al. (2021). *Package 'gimme.'* https://CRAN.R-project.org/package=gimme

Lane, S. T., Gates, K. M., Molenaar, P., Hallquist, M., & Pike, H. (2016). *Gimme: Group iterative multiple model estimation.* [Computer software]. https://CRAN.R-project.org/package=gimme.

Lane, S. T., Gates, K. M., Pike, H. K., Beltz, A. M., & Wright, A. G. C. (2019). Uncovering general, shared, and unique temporal patterns in ambulatory assessment data. *Psychological Methods, 24*(1), 54–69.

Luo, L., Fisher, Z. F., Arizmendi, C., Molenaar, P. C. M., Beltz, A., & Gates, K. M. (2023). Estimating both directed and undirected contemporaneous relations in time series data using hybrid-group iterative multiple model estimation. *Psychological Methods, 28*(1), 189–206.

McCleary, R., Hay, R., Meidinger, E., & McDowall, D. (1980). *Applied time series analysis for the social sciences.* Sage.

Mischel, W., & Shoda, Y. (1995). A cognitive-affective system theory of personality: Reconceptualizing situations, dispositions, dynamics, and invariance in personality structure. *Psychological Review, 102*(2), 246.

Moeller, J. (2021). Averting the next credibility crisis in psychological science: Within-person methods for personalized diagnostics and intervention. *Journal for Person-Oriented Research, 7*(2), 53–77.

Molenaar, P. C. M. (2004). A manifesto on psychology as idiographic science: Bringing the person back into scientific psychology, this time forever. *Measurement: Interdisciplinary Research and Perspectives, 2*(4), 201–218.

Ong, A. D., & Ram, N. (2017). Fragile and enduring positive affect: Implications for adaptive aging. *Gerontology, 63*(3), 263–269.

Piccirillo, M. L., Beck, E. D., & Rodebaugh, T. L. (2019). A clinician's primer for idiographic research: Considerations and recommendations. *Behavior Therapy, 50*(5), 938–951.

Renner, K. H., Klee, S., & von Oertzen, T. (2020). Bringing back the person into behavioural personality science using big data. *European Journal of Personality, 34*(5), 670–686.

Robinaugh, D. J., Hoekstra, R. H. A., Toner, E. R., & Borsboom, D. (2020). The network approach to psychopathology: A review of the literature 2008–2018 and an agenda for future research. *Psychological Medicine, 50*(3), 353–366. Cambridge Core.

Rüegger, D., Stieger, M., Nißen, M., Allemand, M., Fleisch, E., & Kowatsch, T. (2020). How are personality states associated with smartphone data? *European Journal of Personality, 34*(5), 687–713.

Ryan, O., Kuiper, R. M., & Hamaker, E. L. (2018). A continuous-time approach to intensive longitudinal data: What, why, and how? In K. van Montfort, J. H. L. Oud, & M. C. Voelkle (Eds.), *Continuous time modeling in the behavioral and related sciences* (pp. 27–54). Springer.

Sherman, R. A., Rauthmann, J. F., Brown, N. A., Serfass, D. G., & Jones, A. B. (2015). The independent effects of personality and situations on real-time expressions of behavior and emotion. *Journal of Personality and Social Psychology, 109*(5), 872–888.

Simonsohn, U., Simmons, J. P., & Nelson, L. D. (2020). Specification curve analysis. *Nature Human Behaviour, 4*(11), 1208–1214.

Snijders, T. A. B. & Bosker, R. J. (2011). *Multilevel Analysis: An introduction to basic and advanced multilevel modeling.* Sage.

Steegen, S., Tuerlinckx, F., Gelman, A., & Vanpaemel, W. (2016). Increasing transparency through a multiverse analysis. *Perspectives on Psychological Science, 11*(5), 702–712.

Stone, A. A., Smyth, J. M., Pickering, T., & Schwartz, J. (1996). Daily mood variability: Form of diurnal patterns and determinants of diurnal patterns. *Journal of Applied Social Psychology, 26*(14), 1286–1305.

Tibshirani, R. (1996). Regression shrinkage and selection via the lasso. *Journal of the Royal*

Statistical Society: Series B (Methodological), 58(1), 267–288.

Wang, L. (Peggy) & Maxwell, S. E. (2015). On disaggregating between-person and within-person effects with longitudinal data using multilevel models. *Psychological Methods, 20*(1), 63–83.

Wang, W., Harari, G. M., Wang, R., Müller, S. R., Mirjafari, S., Masaba, K., & Campbell, A. T. (2018). Sensing behavioral change over time: Using within-person variability features from mobile sensing to predict personality traits. *Proceedings of the ACM on Interactive, Mobile, Wearable and Ubiquitous Technologies, 2*(3), 1–21.

Wild, B., Eichler, M., Friederich, H.-C., Hartmann, M., Zipfel, S., & Herzog, W. (2010). A graphical vector autoregressive modelling approach to the analysis of electronic diary data. *BMC Medical Research Methodology, 10*(1), 28.

Winter, D. G., & Barenbaum, N. B. (1999). History of modern personality theory and research. In O. P. John, R. W. Robins, & L. A. Pervin (Eds.), *Handbook of personality: Theory and research* (2nd ed., pp. 3–27). Guilford Press.

Wood, D., Spain, S. M., & Harms, P. D. (2017). Functional approaches to representing the interplay of situations, persons, and behavior. In J. F. Rauthmann, R. A. Sherman, & D. C. Funder (Eds.), *The Oxford handbook of psychological situations* (pp. 179–202). Oxford University Press.

Wright, A. G. C., Gates, K. M., Arizmendi, C., Lane, S. T., Woods, W. C., & Edershile, E. A. (2019). Focusing personality assessment on the person: Modeling general, shared, and person specific processes in personality and psychopathology. *Psychological Assessment, 31*(4), 502–515.

Wright, J. C., & Mischel, W. (1987). A conditional approach to dispositional constructs: The local predictability of social behavior. *Journal of Personality and Social Psychology, 53*(6), 1159–1177.

Wrzus, C., Wagner, G. G., & Riediger, M. (2016). Personality-situation transactions from adolescence to old age. *Journal of Personality and Social Psychology, 110*(5), 782–799.

Wundt, W. M. (1911). *Völkerpsychologie: Bd. Die Sprache* (Vol. 1). Engelmann.

Zuckerman, M. (1979). Traits, states, situations, and uncertainty. *Journal of Behavioral Assessment, 1*(1), 43–54.

CHAPTER 17

Machine Learning for Mobile Sensing Data

Andreas M. Brandmaier

CHAPTER OVERVIEW

From the perspective of traditional statistics as taught in the behavioral and social sciences, machine learning reflects a paradigm shift from explanation to prediction. With machine learning, we can leverage flexible forms of regression that allow us more freedom in discovering patterns of associations between potentially large numbers of independent and dependent variables. A particular focus is placed on ensuring the generalizability of results to new samples. This chapter summarizes various fundamental machine learning approaches such as decision trees, regularized regression, quadratic discriminant analysis, naïve Bayes, and support vector machines. Feature generation, model selection, and model evaluation are considered from a practical perspective. The utility of the various learning approaches is illustrated by using the different methods to predict daily life activities from smartphone data.

Introduction

Machine learning is a central part of the broader field of artificial intelligence. It is concerned with algorithms that give computers the ability to learn to solve a well-defined task without being explicitly programmed to do so. The idea can be traced back to early computer pioneers such as Alan Turing. In 1950, Turing proposed substituting the philosophical question "Can machines think?" by a behavioristic definition of the problem, namely, that one can assent to the question if a machine *behaves* as if it could think (Turing, 1950). In his chapter "Learning Machines," Turing imagined a program that matches the "output" of human intelligence and noted that we should strive for a "child program" that learns to solve any task by learning instead of by being programmed.

Meanwhile, machine learning has arrived in everyday technology, in industry, as well as in scientific research. I vividly recall the question posed by a scientist during the discussion of a lecture on the benefits of machine learning for neuroscience research; he asked: "What do these machines know better about dealing with my data than I do?" I appreciated the question because it shows the necessary level of skepticism that we should maintain when encountering such learning machines and their powerful promises. From the perspective of traditional statistics as taught in the behavioral and social sciences, machine learning is a paradigm shift from explanation to prediction that uses flexible forms of regression allowing us more freedom in discovering patterns of associations between potentially large numbers of independent and dependent variables (with a particular focus on ensuring generalization to new samples; Berk, 2008). By the term *prediction* I generally mean the estimation of an outcome regardless of whether it represents a present or future state. However, there is no shortcut from a well-predicting model with practical utility to a novel psychological theory. Still, prediction itself is often a valuable goal and the fact that a predictive model outperforms the most recent theoretical model can say a lot about the value of the theory (see the discussion in Brandmaier, Prindle, McArdle, & Lindenberger, 2016). Machine learning is particularly useful when human expertise either does not exist or is difficult to formalize into a predictive model. In mobile sensing data, machine learning promises to be highly useful because it is often difficult to handcraft models for large and complex datasets for which purely theory-based approaches become unfeasible. We may be able to derive simple rules, for example, derive the orientation of a phone from its accelerometer readings (because we know that gravity exerts a constant force on the spring inside the sensor) or infer a person's wake–sleep level by forming rules based on time of day, upper body orientation, and overall activity level of an accelerometer owing to our common knowledge (i.e., when people sleep, it tends to be nighttime and they usually lie horizontally while hardly moving). However, the larger the number of sensors, the larger the diversity of recorded signals, and with more complicated decision and prediction problems, it will soon become impossible to handcraft such rules. This is where machine learning approaches show their full strength.

Machine learning is usually divided into three major areas, all of which deal with learning structure and regularities from observed data. These areas are *supervised learning*, *unsupervised learning*, and *reinforcement learning*, and they are distinguished by the assumptions made about the environment and the structure of the learning task. In supervised learning, the goal is to predict continuous outcomes (regression) or discrete outcomes (classification), and we assume the existence of a dataset from which we can infer the associations of features and known target values or classes. The models that perform classification tasks are typically referred to as *classifiers*. In *unsupervised learning*, there are no outcomes, and the goal is to find underlying patterns such as simple features or clusters in the data (see Chapter 19, this volume). *Reinforcement learning* deals with approaches that learn to make optimal sequences of decisions as reactions to an observable environment in order to achieve a certain goal. These algorithms are most useful in robotics, self-driving cars, or computer games, for example. This chapter gives a brief overview of fundamental ideas of *supervised learning* in the context of mobile sensor data and gives pointers to relevant literature in which these concepts can be examined in more detail.

I mostly illustrate supervised learning approaches to predict everyday activities from accelerometry, but the algorithms and challenges presented here generalize to a broader class of prediction problems in which we would like to predict discrete outcomes from continuous sensor data (e.g., depression status; Elhai et al., 2018). I discuss algorithms and ideas at a conceptual level, so that readers can get an overview of possible approaches to classification and regression from a machine learning perspective. This requires simplification of some problems, sacrificing depth and detail for the sake of the bigger picture. Readers interested in more detailed information should consult the original articles on the presented approaches and foundational books on machine learning. Researchers who present useful overviews include Hastie, Tibshirani, and Friedman (2009), Bishop (2006), and Murphy (2012). Also, I would like to recommend Berk (2008) and James, Witten, Hastie, and Tibshirani (2013) for their emphasis on practical applications and hands-on R codes.

Most examples presented in this chapter are based on open data from the WISDM Smartphone and Smartwatch Activity and Biometrics Dataset (Weiss, Yoneda, & Hayajneh, 2019), which can be downloaded from the UCI Machine Learning Database (https://archive.ics.uci.edu). This dataset comprises data from 51 participants, each performing 18 activities (e.g., walking, sitting, eating soup, eating pasta, writing, or folding clothes) for 3 minutes per activity. The sensor data were collected at a rate of 20 Hz from accelerometers and gyroscopes of both a smartwatch and a smartphone. The regression and classification approaches I present are predominantly based on time window approaches that capture local properties of time series. I briefly discuss how these approaches can be extended to models that explicitly model temporal dependency in sequential data. The methods presented here are implemented in various well-documented R packages. Comprehensive interfaces to various algorithms are provided by `caret` (Kuhn, 2020) and `tidymodels` (Kuhn & Wickham, 2020). The decision tree was estimated with `partykit` (Hothorn & Zeileis, 2015), and the regularized regression with `glmnet` (Friedman, Hastie, & Tibshirani, 2010).

Features

A *feature* is a measurable property of a phenomenon of interest. The predominant approach to making inferences about sensor data, such as recognizing activities from smartwatch data, is a window-based *feature engineering* and *feature selection* approach because many models profit from transforming raw sensor data into more meaningful and less noisy features (Fukazawa et al., 2020; Stachl et al., 2020). In this approach, we first manually generate ("engineer") meaningful features from raw sensor recordings in small time windows. For example, we compute average acceleration in one direction or the number of apps opened on a smartphone. Then we select a model to make predictions based on these features. The optimal choice of window size depends primarily on the type of sensor, the derived features, the outcome, and the sampling frequency (Bao & Intille, 2004). Typical window sizes cover several seconds, such that a given activity (or major components of it) are included (but also see motion-primitive-based approaches for shorter components, e.g., Zhang & Sawchuk, 2012). The WISDM dataset has a fixed window size of 10 seconds sampled at 20 Hz, such that each window covers 200 data points from which features were generated.

It is also possible to classify directly on the raw sensor values. However, the more prior knowledge we impart to the classifier by creating high-level features, the more successfully it will perform (in the sense of both accuracy and robustness). Yet, the more uninformative information we provide, the less successful the classifier will tend to be (we will return to this thought later). A variety of features computed from raw values have proven useful in empirical applications. Most commonly, standard distributional characteristics of sensor readings are used as features, such as the mean, standard deviation, skewness, and kurtosis. For example, in accelerometer data, the mean and variance already bear a lot of information about physical activity (see Figure 17.1). The mean captures the average deflection of the proof mass in the sensor and, thus, directly translates to the orientation of the device in space and may help to infer posture. The variance directly captures the magnitude of activity over a given period of time and may help to derive the motion and intensity of activity. Numerous other features have proven to work well with different types of sensors. For example, from video images, we may derive centroid, edge, and optical flow features; from GPS, it may be location and speed; from speech snippets, it may be overall signal power (i.e., loudness) or power in selected frequency bands (see Fukazawa et al., 2020, for a survey on features used to predict the user's mental state). Thoughtful feature engineering often already solves the prediction problem to a large extent. In contrast, even the best predictive algorithm will fail if features are mostly uninformative about the prediction goal. When choosing among predictive algorithms, we may prefer those that perform some sort of implicit or explicit feature selection, sometimes also referred to as variable selection (performed by algorithms such as decision trees or regularization). Often, more parsimonious models with fewer selected

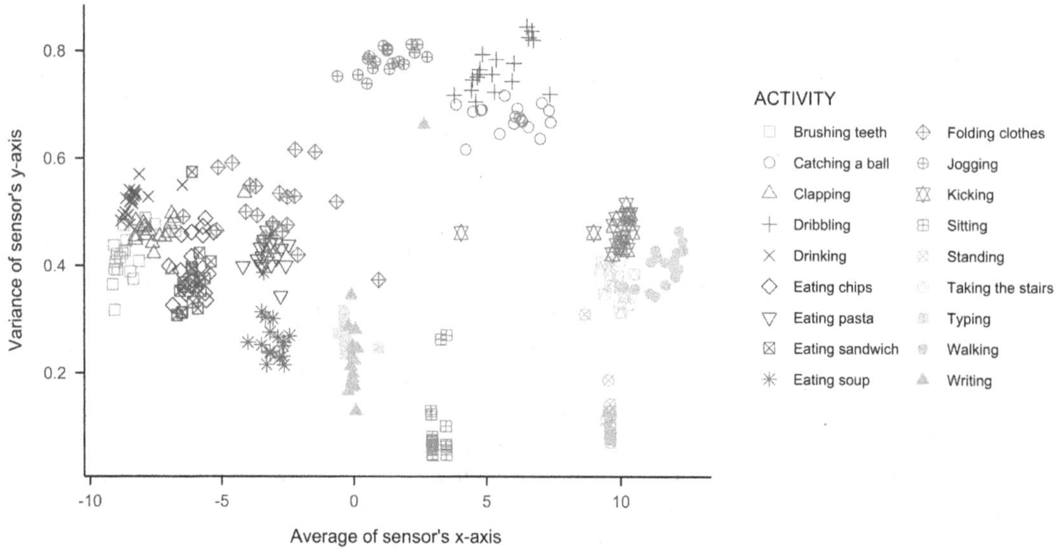

FIGURE 17.1. A two-dimensional feature space for activity classification. Observations of different activities (shown in different shapes) are plotted with the empirical average deflection measured on the x-axis of the accelerometer in a smartwatch (which partly reflects rotation of the arm in one axis) against the variance of activity on the y-axis (reflecting physical activity in one direction). A typical classification problem is to predict a person's activity from such features. As can be seen, these two features alone are already quite informative for distinguishing various activities. This figure is available at https://github.com/brandmaier/mobile-sensing-figures under a CC-BY4.0 license.

features are found to be more accurate and to generalize better because they safeguard against overfitting to noise in the data. In time-critical applications (e.g., when predictions are to be made very fast, or computational power or also battery power is limited on a wearable device), decreasing the number of features may increase the efficiency of the algorithm or decrease costs by relying on the deployment of fewer measurement devices or on cheaper hardware requirements (Guyon & Elisseeff, 2003).

Algorithms

Instance-Based Learning

A simple and intuitive idea for implementing a learning machine is to let it memorize all observations and then make predictions based on how similar a novel observation will be to what it has memorized. This idea is known as *instance-based learning* or *lazy learning.* In this paradigm, learning degrades to a simple storage process, and no explicit model will emerge that could then provide explanations about the phenomena of interest. The most widely known algorithm implementing this idea is *k-nearest neighbors* (kNN; Altman, 1992). To predict a new observation, the algorithm searches all known observations and retrieves the *k*-nearest neighbors in feature space, given some distance metric (typically, Euclidean distance for continuous features). Then, it predicts the majority class (in classification problems) or the mean (in regression problems) of the target variable of these neighbors. An illustration of kNN-based decision boundaries in a two-dimensional feature space is given in Figure 17.2. It shows how kNN partitions the feature space into neighborhoods of activities. The smoothness of the partition depends on the choice of *k*. As *k* goes up, smoothness increases.

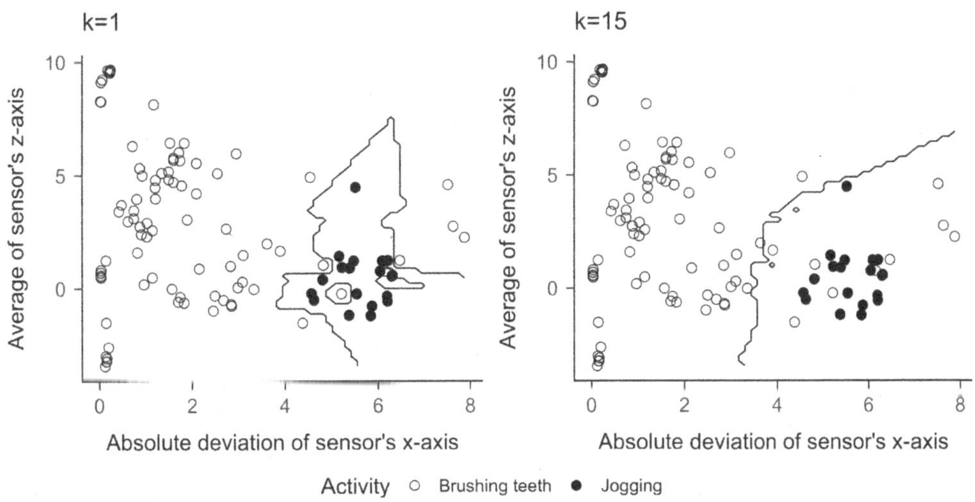

FIGURE 17.2. Decision boundaries of *k*-nearest neighbor classification with $k = 1$ (left) and $k = 15$ (right) shown in black lines. The graph axes correspond to the absolute deviation of the sensor's *x*-axis (shown on the graph's *x*-axis) and the mean of the sensor's *z*-axis (shown on the graph's *y*-axis) for classifying the activities of *jogging* versus *brushing teeth.* With increasing *k*, the smoothness of the decision boundaries increases. This figure is available at https://github.com/brandmaier/mobile-sensing-figures under a CC-BY4.0 license.

kNN is attractive because it almost works "out of the box," and with enough observations, it can learn quite complex decision boundaries. It is fast in the learning phase but may require excessive amounts of storage space, and may be time-consuming when making predictions. This is because naive implementations have to search all stored data points to retrieve the nearest neighbors. kNN has several other problems in practice. With Euclidean distances, features with a larger range will dominate the remaining features to the extreme that a single feature may dominate all others. Therefore, it is advisable to standardize all variables before using kNN. Furthermore, the Euclidean distance is particularly sensitive to outliers because extreme values greatly impact the squared difference between observations. This is why the Manhattan distance (the sum of absolute differences) may yield more robust results in high-dimensional spaces.

Probably most importantly, kNN has no feature-reduction mechanism; that is, all features contribute to the (dis)similarity of data points. If the prediction task really depends only on a few of many features, the true nearest neighbors may actually be not near but far away from each other in the space spanned by the features. Or put differently, as we add uninformative predictors, sparsity of the feature space increases (the same number of observations will reside in a larger space), making neighbors less similar to each other, and decreasing the predictive accuracy of our model. For example, imagine that our data points cover the observed space randomly and uniformly. Let us assume that the observed space is one-dimensional (there is only one feature). If we zoom into a neighborhood that covers only 10%, we will find about 10% of the observed points there. In a cubic space (three features), we will find only $0.1^3 = 0.1\%$ of points in a neighborhood that covers 10% of each dimension. In other words, the more dimensions in our feature space, the less likely it is to find a nearest neighbor that is close by and the more difficult it is to infer general rules. To some extent, we can solve this problem with more data, but we also need to be aware of this fundamental limitation of learning from data. Machine learning is often applied in high-dimensional feature spaces (that is, when the number of features is large) because it is typically difficult to build theory-based models in these scenarios (Brandmaier et al., 2016; Stachl et al., 2020). Therefore, in practice, we may want to switch to other algorithms that implicitly or explicitly perform feature selection. Also, if we can exclude features based on theoretical considerations, we should always do so prior to running a machine learning analysis to improve its chances of finding a generalizable solution.

Linear Discriminant Analysis, Quadratic Discriminant Analysis, and Naive Bayes

When discussing kNN, we realized that storing all observed examples is an inefficient way of learning because it neither scales well nor provides an interpretable model. What if we abstracted from the individual instances by modeling the observed distribution over instances? By adding distributional assumptions about the features, we should be able to obtain a more robust model that is also amenable to further inspection, allowing us to access the mechanics of the classifier (e.g., which features are most important for predictions). For example, assuming a multivariate normal distribution of features per class, it will be sufficient to store the parameters of the normal distribution instead of the individual observations. A multivariate normal distribution in k dimensions (i.e., when there are k features) has k mean parameters and $(k^2 + k)/2$ in the covariance matrix. If we have a total of m different classes in a prediction task, we need to estimate $m \cdot (k^2 + 3k)/2$ parameters. For example, if we have two features and four classes, we need to estimate 20 model parameters (see Figure 17.3). With this probabilistic representation, prediction will now be much more rapid because we do not have to search all observations as in kNN, but rather we compute the likelihood of a new observation under the class-conditional distributions. If Y represents the class to be predicted and X the feature vector, our machine learning challenge can be formalized as learning the probability of observing Y given X, denoted as $P(Y|X)$. Using Bayes's theorem, we can rewrite this as

$$P(Y \mid X) = \frac{P(Y)P(X \mid Y)}{P(X)}$$

From this, we can deduce that we need to obtain two types of information: the prior probabilities $P(Y)$ for each class Y and the probability densities of X within each class Y denoted as $P(X|Y)$. The term $P(X)$ is treated as a constant irrelevant for deciding between classes. If we perfectly knew priors and the class-conditional densities, we could derive an optimal classifier, the so-called *Bayes optimal classifier*, from this. No other classifier could do better because the only error this classifier makes is due to irreducible noise (e.g., measurement error or inherent randomness). Note that in practice, the normality assumption might be oversimplified; and even if we knew the correct type of distribution, we would need to estimate parameters from limited and unreliable data, both of which lead to loss of accuracy in prediction.

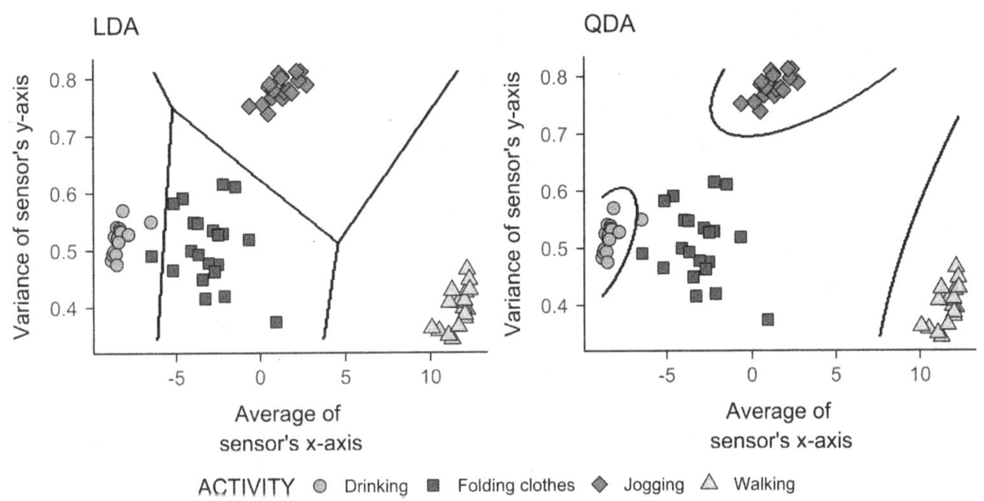

FIGURE 17.3. Two-dimensional feature space spanned by the sensor's average x-axis value (plotted on the graph's x-axis) and the variance of the y-axis of the accelerometer in a smartwatch (plotted on the graph's y-axis). Data points represent four activity classes (jogging, walking, folding clothes, and drinking). Left: Linear discriminant analysis (LDA) fits a set of linear decision boundaries in this space. Right: Quadratic discriminant analysis (QDA) fits a set of quadratic decision boundaries into the space. Here, neither approach perfectly separates the training set into the labeled classes. This figure is available at https://github.com/brandmaier/mobile-sensing-figures under a CC-BY4.0 license.

This probabilistic approach assuming Gaussian feature distributions is typically referred to as *quadratic discriminant analysis* (QDA; Hastie et al., 2009). Linear discriminant analysis (LDA) is a special case of QDA in which the variances and covariances are assumed to be identical across all classes. LDA leads to fewer parameters to estimate, with each parameter estimated from a larger number of data points; that is, the variance and covariance estimates will be more precise. Assume we have 50 features and 4 classes, then we would need to estimate $p \cdot (p + 1)/2 = (50 \cdot 51)/2 = 1{,}275$ free parameters in the covariance matrix for an LDA, respectively, $k \cdot p \cdot (p + 1)/2 = 4 \cdot 1{,}275 = 5{,}100$ parameters in the covariance matrix for a QDA. At the same time, we increase the chance of misspecification when using LDA because identical feature covariances across classes are typically a severe oversimplification of reality. Figure 17.3 illustrates the class-conditional distributions in a two-dimensional feature space as estimated by LDA and QDA. As can be seen, LDA leads to linear decision boundaries and QDA leads to quadratic decision boundaries (hence their names). A further simplification of the model (further trading fidelity for simplicity and robustness) is the naive Bayes classifier in which we assume independence of the class-conditional features and thus simply ignore all covariances to drastically reduce the number of parameters estimated—in the above example, reducing the number of estimated parameters in the covariance matrices to $3 \cdot 50 = 150$ variance estimates.

The LDA model can be reexpressed such that the ratio of the log-posterior odds for the predicted classes is a linear model. This is true for the logistic regression, too, and one may wonder whether they are identical. In fact, their form is identical, but they optimize different loss functions and one may say that the logistic regression makes fewer assumptions. Ultimately, this means that if observations are really Gaussian, LDA will be more efficient; however, if class-conditional distributions are non-Gaussian or distorted by heavy outliers, logistic regression may perform better. Hastie and colleagues (2009) argue that, in practice, both models often yield similar results. But what if we are not willing to make parametric assumptions about the features while allowing for the generation of interpretable prediction rules? The next section covers an entirely nonparametric approach to prediction using decision trees.

Decision Trees

Decision trees are nonparametric models for classification and regression that are widely used across many domains because they yield interpretable models in the form of if–else decision rules. Figure 17.4 shows a decision tree. These decision rules are created hierarchically such that the collection of rules can be represented as a tree. Each inner node (shown as circles here) has a logical decision rule that assigns observations uniquely to one of its child nodes. Starting from the root node (top node) and following the respective branches of each decision node, one arrives at a leaf node (also, terminal node) that makes a prediction about the outcome. Learning decision trees from data is done by recursive partitioning, that is, by choosing splits of the data over and over again that maximally reduce uncertainty about the outcome. For classification, entropy is a general measure to quantify uncertainty. Entropy of a random variable with probabilities p_i for the ith of M discrete states is computed as

$$H = -\sum_{i=1}^{M} p_i \log p_i$$

For regression problems, trees typically maximize a variance-explained criterion. Trees recursively divide the feature space by axis-parallel splits because every smaller-than-x relation divides the feature space into a "left" and "right" subspace. This is illustrated in Figure 17.4 using a prediction task from smartwatch data. The resulting axis-parallel splits implied by the decision nodes are given in Figure 17.5. With this in mind, decision trees can be seen as adaptive nearest neighbor algorithms because (1) a large number of potential neighborhoods are searched before an actual neighborhood is defined and (2) the resulting terminal node neighborhoods are defined by different sets of features. A given predictor may help to define one neighborhood but may be irrelevant for another. Because searching all possible trees for a given set of predictors is computationally infeasible, trees are grown using a *greedy* model search procedure called *recursive partitioning:* Best splits are always chosen as being locally optimal, which does not guarantee finding the globally best tree but often yields reasonable and interpretable results in practice.

Decision trees are simple yet powerful methods because they adapt to the complexity of the data as much as the available information affords it. At the same time, they are notorious for being unstable (Strobl, Malley, & Tutz, 2009). Small perturbations to the training data (such as adding or removing a few cases, for example, by changing an outlier correction procedure or continuing to sample) sometimes drastically change a decision tree because different splits selected further up the tree lead to ever larger subsequent

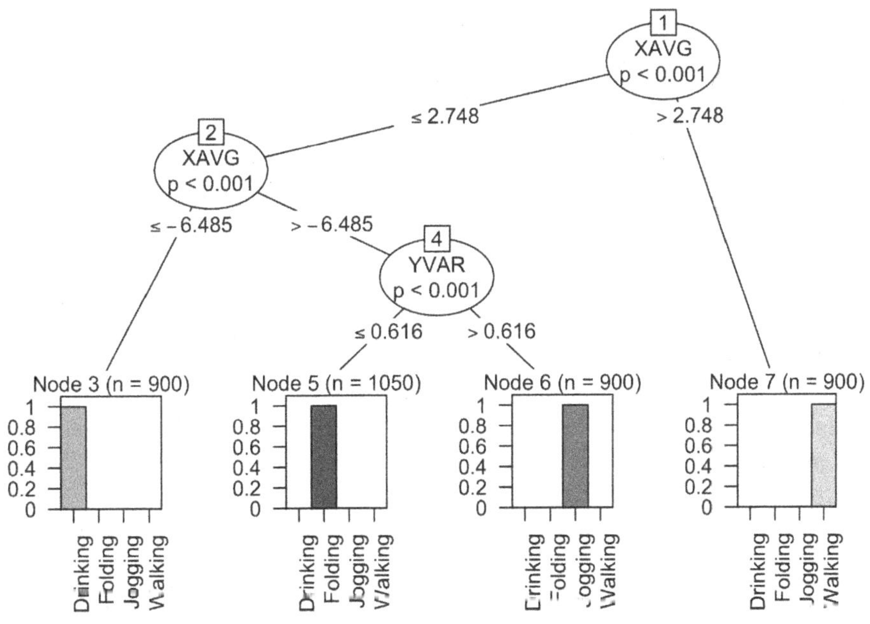

FIGURE 17.4. A decision tree for classifying smartwatch accelerometer data into one of four activities (jogging, walking, folding clothes, and drinking). The tree selected the average of the x-axis (XAVG) as the two first splits that reduce entropy about the outcome maximally. This corresponds to the orientation of the arm on which the watch is worn. To further discriminate between folding clothes and jogging, the variance (corresponding to vigor of activity) in the y-axis (YAVG) is most discriminative. The p values correspond to a test of no association between a given feature and the outcome. This figure is available at https://github.com/brandmaier/mobile-sensing-figures under a CC-BY4.0 license.

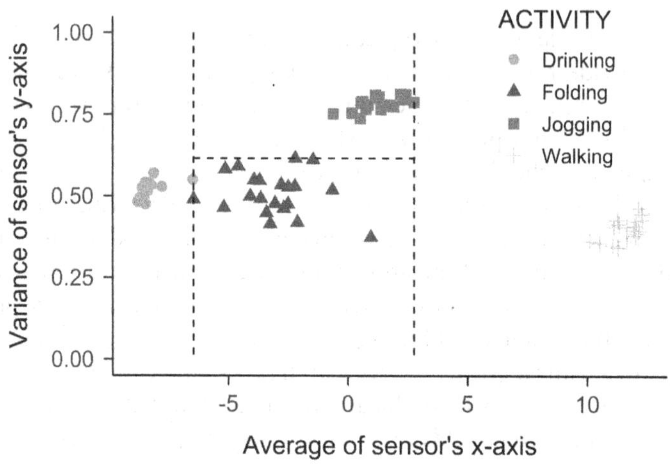

FIGURE 17.5. Axis-parallel splits in feature space based on the tree shown in Figure 17.4. The two features selected by the tree are the average of the x-axis of a smartwatch accelerometer (shown on the x-axis of the plot) and the average of the y-axis of a smartwatch accelerometer (shown on the y-axis of the plot). This figure is available at https://github.com/brandmaier/mobile-sensing-figures under a CC-BY4.0 license.

changes in the conditionally selected splits. This is particularly true if predictors are highly correlated. To not only acknowledge but leverage this problem, Breiman (2001) introduced *random forests* as a principled way to make predictions by using ensembles of trees. The core idea is to combine several "weak" learners and combine their individual predictions to an ensemble prediction by either taking the mean of all predictions (regression) or a majority vote (classification). One can show that averaging predictions of independent learners can lower the variance while maintaining the bias of the learners. The beneficial effect of averaging is decreased by the degree of correlation among the learners. Therefore, random forests force individual trees in the forests to become independent by building the trees based on randomization of the original data. In random forests, each tree is built on a random sample of the training data (either by bootstrapping, that is, sampling with replacement, or subsampling, that is, sampling without replacement). Random forests trade the straightforward interpretability of simple trees for higher robustness and increased predictive power, and they belong to the most successful prediction algorithms across a variety of problems (Fernández-Delgado, Cernadas, Barro, & Amorim, 2014). To examine which features have played a role in predictions of a random forest, we can compute measures of variable importance averaged over all trees. The current best practice is to compute permutation-based *conditional variable importance* (Strobl, Boulesteix, Kneib, Augustin, & Zeileis, 2008). By permuting one predictor at a time, the drop in the predictive performance of the model is taken as a proxy for the importance of that predictor. Figure 17.6 illustrates estimated variable importance derived from conditional variable importance for the acceleration data used in the classification example (with activities drinking, folding, jogging, and walking). Of note is the finding by Strobl and colleagues (2008) that earlier but still widely used (marginal) variable importance measures are biased toward correlated predictor variables and should be avoided.

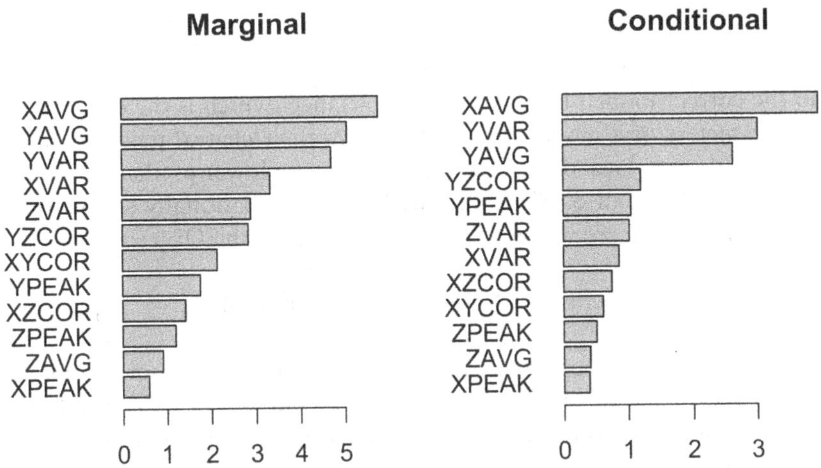

FIGURE 17.6. Variable importance as derived from random forests based on predicting four different activities (jogging, walking, folding clothes, other) based on mean (AVG), peak (PEAK), and variance (VAR) of x-, y-, and z-axis accelerometer readings, and their correlations (COR). Left: Marginal variable importance (potentially biased by correlated variables). Right: Conditional variable importance. This figure is available at https://github.com/brandmaier/mobile-sensing-figures under a CC-BY4.0 license.

Decision trees and random forests can be extended beyond univariate regression and classification problems to multivariate outcomes. These multivariate outcomes can either be model-based, as they are in *structural equation model trees* and *forests* (Brandmaier et al., 2016; Brandmaier, von Oertzen, McArdle, & Lindenberger, 2013), or model-free, such as in multivariate tree boosting (Miller, Lubke, McArtor, & Bergeman, 2016).

Regularization

Earlier, I briefly discussed that implicitly or explicitly, we are often interested in feature selection. This is not only because we may be looking for a solution that is cheap to implement (using fewer sensors) but also because simpler models often seem to perform better. A simple heuristic is to sequentially add or remove features. These approaches are subsumed under *best subset selection* but are notoriously unstable, depend on order effects, and are prone to overfit (but see recursive feature elimination as a model-agnostic, useful approach; Guyon, Weston, Barnhill, & Vapnik, 2002). A more elegant approach is *regularization*, also known as *shrinkage* or *penalization*. Regularized regression solves the variable-selection problem by adding a penalty term to the least-squares fit function that penalizes solutions for the magnitude of their regression coefficients. This favors sparse solutions in which only few predictors are allowed to be "active." By adding the penalty term, we constrain our model to be simpler than what the data "say" and thus force noisy estimates of unimportant variables to become zero. This works particularly well when the number of features is large, the sample size is rather small, and the true model is sparse. In these cases, chances are great that ordinary least squares (OLS) regression will tend to overfit the data, capturing noise in the training data, while regularized models will be less susceptible to this noise and generalize better to new data. However, this also means that our regularized regression coefficients will become biased estimates of the true values (if we had the correct model) but because the variance (which is the extent to which the estimated parameters of a model will deviate from their central tendency across different samples) of our estimates decreases, we can expect a lower prediction error from this approach (see also Yarkoni & Westfall, 2017). A computationally simple optimization function that yields *ridge regression* is given by extending the OLS equation:

$$\min_{(\beta_0,\beta)\in\mathbb{R}^{p+1}} \frac{1}{N}\sum_{i=1}^{N}(y_i - \beta_0 - x_i^T\beta)^2 + \lambda\|\boldsymbol{\beta}\|_2^2$$

where x_i are some features of observation i (of a total of N observations) and y_i the outcome; $\boldsymbol{\beta}$ is the vector of regression coefficients, and λ is a weight that governs the strength of the regularization term, which is added to the common OLS loss function. The regularization term $\|\boldsymbol{\beta}\|_2^2$ is the so-called L_2 norm of $\boldsymbol{\beta}$ and is computed as the sum of the squared regression coefficients. Note that features should be standardized, such that the penalty does not depend on the scale of the features. A more effective penalization is acquired by the *least absolute shrinkage and selection operator* (LASSO), which uses the sum of the absolute regression coefficients as the penalty (L1 norm). LASSO's absolute shrinkage pulls regression coefficients more strongly to zero than the relative shrinkage of the ridge. The elastic net combines both penalties and introduces a mixture parameter, α, that governs the relative impact of the penalties. Both λ and α typically need to be determined either by model selection criteria (such as the Bayesian information criterion, BIC) or by cross-validation (see the section "Model Selection" later in this chapter).

Figure 17.7 shows an application of regularization to a logistic regression model classifying the activities "walking" and "jogging" based on smartwatch accelerometer data. The initial model has 21 predictors, of which only 12 survive after regularization. The strongest predictors are the average activity of the x-axis (potentially reflecting a different hand orientation on average) and indicators of activity intensity (absolute deviation and standard deviation of the y-axis), whereas neither other activity indicators (such as variance of all axes) nor frequency components (Mel-frequency cepstral coefficients, MFCC) are retained.

Support Vector Machine

The linear model has proved successful across many areas because its simplicity makes it robust. We have seen that we can estimate its parameters with different optimization goals in mind, such as least squares, LDA, or regularization. But at least one more optimization goal is worth discussing: the principle of *maximum margin*. This simple yet convincing principle is implemented by the *support vector machine* (SVM; Boser, Guyon, & Vapnik, 1992; Schölkopf & Smola, 2002). The idea behind SVM is to find a (linear) decision boundary between two classes that maximizes the separability of the observations from the two classes. To this end, we try to find the maximal gap—the so-called *margin*—between the observations from two classes and place a separating hyperplane right into the middle. Intuitively, this makes a lot of sense because only a few data points then determine the margin, and extreme values become less influential. Support vectors are those data points that are closest to the separating hyperplane and determine its position and orientation. Figure 17.8 illustrates a two-class problem and the support vectors

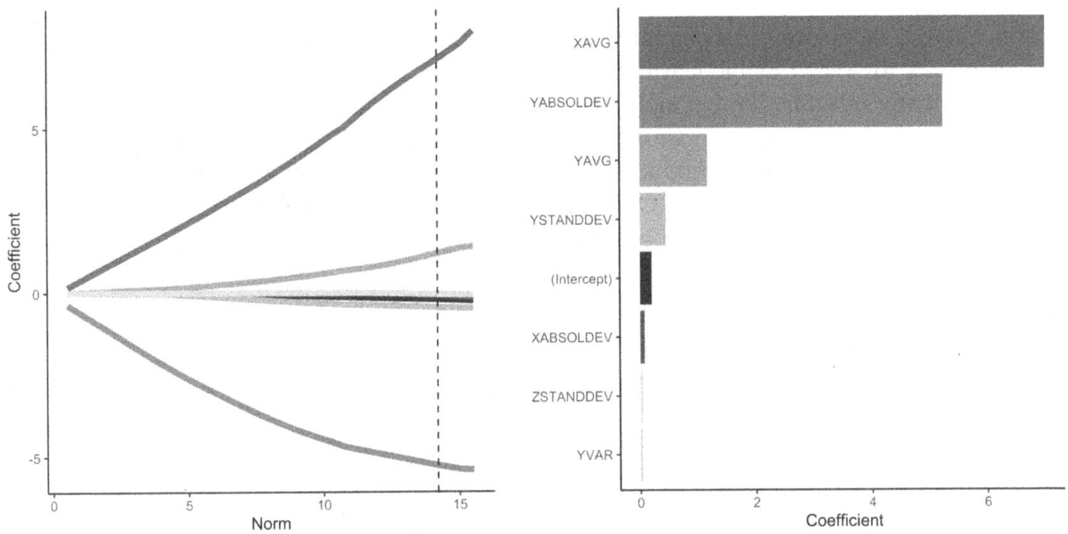

FIGURE 17.7. Results from a regularized logistic regression model with LASSO penalty. Only the most influential values are shown. Left plot: on the x-axis, the L1 norm of the coefficients (i.e., the sum of the absolute values of the regression coefficients) is shown. The y-axis shows the regularized regression coefficients. The lines represent the regression coefficients as they are gradually shrunken toward zero. The dashed line indicates the best model as found by cross-validation. Right plot: The absolute regularized coefficients of the "surviving" variables according to cross-validation. This figure is available at https://github.com/brandmaier/mobile-sensing-figures under a CC-BY4.0 license.

that define the margin. One can show that maximizing the margin boils down to minimizing a quadratic function in the regression coefficients (under additional constraints to guarantee correct classification results). A variety of quadratic solvers can solve this problem efficiently and accurately. However, model fitting involves inverting a matrix, which has a runtime that is cubic in the number of features, and thus SVM becomes unfeasible for very large datasets.

What if the data points are not linearly separable? For example, there may be highly noisy measurements, or the true decision boundary may be nonlinear. SVMs leverage two further ideas to flexibly handle a variety of classification and regression tasks efficiently. First, we abandon the idea of a *hard margin* in favor of a *soft margin* that allows some observations to be "not exactly right"; that is, they may lie within the margin or even on the wrong side of the margin. To handle these cases, we introduce slack variables for each observation that can be thought of as something like a misfit indicator for each observation. It allows for observations on the wrong side of the margin or inside the margin. The larger the total slack, the more we are willing to accept linear decision boundaries even though perfect separation is impossible. So, our new objective becomes: Minimize the slack while maximizing the margin. The tradeoff between complexity and (mis)fit is again governed by a regularization parameter, often called *cost parameter C*.

Finally, the SVM owes much of its success to the *kernel trick*. The kernel trick allows SVM to fit linear decision boundaries in feature spaces that have more dimensions than the original space. Selecting a kernel is akin to an explicit (nonlinear) feature transformation, even though the features are actually never projected into this high-dimensional space. This allows for very flexible learning approaches that remain mathematically tractable and efficiently solvable. For example, the quadratic kernel solves the learning problem in a space in which the feature dimensions are all original features and all pairwise products of all features (including the product of each feature with itself). The linear kernel simply retains the original feature space. One of the most widely used is the radial basis function (RBF) kernel (often the default in software implementations). This kernel can be seen as

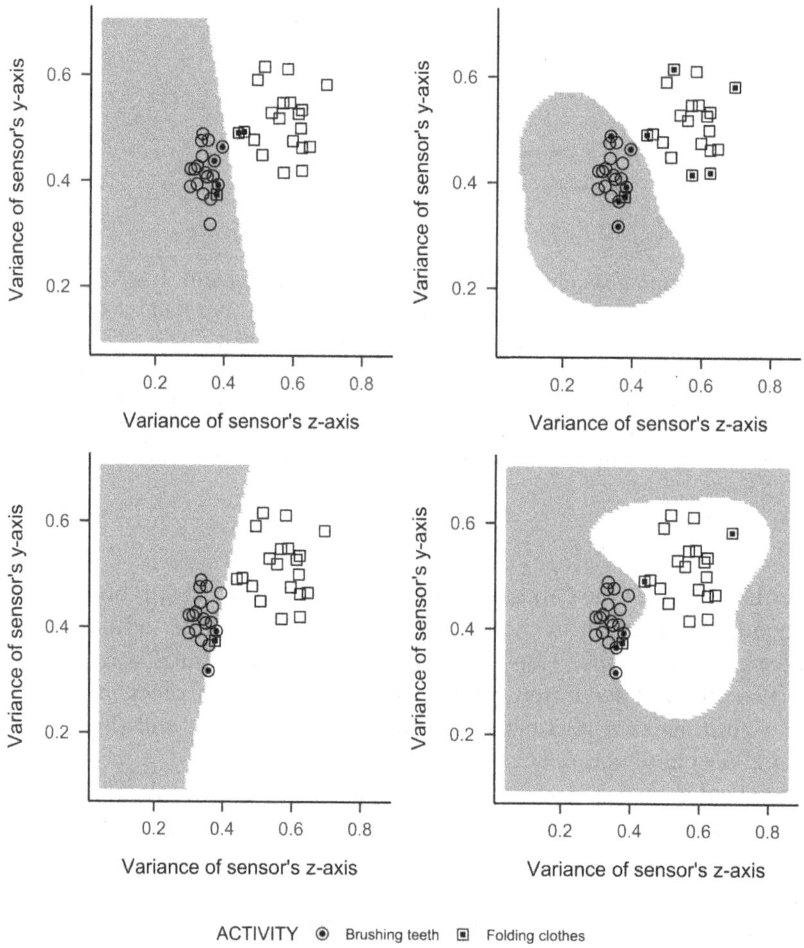

FIGURE 17.8. Two-dimensional feature space for classifying two activities based on the accelerometer features *variance of z-axis* and *variance of the y-axis*. Observations are shown as circles or rectangles either representing the activity *brushing teeth* or *folding clothes*. Support vectors are indicated by black dots inside the observations. The top panels have a large margin (more support vectors), and the lower panels a small margin (fewer support vectors) based on different cost parameters (0.1 vs. 100). Note the outlying rectangle close to the cloud of circles, which has a high influence with hard margins. Softer margins reduce the impact of this outlier. The left-hand panels show linear kernels, and the right-hand panels, radial basis function (RBF) kernels. The learned decision boundary is the border between the gray and white areas. This figure is available at https://github.com/brandmaier/mobile-sensing-figures under a CC-BY4.0 license.

a smooth version of the nearest neighbor or rather the nearest centroid approach because it fits Gaussian distributions to every point to define important neighborhoods in the feature space. The choice of kernel becomes a further tuning parameter and determines the possible shapes of the decision boundary.

Figure 17.8 illustrates linear and nonlinear decision boundaries from four different SVM models based on different combinations of kernels (linear and RBF) and cost parameters (little and much slack). Note that all four panels show the same two-dimensional feature space with identical observations (shown as circles). In the left-hand plots, a linear kernel was chosen, and on the right, an RBF kernel was selected. In SVM, C trades off the costs of misfit and the costs of allowing for slack. A low-cost C means that allowing for slack is relatively cheap compared to increases in misfit. In the top panels, the cost parameter was chosen to be low (allowing for rather more slack, *soft margin*) whereas the cost parameter in the bottom panel was chosen to be high (allowing for little slack, *hard margin*). We can see that the SVM approach can lead to decidedly different decision boundaries that lead to very different generalizations. Deciding between the optimal kernel and cost is usually an empirical problem and is, as with all other approaches we have seen so far, best treated as a model selection problem (see the section "Model Selection" in this chapter). For example, in Figure 17.8, the RBF kernel with a small margin has the lowest cross-validated error estimate (no misclassification), whereas all others make one misclassification error on average.

Sequence Learning

We have looked at classification and regression approaches that were devised for independent observations; that is, any temporal dependencies among observations beyond the current windows were ignored. In many mobile sensing applications, we are dealing with continuous streams of data with informative temporal structure. We have avoided explicitly modeling the continuous nature of time by generating features that model local properties of the time series (such as mean, variance, or dominant frequency). However, this requires at least some prior knowledge of which of these properties carry information; in particular, it does not allow us to model dependencies over time scales that go beyond these local windows. A further problem is that we often train these window-based classifiers on clean data (maybe obtained in a lab under well-controlled conditions) with clear start and endpoints, whereas realistic sensor readings may be much noisier and activities do not show clear boundaries. Ultimately, all this leads us to recognize the necessity of models that explicitly model time or at least consider larger time scales in one way or another. One very general class of models—(deep) recurrent neural networks—can efficiently learn compressed representations of time series directly from the raw sensor values. Understanding the theory and details of technical implementations of these networks requires a level of sophistication that is beyond the scope of a few paragraphs, and this is why this volume dedicates an entire chapter to deep neural networks (see Arizmendi et al., Chapter 18, this volume).

In Chapter 19 (this volume), I discuss hidden Markov models (HMMs), which are simple probabilistic models for the segmentation of sequential data. HMMs can also be used as classifiers. HMMs are very similar to LDA, QDA, and naive Bayes with respect to how they model observations probabilistically—with the difference that HMMs explicitly model temporal dependency by assuming an underlying sequence of states. For classification tasks, one HMM is then used for each target class (e.g., activity), and a given sequence of observations is labeled with the associated class of the HMM that has the highest likelihood of having produced the observed sequence (Wang, Chen, Sun, She, & Wu, 2011). The individual HMMs thus learn the feature sequences within an activity, and we can expect them to outperform static, window-based classification techniques, particularly when activities are complex conjunctions of simpler primitive motions. Also, we should expect that explicitly modeling the hierarchical nature of activities should produce even better results (e.g., Ronao & Cho, 2014). Similarly, if information about the sequential dependence of activities is available, one would ideally also model a second-order Markov process that describes the transition between states (e.g., that it is very unlikely to transition from "taking the stairs" to "asleep" but likely to transition from "sitting" to "eating") to improve classification. As with all classification algorithms, HMM will also profit from a careful selection of meaningful features. If handcrafting the features is difficult, classification approaches can be used as a first variable selection approach. For example, a random forest approach could be used to select optimal features for static classification with the hope that they will also prove useful for a dynamic model. Alternatively, one could also use model selection approaches (such as cross-validation or information criteria) to select the best features among a candidate set of features, but this may quickly become unfeasible because of the exponentially large search space.

Performance Metrics

How do we know how well our preferred prediction algorithm solves a given problem? To evaluate the predictive performance of regression problems, we can resort to the common metrics we know from linear regression, such as root mean squared error, mean absolute error, or R^2. For classification problems, there are a variety of different performance metrics. The simplest metric for classification tasks is *accuracy*, which counts the proportion of correct predictions among all predictions. Accuracy seems intuitive to understand but may be misleading when classes are imbalanced. Assume that a classifier is supposed to predict a dangerous fall from continuous accelerometer data in a smartwatch in order to automatically send out a distress call. If, in a training set, the number of dangerous falls is only 0.01%, any classifier that always predicts the majority class of "no dangerous fall" will have an accuracy of 99.99%. To communicate the average performance per class considering unequal proportions of cases in each class, we should rather report *balanced accuracy*. This assumes that the proportion of errors in each class matters instead of the absolute number of errors overall. To more closely inspect the type of errors a classifier makes, we can compute a confusion matrix. A confusion matrix is a table that shows the absolute number of cases for which a given class was predicted for each true class. It allows us to understand which class labels a classifier confuses when it makes incorrect predictions.

In two-class problems, further measures that are often reported are *precision* and *recall*. They are typically used in information retrieval to quantify how relevant query results are to the actual query. Precision (also known as *positive predictive value*) is the proportion of retrieved relevant results from all retrieved results, and recall is the proportion of retrieved relevant results from all relevant results (Murphy, 2012). Suppose a classifier for recognizing night sleep phases from continuous accelerometry data identifies eight sleep phases in a dataset containing 14 true sleep phases and some wake phases. Of the eight phases identified as sleep phases, seven were indeed sleep phases (true positives), while the remaining one was actually a wake phase (false positive). The classifier's precision is 7/8 = 87.5%, and its recall is 7/14 = 50%. It misses half of the phases (low recall), but those that it detects are mostly correctly classified (high precision). Because we want a classifier to maximize both recall and precision, it seems useful to evaluate the average of precision and recall (note that the average of rates is computed with the harmonic mean), and this is known as the F-measure or F_1 score (Murphy (2012):

$$F = \frac{2}{\frac{1}{precision} + \frac{1}{recall}} = 2 \cdot \frac{precision \cdot recall}{precision + recall}$$

Model Selection

How should we select among the various available classifiers to solve a specific data-analytic problem? The *"no free lunch" theorem* (Wolpert, 1996) has something important to say about this question: There is no universal best classifier for all possible problems. However, this is no reason to throw in the towel. In restricted problem spaces, there may very well be classes of optimal classifiers. Fernández-Delgado and colleagues (2014) have shown that across a variety of prediction problems, random forests performed best, closely followed by SVM and boosting approaches. Which classifier is best for a particular problem depends on many factors, including the type of sensors, the chosen features, population characteristics, the classification goal, and our domain knowledge. A general rule of thumb is to choose classifiers with a high bias (that is, simple models) when sample size is low and many features are in question. Ultimately, the question of what works best is an empirical question; that is, we need to select the best classifier based on estimates of its expected performance. If researchers try out different approaches, I recommend reporting all of them (e.g., as supplementary materials). Note that when selecting among a set of candidate classifiers, it is important to never use the same data for parameter estimation, model evaluation, and model selection—unless one employs corrections for model complexity (see Burnham & Anderson, 2002). Otherwise, our estimates of model performance will be biased toward more complex models because complex models will always seem to fit better on the data they were trained on. This is obvious in simple regression models. Just adding predictors (even though they may be pure noise and bear no information about the outcome) will increase the model fit to the training data (such as R^2). Thus, instead of *in-sample* model fit, we should rather evaluate *out-of-sample* model fit, that is, the expected error on new, previously unseen data.

Ideally, we should keep separate datasets sampled from the same population to train a model (i.e., estimating parameters) and to test a model (that is, evaluating its performance). The test set is kept separate until all data- and modeling-related decisions are fixed and only then is the test set used to estimate the performance of the final model. If there is no dedicated test set, one can simply split the initially available sample into a training and a test set. Particularly when the sample size is small, there may sometimes be considerable variability in the performance estimate across different random partitions into a training and test set. To reduce this variability, one may resort to cross-validation, which allows all data to be used in turn for both training and testing. In k-fold cross-validation, data are split into k partitions. Then, in k rounds, every partition is the test set once while the remaining partitions form the training set. Finally, the resulting k test set error estimates are averaged to obtain a cross-validation-based estimate of prediction error. With n data points, the largest choice of k is n, yielding n-fold cross-validation, typically referred to as *leave-one-out cross-validation*. The choice of the number of folds trades off various properties of the estimator, such as bias, variance, and computation time. Established approaches are 5-fold and 10-fold cross-validation, which work well in practice.

It is important to emphasize the distinction between estimates of expected prediction errors from a hold-out set and from cross-validation. The hold-out set estimates the error we can expect from the model trained from the training data at hand; that is, the error is conditioned on the (fixed) training set and the parameters of the model. In cross-validation, we simulate repeated random draws from the population (the folds) and, thus, estimate the expected error of the method when trained on a new sample (of the same size) from the population; that is, the training set is treated as a random variable over which we integrate. In other words, the difference lies in whether we estimate the expected error from the given model (with given parameters) or from the given model class.

Finally, I would like to briefly point out some typical pitfalls in evaluating and selecting models. First of all, I would like to reiterate the need to ensure that there is no flow of information between training and test set. A common mistake is to perform some variable selection on the complete dataset before splitting into the training and test set. This seems to make good sense because we expect models to be more robust if we feed only informative variables into the model. While the robustness argument is valid, this approach leads to bias when subsequent model selection is done on cross-validation or the split-sample hold-out set approach because information from the test set has already leaked into the training data. The rule of thumb is to restrict all decisions regarding data processing that depend on the actual observations on the basis of the training set and not on all available data (e.g., data transformation, outlier exclusion, feature selection, and feature extraction).

Figure 17.9 illustrates the biases we may face when we do not carefully choose unbiased model selection and evaluation strategies. In this example, I randomly generated five uninformative features with 100 observations each and repeated the simulation 200 times. I independently generated a random dichotomous outcome, such that the expected accuracy should be 50%, as any classifier can do no better than guess. I trained an LDA on the training set and evaluated it on a hold-out set. Across the simulated trials, we obtain an unbiased estimate of its chance performance (dashed darker curve), with some deviations around it based on the uncertainty incurred by the small, noisy sample. Now, if we evaluate the performance on the training set (the *in-sample* error), we obtain the solid darker curve, which is considerably more optimistic and will be increasingly so with growing model complexity (we used the same data for model estimation and evaluation). If we evaluated accuracy on a hold-out set but selected the best among five competing classifiers (we use the same training data for model evaluation and selection), we would obtain the lighter dashed curve. If we selected the best among five classifiers and used the best classifier's training set error estimate, we would observe the largest overoptimism

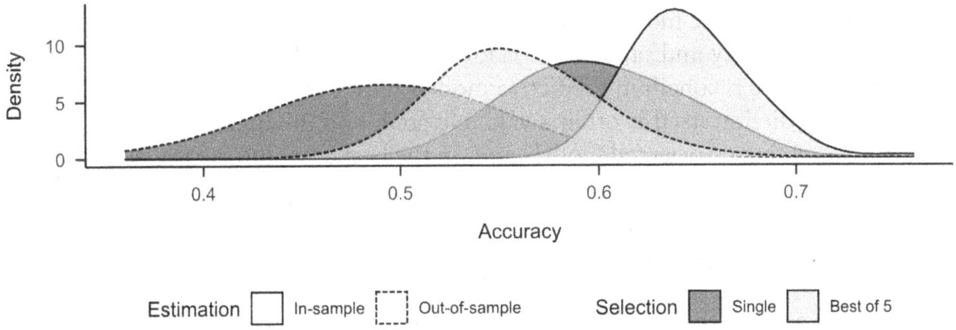

FIGURE 17.9. Bias in model evaluation and selection as a function of training versus test set evaluation and of take-the-best versus single classifier. The Bayes optimal classification rate is the chance level. Using the same model for model fitting and model evaluation leads to overoptimistic results (in-sample error). Instead, out-of-sample error yields unbiased estimates—unless model selection is also performed using the out-of-sample error (best of 5). This figure is available at https://github.com/brandmaier/mobile-sensing-figures under a CC-BY4.0 license.

(same data for estimation, evaluation, and selection; solid lighter curve). Note that under all conditions, there was nothing to learn and classifiers could only perform at chance level.

Conclusions and Future Directions

Machine learning approaches provide us with flexible modeling techniques that allow us to find multivariate and nonlinear functions in high-dimensional data that promise good prediction and generalization to unseen data. Machine learning methods tend to be more complex than classical statistical approaches. This is because they typically allow for more complex functions and thus have a larger number of model parameters and tuning parameters. This increases the danger of overfitting, thereby jeopardizing the utility of the resulting model. Typically, we need not only to estimate the best parameters from a model but also to select the best model from a model family. And often, we even compare different model families to each other, which again necessitates more data or intricate selection and evaluation schemes such as nested cross-validation (e.g., Karch, Sander, von Oertzen, Brandmaier, & Werkle-Bergner, 2015; Stachl et al., 2020). However, machine learning approaches particularly focus on the problem of overfitting, and proper model evaluation and selection increase the chances that models generalize to new data. Ideally, a set of candidate models is selected based on theoretical considerations and is then subjected to optimization, under the condition that the same data should never be used for model estimation, model selection, and model evaluation. Furthermore, we need to bear in mind that predicting well is not necessarily the same as explaining well. The usual caveats of causality also apply to machine learning algorithms that mostly exploit correlational associations. Finally, when selecting among models that predict best, we may not necessarily pick the model that yields the closest representation of reality. Even if the true model is contained in a pool of models from which we select the best predicting model, we may pick a too simple model because it makes better predictions (for example, when measurements are noisy and sample size is low; Shmueli, 2010). Therefore, we need to be careful when we are reconciling predictive models with our theorizing about the subject matter. Still, prediction itself is often a valuable goal, and predictive models can provide a benchmark for theory-oriented models and, in the best case, inform the development of existing theories (Brandmaier et al., 2016).

Taking Machine Learning Out of the Laboratory

A major challenge for the application of machine learning algorithms for mobile sensing is the careful collection of training data representative of the target task. The first issue is ecological validity. The environment from which annotated training data are gathered may differ from the deployment environment (a problem also known as *data shift* [Quiñero-Candela, Sugiyama, Schwaighofer, & Lawrence, 2009] or *concept drift* [Stachl et al., 2020]). For example, selecting the best classifier for activity recognition from lab-based training data may not necessarily yield a robust classifier for deployment outside the lab because activities such as walking might be less natural and more homogeneous under laboratory conditions. Second, we may expect gradual or sudden shifts in how features are predictive of the selected targets. For example, sensors may gradually slip out of place or participants may suddenly change the way they perform certain activities. Third, obtaining reliable and valid training data is time-consuming and expensive. Taken together, it seems advisable to regard the training set as a constantly changing, dynamic pool of information that needs to be monitored. Our algorithms may therefore need to be (re-)calibrated accordingly when deployed for longer periods of time. Some algorithms presented here can be used for novelty detection, such that they indicate that new observations are dissimilar to the training data. Take, for example, a person who starts a new sport in which the observed activity patterns no longer match any of the previously observed ones. Novelty detection could be leveraged to detect such new observations and request manual labeling. One further general approach that has proven useful in these settings is active learning. There, the learning algorithm actively suggests which as yet unlabeled observations (from a large pool of observations) need to be labeled to improve predictions best (Settles & Craven, 2008). On the level of model selection, it also seems advisable to keep multiple models and track their performances over time to investigate which model class will continue performing well.

Implicitly, we have been assuming that the cost of misclassification is symmetric. That is, no matter whether a classifier confuses “walking” with “running” or “walking” with “sleeping,” the cost of misclassification is the same. For example, if we were planning to prompt people to rate their affect in an experience sampling study and used a classifier to determine whether they were awake before prompting them, it would be costlier to falsely predict “awake” when they really were asleep (jeopardizing the participant’s willingness to further participate in this disruptive study) than to predict “asleep” when they were actually awake (missing an opportunity to sample affect). In these cases, one should include this weighting into the cost function. This is particularly straightforward in decision trees and random forests because they allow us to specify cost functions directly. A related problem is class imbalance. For example, when predicting suicidal ideation from smartphone usage, we will likely have only a few cases in the training data, and a classifier will, most likely, always end up predicting the majority class ("no suicidal ideation") for all cases. This is because the simplest model does not make an error most of the time. A more complex model may trade off false positives and false negatives but is not likely to reduce total errors. In practice, one then typically resorts to methods of resampling the training data, such as undersampling the majority class, oversampling the minority class, generating synthetic cases, or all these options at once (e.g., with the Synthetic Minority Over-sampling TEchnique [SMOTE]; see Chawla, Bowyer, Hall, & Kegelmeyer, 2002).

Person-Specific Models

As a final remark, I would like to emphasize that we tacitly assumed that optimal classification algorithms hold across individuals; that is, we have not explicitly accounted for individual differences in the link between features and outcomes. For classification problems, such as activity recognition, this works as long as the variation within classes (i.e., activities) does not exceed between-class variation. To assess the extent to which we can expect a classifier trained across multiple persons to generalize to a previously unseen person, we can use leave-one-person-out cross-validation. If interindividual differences are large (an assumption that is often plausible in human behavior), there may be a need for person-specific models (Karch et al., 2015) or at least subgroup-specific models. These models will likely require larger amounts of training data and will thus pose additional challenges in implementation. Future work needs to address how both group-specific and person-specific models can be combined to solve classification and regression tasks in mobile sensing applications most efficiently and accurately.

ACKNOWLEDGMENTS

I would like to thank Julia Delius for editorial help on the manuscript. Also, I am grateful to Michael Eid, Maximilian Ernst, Aaron Peikert, Anna Elisabeth Riha, and Cornelia Wrzus for providing comments on an earlier version. All figures and their source code are available under free licenses at https://github.com/brandmaier/mobile-sensing-figures.

REFERENCES

Altman, N. S. (1992). An introduction to kernel and nearest-neighbor nonparametric regression. *American Statistician, 46*(3), 175–185.

Bao, L., & Intille, S. S. (2004). Activity recognition from user-annotated acceleration data. In A. Ferscha & F. Mattern (Eds.), *Pervasive computing* (pp. 1–17). Springer.

Berk, R. A. (2008). *Statistical learning from a regression perspective* (Springer Texts in Statistics, Vol. 14). Springer.

Bishop, C. M. (2006). *Pattern recognition and machine learning*. Springer.

Boser, B. E., Guyon, I. M., & Vapnik, V. N. (1992). A training algorithm for optimal margin classifiers. In *Proceedings of the Fifth Annual Workshop on Computational Learning Theory* (pp. 144–152). ACM.

Brandmaier, A. M., Prindle, J. J., McArdle, J. J., & Lindenberger, U. (2016). Theory-guided exploration with structural equation model forests. *Psychological Methods, 21*(4), 566–582.

Brandmaier, A. M., von Oertzen, T., McArdle, J. J., & Lindenberger, U. (2013). Structural equation model trees. *Psychological Methods, 18*(1), 71–86.

Breiman, L. (2001). Random forests. *Machine Learning, 45*(1), 5–32.

Burnham, K. P., & Anderson, D. R. (2002). *Model selection and multimodel inference: A practical information-theoretic approach.* Springer.

Chawla, N. V., Bowyer, K. W., Hall, L. O., & Kegelmeyer, W. P. (2002). SMOTE: Synthetic minority over-sampling technique. *Journal of Artificial Intelligence Research, 16*, 321–357.

Elhai, J. D., Tiamiyu, M. F., Weeks, J. W., Levine, J. C., Picard, K. J., & Hall, B. J. (2018). Depression and emotion regulation predict objective smartphone use measured over one week. *Personality and Individual Differences, 133*, 21–28.

Fernández-Delgado, M., Cernadas, E., Barro, S., & Amorim, D. (2014). Do we need hundreds of classifiers to solve real world classification problems? *Journal of Machine Learning Research, 15*(1), 3133–3181. http://jmlr.org/papers/v15/delgado14a.html

Friedman, J., Hastie, T., & Tibshirani, R. (2010). Regularization paths for generalized linear models via coordinate descent. *Journal of Statistical Software, 33*(1), 1–22.

Fukazawa, Y., Yamamoto, N., Hamatani, T., Ochiai, K., Uchiyama, A., & Ohta, K. (2020). Smartphone-based mental state estimation: A survey from a machine learning perspective. *Journal of Information Processing, 28*, 16–30.

Guyon, I., & Elisseeff, A. (2003). An introduction to variable and feature selection. *Journal of Machine Learning Research, 3*, 1157–1182. www.jmlr.org/papers/v3/guyon03a.html

Guyon, I., Weston, J., Barnhill, S., & Vapnik, V. (2002). Gene selection for cancer classification using support vector machines. *Machine Learning, 46*(1–3), 389–422.

Hastie, T., Tibshirani, R., & Friedman, J. (2009). *The elements of statistical learning* (2nd ed.). Springer.

Hothorn, T., & Zeileis, A. (2015). partykit: A modular toolkit for recursive partytioning in R. *Journal of Machine Learning Research, 16*, 3905–3909. http://jmlr.org/papers/v16/hothorn15a.html

James, G., Witten, D., Hastie, T., & Tibshirani, R. (2013). *An introduction to statistical learning.* Springer.

Karch, J. D., Sander, M. C., von Oertzen, T., Brandmaier, A. M., & Werkle-Bergner, M. (2015). Using within-subject pattern classification to understand lifespan age differences in oscillatory mechanisms of working memory selection and maintenance. *NeuroImage, 118*, 538–552.

Kuhn, M. (2020). *caret: Classification and regression training.* https://CRAN.R-project.org/package=caret

Kuhn, M., & Wickham, H. (2020). *tidymodels: A collection of packages for modeling and machine learning using tidyverse principles.* www.tidymodels.org

Miller, P. J., Lubke, G. H., McArtor, D. B., & Bergeman, C. (2016). Finding structure in data using multivariate tree boosting. *Psychological Methods, 21*(4), 583–682.

Murphy, K. P. (2012). *Machine learning: A probabilistic perspective.* MIT Press.

Quiñero-Candela, J., Sugiyama, M., Schwaighofer, A., & Lawrence, N. D. (Eds.). (2009). *Dataset shift in machine learning.* MIT Press.

Ronao, C. A., & Cho, S.-B. (2014). Human activity recognition using smartphone sensors with two-stage continuous hidden Markov models. In *2014 10th International Conference on Natural Computation (ICNC)* (pp. 681–686). IEEE.

Schölkopf, B., & Smola, A. J. (2002). *Learning with kernels: Support vector machines, regularization, optimization, and beyond.* MIT Press.

Settles, B., & Craven, M. (2008). An analysis of active learning strategies for sequence labeling tasks. In *EMNLP '08: Proceedings of the Conference on Empirical Methods in Natural Language Processing* (pp. 1070–1079). Association for Computational Linguistics.

Shmueli, G. (2010). To explain or to predict? *Statistical Science, 25*(3), 289–310.

Stachl, C., Pargent, F., Hilbert, S., Harari, G. M., Schoedel, R., Vaid, S., et al. (2020). Personality research and assessment in the era of machine learning. *European Journal of Personality, 34*, 613–631.

Strobl, C., Boulesteix, A.-L., Kneib, T., Augustin, T., & Zeileis, A. (2008). Conditional variable importance for random forests. *BMC Bioinformatics, 9*(1), Article No. 307.

Strobl, C., Malley, J., & Tutz, G. (2009). An introduction to recursive partitioning: Rationale, application, and characteristics of classification and regression trees, bagging, and random forests. *Psychological Methods, 14*(4), 323–348.

Turing, A. M. (1950). Computing, machinery and intelligence. *Mind, 59*(236), 433–460.

Wang, J., Chen, R., Sun, X., She, M. F., & Wu, Y. (2011). Recognizing human daily activities from accelerometer signal. *Procedia Engineering, 15*, 1780–1786.

Weiss, G. M., Yoneda, K., & Hayajneh, T. (2019). Smartphone and smartwatch-based biometrics using activities of daily living. *IEEE Access, 7*, 133190–133202.

Wolpert, D. H. (1996). The lack of a priori distinctions between learning algorithms. *Neural Computation, 8*(7), 1341–1390.

Yarkoni, T., & Westfall, J. (2017). Choosing prediction over explanation in psychology: Lessons from machine learning. *Perspectives on Psychological Science, 12*(6), 1100–1122.

Zhang, M., & Sawchuk, A. A. (2012). Motion primitive-based human activity recognition using a bag-of-features approach. In *Proceedings of the 2nd ACM SIGHIT International Health Informatics Symposium* (pp. 631–640). ACM.

CHAPTER 18

Deep-Learning Methods for Mobile Sensing

Cara J. Arizmendi, Christopher J. Urban,
and Kathleen M. Gates

CHAPTER OVERVIEW

Deep learning includes a broad class of nonlinear statistical models that are useful for handling the kind of high-dimensional time-series data often encountered in mobile sensing research. Researchers can use deep learning for a variety of modeling tasks, including classifying individuals based on patterns collected from a mobile device and making predictions about future actions by a participant based on previous actions. This chapter provides an overview of deep-learning methods for mobile sensing data. We specifically focus on time-series data since most mobile sensing data are collected as a temporally ordered series of observations. We first provide example applications of deep learning to psychological and mobile sensing data. We continue with a general overview of deep learning and then provide descriptions of some successful deep-learning models: convolutional neural networks (CNNs) and long short-term memory (LSTM) neural networks. Finally, we describe two empirical examples from the literature in depth.

Introduction

Deep-learning methods are powerful analytic tools for psychological researchers and clinicians who collect mobile sensing data. Current deep-learning methods have their origin in mid-20th-century models of biological learning called artificial neural networks (ANNs). What makes a method "deep" is that the original input data are processed sequentially through a number of steps called layers that are intended to transform the data in such a way that they can be used to accurately predict an outcome of interest; we will describe this process in detail below. While initially motivated by biological and neural science pursuits, deep learning can be applied to an array of data types and attend to varied research questions. Among other applications, deep learning allows researchers to (1) classify individuals based on patterns of behaviors and (2) make predictions about future actions by a participant. Here, we provide an overview of deep-learning methods for mobile sensing time-series data. For psychologists, the data may include psychophysiological, ecological momentary assessment (EMA) or the mobile phone accelerometer.

We begin with examples of applications of deep learning to psychological and mobile sensing data. We focus on applications for classifying and forecasting time series, common problems for mobile sensing data. We continue with a general overview of deep learning and then provide descriptions of current state-of-the-art architectures for classification using CNNS and LSTM neural networks. Finally, we describe two empirical examples from the literature in depth (Killian, Passino, Nandi, Madden, & Clapp, 2019; Suhara, Xu, & Pentland, 2017) to provide context for what questions we can answer with deep learning and tips and tricks for making the most of deep-learning methods. As this chapter focuses primarily on applications on mobile data, the interested reader wishing to learn more about deep learning in general is referred to Goodfellow, Bengio, and Courville (2016) for a comprehensive book that includes a brief history of deep learning, foundational concepts in machine learning, and modern methodology.

Applications of Deep Learning to Psychology

Deep-learning methods have been applied to a variety of questions and are now gaining traction outside the field of computer science. Reviews of neural network approaches and tutorials on deep-learning software are being published in behavioral journals (Pang, Nijkamp, & Wu, 2020; Urban & Gates, 2021). In particular, clinical research benefits from the robust classification abilities of deep learning. For example, neuroimaging, a field with high-dimensional data, has found use for deep learning in feature extraction and classification of disease severity; see Vieira, Pinaya, and Mechelli (2017) for a review of recent work in this area. Self-report data have been used in this framework to detect whether or not an individual is depressed (Victor, Aghajan, Sewart, & Christian, 2019), and medical data have been used to predict likelihood of suicide by patients (Sanderson, Bulloch, Wang, Williamson, & Patten, 2020). Additionally, video footage of participants has been used to detect facial microexpressions (Peng, Wang, Chen, Liu, & Fu, 2017). The flexibility of deep-learning approaches to different types of data and the ability of deep learning to handle high-dimensional data in a computationally efficient manner make deep learning approaches useful for mobile sensing data. For time-series data, a common data type in mobile sensing, deep learning is particularly useful for classification and forecasting, especially in data with long-term time dependencies. Feature-based approaches, such as the windowing approaches discussed by Brandmaier in Chapter 17, this volume, can handle time-dependent data but do not handle *long* time dependencies well, thus making deep-learning approaches a useful tool in cases of long-term dependencies.

Classification Applications to Time-Series Data

In addition to the examples mentioned above, deep learning has been used in the field of computer science for classifying time series. In fact, time-series data extracted from wearable sensors is a common data type for computer scientists studying classification. Much of this work has come from collaborations with psychologists. For example, researchers trained a CNN (a model class we explain in more detail later) on wearable sensor data to classify stretches of time indicative of stereotypical motor movement in participants with autism spectrum disorders (Mohammadian Rad et al., 2018). Wearable sensors were also used for predicting sleep quality based on daytime physical activity data (Sathyanarayana et al., 2016). In this case, a CNN outperformed logistic regression.

Much sensor data can be collected without requiring wearable technology. This type of passive sensing data is useful because of its relatively unobtrusive nature. For example, researchers used features from mobile phone data, including audio, Bluetooth, call logs, number of apps the phone was running, text messaging, and conversations to classify stressed and unstressed students. Stress assessments were collected via EMA (Acikmese & Alptekin, 2019). A similar study used GPS features for classification of stressed and unstressed students in passive data combined with survey data (Shaw, Simsiri, Deznaby, Fiterau, & Rahaman, 2019). Speech recognition is another time-series classification problem for which feature extraction methods from mobile data are being developed and advances in CNNs are being made (Baumeister & Montag, 2019). Similarly, methods are being developed for classifying human activity from mobile data, with the goal of being able to detect if someone is walking, running, lying down, climbing stairs, standing, biking, driving, and so on (Hammerla, Halloran, & Plötz, 2016; Lima, Souto, El-Khatib, Jalali, & Gama, 2019; Ronao & Cho, 2016; Wang, Chen, Hao, Peng, & Hu, 2019; Yao, Hu, Zhao, Zhang, & Abdelzaher, 2017).

Forecasting Applications

Although applications of using forecasting on human sensor data are far less common than classification applications, they are becoming more common. Forecasting physiological and behavioral data is quickly emerging as a tool for clinicians. In particular, forecasting is a potentially useful method for clinicians who aim to make real-time decisions of whether an intervention is necessary.

We can understand the potential for this advancement by considering the common applications for forecasting time series. For example, forecasting electricity load demand allows utility companies to provide enough power supply as predicted by future needs while also keeping costs of operation to a minimum (Qiu, Ren, Suganthan, & Amaratunga, 2017). For similar reasons, we may want to forecast internet traffic. More well-known examples are forecasting stock prices, so that stockholders can make decisions on whether to buy, sell, or hold a stock or forecasting weather (Gamboa, 2017). All these examples use forecasting to make decisions based on what we expect to happen in the future. Similarly, we can apply the forecasting function to mobile sensing data collected from humans. For example, researchers provide a deep-learning framework for predicting and intervening prior to onset of psychosis (Koppe, Guloksuz, Reininghaus, & Durstewitz, 2019), predicting future stress based on GPS data (Mikelsons, Smith, Mehrotra, & Musolesi, 2017), and predicting falls in older adults based on accelerometer data (Nait Aicha, Englebienne, Van Schooten, Pijnappels, & Kröse, 2018).

Deep Learning

Deep-learning methods continue to be modified, created, and tested to accommodate new research questions and data types. The goal of this section is to acquaint readers with common foundations for emerging deep-learning methods. We also seek to prime the reader to use these methods in their own work by explaining common steps that can be used in practice when preparing to use deep-learning methods.

Foundations

We now introduce concepts fundamental to understanding the technical aspects of deep learning, focusing on those typically used as foundations for emerging methods. Deep learning has received a lot of hype in recent years (Marcus, 2018). One successful modeling approach for deep learning, artificial neural networks (ANNs), has a much longer history, dating to the mid-20th century (McCulloch & Pitts, 1943; Rosenblatt, 1958). ANNs were initially inspired by biological neural mechanisms (e.g., Rumelhart, Hinton, & Williams, 1986) and aim to consolidate and transfer information, much like how learning proceeds in biological systems. In more modern parlance, ANNs are statistical models for nonlinear regression. Although psychologists often need to carefully select the variables that are to be included in statistical models to obtain accurate predictions, ANNs may avoid this preprocessing step by automatically extracting their own (typically uninterpretable) representations of the data to use for making predictions. This ability has helped deep ANNs produce major breakthroughs in computer vision and natural language processing (LeCun, Bengio, & Hinton, 2015).

Despite all the hype, basic deep-learning models are not mysterious and complicated. In fact, ANNs are very similar to statistical models commonly used by psychologists. ANNs are especially closely related to generalized linear models (GLMs), a family of models that includes linear and logistic regression. We will clarify this relationship with the following example. We begin with a cross-sectional dataset where y_i denotes the observed outcome and $\mathbf{x}_i$ denotes the observed $p \times 1$ vector of predictors for the ith individual, $i = 1, \ldots, N$. For instance, imagine that our data were collected via a large clinical survey designed to measure mental health and substance use. In this setting, y_i could be a binary outcome that is equal to one when individual i meets the criteria for major depressive disorder (MDD) and is equal to zero otherwise, while $\mathbf{x}_i$ could be a 2×1 vector whose elements $x_{i,1}$ and $x_{i,2}$ are binary predictors indicating whether individual i meets the criteria for nicotine use disorder (NUD) and alcohol use disorder (AUD), respectively; a similar (worked) example is considered by Urban and Gates (2021). Our goal is to determine whether meeting MDD criteria can be accurately predicted based on whether an individual meets NUD and AUD criteria. A GLM could be used to predict the outcome as

$$y_i = f(\mathbf{w}^{\mathrm{T}}\mathbf{x}_i + b) + \varepsilon_i \qquad i = 1, \ldots, N \tag{18.1}$$

where $\mathbf{w}$ is a $p \times 1$ vector of regression weights (in our example, $p = 2$), $(\cdot)^{\mathrm{T}}$ denotes the vector transpose, b is an intercept, f is an inverse link function, and ε_i is an error term. Since y_i is a binary outcome in our example, we can conduct a logistic regression by choosing f to be the inverse logistic link or *sigmoid* function $f(z) = 1/(1 + \exp[-z])$. If y_i were a continuous outcome such as age or income, we could conduct a linear regression by choosing f to be the identity function $f(z) = z$.

Unfortunately, the simple GLM described above is not flexible enough to model highly nonlinear relationships between predictors and outcomes. For instance, suppose our dataset was generated as follows:

$$\begin{aligned} x_{i,1} &\sim \text{Bernoulli}(0.5) \\ x_{i,2} &\sim \text{Bernoulli}(0.4) \\ y_i &\sim \text{Bernoulli}\left(f\left(-2 + 4 \cdot \mathrm{I}\left(x_{i,1} = x_{i,2}\right)\right)\right) \end{aligned} \tag{18.2}$$

where $f(\cdot)$ is the sigmoid function and $\mathrm{I}(x_{i,1} = x_{i,2})$ is an indicator function that is equal to one when the ith individual's NUD and AUD diagnoses are the same and is equal to zero when their diagnoses are different. In words, people in our dataset have a 50% and 40% chance of meeting criteria for NUD and AUD, respectively. Additionally, each person's chance of meeting MDD criteria is high when they meet both NUD and AUD criteria or when they meet neither NUD nor AUD criteria, but their chance of meeting MDD criteria is low when they only meet either NUD or AUD criteria. This relationship could not be captured by the GLM in Equation 18.1 unless an interaction term was included in the model *a priori*. Including interactions and other nonlinearities *a priori* might be feasible for small models with only a few predictors (e.g., our example) but becomes increasingly difficult as the number of predictors grows.

Interestingly, the problem of modeling complicated nonlinearities (without needing to specify these nonlinearities *a priori*) can be solved by applying a sequence of GLMs to our predictors where the output of each GLM is used as input to a subsequent GLM. "Stacking" several GLMs in this manner forms the basis of one of the simplest ANN models: the *multilayer perceptron* (MLP) or *feedforward neural network*. The words "multilayer" and "feedforward" are meant to convey that the predictors $\mathbf{x}_i$ are passed through a sequence of processing steps called *layers* before being used to predict the outcome y_i. To understand how an MLP layer processes the input data, suppose we collect p_1 different GLMs, each with its own regression weights $\mathbf{w}_j^{(1)}$ and intercept $b_j^{(1)}$ $j = 1, \ldots, p_1$. Here, the superscript (1) indicates the first layer. If we apply each of our GLMs to the input data separately as follows:

$$h_{i,j}^{(1)} = f^{(1)}\left(\left(\mathbf{w}_j^{(1)}\right)^{\mathrm{T}} \mathbf{x}_i + b_j^{(1)}\right) \qquad j = 1, \ldots, p_1 \tag{18.3}$$

we end up with a set of p_1 different output values $h_{i,j}^{(1)}$, each of which provides a single-number summary of the input data. In analogy with biological neurons, each GLM is called a *neuron* because it produces output by summarizing information in the input data it receives; the set of p_1 different neurons taken together forms an MLP layer of *width* p_1. Note that the width can be the same size of the input layer or larger. If we collect the regression weights into a $p_1 \times p$ matrix $\mathbf{W}^{(1)}$ whose jth row is $(\mathbf{w}_j^{(1)})^{\mathrm{T}}$, stack the intercepts $b_j^{(1)}$ into a $p_1 \times 1$ vector $\mathbf{b}^{(1)}$, and stack the p_1 single-number summaries $h_{i,j}$ into a $p_1 \times 1$ vector $\mathbf{h}_i^{(1)}$, we can write our first MLP layer more concisely as

$$\mathbf{h}_i^{(1)} = f^{(1)}\left(\mathbf{W}^{(1)}\mathbf{x}_i + \mathbf{b}^{(1)}\right) \tag{18.4}$$

The inverse link function $f^{(1)}(\cdot)$ is called an *activation function* in the context of deep learning. Typical choices for MLP activation functions will be discussed further below. The elements of $h_{i,j}^{(1)}$ of $\mathbf{h}_i^{(1)}$ are called *hidden layer* variables because they are not typically visible to the user; rather, they are used as internal representations of the input data that help the model obtain accurate predictions.[1] To make our MLP more flexible, we could increase our model's *depth* by adding more processing layers as follows:

$$\mathbf{h}_i^{(l)} = f^{(l)}\left(\mathbf{W}^{(l)}\mathbf{h}_i^{(l-1)} + \mathbf{b}^{(l)}\right) \quad (18.5)$$

where l is the total number of MLP layers, $\mathbf{W}^{(l)}$ is a $p_l \times p_{l-1}$ weight matrix, $\mathbf{b}^{(l)}$ is a $p_l \times 1$ intercept vector, $f^{(l)}(\cdot)$ is an activation function, and $\mathbf{h}_i^{(l)}$ is a $p_l \times 1$ vector of hidden layer variables. Once the input data have passed all the way through the model, and we have arrived at the final hidden layer vector $\mathbf{h}_i^{(L)}$, the MLP predicts the outcomes using a single neuron:

$$y_i = f^{(L+1)}\left(\left(\mathbf{w}^{(L+1)}\right)^{\mathrm{T}}\mathbf{h}_i^{(L)} + b^{(L+1)}\right) + \varepsilon_i \quad (18.6)$$

where $\mathbf{w}^{(L+1)}$ is a $p_L \times 1$ vector of regression weights, $b^{(L+1)}$ is an intercept, $f^{(L+1)}(\cdot)$ is the final activation function, and ε_i is an error term.

To complement the use of equations, MLPs and other ANNs are often depicted using schematic diagrams. These diagrams are closely related to the path diagrams used to depict variables and their relationships in structural equation modeling. Specifically, ANN schematic diagrams are directed graphs where circles represent variables (observed or hidden) and arrows between circles represent neurons. To continue our example, suppose we wish to use an MLP with two hidden layers of width four to predict MDD. This model can be depicted using the directed graph shown in Figure 18.1. On the left side of the figure, we note that the predictors $\mathbf{x}$ and the outcome y are called the *input layer* and the *output layer*, respectively, while all the intermediate layers are called hidden layers. On the right-hand side, we write the equations corresponding to the diagram.

The number, widths, and types of the hidden layers, as well as the absence or presence of connections between variables (i.e., arrows/neurons), are collectively called the model's *architecture*. The model's activation functions are particularly essential architectural components. Specifically, the hidden layer activation functions $f^{(1)}, \ldots, f^{(L)}$ enable MLPs and other ANNs to approximate complicated nonlinear relationships rather than purely linear relationships (e.g., Cybenko, 1989). A common choice for each $f^{(1)}, \ldots, f^{(L)}$ is the *rectified linear unit* (ReLU) function $f(z) = \max(z, 0)$, which sets all neurons with negative values to zero (Figure 18.2a). ANNs with ReLU hidden layers are often easy to fit and perform well (e.g., Glorot, Bordes, & Bengio, 2011; Jarrett, Kavukcuoglu, Ranzato, & LeCun, 2009; Nair & Hinton, 2010). Another hidden layer activation function that will be useful for the models considered in this chapter is the *hyperbolic tangent* (tanh) function $f(z) = (\exp[2z] - 1)/(\exp[2z] + 1)$, which outputs a value between 1 and –1 (Figure 18.2b). Similar to GLMs, the form of the final activation function $f^{(L+1)}$ depends on the outcome variables. For example, if the outcomes are continuous, we set $f^{(L+1)}$ to the identity function (Figure 18.2c); if the outcomes are binary, we set $f^{(L+1)}$ to the sigmoid function (Figure 18.2d).

Although the activation functions for MLPs and other ANNs are typically fixed *a priori*, the number and widths of the hidden layers are often determined empirically using

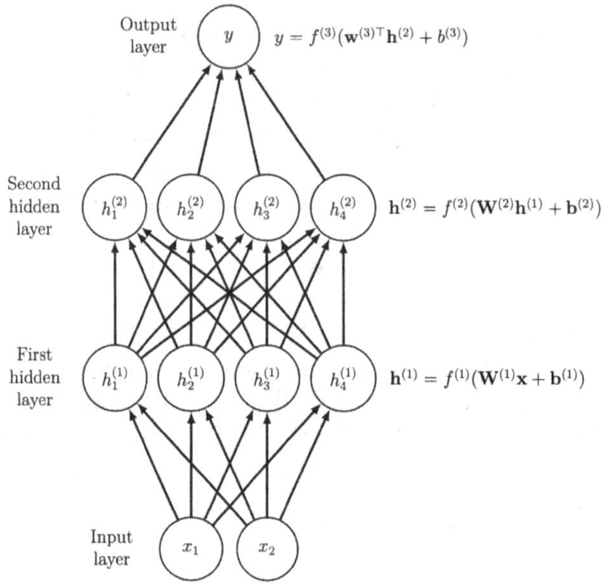

FIGURE 18.1. Schematic representation of a multilayer perceptron with two hidden layers, each of width four. The input data at the bottom of the figure include three different predictors.

the data at hand. However, using a single dataset for model selection typically produces a model that performs well in the sample at hand but performs poorly when applied to new, previously unseen samples. This phenomenon is called *overfitting* and is well known in machine learning (see Brandmaier, Chapter 17, this volume, for a discussion of overfitting). Fortunately, several techniques exist for empirically choosing a well-performing MLP architecture while avoiding overfitting. With large datasets (e.g., $N \geq 2{,}000$), a

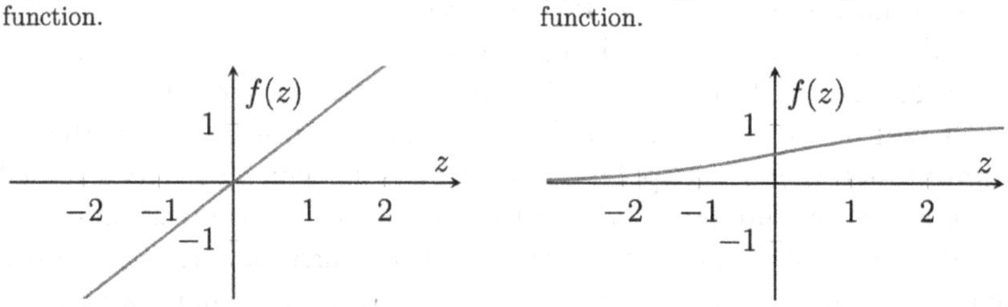

(a) The rectified linear unit activation function.

(b) The hyperbolic tangent activation function.

(c) The identity activation function.

(d) The sigmoid activation function.

FIGURE 18.2. Several common activation functions used to build artificial neural networks.

typical approach in deep learning is to first divide the data randomly into three disjoint subsets called the *training set*, the *validation set*, and the *test set*. Next, several MLPs with different architectural settings are fitted using the training set, and each MLP's performance is evaluated using the validation set (e.g., by computing each MLP's predictive accuracy on the validation set). The MLP with the best validation set performance is selected and refitted on the combined training and validation set data.

Finally, the refitted MLP is evaluated on the test set to get an approximate sense of how the model will perform with new, previously unseen data. With smaller datasets and models, approaches based on *cross-validation* are typically used to prevent overfitting, although this approach is computationally infeasible because of its very large datasets and MLPs, which involve multiple runs of the models with varying subsets of the sample to test and train (see Brandmaier, Chapter 19, this volume, as well as Appendix B in Urban & Gates, 2021, for overviews of cross-validation). For practical guidance regarding choosing model architectures and avoiding overfitting for MLPs, see Heaton (2008, Ch. 8), Bengio (2012), or Smith (2018).

Estimating MLP parameters (i.e., the regression weight matrices and intercepts) is more challenging than estimating GLM parameters. Fitting GLMs is straightforward because GLMs typically have a unique set of parameter values that produce the best-performing model, and fitting procedures are typically guaranteed to come very close to these optimal values. MLPs, on the other hand, have many different sets of parameter values that produce well-performing models (i.e., MLPs are *overparameterized*; see Urban and Gates, 2021, for a discussion of this point), and fitting procedures are not always guaranteed to come close to these optimal values. Fitting in MLPs and other ANNs begins with choosing a loss function to measure model performance. A common loss function for continuous outcomes is the *mean squared error* $\sum_i (y_i - \hat{y}_i)^2$ which is the same loss function used in linear regression and measures the distance between the true outcomes y_i and the outcomes predicted by the model $\hat{y}_i$. A common loss function for binary outcomes is the *binary cross-entropy* $\sum_i y_i \log\hat{y}_i + (1 - y_i)\log(1 - \hat{y}_i)$ which is the same loss function used in logistic regression and measures the distance between the true outcome y_i (which is equal to 1 or 0) and the MLP's predicted probability that the outcome is equal to one given by $\hat{y}_i$. The goal is to find the MLP parameters that minimize the loss function (i.e., to find the best-performing MLP). Fitting in MLPs and other ANNs relies heavily on an algorithm called backpropagation (BP), which is used to efficiently compute the gradients of the loss function with respect to the MLP parameters (Linnainmaa, 1976; Rumelhart et al., 1986). Gradients are multivariate derivatives that provide information about the magnitude and direction in which the MLP parameters should be updated to reduce the loss function by a small amount. Once gradients are obtained using BP, a stochastic gradient (SG) method such as stochastic gradient descent (Robbins & Monro, 1951) or Adam (Kingma & Ba, 2014) combines the gradient with an update rule to change the parameter values a certain amount. BP and the SG method are applied to iteratively update the MLP parameters until adequate performance is achieved on the training set. Since fitting MLPs using SG methods involves a good deal of randomization, in practice we recommend fitting models several times using different random seeds to assess the stability of the model's performance.

To demonstrate the above concepts, we simulated a dataset of size $N = 5{,}000$ according to the example in Equation 18.2 and then used the MLP implemented in the Python package scikit-learn (Version 0.23.1; Pedregosa et al., 2011) to predict MDD using individuals' NUD and AUD diagnoses. Our MLP had two hidden layers of width four as shown in Figure 18.1. We otherwise fitted our MLP using the scikit-learn package defaults, which include ReLU hidden layer activation functions, a sigmoid final activation function, the binary cross-entropy loss, and the Adam SG method. Our fitted MLP obtained an accuracy of 0.87 (i.e., 87% of MDD cases were predicted correctly). This was much higher than the accuracy of 0.56 obtained by a logistic regression classifier (also fitted using scikit-learn), suggesting that unlike the logistic regression classifier, the MLP successfully captured the nonlinear relationship between the predictors and the outcome. We note, however, that unlike logistic regression, the MLP parameters are not directly interpretable due to overparameterization (Urban & Gates, 2021). Code to reproduce this example is available online at https://github.com/cjurban/MobileSensing.

Like Urban and Gates (2021), we now review how our fitted MLP makes predictions using new input data. Suppose we want to use our MLP to predict the MDD diagnosis for an individual who meets NUD criteria but not AUD criteria. We begin with our MLP's first layer, which multiplies our individual's predictor vector $\mathbf{x}$ by the regression weight matrix $\mathbf{W}^{(1)}$ and then adds the intercepts $\mathbf{b}^{(1)}$ to produce a new vector $\mathbf{a}^{(1)}$:

$$\begin{aligned}\mathbf{a}^{(1)} &= \mathbf{W}^{(1)}\mathbf{x} + \mathbf{b}^{(1)} \\ &= \begin{bmatrix} 0.00 & 0.00 \\ 0.00 & 0.00 \\ 1.25 & 1.25 \\ 1.24 & 1.28 \end{bmatrix} \begin{bmatrix} 1 \\ 0 \end{bmatrix} + \begin{bmatrix} -0.64 \\ -0.70 \\ -1.26 \\ 0.00 \end{bmatrix}\end{aligned} \tag{18.7}$$

The vector $\mathbf{a}^{(1)}$ is a modified version of the input data $\mathbf{x}$ and is sometimes called an *activation*. We next apply the ReLU activation function to our activation to compute the first hidden layer vector:

$$\mathbf{h}^{(1)} = f^{(1)}\left(a^{(1)}\right) = [0.00 \quad 0.00 \quad 0.00 \quad 1.29]^{\mathrm{T}} \tag{18.8}$$

which simply sets any negative values in $\mathbf{a}^{(1)}$ to zero. The second MLP layer repeats this process with the first hidden layer vector $\mathbf{h}^{(1)}$ as its input—multiply by the weight matrix $\mathbf{W}^{(2)}$, add the intercepts $\mathbf{b}^{(2)}$, then apply the ReLU activation function $f^{(2)}(\cdot)$:

$$\begin{aligned}\mathbf{h}^{(2)} &= \mathrm{f}^{(2)}(\mathbf{W}^{(2)}\mathbf{h}^{(1)} + \mathbf{b}^{(2)}) \\ &= f^{(2)}\left(\begin{bmatrix} 0.00 & 0.00 & 0.00 & 0.00 \\ 0.00 & 0.00 & 0.00 & 0.00 \\ 0.00 & 0.00 & 0.00 & -2.68 \\ 0.00 & 0.00 & 0.00 & 1.33 \end{bmatrix} \begin{bmatrix} 0.00 \\ 0.00 \\ 0.00 \\ 1.29 \end{bmatrix} + \begin{bmatrix} -0.52 \\ -0.63 \\ -0.50 \\ 0.00 \end{bmatrix}\right) \\ &= [0.00 \quad 0.00 \quad 0.00 \quad 1.72]^{\mathrm{T}}\end{aligned} \tag{18.9}$$

Finally, our MLP predicts the outcome using a single neuron with a sigmoid activation function $f^{(3)}(\cdot)$:

$$\hat{y} = f^{(3)}\left(\left(\mathbf{w}^{(3)}\right)^{\mathrm{T}} \mathbf{h}^{(2)} + b^{(3)}\right)$$
$$= f^{(3)}\left(\begin{bmatrix} 0.00 & 0.00 & 0.00 & -2.31 \end{bmatrix} \begin{bmatrix} 0.00 \\ 0.00 \\ 0.00 \\ 1.71 \end{bmatrix} - 1.81\right) = f^{(3)}(-2.14) = 0.11 \quad (18.10)$$

The value 0.11 is the predicted probability that the individual has been diagnosed with MDD.

Although MLPs are very flexible in theory, in many practical settings they perform worse than specialized ANNs that have been designed to model specific kinds of data (e.g., image data or time-series data). However, understanding MLPs and their associated terminology (e.g., hidden layers, activation functions) is an important first step toward understanding the state-of-the-art, specialized ANNs used to solve challenging real-world problems. As described above, MLPs may be thought of as "stacks" of GLMs. Rather than stacking GLMs, other ANNs stack different transformations that can be layered together in a variety of complicated ways. In the next section, we describe specialized ANN architectures that have been successfully used for processing sequential data (e.g., time series).

Common NN Architectures for Sensor Data

Long Short-Term Memory

LSTMs are a special case of a type of ANN called a *recurrent neural network* (RNN). While GLMs and MLPs typically aim to model cross-sectional data where observations are assumed to be independent, RNNs aim to account for the dependencies between observations that arise in time-series data (Ordóñez & Roggen, 2016). RNNs maintain a hidden state that is updated at each time point based on the hidden state values at the previous time point as well as the current observed variable values. In this sense, RNNs are closely related to classical time-series approaches such as dynamic factor analysis (Molenaar, 1985) that model the relationships between latent variables over time (Urban & Gates, 2021). In practice, however, RNNs perform poorly with large numbers of time points (which is often the case for psychological time series) due to vanishing or exploding gradients. In the case of vanishing gradients, the gradient along which estimation occurs becomes so small that the weights are only slightly updated, potentially stopping the estimation process. In the case of exploding gradients, the gradient becomes so large that weights are updated by large amounts that lead to an unstable model, also potentially stopping the estimation process (Fawaz et al., 2019; Hochreiter & Schmidhuber, 1997; Lipton, Berkowitz, & Elkan, 2015).

LSTMs address the shortcomings of traditional RNNs using a special component called a *cell state* in combination with a technique called *gating*. To illustrate these concepts, let's use an example of number of daily recorded steps. The cell state is an extra hidden layer vector that acts like the LSTM's long-term memory, storing important information from previous time points. For our step-count example, this information could include the current trend of increasing, decreasing, or constant steps as well as any lagged processes such as the previous day's step count or the previous 2 days' step count, and so on. This is similar to modeling trends or autoregressive effects in more traditional time-series models.

The cell state differs from the hidden layer in that it is used to store information, while the hidden layer is used to predict the outcome (e.g., number of steps) at each time point. Gating aims to control the flow of information through the model: Instead of allowing information to flow through the model in an unrestricted manner, LSTMs use multiplication factors called *gates* to determine what information to keep, what information to forget, and what information to update. For example, some information may not be predictive of today's step count, while other information is predictive. Maybe knowing that it is a weekend and the participant walked 5,000 steps yesterday is informative, but how many steps they walked on a weekday 4 months ago is not informative. The gating would keep the information about day of week and yesterday's step count but "forget" the information from 4 months ago.

Some LSTM gates are implemented using sigmoid activation functions (see Figure 18.2d). These gates output values between 0 and 1, which are then multiplied by different model components such as the cell state or the hidden layer. Multiplying by 0 lets no input information through, multiplying by 1 lets all input information through, and multiplying by intermediate values lets a fraction of input information through. Continuing with the step-count example, we see that information on the step count on a weekday from 4 months ago would be multiplied by zero, while information that it is a weekday may be multiplied by 1. Perhaps yesterday's step count is only slightly informative, so that information is given an intermediate weight. Other LSTM gates are implemented using tanh activation functions, which output values between –1 and 1 (Figure 18.2b). Multiplying by a tanh gate produces a positive or negative proportion of the input information, which can then be used to add or subtract information from different model components. Using sigmoid and tanh gates permits making small changes to the information transmitted across time points, resulting in more stable gradients and better accounting for long-term dependencies (Acikmese & Alptekin, 2019; Lipton et al., 2015).

Figure 18.3 illustrates a single LSTM layer or *memory cell*. In this figure, $\mathbf{h}_{t-1}$ is the hidden layer vector from the previous time point, and $\mathbf{h}_t$ is the hidden layer vector at time *t*. The hidden layer is used to predict the outcome value at each time point and then

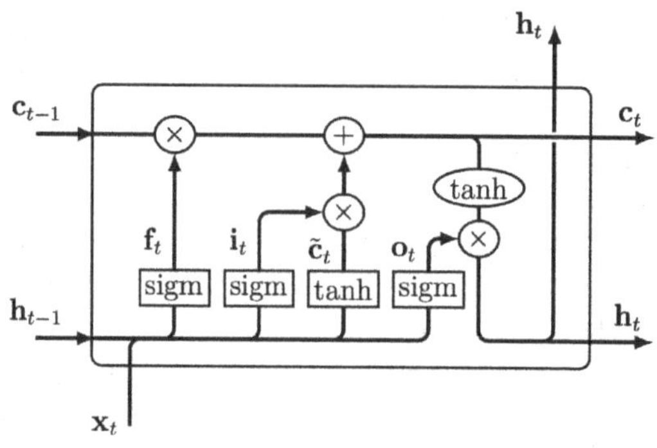

FIGURE 18.3. Schematic representation of a single long short-term memory neural network "cell."

is passed forward to the next time point. $\mathbf{c}_{t-1}$ is the cell state at the previous time point, and $\mathbf{c}_t$ is the cell state at the current time point. The previous hidden layer $\mathbf{h}_{t-1}$ first goes through the *forget gate* to produce the *forget layer* f_t. The forget gate takes information from the previous hidden layer and decides how much information to lose using a sigmoid activation function. The forget layer is *removing* information. The *input layer* $\mathbf{i}_t$ determines which elements of the cell state to update. The input layer is *adding* information. The tanh layer creates a new vector of values based on a candidate cell state $\tilde{\mathbf{c}}_t$. Finally, the last sigmoid layer, $\mathbf{o}_t$ decides which values to output. This then goes to the second tanh layer to standardize values between –1 and 1 (Acikmese & Alptekin, 2019; Lipton et al., 2015; Ordóñez & Roggen, 2016). In equation form, f_t, the forget gate, which decides which information from the prior hidden state to retain, is defined as

$$\mathrm{f}_t = \sigma(\mathbf{W}_\mathrm{f}\mathbf{x}_t + \mathbf{U}_\mathrm{f}\mathbf{h}_{t-1} + \mathbf{b}_\mathrm{f}) \tag{18.11}$$

The input gate, $\mathbf{i}_t$, which dictates what information to keep, is defined as

$$\mathbf{i}_t = \sigma(\mathbf{W}_\mathrm{i}\mathbf{x}_t + \mathbf{U}_\mathrm{i}\mathbf{h}_{t-1} + \mathbf{b}_\mathrm{i}) \tag{18.12}$$

and the output gate, o_t, is defined as

$$\mathrm{o}_t = \sigma(\mathbf{W}_\mathrm{o}\mathbf{x}_t + \mathbf{U}_\mathrm{o}\mathbf{h}_{t-1} + \mathbf{b}_\mathrm{o}) \tag{18.13}$$

where σ is the sigmoid function, $\mathbf{W}_\mathrm{o}$ is a matrix of the weights for the current input, $\mathbf{x}_t$ is the input from the current timepoint, $\mathbf{U}_\mathrm{o}$ is a matrix of the weights for the previous hidden state ($\mathbf{h}_{t-1}$), and $\mathbf{b}_\mathrm{o}$ is a vector of the biases for the given gate.

Therefore, the equation for $\mathbf{h}_t$ is

$$\mathbf{h}_t = (\mathrm{o}_t)\odot\tanh(\mathrm{c}_t) \tag{18.14}$$

where $\mathbf{o}_t$ is the output gate at time t, $\mathbf{c}_t$ is the cell state at time t, and $\odot$ denotes the elementwise product. The equation for the candidate cell state, $\tilde{\mathbf{c}}_t$ is

$$\tilde{\mathbf{c}}_t = \tanh(\mathbf{W}_c\mathbf{x}_t + \mathbf{U}_c\mathbf{h}_{t-1} + \mathbf{b}_c)\odot\tanh(\mathbf{c}_t) = \tanh \tag{18.15}$$

The equation for the current cell state, $\mathbf{c}_t$ is

$$\mathrm{c}_t = f_t\mathrm{c}_{t-1} + i_t\odot\tilde{\mathrm{c}}_t \tag{18.16}$$

(Ordóñez & Roggen, 2016). For a comprehensive and beginner-friendly technical explanation of LSTMs, we recommend readers check out the review by Lipton and colleagues (2015).

Convolutional Neural Networks

CNNs are the most common deep-learning method for classification in general. Made popular for image recognition, CNNs can also work well for time-series classification (Fawaz et al., 2019). CNNs work by applying a filter or "convolving" raw data. During the training of the model, optimal parameters are found for predicting some class of labeled time series (e.g., whether mobile phone accelerometer data indicates standing, sitting, or walking), and during the testing of the model, the class of a time series is predicted based on its filtered characteristics. In the most common case of classifying photographs, a picture passes through a filter, simplifying the data but retaining features important for classifying the image (Michelucci, 2018). For image recognition, CNNs are preferred to feedforward networks because they retain the pixel dependencies of images (i.e., that one pixel is beside some other pixel; Krizhevsky, Sutskever, & Hinton, 2012). In the case of time series, we want to retain the time dependencies of the data, making CNNs an appropriate modeling technique for time series.

A CNN can have multiple layers/filters, with each filter outputting a filtered time series based on the original time series. Typically, a CNN has at least one convolutional layer, one pooling layer, and one fully connected layer. If we are looking at daily step count, the convolutional layers could represent weekday versus weekend relationship, a seasonal fluctuation (e.g., more steps taken in warmer months than colder months), or a general trend (e.g., an increase in daily steps), among other relationships. Typically, the initial convolutional layer extracts general features (e.g., a trend), while additional convolutional layers extract more fine-grained features (e.g., how many steps you take on a Monday when you had 20,000 steps yesterday; Zhao, Lu, Chen, Liu, & Wu, 2017).

CNNs also have at least one pooling layer but can have more than one. Pooling layers reduce the dimensionality of the dataset. Max pooling returns the maximum value for a section of data, and average pooling returns the average value for a section of data. One benefit of pooling methods is noise reduction. For example, if we collect the number of steps taken each minute, we may have additional information/noise. Pooling the data into 1-hour or 1-day windows would reduce the noise and computational load. After the convolutional and pooling layers, we have a fully connected layer. This is where classification occurs. The data are flattened into a single vector, backpropagation, an algorithm used to obtain the gradient for estimation, is performed, and the data are classified (Krizhevsky et al., 2012).

Recently, researchers have argued that the traditional approach of using the RNN framework should be reconsidered (Bai, Kolter, & Koltun, 2018). Extensions of traditional CNNs, such as temporal convolutional neural networks (TCNs), can be used in modeling sequential data. They often outperform LSTMs (a type of RNN) and are simpler to train, requiring less computation. We note here that LSTMs and TCNs are not necessarily mutually exclusive. In fact, some researchers have proposed using combinations of the two frameworks (Ordóñez & Roggen, 2016). Also, TCNs are not a distinct type of architecture from CNNs but instead describe an approach for accounting for long-term dependencies in the CNN architecture (Bai et al., 2018).

Practical Steps and Considerations

Some steps are common across deep-learning techniques. Here we outline practical steps for any research using deep-learning methods. The first three steps—identifying a research question, preparing data, and choosing an analytic model—are best practices for any research project. The final two, choosing tuning parameters and training the model, are more specific to machine learning applications. Information in these steps is not comprehensive but should instead be taken as a starting point for how to set up how you analyze your data using these methods. Two empirical examples will follow, demonstrating these steps in practice.

1. ***Research question.*** Just as is the case with traditional statistical methods, we must develop a question in order to develop a model appropriate for our question. Is the primary goal to predict or forecast when some event will occur, or is it to classify a given event at a given time? If one is trying to identify when (and if) a time-sensitive intervention is warranted, then the goal is to predict when an adverse event (e.g., binging on alcohol use; suicide attempt) may occur so that one might intervene before this happens. Here, the outcome can be a continuous or a categorical variable. However, if the goal is to classify a given state, this would imply a categorical outcome variable. Other considerations might be needed. For example, do you wish to predict an event sometime in the next day or in the next month? Are you interested in classifying people or events (i.e., temporal states)? Clearly stating the research question will help guide the decision points to follow.

2. ***Preprocessing, rescaling, and feature generation.*** Feature extraction is often an exploratory process, especially since these methods and data types are new. Thus, it is not always known what aspects of the data best represent the predictive qualities of the data. Here, background knowledge and information gleaned from prior research are utilized to ensure that useful variables are utilized. Considerations include whether to bin the data to be aggregated within windows of time, and if so, how? Options might be to take the mean, standard deviation, maximum, and minimum of the values in each window of time (e.g., 10-second increments for data continuously gathered). Some researchers may also use raw data if prior theory is not available and computational resources permit. The researcher needs to think critically about which features may be helpful toward investigating their question of interest.

We note here that rescaling is often an important step in preprocessing. Not only does it make the code more efficient, but it also makes the model more stable since models are often sensitive to larger values. This occurs because large values can cause estimated weights to change substantially, making the gradient process more volatile. It is recommended that data are either standardized or rescaled to be in the range of 0 to 1 (Bishop, 1995).

Examples of these decision points will be presented in the empirical examples.

3. ***Choosing a model.*** These final steps are often completed several times until a satisfactory model is discovered. The selection of a modeling framework should be informed by what prior researchers have done, as well as emerging insights into the appropriateness of a given deep-learning method for your specific research question. Researchers must be aware of the relative gains and assumptions when selecting which method to use.

Choosing the number and types of layers is not always straightforward, although there are a variety of recommendations. We recommend Michelucci's (2018) book on applied deep learning and Beysolow's (2017) book on deep learning using R for further information on choosing a network architecture. Beysolow's book contains examples of common architectures, which is often a good starting point for choosing an appropriate architecture.

Sometimes, multiple methods are used to identify which one performs best for a given dataset, or multiple approaches are used in tandem. Care must be taken to avoid overfitting, as discussed extensively in Chapter 17.

4. ***Choosing tuning parameters.*** Parameters often must be tuned, or altered, to identify the final model that reaches the highest accuracy by whatever outcome the researcher uses. Some tuning parameters, referred to as *hyperparameters*, need to be explored by the researcher and will be study-specific and based on a combination of prior theory and model performance. These values cannot be derived or estimated during the modeling approach. Although these values must be indicated prior to starting the analyses, researchers can iterate across these values to identify which ones perform best. As an example, the researcher may wonder if coding the input features in 10-second bins outperforms coding them into 20-second bins. While this decision occurred during the preprocessing stage, one might still consider it a hyperparameter as it is set by the researcher and different values for the length of bins can be used to see which is best. Some algorithms may require the user to either enter a parameter for the model, such as a starting value or the number of nodes to use in a given layer. Although many programs have defaults for these tuning parameters, it is important to consider whether these defaults work for your particular model. Another consideration is the computational time and potential for overfitting in exploring several hyperparameters.

5. ***Training and testing the model.*** A hallmark of machine learning is using one portion of the data to train (or learn) the model and then use the holdout data to test how accurate the prediction or classification is on data not used to inform the model. It is typical to see researchers use 75% of individuals in the training set and the remaining 25% for the testing set. Another approach, called *k-fold cross-validation*, partitions the sample into *k* subsets, and then holds out each subset in turn to identify the generalizability of the predictive model to new data (Stone, 1974).

Selection of a final model occurs by using measures that are the most relevant performance measures for the given research question. For instance, if one is aiming to predict or classify into a binary category, then measures such as sensitivity and specificity, first introduced by Yerushalmy (1947), may be used. Sensitivity assesses the ability to detect an event occurring that really did occur (i.e., true positives), whereas specificity provides the ratio of the number of times an event was coded as zero when it truly was a zero (i.e., true negatives). If one is concerned mostly about correctly classifying an event as occurring when it really did occur, then they may wish to optimize sensitivity and select the model that had the highest sensitivity. This is particularly helpful if the cost of missing an event is high, such as if one wishes to identify a potential suicide attempt. Here, having a high number of false positives (low specificity), or incorrectly predicting this event, might be worth the cost if the prediction of true events is high. On the other hand, if the cost of falsely identifying an event is high, then one might want to optimize specificity. This may be warranted if it is intrusive or expensive to intervene, and the repercussions of not intervening are low.

One measure that balances both false- and true-positive rates is using the area under the receiver–operator characteristic curve (AUC-ROC; Melo, 2013). The ROC curve depicts the balance of sensitivity with the rate of false positives. The false-positive rate is equal to one minus the true negative rate (specificity). Figure 18.4 depicts the ROC curve for an example dataset available in the *AUC* R package (Ballings & Van den Poel, 2013). With sensitivity on the *y*-axis and the false-positive rate on the *x*-axis, one can see if increases in sensitivity come at the cost of an increase in false positives. High sensitivity

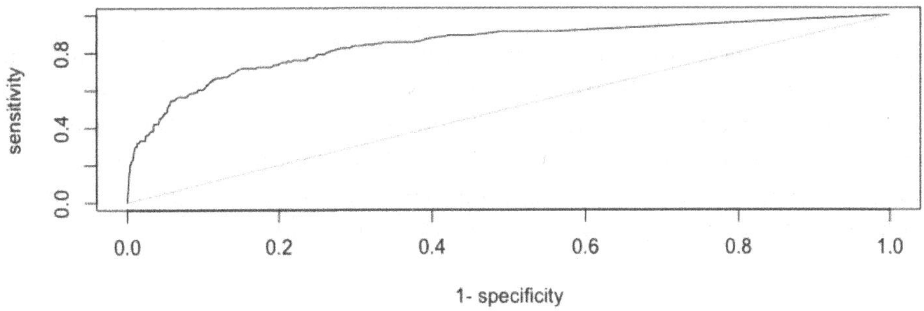

FIGURE 18.4. Example of area under the receiver–operator characteristic curve.

with a low false-positive rate (the left side of this chart) suggests that the detection of true positives occurs at a high rate without the introduction of false positives. If this curve followed the straight diagonal line in the graph, that would indicate that the detection of true positives was equal to that of false positives, which is not ideal. When the curve is above this line, as seen here, that indicates the true positive rate becomes high before the rate of false positives becomes high. For instance, when sensitivity hits .80, the false-positive rate is only about .23, indicating an acceptable specificity rate of .77. The area under this curve can be quantified, with high values indicating better separation of the classes. We can see from the figure that the area under the curve obtained from the data is greater than the area obtained when looking under the straight diagonal line.

This overview of deep learning primes the reader to have a baseline understanding. From this foundation, one can explore emerging methods that are best for specific research questions. We now turn specifically to examples of the use of a couple of deep-learning methods in classification and prediction for psychological inquiry using mobile sensing data. Here we provide more details on the use of these methods and empirical examples.

Empirical Example: Using Deep Learning for Classification

Deep learning addresses the two main issues common to traditional time-series classification methods: efficiency and dimensionality (Fawaz, Forestier, Weber, Idoumghar, & Muller, 2019). Deep-learning algorithms often are both efficient and able to classify multivariate time series. CNNs, presented earlier, are the primary model type for using deep learning for time-series classification. Several extensions of the basic CNN have been proposed and used for time-series classification, and more approaches continue to emerge. In many cases, deep-learning methods outperform other approaches. For example, InceptionTime, an algorithm employing a CNN, outperformed the current state of the art approach of a nearest neighbor algorithm with dynamic time warping (DTW; Fawaz et al., 2019). In another study, a CNN-based approach with DTW outperformed the traditional neural network (NN) combined with DTW across datasets in a large time-series classification archive (Fawaz et al., 2019).

Here, we provide an example of time-series classification from the literature where accelerometer data were used to predict high (>.08) blood alcohol levels. Additionally, researchers wanted to avoid the use of more sensitive personal data, such as location or call data. Accelerometer data are less invasive than location data as they provide information only on movements but not on location. Ultimately, researchers were interested in training a model that uses noninvasive, nonsensitive data and would allow for just-in-time adaptive interventions (JITAI) to prevent heavy drinking.

Data

Data from this study are available at the University of California Irvine Machine Learning Repository (Dua & Graff, 2019). The dataset includes time series from 13 undergraduate students wearing SCRAM (Secure Continuous Remote Alcohol Monitor) ankle bracelets, a wearable device that collects blood alcohol levels transdermally at 30-minute intervals. (Obtaining blood alcohol levels continuously is not feasible, even with transdermal trackers.) These recordings were collected over a 1-day "bar crawl." Cell phone accelerometer data were also collected, with the goal of classifying intoxication over 10-second intervals based on the accelerometer data. Data were collected over an 18-hour period. Although the TAC (transdermal alcohol content) readings were measured as a ratio variable, classification was dichotomized to above or below the legal limit for driving of 0.08.

Method

We break down the process used by the researchers into several steps, which can be applied to your own data.

1. ***Research question.*** Here, the researchers' overarching goal was to infer whether passively collected cell phone accelerometer data are related to the likelihood of intoxication, using SCRAM ankle bracelets as the ground truth. More specifically, they planned to classify 10-second segments of accelerometer data as either not intoxicated or intoxicated in order for the classification system to be applicable to JITAIs.

2. ***Preprocessing, rescaling, and feature generation.*** Prior to conducting any analyses, the researchers filtered the data to remove noisy elements. They also shifted the TAC data by 45 minutes because of the lag between consumption of alcohol and registration of alcohol in the body and segmented the data into 10-second intervals. Researchers ultimately developed 1,215 features from the accelerometer data, which they applied to each 10-second segment of time.

Examples of these features include calculations as simple as the mean or standard deviation of the segment. They also used spectral methods, obtaining the mean of the frequencies or the entropy of energy. Another useful method is to find features from the literature that have shown predictive value. The researchers in the current study did this by including features such as the average time between two steps and the difference between the maximum and minimum of one stride. One novel contribution of the study was the use of mel-frequency cepstral coefficients (MFCC). The researchers note that this feature type is typically used for classifying sound data, but ultimately, they found this feature type improved the accuracy of some of the tested models.

There was no mention of rescaling the data in this study, perhaps because of the methods used for feature generation.

3. ***Choosing a model.*** In this case, the researchers tested multiple models to make comparisons about which features and model parameters predicted high TAC best. Here, we focus on the CNN since it is most relevant to the present topic. The network architecture consisted of six layers: a convolutional layer, a pooling layer, a batch normalization layer, a fully connected layer, a dropout layer, and a fully connected layer. Batch normalization standardizes the output from the previous layer. A batch normalization layer can be used to improve the speed of convergence or avoid unstable gradients (Ioffe & Szegedy, 2015). A dropout layer is a form of regularization, setting the weights of nodes to zero. This is a useful method to prevent overfitting (Srivastava et al., 2014).

4. ***Choosing tuning parameters.*** In the current study, researchers had to decide what an appropriate threshold for intoxication would be, what window length was best for segmenting the data, and how many features to retain. Researchers used a combination of theoretical knowledge and data-driven methods to arrive at an ideal value. They used a grid-based search on each of the three parameters. When choosing the number of features to retain segmentation length, they chose the values that maximized accuracy. However, because the onset of binge drinking, according to the National Institute on Alcohol Abuse and Alcoholism, is defined as a blood alcohol content (BAC) of 0.08, they chose to value interpretability over accuracy.

Other tuning parameters the researcher may want to consider are initial weights and learning rates. Initial weights may be helpful in preventing the convergence of estimated weights at local minima. This is useful if you have an expectation for the weights based on previous research. Learning rates determine the step size in convergence toward the minimum of the loss function. Larger learning rates will converge more quickly but may not be as accurate as a smaller learning rate (Michelucci, 2018).

5. ***Training and testing the model.*** In the study being described, 25% of the sample was randomly chosen to be in the test set. As a reminder, the test set is the set we apply our trained model to in order to see if the model can accurately classify new cases. Researchers trained the CNN using cross-entropy loss and reached 74.3% accuracy, which is a moderate level of accuracy. Researchers tested several segmentation methods and lengths, ultimately finding that a 10-second segment improved classification accuracy (Killian et al., 2019).

Empirical Example: Using Deep Learning for Forecasting

Like classification, a wide range of types of neural networks are used to forecast future values or states. These include deep belief networks (DBNs; Ball, Anderson, & Chan, 2017; Gamboa, 2017; Qiu et al., 2017), event-based deep belief networks (EBDNs; Qiu et al., 2017), deep transformers (Wu, Green, Ben, & O'Banion, 2020), and ensemble methods that forecast based on combinations of learning algorithms (Ball et al., 2017; Gamboa, 2017; Qiu et al., 2014).

Most often, researchers use a variation of either a CNN (Cui, Chen, & Chen, 2016; Qiu et al., 2014), sometimes referred to as a TCN in the context of time series (Chen, Kang, Chen, & Wang, 2020; Yang & Liu, 2019) or an RNN (Gamboa, 2017; Koppe et al., 2019; Lipton et al., 2015; Qiu et al., 2014) because of the models' approaches to handling time-related dependencies. A commonly used variation of the RNN is the long short-term memory (LSTM) neural network (Mikelsons et al., 2017; Mikus et al., 2018; Suhara et al., 2017), described in the introduction to this chapter. TCNs, an extension of CNNs, are current state-of-the-art in deep learning for time-series data (Yang & Liu, 2019).

Like the section on classification, we provide an empirical example so that researchers can better understand the process of using deep-learning methods for forecasting. In the previous example, researchers wanted to classify accelerometer data so that if a person demonstrates behaviors indicative of intoxication, some intervention can be made. With forecasting, there is a similar goal of JITAIs; however, instead of predicting a state given the indicators of that state, the researcher wants to predict future states based on the previous states. More specifically, in the study we explore here, researchers were interested in predicting future depressed mood based on a combination of past reports of depressed mood and behavior in ecological momentary assessment (EMA) data (Suhara et al., 2017).

Data

Researchers collected EMA data from 2,382 individuals who self-reported experiencing depression via a smartphone application over 22 months. To be included in the analyses, participants had to make self-reports on 28 consecutive days. Every morning, afternoon, and evening, participants reported both mood and behavior. Behaviors included going to work, working at home, doing nothing at home, or being sick in bed. In addition, participants reported when they went to bed and when they woke up, medication usage, and hospital attendance.

Method

Many of the steps are like those in the CNN classification example. However, forecasting presents a few additional issues to consider. Additionally, although recent research suggests that temporal extensions of CNNs are preferable to RNNs and LSTMs, there are few examples of TCNs applied to mobile sensing in the literature, likely due to the novelty of the method. In this example, we provide an example that uses RNNs and LSTMs; however, many of the data preparation decision points will carry over to other neural network architectures.

1. ***Research question.*** We know that with forecasting, we are trying to predict future values. We could choose to forecast one observation ahead at a time (iteratively) or as a batch (e.g., predicting 10 future values at once). In the current study, researchers were interested in predicting whether an individual would have one severe depression day in the next *n* days based on reports from the past 14 days. Additionally, they had two

questions they wanted to answer: (a) Can past mood and behavior predict future mood? (b) Does a longer-term history provide better accuracy than modeling based on short-term histories?

2. ***Preprocessing, rescaling, and feature generation.*** Researchers ran the model using two different feature sets. One model predicted future depression based on past depression only. The second model included behavioral features. The labeled dataset was created by dividing user data into 28-day nonoverlapping blocks, in which the first 21 days were used as the user history, and the last 7 days were examined for existence of a severe depressive episode. The current study used 14 days as the user history, but the 21-day user history window was created so that the researchers could test a range of user history periods. Also, the researchers treated the 28-day blocks independently rather than as nested. Allowing for nesting within individuals to be accounted for could potentially improve model accuracy when predicting depressive episodes for a given individual, but that was not explored. Labeling was completed by creating an output variable for each value of *n* in which the researchers were interested.

3. ***Choosing a model.*** Because they were interested in incorporating long-term effects into the model, researchers chose to use an LSTM. The architecture follows the same pattern as described previously in the section on LSTMs. An embedding layer was included to model day-of-the-week effects. An embedding layer is a type of layer that reduces dimensionality. For example, one could reduce categorical variables (in this case, day-of-the-week) to integer values. Finally, there was a fully connected layer with 64 nodes.

4. ***Choosing tuning parameters.*** The outcome, severe depression, was defined as having negative feelings all day combined with physical inactivity. As explained previously, researchers also ran the model across several combinations of *k* (number of days used to predict future depression) and *n* (number of depressive days predicted in the next 10 days). A dropout of 0.1 was chosen. Again, dropout is a method of randomly removing units and their connections during training to prevent overfitting (Srivastava et al., 2014)

5. ***Training and testing the model.*** In this study, the training and test datasets were divided among individuals. Seventy-five percent of individuals were assigned to the training set and 25% of individuals were assigned to the test set. This was done to see if the model could make predictions about individuals that were not in the training set. In forecasting, there are several methods for splitting a training and test set, depending on the goal of the research. In cases where we are forecasting for one person instead of several people, backtesting is recommended. Backtesting is a method for checking how well the model would have performed if it was used on past data (Virdi, 2011). If we only have one individual, we would need to split the training and test set based on observations across time.

Results found that modeling the previous 2 weeks of self-reports was sufficient for forecasting depression. Performance improved substantially from using 1 day of self-reports to 14 days of self-reports but only improved slightly after the 14-day mark.

The feature set that performed best included both mood and behavioral variables, achieving an AUC-ROC of .886. This was only slightly better than using only mood in the feature set (AUC-ROC = .846). The model performed best when predicting at least 1 depressive day occurred out of the next 10 and progressively worsened when more days were predicted.

Conclusions

This chapter summarized current applications of deep learning on mobile sensing data, provided an overview of fundamental deep-learning concepts, and provided two examples from the literature demonstrating classification and forecasting using a CNN and a LSTM. Prior to readily available mobile sensing technologies, psychological data outside the laboratory mostly consisted of daily diary data, initially collected on paper, a collection method that can become laborious for some participants. Passive sensing, as well as some mobile EMA methods, provide a data collection method that lessens the mental burden on participants, allowing researchers to collect data that are more "real-world." These data are typically high-dimensional and are not necessarily linear in nature. Deep learning addresses these concerns and provides a framework for solving classification and forecasting problems efficiently. Just-in-time adaptive interventions are particularly interesting uses of mobile sensing data. Having models that can learn and react efficiently is beneficial to timely interventions.

We reviewed important steps in the process of modeling data using a neural network. Many of these steps will be familiar to researchers using traditional statistical techniques. For example, formulating an appropriate model for your research question is common among all techniques. Many of the questions researchers ask when choosing tuning parameters may seem familiar since some tuning parameters involve defining a theoretically relevant cutoff point. This is also applicable to feature generation and preprocessing steps.

Deep learning is a rapidly developing field, and current state-of-the-art techniques are being updated quickly. CNNs are flexible and are constantly being updated to find new solutions to new problems. However, the literature reviewed here and the empirical examples presented are a good starting point for researchers interested in adding deep learning to their statistics toolkit.

Note

1. MLPs are closely related to methods such as partial least squares (Wold, 1974), which automatically extract the latent variable representation of the predictors that is most helpful for predicting the outcomes. See Urban and Gates (2021) for discussion of the relationship between deep learning and traditional latent variable models.

REFERENCES

Acikmese, Y., & Alptekin, S. E. (2019). Prediction of stress levels with LSTM and passive mobile sensors. *Procedia Computer Science, 159*, 658–667.

Bai, S., Kolter, J. Z., & Koltun, V. (2018). *An empirical evaluation of generic convolutional and recurrent networks for sequence modeling.* http://arxiv.org/abs/1803.01271

Ball, J. E., Anderson, D. T., & Chan, C. S. (2017). Comprehensive survey of deep learning in remote sensing: Theories, tools, and challenges for the community. *Journal of*

Applied Remote Sensing, 11(04). https://arxiv.org/abs/1709.00308

Ballings, M., & Van den Poel, D. (2013). *AUC: Threshold independent performance measures for probabilistic classifiers.* R package version 0.3.0. https://CRAN.R-project.org/package=AUC

Baumeister, H., & Montag, C. (2019). *Digital phenotyping and mobile sensing in psychoinformatics—a rapidly evolving interdisciplinary research endeavor.* Springer.

Bengio, Y. (2012). Practical recommendations for gradient-based training of deep architectures, In G. Montavon, G. B. Orr, & K. R. Müller (Eds.), *Neural networks: Tricks of the trade* (pp.437–478). Springer.

Beysolow, T., II. (2017). *Introduction to deep learning using R.* APRESS.

Bishop, C. M. (1995). *Neural networks for pattern recognition.* Oxford University Press.

Chen, Y., Kang, Y., Chen, Y., & Wang, Z. (2020). Probabilistic forecasting with temporal convolutional neural network. *Neurocomputing, 399,* 491–501. https://arxiv.org/abs/1906.04397

Cui, Z., Chen, W., & Chen, Y. (2016). *Multiscale convolutional neural networks for time series classification.* https://arxiv.org/abs/1603.06995v4

Cybenko, G. (1989). Approximation by superpositions of a sigmoidal function. *Mathematics of Control, Signals, and Systems, 2*(4), 303–314.

Dua, D., & Graff, C. (2019). UCI Machine Learning Repository.

Fawaz, H. I., Lucas, B., Forestier, G., Pelletier, C., Schmidt, D. F., Weber, J., et al. (2019). InceptionTime: Finding AlexNet for time series classification. *Data Mining and Knowledge Discovery, 34*(6), 1936–1962.

Gamboa, J. C. B. (2017). *Deep learning for time-series analysis.* http://arxiv.org/abs/1701.01887

Glorot, X., Bordes, A., & Bengio, Y. (2011). Deep sparse rectifier neural networks. *Proceedings of the Fourteenth International Conference on Artificial Intelligence and Statistics. JMLR Workshop and Conference Proceedings*, pp. 315–323.

Goodfellow, I., Bengio, Y., & Courville, A. (2016). *Deep learning.* MIT Press.

Hammerla, N. Y., Halloran, S., & Plötz, T. (2016). Deep, convolutional, and recurrent models for human activity recognition using wearables. *IJCAI International Joint Conference on Artificial Intelligence*, pp. 1533–1540. https://arxiv.org/abs/1604.08880

Heaton, J. (2008). *Introduction to neural networks with Java.* Heaton Research.

Hochreiter, S., & Schmidhuber, J. (1997). Long short-term memory. *Neural Computation, 9*(8), 1735–1780.

Ioffe, S., & Szegedy, C. (2015). Batch normalization: Accelerating deep network training by reducing internal covariate shift. *32nd International Conference on Machine Learning, ICML 2015*, pp. 448–456. https://arxiv.org/abs//1502.03167

Fawaz, H. I., Forestier, G., Weber, J., Idoumghar, L., & Muller, P. A. (2019). Deep learning for time series classification: a review. *Data Mining and Knowledge Discovery, 33*(4), 917–963.

Jarrett, K., Kavukcuoglu, K., Ranzato, M., & LeCun, Y. (2009). What is the best multistage architecture for object recognition? *2009 IEEE 12th International Conference on Computer Vision*, pp. 2146–2153.

Killian, J. A., Passino, K. M., Nandi, A., Madden, D. R., & Clapp, J. (2019). Learning to detect heavy drinking episodes using smartphone accelerometer data. *CEUR Workshop Proceedings, 2429*, 35–42.

Kingma, D. P., & Ba, J. (2014). *Adam: A method for stochastic optimization.* https://arxiv.org/abs/1412.6980

Koppe, G., Guloksuz, S., Reininghaus, U., & Durstewitz, d. (2019). recurrent Neural Networks in Mobile Sampling and Intervention. *Schizophrenia Bulletin, 45*(2), 272–276.

Krizhevsky, A., Sutskever, I., & Hinton, G. E. (2012). Imagenet classification with deep convolutional neural networks, *Advances in Neural Information Processing Systems, 25*, 1097–1105.

LeCun, Y., Bengio, Y., & Hinton, G. (2015). Deep learning. *Nature, 521*(7553), 436–444.

Lima, W. S., Souto, E., El-Khatib, K., Jalali, R., & Gama, J. (2019). Human activity recognition using inertial sensors in a smartphone: An overview. *Sensors, 19*(14), 14–16.

Linnainmaa, S. (1976). Taylor expansion of the accumulated rounding error. *BIT Numerical Mathematics, 16* (2), 146–160.

Lipton, Z. C., Berkowitz, J., & Elkan, C. (2015). *A critical review of recurrent neural net-*

works for sequence learning. http://arxiv.org/abs/1506.00019

Marcus, G. (2018). *Deep learning: A critical appraisal.* https://arxiv.org/abs/1801.00631

McCulloch, W. S., & Pitts, W. (1943). A logical calculus of the ideas immanent in nervous activity. *Bulletin of Mathematical Biophysics, 5*(4), 115–133.

Melo, F. (2013). Area under the ROC curve. In W. Dubitzky, O. Wolkenhauer, K.-H. Cho, & H. Yokota (Eds.), *Encyclopedia of systems biology* (pp. 38–39). Springer.

Michelucci, U. (2018). *Applied deep learning: A case-based approach to understanding deep neural networks.* APRESS.

Mikelsons, G., Smith, M., Mehrotra, A., & Musolesi, M. (2017). Towards deep learning models for psychological state prediction using smartphone data: Challenges and opportunities. *Proceedings of the NIPS Workshop on Machine Learning for Healthcare 2017,* pp. 1–6. http://arxiv.org/abs/1711.06350

Mikus, A., Hoogendoorn, M., Rocha, A., Gama, J., Ruwaard, J., & Riper, H. (2018). Predicting short term mood developments among depressed patients using adherence and ecological momentary assessment data. *Internet Interventions, 12,* 105–110.

Mohammadian Rad, N., Kia, S. M., Zarbo, C., van Laarhoven, T., Jurman, G., Venuti, P., et al. (2018). Deep learning for automatic stereotypical motor movement detection using wearable sensors in autism spectrum disorders. *Signal Processing, 144,* 180–191. http://arxiv.org/abs/1709.05956

Molenaar, P. C. (1985). A dynamic factor model for the analysis of multivariate time series. *Psychometrika, 50*(2), 181–202.

Nair, V., & Hinton, G. E. (2010). Rectified linear units improve restricted Boltzmann machines. *Proceedings of the 27th International Conference on Machine Learning (ICML-10),* pp. 807–814.

Nait Aicha, A., Englebienne, G., Van Schooten, K. S., Pijnappels, M., & Kröse, B. (2018). Deep learning to predict falls in older adults based on daily-life trunk accelerometry. *Sensors, 18*(5), 1654.

Ordóñez, F. J., & Roggen, D. (2016). Deep convolutional and LSTM recurrent neural networks for multimodal wearable activity recognition. *Sensors, 16*(1).

Pang, B., Nijkamp, E., & Wu, Y. N. (2020). Deep learning with TensorFlow: A review. *Journal of Educational and Behavioral Statistics, 45*(2), 227–248.

Pedregosa, F., Varoquaux, G., Gramfort, A., Michel, V., Thirion, B., Grisel, O., et al. (2011). Scikit-learn: Machine learning in Python. *Journal of Machine Learning Research, 12,* 2825–2830.

Peng, M., Wang, C., Chen, T., Liu, G., & Fu, X. (2017). Dual temporal scale convolutional neural network for micro-expression recognition. *Frontiers in Psychology, 8,* 1–12.

Qiu, X., Ren, Y., Suganthan, P. N., & Amaratunga, G. A. (2017). Empirical mode decomposition based ensemble deep learning for load demand time series forecasting. *Applied Soft Computing Journal, 54,* 246–255.

Qiu, X., Zhang, L., Ren, Y., Suganthan, P., & Amaratunga, G. (2014). Ensemble deep learning for regression and time series forecasting. *IEEE SSCI 2014–2014 IEEE Symposium Series on Computational Intelligence—CIEL 2014: 2014 IEEE Symposium on Computational Intelligence in Ensemble Learning, Proceedings,* pp. 1–6.

Robbins, H., & Monro, S. (1951). A stochastic approximation method. *Annals of Mathematical Statistics,* 400–407.

Ronao, C. A., & Cho, S. B. (2016). Human activity recognition with smartphone sensors using deep learning neural networks. *Expert Systems with Applications, 59,* 235–244.

Rosenblatt, F. (1958). The perceptron: A probabilistic model for information storage and organization in the brain. *Psychological Review, 65*(6), 386.

Rumelhart, D. E., Hinton, G. E., & Williams, R. J. (1986). Learning representations by back-propagating errors. *Nature, 323*(6088), 533–536.

Sanderson, M., Bulloch, A. G., Wang, J. L., Williamson, T., & Patten, S. B. (2020). Predicting death by suicide using administrative health care system data: Can recurrent neural network, one-dimensional convolutional neural network, and gradient boosted trees models improve prediction performance? *Journal of Affective Disorders, 264,* 107–114.

Sathyanarayana, A., Joty, S., Fernandez-Luque, L., Ofli, F., Srivastava, J., Elmagarmid, A., et al. (2016). Sleep quality prediction from wearable data using deep learning. *JMIR mHealth and uHealth, 4*(4), e125.

Shaw, A., Simsiri, N., Deznaby, I., Fiterau, M., & Rahaman, T. (2019). Personalized student stress prediction with deep multitask network. *Proceedings of the 1st Adaptive and Multitask Learning Workshop*. http://arxiv.org/abs/1906.11356

Smith, L. N. (2018). *A disciplined approach to neural network hyper-parameters: Part 1–learning rate, batch size, momentum, and weight decay*. https://arxiv.org/abs/1803.09820

Srivastava, N., Hinton, G. E., Krizhevsky, A., Sutskever, I., & Salakhutidinov, R. (2014). Dropout: A simple way to prevent neural networks from overfitting. *Journal of Machine Learning Research, 15(1), 1929–1958.*

Stone, M. (1974). Cross-validatory choice and assessment of statistical predictions. *Journal of the Royal Statistical Society: Series B (Methodological), 36*(2), 111–133.

Suhara, Y., Xu, Y., & Pentland, A. S. (2017). DeepMood: Forecasting depressed mood based on self-reported histories via recurrent neural networks. *26th International World Wide Web Conference, WWW 2017*, pp. 715–724.

Urban, C., & Gates, K. M. (2021). Deep learning: A primer for psychologists. *Psychological Methods, 26*(6), 743–773.

Victor, E., Aghajan, Z. M., Sewart, A. R., & Christian, R. (2019). Detecting depression using a framework combining deep multimodal neural networks with a purpose-built automated evaluation. *Psychological Assessment, 31*(8), 1019–1027.

Vieira, S., Pinaya, W. H., & Mechelli, A. (2017). Using deep learning to investigate the neuroimaging correlates of psychiatric and neurological disorders: Methods and applications. *Neuroscience & Biobehavioral Reviews, 74*, 58–75.

Virdi, N. K. (2011). A review of backtesting methods for evaluating value-at-risk. *International Review of Business Research Papers*, 7(4), 14–24.

Wang, J., Chen, Y., Hao, S., Peng, X., & Hu, L. (2019). Deep learning for sensor-based activity recognition: A survey. *Pattern Recognition Letters, 119*, 3–11. https://arxiv.org/abs/1707.03502

Wold, H. (1974). Causal flows with latent variables: Partings of the ways in the light of NIPALS modelling. *European Economic Review, 5*(1), 67–86.

Wu, N., Green, B., Ben, X., & O'Banion, S. (2020). *Deep transformer models for time series forecasting: The influenza prevalence case*. http://arxiv.org/abs/2001.08317

Yang, L., & Liu, J. (2019). EEG-based emotion recognition using temporal convolutional network. *Proceedings of 2019 IEEE 8th Data Driven Control and Learning Systems Conference, DDCLS 2019*, pp. 437–442.

Yao, S., Hu, S., Zhao, Y., Zhang, A., & Abdelzaher, T. (2017). DeepSense: A unified deep learning framework for time-series mobile sensing data processing. *26th international world wide web conference, www 2017*, pp. 351–360. https://arxiv.org/abs/1611.01942

Yerushalmy, J. (1947). Statistical problems in assessing methods of medical diagnosis, with special reference to X-ray techniques. *Public Health Reports (1896–1970)*, 1432–1449.

Zhao, B., Lu, H., Chen, S., Liu, J., & Wu, D. (2017). Convolutional neural networks for time series classification. *Journal of Systems Engineering and Electronics, 28*(1), 162–169.

CHAPTER 19

Big Data Dimensionality Reduction Methods

Andreas M. Brandmaier

CHAPTER OVERVIEW

Getting a grasp of time series in the context of mobile sensing is challenging. Datasets are typically large, heterogeneous (including, for example, GPS, accelerometry, ambient light, or audio), and it is often difficult to come up with exact, testable theories. *Unsupervised learning* approaches can help us to reduce data dimensionality by decreasing either the number of variables or the number of observations. The former category encompasses approaches such as principal and independent component analysis, and the latter category comprises various clustering approaches that reduce observations to a few underlying groups. A special focus is on clustering approaches for time series, such as permutation distribution clustering and dynamic time warping. Hidden Markov models are also discussed, which allow for the reduction of complex time series, the determination of event boundaries, or prediction. All of these approaches make large datasets easier to handle, easier to visualize, and easier to model.

Introduction

Making sense of multivariate time series such as those arising from mobile sensing in psychology is challenging for several reasons. Datasets are typically large (in the sense of hundreds and thousands of repeated observations across multiple variables and people), they arise from quite different sources (such as GPS, accelerometry, light, temperature, audio, video, or information about nearby devices), and it is difficult, if not impossible, to come up with comprehensive, testable theories that reflect all dependencies and intricacies of the constructs of interest and the instruments that measured them. Irrespective of whether we believe we have a good theory to start modeling with or whether we opt for an exploratory machine learning approach, we face the challenge of finding and representing simple yet informative patterns in our data. The sheer volume of data can make it difficult to explore, visualize, and understand them. They also challenge modeling approaches because it is more likely that we violate model assumptions (such as independence of predictors or certain distributional assumptions) or that we accidentally pick up seemingly informative patterns that actually arose by chance alone, which is usually referred to as *overfitting*. Furthermore, large datasets may not fit into the computer's memory, or the required computation time of a given analysis may make it impractical. And, finally, we face the curse of dimensionality (see Chapter 17, this volume) that essentially tells us that high-dimensional data often make it difficult to glean knowledge of general rules. This is where *dimensionality reduction* (Vlachos, 2010) may come to the rescue. Dimensionality reduction approaches select variables or combinations of variables, such that we retain a smaller and simpler, but similarly information-rich dataset that is easier to store, handle, visualize, and understand, and promises more robust and generalizable inferences for a given problem.

Chapters 17 and 18 (this volume) have focused primarily on supervised learning approaches to modeling time-series data arising from mobile sensing applications. In supervised learning, the primary challenge was to best predict an outcome in regression or classification tasks by learning from examples that were assumed to be correctly labeled. In these scenarios, we can use the known outcomes from a given training set to inform our dimensionality reduction. But what if such labels do not exist? In this case, we can resort to techniques that are described under the umbrella term of *unsupervised learning* and help us reduce data dimensionality by decreasing either the number of variables or the number of observations. In this chapter, I summarize projection-based methods (e.g., principal components analysis) that assume that data arise from unobserved sources we aim to recover in order to obtain a few informative and predictive features. Next, I describe various approaches to clustering with a particular emphasis on time-series clustering. Clustering may help us reduce data dimensionality with respect to the number of observations by mapping potentially many observations to a few underlying clusters. Last, I show how sequences of observations can be reduced to sequences of latent discrete states, which is particularly useful for time-series segmentation. All approaches described here serve the goal of making large datasets easier to handle and easier to visualize. A further goal is to make the results of subsequent confirmatory modeling or predictive modeling approaches simpler, computationally less demanding, and more robust (by reducing the chance of overfitting).

Projection Methods

Projection methods aim to find a mapping of a large number of variables to a smaller number of variables with the hope that the resulting components (i.e., the projected variables) retain most of the information but are a simpler representation. There are various projection methods that mostly try to achieve two goals at the same time. They try to minimize redundancy in the resulting components while trying to maximize the information in them. If we succeed with this approach, we can retain only a small set of components that retain most of the information of the original variables, and subsequent data analysis will become easier to handle and potentially even more robust. The classic and most widely used projection method is *principal component analysis* (PCA; Jolliff, 1986). PCA assumes that important information is in the variances and covariances of the observed variables. It captures information as variability and aims at preserving as much of it as possible. Redundancy is captured as covariation, and projected components are chosen to be uncorrelated. Finally, PCA assumes that the observed variables are linear combinations of the components. Finding such new variables, the principal components (PCs), reduces to solving an eigenvector problem, and the literature describing this approach dates back at least to Hotelling (1933) and Pearson (1901). If we want to use a stronger criterion of nonredundancy, we could choose a projection onto sources that are not only uncorrelated but statistically independent. This leads to *independent component analysis* (ICA; Jutten & Herault, 1991). Statistical independence of two random variables means that information about one random variable does not change our knowledge about the other. In general, if two random variables are independent, they are also uncorrelated but not vice versa.

With most projection methods, the resulting components are linear combinations of many, if not all, original variables. Consequently, few to none of the original variables can be entirely discarded (e.g., in future data collection), even though simpler models are often more accurate and more interpretable (Ma & Huang, 2008). Other than removing items with low loadings, a formal solution to this problem is to employ sparse variants of projection methods (similar to rotation to simple structure in factor models), which enforce components that are simple combinations of the observed variables. In the following sections, I briefly describe the two most common projection approaches, PCA and ICA, and some of their variants.

Principal Component Analysis

PCA is the standard approach to dimensionality reduction (Jolliff, 1986). Principal components are new variables that are linear projections of the original variables. They are chosen such that components are uncorrelated (i.e., redundancy is minimized) and sorted in order of variance explained in the original data (i.e., information is maximized). PCA is fast to compute and yields simple projections of complex data across many situations. Importantly, it has no tuning parameter and thus is straightforward to use. PCA assumes that data are generated from uncorrelated sources that are observed as linear mixtures.

Features obtained from a PCA projection have several useful properties. First of all, they are uncorrelated, which solves problems with algorithms that cannot handle correlated features well. Second, the projected features will be ranked by the magnitude of explained variance in the original space, such that the first component explains most of the variance. PCA is quite similar to classic factor analysis (FA) models. Both assume that the essential information in observed signals is in the variances and covariances and that the observations are linear combinations of the sources.

PCA can be regarded as a special case of exploratory factor analysis in which the observed variables are indeed projected onto uncorrelated latent sources, but there is no explicit measurement model. If a projection on few PCA components is chosen, the resulting residual errors are typically not orthogonal (other than in typical FA). Exploratory FA encompasses a variety of other choices for determining the optimality of the projection (e.g., the option of correlated latent sources, or various rotations to simple structure). Confirmatory FA may be favorable if there is a theory-driven model available that prescribes a particular measurement model or structural relationships (see Chapter 14, this volume).

Because principal components are ordered by decreasing magnitude of explained variance, PCA can be used to select only a few of the resulting components as features for subsequent classification or regression tasks, or for visualization, thus allowing us to trade off simplicity for fidelity. Figure 19.1 shows the first two principal components (PC1 and PC2) of a set of features derived from accelerometry in a smartwatch (see Chapter 17, this volume, for a description of the WISDM dataset used here). The original features are shown as arrows and are the average activity (XAVG, YAVG, and ZAVG), the dominant frequency (XPEAK, YPEAK, and ZPEAK), and average absolute deviations from the mean of the sensor readings (XABSDEV, YABSDEV, and ZABSDEV) in each of the three dimensions. For example, we can see that the average of the *y*-axis sensor and the absolute deviations from the mean of the *y*-axis are projected onto the same axis, while they are almost perpendicular to the average of the *x*-axis. The resulting projected two-dimensional space separates the observations of the different activities well and may serve as a useful starting point for further supervised learning tasks (see Chapters 17 and 18, this volume).

It is common practice to apply PCA to noncontinuous scales (such as rating scale items), but strictly this is in violation of the PCA assumptions. It is advisable rather to perform a PCA on a polychoric correlation matrix for ordinal variables or tetrachoric correlation matrix for binary variables, or to resort to approaches tailored to other distributions. For example, Linting, Meulman, Groenen, and van der Kooij (2007) proposed

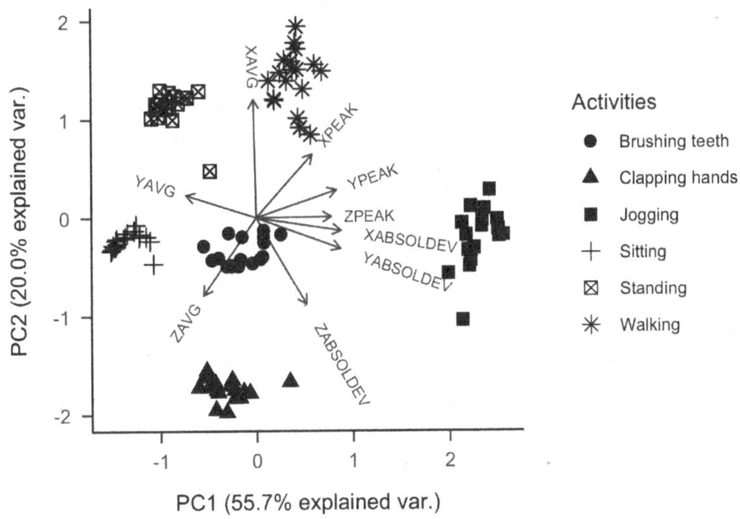

FIGURE 19.1. Latent-space representation of various activities (brushing teeth, clapping hands, jogging, sitting, standing, or walking) derived from features of smartphone accelerometry in the WISDM dataset. The plot axes represent the first two principal components of a feature space spanned by the sensor's average *x*-, *y*-, and *z*-readings (XAVG, YAVG, and ZAVG); the sensor's dominant frequency in *x*-, *y*-, and *z*-axes (XPEAK, YPEAK, and ZPEAK); and the sensor's absolute deviations in *x*-, *y*-, and *z*-axes (XABSOLDEV, YABSOLDEV, and ZABSOLDEV). The first principal component (*x*-axis) explains 56% of the variance, and the second principal component explains 20% of the variance. Arrows indicate the projection of the features onto the two-dimensional space. For example, we can see that in the projection, XAVG and YAVG are almost orthogonal, whereas YPEAK, ZPEAK, XABSOLDEV, and YABSOLDEV are highly dependent. This figure is available at https://github.com/brandmaier/mobile-sensing-figures under a CC-BY4.0 license.

a nonlinear PCA approach that can deal with variables at their appropriate measurement level. A disadvantage of PCA may be that the resulting components (even though only one or only a few are selected) are each linear combinations of all original variables. This means that a potentially large set of features need to be gathered that are then projected to the underlying source space. If we assume that not all observations are influenced by all sources, the PCA model will likely overfit to some degree. To enforce a sparse solution, we can resort to sparse PCA (Zou, Hastie, & Tibshirani, 2006), which constrains the number of nonzero coefficients in the projection using regularization (see Chapter 17, this volume). However, ensuring sparsity and orthogonality is not trivial, and there are several approaches to estimate sparse PCA (see Zou & Xue, 2018, for an overview).

Independent Component Analysis

In PCA, we assumed that each source is uncorrelated with all others and the sources linearly mix to a set of observed signals. The goal was to find a few sources with little redundancy. Redundancy was captured in a correlation metric and was thus limited to second-order moments. If we want to capture redundancy as statistical independence, thus accounting for higher-order moments, we can use ICA (Jutten & Herault, 1991). ICA retrieves the source signals by maximizing the statistical independence of the sources. ICA algorithms differ by how they estimate the projection. This can be achieved by choosing the projection such that either the non-Gaussianity of the resulting sources is maximized or their mutual information is minimized (Hyvärinen & Oja, 2000). Both PCA and ICA assume linearity of components. However, the projected space recovered by PCA is identified only up to rotation. ICA uses the higher-order moments to identify the best rotation to obtain independent sources. Note that the algorithm cannot recover the scale of the independent sources; that is, the amplitude of the signal is arbitrary. Also, unlike the case in PCA, the estimated sources are returned in no particular order.

ICA is typically used as a computational method for separating a multivariate signal into additive, mutually independent subcomponents, with the goal of recovering the true underlying signals (and not only the original subspace as in PCA, which may still be rotated). Commonly, the cocktail-party problem is used to illustrate the goal of an ICA: Given a room full of speakers (at a cocktail party), can you isolate the speech signals of the individual speakers? Similar problems are often encountered in the analysis of mobile sensing data. For example, Kobana, Takahashi, Kitsunezaki, Tobe, and Lopez (2014) used ICA to separate continuous multidimensional accelerometer readings of cyclists into a "road signal" and a pedaling signal. Then they used the unmixed "road signal" in order to classify road conditions. Mantyjarvi, Himberg, and Seppanen (2001) used two triaxial accelerometers, one each attached to the left and right hip of the participant. They showed that classification of activities improved considerably and best when ICA sources were used for subsequent classification instead of the raw sensor values.

Clustering

Clustering encompasses *unsupervised learning* approaches to group similar objects together while dissimilar objects are placed far apart from each other, with the goal of discovering latent similarity structure (Murphy, 2012). As input, clustering algorithms usually take a feature matrix, with one or more features per object and a function to compute their similarity. The goal is to form groups, that is, clusters, of objects. These clusters can either be flat (also called *partitional clustering*) or arranged in a hierarchical structure. Partitional clustering algorithms typically require specification of the number of clusters prior to the analysis. Hierarchical clustering, in contrast, provides an entire hierarchy of grouping relationships at various levels at a glance. Unlike in *supervised learning approaches* (see Chapter 17, this volume), no well-defined optimization goal exists because there is no specified outcome that is to be predicted. Without a given ground truth, there is no objective loss function that can be optimized. This is why some regard clustering as an ill-defined problem. However, one can still see clustering as a useful approach to make sense of data. We can use it as a technique to reduce the complexity of the data by reducing many observations to a few representative clusters if we can find a meaningful or theoretically plausible similarity function that allows us to interpret the results.

Clustering Algorithms

A variety of approaches exist to compute a clustering from a given dissimilarity matrix. Here, I will only describe the two most common algorithms, *hierarchical clustering* (Johnson, 1967) and *k-means* (MacQueen, 1967). Other clustering algorithms that have practically useful properties are density-based clustering (Ester, Kriegel, Sander, & Xu, 1996) or spectral clustering (von Luxburg, 2007).

Hierarchical Clustering

Sequential agglomerative hierarchical nonoverlapping clustering (Johnson, 1967) creates a hierarchical structure of clusters by sequentially merging objects to clusters until a single cluster with all objects is obtained. Initially, each object is its own cluster. Based on a chosen dissimilarity measure, the hierarchical clustering is obtained by repeatedly merging the two closest clusters. This leads to a tree-like structure of clusters where the root of the tree is the top-level cluster with all members and the leaves are the individual objects. To compute the dissimilarity of two clusters, we need a cluster dissimilarity measure as a function of the dissimilarity measure of objects. There are three common linkage functions to achieve this computation. *Complete linkage* defines cluster distance as the smallest maximum pairwise distance of cluster members and is rather sensitive to outliers. *Single linkage* computes distances as the smallest minimum pairwise distance and tends to form long chains rather than compact subgroups. *Average linkage* computes the cluster distance as the average distance of all combinations of pairs of members from each cluster and is a compromise between the two former approaches. An example of hierarchical clustering on accelerometer raw data based on the Euclidean distance is given in Figure 19.2. Here, we see that clustering the raw sensor data of a single axis of an accelerometer already yields clusters of "walking" activity and "jogging" activity that can be well separated.

K-Means Clustering

K-means clustering (also known as Lloyd's algorithm; MacQueen, 1967) is a simple clustering algorithm that produces a predefined number *k* of clusters. The clustering solution is represented by cluster centers, and all objects are members of the cluster with the closest center. The idea of the approach resembles the nearest neighbor notion in classification (see Chapter 17, this volume). The algorithm starts with random cluster centers

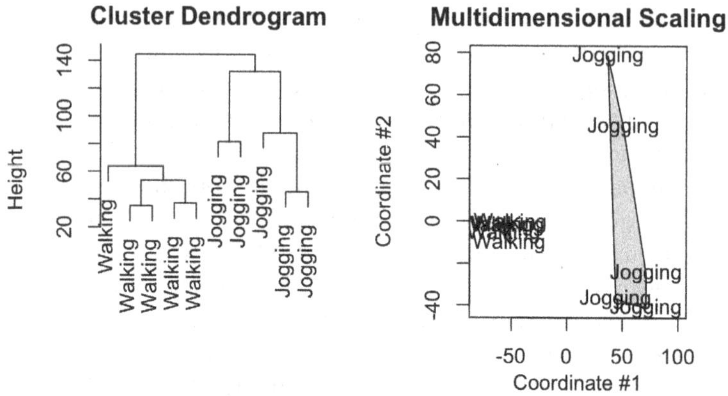

FIGURE 19.2. Clustering of raw sensor signals of a single axis of an accelerometer in the WISDM dataset. The clustered objects are time-series segments of 5 seconds in length recorded from a participant performing the activities "walking" and "jogging." Similarity was computed by the Euclidean distance. Segments are well separated according to their activity. Left: The cluster dendrogram representing the hierarchical clustering with complete linkage. Height represents dissimilarity of segments. Right: Multidimensional scaling to a two-dimensional space. In both representations, we can see that walking segments are more similar to each other than jogging segments are to each other. This figure is available at https://github.com/brandmaier/mobile-sensing-figures under a CC-BY4.0 license.

and iterates between two steps (a classic expectation–maximization algorithm). First, it computes the nearest cluster center for every member and then moves the cluster center to the center of all members. Obviously, the solution of the algorithm depends on the initial randomly assigned cluster centers, and results may differ across runs. Furthermore, the number of clusters must be chosen *a priori*, and it is difficult to check the appropriateness of the number of clusters. If k cannot be determined *a priori*, one must resort to heuristics, such as the elbow method (similar to a scree plot in exploratory factor analysis), cross-validation of the squared distance to cluster centers, or an internal validity heuristic (see the section "Evaluating Clustering Algorithms" below). The cluster centers in k-means are geometric cluster centers and, thus, are also referred to as centroids. Because they are averages, cluster centers almost never represent an observed object; instead they represent a hypothetical average object. K-medoids (Kaufman & Rousseeuw, 1987) is a variant of k-means in which cluster centers are always observed objects.

DBSCAN

Density-based spatial clustering of applications with noise (DBSCAN; Ester et al., 1996; Schubert, Sander, Ester, Kriegel, & Xu, 2017) clusters together points in dense neighborhoods. It can be considered a nonparametric density estimator that marks densely populated regions as clusters. The algorithm classifies observations as either core points, directly reachable points, or outliers. For this classification, it has two hyperparameters—the neighborhood radius ϵ and the minimum number of neighbors p—for an observation to be a core point. A cluster is then defined as all observations (core points or noncore points) that are reachable from any of its members. Any remaining nonreachable point is an outlier. The advantage of DBSCAN over k-means is that the nonparametric density estimation of the clusters allows for complex cluster shapes, whereas k-means always forms spherical shapes.

Instead of having to specify the number of clusters in advance, DBSCAN has the cluster density as the central parameter. It is often considered an advantage that the number of clusters does not have to be chosen, yet in practice it is usually just as difficult to choose the density.

Measures of Dissimilarity

The most important decision in the application of clustering algorithms is the choice of dissimilarity measure (typically, a distance metric). The dissimilarity measure formalizes what we mean when we say two objects are similar or are not. It principally determines our substantial interpretation of the clustering results. A particular clustering solution is thus hardly ever right or wrong but rather represents a structuring of a dataset given a chosen formalization of similarity. The very same dataset may be clustered in different ways, and each of these solutions may be insightful and useful for a different group of researchers, at a different time, or in different applications. For non-time-series data, often, the Euclidean distance is used. A generalization for the dissimilarity between two objects x and y with p features is the Minkowski metric (Hennig, 2020):

$$d(x,y) = \left(\sum_{j=1}^{p} | x_j - y_j |^m\right)^{1/m}$$

which becomes the Manhattan distance (sum of absolute differences of all p features) for $m = 1$, the Euclidean distance (sum of squared distance of all p features) for $m = 2$, or the Chebyshev distance (maximum of all feature distances) for $m = \infty$.

In high-dimensional spaces (that is, when the number of features is large), unsupervised approaches such as clustering suffer from the curse of dimensionality just like supervised approaches (see Chapter 17, this volume). Here, the curse of dimensionality means that as the number of features increases, there is a loss of meaningful distinction between similar and dissimilar objects. One solution to perform clustering in high dimensions effectively and efficiently is to first apply ideas of feature selection and extraction, for example, selecting variables and/or performing a projection to a few principal components (Assent, 2012). As alternatives to such global dimensionality reduction, there are approaches to find clusters with locally lower dimensionality (for an overview, see Steinbach, Ertöz, & Kumar, 2004).

Multidimensional Scaling

Dimensionality reduction techniques project high-dimensional observations onto a lower-dimensional space that may be easier to work with, easier to plot, or easier to understand. In the context of clustering, objects are typically given by their distances or dissimilarities in a chosen metric. Given a distance matrix with all pairwise distances of a set of objects, multidimensional scaling (MDS) places each object into an N-dimensional space (with N being chosen by the user, typically, $N = 2$), such that the distances in the original space are preserved as well as possible in the embedded space. For example, we may be given a list of cities in Germany and a matrix of their aerial distances. MDS can be used to place the cities into a two-dimensional space, such that the distance matrix of the resulting two-dimensional coordinates of the cities is as close as possible to the input distance matrix. In this example, the embedding will mostly work without loss of precision (with little loss of fit induced by the curvature of Earth). In other examples, objects may actually reside in high-dimensional spaces, and a projection to low dimensions may incur a large loss of fidelity. This loss is usually referred to as *strain*. A simple way to define strain is the metric MDS approach, in which we use the sum of the Euclidean distance of distances in the original space and the projected space:

$$\text{Strain} = \sum_{i<j} \left(d_{i,j} - z_{i,j}\right)^2$$

with $d_{i,j}$ being the distance between object i and j in the original space and $z_{i,j}$ the distance between objects i and j in the projected space. It is easy to compute a gradient and apply standard optimization algorithms to solve this problem. Note that the optimized solution lays out objects in the projected space relative to each other, so the solution is optimal up to rotation and mirroring. Examples of MDS are shown in Figures 19.2 and 19.5. Alternative projection approaches have gained a lot of traction in the field of machine learning, such as *t*-distributed stochastic neighborhood embedding (*t*-SNE; van der Maaten & Hinton, 2008). This approach does not optimize the projection error in the distances of all objects but in local neighborhoods and can thus create compelling visualizations in complex datasets.

Time-Series Clustering

When time series are subject to clustering, we need to select distance measures that capture temporal structure of the time series. In principle, we could simply treat a time series as a high-dimensional data point (with as many dimensions as the length of the time series) and use the Euclidean distance to evaluate their dissimilarity. In fact, this is often done to produce satisfactory results (e.g., see the example in Figure 19.2). However, one may encounter some problems with this approach (see Brandmaier, 2015). First, we would lose important information about the temporal dependency of measurements because we would treat all dimensions (i.e., time points) as independent. Second, we would not be able to compare time series of different lengths. Third, we would limit our notion of similarity to absolute quadratic differences among pairs of identical time points across objects. Even only slight lags, drift, outliers, or differences in process noise may easily obscure true similarities. Therefore, a host of different approaches have been suggested to model the similarity of time series (Liao, 2005; Montero & Vilar, 2014). Roughly, we can group them into different types of approaches: clustering based on a parametric time-series model (e.g., similarity of autoregressive process parameters), similarity in shape (e.g., the Euclidean distance), or structure (e.g., Fourier coefficients; Faloutsos, Ranganathan, & Manolopoulos, 1994), or clustering based on relative complexity (e.g., permutation distribution clustering; Brandmaier, 2015). A variety of dissimilarity measures have been proposed in the literature, and it is impossible to list them all (but see Liao, 2005; Montero & Vilar, 2014). Here, I list a selection of metrics that have useful properties for clustering mobile sensing data and seem to work well across different domains.

Dynamic Time Warping

The Euclidean distance is not robust against shifts in the time series. A simple one-lag shift of one time series versus another may result in very large dissimilarity estimates. In particular, such shifts may not only be global but also local, for example, if two time series are identical up to some local accelerations or decelerations of one of the two. This calls for elastic dissimilarity measures that can handle local and global distortions in time. Dynamic time warping (DTW; Berndt & Clifford, 1994) was designed to be invariant to those elastic differences. It is an algorithm matching each observation of one time series to an observation in the other time series in a monotonically increasing way, which means that several indices of one time series can be matched to a single one in the other time series (representing a local time warp) and no pair of matchings can cross. At the same time, the first indices and last indices always match. Figure 19.3 illustrates the difference between a Minkowski-type error measure (such as Euclidean distance) and DTW. The bottom time series was derived from the top time series by shifting it down by five units and by accelerating the signal between the third and sixth measurement. The DTW algorithm finds the optimal match satisfying all the restrictions with minimal cost, where the cost is the sum of absolute differences, for each matched pair of indices. Sometimes, DTW finds an optimal matching with extreme warps, such that most time points of one series are matched to only a few time points of the other. Extensions of the algorithm have been designed to avoid extreme warps by restricting warps to a maximum length (Sakoe & Chiba, 1978).

Symbolic Representations

Continuous time series may also be transformed into symbolic representations with the hope that symbolic analysis approaches can be exploited to find structure in these data, such as those from text mining or bioinformatics (e.g., hashing, Markov models, or prefix trees; Lin, Keogh, Wei, & Lonardi, 2007). Deriving symbolic representations from continuous observations is also called tokenization, quantization, or discretization, and there are a host of different approaches to choose from (Daw, Finney, & Tracy, 2003). Lin and colleagues (2007) have proposed a symbolic time-series representation called SAX to

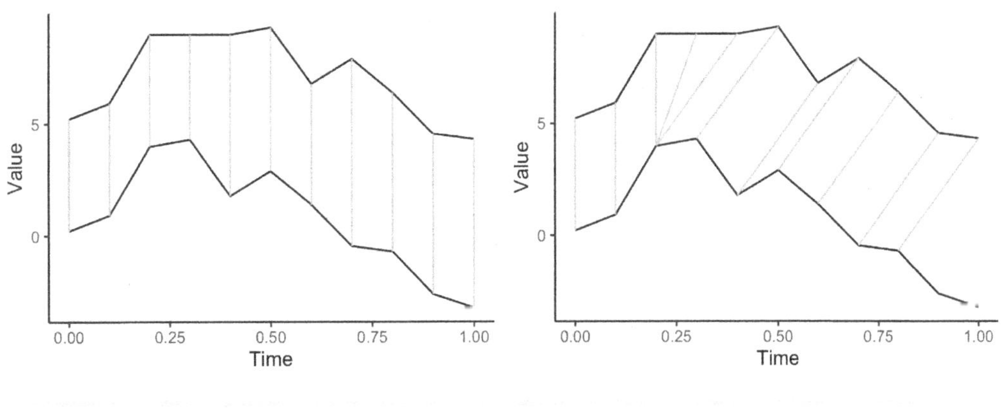

FIGURE 19.3. Schematic distances between time series. Left: A one-to-one mapping based on the distance of corresponding time points. The sum of the light gray lines corresponds to Manhattan distance, and the sum of the squared distances corresponds to the Euclidean distance. Right: Dynamic time-warping distance based on time-warped matching. The gray lines indicate how the upper time series is to be warped to best match the lower time series. This figure is available at https://github.com/brandmaier/mobile-sensing-figures under a CC-BY4.0 license.

allow for clustering, anomaly detection, motif discovery, and visualization of continuous time series in a symbolic space. First, the time series is divided into segments, and each segment is replaced by the average of its data points. This is called the piecewise approximate aggregation (PAA) of the time series. Then, the value of each segment is replaced by a symbol such that the "breakpoints" will produce equal-sized areas under a Gaussian curve. Using the algorithm requires choosing both the number of resulting symbols and the window size of the PAA.

Symbolic representations allow various techniques for matching strings. For example, longest common subsequence (LCS) finds the longest subsequence shared by two strings. For two strings ABDCBDBABCB and BBBDBAAAABC, the LCS is BDBA, and thus the similarity is the length of that common sequence, 4. This measure can be standardized to range between zero and one by dividing the subsequence length by the maximum of the length of each time series. Finally, one typically converts the standardized similarity metric into a dissimilarity metric by computing one minus the standardized length. Furthermore, some extensions to continuous time series use a threshold model to determine whether or not two observations match (Vlachos, Kollios, & Gunopulos, 2002). LCS belongs to the class of edit distance measures. Edit distances are those distances that compute the cost for turning one string into another by allowing insertions, deletions, and substitutions. LCS can be seen as an edit distance that allows deletions and insertions but no substitutions (to find the common substrings). Other well-known edit distances are the Hamming distance that counts the number of positions at which two strings are different (thus, it only allows substitutions to compute matching cost) and the Levenshtein distance that is successfully used in spelling correction, allowing all three operations to compute matching cost.

Permutation Distribution Clustering

To measure the complexity of a time series, Bandt and Pompe (2002) proposed *permutation entropy*—a single number that tells us the predictability of a time series based on the frequency of observed order patterns of a given length, *m*. The order pattern is simply the order of observed values (obtained as the sorting indices of the observed values) in windows of length *m* (see Figure 19.4). If we observe the values 5, 10, 8, 2, 1, the order pattern is 5-4-1-3-2. (The fifth value is the lowest, the fourth value is the second-lowest,

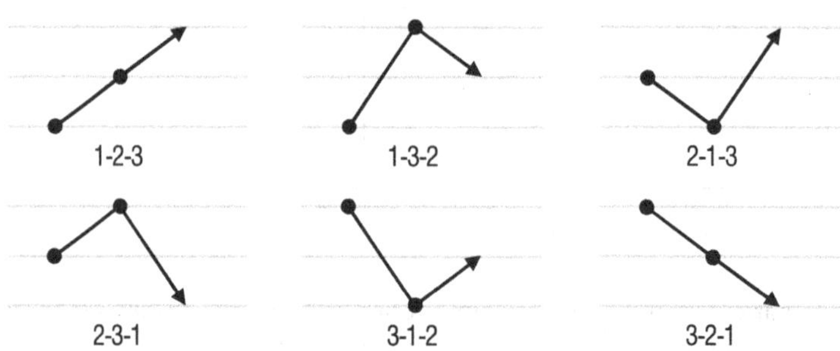

FIGURE 19.4. All six order patterns for embedding dimension 3. The panels show the schematic orders of three different values and the respective order pattern below. This figure is available at https://github.com/brandmaier/mobile-sensing-figures under a CC-BY4.0 license.

the first is the third-lowest, and so forth.) For windows of length m there are $m!$ different order patterns. The entropy of the order patterns yields an informative measure about the local predictability of a time series with some interesting properties. It is invariant to monotonous transformations of the time series, such as a changing mean or variance. In particular, the order patterns will be unchanged whether or not we normalize the time series. Also, extreme outliers play a much smaller role because no matter how far away they are, they only change a few local order patterns (if at all). Lastly, the order patterns can be computed in a single pass over the time series, which makes the approach highly efficient. Brandmaier (2015) proposed computing dissimilarities between permutation distributions to assess complexity-based similarity between time series resulting in *permutation distribution clustering* (PDC). To choose optimal values of the embedding dimension m and possibly a time lag t between observations, PDC provides an entropy-based heuristic. The entropy heuristic selects the embedding dimension such that the entropy of the resulting distributions is maximal. The result of PDC is a dissimilarity matrix based on the relative complexity of time series and is typically rendered as a hierarchical clustering diagram.

Differences between selected clusters can also be tested using a hypothesis testing framework based on multinomial likelihood ratio tests. Figure 19.5 shows an application of PDC to the raw sensor readings of accelerometer data from different activities. This is similar to the example given in Figure 19.2, in which the Euclidean distance was used to form clusters based on shape features of the time series. Here, however, the time series are clustered with respect to their similarity in permutation distributions. In this example, all activities (e.g., writing, standing, sitting, brushing teeth) were subject to clustering. As can be seen from both the dendrogram and the MDS, all eating- and drinking-related activities are close to each other (shown as polygons on the MDS plot), and the activities with low intensity are clustered together (e.g., sitting, standing, writing), even though the clustering algorithm was not exposed to this information.

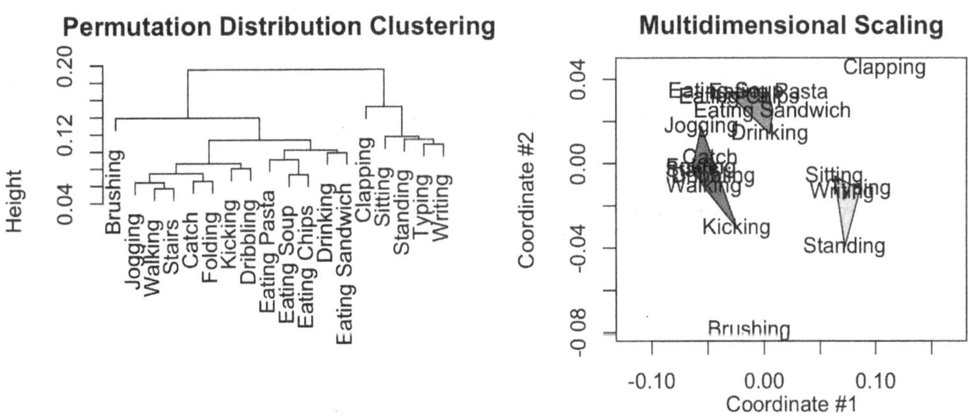

FIGURE 19.5. Left: Hierarchical clustering solution of everyday activities using permutation distribution clustering of one-dimensional accelerometer data from the WISDM dataset. Right: MDS projection of the solution on the left-hand side reveals compact clusters (polygons correspond to types of activity). This figure is available at https://github.com/brandmaier/mobile-sensing-figures under a CC-BY4.0 license.

Evaluating Clustering Algorithms

To evaluate cluster solutions, we can either resort to measures of internal or external validity. Measures of internal validity are heuristics that mostly relate the average similarity of cluster members to the average dissimilarity of members from different clusters. Internal validity is high if the average similarity among cluster members is high and their similarity to members of other clusters is low. However, these measures always remain heuristics because clusters, even though well separated, may not be useful for a given task. Measures of external validity evaluate how well a given clustering matches a known ground truth. Usually, we do not know the ground truth (this is why we apply unsupervised learning approaches after all) and measures of external validity are mostly important for studying the behavior of clustering in simulation studies or comparative studies. If some ground truth is available in practical applications (e.g., some labels are known in a dataset), one should rather switch to supervised learning approaches (see Chapter 17, this volume) than clustering. Finally, one may also be interested in the stability of a clustering algorithm, which can be assessed by the variability of the clustering solution over subsets (e.g., Ben-Hur, Elisseeff, & Guyon, 2001). In the following, I describe two heuristics for evaluating internal validity and three measures for evaluating external validity.

Internal Validity

The *silhouette width* is a measure of how similar an object is to members of its own cluster compared to members of other clusters and thus combines a measure of separation and compactness. Computation of silhouette requires computation of two interim values. For each object, we first compute the average distance to all members in its own cluster, $a(i)$. Second, we compute the average distance to all members of clusters it does not belong to, $b(i)$. Then, we define silhouette width as

$$s(i) = \frac{b(i) - a(i)}{\max\left[a(i), b(i)\right]}$$

Based on this definition, $s(i)$ ranges between –1 (object is well matched to its neighbors), and +1 (object is badly matched to its neighbors). For each cluster, we obtain the silhouette value as the average over the $s(i)$ values of its members. Like most distance-based measures, silhouette prefers spherical clusters; a recent extension promises to reduce this preference by emphasizing compactness over connectedness (Lengyel & Botta-Dukát, 2019).

Dunn Index

The *Dunn index* (Dunn, 1974) is defined as the ratio between the minimal intercluster distance to maximal intracluster distance. The goal of this index is to identify both dense and well-separated clusters. The index ranges between zero and infinity, and higher values indicate clustering solutions that are well separated. For each clustering solution, the Dunn index is calculated as follows:

$$D = \frac{\min\limits_{1 \le i \le j \le n} d_{\text{between}}(i, j)}{\max\limits_{1 \le i \le n} d_{\text{within}}(i)}$$

where $d_{\text{between}}(i, j)$ represents the intercluster distance between two clusters i and j of n clusters, and $d_{\text{within}}(i)$ is a measure of the intracluster distance. Both can be defined in various ways. A common choice is the distance of the cluster centroids for d_{between} and the maximal distance of any pair of members within a cluster as d_{within}.

External Validity

Good scores on an internal criterion do not necessarily translate into effectiveness for a given task, particularly because the same data may show different *interesting* clustering solutions. An alternative to the evaluation of internal criteria is a direct evaluation of a given problem for which ground truth is known. Cluster effectiveness can then be given with measures of external validity.

Purity

Assume we know the true clustering of objects into clusters. For a given clustering solution, let N_{ij} be the number of objects in cluster i that belong to true cluster j. Let N_i be the total number of objects in cluster i. Then, we can define the purity of a cluster as

$$p_i = \max_j \frac{N_{ij}}{N_i}$$

—that is, the proportion of cases in the majority class in the cluster. Then, let overall purity be the weighted sum of the cluster purities:

$$\text{Purity} = \sum_i \frac{N_i}{N} p_i$$

Purity ranges between 0 for bad clusterings and 1 for perfect clusterings. Note, however, that the trivial clustering (each object is its own cluster) always achieves perfect purity.

Rand Index

Another common summary statistic to quantify the overlap of partitions is the *Rand index* (Rand, 1971), also known as the *simple matching coefficient.* It can be used to assess the (dis)similarity of different clustering solutions or of a given clustering solution and a known ground truth. For a pair of clustering solutions X and Z, we first create a 2×2 contingency table. The following terminology assumes that Z is a ground truth reference, but the index can be applied to any set of two clusterings. Now, we count the number of pairs of objects that are in the same cluster in both X and Z (true positives [TP]); the number of pairs that are not in the same cluster in both X and Z (true negatives [TN]); the number of pairs that are in different clusters in X but in the same cluster in Z (false negatives [FN]); and the number of pairs that are in the same cluster in X but in different clusters in Z (false positives [FP]). Then, we compute the accuracy of the decisions to cluster pairs of objects correctly into the same or different clusters:

$$R = \frac{TP + TN}{TP + FP + FN + TN}$$

Like accuracy in classification, *TP* and *TN* are weighted equally, and other measures of classification performance such as the F-score can be employed (see Chapter 17, this volume). The Rand index is zero if both *TP* and *TN* are zero (and thus similar objects are never together in any cluster and only dissimilar objects are clustered together). The adjusted Rand index is also sometimes reported, where the Rand index is adjusted for the expected similarities based on a random model. Another related measure is the *Jaccard* index (Jaccard, 1912), which is similar to *R* but removes the *TN* from both numerator and denominator. Thus, the Jaccard index does not reward correctly putting dissimilar objects into dissimilar clusters (as measured by *TN*). This may be particularly useful when clusters are many and small.

Leave-One-Out Cross-Validation

To evaluate the clustering performance of an algorithm when a ground truth clustering is known, leave-one-out cross-validation (LOO-CV) is a robust method to assess the inherent structure of a dissimilarity matrix (Stone, 1974). LOO-CV iterates over the rows of a dissimilarity matrix, finds the closest neighbor for each object, and counts the frequency of matches, that is, the proportion of objects that have the same true group identity as their nearest neighbor.

Hidden Markov Models

In this chapter, we have regarded clustering methods to find patterns of similarity in time series. In mobile sensing applications, it can be useful to use the concept of dissimilarity in time series for time-series segmentation—most importantly, to find event boundaries, such as the beginning or end of an activity. A widely used approach for modeling streams of observations in applications such as speech recognition or activity recognition are *hidden Markov models.* A Markov chain describes the way a system moves through different discrete states over time. To form a Markov chain, we start by defining a finite set of states, for example, a set of different activities of interest (such as "walking" or "sleeping"). Markov models are probabilistic models that model dependence over time with the simplifying assumption that dependence on only the previous state is sufficient to model the process of interest. For a complete definition, we also need an initial state (or a distribution representing the probability of each state being the initial state) and a transition matrix that describes the probabilities with which the system either stays in the current state or moves to a given different state. Such Markov chains can be estimated by observing a system long enough (even though this only permits estimation of a single initial state) or by gathering multiple observations of the same system (allowing one to estimate a distribution over initial states). In both cases, we can estimate the transition matrix from data if the observed process is ergodic (which in this context roughly corresponds to the intuition that the process must not "get stuck" in some subchain and never return to the other states). All this assumes that we can directly observe the state of a system (e.g., a given activity).

Whenever the states are not directly observable, we can resort to *hidden Markov models* (HMMs). In HMMs, we still assume that the Markov assumption is true (the probability of transitioning from one state to another depends only on the current state), but the states are only indirectly measured with stochastic measurements. Each discrete state is associated with a probability density function that determines the likelihood of an observation (which may be multivariate), given that the system is in that state. For example, when the hidden states represent activity classes such as walking or sleeping, the observations could be the continuous sensor readings of a smartphone.

HMMs are similar to latent mixture models with the mixture components coupled over time. Assuming that the observations come from a multivariate normal distribution, an HMM is identical to a Gaussian mixture model in which we postulate that the system occasionally jumps from one state (that is, mixture component) to another as time evolves. Based on the Markov assumptions, we further assume that these jumps (or rather their probabilities) are fully described by a transition matrix.

In unsupervised learning challenges, we can use an HMM to infer underlying and unobserved states from a multivariate time series. For example, when we have no labels but only raw sensor data, we can use an HMM to infer the most likely sequence of underlying states. These states then represent a lower-dimensional representation than the observed, potentially multivariate signals, and they may be used as the primary unit for further analyses (see Figure 19.6). For example, we may then label the states post-hoc

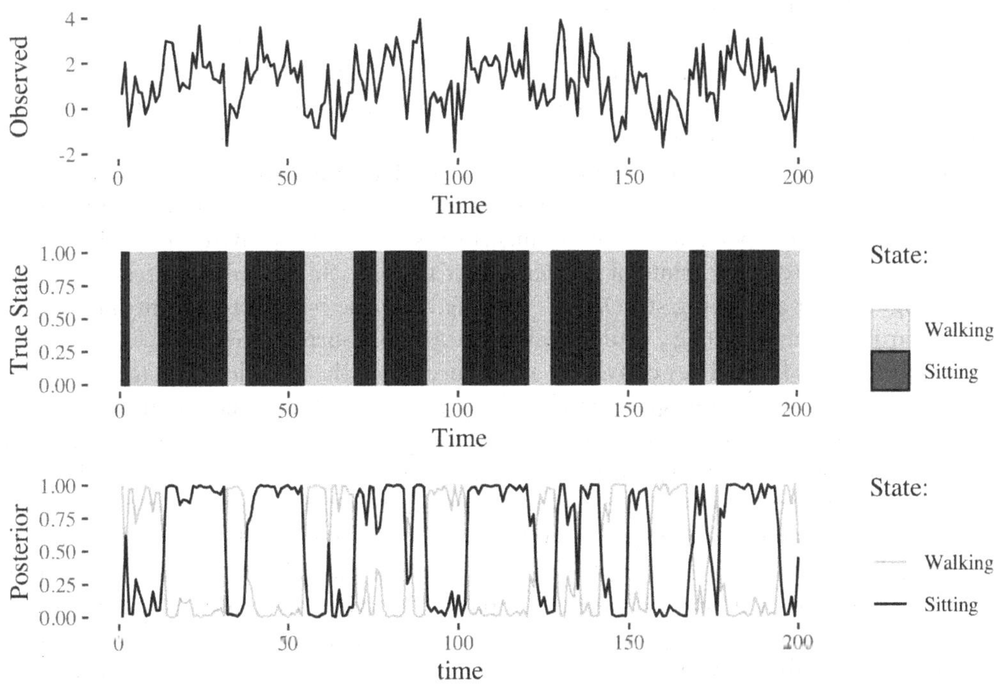

FIGURE 19.6. Estimated sequence of states from a hidden Markov model on a sequence of simulated, continuous sensor readings. The top row shows simulated sensor readings that were generated from a Gaussian distribution with a mean difference of two units between the two activities. The middle row shows the true states that were randomly drawn with a state switching probability of 90%. The bottom row shows the estimated posterior probabilities of being in the respective states. This figure is available at https://github.com/brandmaier/mobile-sensing-figures under a CC-BY4.0 license.

based on participants' self-reports or raters, or we may simply use them as a sparser level of description or make inferences about the (un)predictability of the person. A critical question is then the choice of the number of states because it cannot be directly inferred from the data (larger number of states will always lead to better fit on the training data). As usual, we may want to use some generalization criterion like the Bayesian information criterion (BIC) or cross-validation to determine the optimal number of states in an HMM (Murphy, 2012).

A recent extension of the HMM model allows for modeling non-Markovian dwell times in a given state. This can be achieved by modeling the dwell time in each state with a Poisson process, which is appropriate for modeling the number of events occurring in a fixed interval of time. Because the Poisson assumption makes the hidden state process non-Markovian, the resulting model class is called the hidden semi-Markov model (Yu, 2010).

Applications

A variety of research studies have been published involving mobile sensing data that use clustering, and some examples are presented here. For many applications, locating the user is valuable to infer their daily routines (e.g., whether they went shopping, went to work, or went out for sports) and their potential impact on psychological variables such as well-being or affect. While GPS and the signal strength of nearby routers provides spatial information, its inaccuracy ranges between 10 and 100 meters (up to about 110 yards) and makes it impossible to decide whether the device owner is, say, in a coffee shop or in the next-door clothing store. The SurroundSense approach (Azizyan, Constandache, & Roy Choudhury, 2009) uses ambient fingerprinting by leveraging sound, light, color, and movement patterns to obtain fingerprints of the user's environment. They used clustering to create fingerprints of accelerometer traces yielding three clusters of sitting, browsing (e.g., in a clothing store), and walking. Because users often point their phone downward while using it (e.g., while checking messages), SurroundSense takes pictures of the environment's floor. They converted all pictures from the same location (e.g., store) to a hue-luminance-saturation space and used *k*-means clustering to create ambient color-light fingerprints of places using the cluster centroids and sizes. To better understand users' movement and mobility patterns, Wang and colleagues (2018) used the DBSCAN algorithm to cluster the sampled coordinates during a day. The resulting clusters represented the users' significant locations and dwell times. Saeb and colleagues (2015) used a cluster analysis approach to determine places where the participants of their study spent most of their time, such as home, office, or park. They first divided GPS-based location data into stationary and transitional states based on estimates of movement speed (at a 1 kilometer/hour threshold). Then, they used *k*-means clustering to identify the clusters. To determine the number of clusters, starting with $k = 1$, they increased the number of clusters until the distance of the farthest point in each cluster to its cluster center fell below 500 meters. The number of clusters was then used as a feature for a subsequent prediction task, classifying people into depressed and nondepressed people. The best predictor of depression was roaming entropy, an index of the variability of the time participants spent at a given location. Roaming entropy was previously shown to be an excellent marker of developmental differences in both brain and behavior in an animal model (Freund et al.,

2013). To assess the social behavior of students on campus, Wang, Harari, Hao, Zhou, and Campbell (2015) investigated the partying versus nonpartying behavior of students by applying k-means clustering to audio signals (e.g., presence of music or chatter) and activity recordings (e.g., dancing). Based on the clustering solution, they conjectured that the audio features alone were sufficiently informative to discriminate party versus non-party times in the dataset.

DTW is typically applied to handwriting classification or speech recognition. Pham, Plötz, and Olivier (2010) demonstrated that DTW can be used to classify various low-level food preparation activities (such as chopping, peeling, slicing, dicing, scraping, shaving, scooping, stirring, coring, or spreading), while DTW can adjust for the individual differences in the speed with which these activities are executed (e.g., chopping vegetables fast versus slow).

Dobbins and Rawassizadeh (2018) used feature selection to refine accelerometer data in order to detect physical activity, arguing that smaller feature sets are computationally more efficient and thus more energy efficient on a mobile device. They used heuristics based on PCA and correlational statistics to select only those variables that largely contribute to the first principal components and remove those that are highly correlated with others to remove redundancy. Then, they evaluated *k*-means, hierarchical clustering, and DBSCAN on the selected features. Biswas and colleagues (2015) also used *k*-means clustering for preprocessing features for a subsequent classification task of fundamental human forearm movements using a wrist-worn sensor. For segmenting continuous data streams from wearable accelerometers, Kuppevelt and colleagues (2019) used hidden semi-Markov models, which they claim are much easier to interpret than complex temporal learning approaches such as deep neural networks.

R Packages

There are various R packages that implement unsupervised learning approaches. PCA is available as function `prcomp()` from the stats package, which is part of the base R installation (R Core Team, 2021). Various ICA implementations are available from the package `ica` (Helwig, 2018). The stats package also offers k-means clustering with the function `kmeans()` and hierarchical clustering with the function `hclust()`. The Comprehensive R Archive Network (CRAN) has a taskview that lists all major packages for clustering (*https://cran.r-project.org/web/views/Cluster.html*). The package `TSclust` (Montero & Vilar, 2014) offers various dissimilarity metrics for clustering time series, including an interface to permutation distribution clustering from package `pdc` (Brandmaier, 2015). The HMM in Figure 19.6 was estimated with the R package `depmixS4` (Visser & Speekenbrink, 2010).

Summary

This chapter reviews a variety of approaches that can be subsumed under the umbrella of time-series data mining or knowledge discovery in databases (Fayyad, Piatetsky-Shapiro, & Smyth, 1996). These approaches are useful to make sense of multivariate, intensive, and complex time-series data or features that were derived from time series (such as

Fourier coefficients, mean signal, or signal power). I would like to stress that there is no single best approach that promises success in all situations. The approaches presented in this chapter all make different assumptions about the data-generating process and need to be carefully chosen in accordance with the respective project and data-analytic goal. I reviewed approaches for dimensionality reduction that help to project multivariate datasets, and specifically those with time series, to lower dimensions, as well as clustering approaches that group together individual observations into those that are similar to each other in their inherent structure. Both groups of methods can be regarded as methods that aim to reduce the complexity of observed data such that we obtain simpler representations. Projection methods obtain simpler representations by reducing the complexity in the number of variables, and clustering methods obtain simpler representations by reducing the complexity in the number of observations. If we imagine our data arranged in a cube, we can also reduce complexity in a third dimension, namely, time. Those algorithms that define similarities between time series almost always implicitly reduce the complexity in time to solve the clustering problem. We can also explicitly use those algorithms to find simpler representations of time (for example, symbolic representations or order patterns). The hope is that simpler representations aid us in *understanding* the data by means of either inspection (such as visualization) or modeling, which may profit from simpler representations in terms of increased robustness and generalizability.

ACKNOWLEDGMENTS

I thank Julia Delius for editorial help on the manuscript and Michael Eid, Matthias Mehl, and Anna Elisabeth Riha for providing comments on an earlier version. All figures and their source code are available under free license at *https://github.com/brandmaier/mobile-sensing-figures.*

REFERENCES

Assent, I. (2012). Clustering high dimensional data. *Wiley Interdisciplinary Reviews: Data Mining and Knowledge Discovery, 2*(4), 340–350.

Azizyan, M., Constandache, I., & Roy Choudhury, R. (2009). Surroundsense: Mobile phone localization via ambience fingerprinting. In *Proceedings of the 15th Annual International Conference on Mobile Computing and Networking* (pp. 261–272). ACM.

Bandt, C., & Pompe, B. (2002). Permutation entropy: A natural complexity measure for time series. *Physical Review Letters, 88*(17), Article No. 174102.

Ben-Hur, A., Elisseeff, A., & Guyon, I. (2001). A stability based method for discovering structure in clustered data. In *Pacific Symposium on Biocomputing* (Vol. 7, pp. 6–17). World Scientific.

Berndt, D. J., & Clifford, J. (1994). Using dynamic time warping to find patterns in time series. In *Proceedings of the 3rd International Conference on Knowledge Discovery and Data Mining* (pp. 359–370). AAAI Press.

Biswas, D., Cranny, A., Gupta, N., Maharatna, K., Achner, J., Klemke, J., et al. (2015). Recognizing upper limb movements with wrist worn inertial sensors using k-means clustering classification. *Human Movement Science, 40,* 59–76.

Brandmaier, A. M. (2015). pdc: An R package for complexity-based clustering of time series. *Journal of Statistical Software, 67*(5), 1–23.

Daw, C. S., Finney, C. E. A., & Tracy, E. R. (2003). A review of symbolic analysis of experimental data. *Review of Scientific Instruments, 74*(2), 915–930.

Dobbins, C., & Rawassizadeh, R. (2018).

Towards clustering of mobile and smartwatch accelerometer data for physical activity recognition. *Informatics, 5*(2), Article No. 29.

Dunn, J. C. (1974). Well-separated clusters and optimal fuzzy partitions. *Journal of Cybernetics, 4*(1), 95–104.

Ester, M., Kriegel, H.-P., Sander, J., & Xu, X. (1996). A density-based algorithm for discovering clusters in large spatial databases with noise. In *Proceedings of the Second International Conference on Knowledge Discovery and Data Mining* (Vol. 96, pp. 226–231). AAAI Press.

Faloutsos, C., Ranganathan, M., & Manolopoulos, Y. (1994). Fast subsequence matching in time-series databases. In R. T. Snodgrass & M. Winslett (Eds.), *Proceedings of the 1994 ACM SIGMOD International Conference on Management of Data* (Vol. 23, pp. 419–429). ACM.

Fayyad, U. M., Piatetsky-Shapiro, G., & Smyth, P. (1996). Knowledge discovery and data mining: Towards a unifying framework. In *Proceedings of the Second International Conference on Knowledge Discovery and Data Mining* (pp. 82–88). AAAI Press.

Freund, J., Brandmaier, A. M., Lewejohann, L., Kirste, I., Kritzler, M., Krüger, A., et al. (2013). Emergence of individuality in genetically identical mice. *Science, 340*(6133), 756–759.

Helwig, N. E. (2018). *ica: Independent component analysis.* https://CRAN.R-project.org/package=ica

Hennig, C. (2020). Minkowski distances and standardisation for clustering and classification on high-dimensional data. In T. Imaizumi, A. Nakayama, & S. Yokoyama (Eds.), *Advanced studies in behavior metrics and data science: Essays in honor of Akinori Okada* (pp. 103–118). Springer.

Hotelling, H. (1933). Analysis of a complex of statistical variables into principal components. *Journal of Educational Psychology, 24*(6), 417–441.

Hyvärinen, A., & Oja, E. (2000). Independent component analysis: Algorithms and applications. *Neural Networks, 13*(4), 411–430.

Jaccard, P. (1912). The distribution of the flora in the alpine zone. *New Phytologist, 11*(2), 37–50.

Johnson, S. C. (1967). Hierarchical clustering schemes. *Psychometrika, 32*(3), 241–254.

Jolliff, I. (1986). *Principal component analysis.* Springer.

Jutten, C., & Herault, J. (1991). Blind separation of sources, part I: An adaptive algorithm based on neuromimetic architecture. *Signal Processing, 24*(1), 1–10.

Kaufman, L., & Rousseeuw, P. J. (1987). Clustering by means of medoids. In Y. Dodge (Ed.), *Statistical data analysis based on the L_1 norm and related methods* (pp. 405–416). North Holland.

Kobana, Y., Takahashi, J., Kitsunezaki, N., Tobe, Y., & Lopez, G. (2014). Detection of road damage using signals of smartphone-embedded accelerometer while cycling. In *Proceedings of the 2014 International Workshop on Web Intelligence and Smart Sensing* (pp. 1–2). ACM.

Kuppevelt, D. van, Heywood, J., Hamer, M., Sabia, S., Fitzsimons, E., & van Hees, V. (2019). Segmenting accelerometer data from daily life with unsupervised machine learning. *PLoS One, 14*(1), e0208692.

Lengyel, A., & Botta-Dukát, Z. (2019). Silhouette width using generalized mean: A flexible method for assessing clustering efficiency. *Ecology and Evolution, 9*(23), 13231–13243.

Liao, T. W. (2005). Clustering of time series data: A survey. *Pattern Recognition, 38*(11), 1857–1874.

Lin, J., Keogh, E., Wei, L., & Lonardi, S. (2007). Experiencing SAX: A novel symbolic representation of time series. *Data Mining and Knowledge Discovery, 15*(2), 107–144.

Linting, M., Meulman, J. J., Groenen, P. J., & van der Koojj, A. J. (2007). Nonlinear principal components analysis: Introduction and application. *Psychological Methods, 12*(3), 336–358.

Ma, S., & Huang, J. (2008). Penalized feature selection and classification in bioinformatics. *Briefings in Bioinformatics, 9*(5), 392–403.

MacQueen, J. B. (1967). Some methods for classification and analysis of multivariate observations. In M. L. Le Cam & J. Neyman (Eds.), *Proceedings of the Fifth Berkeley Symposium on Mathematical Statistics and Probability* (pp. 281–297). University of California Press.

Mantyjarvi, J., Himberg, J., & Seppanen, T. (2001). Recognizing human motion with multiple acceleration sensors. In *2001 IEEE International Conference on Systems, Man and Cybernetics. e-Systems and e-Man for*

Cybernetics in Cyberspace (Vol. 2, pp. 747–752). IEEE.

Montero, P., & Vilar, J. A. (2014). TSclust: An R package for time series clustering. *Journal of Statistical Software, 62*(1), 1–43.

Murphy, K. P. (2012). *Machine learning: A probabilistic perspective.* MIT Press.

Pearson, K. (1901). LIII. On lines and planes of closest fit to systems of points in space. *London, Edinburgh, and Dublin Philosophical Magazine and Journal of Science, 2*(11), 559–572.

Pham, C., Plötz, T., & Olivier, P. (2010). A dynamic time warping approach to real-time activity recognition for food preparation. In *International Joint Conference on Ambient Intelligence* (pp. 21–30). Springer.

R Core Team. (2021). *R: A language and environment for statistical computing.* R Foundation for Statistical Computing. www.R-project.org

Rand, W. M. (1971). Objective criteria for the evaluation of clustering methods. *Journal of the American Statistical Association, 66*(336), 846–850.

Saeb, S., Zhang, M., Karr, C. J., Schueller, S. M., Corden, M. E., Kording, K. P., & Mohr, D. C. (2015). Mobile phone sensor correlates of depressive symptom severity in daily-life behavior: An exploratory study. *Journal of Medical Internet Research, 17*(7), No. e175.

Sakoe, H., & Chiba, S. (1978). Dynamic programming algorithm optimization for spoken word recognition. *IEEE Transactions on Acoustics, Speech, and Signal Processing, 26*(1), 43–49.

Schubert, E., Sander, J., Ester, M., Kriegel, H. P., & Xu, X. (2017). DBSCAN revisited, revisited: Why and how you should (still) use DBSCAN. *ACM Transactions on Database Systems, 42*(3), Article No. 19.

Steinbach, M., Ertöz, L., & Kumar, V. (2004). The challenges of clustering high dimensional data. In L. T. Wille (Ed.), *New directions in statistical physics: Econophysics, bioinformatics, and pattern recognition* (pp. 273–309). Springer.

Stone, M. (1974). Cross-validatory choice and assessment of statistical predictions. *Journal of the Royal Statistical Society: Series B (Methodological), 36*(2), 111–133.

van der Maaten, L. & Hinton, G. (2008). Visualizing data using t-SNE. *Journal of Machine Learning Research, 9*, 2579–2605.

Visser, I., & Speekenbrink, M. (2010). depmixS4: An R package for hidden Markov models. *Journal of Statistical Software, 36*(7), 1–21.

Vlachos, M. (2010). Dimensionality reduction. In C. Sammut & G. I. Webb (Eds.), *Encyclopedia of machine learning* (pp. 274–279). Springer.

Vlachos, M., Kollios, G., & Gunopulos, D. (2002). Discovering similar multidimensional trajectories. In *Proceedings of the 18th International Conference on Data Engineering* (pp. 673–684). IEEE.

von Luxburg, U. (2007). A tutorial on spectral clustering. *Statistics and Computing, 17*(4), 395–416.

Wang, R., Harari, G., Hao, P., Zhou, X., & Campbell, A. T. (2015). SmartGPA: How smartphones can assess and predict academic performance of college students. In *Proceedings of the 2015 ACM International Joint Conference on Pervasive and Ubiquitous Computing* (pp. 295–306). ACM.

Wang, W., Harari, G. M., Wang, R., Müller, S. R., Mirjafari, S., Masaba, K., & Campbell, A. T. (2018). Sensing behavioral change over time: Using within-person variability features from mobile sensing to predict personality traits. *Proceedings of the ACM on Interactive, Mobile, Wearable and Ubiquitous Technologies, 2*(3), Article No. 141.

Yu, S.-Z. (2010). Hidden semi-Markov models. *Artificial Intelligence, 174*(2), 215–243.

Zou, H., Hastie, T., & Tibshirani, R. (2006). Sparse principal component analysis. *Journal of Computational and Graphical Statistics, 15*(2), 265–286.

Zou, H., & Xue, L. (2018). A selective overview of sparse principal component analysis. *Proceedings of the IEEE, 106*(8), 1311–1320.

PART IV

Mobile Sensing Applications in Psychological Science

CHAPTER 20

Mobile Sensing in Personality Science

Felix Beierle, Sandra C. Matz,
and Mathias Allemand

CHAPTER OVERVIEW

Advances in mobile technology and the ubiquity of the smartphone have allowed a deeper understanding of aspects of personality than is possible with traditional self-report methods. Mobile sensing allows us to track sensor measurements and device usage statistics that describe the environment and the behavior of the user. In this chapter, we give a detailed overview of the types of mobile sensing data available on smartphones and introduce a concrete example of an app showcasing how mobile sensing studies can be conducted in personality science. Furthermore, we give an extensive overview of existing studies, related to both relatively stable personality traits and variable personality states and dynamics. We summarize each study's core results and present an overview of the state of the art in the field. We conclude with a glimpse into future directions in the field of mobile sensing in personality science.

Introduction

Personality research can draw on a wide range of methods and measures to explore and better understand human personality in everyday life as well as in laboratory settings (Allemand & Mehl, 2017; Robins, Fraley, & Krueger, 2007; Wrzus & Mehl, 2015). In addition to traditional self-report questionnaires, recent advances in computational social science have highlighted the potential of predictive technologies that use the digital footprints created by individuals to automatically infer their personality using machine learning. One particular type of predictive technology that holds great promise for complementing the existing toolbox of personality researchers is mobile sensing. *Mobile sensing* refers to the utilization of digital devices (e.g., smartphones, tablets, smartwatches) and mobile sensors to collect data about individuals' daily behaviors and the situations they might encounter. For example, GPS sensors embedded in a variety of devices can provide granular insights into the whereabouts of individuals (e.g., visit to a coffee shop), the likely behaviors associated with specific locations (e.g., chat with friends), as well as the potential situational characteristics associated with these locations (e.g., social atmosphere).

Recent advances in computer technology, computer science, and software development have led to almost unlimited possibilities for mobile sensing when it comes to inferring personal characteristics about the owner and the environment (Boubiche, Imran, Maqsood, & Shoaib, 2019; Laport-López, Serrano, Bajo, & Campbell, 2020; Miller, 2012). Among all sensing devices, smartphones have taken on a particularly prominent role in our everyday lives: The rapid growth in popularity of smartphones across the globe, their increasing availability and decreasing costs have made them the most ubiquitous digital device in today's connected world (Verto Analytics, 2017). Because smartphones are an integral part of people's lives, this digital device is very attractive for collecting large amounts of sensing data in natural as well as laboratory settings. Smartphone sensing allows researchers to study inter- and intraindividual differences in human behavior on a large scale and at high levels of granularity using tools and techniques from computer and information sciences (Baumeister & Montag, 2019; Insel, 2017; Montag, Duke, & Markowetz, 2016; Seifert, Hofer, & Allemand, 2018; Yarkoni, 2012). Similarly, developments in statistical techniques and applications of computational methods such as machine learning—which are well suited to manage and analyze large amounts of data gathered from smartphone sensing studies—have contributed to the increasing interest in smartphone sensing within personality research (Bleidorn & Hopwood, 2019; Brandmaier, Chapter 17, this volume; Stachl, Pargent, et al., 2020).

There are at least two reasons why mobile sensing can meaningfully complement the existing toolbox of personality science. First, mobile sensing provides a unique method to automatically track daily behaviors and experiences across different life situations and contexts without requiring individuals to self-report on their subjective experiences and behaviors. Over time, such momentary assessments allow identification of stable patterns of experiences and behaviors, that is, personality traits. In other words, smartphone sensing is an innovative approach for unobtrusive, passive ambulatory assessments and complements ambulatory self-report assessments (Harari et al., 2016; Miller, 2012; Trull & Ebner-Priemer, 2014). Second, the wide range of built-in mobile sensors on smartphones allows researchers to extract a broad spectrum of potentially interesting person-centric behavioral information (e.g., activities, mobility patterns) and context-centric information (e.g., information about the surroundings and life contexts of the sensed person) (Harari et al., 2016; Laport-López et al., 2020). This gets us closer to the personality triad, which is about assessing persons, situations, and behaviors in concert (Funder, 2006). Moreover, the combination of sensing data with other types of data from personality research (e.g., observer reports, physiological assessments, experimental approaches) may lead to unique and novel perspectives on personality constructs, processes, and dynamics.

Although mobile sensing is an exciting and promising method for personality science, it is important to provide further evidence for the validity and reliability of this method. To ascertain that personality science reaps the full potential of mobile sensing in its endeavor to describe, explain, and predict individual differences, the idiosyncratic opportunities and challenges provided by mobile sensing technologies need to be better understood both theoretically and empirically. For example, it is crucial to show that sensing methods do not just work in isolation but can provide incremental external validity to the existing and established toolbox of personality research.

Scope of This Chapter

The majority of published mobile sensing studies to date have examined associations between smartphone-sensed information and self-reported personality traits. We build on this work to synthesize the existing work on personality traits and foreshadow interesting opportunities for future work focused on personality states. In line with a working definition by Baumert and colleagues (2017), we define personality traits as "relatively stable interindividual differences in the degree of coherent behaviors, thoughts, and feelings" (p. 528). Traits describe basic dimensions on which individuals are typically perceived to differ. These individual differences are often organized within the prominent conceptual framework of the Big Five, which includes five broad traits (cf. John, Naumann, & Soto, 2008): neuroticism (negative emotionality; Soto & John, 2017), extraversion, openness to experience (open-mindedness; Soto & John, 2017), agreeableness, and conscientiousness. In the context of mobile sensing studies, personality traits are typically measured with the help of self-report questionnaires that are administered before, during, or after the study period. In addition to personality traits, we also discuss links between smartphone sensing and how personality traits are expressed or manifested in given situations as states. Personality states reflect "the degree of coherent behaviors, thoughts, and feelings at a particular time" (Baumert et al., 2017, p. 528). Personality states are usually measured repeatedly over short periods of time. Whereas state levels can vary over short time periods, trait levels typically develop slowly or in rather persistent manners. Despite this temporal difference between traits and states, the content of states and traits can be identical. In this chapter, we use the term *personality states* in a broad sense that also includes affective states such as depressive states.

The main purpose of the current chapter is to discuss the potential of mobile sensing for personality science. First, we introduce a conceptual framework for the categorization of contextual sensing data for smartphone applications. Second, we discuss how mobile sensing contributes to personality assessment through behavioral data. Here, we present research on the prediction of individual differences in personality traits with smartphone sensor data as well as smartphone usage data. Third, we discuss the role of mobile sensing for research on personality dynamics such as personality states. Fourth, we illustrate how researchers can integrate mobile sensing into personality research using one smartphone application as an example. Fifth, we discuss the lessons learned from building and implementing such an application and highlight important future directions.

Categorization of Mobile Sensing Data

In computer science, the data that can be collected via mobile sensing are often referred to as context data. Context is typically defined as something that characterizes an entity relevant to the user or application (Dey, 2001). For example, a weather warning application will process the user's geolocation as context data. Context data can be used beyond the purpose of offering services to users. Specific context data sources or a combination of data sources can give insight into the user's behaviors, preferences, or personality traits. For example, the number of pictures taken or the usage of particular apps may yield important information about the user's context. A person taking many pictures and regularly checking Google Maps is likely spending time in a somewhat unfamiliar place that he or she enjoys.

In the following, we present a categorization framework based on context data (Beierle, Tran et al., 2018a, 2020), giving an overview of the types of data available from current Android smartphones (see Table 20.1). iOS devices (iPhones) typically do not make all of these data points available. The four context data categories are (1) physical conditions and activity, (2) device status and usage, (3) core functions usage, and (4) app usage. Furthermore, an additional technical category constitutes the explicit permission by the user to allow an app to access data from the given source.

TABLE 20.1. Context Data Framework for the Categorization of Context Data for Smartphone Applications

	Category				
	Physical	Device	Core functions	Apps	Permission
Location	•				•
Weather	•				(•)
Ambient light sensor	•				
Ambient noise level	•				•
Accelerometer	•				
Gyroscope	•				
Activity	•				
Steps	•				
Screen and lock state		•			
Headphone plug		•			
Battery and charging		•			
Wi-Fi		•			
Bluetooth		•			
Calls metadata			•		•
Music metadata			•		(•)
Photos metadata			•		•
Notifications metadata			•	•	•
App usage				•	•
App traffic				•	•

Note. The last column indicates if an explicit user permission is required (Android).

The category *physical conditions and activity* deals with the physical context of the user that is not related to the interaction with the smartphone. Here, sensors deliver data without the user interacting with the phone, for example, location or step count. The ambient light sensor typically offers data only when the screen is active (i.e., when the user is interacting with the phone). However, as the light sensor's data are related to the physical context (i.e., the light level of the environment of the user), we regard it as part of the physical category. The category *device status and usage* designates data related to the status and the connectivity of the smartphone. This comprises screen/lock state, headphone connection status, battery level and charging status as well as Wi-Fi and Bluetooth connectivity. *Core functions usage* deals with the users' interaction with core functionalities of the phone, regardless of which specific apps they are using for it. The core functions comprise calling, music listening, taking photos, and dealing with notifications. The fourth category, *app usage*, is concerned with data about the usage and traffic of specific apps. Notifications fit both in the core functions and the apps categories because they can be related to either. Overall, the four categories comprise data related to the user's surroundings and everyday behaviors as well as specific behaviors associated with phone usage. The permission column indicates if the user has to confirm an Android system permission to the app. Weather is given in parentheses because it can only be collected if the location is available, so it is bound to the location permission. Music is given in parentheses as well because most major music player apps or music streaming apps automatically broadcast metadata about music that the user is currently listening to. The broadcast events can be received by any app that subscribes as a listener. However, for Spotify, such broadcasting has to be activated manually. The context data sources given in Table 20.1 can be collected in studies conducted in daily life. Additional data can be gathered from mobile phones, (e.g., touch patterns or touch intensity; Carneiro, Pinheiro, & Novais, 2017). However, data points are only available when the developed app itself is in the foreground, not whenever any other app is being used. Such data sources can be used in more controlled lab studies that are specifically designed around a particular device and application (e.g., studying touch intensity).

Various other efforts have been made to categorize the data collected by mobile sensing (e.g., Harari et al., 2016; Laport-López et al., 2020), all of which provide their own unique insights into the nature of contextual sensor data. For example, one categorization framework discusses several types of smartphone sensing data along with their functions, features, and the behaviors they capture (Harari et al., 2016). According to this framework, smartphone data may capture three classes of behaviors including social interactions (e.g., microphone sensor, call log), daily activities (e.g., accelerometer sensor, proximity sensor), and mobility patterns (e.g., GPS scans, Wi-Fi scans).

Mobile Sensing and Personality Traits

The most prominent area of mobile sensing in personality research refers to personality assessment. Interesting research questions examined in past research include: Can individual differences in relatively stable patterns of behaviors and experiences be captured by mobile sensing? What are the sensing correlates of personality traits and other individual differences variables? Can personality traits predict the smartphone usage and the pattern of sensing? Previous work in this area can be discussed along two major lines.

The first line refers to *participatory sensing* and focuses on an active collection, and users' sharing, of data obtained by the sensors (Burke et al., 2006; Laport-López et al., 2020). Here, the user is actively involved in the sensing process and deliberately decides which information can be gathered and how to share it. The second major line of research is *opportunistic sensing* and refers to passive sensing with minimal user involvement (Lane et al., 2010; Laport-López et al., 2020). The user is not involved in the decision process because the sensing system itself decides when to gather and share information. Daily life smartphone studies typically fall in the category of opportunistic sensing, as the smartphone data correlated with psychological aspects about the user are sensed passively in the background.

The scientific exercise of translating mobile sensing data into personality profiles requires multiple steps. First, contextual data collected via smartphones has to be turned into features (a.k.a. predictors) that translate the raw input data (e.g., longitude and latitude coordinates from GPS) into more meaningful variables (e.g., distance traveled). This process can entail simple calculations of distribution parameters (e.g., number of times social networking apps were opened during weekends or average estimated sleep duration), as well as more complex metrics such as routine patterns or usage over time (e.g., the extent to which a user is switching between different apps).

In addition to these contextual data, researchers also need "labels"—or ground truth data—which indicate personality traits and other individual differences. Such data are usually assessed via the existing toolbox of personality researchers, most frequently with established self-reports or observer reports. A typical study, for example, would ask participants to respond to a battery of personality tests and then ask for permission to either retrospectively or prospectively collect their associated smartphone sensor data. Once the two data sources have been collected, researchers can start investigating the relationships between the features obtained by mobile sensing and the label obtained by self-reports or observer reports.

In the following section, we provide an overview of existing studies examining the links between mobile sensing data and personality traits as well as other trait-like characteristics (e.g., depressive tendencies; see Table 20.2). We focus our overview on studies that dealt with relatively stable individual differences in thoughts, feelings, and behaviors (Baumert et al., 2017). Note that the first two studies were conducted with feature phones, before the advent of smartphones (Chittaranjan, Blom, & Gatica-Perez, 2011, 2013). There are some additional studies correlating personality traits and phone usage that did not collect data from feature or smartphones but relied on self-reports of users (Butt & Phillips, 2008).

The data sources given in the table differ in the extent to which they are based on raw sensor data or have been preprocessed into more meaningful latent features. For example, accelerometer data are low-level sensor data, while the current activity (e.g., walking, in car) or a daily step count is higher-level sensor data that utilize accelerometer data. The available data sources depend on the mobile operating systems and on the available libraries and software development kits (SDKs). In the table, we list the sources mentioned in the cited papers. Predicting user's personality often requires that researchers turn lower-level sensor data into more meaningful higher-level features, such as estimating the user's sleep pattern from low-level sensor data like phone lock/unlock events. For overviews related to determining higher-level features from lower-level sensor data, see, for example, Harari and colleagues (2016); Harari, Müller, Aung, and Rentfrow

(2017); Mohr, Zhang, and Schueller (2017). While some of the studies are only interested in specific data types, others track a wider range of data sources.

As the comment column in Table 20.2 shows, the research focus of the studies often varies. Even comparing those studies that seek to predict personality from smartphone sensing data is not as straightforward as one might think. A variety of different statistical and machine learning-based approaches is used, along with different evaluation metrics. For example, sometimes the prediction is made into a binary classification problem (low/high values of each trait), sometimes into a three-class problem (low/medium/high). Another approach is to use regression to predict the score for each trait. In addition, small sample sizes, potentially biased datasets, and use of different data sources make it hard to draw overall conclusions. The studies often vary greatly in their reported accuracies for prediction personality from sensing data. While some report modest prediction success for multiple personality traits, including extraversion, openness, conscientiousness, and some facets of emotional stability (Stachl, Au, et al., 2020), others only report accuracies better than baseline for the trait of extraversion (Mønsted, Mollgaard, & Mathiesen, 2018).

Moving beyond mere predictive accuracies to studying the relationships between individual sensing features and personality traits, we see that research has highlighted the links between extraversion and social behaviors, including increased smartphone usage, receiving more calls (Chittaranjan et al., 2013), and daily screen wakeups (Beierle, Probst, et al., 2020), as well as a higher number of calls and higher use of photography apps (Stachl et al., 2017). Conscientiousness was found to be associated with higher usage of work email, but with lower usage of YouTube, fewer voice calls (Chittaranjan et al., 2013), as well as low usage of gaming apps (Stachl et al., 2017) and a shorter mean session duration of general smartphone usage (Beierle, Probst, et al., 2020). Individuals who score high on agreeableness tended to have more calls in general, while individuals with high emotional stability had a higher number of incoming SMS (Chittaranjan et al., 2013) but a lower number of screen wakeups. Women with high scores on openness demonstrated greater usage of video/audio/music (Chittaranjan et al., 2013).

We want to highlight one of the most recent studies in the context of predicting personality traits from smartphone sensing, which combined a relatively large sample (N = 624) with a broad variety of data sources and features (see Stachl, Au, et al., 2019, 2020). The study found the highest predictability for extraversion (r median = .37), no predictability for agreeableness, and moderate levels of accuracy for the other traits. The features that were most predominantly related to extraversion are related to communication behavior (based on call, message, and communication app usage logs), supporting the social nature of the trait; for openness it was a diverse mix of indicators based on app usage, music listening, and communication behavior, potentially highlighting the fact that openness by definition is associated with a preference for variety. Conscientiousness was related to indicators of daily routine and app usage, which is well aligned with the tendency of conscientious people to favor order over spontaneity. Only some facets of emotional stability (converse of neuroticism/negative emotionality) could be predicted, for example, by indicators related to communication, and among others, usage of email and gaming apps.

In summary, extraversion is the personality trait that has repeatedly been shown to have the strongest correlation with smartphone data. Considering the social nature of the extraversion trait, as well as the fact that many smartphone features were specifically

TABLE 20.2. Overview of Data Sources and Personality Traits/Trait-Like Characteristics (User Information) That Were Correlated in Related Studies

Data source	User information	Reference[b]	Sample size	Comment
Application usage (pre-smartphone), Bluetooth, calling profiles, calls, SMS	Personality traits	Chittaranjan et al. (2011)	83	Predicting personality traits based on smartphone data via SVM; highest classification accuracy for extraversion (75.9%)
Application usage (pre-smartphone), Bluetooth, calling profiles, calls, SMS	Personality traits	Chittaranjan et al. (2013)	117	Feature aggregation for personality prediction; gender-specific classification models
Calls, location, SMS	Personality traits	de Montjoye, Quoidbach, Robic, & Pentland (2013)	69	Predicting personality traits based on CDRs (call data record; data mobile carriers have about their customers)
Calls, SMS	Personality traits	Montag et al. (2014)	49	Calling and SMS usage; extraversion was positively correlated
WhatsApp usage	Age, gender, education, personality traits	Montag et al. (2015)	2,418	WhatsApp accounts for almost 20% of smartphone use; extraversion positively associated with daily WhatsApp use; conscientiousness inverse correlation
Location	Personality traits	Chorley, Whitaker, and Allen (2015)	174	Significant correlations for conscientiousness, openness, and neuroticism and foursquare location venue check-in
Display state, location	Depression	Saeb et al. (2015)	28	Predicting depressive symptoms (PHQ-9) in binary classification with accuracy of 86.5%; regression model has an average error of 23.5%
Installed apps	Personality traits	Xu, Frey, Fleisch, and Ilic (2016)	2,043	Predicting personality traits based on installed apps with 65% higher precision than random guess
Location	Social anxiety	Huang et al. (2016)	18	Development of tracking framework; significant correlation between social anxiety levels and places students visited and location transitions
App usage, Bluetooth, calls, location	Sociability	Eskes, Spruit, Brinkkemper, Vorstman, and Kas (2016)	10	Development of a framework for creating measurements of sociability based on mobile sensing data
Calls, location, SMS	Cooperation attitude	Singh and Agarwal (2016)	54	Mobile sensing data significantly associated with user's cooperation attitudes; mobile sensing predictive model performs significantly better than demography-based model
App usage, notification metadata	Depression	Mehrotra, Hendley, and Musolesi (2016)	25	Using mobile sensing to improve depressive symptom prediction
Technology usage times	Personality traits	Grover and Mark (2017)	62	Temporal patterns of smartphone and PC use; some features highly correlated with personality traits; machine learning model classifies extraversion, openness, agreeableness, and neuroticism

App usage	Personality traits	Stachl et al. (2017)	137	Personality traits predict smartphone use in specific app categories; extraversion, conscientiousness, and agreeableness are better predictors than basic demographic variables
Calls, SMS	Social capital	Singh and Ghosh (2017)	55	Highly accurate inferring of user's bridging, bonding, and overall social capital scores
Calls, location, SMS	Social anxiety	Boukhechba et al. (2017)	54	Assess and predict social anxiety of college students based on mobility and communication patterns; prediction of social anxiety level with an accuracy of up to 85%
Location	Personality traits	Kim, Koo, and Song (2018)	20	Preference for a home location is positively related with extraversion, and negatively related to conscientiousness; preference for home location is negative at night and positive during the daytime for neuroticism
Bluetooth, calls, location, SMS	Personality traits	Mønsted et al. (2018)	636	Only extraversion is predicted significantly better (25.6%) than by a null model, based on classification in three classes (low, medium, high)
Location, microphone (ambient sound, ambient voice), phone usage, physical activity	Personality traits	Wang et al. (2018)	159	Predicting self-reported personality traits with within-person variability in behavioral patterns based on passive mobile sensing data
App usage, calls, location	Sensation seeking	Schoedel et al. (2018)	260	Predicting sensation seeking based on mobile sensing data; limited prediction accuracies
App usage, battery status, Bluetooth, calls, display state, location, photo metadata, SMS, Wi-Fi	Personality traits	Stachl, Au, et al., (2019; 2020)	624	Predicting personality traits and facets based on mobile sensing data; using six categories of behavioral information (communication/social, music, app usage, mobility, phone activity, day- and nighttime activity)
Calls	Personality traits	Montag et al. (2019)	106	Presenting an app for mobile sensing and personality science; validation study with calls and personality; positive association of extraversion and calls; negative association between neuroticism and incoming calls
Calls, media app usage, messaging app usage, SMS	Sociability	Harari et al. (2020)	926[a]	Mapping measured sociability to self-reports
Phone usage	Personality traits	Beierle, Probst, et al. (2020)	526	Conscientiousness negatively associated with mean smartphone usage session duration; extraversion and neuroticism positively associated with frequency of smartphone use
App usage	Personality traits	Peltonen et al. (2020)	739	Category-level aggregated app usage predicts personality traits with up to 86–96% prediction fit

[a]Combined dataset from four studies. [b]The references were sorted chronologically.

designed to facilitate social interactions, this result aligns well with personality theory. The limited predictability of personality traits from smartphone sensing data might be attributed to individual differences in how personality traits are expressed in relation to what the smartphone can capture. Furthermore, smartphones, their sensors, and apps are constantly evolving, which might also explain different results in different studies.

Mobile Sensing and Personality States and Dynamics

While most of the research to date has focused on the prediction of personality traits, mobile sensing also is likely to become more prominent in the study of personality processes and states. Indeed, the fact that smartphones can collect data continuously over time and often capture context that might hold information about the individual's current mindset, make them the ideal candidate for assessing psychological states. Leveraging this technology for momentary assessments of personality experiences opens the door for a whole range of novel research questions: Can mobile sensing be used to reliably and validly capture an individual's momentary behaviors, thoughts, and feelings on a within-person level? Are mobile sensing indicators predictive for variability in personality states? Can information about a person's context provide information about their current psychological state as theorized in the personality triad model developed by Funder (2006)? In contrast to personality traits, personality states are not assessed as a one-time measure but are continuously tracked over short periods of time (e.g., a week) to study fluctuations of personality expressions within individuals.

From a data perspective, this means that in order to predict personality states from sensing data, researchers first need to collect repeatedly labeled data, which make it possible to relate certain activities through mobile sensing to the self-reported subjective experience of that individual in a given moment. For example, imagine a personality dynamics questionnaire that, every evening, lets users reflect on their feelings and experiences from that day or other measures of states with multiple assessments per day (e.g., Finnigan & Vazire, 2018; Horstmann & Ziegler, 2020; Matz & Harari, 2020; Zimmermann et al., 2019). Once these data have been collected, the features extracted from the mobile sensing data for that particular day—or features comparing today's data to those of previous days—can subsequently be used to predict how that individual feels in that moment. For example, do individuals exhibit extraverted behavior when they have spent more or less time in coffee shops? Do they feel more or less agreeable after having chatted with their friends and family? Or do they feel more neurotic on days on which they have spent a large amount of time on online social networks?

Table 20.3 lists currently available studies that investigated the relationships between mobile sensing data and dynamic psychological aspects about the user that change or vary over time. Such change can be over rather short time frames (e.g., momentary thoughts, feelings, and behaviors) to hours, daily changes, or 14-day intervals (some of depression-related studies; e.g., Farhan et al., 2016). With respect to the collection of data, this means that users have to spend more effort on responding to multiple short surveys over time (which effectively is the manual annotation ("labeling") of the collected smartphone context data). Given the extra burden on participants and the additional costs to researchers, it is not surprising that the sample sizes for longitudinal within-person studies of psychological states are lower than those for between-person studies of personality traits. The majority of existing studies in the context of predicting psychological states has focused on mental health and well-being-related constructs such as mood, depression, or stress.

Some of the studies listed in Table 20.3 find strong correlations between smartphone sensing data, and mental health or well-being-related constructs, whereas others find only limited correlations or predictability. The use of different sensor data sources and often modest sample sizes could be two reasons for these differing results. A common theme of interest to several of the listed papers is (improving) the user's automatic recognition of mental states. To the best of our knowledge, only one study so far has explored the links between smartphone sensing indicators and usage logs and within-person variability in state manifestations or expressions of the Big Five traits (Rüegger et al., 2020). A set of behavioral and situational indicators was first compiled based on existing literature. This set of sensing indicators was then applied to an ambulatory assessment dataset ($N = 316$ Android users) consisting of self-reported personality states that were assessed randomly four times per day across one week. The results of machine learning analyses investigating the predictability of personality states from the set of indicators have shown that only for extraversion, smartphone data—specifically ambient noise levels—were informative beyond what could be predicted based on time and day of the week alone (Rüegger et al., 2020).

To summarize, while quite a few studies combine mobile sensing and self-reported levels of depression, stress, mood, and the like, only initial work has been done on the smartphone data and the expression of personality states specifically.

The TYDR Application for Mobile Sensing: A Case Study

In this section, we illustrate how this all works using one specific mobile sensing application. The Track Your Daily Routine (TYDR) app combines mobile sensing and personality assessment (Beierle, Tran, et al., 2018b; 2020). From a user perspective, TYDR's core ideas are to provide descriptive statistics about the sensing data that are collected via the app and to visualize the results of personality traits and states questionnaires. TYDR is available on Google Play for Android smartphones.[1] The focus on Android devices is a result of the more generous permissions for data collection compared to iOS. However, given that there are only marginal differences in personality between Android and iOS users (Götz, Stieger, & Reips, 2017), the general tendencies and relationships reported for Android users are likely to generalize to iOS users. Researchers should keep in mind, however, that the data volume needed to train robust predictive models for individuals or groups of individuals might be harder to achieve for iOS users.

Several important aspects should be considered when developing a mobile sensing app like TYDR. The more individuals can be attracted to use an application and the more data these individuals generate on a continuous basis, the more reliable the results about the relationship between smartphone data and the user's personality will be. Consequently, the app should have an appealing interface and provide value for the users, not just the researchers. This can often happen in the form of feedback that allows users to make sense of the data they generate and to better understand themselves and their daily

TABLE 20.3. Studies of the Relationships Between Mobile Sensing Data and Dynamic Psychological User Aspects That Change or Vary Over Time

Data source	User information	Reference[a]	Sample size	Comment
Accelerometer, Bluetooth, location	Emotions/ affective states	Rachuri et al. (2010)	12	Showcases mobile phone software; recognizes user's emotions by locally running classifiers
App usage, calls, email, location, SMS, websites	Mood/affective states	LiKamWa, Liu, Lane, & Zhong (2013)	32	Smartphone app that infers the user's mood based on sensing data; initial accuracy of 66%; with a personalized model and 2 months data 93% accuracy
Bluetooth, calls, SMS, weather	Daily stress	Bogomolov, Lepri, Ferron, Pianesi, & Pentland (2014)	117	Daily stress level recognition; person-independent multifactorial statistical model with accuracy score of 72.28% for a two-class problem
Location	Depressive states	Canzian & Musolesi (2015)	28	Significant correlation between mobility trace characteristics and depressive mood; successfully predicting changes in depressive mood
Calls, location, SMS	Stress, depression, loneliness	Ben-Zeev, Scherer, Wang, Xie, and Campbell (2015)	47	Association between sensing data and daily stress levels, changes in depression, changes in loneliness
App usage, calls, display state, light sensor, microphone, network, traffic, physical activity, SMS	Stress	Stütz et al. (2015)	15	Significant correlations between smartphone sensing data and stress scores
Accelerometer, app usage, calls, display state, SMS	Mood/affective states	Becker et al. (2016)	27	Predicting mood with mobile sensing data; prediction performance increases with personalized models; only slightly better performance than a mean model
Accelerometer, app usage, calls, display state, photo metadata, SMS	Mood/affective states	Asselbergs et al. (2016)	27	Predicting 55–76% of EMA mood scores; performance significantly inferior to naive benchmark models
Location, physical activity	Depressive states	Farhan et al. (2016)	79	Prediction of clinical depression with good accuracy; best accuracy by combining sensing data and PHQ-9 scores
App usage, calls, display	Depressive states, anxiety, stress	Hung, Yang, Chang, Chiang, and Chen (2016)	18	Predicting negative emotions with mobile sensing with an accuracy of 86.17%

Location	Depressive states	Saeb, Lattie, Schueller, Kording, and Mohr (2016)	48	Location features were significantly correlated with PHQ-9 scores; stronger relationship for weekend compared to weekday
Accelerometer, keypress entry time	Depressive states	Cao et al. (2017)	20	Measuring typing behavior of users with bipolar affective disorder; 90.31% prediction accuracy on the depression score for typing sessions
App usage, Bluetooth, calls, location, physical activity, SMS, Wi-Fi	Emotions/affective states	Sun, Ma, Zhang, Liu, and Liu (2017)	10	Detection of the user's emotions based on sensing data; addressing the cold-start problem (having no data about new users); by employing transfer learning, a high accuracy with few labeled samples is achieved
Location, notification metadata, physical activity	Mood/affective states	Mehrotra, Tsapeli, Hendley, and Musolesi (2017)	28	Study shows causal impact emotions have on phone use; use of specific apps reflects user context and in turn impacts happiness and stress levels
Accelerometer, app usage, calls, compass, display state, gyroscope, light sensor, location, microphone, Wi-Fi, SMS	Compound emotion/ affective states	Zhang, Li, Chen, and Lu (2018)	30	Compound emotion (set of multiple basic emotions) detection via smartphone sensors; self-reported emotional states show high correlation with sensing data; app that recognizes the user's compound emotion in 76% of cases
Accelerometer, app usage, display state, light sensor, microphone, Wi-Fi	Mood instability/ affective states	Zhang et al. (2019)	68	Detecting mood instability via sensing with minimal user effort; employing classifier trained with data from study; outperforming baseline classifiers
Location	Stress	Pryss et al. (2019)	77	Presents app for mobile crowdsourcing of stress levels; predicts stress based on GPS location data
Accelerometer, Bluetooth, calls, location, microphone	Personality states	Rüegger et al. (2020)	316	Prediction of personality states from sensing data; only extraversion benefits from sensing data in prediction model, compared to using time and day of week alone
Location	Mood, affect, depression, loneliness	Müller, Peters, Matz, Wang, and Harari (2020)	1,765	Movement patterns and places visited are associated with subjective well-being at the between- and within-person levels; distance traveled is related to anxiety, affect, and stress; irregularity is related to depression and loneliness; spending time in social places is negatively associated with loneliness

[a]The references were sorted chronologically.

experiences. When developing for a mobile device, it is important to consider the restrictions these devices pose, including battery capacity and space limitations. In the following, we detail how TYDR makes the data tracking its core feature by processing and visualizing resulting insights for the user. The three main components of TYDR's user interface are the main screen, the questionnaires the users can fill out and their results, and the permanent notification.

The first main component of TYDR is its main screen. Figure 20.1a shows the main screen after TYDR is started for the first time. The tile-based design gives the user an immediate overview of the data for the current day. The gray overlay with the "Grant Permission" buttons indicates missing permissions that the user has to give in order to see more statistics, giving the user full control in deciding which data they are willing to share in return for additional insights. Each tile can be touched to slide open a bigger tile with a more detailed view of the data. Figure 20.1b shows more detailed information on location data after touching the corresponding tile. The visited locations are visualized on a map. The stay points (i.e., staying more than 20 minutes at one place) are indicated by a marker. Pressing the "Full Map" button shows the full-screen view of the day's location history and related data such as weather (see Figure 20.1c). Figure 20.1d shows the usage times for the past week. This tile is shown after the small "Usage" tile on the main screen is touched. Similarly, Figure 20.1e shows the number of photos taken, distinguished by front and back camera screens. Figure 20.1f shows how persons using the calendar function can access data from previous days (the top-right icon of the main screen). Not shown in these screenshots are additional tiles related to call statistics, music statistics, steps taken, the most used apps, apps with most traffic, and the number of notifications per app. The related statistics are visualized in a similar way as the shown examples.

The second main component of TYDR is the personality assessment. Via the self-report questionnaire, the collected context data are labeled with personality information given by the user. TYDR can be used to study both personality traits and personality dynamics as the state expression of personality traits. TYDR contains three self-report questionnaires. The first one is a demographic questionnaire asking for age, gender, level of education, and so on. The second one assesses personality traits. For this questionnaire, the Big Five Inventory 2 (BFI-2) questionnaire (Soto & John, 2017) is used, consisting of 60 items. Each of the five traits is assessed with 12 items based on a 5-point Likert scale, ranging from 1 (*strongly disagree*) to 5 (*strongly agree*). For researching personality dynamics, TYDR integrates a personality states questionnaire. TYDR utilizes the PDD (Personality Dynamics Diary) questionnaire, which captures the user's experience of daily situations and behaviors (Zimmermann et al., 2019). The PDD questionnaire can be regarded as an example for conducting personality dynamics studies. PDD could be replaced with any other state-related questionnaire assessing personality states (Finnigan & Vazire, 2018; Horstmann & Ziegler, 2020) and other state-like aspects about the user or the context (Matz & Harari, 2020).

TYDR displays only one question at a time, which avoids scrolling. Users can switch between apps or turn off the screen and continue where they left off when resuming TYDR. A progress bar indicates how much of the current questionnaire is already filled out. The incentive for the user to fill out the personality questionnaires is to see their results in the related tile. Figure 20.2a shows the questionnaire interface. Figure 20.2b

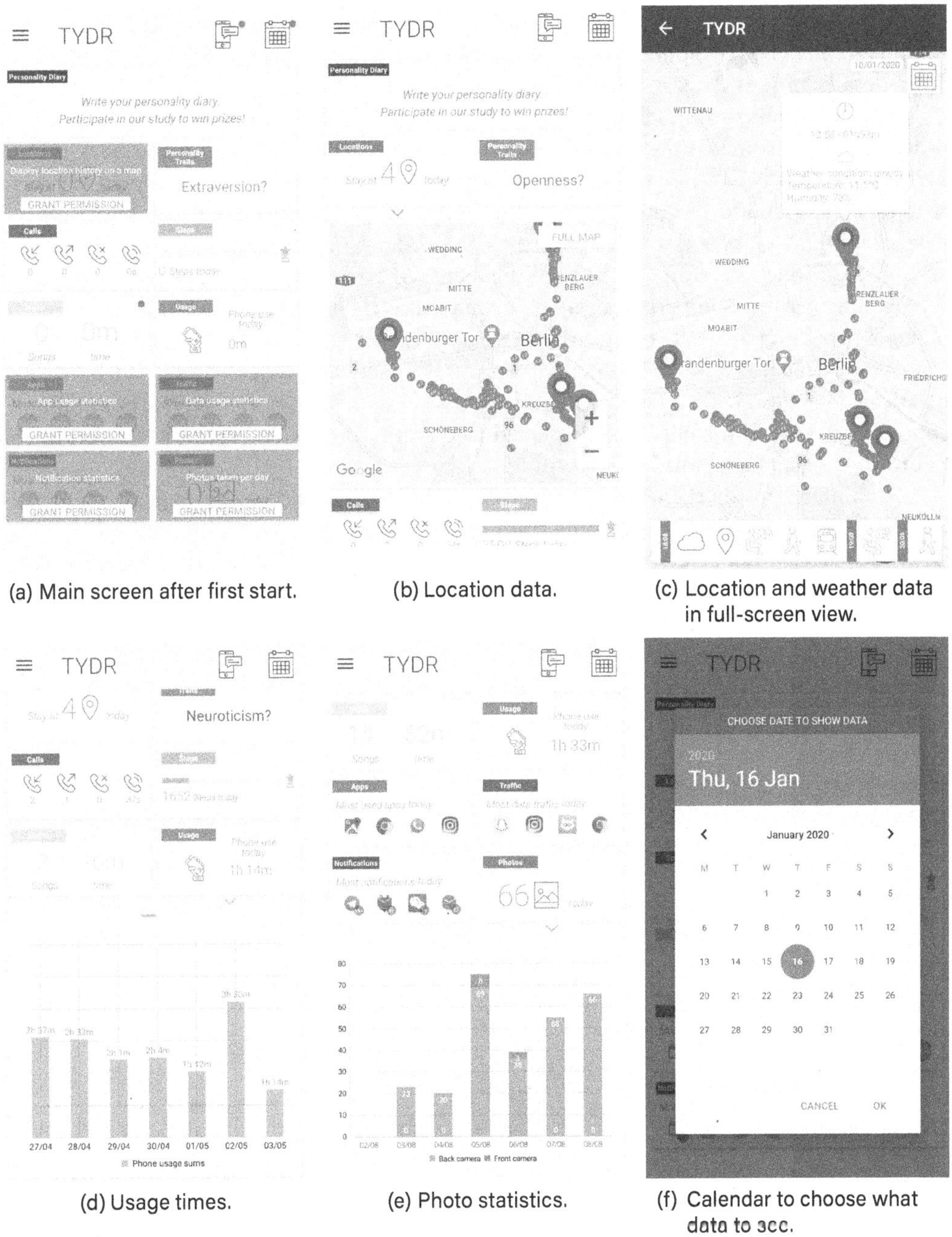

(a) Main screen after first start.

(b) Location data.

(c) Location and weather data in full-screen view.

(d) Usage times.

(e) Photo statistics.

(f) Calendar to choose what data to see.

FIGURE 20.1. TYDR main screen and sensor and usage statistics. (a) Main screen after first start; (b) location data; (c) location and weather data in full-screen view; (d) usage times; (e) photo statistics; (f) calendar to choose what data to see.

shows the extended tile shown after completing the questionnaire and touching the "Personality Traits" tile. Tapping on the "More Details" button opens a full-screen view with more details about the user's personality; see Figure 20.2c.

The third main component of TYDR is the customizable permanent notification. In order to collect some of the context data, TYDR has to be running in the background permanently. This can be a nontrivial challenge from a software development perspective, especially due to fragmentation, which refers to the multitude of different Android devices with different software and hardware specifications. One way to help ensure that an app is not being terminated is to implement a permanent notification that means a TYDR notification will permanently be displayed to the user in the notification area. To make it appealing, TYDR follows the same approach as that for the main screen: showing the user meaningful and informative figures based on processed context data. The notification is designed to be adaptive to the user's interests by offering the possibility of configuring what information is displayed (see Figure 20.3). The Preview section in the figure shows what the notification will look like.

A similar app for the combination of mobile sensing and psychological research is Insights.[2] Similar to TYDR, Insights tracks a variety of data sources (contact list, calls, SMS, display state, battery state, installed apps, app usage, location, and data traffic; Montag et al., 2019). In addition, researchers have developed software frameworks or libraries that aid other researchers in implementing apps for conducting studies related to the collection of mobile context data. Sensus (Xiong, Huang, Barnes, & Gerber, 2016), LiveLabs (Jayarajah, Balan, Radhakrishnan, Misra, & Lee, 2016), and AWARE (Ferreira, Kostakos, & Dey, 2015) are some examples.

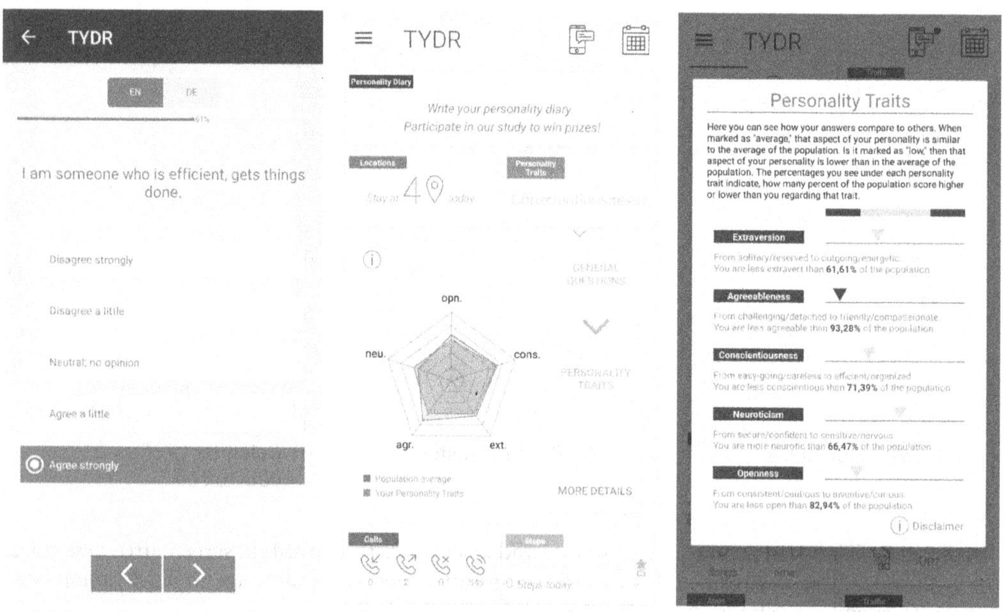

(a) Questionnaire interface. (b) Personality traits questionnaire results—extended tile. (c) Personality traits questionnaire results—detailed view.

FIGURE 20.2. TYDR questionnaire interface and results.

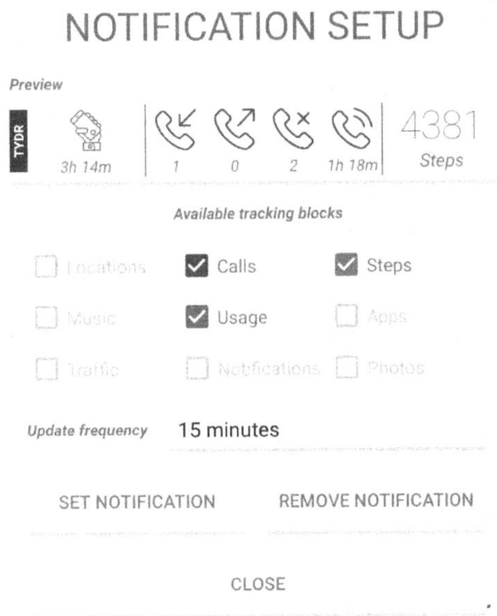

FIGURE 20.3. The user can configure the notification. The preview section shows what the notification will look like.

Lessons Learned and Future Directions

Based on the research with TYDR, we discuss challenges researchers will likely face when running mobile sensing studies. The first challenge concerns the extent to which researchers can assure sufficient levels of privacy in mobile-sensing-related apps. The second concerns the development and maintenance of mobile sensing apps. The third concerns user retention, that is, to what extent researchers can engage users to continuously participate in studies. The fourth deals with the limits of personality predictability.

Safeguarding Participants' Privacy

The collection and use of mobile sensing data raise important ethical questions with regard to privacy (Harari, 2020). This is true for companies that use sensing data to improve the functionality of their services, but it is also true for researchers who aim to gain insights into the human psyche by tracking human behavior. Privacy concerns need to be at the core of any consideration, whether this means developing one's own application or using an existing application for research purposes. *Merriam-Webster* defines privacy as "the state of being apart from company or observation" and "freedom from unauthorized intrusion."[3] This can seem quite fuzzy when applied in the context of mobile data collection. Regional data protection regulations such as the GDPR (General Data Protection Regulation) try to make privacy measures more concrete. However, uncertainties remain regarding the specifics on how to comply to those regulations (Filippo, 2018). About two-thirds of the papers reviewed above give only partial information about how privacy was considered when conducting the research presented. A recent review of mobile sensing systems found that only 13% of the studies included had implemented privacy measures (Laport-López et al., 2020).

Recently, we proposed the privacy model for mobile data collection applications (PM-MoDaC; Beierle, Tran, et al., 2018a, 2020). PM-MoDaC comprises nine concrete privacy measures (PMs) that can be implemented in the context of mobile sensing studies (including informed consent, anonymization of data, and usage of metadata). After collecting data with TYDR, we analyzed how users interacted with our privacy model and what data the users were willing to share (Beierle, 2021; Beierle, Tran, et al., 2020). Overall, we found that 95% of the users that, according to Google, installed the app, accepted the terms and conditions and the privacy policy. For some of the users (778), we could access their app usage statistics and see that they only spend 10 seconds (median) reading the terms and policies before accepting them. Convenience seems to trump privacy concerns. Regarding the data users are willing to share, we found that overall, female users and younger users were less likely to give all system permissions, confirming findings made by López, Marín, and Calderón (2017).

Development of Mobile Sensing Apps

When planning to conduct a mobile sensing study with a smartphone app, several options are possible. A new app could be built from the ground up, or a new app could be built on the basis of an existing software framework. A third option is to seek collaboration with an existing application that can conduct additional studies. The option to choose depends on the goals and scope of the project. Developing or even simply maintaining a mobile sensing app for personality research is a challenging endeavor. With its 4,000 installations, we already identified more than 600 different devices using TYDR. Optimizing an app for all these devices is no trivial matter, and additionally, the underlying operating system keeps evolving and changing. Likely driven by public discussions about privacy, the provided programming interfaces of the relevant mobile operating systems tend to become more restrictive over time. This means that it will get harder to retrieve and track the same amount of smartphone sensing data. Not only from a technical side, also from a regulatory side, mobile sensing apps might become more difficult to develop and maintain. We expect the regulations regarding mobile apps to increase. Germany, for example, introduced a regulation that makes it possible to register an app as a medical product. Institutional review boards might require compliance to this regulation, which is associated with large efforts (Vogel, Pryss, Schobel, Schlee, & Beierle, 2021).

User Retention

TYDR includes the daily PDD questionnaire. While about 20% of all users who installed the app filled out the BFI-2 questionnaire, there were many fewer users who consistently filled out PDD. Only about 7% filled out PDD once, and only 2% filled it out for 21 days. This issue of users dropping out of using a mobile sensing app is commonly referred to as a lack of *user retention* or *adherence*. This is a common issue for apps in general. What makes it so relevant for personality science is that in order to analyze relationships between different personality states and sensing data, many users would have to be willing to install and consistently use the app. Only then can a diverse set of situations and experiences be recorded. For example, specific emotions might only be experienced in specific situations and might show high predictability from sensing data. However, if the user retention is too low and each user only answers a few self-reports, such situations might not be recorded at all. Future work will be to create the right incentives while at the same time recognizing the biases that these incentives will create. Typical approaches to increase user retention are individualized feedback or gamification (Onnela, 2021).

Prediction Ceiling

Another point that future work will show is where the "ceiling" of personality predictability lies. Hypothetically, given all the data from the best sensors recorded at the highest frequencies, and given unlimited computing power for machine learning, predicting personality traits or states might still only be possible to some extent. Different people might express the same personality trait/state in different ways with respect to what the smartphone's sensors can capture.

Conclusion

In this chapter, we explored the potential of mobile sensing technology in the context of personality science. The ability to passively collect granular behavioral data *in vivo* and connect these data with self-reported personality trait and state assessments makes it possible to better understand how personality gets expressed in everyday life. As psychologists, we are concerned with one of the most fascinating questions there is: Why do people do what they do? Yet, we rarely study natural human behavior as it unfolds in daily life, but instead we rely on retrospective reports of behavior or observe behavioral responses in highly controlled laboratory settings. As the personality psychologist David Funder noted: "the cumulative result is an uneven and unrepresentative map of the behavioral terrain" (2009, p. 340). Mobile technology offers a promising way to change this.

Importantly, just like any other methodology in the psychological toolkit, mobile sensing is not without serious challenges that pertain to data quality, analytical skills, and user privacy. We encourage researchers who are interested in using mobile sensing in their own research to familiarize themselves with the underlying technology and to get a good understanding of how to avoid potential pitfalls that could undermine the promise of such technological advances. Collectively, we have an opportunity to use mobile sensing as a means to dive deeper into people's everyday psychology and to ask questions that to date were impossible to answer. But we should all be compelled to ensure that this noble endeavor does not infringe on the rights of our participants.

The use of mobile sensing in the social sciences is still in its infancy. While the research to date has predominantly focused on smartphone devices, the possibilities are almost endless. Wearable devices and connected smart homes are already collecting vast amounts of behavioral data today, and the future is likely to see an even stronger integration of people's everyday lives with technology. We might soon have micro devices embedded in our bodies that continuously monitor changes in our health and report back our blood sugar, cholesterol, heart rate, and potential anomalies in real time. Companies are already working on contact lenses that capture everything that is happening in our environment and feedback information directly to our retina. While these sensing technologies come with tremendous ethical challenges, they can also provide us with an even deeper understanding of who we are. Scholars in computer science and engineering are at the forefront of this technological development. As psychologists, we should be ready to have a seat at the table and make sure that the human element of mobile technologies is not overlooked and becomes the center piece of inquiry.

Notes

1. https://www.tydr.de.
2. Android app; more info at https://www.insightsapp.org
3. https://www.merriam-webster.com/dictionary/privacy

REFERENCES

Allemand, M., & Mehl, M. R. (2017). Personality assessment in daily life: A roadmap for future personality development research. In J. Specht (Ed.), *Personality development across the lifespan* (pp. 437–454). Elsevier.

Asselbergs, J., Ruwaard, J., Ejdys, M., Schrader, N., Sijbrandij, M., & Riper, H. (2016). Mobile phone-based unobtrusive ecological momentary assessment of day-to-day mood: An explorative study. *Journal of Medical Internet Research, 18*(3), e72.

Baumeister, H., & Montag, C. (Eds.). (2019). *Digital phenotyping and mobile sensing: New developments in psychoinformatics*. Springer.

Baumert, A., Schmitt, M., Perugini, M., Johnson, W., Blum, G., Borkenau, P., et al. (2017). Integrating personality structure, personality process, and personality development. *European Journal of Personality, 31*, 503–528.

Becker, D., Bremer, V., Funk, B., Asselbergs, J., Riper, H., & Ruwaard, J. (2016). How to predict mood? Delving into features of smartphone-based data. *Proceedings of the 22nd Americas Conference on Information Systems (AMCIS)*, pp. 1–10.

Beierle, F. (2021). *Integrating psychoinformatics with ubiquitous social networking: advanced mobile-sensing concepts and applications*. Springer.

Beierle, F., Probst, T., Allemand, M., Zimmermann, J., Pryss, R., Neff, P., et al. (2020). Frequency and duration of daily smartphone usage in relation to personality traits. *Digital Psychology, 1*(1), 20–28.

Beierle, F., Tran, V. T., Allemand, M., Neff, P., Schlee, W., Probst, T., et al. (2018a). Context data categories and privacy model for mobile data collection apps. *Procedia Computer Science, 134*, 18–25.

Beierle, F., Tran, V. T., Allemand, M., Neff, P., Schlee, W., Probst, T., et al. (2018b). TYDR—Track Your Daily Routine. Android app for tracking smartphone sensor and usage data. In *IEEE/ACM 5th International Conference on Mobile Software Engineering and Systems (MOBILESoft)* (pp. 72–75). ACM.

Beierle, F., Tran, V. T., Allemand, M., Neff, P., Schlee, W., Probst, T., et al. (2020). What data are smartphone users willing to share with researchers? *Journal of Ambient Intelligence and Humanized Computing, 11*, 2277–2289.

Bleidorn, W., & Hopwood, C. J. (2019). Using machine learning to advance personality assessment and theory. *Personality and Social Psychology Review, 23*(3), 190–203.

Ben-Zeev, D., Scherer, E. A., Wang, R., Xie, H., & Campbell, A. T. (2015). Next-generation psychiatric assessment: Using smartphone sensors to monitor behavior and mental health. *Psychiatric Rehabilitation Journal, 38*(3), 218–226.

Bogomolov, A., Lepri, B., Ferron, M., Pianesi, F., & Pentland, A. S. (2014). Daily stress recognition from mobile phone data, weather conditions and individual traits. In *Proceedings of the 2nd ACM International Conference on Multimedia* (pp. 477–486). ACM.

Boubiche, D. E., Imran, M., Maqsood, A., & Shoaib, M. (2019). Mobile crowd sensing – Taxonomy, applications, challenges, and solutions. *Computers in Human Behavior, 101*, 352–370.

Boukhechba, M., Huang, Y., Chow, P., Fua, K., Teachman, B. A., & Barnes, L. E. (2017). Monitoring social anxiety from mobility and communication patterns. In *Proceedings of the 2017 ACM International Joint Conference on Pervasive and Ubiquitous Computing and Proceedings of the 2017 ACM International Symposium on Wearable Computers* (pp. 749–753). ACM.

Burke, J., Estrin, D., Hansen, M., Parker, A., Ramanathan, N., Reddy, S., et al. (2006). Participatory sensing. In *Workshop on World-Sensor-Web (WSW'06): Mobile device centric sensor networks and applications* (pp. 117–134). ACM.

Butt, S., & Phillips, J. G. (2008). Personality and self-reported mobile phone use. *Computers in Human Behavior, 24*(2), 346–360.

Canzian, L., & Musolesi, M. (2015). Trajectories of depression: Unobtrusive monitoring of depressive states by means of smartphone mobility traces analysis. In *Proceedings of the 2015 ACM International Joint Conference on Pervasive and Ubiquitous Computing* (pp. 1293–1304). ACM.

Cao, B., Zheng, L., Zhang, C., Yu, P. S., Piscitello, A., Zulueta, J., et al. (2017). DeepMood: Modeling mobile phone typing dynamics for mood detection. In *Proceedings of the 23rd ACM SIGKDD International Conference on Knowledge Discovery and Data Mining* (pp. 747–755). ACM.

Carneiro, D., Pinheiro, A. P., & Novais, P. (2017). Context acquisition in auditory emotional recognition studies. *Journal of Ambient Intelligence and Humanized Computing, 8*(2), 191–203.

Chittaranjan, G., Blom, J., & Gatica-Perez, D. (2011). Who's who with Big-Five: Analyzing and classifying personality traits with smartphones. In *Proceedings of the 15th Annual International Symposium on Wearable Computers* (pp. 29–36). IEEE.

Chittaranjan, G., Blom, J., & Gatica-Perez, D. (2013). Mining large-scale smartphone data for personality studies. *Personal and Ubiquitous Computing, 17*(3), 433–450.

Chorley, M. J., Whitaker, R. M., & Allen, S. M. (2015). Personality and location-based social networks. *Computers in Human Behavior, 46*(Suppl. C), 45–56.

de Montjoye, Y.-A., Quoidbach, J., Robic, F., & Pentland, A. S. (2013). Predicting personality using novel mobile phone-based metrics. In A. M. Greenberg, W. G. Kennedy, & N. D. Bos (Eds.), *Social computing, behavioral-cultural modeling and prediction* (pp. 48–55). Springer.

Dey, A. K. (2001). Understanding and using context. *Personal Ubiquitous Computing, 5*(1), 4–7.

Eskes, P., Spruit, M., Brinkkemper, S., Vorstman, J., & Kas, M. J. (2016). The sociability score: App-based social profiling from a healthcare perspective. *Computers in Human Behavior, 59*, 39–48.

Farhan, A. A., Yue, C., Morillo, R., Ware, S., Lu, J., Bi, J., et al. (2016). Behavior vs. introspection: Refining prediction of clinical depression via smartphone sensing data. In *IEEE Wireless Health (WH)* (pp. 1–8). IEEE.

Ferreira, D., Kostakos, V., & Dey, A. K. (2015). AWARE: Mobile context instrumentation framework. *Frontiers in ICT, 2*, Article No. 6.

Filippo, A. R. (2018). Innovating in uncertainty: Effective compliance and the GDPR. *Harvard Journal of Law and Technology*. https://jolt.law.harvard.edu/digest/innovating-in-uncertainty-effective-compliance-and-the-gdpr

Finnigan, K. M., & Vazire, S. (2018). The incremental validity of average state self-reports over global self-reports of personality. *Journal of Personality and Social Psychology, 115*(2), 321–337.

Funder, D. (2006). Towards a resolution of the personality triad: Persons, situations, and behaviors. *Journal of Research in Personality, 40*(1), 21–34.

Götz, F. M., Stieger, S., & Reips, U.-D. (2017). Users of the main smartphone operating systems (iOS, Android) differ only little in personality. *PLoS One, 12*(5), e0176921.

Grover, T., & Mark, G. (2017). Digital footprints: Predicting personality from temporal patterns of technology use. In *Proceedings of the 2017 ACM International Joint Conference on Pervasive and Ubiquitous Computing and Proceedings of the 2017 ACM International Symposium on Wearable Computers* (pp. 41–44). ACM.

Harari, G. M. (2020). A process-oriented approach to respecting privacy in the context of mobile phone tracking. *Current Opinion in Psychology, 31*, 141–147.

Harari, G. M., Lane, N. D., Wang, R., Crosier, B. S., Campbell, A. T., & Gosling, S. D. (2016). Using smartphones to collect behavioral data in psychological science: Opportunities, practical considerations, and challenges. *Perspectives on Psychological Science, 11*(6), 838–854.

Harari, G. M., Müller, S. R., Aung, M. S., & Rentfrow, P. J. (2017). Smartphone sensing methods for studying behavior in everyday life. *Current Opinion in Behavioral Sciences, 18*(Suppl. C), 83–90.

Harari, G. M., Müller, S. R., Stachl, C., Wang, R., Wang, W., Bühner, M., et al. (2020). Sensing sociability: Individual differences in young adults' conversation, calling, texting, and app use behaviors in daily life. *Journal of Personality and Social Psychology, 119*(1), 204–228.

Horstmann, K. T., & Ziegler, M. (2020). Assessing personality states: What to consider when constructing personality state measures. *European Journal of Personality, 34*(6), 1037–1059.

Huang, Y., Xiong, H., Leach, K., Zhang, Y., Chow, P., Fua, K., et al. (2016). Assessing social anxiety using GPS trajectories and point-of-interest data. In *Proceedings of the 2016 ACM International Joint Conference on Pervasive and Ubiquitous Computing* (pp. 898–903). ACM.

Hung, G. C.-L., Yang, P.-C., Chang, C.-C., Chiang, J.-H., & Chen, Y.-Y. (2016). Predicting negative emotions based on mobile phone usage patterns: An exploratory study. *JMIR Research Protocols, 5*(3), e160.

Insel, T. R. (2017). Digital phenotyping: Technology for a new science of behavior. *JAMA, 318*(13), 1215–1216.

Jayarajah, K., Balan, R. K., Radhakrishnan, M., Misra, A., & Lee, Y. (2016). LiveLabs: Building in-situ mobile sensing & behavioral experimentation TestBeds. In *Proceedings of the 14th Annual International Conference on Mobile Systems, Applications, and Services* (pp. 1–15). ACM.

John, O. P., Naumann, L. P., & Soto, C. J. (2008). Paradigm shift to the integrative Big Five trait taxonomy: History, measurement, and conceptual issues. In O. P. John, R. W. Robins, & L. A. Pervin (Eds.), *Handbook of personality: Theory and research* (3rd ed., pp. 114–158). Guilford Press.

Kim, S. Y., Koo, H. J., & Song, H. Y. (2018). A study on estimation of human personality from location visiting preference. *Journal of Ambient Intelligence and Humanized Computing, 9*(3), 629–642.

Lane, N. D., Miluzzo, E., Lu, H., Peebles, D., Choudhury, T., & Campbell, A. T. (2010). A survey of mobile phone sensing. *IEEE Communications Magazine, 48*(9), 140–150.

Laport-López, F., Serrano, E., Bajo, J., & Campbell, A. T. (2020). A review of mobile sensing systems, applications, and opportunities. *Knowledge and Information Systems, 62*, 145–174.

LiKamWa, R., Liu, Y., Lane, N. D., & Zhong, L. (2013). MoodScope: Building a mood sensor from smartphone usage patterns. In *Proceeding of the 11th Annual International Conference on Mobile Systems, Applications, and Services* (pp. 389–402). ACM.

López, G., Marín, G., & Calderón, M. (2017). Human aspects of ubiquitous computing: A study addressing willingness to use it and privacy issues. *Journal of Ambient Intelligence and Humanized Computing, 8*(4), 497–511.

Matz, S. C., & Harari, G. M. (2020). Personality–place transactions: Mapping the relationships between Big Five personality traits, states, and daily places. *Journal of Personality and Social Psychology, 120*(5), 1367–1385.

Mehrotra, A., Hendley, R., & Musolesi, M. (2016). Towards multi-modal anticipatory monitoring of depressive states through the analysis of human-smartphone interaction. In *Proceedings of the ACM International Joint Conference on Pervasive and Ubiquitous Computing: Adjunct* (pp. 1132–1138). ACM.

Mehrotra, A., Tsapeli, F., Hendley, R., & Musolesi, M. (2017). MyTraces: Investigating correlation and causation between users' emotional states and mobile phone interaction. In *Proceedings of the ACM on Interactive, Mobile, Wearable and Ubiquitous Technologies, 1*(3), 1–21.

Miller, G. (2012). The smartphone psychology manifesto. *Perspectives on Psychological Science, 7*, 221–237.

Mohr, D. C., Zhang, M., & Schueller, S. M. (2017). Personal sensing: Understanding mental health using ubiquitous sensors and machine learning. *Annual Review of Clinical Psychology, 13*, 23–47.

Mønsted, B., Mollgaard, A., & Mathiesen, J.

(2018). Phone-based metric as a predictor for basic personality traits. *Journal of Research in Personality, 74*, 16–22.

Montag, C., Baumeister, H., Kannen, C., Sariyska, R., Meßner, E.-M., & Brand, M. (2019). Concept, possibilities and pilot-testing of a new smartphone application for the social and life sciences to study human behavior including validation data from personality psychology. *[stet]Multidisciplinary Scientific Journal, 2*(2), 102–115.

Montag, C., Błaszkiewicz, K., Lachmann, B., Andone, I., Sariyska, R., Trendafilov, B., et al. (2014). Correlating personality and actual phone usage. *Journal of Individual Differences, 35*(3), 158–165.

Montag, C., Błaszkiewicz, K., Sariyska, R., Lachmann, B., Andone, I., Trendafilov, B., et al. (2015). Smartphone usage in the 21st century: Who is active on WhatsApp? *BMC Research Notes, 8*(1), 331.

Montag, C., Duke, É., & Markowetz, A. (2016). Toward psychoinformatics: Computer science meets psychology. *Computational and Mathematical Methods in Medicine, 2016*, 1–10.

Müller, S. R., Peters, H., Matz, S. C., Wang, W., & Harari, G. M. (2020). Investigating the Relationships between mobility behaviours and indicators of subjective well-being using smartphone-based experience sampling and GPS Tracking. *European Journal of Personality, 34*(5), 714–732.

Onnela, J.-P. (2021). Opportunities and challenges in the collection and analysis of digital phenotyping data. *Neuropsychopharmacology, 46*(1), 45–54.

Peltonen, E., Sharmilla, P., Asara, K. O, Visuri, A., Lagerspetz, E., & Ferreira, D. (2020). When phones get personal: Predicting Big Five personality traits from application usage. *Pervasive and Mobile Computing, 69*, 101269.

Pryss, R., John, D., Reichert, M., Hoppenstedt, B., Schmid, L., Schlee, W., et al. (2019, July). Machine learning findings on geospatial data of users from the TrackYourStress mHealth Crowdsensing Platform. *Proceedings of the 2019 IEEE 20th International Conference on Information Reuse and Integration for Data Science (IRI)*, pp. 350–355.

Rachuri, K. K., Musolesi, M., Mascolo, C., Rentfrow, P. J., Longworth, C., & Aucinas, A. (2010). EmotionSense: A mobile phones-based adaptive platform for experimental social psychology research. In *Proceedings of the 12th ACM International Conference on Ubiquitous Computing* (pp. 281–290). ACM.

Robins, R. W., Fraley, R. C., & Krueger, R. F. (Eds.). (2007). *Handbook of research methods in personality psychology*. Guilford Press.

Rüegger, D., Stieger, M., Nißen, M., Allemand, M., Fleisch, E., & Kowatsch, T. (2020). How are personality states associated with smartphone data? *European Journal of Personality, 34*, 687–713.

Saeb, S., Lattie, E. G., Schueller, S. M., Kording, K. P., & Mohr, D. C. (2016). The relationship between mobile phone location sensor data and depressive symptom severity. *PeerJ, 4*, e2537.

Saeb, S., Zhang, M., Karr, C. J., Schueller, S. M., Corden, M. E., Kording, K. P., et al. (2015). Mobile phone sensor correlates of depressive symptom severity in daily-life behavior: An exploratory study. *Journal of Medical Internet Research, 17*(7), e175.

Schoedel, R., Au, Q., Völkel, S. T., Lehmann, F., Becker, D., Bühner, M., et al. (2018). Digital footprints of sensation seeking. *Zeitschrift für Psychologie, 226*(4), 232–245.

Seifert, A., Hofer, M., & Allemand, M. (2018). Mobile data collection: Smart, but not (yet) smart enough. *Frontiers in Neuroscience, 12*, Article No. 971.

Singh, V. K., & Agarwal, R. R. (2016). Cooperative phoneotypes: Exploring phonebased behavioral markers of cooperation. In *Proceedings of the ACM International Joint Conference on Pervasive and Ubiquitous Computing* (pp. 646–657). ACM.

Singh, V. K., & Ghosh, I. (2017). Inferring individual social capital automatically via phone logs. *Proceedings of the ACM on Human-Computer Interaction, 1*(CSCW), 1–12.

Soto, C. J., & John, O. P. (2017). The next Big Five Inventory (BFI-2): Developing and assessing a hierarchical model with 15 facets to enhance bandwidth, fidelity, and predictive power. *Journal of Personality and Social Psychology, 113*(1), 117–143.

Stachl, C., Au, Q., Schoedel, R., Buschek, D., Völkel, S., Schuwerk, T., et al. (2019). *Behavioral patterns in smartphone usage predict Big Five personality traits*. PsyArXiv. https://psyarxiv.com/ks4vd

Stachl, C., Au, Q., Schoedel, R., Gosling, S. D., Harari, G. M., Buschek, D., et al. (2020). Predicting personality from patterns of behavior collected with smartphones. *Proceedings of the National Academy of Sciences, 117*(30), 17680–17687.

Stachl, C., Hilbert, S., Au, J.-Q., Buschek, D., De Luca, A., Bischl, B., et al. (2017). Personality traits predict smartphone usage. *European Journal of Personality, 31*(6), 701–722.

Stachl, C., Pargent, F., Hilbert, S., Harari, G. M., Schoedel, R., Vaid, S., et al. (2020). Personality research and assessment in the era of machine learning. *European Journal of Personality 34*, 613–631

Stütz, T., Kowar, T., Kager, M., Tiefengrabner, M., Stuppner, M., Blechert, J., et al. (2015). Smartphone based stress prediction. In F. Ricci, K. Bontcheva, O. Conlan, & S. Lawless (Eds.), *User modeling, adaptation and personalization* (pp. 240–251). Springer.

Sun, B., Ma, Q., Zhang, S., Liu, K., & Liu, Y. (2017). iSelf: Towards cold-start emotion labeling using transfer learning with smartphones. *ACM Transactions on Sensor Networks, 13*(4), 1–22.

Trull, T. J., & Ebner-Priemer, U. (2014). The role of ambulatory assessment in psychological science. *Current Directions in Psychological Science, 23*, 466–470.

Verto Analytics (2017, October 11). *Consumer device use: Which gadgets get used most frequently?* https://vertoanalytics.com/chart-of-the-week-which-devices-are-used-most-often

Vogel, C., Pryss, R., Schobel, J., Schlee, W., Beierle, F. (2021). Developing apps for researching the COVID-19 pandemic with the TrackYourHealth Platform. In *IEEE/ACM 8th International Conference on Mobile Software Engineering and Systems (MOBILESoft)* (pp. 65–68). IEEE.

Wang, W., Harari, G. M., Wang, R., Müller, S. R., Mirjafari, S., Masaba, K., et al. (2018). Sensing behavioral change over time: Using within-person variability features from mobile sensing to predict personality traits. In *Proceedings of the ACM on Interactive, Mobile, Wearable and Ubiquitous Technologies (IMWUT),2*(3), 1–21.

Wrzus, C., & Mehl, M. R. (2015). Lab and/or field? Measuring personality processes and their social consequences. *European Journal of Personality, 29*, 250–271.

Xiong, H., Huang, Y., Barnes, L. E., & Gerber, M. S. (2016). Sensus: A crossplatform, general-purpose system for mobile crowdsensing in human-subject studies. In *Proceedings of the ACM International Joint Conference on Pervasive and Ubiquitous Computing (UbiComp 2016)* (pp. 415–426). ACM.

Xu, R., Frey, R. M., Fleisch, E., & Ilic, A. (2016). Understanding the impact of personality traits on mobile app adoption—Insights from a large-scale field study. *Computers in Human Behavior, 62*(Suppl. C), 244–256.

Yarkoni, T. (2012). Psychoinformatics: New horizons at the interface of the psychological and computing sciences. *Current Directions in Psychological Science, 21*(6), 391–397.

Zhang, X., Li, W., Chen, X., & Lu, S. (2018). MoodExplorer: Towards compound emotion detection via smartphone sensing. *Proceedings of the ACM on Interactive, Mobile, Wearable and Ubiquitous Technologies (IMWUT), 1*(4), 1–30.

Zhang, X., Zhuang, F., Li, W., Ying, H., Xiong, H., & Lu, S. (2019). Inferring mood instability via smartphone sensing: A multi-view learning approach. In *Proceedings of the 27th ACM International Conference on Multimedia* (pp. 1401–1409). ACM.

Zimmermann, J., Woods, W. C., Ritter, S., Happel, M., Masuhr, O., Jaeger, U., et al. (2019). Integrating structure and dynamics in personality assessment: First steps toward the development and validation of a personality dynamics diary. *Psychological Assessment, 31*(4), 516–531.

CHAPTER 21

Mobile Sensing Applications in Moral Psychology

Farzan Karimi-Malekabadi, Mohammad Atari, and Morteza Dehghani

CHAPTER OVERVIEW

How often do people download or use a religious app on their smartphone? How fiercely do people try to signal to others in social media, say Facebook, that they donated to a charitable cause? Are men or women more likely to secretly check their partner's social media activities and chats? Questions like these are morally laden but were not in antiquity. Philosophers have relentlessly argued over the concept of "right" and "wrong" for thousands of years, but Aristotle and Plato never discussed the morality underlying sharing a "nude pic" or going over the logs of someone else's chat. New phenomena require new tools in order to be explained adequately, and the science of morality requires new methods, beyond hypothetical moral dilemmas and self-report questionnaires, to address morally relevant questions in the 21st century. Indeed, that is not to say that principles of moral cognition are not applicable in novel contexts such as social media, but that our theoretical views and methodological apparatuses should be adapted to the environment in which new inquiries are made.

Since the birth of moral psychology as an empirical science, psychological foundations of morality have been studied via survey-based methods such as self-reported questionnaires or laboratory experiments such as the trolley problem (Ellemers, van der Toorn, Paunov, & van Leeuwen, 2019). More recently, however, researchers have incorporated ambulatory assessment methods (e.g., daily diary methods, experience sampling, and ecological momentary assessment) to study moral judgments and moral concerns as they naturally unfold in the context of daily life (e.g., Bollich et al., 2016; Newman, Schwarz, Graham, & Stone, 2019). In addition to these developments, a parallel line of research has advanced computational methods to capture moral concerns from natural language data (Iliev, Dehghani, & Sagi, 2015; Kennedy et al., 2021; Sagi & Dehghani,

2014). In this chapter, we review these recent methodological developments in moral psychology, with an emphasis on ambulatory assessment and language analysis methods. Then, we focus on the applications, promises, and pitfalls of mobile sensing methods (MSMs; Harari et al., 2016; Lane et al., 2010) in moral psychology.

Morality: What Is It and Who Cares?

Not all scientists and philosophers agree upon a unified definition of "morality." However, questions concerning what is the "right" and "wrong" way to behave and what characters are "virtuous" or "vicious" have occupied philosophers since classical antiquity. Morality describes the way people think about themselves, interact with others, live and work together in groups, and relate to other groups in society. More recently, the interdisciplinary science of morality has become a popular area of study (Graham, 2014). Social scientific approaches to moral psychology bring experimental methods to bear on topics such as moral emotions, moral motivations, moral character development, and evolution of moral capacities.

In a broad sense, moral psychology focuses on the set of interconnected values, practices, institutions, and evolved psychological mechanisms that make social life possible (Haidt, 2008). To emphasize the importance of everyday morality in humans' social life, Gintis, Henrich, Bowles, Boyd, and Fehr (2008) argued that ethical behavior was, in evolutionary terms, fitness-enhancing in the years marking the emergence of *Homo sapiens*. The root of this argument is that groups with many altruists functioned better than groups with many selfish individuals, and the fitness losses sustained by altruists were more than compensated by the better performance of the groups they belonged to.

In the last few decades, different areas of psychological science have relied on their area-specific set of tools to examine different aspects of morality. Social psychologists, for example, have weighed in on intra- and intergroup processes (e.g., Day, Fiske, Downing, & Trail, 2014; Kouchaki, 2011) as well as social structures as important factors in shaping moral cognition. Developmental psychologists, on the other hand, have uncovered developmental processes in moral capacities such as how infants represent fairness and how they forgive transgressions (e.g., Amir, Ahl, Parsons, & McAuliffe, 2021; Sloane, Baillargeon, & Premack, 2012). Cultural psychologists have examined culture-specific and culturally universal aspects of morality (e.g., Haidt & Joseph, 2004; Saucier, 2018). Evolutionary psychologists and anthropologists have examined evolutionary and ecological origins of morality as well as cross-cultural differences in moral values (e.g., Krasnow, 2017; Purzycki et al., 2018). Neuroscientists have explored the neural circuits underlying moral decision making (e.g., Crockett, Siegel, Kurth-Nelson, Dayan, & Dolan, 2017; Hackel & Amodio, 2018). These insightful lines of inquiry have provided an unprecedented amount of evidence about how the human mind generates and navigates notions of right and wrong which may collectively be called the field of moral psychology.

Recently, Ellemers and colleagues (2019) analyzed empirical studies in moral psychology published from 1940 through 2017, and categorized research questions in moral psychology into five principal research themes: (1) moral reasoning, (2) moral judgments, (3) moral behavior, (4) moral emotions, and (5) moral self-views. Moral reasoning research explores people's choices in hypothetical dilemmas, their positions on specific issues (e.g., gay adoption, abortion, animal rights), and which values (e.g., loyalty) they endorse as most important in their life as a moral person. Studies of moral judgments consider the ways in which we assign moral traits (e.g., humble, honest, trustworthy) to other individuals or groups. Moral behaviors are implicated in questions studying self-reported past behavior or behavioral intentions, as well as reports of cooperative behavior in real life (e.g., volunteering, donating money, forgiving). Moral emotions research consists of probing emotional responses people experience in relation to morally relevant issues or situations (e.g., guilt, shame, disgust). Finally, moral self-views research focuses on the ways in which different aspects of people's self-views relate to each other (e.g., personality characteristics with self-stated inclinations to display moral behavior), as well as the way experimentally induced situations relate to people's self-views.

Ellemers and colleagues (2019) suggest that while there is a large body of work about moral reasoning and judgment, much less is known about moral behavior. This asymmetry in empirical morality research is due partly to the questionable assumption that moral reasoning and judgments of others are seen to inform the choices people make in their own moral behaviors (Bostyn, Sevenhant, & Roets, 2018). In addition, the measures in moral psychology largely rely on subjective self-reports of general dispositions (or overall preferences) and intentions (or laboratory experiments). These methods aim to approximate real-world, morally relevant phenomena, but we need objective data to understand and interpret subjective experience, and widespread reliance on these methods has raised concerns regarding the external validity of morality research (Graham, Meindl, & Beall, 2012; Kahane, Everett, Earp, Farias, & Savulescu, 2015). In addition, most empirical research in morality has been conducted with undergraduates in decontextualized laboratory settings, which do not adequately address (1) the diversity of moral values across populations and (2) the dynamic aspects of morality in everyday life.

Recent methodological advances in the social and behavioral sciences have given moral psychologists the opportunity to address some of the ecological-validity concerns in the field. In particular, *ambulatory assessment* methods and *language analysis* tools provide a new horizon for researchers to explore morality "in the wild" (Hoover, Dehghani, Johnson, Iliev, & Graham, 2018). Of note, other methodological developments in moral psychology (e.g., social network analysis, agent-based modeling) can be used to answer a host of important questions about daily manifestations of morality, but they are outside the scope of this chapter. In what follows, we briefly review the emerging lines of work answering real-world questions about moral concerns using these methodological tools.

Ambulatory Assessment in Moral Psychology

The term *ambulatory assessment* encompasses a wide range of methods used to study people in their natural environment, including experience sampling methods (ESMs), ecological momentary assessment (EMA), observational (e.g., audio recording such as electronically activated recorder [EAR]), and physiological (e.g., cardiac and respiratory activity assessed using physiological sensors worn by participants; Trull & Ebner-Priemer, 2014). Note that ESMs and EMA are often used interchangeably, although their historical antecedents and original aims differ (Shiffman, Stone, & Hufford, 2008). Ambulatory assessment may be considered the broad term encompassing all the methods mentioned above. ESMs and EMA overlap considerably, but specifically, ESMs emphasize random sampling schemes and often use paper-and-pencil diaries and beepers, while

EMA is often used to collect momentary self-report using electronic diaries. In that sense, these methods are "active" in their assessment. On the other hand, EAR uses a "passive" mode of assessment by intermittently recording snippets of ambient sounds while participants go about their lives (Mehl, 2017). Below, we briefly review recent applications of ESMs and EAR in morality research.

Experience Sampling Methods

Experience sampling methods have provided insightful results regarding daily manifestations of moral concerns. In addition to providing a way of assessing cross-situational consistency, this form of assessment provides a way of overcoming the limitations of laboratory studies and standard assessments (Bolger & Laurenceau, 2013). In an application of ESM in probing the temporal dynamics of (im)moral acts, Hofmann, Wisneski, Brandt, and Skitka (2014) asked participants five times daily on their smartphone whether they committed, were the target of, witnessed, or learned about a moral or immoral act. They demonstrated that 28.9% of daily experiences for American and Canadian participants are morally relevant, suggesting that moral experiences are relatively frequent in daily life, at least in these two countries.

Next, Hofmann and colleagues (2014) probed the content of daily moral experiences. They built upon an influential, descriptive taxonomy of moral dimensions, moral foundations theory (MFT; Graham et al., 2013), to account for descriptive content and to examine whether everyday moral experiences highlight understudied dimensions of morality. According to MFT, the moral domain can be mapped to the following five moral foundations: care (basic concerns for the suffering of others, including caring and compassion); fairness (concerns about unfair treatment, inequality, and more abstract notions of justice); loyalty (concerns related to obligations of group membership, such as loyalty, self-sacrifice, and vigilance against betrayal); authority (concerns related to social order and the obligations of hierarchical relationships such as obedience, respect, and proper role fulfillment); and purity (concerns about physical and spiritual contagion, including virtues of chastity, wholesomeness, and control of desires). Hofmann and colleagues also added the concern for liberty, a newly added moral foundation (Iyer, Koleva, Graham, Ditto, & Haidt, 2012), and two additional categories of "honesty" and "self-discipline" derived from their own data. The results revealed that for moral acts, 70% of responses were about care, 10% about fairness and honesty, and less than 5% about loyalty, authority, purity, liberty, and self-discipline.

The descriptive findings of Hofmann and colleagues (2014) also showed that liberals mentioned events related to fairness, liberty, and honesty more frequently than their conservative counterparts, whereas conservatives mentioned daily events related to loyalty, authority, and purity more frequently than did liberals. Hence, liberal–conservative differences in this everyday-life framework largely corroborate the idea that political ideology relates to different moral foundations (Graham, Haidt, & Nosek, 2009). Finally, these authors found evidence for both "moral contagion," a phenomenon where becoming the target of a moral act increases the likelihood of committing a moral act later, and "moral licensing," where committing a moral act earlier in the day may increase the possibility of a subsequent immoral act.

In a similar vein, ESMs can be used to investigate moral emotions as experienced in daily life. For instance, Nakamura (2013) asked 518 American parents to complete a questionnaire addressing participants' work and family life (e.g., work benefits and household division of labor) and to describe their feelings when signaled. In this ESM study, participants carried response forms and a paging device programmed to signal several times a day. When signaled, they were instructed to report what they were thinking and doing, where they were, whom they were with, and how they were feeling. Researchers investigated pride as a moral emotion, aiming to explore to what extent daily experiences of pride are associated with achievement, as compared to prosocial behavior and praise. Results suggested that being with one's children and working with clients are more closely related to the momentary experience of pride in family and work contexts, respectively.

In another study, the relationship between self-reported empathy and actual social interactions was examined using ESMs (Grühn, Rebucal, Diehl, Lumley, & Labouvie-Vief, 2008). Participants were instructed to carry the handheld computer device for a week and to respond to questions when prompted. Each time participants received a beep, they were instructed to report on their social interactions since the last beep. Positive and negative interactions were assessed by asking participants two questions: "Did you have a positive interaction with another person since the last beep?" and "Did you have a negative interaction with another person since the last beep?" The results demonstrated that individuals with high self-reported empathy display behaviors that make it easier for others to relate to them. For example, others may perceive empathic individuals as more understanding, more caring, and more concerned about how they feel and what they may think.

ESMs have also been employed to examine eudaimonia and compassion as important moral virtues. Eudaimonia is well-being analyzed in terms of life purpose, meaning, a sense of personal growth, and contribution to the lives of others. Runyan and colleagues (2019) found that compassion predicts eudaimonia. Moreover, while not impervious to situational factors such as relationship status and stress levels, considerable consistency was observed in the relationship between compassion and eudaimonia. Moreover, compassion, along with eudaimonia, predicted donating behavior, which standard assessments did not.

To discover patterns between trait morality and the manifestation of moral behaviors, researchers studied individual differences in moral behavior and determined whether those differences were consistent over time, using an experience sampling questionnaire which was designed to assess the extent to which actions and thoughts in the past 3 hours were in line with the four virtues of honesty, compassion, fairness, and moral courage (Meindl, Jayawickreme, Furr, & Fleeson, 2015). Results showed that moral behavior is consistent in many different ways, suggesting that individual differences in moral values substantially drive moral behavior. Multiple analyses revealed that individual differences in moral behavior appear to be robustly consistent; that is, people who are relatively moral on one occasion (or across one set of occasions) tend to be relatively moral on other occasions (or across another set of occasions), across a 9-day period.

Finally, ambulatory assessment methods offer a unique opportunity to investigate the relationship between daily religious involvement, spirituality, and moral emotions. Hardy, Zhang, Skalski, Melling, and Brinton (2014) sent participants a daily survey to measure self-reported levels of religious activity, spiritual experience, and moral emotions (empathy, gratitude, and forgiveness) for up to 50 days. Researchers found that on days that people engaged in more religious activity, they also had more spiritual experiences, and on days when they had more spiritual experiences, they also reported feeling more empathy, gratitude, and forgiveness.

Electronically Activated Recorder

From a methodological perspective, momentary and standard self-reports both derive their data from participants' reports of their introspections and perceptions; therefore, some of the limitations of traditional self-report methods such as impression management and self-deceptive enhancement also apply to momentary self-reports (Paulhus, 1986; Schwarz, 1999). Thus, to enrich the researcher's methodological toolkit, it would be beneficial to complement momentary self-report data with momentary observational data. The main distinction between ESMs and momentary observational methods is that they adopt different assessment perspectives: active measure for ESMs and passive assessment for momentary observational methods.

In earlier EAR studies, participants would attach an EAR device to their belts or carry it in a purse-like bag while going about their daily lives (Mehl, Pennebaker, Crow, Dabbs, & Price, 2001). Although the function of the EAR—to acoustically sample social environments—has remained consistent since 2001, the technology used to make the recordings has evolved exponentially. The EAR has progressed from digital tape recorders to the current "iEAR" app that can be conveniently downloaded and effortlessly used on participants' smartphones (Mehl, 2017).

EAR has been incorporated in a number of areas in psychology, ranging from the assessment of subclinical depression (Mehl, 2006) to narcissism (Holtzman, Vazire, & Mehl, 2010). In the realm of morality, Bollich and colleagues (2016) examined the stability of everyday moral behaviors using EAR and provided evidence that there are stable individual differences in moral behaviors. In their study, 19,063 EAR files containing audible speech were coded for everyday moral behaviors (e.g., showing sympathy, gratitude) and morally neutral comparison language behaviors (e.g., use of prepositions, articles) and transcribed by trained research assistants. Then, EAR transcripts were analyzed using the Linguistic Inquiry and Word Count (LIWC; Pennebaker, Booth, & Francis, 2007) text analysis program. They selected word categories that (1) were evaluatively neutral (i.e., they had no or minimal positive or negative connotation) and (2) had relatively similar base rates to moral behaviors. Results indicated that stable individual differences in moral behavior can be systematically observed in daily life. The implication of this research is that individual differences in moral behavior are as stable as individual differences in neutral language behaviors. Indeed, these authors argued that analyzing neutral language can be recognized as a high benchmark for gauging the stability of moral behaviors.

In a recent study, Atari and colleagues (2023) coded tens of thousands of EAR recordings based on the typology of moral concerns by MFT, that is, care, fairness, loyalty, authority, and purity. These authors examined (1) what percentage of daily language behaviors is essentially moral and (2) what moral categories are most talked about in daily life. This study was therefore a conceptual replication of Hofmann and colleagues (2014) except that it used a passive EAR framework, as opposed to an active ESM framework. Interestingly, and in contrast to Hofmann and associates, only 1.2 to 6.1% of daily interactions consisted of some sort of moral content across four different samples. Breaking down these percentages based on moral categories, care and purity values were consistently and robustly more prevalent in daily interactions, compared with the other three moral foundations. The much smaller percentage of moral content in everyday interactions found in this study, in contrast to that of Hofmann and colleagues, may be attributed to its passive methodology. Indeed, consistent with the general principle that "questions shape the answers" (Schwarz, 1999), the questions in ESM studies remind participants of moral phenomena, and hence, participants might overestimate the significance of moral content in their answers. Passive assessment of morality based on natural language, on the other hand, takes an observational standpoint and is more robust to self-report biases. Hence, statistics based on this method might be closer to an objective frequency of moral transactions in everyday life.

Language Analysis in Moral Psychology

While much of psychology research has historically focused on understanding moral cognition using survey-based and experimental methods, the explosion of naturally occurring communication data available to researchers through digital media (e.g., blogs, email, text messaging, and social media posts) has led to renewed interest in assessing text for capturing social dynamics and moral concerns (Hoover et al., 2018). Language analysis allows psychologists to link features of what people say and subtleties in their linguistic styles to personality traits, temporal and situational fluctuations, and attitudinal preferences (Boyd & Schwartz, 2020; Pennebaker, Mehl, & Niederhoffer, 2003).

People across cultures—especially politicians—tend to frame their positions as fundamental moral beliefs about right and wrong. This use of *moral rhetoric* via language is evident in a broad range of social issues. For example, in the United States, both opponents and proponents of government aid frame their case in terms of some moral issue, for example, by focusing on deservingness (i.e., "judgment of who is deserving, as opposed to what is most effective"). The efficacy and rise of the use of moral rhetoric may perhaps be traced back to the idea that "morality does the work of politics" (Clifford & Jerit, 2013). In support of this idea, language analysis of party manifestos has revealed that moral rhetoric mobilizes copartisan voters by activating positive emotions about their partisan preference (Jung, 2020). These developments have rendered language analysis a fruitful and dynamic methodological tool in moral psychology (Sagi & Dehghani, 2014; Weber et al., 2018). Recent computational studies in morality research have used a diverse set of methodologies, but broadly, language analysis in moral psychology could be divided into three categories: (1) dictionary-based assessment, (2) distributed-representation assessment, and (3) human-annotation-based assessment (Atari & Dehghani, 2022).

Dictionary-Based Assessment of Moral Language

The first modern empirical attempt to provide moral psychological language analysis was the Moral Foundations Dictionary (MFD) by Graham and colleagues (2009) as a part of their work on MFT (Graham et al., 2013). The MFD consists of 295 words and word stems related to each of the virtues and vices of moral foundations, originally designed to work with the Linguistic Inquiry and Word Count (LIWC) program. Graham and colleagues used MFD to analyze sermons delivered in conservative and liberal churches. Consistent with their previous experiments in which they used the Moral Foundations Questionnaire (MFQ; Graham et al., 2011), they demonstrated that sermons given at liberal churches tend to focus more on issues related to care and fairness compared to conservative churches, which tend to focus more on issues related to authority and purity.

Kennedy and colleagues (2021), whose research combined people's social media posts and their self-reported moral values measured through MFQ, investigated the relationship between people's moral values and their Facebook status updates. These authors used MFD and LIWC dictionaries in addition to machine learning methods to quantify the associations each moral foundation had with everyday concerns observed in social media language. A reliable, but small, relationship was established between individual differences in endorsement of moral foundations and everyday language. In other words, people's responses to the MFQ could be predicted using their Facebook status updates. This link was found to be robust using a battery of methods, including the MFD, LIWC dictionaries, and machine learning methods, although the magnitude of the effect varied substantially across the methodologies. They also found that moral concerns are not necessarily "everyday concerns," manifested in the usage of moral language in everyday contexts. This was in fact the case for care and purity, as individuals with higher scores on the MFQ used both care- and purity-based language with much higher frequency, but interestingly, in the case of fairness, loyalty, and authority, this was not found.

Recent work using MFD and other dictionary-based methods have demonstrated that morally laden messages play an instrumental role in fomenting moral outrage online (Brady & Crockett, 2019) and that moral framing can exacerbate political polarization (Brady, Wills, Jost, Tucker, & Van Bavel, 2017). Indeed, moral words have a unique influence on emotional and cognitive processing. Day and colleagues (2014) suggested that framing issues using moral foundations may change political attitudes in at least two ways: (1) *entrenching*: Relevant moral foundations strengthen existing political attitudes when framing pro-attitudinal social issues (e.g., conservatives exposed to a free-market economic stance) and (2) *persuasion*: The mere presence of relevant moral foundations may alter political attitudes in counter-attitudinal directions in the context of social issues (e.g., conservatives exposed to an economic regulation stance).

Distributed-Representation Assessment of Moral Language

Dictionaries are (1) unlikely to include all of the words that may be relevant to a given category, especially when word usage is context-dependent; (2) unlikely to capture temporally dynamic semantic structures as the meaning of words change in time (e.g., the word *gay* has changed meaning from "cheerful" to "homosexual"); and (3) unlikely to capture sociolects across races, ethnicities, gender identities, and social classes (e.g., English spoken by African Americans may include words, moral in nature, that are not recognized in other types of English usage; Sap, Card, Gabriel, Choi, & Smith, 2019). One possible answer is to consider the semantic similarity (referencing the underlying meaning of words) rather than the morphological similarity (referencing the surface-level differences among words), as in dictionary-based methods (Bhatia, Richie, & Zou, 2019; Garten et al., 2018).

Using a distributed-representation technique to quantify moral language, Dehghani and colleagues (2016) investigated which types of moral similarities (based on moral foundations) influence tie formations in social networks. These authors investigated the idea that moral homophily (love of the same) plays a crucial role in the formation of social networks, hypothesizing that the distance between two people in a social network could be predicted by the differences in their moral purity. Indeed, these authors found that the distance between two individuals in a social network can be predicted based on their similarity in purity language (e.g., language related to religiosity and sanctity).

Mokhberian, Abeliuk, Cummings, and Lerman (2020) proposed a framework to quantify the moral framing of news stories based on distributed representations. This framework leverages a large corpus of tweets annotated with regard to moral sentiment based on the MFT typology (Hoover et al., 2020). These authors used distributed representations (embeddings) of text as features to train a classifier to predict the scores of text corresponding to the moral frames. This work shows that moral frames significantly improve the prediction of the partisanship of news based on the headlines and showcases the feasibility of automatically classifying the moral framing and political partisanship of news sources on social media platforms.

Human-Annotation-Based Assessment of Moral Language

Other than dictionary-based assessment of moral language (e.g., MFD) and contextualized assessment of moral language using distributed representations, a new methodology is being widely adopted by psychologists: manual annotation of moral language as ground truth for training machine learning algorithms. In this method, researchers agree on a theoretical framework with which they code signals for moral rhetoric. Then, a number of trained annotators code textual data for the presence of morally relevant information based on an *a priori*, theoretically justified typology (e.g., MFT). An implicit presupposition of this approach is that moral language is complex and context-dependent, thus, human judges can best capture the nuances and complexities of moral rhetoric in language data.

Mooijman, Hoover, Lin, Ji, and Dehghani (2018) conducted an observational study of the relationship between online moral rhetoric and real-world indicators of violent protest during the 2015 Baltimore protests that erupted following the death of Freddie Gray at the hands of the police, and they manually labeled about 5,000 tweets on the protests. The embeddings of these tweets and their moral labels were then passed on to a long short-term memory algorithm (LSTM; Hochreiter & Schmidhuber, 1997). This model was used to predict binary "moral" or "nonmoral" labels for 18 million tweets that were posted during the civic disturbance in cities where a protest responding to the death of Freddie Gray took place. Using these predicted labels, the researchers showed that days with violent protests have higher counts of moral tweets. Not only did the degree of moral rhetoric used on social media increase on days with violent protests, but also the hourly frequency of morally laden tweets predicted the future counts of arrests during violent protests, indicating a dynamic association between moralization and protest violence. These authors argued that the combination of moral outrage (see Salerno & Peter-Hagene, 2013) and perceived moral homogeneity contribute to violent protests.

As another example, Atari and colleagues (2022) recently investigated how morally homogeneous environments in two social networks (a social media site called Gab and a sub-Reddit called Incels) are conducive to hateful rhetoric. These authors relied on MFT and handcoded a large subset of posts from these two platforms, one of which is known to be highly popular among alt-right individuals (Gab) and the other which is a banned sub-Reddit known for disseminating misogynist content (Incels). These authors followed the human-annotation-based assessment framework to annotate moral rhetoric in these radicalized social networks. By relying on MFT, annotating more than 8,000 posts from these platforms, training neural-network models, automatically labeling millions of Gab and Incels posts, and performing cluster analysis based on network characteristics, these authors found that users who were more fused to their cluster in terms of moral language were more likely to disseminate more hateful, outgroup-derogatory language.

In an attempt to provide a resource for studying moral norms in language, Forbes, Hwang, Shwartz, Sap, and Choi (2020) lay out a conceptual formalism for studying people's everyday social norms and moral judgments over a rich spectrum of real-life situations as described in natural language. In doing so, they recorded participants' judgments, including social judgments of good and bad, moral foundations, expected cultural pressure, and assumed legality, based on "social rules of thumb." By relaying on the provided data on ethical assessments, these authors trained a computational language model, which can reason about social norms in new situations.

More accurate predictions of moral concerns in language are expected as the natural language processing models for text representation evolve and become publicly accessible. However, the fairness, transparency, and accountability concerns of such models shed doubt on their ethical application for assessing moral language. Issues concerning data selection, language annotation, and model training processes can lead to biased models with disproportionate capabilities in understanding specific language, generated by or directed to particular social groups (Mehrabi, Morstatter, Saxena, Lerman, & Galstyan, 2019). Particularly for evaluating moral language, researchers should consider the subjectivity of annotators in coding moral concerns as a critical barrier to achieve unbiased predictions for controversial or unconventional textual data.

Opportunities for Application of Mobile Sensing in Moral Psychology

MSMs capitalize on embedded sensors in digital media devices to capture an individual's experiences as well as their environments. MSMs offer a new opportunity to record and track behavior on repetitive occasions at the same time, such as tracking calls and social network activities (Ganti, Ye, & Lei, 2011; Gosling & Mason, 2015; Miller, 2012). These methods use sensor-rich devices, such as smartphones, wearables (e.g., smartwatches), and household appliances (e.g., smart thermostats) that are interconnected (Allemand & Mehl, 2017). The microphone, accelerometer, global positioning system (GPS), Bluetooth radio, Wi-Fi scans, ambient light sensor, gyroscope, and thermometer are the most common mobile sensors (Miller, 2012). Other types of data such as visual data (e.g., photos taken by camera), device use logs (e.g., battery status), and app use logs (e.g., text messages, calls, calendar entries) could be entered into a multimodal data processing pipeline to capture information about a broad range of features that characterize human behavior and the surrounding environment.

One recent study examined the extent to which individuals' personality traits can be predicted on the basis of six different classes of behavioral information collected via sensor and log data harvested from smartphones. Using a machine learning method, Stachl and colleagues (2020) successfully predicted facet-level personality traits (some of which were morally laden, such as sense of duty and discipline) based on behavioral data collected from 624 volunteers over 30 consecutive days (25,347,089 logging events). These findings revealed that specific patterns in behaviors in the domains of (1) communication and social behavior, (2) music consumption, (3) app usage, (4) mobility, (5) overall phone activity, and (6) day- and nighttime activity are distinctively predictive of personality traits. According to Stachl and colleagues, the accuracy of these machine learning models is similar to that found for predictions based on digital footprints from social media platforms and demonstrates the possibility of obtaining information about individuals' traits from behavioral patterns passively collected from their smartphones. All in all, this study points to both the benefits (e.g., in research settings) and dangers (e.g., privacy implications) presented by the widespread collection and modeling of behavioral data obtained from smartphones.

MSMs can assist morality research in novel and creative ways. By facilitating a hybrid methodology in which all aspects of morality could be examined simultaneously, instead of studying them in isolation, MSMs offer high ecological validity. In particular, since there is relatively little insight into how moral behavior, emotions, and self-views turn out in everyday life, MSMs are able to capture reliable measurement of morality by automating through use of smartphone apps, text messages, or emails. Language data collected by mobile sensors (e.g., spoken conversations) and device logs (e.g., text messages) could then reveal moral behavior, emotions, and judgments using the methods we outlined.

At the time of writing, MSMs have not been widely adopted by moral psychologists. In one early study, Youyou, Kosinski, and Stillwell (2015) examined the relationship between Facebook "likes" and basic human values (Schwartz, 1992; Schwartz & Bilsky, 1987). Schwartz's model of basic values includes achievement (personal success through demonstrating competence according to social standards), benevolence (preserving and enhancing the welfare of those with whom one is in frequent personal contact), conformity (restraint of actions, inclinations, and impulses likely to upset or harm others and violate social expectations or norms), hedonism (pleasure and sensuous gratification for oneself), power (social status and prestige, control or dominance over people and resources), security (safety, harmony, and stability of society, relationships, and self), self-direction (independent thought and action; choosing, creating, exploring), stimulation (excitement, novelty, and challenge in life), tradition (respect, commitment, and acceptance of the customs and ideas that traditional culture or religion provide the self), and universalism (understanding, appreciation, tolerance, and protection for the welfare of all people and for nature). Youyou and colleagues found that basic values can be linked to Facebook likes but did not provide much information about the interpretation of this finding.

In an exceptional effort to explore the link between digital behavioral records and moral values, Kalimeri, Beiró, Delfino, Raleigh, and Cattuto (2019) collected self-reported moral values through questionnaires from more than 7,600 individuals in the United States and combined these scores with multimodal digital data from participants' Web browsing behavior and smartphone usage, hence bridging the offline and online worlds in the moral domain. Upon acceptance of the study's privacy policy, all participants were asked to complete several questionnaires and were allowed access to either their basic mobile or desktop traffic data for a period of 1 month. For the participants who permitted the logging of their desktop Web-browsing data, the following information was recorded: the domain names, the time spent online, and the number of visits per day for each domain. Participants who allowed access to their mobile data were asked to download an application that logged their Web-browsing activity and app usage. The digital behaviors were then used to predict participants' demographic characteristics and moral values obtained via self-report. Results suggested that the Web domains from Desktop browsing were more informative than mobile data in predicting moral values.

Specifically, the top five websites emerging as the best predictors of moral foundations were google.com, foxnews.com, dailykos.com, yelp.com, and imdb.com. Using apps such as FOX News and Bible were also predictive of participants' self-reported moral values. Visiting websites and apps such as Snapchat, Bible, FOX News, Fantasy Sports, WhatsApp, Spotify, and YouTube were predictive of basic values (Schwartz, 1992). Overall, the prediction of Schwartz's basic values proved to be a more difficult classification problem than that of moral foundations. In other words, the five moral foundations were more robustly related to digital behavioral fingerprints, compared with the 10 basic values. The average classification metrics (wherein 50% indicates chance and 100% indicates perfect classification) for moral foundations and Schwartz's basic values were about 63% and 58%, respectively. According to Kalimeri and colleagues (2019), the results obtained for moral foundations and Schwartz values indicate that online behaviors are somewhat informative of people's moral values, but the poor-to-medium prediction accuracies may be related to the complexity of the moral values that are often expressed in subtle ways in everyday life, and only occasionally in a more intense, explicit manner in the digital world. Much like the link between social media language and moral foundations examined by Kennedy and colleagues (2021), the connection between digital behaviors and morality is characterized by complex dynamics, and these may not have been accessible to the authors in this study.

In a different domain, namely, health and fitness, moral values have also been linked to digital behaviors. Mejova and Kalimeri (2019) collected a demographically representative sample of over 15,000 U.S. participants and combined technology usage logs with surveys on moral foundations, Schwartz's basic values, as well as emotional contagion (i.e., the tendency to feel emotions, such as happiness, or sadness, triggered by the feelings expressed by the people with whom one interacts). Combining digital behaviors and self-reports similar to those of Kalimeri and colleagues (2019) showed that users who score higher on purity but lower on values of conformity, hedonism, and security are more likely to use health and fitness mobile applications.

Many smartphone data sources (e.g., accelerometer, GPS, light sensors) have not been fully used thus far in the moral psychology literature. However, MSMs do offer a unique opportunity for psychological research on morality. The value of MSMs for research on moral behavior is derived from their ability to assess actual daily behavior unobtrusively and continuously. One of the clearest opportunities is the prospect of obtaining a descriptive understanding of how moral values manifest in daily lives of people (see Atari & Colleagues, 2023; Hofmann et al., 2014). Indeed, a large number of open questions in moral psychology are best answered using new methodological advances such as MSMs. In particular, we argue that MSMs are well suited to address two open questions, among others, in contemporary science of morality: (1) *everyday relevance*: how relevant are moral values in everyday life and what kinds of moral behavior are most prevalent? and (2) *social influence*: how are moral attitudes, beliefs, or behavior modified by the presence or action of others?

Everyday Relevance

MSMs hold much promise as assessment tools for measuring moral behavior in daily life. Specifically, MSMs address the limitations of surveys and lab experiments for quantifying behavior by allowing the naturalistic observation of daily behaviors without the experimenter's interference (e.g., social interactions, chatting with friends, online donations). Hofmann and colleagues (2014) and Atari and colleagues (2023) both tackled the topic of "morality in everyday life" and got somewhat different results with regard to the primacy of morality in everyday life. These discrepancies could perhaps be due to their different methodologies, ESMs versus EAR. MSMs could further inform our understanding of the relevance of morality in everyday life, an ancient yet open question.

MSMs are promising for moral psychology as they can be used to obtain objective and automated measures of behavior. In addition, they permit researchers to collect data from traditionally hard-to-reach populations around the world. MSMs could expand our understanding of the moral domain in different cultures by permitting easier recruitment of individuals from different societies into research studies. Today, people around the world use a variety of sensing technologies, and the adoption rates will continue to increase as the technology becomes more affordable. The widespread usage of sensing technologies permits researchers to recruit participants from around the world, for instance, by having them download sensing software to their own personal devices, which can then be used to conduct theoretically informed psychological studies.

Using these methods can shed light on how morality shapes (and is shaped by) everyday interactions. For example, today it remains unclear what specific classes of digital behavior (e.g., app usage, music consumption, communication, mobility behavior, overall phone activity) are differentially informative about moral values. Other open questions in the domain of morality include: What do smartphones reveal about people's moral intuitions? To what extent do digital behaviors capture patterns of stability and variability in people's everyday thoughts, feelings, and behaviors in the moral domain? What can digital behaviors inform us about with regard to the extent to which people differ from one another and from themselves over and across time? These questions not only clarify past questions in moral psychology, but also help us better develop and refine theories (see Harari et al., 2020; Muthukrishna & Henrich, 2019).

Social Influence

Due to a high level of abstraction in moral cognition, moral values may be better captured by verbal rather than nonverbal behaviors. This further emphasizes the role of language analysis in moral psychology, but that is not to say that nonverbal behaviors do not have meaningful associations with morality (e.g., Stachl et al., 2020). MSMs hold a great deal of promise in exploring the much-studied link between social interactions and morality (see Rai & Fiske, 2011), which can be broken into two categories of face-to-face encounters and computer-mediated communication (Harari, Müller, Aung, & Rentfrow, 2017).

Face-to-face encounters refer to social interactions carried out in person without a mediating technology (Harari et al., 2017). Face-to-face encounters are typically captured by using microphone sensors and Bluetooth data. Microphones assess whether a person is engaged in conversation, the frequency of conversations, their duration, the content of conversations, and turn-taking in conversations (e.g., Miluzzo et al., 2008). Moreover, microphones provide information about features of speech during in-person conversations such as a speaker's voice pitch, voice frequencies, and speaking rates (Lu et al., 2012). Such social encounters may be analyzed, translating raw data across modalities and partners into structured data, by applying machine learning algorithms to microphone data, for example determining when a face-to-face conversation takes place or transcribing audio into written speech (Timmons et al., 2017). Secondary algorithms can be used to extract meaning from language data in these conversations as described in the language analysis section in this chapter. Bluetooth data may also be used to infer whether someone is physically isolated, the number of other co-present people, and the number of unique and repeated interaction partners (Chen et al., 2014). In addition, Wi-Fi data have been used to identify the size of co-present groups and the duration of such encounters (Vanderhulst, Mashhadi, Dashti, & Kawsar, 2015).

Computer-mediated communication refers to social interactions carried out through an electronic device (Harari et al., 2017). Computer-mediated communications are often quantified using data from smartphone application-use logs. App use logs can assess the frequency and duration of incoming and outgoing calls, the frequency and content of text messages, and the number of unique and repeated interaction partners a person communicates with (Boase & Ling, 2013; Kobayashi, Boase, Suzuki, & Suzuki, 2015). Furthermore, app use logs assess the frequency of using email and other communication applications (e.g., Facebook, Twitter) to interact with others (e.g., Mehrotra et al., 2017). Such communication measures have been used to understand people's social, family, and work networks (Min, Wiese, Hong, & Zimmerman, 2013) and predict personality traits (Chittaranjan, Blom, & Gatica-Perez, 2013), stress levels (Ferdous, Osmani, & Mayora, 2015), and sleeping patterns (Murnane, Abdullah, Matthews, Choudhury, & Gay, 2015).

These developments further highlight how MSMs can be helpful in answering an important psychological question: Can social context and conformity influence morality? Despite the ubiquity and gravity of moral judgment in our everyday lives, scant research exists on the role of conformity in moral judgment outside strictly experimental settings. In a classic study, Crutchfield (1955) tested the impact of majority opinion on judgments in a variety of different domains, including agreement with morally relevant statements and found that only 19% of participants agreed with such statements when alone, but 58% agreed when confronted with a unanimous group who endorsed the statements. Aramovich, Lytle, and Skitka (2012) assessed prior beliefs concerning the acceptability of torture, along with their prior moral commitments and sociopolitical attitudes. Then, participants took part in an allegedly group discussion concerning the use of torture via a computer-simulated chat room; the participants believed they were discussing the topic with fellow students. During the simulated group discussion, 80% of the participants reported less opposition to torture than they had reported at pretest, but strength of moral conviction about torture was negatively associated with degree of pro-torture attitude change. These results suggest that moral judgments in everyday life are susceptible to conformity pressures (Kundu & Cummins, 2013). MSMs offer great opportunity to test and expand these ideas beyond the lab in face-to-face encounters and computer-mediated communication.

Pitfalls and Future Directions of Mobile Sensing in Moral Psychology

Although MSMs offer a unique opportunity to explore different aspects of human morality, challenges in employing such methods persist. The rest of this chapter will focus on describing these drawbacks and explaining how researchers can potentially address them.

Interdisciplinary Issues

While MSMs offer many methodological benefits for psychological research, relatively few studies use such methods. This is potentially because researchers interested in using MSMs have to assemble a multidisciplinary team. The creation or modification of sensing software requires skills in computer programming and familiarity with setting up physical or cloud-based servers. Also, the continuous and fine-grained nature of sensor data collection results in massive datasets that can easily reach several gigabytes per participant, depending on the types of data collected. These datasets require skills in database management and advanced analytic techniques. Hence, mobile sensing is essentially a "team science" effort.

A group that is composed of only psychologists (or other social scientists) may not fully utilize the potential of MSMs due to technical barriers. On the other hand, a group of researchers without knowledge of the subject matter will fail to understand a sociopsychological phenomenon, no matter how advanced their methodological apparatus is. Thus, conducting a mobile sensing study requires engaging interdisciplinary collaborations ranging from psychologists and computational social scientists to computer scientists. As we have discussed, this promising methodology may be worth the effort since it can address questions that are otherwise impossible to answer. On the one hand, efforts to capture moral judgments, emotions, and behaviors with technical sophistication per se can fail to consider the nuances of moral cognition and its long history in philosophy and social sciences. On the other hand, highly theory-driven efforts may not fully actualize the state-of-the-art technologies that outperform traditional methods. In that sense, theory and methods coevolve best in team efforts by integrating the theoretical insights of moral psychology and the methodological advances of MSMs.

WEIRD Issues

Although people across the globe have much in common, research demonstrates that many aspects of psychology, including basic perceptual and cognitive functioning, differ depending on social and cultural context. However, samples in studies of moral psychology have been drawn mainly from Western, educated, industrialized, rich, and democratic (WEIRD; Henrich, Heine, & Norenzayan, 2010) societies since the 1940s to the present day (Ellemers et al., 2019). An unusual 5% of the world's population cannot continue to stand in for all of humanity if psychologists wish to have an ethical, empirically sound science that is useful to increasingly polyethnic societies and a globally connected world. For the years 2014–2018, the proportional representation of authors and samples from the United States decreased and that of other English-speaking and Western European countries increased, thereby improving the internationalization of psychology to an extent. However, the participation of the majority of countries has not meaningfully increased (Thalmayer, Toscanelli, & Arnett, 2020). To our knowledge, most existing work using MSMs (as well as ambulatory and language analysis) focus on WEIRD populations, neglecting a large slice of human diversity. First, we argue how morality research can benefit from studying a non-WEIRD society according to one recent study. Second, we discuss how WEIRD issues can impact applications of MSMs in moral psychology.

Morality can be described as a culturally transmitted set of normative values and rules that enable people to live together (more or less) in harmony. As such, moral concerns might be known to researchers only by their WEIRD manifestations if their sample is largely drawn from WEIRD cultures such as the United States. However, as one of the few existing examples of studying morality in a non-WEIRD society, Atari, Graham, and Dehghani (2020) evaluated the utility of MFT in Iran, a non-Western, Muslim-majority, understudied cultural setting. Across five qualitative and quantitative studies, these authors reported that although MFT is a useful framework, it may not fully reflect the foundations of morality (possibly, a new "moral foundation"; see Graham et al., 2013) in Iran. Specifically, qualitative studies uncovered a new dimension of morality in the Farsi language, "Qeirat," which comprises the guarding and protectiveness of female kin, romantic partners, broader family, and country. These studies clearly show that moral psychological research should investigate, as well as be informed by, cultural and linguistic diversity.

As a new technique for capturing psychological phenomena in the wild, MSMs depend on widespread use of smartphones. MSMs could help with the WEIRDness of moral psychology by permitting easier recruitment of individuals from non-WEIRD societies into research studies. These days, people across cultures use a variety of sensing technologies, and smartphones are very widespread, and the adoption rates are expected to continue to increase as the technology becomes more affordable and equitable. The widespread usage of sensing technologies permits researchers to recruit participants from previously neglected populations, which in turn can be used to develop more inclusive theories of human morality. It is thus imperative to promote and conduct cross-cultural studies using MSMs. International collaboration and technology transfer (e.g., sharing needed technical skills to set up the sensing software and data processing tools) may immensely improve such investigation.

Ethical Issues

Article 12 of the United Nations Universal Declaration of Human Rights recognizes the protection of privacy as a central human right. Specifically, within the psychological research community, the protection of personal data has already been considered as a top priority. In this sense, MSMs raise more privacy concerns regarding the collection, transfer, processing, storage, potential release, or final deletion of data. The term *psychological targeting* has been coined to describe the practice of influencing the behavior of large groups of people through interventions that are psychologically tailored. This kind of targeting is defined by two components that carry their unique challenges when it comes to privacy issues: (1) *psychological profiling* refers to the automated assessment of psychological characteristics from digital footprints and (2) *psychologically informed interventions* describe the attempt to influence people's attitudes and behaviors based on their psychological motivations (Matz, Appel, & Kosinski, 2020).

The concept of psychological targeting gained global infamy during the U.S. presidential election of 2016, after a company named Cambridge Analytica inappropriately collected data from approximately 87 million Facebook users to target them with psychologically tailored advertising, allegedly aimed to influence people's voting preferences in the 2016 U.S. presidential election. Scandals such as Cambridge Analytica often result in calls for stronger regulation and governmental oversight, even though individuals might consider themselves immune to psychologically tailored ads (Hinds, Williams, & Joinson, 2020). The European Union's General Data Protection Regulation (GDPR) is among the strictest data protection regulations around the globe and the first to mention the concept of profiling and its use in automated decision making (Matz et al., 2020). GDPR's basic principle of transparency mandates that companies have to disclose—in clear and simple terms—not only what type of data is collected, but also for which purposes and whether it will be shared with third parties. Privacy issues are particularly important in moral psychology studies, as morality is closely related to political attitudes (Voelkel, Mernyk, & Willer, 2023), and these political attitudes are often the target of psychological profiling.

Privacy behaviors are culture- and context-dependent, which makes the dilemma of what to share and what to keep private, across societies and over time, a perplexing issue. The task of navigating contextual nuances and the consequences of mismanaging them have grown increasingly complicated in the information age, to the point that natural human instincts do not seem to be nearly adequate (Acquisti, Brandimarte, & Loewenstein, 2015). In short, transparency and accountability are needed in terms of describing how sensing software is sampled (e.g., what and how often sensors will activate) and also, assuring individuals that any data collected, stored, and shared are handled using secure practices. These protocols include using industry-standard techniques for data transfer and use of password-protected platforms for secure data storage and sharing. These ethical issues are even more pronounced in moral psychology research as the very subject of study is about people's judgment of right and wrong.

Conclusion

Human morality is an ancient area of inquiry in philosophy and, more recently, in psychology. As humans' social lives evolve into complicated forms intertwined with technology use, it is important to understand how human morality interacts with technology use as well as, conversely, how technology use can affect moral concerns. Mobile sensing methods offer a collection of methodological advancements that can help understand morality. However, few studies have used such methods to collect objective measures of moral behavior as they transpire in daily life, out in the real world. In this chapter, we provided a review of recent studies focused on ambulatory assessment and language analysis in moral psychology, and then we reviewed the opportunities for applying MSMs in moral psychology research by integrating these lines of research. We argue that moral psychology in the domain of everyday relevance and social influence can particularly benefit from these new methods. Finally, we draw attention to the issues and barriers in the field, namely, the issues of interdisciplinarity and overreliance on Western samples in MSM research, and ethical pitfalls in collecting, saving, and sharing digital fingerprints.

REFERENCES

Acquisti, A., Brandimarte, L., & Loewenstein, G. (2015). Privacy and human behavior in the age of information. *Science, 347*(6221), 509–514.

Allemand, M., & Mehl, M. R. (2017). Personality assessment in daily life: A roadmap for future personality development research. In J. Specht (Ed.), *Personality development across the lifespan* (pp. 437–454). Elsevier.

Amir, D., Ahl, R., Parsons, W. S., & McAuliffe, K. (2021). Children are more forgiving of accidental harms across development. *Journal of Experimental Child Psychology, 205*, 105081.

Aramovich, N. P., Lytle, B. L., & Skitka, L. J. (2012). Opposing torture: Moral conviction and resistance to majority influence. *Social Influence, 7*(1), 21–34.

Atari, M., Davani, A. M., Kogon, D., Kennedy, B., Ani Saxena, N., Anderson, I., & Dehghani, M. (2022). Morally homogeneous networks and radicalism. *Social Psychological and Personality Science, 13*(6), 999–1009.

Atari, M., & Dehghani, M. (2022). Language analysis in moral psychology. In M. Dehghani & R. Boyd (Eds.), *Handbook of language analysis in psychology* (pp. 207–228). Guilford Press.

Atari, M., Graham, J., & Dehghani, M. (2020). Foundations of morality in Iran. *Evolution and Human Behavior, 41*(5), 367–384.

Atari, M., Mehl, M. R., Graham, J., Doris, J. M., Schwarz, N., Davani, A. M., . . . Dehghani, M. (2023). The paucity of morality in everyday talk. *Scientific Reports, 13*(1), 5967.

Bhatia, S., Richie, R., & Zou, W. (2019). Distributed semantic representations for modeling human judgment. *Current Opinion in Behavioral Sciences, 29*, 31–36.

Boase, J., & Ling, R. (2013). Measuring mobile phone use: Self-report versus log data. *Journal of Computer-Mediated Communication, 18*(4), 508–519.

Bolger, N., & Laurenceau, J.-P. (2013). *Intensive longitudinal methods: An introduction to diary and experience sampling research.* Guilford Press.

Bollich, K. L., Doris, J. M., Vazire, S., Raison, C. L., Jackson, J. J., & Mehl, M. R. (2016). Eavesdropping on character: Assessing everyday moral behaviors. *Journal of Research in Personality, 61*, 15–21.

Bostyn, D. H., Sevenhant, S., & Roets, A. (2018). Of mice, men, and trolleys: Hypothetical judgment versus real-life behavior in trolley-style moral dilemmas. *Psychological science, 29*(7), 1084–1093.

Boyd, R. L., & Schwartz, H. A. (2020). Natural language analysis and the psychology of verbal behavior: The past, present, and future states of the field. *Journal of Language and Social Psychology, 40*(1), 21–41.

Brady, W. J., & Crockett, M. J. (2019). How effective is online outrage? *Trends in Cognitive Sciences, 23*(2), 79–80.

Brady, W. J., Wills, J. A., Jost, J. T., Tucker, J. A., & Van Bavel, J. J. (2017). Emotion shapes the diffusion of moralized content in social networks. *Proceedings of the National Academy of Sciences, 114*(28), 7313–7318.

Chen, Z., Chen, Y., Hu, L., Wang, S., Jiang, X., Ma, X., et al. (2014). Contextsense: Unobtrusive discovery of incremental social context using dynamic Bluetooth data. *Proceedings of the 2014 ACM International Joint Conference on Pervasive and Ubiquitous Computing: Adjunct Publication*, pp. 23–26.

Chittaranjan, G., Blom, J., & Gatica-Perez, D. (2013). Mining large-scale smartphone data for personality studies. *Personal and Ubiquitous Computing, 17*(3), 433–450.

Clifford, S., & Jerit, J. (2013). How words do the work of politics: Moral foundations theory and the debate over stem cell research. *The Journal of Politics, 75*(3), 659–671.

Crockett, M. J., Siegel, J. Z., Kurth-Nelson, Z., Dayan, P., & Dolan, R. J. (2017). Moral transgressions corrupt neural representations of value. *Nature Neuroscience, 20*(6), 879.

Crutchfield, R. S. (1955). Conformity and character. *American Psychologist, 10*(5), 191.

Day, M. V., Fiske, S. T., Downing, E. L., & Trail, T. E. (2014). Shifting liberal and conservative attitudes using moral foundations theory. *Personality and Social Psychology Bulletin, 40*(12), 1559–1573.

Dehghani, M., Johnson, K., Hoover, J., Sagi, E., Garten, J., Parmar, N. J., et al. (2016). Purity homophily in social networks. *Journal of Experimental Psychology: General, 145*(3), 366.

Ellemers, N., van der Toorn, J., Paunov, Y., & van Leeuwen, T. (2019). The psychology of morality: A review and analysis of empirical studies published from 1940 through 2017. *Personality and Social Psychology Review, 23*(4), 332–366.

Ferdous, R., Osmani, V., & Mayora, O. (2015). Smartphone app usage as a predictor of perceived stress levels at workplace. *2015 9th International Conference on Pervasive Computing Technologies for Healthcare (Pervasivehealth)*, pp. 225–228.

Forbes, M., Hwang, J. D., Shwartz, V., Sap, M., & Choi, Y. (2020, November). Social chemistry 101: Learning to reason about social and moral norms. *Proceedings of the 2020 Conference on Empirical*

Methods in Natural Language Processing (EMNLP), pp. 653–670. www.aclweb.org/anthology/2020.emnlp-main.48

Ganti, R. K., Ye, F., & Lei, H. (2011). Mobile crowdsensing: Current state and future challenges. *IEEE Communications Magazine, 49*(11), 32–39.

Garten, J., Hoover, J., Johnson, K. M., Boghrati, R., Iskiwitch, C., & Dehghani, M. (2018). Dictionaries and distributions: Combining expert knowledge and large scale textual data content analysis. *Behavior Research Methods, 50*(1), 344–361.

Gintis, H., Henrich, J., Bowles, S., Boyd, R., & Fehr, E. (2008). Strong reciprocity and the roots of human morality. *Social Justice Research, 21*(2), 241–253.

Gosling, S. D., & Mason, W. (2015). Internet research in psychology. *Annual Review of Psychology, 66*, 877–902.

Graham, J. (2014). Morality beyond the lab. *Science, 345*(6202), 1242.

Graham, J., Haidt, J., Koleva, S., Motyl, M., Iyer, R., Wojcik, S. P., et al. (2013). Moral foundations theory: The pragmatic validity of moral pluralism. In *Advances in experimental social psychology* (Vol. 47, pp. 55–130). Elsevier.

Graham, J., Haidt, J., & Nosek, B. A. (2009). Liberals and conservatives rely on different sets of moral foundations. *Journal of Personality and Social Psychology, 96*(5), 1029.

Graham, J., Meindl, P., & Beall, E. (2012). Integrating the streams of morality research: The case of political ideology. *Current Directions in Psychological Science, 21*(6), 373–377.

Graham, J., Nosek, B. A., Haidt, J., Iyer, R., Koleva, S., & Ditto, P. H. (2011). Mapping the moral domain. *Journal of Personality and Social Psychology, 101*(2), 366.

Grühn, D., Rebucal, K., Diehl, M., Lumley, M., & Labouvie-Vief, G. (2008). Empathy across the adult lifespan: Longitudinal and experience-sampling findings. *Emotion, 8*(6), 753.

Hackel, L. M., & Amodio, D. M. (2018). Computational neuroscience approaches to social cognition. *Current Opinion in Psychology, 24*, 92–97.

Haidt, J. (2008). Morality. *Perspectives on Psychological Science, 3*(1), 65–72.

Haidt, J., & Joseph, C. (2004). Intuitive ethics: How innately prepared intuitions generate culturally variable virtues. *Daedalus, 133*(4), 55–66.

Harari, G. M., Lane, N. D., Wang, R., Crosier, B. S., Campbell, A. T., & Gosling, S. D. (2016). Using smartphones to collect behavioral data in psychological science: Opportunities, practical considerations, and challenges. *Perspectives on Psychological Science, 11* (6), 838–854.

Harari, G. M., Müller, S. R., Aung, M. S., & Rentfrow, P. J. (2017). Smartphone sensing methods for studying behavior in everyday life. *Current Opinion in Behavioral Sciences, 18*, 83–90.

Harari, G. M., Vaid, S. S., Müller, S. R., Stachl, C., Marrero, Z., Schoedel, R., et al. (2020). Personality sensing for theory development and assessment in the digital age. *European Journal of Personality, 34*(5), 649–669.

Hardy, S. A., Zhang, Z., Skalski, J. E., Melling, B. S., & Brinton, C. T. (2014). Daily religious involvement, spirituality, and moral emotions. *Psychology of Religion and Spirituality, 6*(4), 338.

Henrich, J., Heine, S. J., & Norenzayan, A. (2010). Most people are not weird. *Nature, 466*(7302), 29.

Hinds, J., Williams, E. J., & Joinson, A. N. (2020). "It wouldn't happen to me": Privacy concerns and perspectives following the Cambridge Analytica scandal. *International Journal of Human-Computer Studies, 143*, 102498.

Hochreiter, S., & Schmidhuber, J. (1997). Long short-term memory. *Neural Computation, 9*(8), 1735–1780.

Hofmann, W., Wisneski, D. C., Brandt, M. J., & Skitka, L. J. (2014). Morality in everyday life. *Science, 345*(6202), 1340–1343.

Holtzman, N. S., Vazire, S., & Mehl, M. R. (2010). Sounds like a narcissist: Behavioral manifestations of narcissism in everyday life. *Journal of Research in Personality, 44*(4), 478–484.

Hoover, J., Dehghani, M., Johnson, K., Iliev, R., & Graham, J. (2018). Into the wild: Big Data analytics in moral psychology. In K. Gray & J. Graham (Eds.), *Atlas of Moral Psychology* (pp. 525–536). Guilford Press.

Hoover, J., Portillo-Wightman, G., Yeh, L., Havaldar, S., Davani, A. M., Lin, Y., et al.

(2020). Moral foundations twitter corpus: A collection of 35k tweets annotated for moral sentiment. *Social Psychological and Personality Science, 11*(8), 1057–1071.

Iliev, R., Dehghani, M., & Sagi, E. (2015). Automated text analysis in psychology: Methods, applications, and future developments. *Language and Cognition, 7*(2), 265–290.

Iyer, R., Koleva, S., Graham, J., Ditto, P., & Haidt, J. (2012). Understanding libertarian morality: The psychological dispositions of self-identified libertarians. *PloS One, 7*(8), e42366.

Jung, J.-H. (2020). The mobilizing effect of parties' moral rhetoric. *American Journal of Political Science, 64*(2), 341–355.

Kahane, G., Everett, J. A., Earp, B. D., Farias, M., & Savulescu, J. (2015). "Utilitarian"judgments in sacrificial moral dilemmas do not reflect impartial concern for the greater good. *Cognition, 134*, 193–209.

Kalimeri, K., Beiró, M. G., Delfino, M., Raleigh, R., & Cattuto, C. (2019). Predicting demographics, moral foundations, and human values from digital behaviours. *Computers in Human Behavior, 92*, 428–445.

Kennedy, B., Atari, M., Davani, A. M., Hoover, J., Omrani, A., Graham, J., & Dehghani, M. (2021). Moral concerns are differentially observable in language. *Cognition, 212*, 104696.

Kobayashi, T., Boase, J., Suzuki, T., & Suzuki, T. (2015). Emerging from the cocoon?: Revisiting the tele-cocooning hypothesis in the smartphone era. *Journal of Computer-Mediated Communication, 20*(3), 330–345.

Kouchaki, M. (2011). Vicarious moral licensing: The influence of others' past moral actions on moral behavior. *Journal of Personality and Social Psychology, 101*(4), 702.

Krasnow, M. M. (2017). An evolutionarily informed study of moral psychology. In B. G. Voyer & T. Tarantola (Eds.), *Moral Psychology: A Multidisciplinary Guide* (pp. 29–41). Springer.

Kundu, P., & Cummins, D. D. (2013). Morality and conformity: The Asch paradigm applied to moral decisions. *Social Influence, 8*(4), 268–279.

Lane, N. D., Miluzzo, E., Lu, H., Peebles, D., Choudhury, T., & Campbell, A. T. (2010). A survey of mobile phone sensing. *IEEE Communications Magazine, 48*(9), 140–150.

Lu, H., Frauendorfer, D., Rabbi, M., Mast, M. S., Chittaranjan, G. T., Campbell, A. T., et al. (2012). Stresssense: Detecting stress in unconstrained acoustic environments using smartphones. *Proceedings of the 2012 ACM Conference on Ubiquitous Computing*, pp. 351–360.

Matz, S. C., Appel, R. E., & Kosinski, M. (2020). Privacy in the age of psychological targeting. *Current Opinion in Psychology, 31*, 116–121.

Mehl, M. R. (2006). The lay assessment of subclinical depression in daily life. *Psychological Assessment, 18*(3), 340.

Mehl, M. R. (2017). The electronically activated recorder (EAR): A method for the naturalistic observation of daily social behavior. *Current Directions in Psychological Science, 26*(2), 184–190.

Mehl, M. R., Pennebaker, J. W., Crow, D. M., Dabbs, J., & Price, J. H. (2001). The electronically activated recorder (EAR): A device for sampling naturalistic daily activities and conversations. *Behavior Research Methods, Instruments, and Computers, 33*(4), 517–523.

Mehrabi, N., Morstatter, F., Saxena, N., Lerman, K., & Galstyan, A. (2019). A survey on bias and fairness in machine learning. *ACM Computing Surveys (CSUR), 54*(6), 1–35.

Mehrotra, A., Müller, S. R., Harari, G. M., Gosling, S. D., Mascolo, C., Musolesi, M., et al. (2017). Understanding the role of places and activities on mobile phone interaction and usage patterns. *Proceedings of the ACM on Interactive, Mobile, Wearable and Ubiquitous Technologies, 1*(3), 1–22.

Meindl, P., Jayawickreme, E., Furr, R. M., & Fleeson, W. (2015). A foundation beam for studying morality from a personological point of view: Are individual differences in moral behaviors and thoughts consistent? *Journal of Research in Personality, 59*, 81–92.

Mejova, Y., & Kalimeri, K. (2019). Effect of values and technology use on exercise: implications for personalized behavior change interventions. *Proceedings of the 27th ACM Conference on User Modeling, Adaptation and Personalization*, pp. 36–45.

Miller, G. (2012). The smartphone psychology manifesto. *Perspectives on Psychological Science, 7*(3), 221–237.

Miluzzo, E., Lane, N. D., Fodor, K., Peterson, R., Lu, H., Musolesi, M., et al. (2008). Sensing meets mobile social networks: The design, implementation and evaluation of the cenceme application. *Proceedings of the 6th ACM Conference on Embedded Network Sensor Systems*, pp. 337–350.

Min, J.-K., Wiese, J., Hong, J. I., & Zimmerman, J. (2013). Mining smartphone data to classify life-facets of social relationships. *Proceedings of the 2013 Conference on Computer Supported Cooperative Work*, pp. 285–294.

Mokhberian, N., Abeliuk, A., Cummings, P., & Lerman, K. (2020). Moral framing and ideological bias of news. *International Conference on Social Informatics*, pp. 206–219.

Mooijman, M., Hoover, J., Lin, Y., Ji, H., & Dehghani, M. (2018). Moralization in social networks and the emergence of violence during protests. *Nature Human Behaviour, 2*(6), 389–396.

Murnane, E. L., Abdullah, S., Matthews, M., Choudhury, T., & Gay, G. (2015). Social (media) jet lag: How usage of social technology can modulate and reflect circadian rhythms. *Proceedings of the 2015 ACM International Joint Conference on Pervasive and Ubiquitous Computing*, pp. 843–854.

Muthukrishna, M., & Henrich, J. (2019). A problem in theory. *Nature Human Behaviour, 3*(3), 221–229.

Nakamura, J. (2013). Pride and the experience of meaning in daily life. *The Journal of Positive Psychology, 8*(6), 555–567.

Newman, D. B., Schwarz, N., Graham, J., & Stone, A. A. (2019). Conservatives report greater meaning in life than liberals. *Social Psychological and Personality Science, 10*(4), 494–503.

Paulhus, D. L. (1986). Self-deception and impression management in test responses. In A. Angleitner & J. S. Wiggins (Eds,), *Personality assessment via questionnaires* (pp. 143–165). Springer.

Pennebaker, J. W., Booth, R. J., & Francis, M. E. (2007). *Linguistic inquiry and word count: LIWC* [Computer software]. LIWC.net.

Pennebaker, J. W., Mehl, M. R., & Niederhoffer, K. G. (2003). Psychological aspects of natural language use: Our words, our selves. *Annual Review of Psychology, 54*(1), 547–577.

Purzycki, B. G., Henrich, J., Apicella, C., Atkinson, Q. D., Baimel, A., Cohen, E., et al. (2018). The evolution of religion and morality: A synthesis of ethnographic and experimental evidence from eight societies. *Religion, Brain and Behavior, 8*(2), 101–132.

Rai, T. S., & Fiske, A. P. (2011). Moral psychology is relationship regulation: Moral motives for unity, hierarchy, equality, and proportionality. *Psychological Review, 118*(1), 57.

Runyan, J. D., Fry, B. N., Steenbergh, T. A., Arbuckle, N. L., Dunbar, K., & Devers, E. E. (2019). Using experience sampling to examine links between compassion, eudaimonia, and pro-social behavior. *Journal of Personality, 87*(3), 690–701.

Sagi, E., & Dehghani, M. (2014). Measuring moral rhetoric in text. *Social Science Computer Review, 32*(2), 132–144.

Salerno, J. M., & Peter-Hagene, L. C. (2013). The interactive effect of anger and disgust on moral outrage and judgments. *Psychological Science, 24*(10), 2069–2078.

Sap, M., Card, D., Gabriel, S., Choi, Y., & Smith, N. A. (2019). The risk of racial bias in hate speech detection. *Proceedings of the 57th Annual Meeting of the Association for Computational Linguistics*, pp. 1668–1678.

Saucier, G. (2018). Culture, morality and individual differences: Comparability and incomparability across species. *Philosophical Transactions of the Royal Society B: Biological Sciences, 373*(1744), 20170170.

Schwartz, S. H. (1992). Universals in the content and structure of values: Theoretical advances and empirical tests in 20 countries. *Advances in Experimental Social Psychology, 25*(1), 1–65.

Schwartz, S. H., & Bilsky, W. (1987). Toward a universal psychological structure of human values. *Journal of Personality and Social Psychology, 53*(3), 550.

Schwarz, N. (1999). Self-reports: how the questions shape the answers. *American Psychologist, 54*(2), 93.

Shiffman, S., Stone, A., & Hufford, M. (2008). Ecological momentary assessment. *Annual Review of Clinical Psychology, 4*, 1–32.

Sloane, S., Baillargeon, R., & Premack, D. (2012). Do infants have a sense of fairness? *Psychological Science, 23*(2), 196–204.

Stachl, C., Au, Q., Schoedel, R., Gosling, S. D., Harari, G. M., Buschek, D., et al. (2020). Predicting personality from patterns of behavior collected with smartphones. *Proceedings of the National Academy of Sciences, 117*(30), 17680–17687.

Thalmayer, A. G., Toscanelli, C., & Arnett,

J. J. (2020). The neglected 95% revisited: Is American psychology becoming less American? *American Psychologist, 76*(1), 116–129.

Timmons, A. C., Baucom, B. R., Han, S. C., Perrone, L., Chaspari, T., Narayanan, S. S., et al. (2017). New frontiers in ambulatory assessment: Big data methods for capturing couples' emotions, vocalizations, and physiology in daily life. *Social Psychological and Personality Science, 8*(5), 552–563.

Trull, T. J., & Ebner-Priemer, U. (2014). The role of ambulatory assessment in psychological science. *Current Directions in Psychological Science, 23*(6), 466–470.

Vanderhulst, G., Mashhadi, A., Dashti, M., & Kawsar, F. (2015). Detecting human encounters from wifi radio signals. *Proceedings of the 14th International Conference on Mobile and Ubiquitous Multimedia*, pp. 97–108.

Voelkel, J. G., Mernyk, J. S., & Willer, R. (2023). Moral reframing increases support for economically progressive candidates. *PNAS Nexus, 2*(6), pgad154.

Weber, R., Mangus, J. M., Huskey, R., Hopp, F. R., Amir, O., Swanson, R., et al. (2018). Extracting latent moral information from text narratives: Relevance, challenges, and solutions. *Communication Methods and Measures, 12*(2–3), 119–139.

Youyou, W., Kosinski, M., & Stillwell, D. (2015). Computer-based personality judgments are more accurate than those made by humans. *Proceedings of the National Academy of Sciences, 112*(4), 1036–1040.

CHAPTER 22

Mobile Sensing in Relationship Research

Andrea B. Horn and Adela C. Timmons

CHAPTER OVERVIEW

Mobile sensing technologies provide a unique opportunity for investigating relational processes. In this chapter, first, generic views on what constitutes social relationships are introduced that help to organize the richness of data resulting from sensing social interactions. This is followed by a short introduction to existing frameworks when dealing with interdependent data streams of dyads (like a romantic couple or two friends). We then present a relevant selection of relational constructs and their corresponding sensor measures in the literature. Two innovative studies—the Couple Mobile Sensing Project and the Co-Sense Study—are then discussed in more detail as examples of sensing studies in the field of couple research. The chapter concludes with a discussion of the opportunities and remaining challenges of relationship sensing research.

Why Use Mobile Sensing in Relationship Research?

Mobile sensing technologies afford several unique opportunities for enhancing research on couples and families. First, couples and families who are in a laboratory setting are more likely to censor or change their behavior than those who are in their home environments. Thus, the intensity of arguments or other negative behaviors, such as blaming or criticizing, may be blunted as participants attempt to limit undesirable behaviors while being viewed by strangers. Second, data collected in laboratory settings often require researchers to put arbitrary limitations on the length of the interactions, and thus, critical information regarding the time scale of relationship phenomena is lost. In the case of conflict, for example, lab-based paradigms cannot typically determine how long a conflict would have lasted had it not been stopped and cannot determine how frequently such conflicts would occur. Third, mobile sensing methods allow researchers to model how contextual factors and events may impact relationship processes. External factors such as everyday stressors (e.g., a bad day at work, a broken dishwasher, a sick child) can affect how couples and families relate to one another, possibly triggering conflict or other maladaptive interactional patterns if stress enters the family system and impacts individual family members' mood (e.g., Repetti, Wang, & Saxbe, 2009). Finally, constructs and theories central to relationship research—such as conflict escalation, co-regulation, and attachment—require modeling of multimodal (e.g., physiology, language, tone), cross-person (e.g., parent-to-parent or parent-to-child), time-lagged response contingencies. Mobile sensing technologies (i.e., smartphones and wearable sensors), combined with statistical techniques such as multilevel modeling, dynamical systems modeling, and machine learning, may be especially well suited for modeling relationship processes (e.g., Ferrer & Helm, 2013).

In this chapter, we provide a short introduction to the conceptual foundations of close relationships and their characteristics. We then proceed to give examples of mobile sensing solutions, assessing these constructs in romantic relationships. Finally, we finish with an outlook and critical reflection on the opportunities and pitfalls of mobile sensing in relationship research.

Models of Relationships: A Short Introduction

Humans, as Aristotle says in his *Politeia*, are social animals who are characterized by their *need to belong* (Baumeister & Leary, 1995). Accordingly, lack of social connection and loneliness have become public health issues, as they are associated with physical (Valtorta, Kanaan, Gilbody, Ronzi, & Hanratty, 2016) and mental health problems (Beutel et al., 2017) and even predict mortality (Holt-Lunstad, Smith, & Layton, 2010). In adulthood, the quality of the romantic relationships plays a prominent role in adult health and well-being (Robles, Slatcher, Trombello, & McGinn, 2014), coping with disease (Horn, Boettcher, et al., 2019), and healthy aging (Horn & Röcke, 2020).

Given the importance of relational processes, one might wonder why an interpersonal perspective has been underrepresented in psychological investigations. Investigating interactive relationship processes is challenging. It requires methods that provide frameworks for dyadic data analysis, that is, considering both interaction partners in the data analysis to tap truly interactive processes. More importantly, data on social interactions need to be collected on the time scale at which they naturally unfold and in the context in which they occur. As an example, conflict has been of interest in couple research for a long time. However, it has mostly been studied in instructed lab situations with all its limitations regarding ecological validity. Mobile sensing is particularly promising in this regard, for it offers an economic way to passively and in a "just-in-time" manner assess relational variables around how couples and families interact in a synchronized way.

For a framework to interpret relational variables with mobile sensing, it is recommended that earlier theories attempting to provide generic frameworks of conceptualizing dyadic relationships be acknowledged. A dyad consists of two interacting individuals that can represent different types of relationships—for example, mother and child, two strangers, acquaintances, romantic partners, and sports buddies. However, within these types of dyads, great differences in terms of their psychological characteristics can be found (Berscheid, 1994); as an example, labeling a relationship with "friendship" can represent different things to different people. As one solution, generic views on the qualities of *close relationships* have been introduced suggesting that relationships can be characterized by the level of interdependence of two individuals' actions, thoughts, and feelings (Berscheid, 1994; Neyer & Lang, 2003; Neyer, Wruz, Wagner, & Lang., 2011; Reis, Collins, & Berscheid, 2000) and the interconnection of cognitive representations of the self and the partner (Aron et al., 2004). Blending the resources of both partners opens up compensatory and uniquely relational resources when coping with adversities (Bodenmann, 1997; Fergus, 2015) such as diseases (Rohrbaugh, Mehl, Shoham, Reilly, & Ewy, 2008) and different forms of stress and trauma (Maercker & Horn, 2013). The establishment of psychological representations of the properties of this interdependence, or *psychological intimacy,* is a core feature defining the quality, rather than the type, of a given relationship (Reis & Shaver, 1988). From a developmental perspective, a highly influential model on the function of relationships is the *attachment model*, which assumes that early caregiver–infant interactions represent a formative experience of *co-regulation* of needs and affect (Bowlby, 1996). Recent models of adult psychological regulation suggest that *co-regulation* remains in default over the life span and underlines the importance of *social proximity* as a cue for a predictable, safe environment for human functioning (Coan & Sbarra, 2015).

These conceptual foundations of close relationships informed the development of methodological frameworks that were fundamental to the development in the area. The assumption that relationships are constituted by the interdependence of both interaction partners' behaviors leads to statistical frameworks empirically quantifying and controlling for these interdependencies and calling for the reliance on dyadic data when investigating relationships. The *actor–partner interdependence model* (APIM) controls for interdependencies and quantifies *mutual influences within and across partners* of a dyad (Kenny, Kashy, & Cook, 2006). The APIM framework has been highly influential in recent research on relationships. As an example, it allowed the investigation of *interpersonal emotion regulation*, that is, how the behavior of one partner shows effects on the other with respect to the unfolding of the momentary affect of both partners—considering the interdependencies and the effects of one's own regulatory behavior on their affect (Debrot, Schoebi, Perrez, & Horn, 2013; Horn, Samson, Debrot, & Perrez, 2019). Furthermore, it allows addressing the predictors and outcomes of *conflict situations* in couples and families within and across partners (Saxbe, Ramos, Timmons, Rodriguez, & Margolin, 2014).

In contrast, the *common fate model* (Ledermann & Kenny, 2012) and the recent *dyadic score model* (Iida, Seidman, & Shrout, 2018) focus on quantifying the effects of overlapping genuinely *dyadic features* on other variables in the dyad. Here the dyad is the analytical unit. For the common fate model, one latent variable is derived, for example, from the perspectives of both interaction partners in one communication episode. The dyadic parameters derived from the dyadic score model are the difference and mean of the two perspectives of a shared process (e.g., expressions of affection in a support episode). By considering both dyadic parameters simultaneously in the model, level differences are accounted for when looking at the role of the asymmetric reporting of dyadic processes. The most intuitive, straightforward way of quantifying interdependencies is to assess *synchronization* of behaviors (Butler & Randall, 2012; Coutinho et al., 2019; Ireland et al., 2011; Tschacher, Ramseyer, & Koole, 2018) and physiology (Saxbe & Repetti, 2010; Thorson, West, & Mendes, 2018; Timmons, Margolin, & Saxbe, 2015). A dynamic framework considering dampening and escalating over time within an episode in dyads provides the *temporal interpersonal systems* framework on emotions (Butler, 2017; Butler et al., 2017). An example for an escalating dynamic pattern would be the cyclical buildup of negative affect over time in both interaction partners during a conflict.

With regard to investigating close relationship processes with mobile sensing, these frameworks are useful for structuring and interpreting the data streams at hand. As depicted in Figure 22.1, first, *interactive behavior and shared contexts* can be gathered, as, for example, the number of phone calls, encounters, or conflicts or the couple's time spent together per day. This information represents dyad-level information in a multilevel framework; in other words, interactive behavior and shared contexts are always identical for both interaction partners. This genuinely dyadic information is often assessed, for example, via separate logfiles of both partners' mobile phones and thus is combined from two nonidentical data sources with distinct measurement errors. Furthermore, individual perceptions regarding the same event might differ; for example, one partner might assess an encounter as a conflict and the other not. Second, synchronously sensed *individual behavior and physiology* allow investigation of relationship processes by analyzing interdependencies (like synchronization) and mutual influences.

Sensing Measures in Relationship Research: Mobile Sensing Research on Couples

In this section, we provide an overview of parameters based on sensing information used in relationship research. In adulthood, the closest and most relevant relationship tends to be the romantic one (Reis et al., 2000). We focus on relevant examples of parameters in the research of romantic relationships. However, as described above, a generic view on

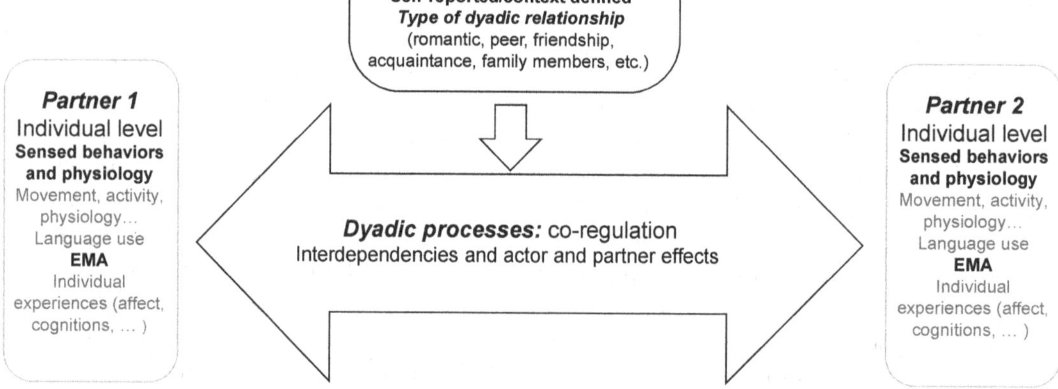

FIGURE 22.1. Sensing dyadic interactions and processes in close relationships: A conceptual framework.

relationship closeness bridges conceptually to other kinds of dyadic relationships; most of the parameters described in the following are not limited to romantic relationships. Therefore, the presented examples could inform research in other types of relationships, for example, acquaintances or friendships.

Sensing Social Proximity: Time Spent Together and Spatial Synchronization

Social proximity, time spent together, and interaction frequencies are relevant context factors in psychological research of close and romantic relationships that had been assessed mainly by self- and partner-report (Milek, Butler, & Bodenmann, 2015; Rauers, Blanke, & Riediger, 2013). Mobile sensing offers an unobtrusive way of assessing these constructs. Most research in this young area relies on two mobile phone sensors: GPS or Bluetooth. From logs of Bluetooth enter/exit signals and the corresponding IDs, relational variables can be derived (Matusik et al., 2019). Furthermore, synchronously assessed accelerometer data can be used to assess shared physical mobility in dyads, often in combination with Bluetooth information of the activity partner's presence (Dlugonski, Wood, DuBose, Rider, & Schoemann, 2019; Kuzik & Carson, 2018).

Another variant of Bluetooth sensor information—*Bluetooth low-energy beacons*—are commonly used in commercial contexts. Besides beacons found in places of interest like homes, mobile phones can be used as a virtual beacon that allows study of the proximity of different smartphones as a proxy for social proximity; algorithms have been developed to extract more precise distance measures from the information (Girolami, Mavilia, & Delmastro, 2020; see also Co-Sense Study). Moreover, dyadic location identification by GPS signals from both partners of a dyad allows detecting corresponding mobility patterns, distance between couples, and more or less correspondence regarding spatial patterns (Timmons, Chaspari, et al., 2017).The Co-Sense study is presented later in this chapter as a further example of the reliance of relationship research on sensing.

GPS- or beacon-sensor information of location can be used as a situational cue of proximity for initiating ecological momentary assessments (EMAs; Boateng, Santhanam, Lüscher, Scholz, & Kowatsch, 2019; Timmons, Chaspari, et al., 2017) or digital ecological momentary interventions (EMIs; Heron & Smyth, 2010). As an example, a recent study (Durbin, Debrot, Karremans, & van der Wal, 2020) implemented a couples intervention in the form of text messages to the romantic partners which called them to show physical affection. These text message interventions were triggered by the sensed presence of the romantic partner. Sensing-based assessment and intervention of social behavior is also a promising tool in management of physical disease. As an example, *DyMand*, a mobile, wearable system, has been developed to monitor and possibly intervene in common dyadic coping and support processes in couples facing a chronic disease (Boateng et al., 2019). The system combines dyadic assessment of mobile sensing with EMA and EMI triggered by the proximity of the couples (based on Bluetooth sensor information).

GPS sensing can also be used as an automatic indicator of the location of the romantic partner for long-distance couples, as studied with the application *CoupleVibe* (Bales, Li, & Griwsold, 2011). Couples can choose locations (e.g., home, work/school, fitness studio), and as soon as the partner arrives there they will receive a distinct vibration signal on the mobile phone. The authors report that the participating couples in the study interpreted the signals as a proxy for the partner's availability and also as a safety signal (*he arrived home safely*). Sharing sensor information of their romantic partners' mobile phones, including GPS-based estimates of distance from home, have been interpreted as computer-assisted augmentation of the couple communication and fostering closeness in this field (Griggio, Nouwens, McGrenere, & Mackay, 2019). As introduced above, couple relationships are constituted by interdependence and shared construal of the self, the "we" and the world. However, a balance between needs for autonomy and interdependence is a dilemma that requires constant recalibration of romantic relationships (Willi, 1985). Automatic sharing of mobile sensing data illustrates possible caveats of sensor-informed intervention programs. As an example, the interest of increasing closeness and interdependence in the couple by "spying" via sensing information what the other is doing 24/7 might be in conflict with the interest of the partner's autonomy and privacy. It requires a very sensitive process of establishing informed and shared consent in both interaction partners involved.

Sensing Digital Communication

Mobile devices can provide detailed information about how couples communicate digitally. Using phones, one can track a variety of metrics, including the number of communications or length of communications sent between partners, via either emails, text messages, or social media posts. It is also possible to analyze the content and quality of these communications through linguistic analysis (e.g., the frequency of words in specific language categories using programs such as the Linguistic Inquiry and Word Count [LIWC]; Pennebaker, Boyd, Jordan, & Blackburn, 2015) or through extraction of measures of vocal quality or tone (e.g., fundamental frequency; Weusthoff, Baucom, & Hahlweg, 2013). These data provide basic information about connectivity between people in relationships in real life and how the quality of these communications relates to or impacts relationship functioning. In one study by Slatcher and Pennebaker (2006), for example, researchers examined the content of instant messages sent between dating couples. Results showed that pronoun and emotion word use in instant messages predicted greater relationship satisfaction and stability. More studies followed in this area investigating social behavior by linguistic analyses of digital communication (Underwood, Ehrenreich, More, Solis, & Brinkley, 2015; Underwood, Rosen, More, Ehrenreich, & Gentsch, 2012), opening the door for this promising area of sensing research.

Additionally, these kinds of methods can provide information about how digital communication might help or harm relationships. Although digital communication affords opportunities to connect and stay in touch, it might also impede connection and closeness if such communications take the place of in-person interaction (Sbarra, Briskin, & Slatcher, 2019). Digital communication lacks aspects of interaction that are central components of bonding in relationships, such as physical touch, which may therefore limit its positive impact relative to in-person interactions. Furthermore, the impact of digital communications on relationship functioning likely depends on how the communications are used, for example, whether digital messages are used to express affection or to criticize and express discontent (e.g., Luo & Tuney, 2015; Schade, Sandberg, Bean, Busby, & Coyne, 2013). The challenges of sensing digital communication include privacy issues and informed consent of communicating individuals. Thus, many studies rely on romantic couples, with both partners participating in the research project and giving consent. Another strategy to avoid privacy and data security issues is to include a language analysis algorithm into the app that logs the communication; this only allows downloading and analyzing quantified parameters (e.g., percentage of certain word categories as assessed by the LIWC) without relying on personal information possibly without consent.

Sensing Daily Conversations of Couples

The sensing of acoustic signals via ambient audio recording has been established in psychological research through the electronically activated recorder (EAR), even before the smartphones were invented (for a review, see Mehl, 2017). In the meantime, its potential for research on relationship processes has been shown in several dyadic studies using the EAR method (e.g., Karan, Wright, & Robbins, 2017; Robbins, Karan, López, & Weihs, 2018; Robbins, López, Weihs, & Mehl, 2014; Robbins, Mehl, Smith, & Weihs, 2012). In these studies, the EAR is applied in parallel to both partners of a dyad, with most studies investigating the daily life of couples coping with cancer. After the presence of the partner is identified in the recording, couple conversations can be analyzed through ratings and analyses of language use. This increases ecological validity as compared to the prevailing analog couple conversation paradigms (Gottman, Markman, & Notarius, 1977), where couples are video-recorded in the lab talking about a topic of conflict or support. There has long been a call in couple research for more ecologically valid assessment of couple conversation. Gottman introduced the *dinnertime conversation* (back then, still in the lab) and provided a coding scheme to rate naturalistic couple conversations (Driver & Gottman, 2004).

Although the EAR method overcomes ethical and privacy concerns by sampling only short sound bites of daily conversations, it is not suitable for capturing an entire conversational sequence. If couples or families are at home and are not meeting bystanders, all can give consent to a "day in the life" paradigm that assesses continuous audio or even video recordings during a whole day or even longer. This methodology has been employed and extended by several groups of researchers, including the UCLA Center on the Everyday Lives of Families, which has employed detailed, ethnographic methods to capture the home lives of families (Campos, Graesch, Repetti, Bradbury, & Ochs, 2009) and couples coping with cancer diagnoses (e.g., Reblin et al., 2018, 2020; Reblin, Sutton, Vadaparampil, Heyman, & Ellington, 2019). Recently, the use of anger words of audio sensings of naturalistic couple conversations and EMA reported annoyance revealed insight into the role of family-of-origin aggression in daily conflict (Han et al., 2020).

Audio recordings allow further automatic analyses of the voice; so far, it has been used mostly for detecting emotional responses in (high-quality) lab recordings of couple conversations addressing conflict and support topics (e.g., Boateng, Sels, Kuppens, Hilpert, & Kowatsch, 2020). In spite of these promising developments, thorough psychometrical investigations continue to reveal the questionable validity of the automatically extracted emotional features in daily life (Weidman et al., 2020).

One primary challenge related to collecting audio conversations in daily life relates to privacy and ethical concerns. Researchers must take care to avoid collecting data on unconsented persons and to establish procedures for reviewing and responding to risk incidents that might be captured by audio recordings. Challenges also relate to processing the large amount of audio that is collected; researchers typically obtain many files that do not contain speech (e.g., TV). They must therefore spend significant time locating meaningful interactions and then transcribing or coding them. Furthermore, it is difficult to control the quality of recordings obtained in daily life, sometimes leading to uncodable files and limiting the accuracy of vocal measures extracted from them.

Sensing Conflict and Aggression in Dyadic Interactions

Mobile sensing might also provide valuable information regarding couple and family conflict and aggression escalation. Conflicts in close relationships often start quickly and inexplicably with little warning, resulting from subtle triggers that initiate well-ingrained feedback loops and behavioral response contingencies (e.g., Patterson, 1982). In these response loops, one person's negative affect and tone are met with increased negative affect and tone in the other person, which can escalate over time into full-blown aggressive episodes (Gottman, Coan, Carrere, & Swanson, 1998). Unlike lab-based conflict tasks, mobile sensing provides a unique opportunity to capture naturalistic triggers of conflict episodes, to measure how long conflict lasts, and to identify factors related to the eventual deescalation of the conflict. Furthermore, researchers can obtain information about how frequently the conflict occurred and how the intensity and frequency of real-life conflicts relate more generally to relationship satisfaction and relationship functioning. Through these methods, it is also possible to study how naturalistically occurring external events might contribute to conflict and aggression within family systems. For example, does conflict occur at a certain time of day or day of the week? What is the optimal level of conflict for maximizing relationship satisfaction? Is conflict more likely to occur when family members are under stress (e.g., a child misbehaves or the car breaks down)?

A number of studies to date have used mobile sensing methodologies to better understand conflict processes in close relationships. In some of the earliest studies examining conflict in naturalistic settings, researchers used daily diary data to measure conflict on an hourly or daily basis and to test how various occupational stressors or other types of stress impact marital and family functioning (e.g., Almeida, Wethington, & Chandler, 1999; Bolger, DeLongis, Kessler, & Wethington, 1989; Story & Repetti, 2006; Timmons, Arbel, & Margolin, 2017; Timmons & Margolin, 2015). The results of these studies generally show that families exhibiting high levels of aggression showed increased levels of spillover, a process whereby negative moods and daily stressors increase the likelihood of family conflicts occurring on the same day or even the next day.

Beyond daily diary EMA data, new technologies and sensing systems are being increasingly incorporated to study conflict processes in real life. For example, in one study conducted by our research team, we captured levels of electrodermal activity using wearable sensors during naturally occurring periods of relationship distress. Women with higher levels of family-of-origin aggression and a history of dating aggression perpetration showed greater physiological reactivity in daily life when feeling annoyed at their romantic partners. Moreover, heightened physiological reactivity in daily life mediated the association between family-of-origin aggression and dating aggression among women (Timmons et al., 2019). Another study conducted by our team examined how language use changes during periods of naturally occurring conflict in couples with high versus low levels of aggression. Results showed that couples with high levels of aggression switched to using more symmetrical "you" speech (where both partners simultaneously used second-person singular pronouns) when feeling annoyed at each other, suggesting increased blaming and focus toward the other person's actions and behaviors (Timmons et al., 2021).

A challenge when conducting research aimed at capturing conflict processes is ensuring conflict episodes are captured by the recordings and then having procedures for locating them in the large number of audio recordings obtained. Researchers conducting this work must ensure that they sample frequently enough to capture conflicts that do occur and to sample for a long enough duration that they obtain enough instances of conflict to meaningfully model the processes of interest. Additionally, it is critical to develop strategies for finding conflicts in the files: Listening to all audio recordings obtained to locate conflicts can be highly time intensive. Some strategies include using EMA surveys or exit interviews to identify likely instances of conflict to reduce the number of files that must be reviewed.

Synchronized Bodies: Sensing Physiological Linkage and Physical Health

One interesting application in mobile sensing research includes capturing synchronization in physiological arousal across people in daily life. To date, a small but growing body of research has shown that people in close relationships, including family members and romantic partners, demonstrate covariation in their levels of physiological arousal over time. This covariation, also known as co-regulation, has been linked to a variety of indices of relationship functioning, such as relationship satisfaction, attachment style, and conflict (Butler & Randall, 2012; Saxbe & Repetti, 2010; Sbarra & Hazan, 2008; Timmons, Margolin, & Saxbe, 2015). However, specific results have varied depending on the context in which linkage occurs and on the physiological response system measured. Importantly, mobile sensing methods provide several unique opportunities to study physiological linkage. Of note is the ability to study linkage over time frames longer than a standard lab visit, which is typically limited to several hours. Moreover, these methods allow researchers to model how physiological linkage varies across contexts and how naturally occurring events or stressors might amplify or dampen these processes.

A related promising application for mobile sensing research includes studying how relationship processes impact physical health. Individuals exposed to high levels of interpersonal aggression exhibit increased stress responding, resulting in repeated activation of the fight-or-flight response that triggers inflammatory responses, which causes wear and tear on the body over time (Repetti, Robles, & Reynolds, 2011; Wilson, Bailey, Malarkey, & Kiecolt-Glaser, 2021). This repeated and cumulative wear and tear may then put individuals at risk for a variety of negative health outcomes over the life course (Burman, & Margolin, 1992). Although much research focuses on the impact of large-scale stressors and events, it has been theorized that small, quotidian interactions between people in close relationships can have insidious impacts on regulatory response systems (Repetti, Wang, & Saxbe, 2011). Mobile sensing methods provide a unique methodology to test how small-scale behaviors in close relationships impact later health outcomes. For example, in one paper examining heart rate in couples in daily life, results showed that women's feelings of annoyance toward their dating partners were linked to heightened heart rate in their male romantic partners while sleeping that same night. Conversely, women's feelings of closeness were associated with lower overnight heart rate in their male partners (Schacter et al., 2020). Given that sleep is a restorative process, heart rate when sleeping might serve as a critical surrogate endpoint for determining how short-term relationship dynamics relate to short-term health processes and thereby influence long-term health.

Although capturing fine-grained physiological data in daily life can provide important insights into couple processes and health, data collected in daily life can lack experimental control. Various external factors (e.g., exercise, watching a scary movie, going outside into the heat) can impact physiological signals and contribute to high levels of noise and artifacts in the signal obtained. Care must be taken to collect detailed measures of contextual activities (e.g., using EMAs or automated sensors to track exercise) and to statistically adjust for confounding variables. Participants must also agree and be comfortable with wearing sensors for an extended time. Participants may forget to wear devices or take them off for a variety of reasons (e.g., discomfort, attending a party), potentially leading to nonrandom missingness that could bias analyses.

Two Examples of Psychological Research on Couples Using Mobile Sensing

The Couple Mobile Sensing Project: 24 Hours of 109 Couples

The Couple Mobile Sensing Project provides one example of how mobile sensing can be incorporated into relationship research (Timmons, Chaspari, et al., 2017). In this project, our team used mobile phones and wearable devices to track ongoing relationship functioning in real time and real life. As part of the project, dating couples visited the laboratory at 10:00 A.M. and were outfitted with a chest monitor, electrodermal activity (EDA) sensor, heart rate monitor, and smartphones. The phones took surveys, tracked GPS, and also took 3-minute audio recordings every 6 minutes. Couples carried the phones for a 24-hour period and responded to hourly surveys regarding their moods, the quality of their interactions, and other factors, such as whether they interacted, exercised, used drugs, and so on. After 24 hours, couples returned to the lab where they completed an exit interview to record their activities for each hour of the day and to complete a questionnaire reporting the extent to which they changed their behavior as a result of the study procedures.

Once the data were collected, we created a file linking all data streams obtained over the 24-hour study period. Measures captured from the mobile devices include hourly survey reports, electrodermal activity, movement, body temperature, heart rate, GPS, and audio files. Research assistants (1) manually transcribed all audio files to obtain measures of linguistic content and (2) coded the files to obtain metrics of communication quality and tone (e.g., criticism, validation). We further processed audio files by extracting fundamental frequency to determine couples' vocal pitch when speaking to each other (e.g., Weusthoff et al., 2013). Using these data, we have been able to examine covariation across different data stream modalities (e.g., hourly self-reports of couple conflict linked to physiological activity, communication patterns, language use, and vocal tone). Furthermore, we have been able to test (1) linkages in responding across dating partners over a variety of time scales (ranging from seconds to minutes), (2) how concurrent contextual events (e.g., events occurring in that same hour) impact linkages across people and across data modalities, and (3) how global factors (e.g., dating aggression or relationship satisfaction) impact these processes.

In one example paper resulting from this project, we tested whether romantic partners showed covariation in their levels of electrodermal activity over the course of one day (Timmons, Chaspari, et al., 2017). Results showed that romantic partners evidence similarity in their levels of physiological arousal over time, but only when they are physically together. Moreover, linkage in levels of physiological arousal was greater in people with anxious and avoidant attachment, suggesting increased interpersonal reactivity among those individuals with insecure attachment styles. In another example paper, our team used the multimodal data streams as input features in machine learning algorithms aiming to detect conflict in couples (Timmons, Arbel, et al., 2017). Results showed that using data such as vocal content and physiological arousal, we could detect when couples were having relationship conflicts within a 1-hour time frame with 79% accuracy.

In total, this project demonstrates how mobile methods can be utilized on multiple time scales, multiple levels of analysis, across people, across time, and across modalities to obtain rich and time-sensitive data. However, several challenges related to collecting such data should be considered. First, recruiting research participants willing to provide such detailed data about their daily lives can be difficult and potentially lead to sampling biases. Second, collecting and processing such data can require a significant time investment. Researchers must write scripts and programs for processing, cleaning, and extracting the vast amounts of physiological and audio signals obtained. Transcribing and coding audio files is also highly time intensive. In our study, which included 24 hours of data, our team spent 4 years transcribing audio files and 5 years coding them. Automated transcription software has evolved significantly in recent years and can now assist in such efforts; however, such software can still output significant numbers of errors that require human inspection and revision. Care must also be taken to combine data streams that are obtained from multiple sources (e.g., sensors, phones) and on different time scales (e.g., physiological data, EMAs) prior to conducting analyses. Although mobile sensing research is intensive, requiring significant effort to collect, clean, process, and assemble the data streams, it also provides high precision and flexibility for capturing dynamic features of real-life relationship functioning.

The Co-Sense Study: Co-Regulation in Younger and Older Couples

The Co-Sense study is another example of psychological relationship research incorporating sensing measures. The goal of the Co-Sense study is to investigate interpersonal emotion-regulation strategies in daily life as an important pathway between relational processes and individual well-being and health (Horn, Holzgang, & Rosenberger, 2021). Social proximity is seen as constituting relational resources for regulating affective responses (Coan & Sbarra, 2015). So far, most studies in this context have been conducted in the lab, with handholding as a proxy for social proximity. Even less is known about the role of daily social regulational resources over the lifespan: Do older couples benefit more or less from time spent together given the known tendency to prioritize pleasant social experiences as confronted with a limited time horizon (Carstensen, Isaacowitz, & Charles, 1999)? Are individuals with higher depression risk benefiting less from social proximity given the interpersonal patterns that have been linked with depression risk (Joiner & Coyne, 1999)?

To get insight into the role of social proximity in daily life, mobile sensing of the physical presence of the partner (or, to be precise, the partner's smartphone) by beacon-based low-energy *Bluetooth sensing* offers exciting new possibilities in this research area. It builds upon existing EMA studies, underlining the regulatory function of self-reported perceptions of *psychological* closeness in couples' daily lives (Debrot et al., 2013; Horn, Samson, et al., 2019; Laurenceau, Barrett, & Pietromonaco, 1998).

Furthermore, audio sensing of couple conversations allowed the assessment of real-life communication in the couple. To investigate sequences of conversations in their entirety, couples initiated the sensing when they were alone and anticipated time together talking. As mentioned earlier, a way of assessing *we-ness* (Karan, Rosenthal, & Robbins, 2019) and relational dynamics in couples' language indicators has been established in relationship research (for an overview, see Horn & Meier, 2022). This opens the door for investigating relational processes in verbal couple communications at scale.

The core of the Co-Sense study was a dyadic 3-week mobile sensing and EMA (three times a day) period relying on the Movisens app (Movisens, 2018). To assess individual moderators of these daily interactions, couples were invited into the lab to test their cognitive functioning (via cognitive testing), mental health history, and current adjustment challenges (via clinical interview). Furthermore, individual and relational characteristics were assessed by an online questionnaire prior to and 3 months after the mobile sensing period. In total, N = 116 German-speaking Swiss opposite-sex couples participated in the study aged between 18 and 33 and 60 and 83 years. For analyzing the data, daily "time spent together" corresponding to the three EMA reports (morning, midday, end of the day) was derived from the logged "enter"/"exit" signals of Bluetooth connections of both partners, which required artifact cleaning. EMA self-reports of time spent together were helpful to clean contradictory information from the partner's sensing logs. In our study, the raw data of both partners showed inconsistencies and rapid fluctuation (possibly due to technical conditions like low battery, etc.). In general, the advantage of dyadic sensing, that is, relying on cell phone sensor information of both partners is that both sources of information can be used and aggregated, and thus possible nonsystematic measurement errors can be reduced. We additionally used information reported in the EMA (e.g., whether partners report to have had any contact with the partner) to identify artifacts.

Audio-recorded conversations were transcribed manually and analyzed using the validated German version of LIWC (Meier et al., 2019). First analyses reveal a robust coupling of fluctuations of sensed physical closeness and perceived psychological closeness for all couples, regardless of whether they are old or young or at risk of depression (Horn, Meier, & Huber, 2021). Furthermore, daily conversations about mundane topics reveal differences in language use between older and younger couples: Younger couples' language indicates more focus on the individuals in the relationship (as indicated by "you" and "I" pronoun usage), while older couples showed more communal orientation (as indicated by more "we" pronouns) and words indicating less high-arousal emotion (Meier et al., 2021). Furthermore, it was possible to extract topics raised in daily communication indicating more complex and abstract social references in older couples' conversations and more concrete mundane topics in younger couples.

Future Directions in Couple Mobile Sensing Research

Methods in mobile sensing research are advancing quickly, in line with innovations in industry and health care that seek to utilize novel technologies as a way to respond to societal challenges and to promote mental and physical health. One exciting application on the horizon includes the integration of machine learning methods for passive and automatic measurement of relationship processes using mobile sensors in daily life. Given the identified individual and societal costs of dysfunctional relationships and lack of social integration taking advantage of the potential of personalized interpersonal EMIs (Heron & Smyth, 2010) based on mobile sensing seems particularly relevant. Passive and automatic sensing may be particularly beneficial in the context of couple and parent–child interaction therapies. For example, systems such as these could be used to predict conflict or shifts in emotions and to send interventions in moments of critical need. Adaptive and remote sensing that is dynamically responsive to shifting contexts could be used to augment therapy gains and to increase the reach and impact of mental health care. Relatedly, such interpersonal intervention systems could be personalized for increased therapeutic efficacy. Specific groups of people (e.g., people with high aggression or specific attachment styles) may evidence particular patterns (e.g., increased conflict during stress) of relationship functioning. Through machine learning, it may be possible to learn couple- or family-specific patterns and to learn which interventions work for which couples and families. Moreover, sensing solutions promise to reduce the burden of the assessment of relevant variables dramatically; this could allow access to populations that are hard to reach and for various reasons are not able to comply with demanding study designs. Often, these difficult to reach groups are already facing adversities, including disease, stressful life events, or trauma, which in turn affect not only the individual but also close relationships. Sensing solutions might open the door to the necessary scientific groundwork for developing supporting interventions for these challenged social systems. Research in this domain will require careful consideration of ethical and privacy practices; nonetheless, applying mobile sensing technologies to the development of new personalized care and precision medicine models holds immense potential for intervening upon maladaptive relationship processes and for improving health care applications for couples and families generally.

REFERENCES

Almeida, D. M., Wethington, E., & Chandler, A. L. (1999). Daily transmission of tensions between marital dyads and parent-child dyads. *Journal of Marriage and the Family, 61*(1), 49–61.

Aron, A., McLaughlin-Volpe, T., Mashek, D., Lewandowski, G., Wright, S. C., & Aron, E. N. (2004). Including others in the self. *European Review of Social Psychology, 15*(1), 101–132.

Bales, E., Li, K. A., & Griwsold, W. (2011). Couplevibe: Mobile implicit communication to improve awareness for (long-distance) couples. In P. Hinds (Ed.), *Proceedings of the ACM 2011 Conference on Computer Supported Cooperative Work* (p. 65). ACM.

Baumeister, R. F., & Leary, M. R. (1995). The need to belong: Desire for interpersonal attachments as a fundamental human motivation. *Psychological Bulletin, 117*(3), 497–529.

Berscheid, E. (1994). Interpersonal relationships. *Annual Review of Psychology, 45*(1), 79–129.

Beutel, M. E., Klein, E. M., Brähler, E., Reiner, I., Jünger, C., Michal, M., et al. (2017). Loneliness in the general population: Prevalence, determinants and relations to mental health. *BMC Psychiatry, 17*(1), 97.

Boateng, G., Santhanam, P., Lüscher, J., Scholz, U., & Kowatsch, T. (2019). Poster: DyMand—An open-source mobile and wearable system for assessing couples' dyadic management of chronic diseases. In S. Agarwal (Ed.), *ACM Digital Library, The 25th Annual International Conference on Mobile Computing and Networking* (pp. 1–3). ACM.

Boateng, G., Sels, L., Kuppens, P., Hilpert, P., & Kowatsch, T. (2020). Speech emotion recognition among couples using the peak-end rule and transfer learning. In K. Truong, D. Heylen, M. Czerwinski, N. Berthouze, M. Chetouani, & M. Nakano (Eds.), *Companion publication of the 2020 International Conference on Multimodal Interaction* (pp. 17–21). ACM.

Bodenmann, G. (1997). Dyadic coping-a systematic-transactional view of stress and coping among couples: Theory and empirical findings. *European Review of Applied Psychology, 47*, 137–140.

Bolger, N., DeLongis, A., Kessler, R. C., & Wethington, E. (1989). The contagion of stress across multiple roles. *Journal of Marriage and the Family, 51*(1), 175–183.

Bowlby, J. (1996). *A secure base: Parent-child attachment and healthy human development.* Routledge.

Burman, B., & Margolin, G. (1992). Analysis of the association between marital relationships and health problems: An interactional perspective. *Psychological Bulletin, 112*(1), 39.

Butler, E. A. (2017). Emotions are temporal interpersonal systems. *Current Opinion in Psychology, 17*, 129–134.

Butler, E. A., Guan, J., Predoehl, A., Brau, E., Simek, K., & Barnard, K. (2017). Computational temporal interpersonal emotion systems. In R. R. Vallacher, S. J. Read, & A. Nowak (Eds.), *Computational Social Psychology* (pp. 127–143). Routledge.

Butler, E. A., & Randall, A. K. (2012). Emotional coregulation in close relationships. *Emotion Review, 5*(2), 202–210.

Campos, B., Graesch, A. P., Repetti, R., Bradbury, T., & Ochs, E. (2009). Opportunity for interaction? A naturalistic observation study of dual-earner families after work and school. *Journal of Family Psychology, 23*(6), 798–807.

Carstensen, L. L., Isaacowitz, D. M., & Charles, S. T. (1999). Taking time seriously: A theory of socioemotional selectivity. *American Psychologist, 54*(3), 165–181.

Coan, J. A., & Sbarra, D. A. (2015). Social baseline theory: The social regulation of risk and effort. *Current Opinion in Psychology, 1*, 87–91.

Coutinho, J., Oliveira-Silva, P., Fernandes, E., Gonçalves, O. F., Correia, D., Perrone McGovern, K., et al. (2019). Psychophysiological synchrony during verbal interaction in romantic relationships. *Family Process, 58*(3), 716–733.

Debrot, A., Schoebi, D., Perrez, M., & Horn, A. B. (2013). Touch as an interpersonal emotion regulation process in couples' daily lives: The mediating role of psychological intimacy. *Personality and Social Psychology Bulletin, 39*(10), 1373–1385.

Dlugonski, D., Wood, A. P., DuBose, K. D., Rider, P., & Schoemann, A. M. (2019). Validity and reliability of proximity detection with Bluetooth-enabled accelerometers among adults. *Measurement in Physical Education and Exercise Science, 23*(3), 272–279.

Driver, J. L., & Gottman, J. M. (2004). Daily marital interactions and positive affect during marital conflict among newlywed couples. *Family Process, 43*(3), 301–314.

Durbin, K. B., Debrot, A., Karremans, J., & van der Wal, R. (2020). Can we use smart-phones to increase physical affection, intimacy and security in couples?: Preliminary support from an attachment perspective. *Journal of Social and Personal Relationships*, 1035–1045.

Fergus, K. (2015). Theoretical and methodological underpinnings of resilience in couples: locating the "we." In K. Skerrett & K. Fergus (Eds.), *Couple resilience: Emerging perspectives* (pp. 23–42). Springer.

Ferrer, E., & Helm, J. L. (2013). Dynamical systems modeling of physiological coregulation in dyadic interactions. *International Journal of Psychophysiology, 88*(3), 296–308.

Girolami, M., Mavilia, F., & Delmastro, F. (2020). Sensing social interactions through BLE beacons and commercial mobile devices. *Pervasive and Mobile Computing, 67*, 101198.

Gottman, J. M., Coan, J., Carrere, S., & Swanson, C. (1998). Predicting marital happiness and stability from newlywed interactions. *Journal of Marriage and the Family, 60*(1), 5–22.

Gottman, J. M., Markman, H., & Notarius, C. (1977). The topography of marital conflict: A sequential analysis of verbal and nonverbal behavior. *Journal of Marriage and the Family, 39*(3), 461.

Griggio, C. F., Nouwens, M., McGrenere, J., & Mackay, W. E. (2019). Augmenting couples' communication with lifelines. In S. Brewster, G. Fitzpatrick, A. Cox, & V. Kostakos (Eds.), *CHI 2019: Proceedings of the 2019 CHI Conference on Human Factors in Computing* (pp. 1–13). ACM.

Han, S. C., Schacter, H. L., Timmons, A. C., Kim, Y., Sichko, S., Pettit, C., et al. (2020). Feelings of annoyance and spoken anger words in couples' everyday lives: The role of family-of-origin aggression. *Social Psychological and Personality Science, 12*(6), 898–907.

Heron, K. E., & Smyth, J. M. (2010). Ecological momentary interventions: Incorporating mobile technology into psychosocial and health behaviour treatments. *British Journal of Health Psychology, 15*(1), 1–39.

Holt-Lunstad, J., Smith, T. B., & Layton, J. B. (2010). Social relationships and mortality risk: A meta-analytic review. *PLoS Medicine, 7*(7), e1000316.

Horn, A. B., Boettcher, V. S., Holzer, B. M., Siebenhuener, K., Maercker, A., Battegay, E., et al. (2019). Couples adjusting to multimorbidity: A Dyadic study on disclosure and adjustment disorder symptoms. *Frontiers in Psychology, 10*, 2499.

Horn, A. B., Holzgang, S., & Rosenberger, V. (2021). Couples' adjustment to the transition to retirement: the interplay of intra-and interpersonal emotion regulation in daily life. *Frontiers in Psychology, 12*, 654255.

Horn, A. B., & Meier, T. (2022). Language in close relationships. In M. Dehghani & R. L. Boyd (Eds.), *Handbook of language analysis in psychology* (pp. 102–124). Guilford Press.

Horn, A. B., Meier, T., & Huber, Z. (2021). Social proximity and psychological intimacy: A dyadic ambulatory assessment sensing study with young and old couples with and without depression risk. In International Association of Relationship Research (Chair), *Conference 2021*, London.

Horn, A. B., & Röcke, C. (2020). Aging dyads and health. *GeroPsych, 33*(3), 117–123.

Horn, A. B., Samson, A. C., Debrot, A., & Perrez, M. (2019). Positive humor in couples as interpersonal emotion regulation: A dyadic study in everyday life on the mediating role of psychological intimacy. *Journal of Social and Personal Relationships, 36*(8), 2376–2396.

Iida, M., Seidman, G., & Shrout, P. E. (2018). Models of interdependent individuals versus dyadic processes in relationship research. *Journal of Social and Personal Relationships, 35*(1), 59–88.

Ireland, M. E., Slatcher, R. B., Eastwick, P. W., Scissors, L. E., Finkel, E. J., & Pennebaker, J. W. (2011). Language style matching predicts relationship initiation and stability. *Psychological Science, 22*(1), 39–44.

Joiner, T. E., & Coyne, J. C. (Eds.) (1999). *The interactional nature of depression: Advances in interpersonal approaches*. American Psychological Association.

Karan, A., Rosenthal, R., & Robbins, M. L. (2019). Meta-analytic evidence that we-talk predicts relationship and personal functioning in romantic couples. *Journal of Social and Personal Relationships, 36*(9), 2624–2651.

Karan, A., Wright, R. C., & Robbins, M. L. (2017). Everyday emotion word and personal pronoun use reflects dyadic adjustment among couples coping with breast cancer. *Personal Relationships, 24*(1), 36–48.

Kenny, D. A., Kashy, D. A., & Cook, W. L. (2006). *Dyadic data analysis*. Guilford Press.

Kuzik, N., & Carson, V. (2018). Accelerometer Bluetooth proximity validation in parents and early years children. *Measurement in Physical Education and Exercise Science, 22*(4), 287–293.

Laurenceau, J.-P., Barrett, L. F., & Pietromonaco, P. R. (1998). Intimacy as an interpersonal process: The importance of self-disclosure, partner disclosure, and perceived partner responsiveness in interpersonal exchanges. *Journal of Personality and Social Psychology, 74*(5), 1238–1251.

Ledermann, T., & Kenny, D. A. (2012). The common fate model for dyadic data: Variations of a theoretically important but underutilized model. *Journal of Family Psychology, 26*(1), 140–148.

Luo, S., & Tuney, S. (2015). Can texting be used to improve romantic relationships?—The effects of sending positive text messages on relationship satisfaction. *Computers in Human Behavior, 49*, 670–678.

Maercker, A., & Horn, A. B. (2013). A socio-interpersonal perspective on PTSD: The case for environments and interpersonal processes. *Clinical Psychology and Psychotherapy, 20*(6), 465–481.

Matusik, J. G., Heidl, R., Hollenbeck, J. R., Yu, A., Lee, H. W., & Howe, M. (2019). Wearable bluetooth sensors for capturing relational variables and temporal variability in relationships: A construct validation study. *Journal of Applied Psychology, 104*(3), 357–387.

Mehl, M. R. (2017). The electronically activated recorder (EAR): A method for the naturalistic observation of daily social behavior. *Current Directions in Psychological Science, 26*(2), 184–190.

Meier, T., Boyd, R., Pennebaker, J., Mehl, M., Martin, M., Wolf, M., et al. (2019). *DE-LIWC2015*. Open Science Framework.

Meier, T., Dworakowski, O., Huber, Z., Haase,

C. M., Martin, M., & Horn, A. B. (2021). *Shared positivity in daily life of younger and older couples: Links between we-ness and positive emotions.* Symposium conducted at the annual meeting of The Gerontological Society of America, Phoenix, AZ.

Milek, A., Butler, E. A., & Bodenmann, G. (2015). The interplay of couple's shared time, women's intimacy, and intradyadic stress. *Journal of Family Psychology*, 831–842.

Movisens. (2018). MovisensXS [Computer software]. Movisens GmbH.

Neyer, F. J., & Lang, F. R. (2003). Blood is thicker than water: Kinship orientation across adulthood. *Journal of Personality and Social Psychology, 84*, 310–321.

Neyer, F. J., Wruz, C., Wagner, J., & Lang, F. R. (2011). Principles of relationship differentiation. *European Psychologist*, 1–11.

Patterson, M. L. (1982). A sequential functional model of nonverbal exchange. *Psychological Review, 89*(3), 231.

Pennebaker, J. W., Boyd, R. L., Jordan, K. N., & Blackburn, K. (2015). *The development and psychometric properties of LIWC2015*. University of Texas at Austin.

Rauers, A., Blanke, E., & Riediger, M. (2013). Everyday empathic accuracy in younger and older couples: Do you need to see your partner to know his or her feelings? *Psychological Science, 24*(11), 2210–2217.

Reblin, M., Heyman, R. E., Ellington, L., Baucom, B. R. W., Georgiou, P. G., & Vadaparampil, S. T. (2018). Everyday couples' communication research: Overcoming methodological barriers with technology. *Patient Education and Counseling*, 101(3), 551–556.

Reblin, M., Otto, A. K., Ketcher, D., Vadaparampil, S. T., Ellington, L., & Heyman, R. E. (2020). In-home conversations of couples with advanced cancer: Support has its costs. *Psycho-Oncology*, 1280–1287.

Reblin, M., Sutton, S. K., Vadaparampil, S. T., Heyman, R. E., & Ellington, L. (2019). Behind closed doors: How advanced cancer couples communicate at home. *Journal of Psychosocial Oncology, 37*(2), 228–241.

Reis, H. T., Collins, W. A., & Berscheid, E. (2000). The relationship context of human behavior and development. *Psychological Bulletin, 126*(6), 844–872.

Reis, H. T., & Shaver, P. (1988). Intimacy as an interpersonal process. In S. Duck, D. F. Hay, S. E. Hobfoll, W. Ickes, & B. M. Montgomery (Eds.), *Handbook of personal relationships: Theory, research and interventions* (pp. 367–389). Wiley.

Repetti, R. L., Robles, T. F., & Reynolds, B. (2011). Allostatic processes in the family. *Development and Psychopathology, 23*(3), 921–938.

Repetti, R., Wang, S., & Saxbe, D. (2009). Bringing it all back home: How outside stressors shape families' everyday lives. *Current Directions in Psychological Science, 18*, 106–111.

Repetti, R. L., Wang, S. W., & Saxbe, D. E. (2011). Adult health in the context of everyday family life. *Annals of Behavioral Medicine, 42*(3), 285–293.

Robbins, M. L., Karan, A., López, A. M., & Weihs, K. L. (2018). Naturalistically observing noncancer conversations among couples coping with breast cancer. *Psycho-Oncology*, 27(9), 2206–2213.

Robbins, M. L., López, A. M., Weihs, K. L., & Mehl, M. R. (2014). Cancer conversations in context: Naturalistic observation of couples coping with breast cancer. *Journal of Family Psychology, 28*(3), 380–390.

Robbins, M. L., Mehl, M. R., Smith, H. L., & Weihs, K. L. (2012). Linguistic indicators of patient, couple, and family adjustment following breast cancer. *Psycho-Oncology, 22*(7), 1501–1508.

Robles, T. F., Slatcher, R. B., Trombello, J. M., & McGinn, M. M. (2014). Marital quality and health: A meta-analytic review. *Psychological Bulletin, 140*(1), 140–187.

Rohrbaugh, M. J., Mehl, M. R., Shoham, V., Reilly, E. S., & Ewy, G. A. (2008). Prognostic significance of spouse we talk in couples coping with heart failure. *Journal of Consulting and Clinical Psychology, 76*(5), 781–789.

Saxbe, D. E., Ramos, M. R., Timmons, A. C., Rodriguez, A. R., & Margolin, G. (2014). A path modeling approach to understanding family conflict: Reciprocal patterns of parent coercion and adolescent avoidance. *Journal of Family Psychology, 28*(3), 415–420.

Saxbe, D., & Repetti, R. L. (2010). For better or worse?: Coregulation of couples' cortisol levels and mood states. *Journal of Personality and Social Psychology, 98*(1), 92–103.

Sbarra, D. A., Briskin, J. L., & Slatcher, R. B. (2019). Smartphones and close relationships: The Case for an evolutionary mismatch. *Per-*

spectives on Psychological Science, 14(4), 596–618.

Sbarra, D. A., & Hazan, C. (2008). Coregulation, dysregulation, self-regulation: An integrative analysis and empirical agenda for understanding adult attachment, separation, loss, and recovery. *Personality and Social Psychology Review, 12*(2), 141–167.

Schacter, H. L., Pettit, C., Kim, Y., Sichko, S., Timmons, A. C., Chaspari, T., et al. (2020). A matter of the heart: Daytime relationship functioning and overnight heart rate in young dating couples. *Annals of Behavioral Medicine, 54*(10), 794–803.

Schade, L. C., Sandberg, J., Bean, R., Busby, D., & Coyne, S. (2013). Using technology to connect in romantic relationships: Effects on attachment, relationship satisfaction, and stability in emerging adults. *Journal of Couple and Relationship Therapy, 12*(4), 314–338.

Slatcher, R. B., & Pennebaker, J. W. (2006). How do i love thee? Let me count the words: The social effects of expressive writing. *Psychological Science, 17*(8), 660–664.

Story, L. B., & Repetti, R. (2006). Daily occupational stressors and marital behavior. *Journal of Family Psychology, 20*(4), 690.

Thorson, K. R., West, T. V., & Mendes, W. B. (2018). Measuring physiological influence in dyads: A guide to designing, implementing, and analyzing dyadic physiological studies. *Psychological Methods, 23*(4), 595–616.

Timmons, A. C., Arbel, R., & Margolin, G. (2017). Daily patterns of stress and conflict in couples: Associations with marital aggression and family-of-origin aggression. *Journal of Family Psychology, 31*(1), 93.

Timmons, A. C., Chaspari, T., Han, S. C., Perrone, L., Narayanan, S. S., & Margolin, G. (2017). Using multimodal wearable technology to detect conflict among couples. *Computer, 50*(3), 50–59.

Timmons, A. C., Han, S. C., Chaspari, T., Kim, Y., Pettit, C., Narayanan, S., et al. (2019). Family-of-origin aggression, dating aggression, and physiological stress reactivity in daily life. *Physiology and Behavior, 206*, 85–92.

Timmons, A. C., Han, S. C., Kim, Y., Pettit, C., Perrone, L., Power, K., et al. (2021). Fluctuations in pronoun use in daily life: Couple aggression in context. *Journal of Family Psychology, 35*, 149–159.

Timmons, A. C., & Margolin, G. (2015). Family conflict, mood, and adolescents' daily school problems: Moderating roles of internalizing and externalizing symptoms. *Child Development, 86*(1), 241–258.

Timmons, A. C., Margolin, G., & Saxbe, D. E. (2015). Physiological linkage in couples and its implications for individual and interpersonal functioning: A literature review. *Journal of Family Psychology, 29*(5), 720–731.

Tschacher, W., Ramseyer, F., & Koole, S. L. (2018). Sharing the now in the social present: duration of nonverbal synchrony is linked with personality. *Journal of Personality, 86*(2), 129–138.

Underwood, M. K., Ehrenreich, S. E., More, D., Solis, J. S., & Brinkley, D. Y. (2015). The BlackBerry project: The hidden world of adolescents' text messaging and relations with internalizing symptoms. *Journal of Research on Adolescence, 25*(1), 101–117.

Underwood, M. K., Rosen, L. H., More, D., Ehrenreich, S. E., & Gentsch, J. K. (2012). The BlackBerry project: Capturing the content of adolescents' text messaging. *Developmental Psychology, 48*(2), 295–302.

Valtorta, N. K., Kanaan, M., Gilbody, S., Ronzi, S., & Hanratty, B. (2016). Loneliness and social isolation as risk factors for coronary heart disease and stroke: Systematic review and meta-analysis of longitudinal observational studies. *Heart, 102*(13), 1009–1016.

Weidman, A. C., Sun, J., Vazire, S., Quoidbach, J., Ungar, L. H., & Dunn, E. W. (2020). (Not) hearing happiness: Predicting fluctuations in happy mood from acoustic cues using machine learning. *Emotion, 20*(4), 642–658.

Weusthoff, S., Baucom, B. R., & Hahlweg, K. (2013). The siren song of vocal fundamental frequency for romantic relationships. *Frontiers in Psychology, 4*, 439.

Willi, J. (1985). *Koevolution: die Kunst gemeinsamen Wachsens: [Co-evolution: the art of communal growth]*. Rowohlt.

Wilson, S. J., Bailey, B. E., Malarkey, W. B., & Kiecolt-Glaser, J. K. (2021). Linking marital support to aging-related biomarkers: Both age and marital quality matter. *Journals of Gerontology: Series B, 76*(2), 273–282.

CHAPTER 23

Wearable Technologies in the Workplace

Sensing to Create Responsive Industrial and Occupational Environments Optimized for Health

Jacob N. Hyde, Johnny R. Runyon, Altaf Engineer, Beth Kramer, Casey M. Lindberg, and Esther M. Sternberg

CHAPTER OVERVIEW

The world that surrounds us affects our health, well-being, interactions, and performance in myriad ways. Modern-day sensing technologies are now able to help quantify, monitor, and quickly analyze multiple environmental aspects that affect our lives, and the data provided allow for the design and implementation of countermeasures to issues that degrade the performance and capability of individuals. In the future, designing workplace environments that can automatically assess and respond to human comfort needs, to optimize environments for both physical health and emotional well-being, will be the next step in enhancing the productivity and safety of workers. This chapter reviews some of the most salient and novel work in this area and appraises how new technologies, sensors, and human–environment interactions can inform each other. We provide an overview of data derived from wearable sensors that have been used in workplace settings to assess the impacts of various built environment attributes on stress and health behaviors. In this context, we review how environmental features such as the physical layout of the workplace, light, sound, temperature/humidity, and indoor air quality (IAQ), including carbon dioxide (CO_2) and volatile organic compounds (VOCs), may be measured, monitored, and modified to optimize both physical and emotional health. Finally, we review evidence for the impact of such data-driven design for health and the likely high return on investment for both the organization and worker.

Introduction

Our surroundings impact all aspects of health, including physical health, emotional well-being, health-related behaviors, and psychosocial interactions. Sensing technologies are now available to objectively measure and assess the impact of many aspects of the environment on many aspects of health. Figure 23.1 presents a conceptual layering of the elements of the environment, both built and natural, which impact health and well-being. Measurable variables at each of these layers, such as air quality, airflow, temperature and humidity, light, sound, and elements of natural environments, impact aspects of health at all levels, including social, behavioral, psychological, physiological, and molecular.

The proliferation of noninvasive wearable and stationary technologies measuring both health and environmental factors in real or near-real time has brought environmental psychology to a turning point, in which objective and quantifiable information can inform the rich interplay between individuals and their surroundings. Data analytics has advanced to the point that these complex interactions can be teased apart to elucidate which elements of the environment, alone or in combination, affect which elements of health and well-being. In turn, these data can be used to design and operate environments to optimize health, well-being, and performance.

This chapter reviews some of the most salient and novel work that relates human health, well-being, and performance to variables in the built environment, and how new technologies, sensors, and human–environment interactions can inform each other. It provides an overview of data derived from wearable sensors that have been used in workplace settings to assess the impacts of various built environment attributes on stress and health behaviors, such as physical activity and sleep. In this context, this chapter reviews how environmental features such as the physical layout of the workplace, light, sound, temperature and humidity, and IAQ, including CO_2, and VOCs, may be measured, monitored, and modified to optimize both physical and emotional health. We also review evidence for the impact of such data-driven design for health on a high return on investment for both the organization and the worker. In the future, designing workplace environments that can automatically assess and respond to human comfort needs, to optimize environments for both physical health and emotional well-being, will be the next step in enhancing the productivity and safety of workers.

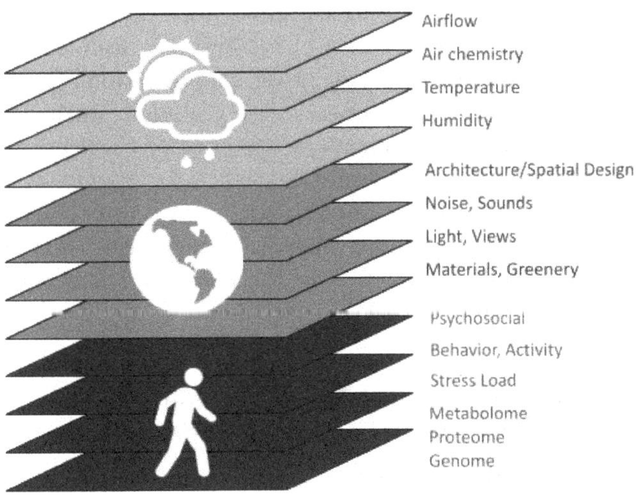

FIGURE 23.1. Environmental attributes affecting health. From Engineer et al. (2021). Reprinted with permission from Elsevier.

Impacts of Elements of the Built Environment on Stress and Relaxation Responses

Many elements of the built environment can induce stress, while others can ameliorate it. Lighting, glare, noise, temperature and humidity extremes, and noxious odors are all elements of the environment that can stimulate stress responses and alter thinking, performance, and subjective and objective well-being. As an example, military personnel working on airplane tarmacs may be tasked with rapidly servicing, fueling, and loading payload onto an attack aircraft, all while floating on an aircraft carrier. This type of work requires precision, dexterity, split-second timing, rapid reaction time, and complex routines spread across multiple people, with deadly consequences for errors. Often, personnel performing these types of tasks on an aircraft carrier are inundated with high winds, cold and humid air, high levels of sun exposure, and noxious fumes, and they are dealing with equipment that is explosive, biologically deadly, and expensive. This combination of job tasks can be made challenging by both built and natural environment elements and, while extreme examples, reflect typical stressors that all workers face in less extreme occupational settings. Conversely, aspects of the environment that can alleviate the stress response include diffuse light, which follows the tempo of the sun, nature sounds and soft music, temperature and humidity within a comfortable range, and access to windows with views of natural environments. Hospitals have recently begun incorporating nature scenes, variable lighting, and access to natural environments (e.g., atriums, courtyards) within their facilities to enhance healing and positive mood during hospitalization.

In occupational environments, environmental attributes such as noise, lighting, and ventilation have been linked to job satisfaction (Veitch, Charles, Farley, & Newsham, 2007), and productivity has been shown to be linked with well-being, degree of autonomy, and quality of coworker interaction (Adams, 2019). While such subjective data are informative of individuals' perceptions of their experience, it may not accurately reflect aspects of the environment that contribute to different aspects of health and well-being. Quantitative objective measurement of health outcomes is therefore important to provide accurate and actionable insights into aspects of the built environment that impact health and to inform design and operations of the built environment to optimize occupant health. Such quantitative data can provide design professionals, employers, occupational therapists, and human factors engineers with granular information regarding the design and operation of built environments to optimize physical health and emotional well-being. The recent proliferation of wearable devices for monitoring many aspects of health, combined with recent technologies allowing continuous monitoring of environmental attributes, such as workplace noise, lighting, temperature, humidity, and ventilation, have allowed for objective evaluation of the complex interactions between these many variables.

Rationale for Using Wearable Devices to Measure Impacts of the Built Environment on Health in the Workplace

Estimates indicate that people spend 90% of their time indoors (U.S. Environmental Protection Agency, 1989) and, pre-SARS-CoV-2, about one-third of their waking hours at their workplace (Conrad, 1988). Maximizing the health, well-being, and performance of workers is essential to both the individual and organization. Most occupational health monitoring has typically focused on exposures to various work hazards such as chemicals, gasses, and environmental conditions, which are monitored to reduce such hazards and mitigate safety risks. Wearable health devices, however, do not monitor such exposures. Most currently available wearable health devices measure physical activity, posture, and heart rate, from which measures of the stress and relaxation responses and sleep quality can be derived (see the section "Heart Rate Variability"). Such health outcome measures provide a different kind of insight into the impacts of the built environment on health, beyond the impacts of environmental hazards that cause disease, and shed light on the role of elements of the built environment in enhancing both physical health and emotional well-being.

Need for Objective Measures of Health in the Workplace

To begin to objectively and noninvasively measure objective worker performance and well-being in the industrial and occupational environment, a combination of measurement techniques that gather data at various resolutions would be preferable to subjective surveys and behaviorally anchored rating scales. Self-report and similar tools rely on subjectivity for ratings, thus creating multiple shortfalls in accurate collection of real-time data of worker health and well-being. While self-report can be an extremely useful tool for uncovering emotions and preferences, it has shortcomings in some circumstances, particularly where affect and emotion concealment are strong motivators in certain occupations. Military service members and law enforcement officers are two such groups, with multiple reasons to conceal reports of health and well-being in occupational environments where they are compelled to remain mission capable, to evade the perceived stigma of mental health dysfunction, and to maintain the stoic persona typical in this population (Hoge et al., 2004). While these are two examples of specific and often extreme work environments, in general work settings, objective measures using wearable devices can help to add a layered understanding to augment the shortcomings of self-report. In occupational settings, accurate, quantifiable data derived from wearable devices can provide both the worker and the employer valuable information regarding readiness for task performance and need for appropriate health interventions should work readiness be suboptimal.

Health and Environmental Monitoring Devices in the Workplace

Wearable Devices: Physiological Responses

A review of the latest state-of-the-art wearable health-sensing devices reveals several innovative technologies that are both available in the marketplace and in development. Wearable sensor-based health monitoring systems include sensors that can be integrated into textile fibers in clothing, elastic bands that attach to the body, or sensors that can be directly placed on the body and/or skin through deformable sensors. These sensors can measure physiological health metrics such as electrocardiogram (ECG), electromyography (EMG), heart rate (HR), body temperature, electrodermal activity (EDA), arterial oxygen saturation (SpO_2), blood pressure (BP), and respiration rate (RR), all of which can be monitored and transmitted in real time (Majumder, Mondal, & Deen, 2017).

Heart Rate Variability

Most wearable health devices measure a combination of heart rate (either ECG or pulse-based), heart rate variability (based on beat-to-beat intervals), physical activity (actigraphy), and posture. From this raw data, several physiological measures can be derived. Heart rate variability (HRV), based on the variability of time intervals between beats, gives an indication of the status of the autonomic nervous system response—the balance between the sympathetic stress response and parasympathetic relaxation response. HRV can be analyzed in the time or frequency domains, and measures that are derived include *SDNN* (standard deviation of normal-to-normal RR intervals) and *RMSSD* (root mean square of successive differences between normal heartbeats) (Thayer & Sternberg, 2006). The former is generally thought to reflect the sympathetic adrenergic response and the latter reflects a combination of the sympathetic and parasympathetic responses. Since these two modes of analysis reflect different aspects of the autonomic nervous system response, they may not concordantly change in response to different stressors (Williams et al., 2019). Generally, a decrease in HRV indicates an increased stress response, while an increase is associated with an enhanced relaxation response (Thayer & Sternberg, 2006). Combinations of these measures have been derived further to reflect other aspects of health (e.g., sleep quality). Thus, algorithms combining physical activity, HRV, and posture, have been developed to derive information regarding sleep quality from some wearable sensors, including sleep latency (time to fall asleep), sleep duration, postures during sleep, light sleep, deep sleep, and even rapid eye movement (REM). These algorithms have been compared to gold-standard sleep quality data collected in the sleep lab (Lee et al., 2018).

Wearable Devices: Social Interactions

Other aspects of health that can be measured in the workplace include psychosocial interactions, based on collections of snippets of ambient sounds and human speech using devices such as the electronically activated recorder app (EAR; Mehl, 2017) and sociometric badges (Kim, McFee, Olguin, Waber, & Pentland, 2012). In the latter, employees wear sociometric badges like identification badges; these badges measure fine-scale speech patterns known to correlate with social behavior (e.g., speaking time, speed, and energy). These badges also use an accelerometer to measure body movement to analyze social dynamics between badge wearers (e.g., gestures, posture, mimicry of others' body movements). Because these devices collect data over longer periods of time (hours or days), they are capable of more accurately reflecting social interactions and emotional responses during those interactions.

Experience sampling (covered in greater detail in Chapter 13, this volume) is another approach to collecting such data as well as data related to perceived stress and mood. Experience sampling can be carried out in three ways: time-contingent, in which questions are sent to a participant's smartphone/device several times per day, event-contingent, which relies on the individual taking the initiative to report a salient event, and location-contingent, which relies on the participant reporting a salient event in given locations (Mehl & Conner, 2012). All these methods rely on prompts: in the case of time-contingent, they ping to the smartphone; in the case of event-contingent, the event itself; and in the case of location-contingent, a prompt, usually visual, is provided as the participant enters the location that is being evaluated. In all these cases, the subjective survey data can be linked through time or location stamps to the other data streams being collected (e.g., HRV or physical activity).

Wearable Devices: Environmental Monitoring Devices

Numerous environmental monitoring devices are available to measure air quality, VOCs, CO_2, airflow and turbulence, light of varying wavelengths and intensities, glare, sound at levels ranging from low (<30 decibels) to high (>90 decibels), and temperature and relative humidity (Al-Mamun & Yuce, 2019). Most environmental monitoring devices are stationary, wall-mounted, movable, placed on desks or furniture, or handheld. A few wearable environmental monitoring devices have been developed for selected environmental attributes. The most well-established devices measure light intensity and/or circadian light (e.g., Philips Actiwatch) and a combination of light and activity measured by the Dimesimeter, which is a light and activity sensor (Rea, Figueiro, Bierman, & Bullough, 2010). Some wearable environmental monitors have been developed for research purposes to measure a limited number of attributes, including sound, temperature, CO_2, and light (Ghahramani et al., 2018). Others detect speech and nonspeech-related sounds (EAR).

Environmental monitoring technology is expanding to include self-powered wearable monitoring devices. These devices harvest energy from body heat and body motion to power monitoring. By leveraging nanotechnology to build flexible, self-powered, multimodal wearable sensing devices, personal health and environmental exposure can now be monitored with maximum comfort and a longer system life (Misra et al., 2015). This sensing technology uses nanowires for environmental monitoring such attributes as toxic gas exposure. There is a strong association of exposure to toxic gasses such as ozone in the environment with health responses such as wheezing and EKG (Misra et al., 2015). Other new technology uses capacitive micromachined ultrasonic transducers (CMUTs) to monitor VOCs. The mechanism for sensing VOCs is through the CMUT. When the device is exposed to VOCs, the additional mass of the absorbed analyte on the resonate structure causes a shift in the resonant frequency (Misra et al., 2015). This technology can be expanded to include several environmental VOCs to detect levels that can impact health negatively.

Depending on the environmental attribute being measured, wearable environmental monitoring devices pose challenges that may impact data validity when worn by working populations in the field, rather than in closely monitored lab settings. These are intuitive, but unless carefully instructed and monitored, study participants may neglect to follow optimal practice. Thus, light monitors, whether worn on the wrist, pendant, or forehead, must be worn over clothing, so as not to obscure the light. CO_2 monitors, if worn close to the mouth or within the CO_2 bubble (see the section "Air Quality") may give falsely high readings regarding ambient room air, while accurately measuring CO_2 levels in the person's immediate breathing zone. Similarly, wearable temperature monitors may measure skin and body temperature rather than ambient air temperature.

Combining Health and Environmental Monitoring Devices

The health impacts of built environments may be measured holistically—that is, by examining the impact of a total environment on various health outcomes, or individually, in which single or several environmental attributes may be monitored and linked alone or in combination to selected health outcomes. Two classic examples of holistic measures are the landmark study by Roger Ulrich (1984), in which health outcomes were compared in hospital patients recovering from gall bladder surgery. Those patients whose windows had a view of a grove of trees needed less pain medication, had better mood, and left the hospital a day sooner than those with a view of a brick wall. Similarly, Kuo and Sullivan (2001) showed that persons in an inner-city Chicago housing project who were randomly assigned to apartments with a view of trees had better moods and less aggressive behaviors than those with a view of a blacktop. While these studies were carried out prior to the era of sophisticated health and environmental monitoring, they indicate that the built environment, and at least a view of nature, does impact physical health and emotional well-being. With the advent of technologies to measure health, and specifically stress outcomes more quantitatively, it has become possible to carry out similar studies measuring the holistic impact of a built office environment on stress measures.

Thayer, Verkuil, and colleagues (2010) took advantage of a retrofit of a U.S. federal building to monitor the stress response of personnel at a hormonal and neuronal scale. Salivary cortisol and heart rate variability were measured for 3 days over the course of 17 months in 60 U.S. federal government office workers while they occupied legacy space and after they moved into the same space that had been retrofitted. The legacy office space had dim lighting, high-wall cubicles, higher mechanical noise, and poorer ventilation compared to the remodeled space with better ventilation, brighter and more natural lighting, lower mechanical noise, and open office design with greater visibility and better views. Results showed that workers in the new space had both lower neuronal stress response (as measured by HRV) and lower hormonal stress response, with lower morning cortisol rises compared to those working in the legacy office space. The HRV changes carried over as well through the night, during sleep. Importantly, subjective questionnaires did not reveal any significant differences in participants' perceptions of their stress levels, indicating that subjective questionnaires alone, while informative of the individual's experience, may miss the physiologically important stress impacts of the built environment.

While these studies confirm that the built environment does impact at least one aspect of health—the physiological stress response—and, in the older studies, that the built environment also impacts mental health and clinical health outcomes, they do not address which elements of the built environment impact which aspects of health, either alone or in combination. More sophisticated studies are required to address that question, monitoring multiple environmental attributes simultaneously and in real time, and linking them through Big Data analytics to multiple physical and emotional health outcomes.

Monitoring the Impact of Multiple Environmental Attributes on Health Outcomes

The U.S. General Services Administration's Wellbuilt for Wellbeing study (WB2), carried out with the University of Arizona, Baylor College of Medicine, and Aclima, Inc. (Lindberg et al., 2018), provides a template for linking multiple environmental attributes with multiple health outcomes. In this study, 231 office workers in four federal buildings were fitted with a wearable chest-worn sensor EcgMove 3 (Movisens, Karlsruhe, Germany) that tracked HRV, posture, and physical activity. Time-contingent experience sampling was also carried out, with questions regarding mood and stress sent to the participants' smartphones randomly every hour and at least 30 minutes apart. At the same time, wall nodes (Aclima, Inc.) were used to continuously measure up to 11 environmental attributes, including light, sound, temperature, relative humidity, CO_2, and VOCs. Participants also wore a chest-worn environmental monitor that tracked a subset of environmental attributes continuously and in real time, including light, temperature, relative humidity, and CO2. Timestamped data from the environmental and health monitors and experience sampling data streamed together with HRV data via the Movisens monitors allowed for coordination of health events with environmental variations during subsequent data analytics. Finally, office design and spatial characteristics were measured and linked to health outcomes, including stress responses (HRV), physical activity, sleep quality, and fatigue.

An essential component of such studies is the application of complex data analytics to statistically isolate the impact of each environmental attribute on multiple health outcomes. In addition to linking environmental attributes to these basic health outcomes—stress response, physical activity, posture, and subjective experience—further analyses were carried out to derive sleep quality from the raw Movisens HRV, posture, and physical activity data. These data were compared to data collected from individuals in a fully equipped sleep lab to validate the wearable Movisens device data for sleep quality (Lee et al., 2018).

Two approaches can be taken to analyzing such data, collected in real-world settings: discovery-driven and hypothesis-driven, or a combination of the two. A first-pass discovery approach, where data are analyzed without a hypothesis, can provide insights into relationships that can then be explored in more detail using a hypothesis-driven approach, or in controlled settings where individual environmental attributes are experimentally modified to discover their impacts on selected health outcomes.

Using this combined and sequential approach, the WB2 data revealed several novel findings. The findings showed that workers in open office-designed settings, with bench seating and many choices for larger and smaller meeting areas, were 32% more active than workers in private offices and 20% more active than those in cubicles (Lindberg et al., 2018). Additionally, those who were more active during the day had 14% lower stress levels as measured by HRV (*SDNN*) in after-work hours. Further analysis revealed that the more active workers in open office settings had better sleep quality than those in cubicles or private offices (Lee et al., 2018). Finally, those workers with better sleep quality reported less daytime fatigue (Goel et al., 2021).

Temperature and humidity evaluation revealed that relative humidity had an impact on health outcomes, while temperature alone did not. Specifically, in this cross-sectional, exploratory study, Razjouyan and colleagues (2019) found that individuals who spent more than 50% of their time outside the 30–60% relative humidity (RH) conditions exhibited a 25% higher stress response, as measured by HRV (*SDNN*). The optimal RH for reduced stress response was closer to 45 +/– 5%. Further analysis also revealed an indirect effect of RH on objectively measured sleep quality. This evidence supports the 30–60% RH range included in the earlier version of the U.S. standard for indoor air quality, the ASHRAE 55-1989 thermal comfort standard. In a recent study, Altomonte and colleagues (2020) also emphasized that temperature variability in the workplace influences cognitive performance and may cause a loss in concentration and an increase in drowsiness. Of particular importance during pandemic conditions, low RH in the precise range that is associated with higher stress levels, that is, less than 30%, is associated with higher rates of viral infections in hospital settings (Taylor & Hugentobler, 2016). This may be because drier conditions may favor the survival of common viruses and pathogens such as the influenza virus on surfaces leading to greater likelihood of transmission. In addition, drier conditions also predispose those exposed to the virus to greater susceptibility to becoming sick due to the drying of mucus membranes.

Risks, Drawbacks, and Considerations in Selecting Different Methods and Devices

Critical to the validity of the conclusions derived from wearable and noninvasive health device studies are the sensitivity and accuracy of the devices being used. While technologies have advanced considerably, many commercially available health monitoring devices still have not been validated against gold-standard measures. Technologies are being upgraded continuously; therefore, before selecting a health monitoring device for research purposes, it is essential to ensure that the devices selected are research grade and have been validated for the outcomes of interest. Finally, another issue for research-grade health monitoring devices is the format of the data collected. Many commercially available devices do not collect data continuously throughout the day but collect only a short period at programmed intervals. To accurately measure the impact of built environment attributes throughout the day and night, devices must be used in which raw data can be collected continuously and downloaded in formats appropriate for data analysis at various scales of resolution.

Impacts of Individual Environmental Attributes on Health Outcomes

Air Quality

Recent studies highlight the role of indoor air quality (IAQ) and air temperature on human performance, health, and productivity. One important and prevalent pollutant within industrial and occupational areas is CO_2, which is a common gas that makes up 0.04% of atmospheric air and is exhaled as we breathe. Various types of industrial environments may expose individuals to dangerously high levels of CO_2 (i.e., firefighters, oil and gas drillers, diesel engine operators; Hawley, Cox-Ganser, & Cummings, 2017). But CO_2 also builds up to levels that impair cognitive performance even in normal office settings, if ventilation and fresh air exchange are too low (Ghahramani et al., 2019). In general, the greater the number of people in an enclosed space, the longer they occupy that space, and the poorer the ventilation, the higher the CO_2 levels will be in that space. The negative impacts of slightly elevated levels of CO_2 on cognitive performance have only recently been identified, with cognitive performance declining approximately 15% at 945 parts per million (ppm) of CO_2 and 50% at 1,400 ppm (Allen et al., 2016). Previous recommendations by the Occupational Safety and Health Administration (OSHA; 2012) and the American Conference of Government Industrial Hygienists previously allowed much higher CO_2 levels, with threshold limit values for CO_2 concentrations over an 8-hr workday being 5,000 ppm. Current OSHA regulations list the ceiling exposure limit of

CO_2 at 30,000 ppm for up to 10 minutes with 40,000 ppm being "immediately dangerous to life and health" (Satish et al., 2012).

In typical work environments, the employees occupying office or industrial spaces are the primary sources of CO_2 buildup. Ghahramani and colleagues (2019) identified a personal "CO_2 bubble" (Figure 23.2), which accumulates around the mouth and the face as people breathe, especially in stagnant air conditions. Levels of CO_2 were as high as 2,200 ppm, with a mean of approximately 1,200 ppm, in the range of levels known to impair cognitive performance by over 50% in occupational settings (Ghahramani et al., 2019; Pantelic et al., 2020). Body posture, the anatomical configuration of a person's nose and mouth, airflow, spatial motions, and furniture placement also can influence the shape and concentration of this bubble of gas. As seen in Figure 23.3, CO_2 measurements in the inhalation zone revealed that the use of even a small-sized portable desk fan to disturb the air around the face significantly reduced the CO_2 concentration in participants' personal spaces.

Current IAQ monitors track a combination of all or any of several IAQ indicators, including but not limited to temperature, humidity, VOCs, particulate matter (PM), CO_2, ozone, and other gasses that impact human health. In addition to these features, some may be able to mechanically filter air automatically in response to its sensors' readings, or on a schedule with a fan or other type of appliance to mitigate a pollutant or stagnant air. Advanced IAQ sensing technologies can be used to analyze the influence of airflow design related to spatial layout and its influence on health and well-being. As discussed in the "Health and Environmental Monitoring Devices in the Workplace" section, this information can be combined with that collected by sensors which monitor different physiological aspects of workers such as heart activity, physical movement, and sleep activity. These objective environmental and physiological data can then be further combined with subjective data in the form of daily survey responses. These types of disparate data streams give researchers rich information to analyze and discover how IAQ in different environments can affect the physical and mental health and well-being of occupants. Office workers are vulnerable to illnesses because of sedentary behavior and the design of their immediate work environments. IAQ research and its findings can

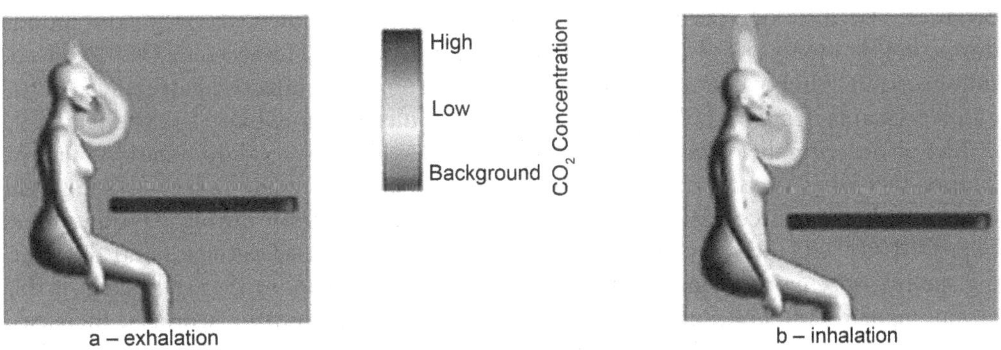

FIGURE 23.2. Respiratory CO_2 concentration in the breathing zone (a: during exhalation, b: during inhalation) forming a bubble. From Ghahramani et al. (2019). Reprinted with permission from Elsevier.

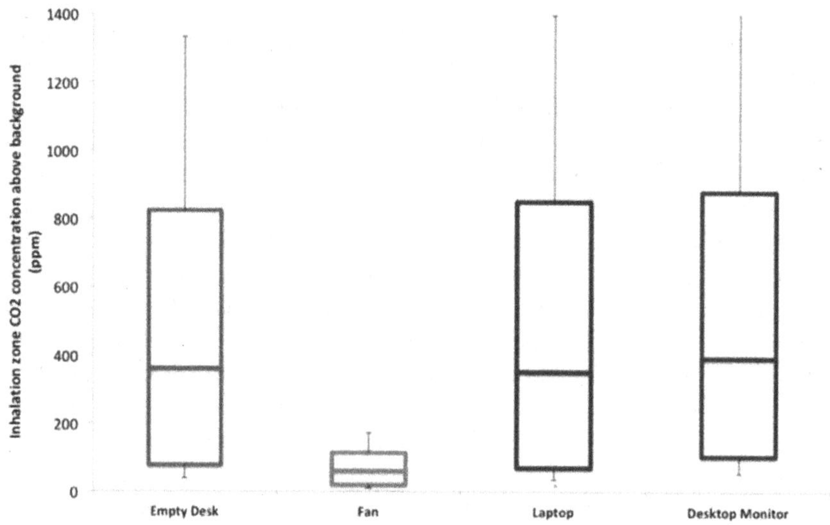

FIGURE 23.3. The CO_2 concentration in the inhalation zone above the room background for the combined effect of breathing, talking, breathing while looking down, and free activity. From Pantelic (2020). Reprinted with permission from Springer.

positively influence worker performance by reducing workplace absenteeism, illnesses, and stress, and improving sleep quality, all of which are directly associated with the work environment.

Light

Daylight influences health, mood, sleep, and circadian rhythms. Heerwagen (1990) found increased satisfaction in office workers who had good visual access to daylight via interior glazing even if the daylight was not in their immediate space. Merely seeing daylight somewhere in their environment also had positive effects. Sunlight in indoor environments is also associated with perceived cheerfulness of the environment and higher levels of positive affect for occupants. Seasonal affective disorder (SAD), a form of depressive disorder related to long periods of low light, which leads to lowered energy and moods during winter months, is also benefited by sunlight exposure (Heerwagen, 1990). Indeed, full spectrum light boxes that mimic sunlight can be almost as effective in treating SAD as antidepressants. Figueiro (2013) found that older adults are more likely to experience circadian disorders in the form of sleep disturbances, possibly due to a combination of many factors, including a less sensitive circadian clock and age-dependent reduced retinal light exposure. Light sources delivering higher circadian stimulation during daytime hours improved sleep quality in older adults and Alzheimer's disease patients, and daylighting the interior environment was found to be highly beneficial to the well-being of this group. Figueiro and colleagues (2017) found similar results in office workers. Increased daylight exposure, especially bright light from 8:00 A.M. to noon, regulated circadian rhythms and improved mood and sleep quality in office workers. The U.S. General Services Administration, with its academic partners, has extensively studied circadian lighting in its offices, which include dynamic lighting solutions using short-wavelength electric light in the morning that changes to longer-wavelength light in the afternoon to test the relationship of this lighting to daytime alertness (Figueiro et al., 2019). This study found greater alertness in office workers via circadian entrainment provided by a new type of light fixture which regulated and delivered appropriate circadian wavelength and intensity of light exposure throughout the day.

Light measurements in our surrounding environment can reveal valuable information, particularly if they are collected over a longer period of time. As discussed in the previous section, this information can be correlated with measures of physical activity, stress, and sleep to understand how light exposure may impact these human health factors. Environmental light sensors such as luxmeters can measure light levels in most indoor and outdoor environments, measuring illuminance in lux (lx) or footcandles (fc). Most commercially available meters can measure high natural lighting levels, which may reach levels up to 100,000 lx or more, or electric lighting levels in workspaces that tend to be around 500–1,000 lx on average. Computer simulations in different types of available software are also able to show the distribution of illuminance or luminance measurements throughout a room in specific daylight conditions, such as overcast, partially cloudy, or sunny. These computer renderings look similar to a heat map displaying their light measurements in lux above the clusters of different light intensities (Velux, n.d.). Information collected from physical light measurements and simulations can be compared to design recommendations for best practices derived from scientific literature, which in turn can ultimately lead to new lighting modifications or strategies for healthy outcomes.

Wearable devices can also be worn around the wrist and measure an individual's light exposure, sleep, and activity levels. In these cases, sensors provide photometric light measures, which measures the light in a way that is experienced by the human eye in the real world. It also records the blue, green, and red-light spectrums separately through three different sensors. This information is particularly useful since certain light spectra can impact circadian cycles differently (Rea & Figueiro, 2018). These kinds of sensors also allow for comparison of various light exposures to sleep quality, physical activity, alertness, changes in mood, and satisfaction.

Sound

The acoustic environment of a place or space is the combination of sounds from all sources that a human can hear (Brown, Gjestland, & Dubois, 2016). These sounds can have positive effects on overall health and well-being or affect individuals negatively by contributing to illness and disease. Noise is described as sound that can cause annoyance and stress that trigger the autonomic nervous system sympathetic stress response and physiological changes contributing to hearing impairment, difficulties in task and cognitive performance, as well as cardiovascular disturbances, including increased systolic blood pressure and heart rate (Goines & Hagler, 2007). Ongoing exposure to stressful noise can lead to a chronic imbalance in the homeostasis of the endocrine system, which directly impacts the cardiovascular system. This chronic imbalance raises the risk of cardiovascular disturbances such as increased blood pressure, blood lipid concentrations, blood viscosity, and blood glucose concentrations. Epidemiological studies have confirmed an increase in the prevalence and incidence of cardiovascular disease (e.g., ischemic heart disease, hypertension) and strokes in highly noise-exposed groups (Basner et al., 2014).

The best described impact of noise exposure on health is hearing impairment. Both intermittent and continuous noise exposure at moderate levels can impact hearing loss. The disruption can cause a temporary shift in the hearing threshold caused by reversible damage to the stereocilia of hair cells in the ear anatomy (Rosati & Jamesdaniel, 2020). The level and characteristics of hearing loss can vary depending on continuous versus intermittent exposure. In addition to hearing loss, noise exposure has also been linked to other hearing disorders, including tinnitus, recruitment, and hyperacusis (Rosati & Jamesdaniel, 2020). These hearing disturbances induced by noise exposure can also impact cognitive functions and lead to mood disorders including anxiety and depression (Bhatt, Bhattacharyya, & Lin, 2017).

Performance can also be affected by an impairment of information processing due to levels of noise exposure and its impact on attention. According to Jafari, Khosrowabadi, Khodakarim, and Mohammadian (2019), noise exposure can reduce cognitive functioning, including performance accuracy, reaction time, attention, memory, intelligence, and concentration.

Tracking and measurement of acoustics in the built environment facilitate data collection that can improve the quality of spaces we occupy. One of the most common acoustical sensing methods is through a smartphone that leverages embedded microphone technology. A mobile sensor called BumpAlert uses acoustical sensing to help improve risk for collision with indoor objects, thus alleviating risks of falls. BumpAlert builds a sonar-like system for detecting nearby obstacles by utilizing a smartphone's built-in microphones and speakers. It further improves detection accuracy since the microphones and speakers are omni directional and are also able to integrate the inertial sensors and camera (Tung, 2018).

Another smartphone technology utilizing acoustical sensing is Echotag. This sensing application uses context-aware computing. Leveraging the microphone on the smartphone, it stores sounds in specific indoor locations by actively rendering acoustic signatures using the phone speakers to transmit sound and phone microphones to sense its reflections (Tung, 2018). This type of acoustical sensing allows for automatic sound muting of the smartphone in specific locations.

Finally, mobile acoustical sensing can be used in mapping indoor spaces through a program known as BatMapper, which measures environment geometries from sound reflection signals and combines it with calibrated user traces to construct maps in a few minutes (Zhou, 2019). Using this acoustical sensing technology designed to map indoor space quickly and accurately also allows for the creation of optimal space usage within the indoor setting.

Return on Investment

The business case for healthy buildings has been extensively reviewed in Allen and Macomber (2020) and will not be covered here. However, the new mobile sensing tools and techniques to measure the impact of the built environment on health, well-being, and performance described in this chapter can be used to obtain quantitative objective data that add power to the business case for return on investment (ROI) of such interventions and enhancements for physical and emotional health. To be effective, ROI planning and budgetary models should provide optimal as well as over-and-above building standards' ranges for ventilation, air quality, thermal health, moisture, dust and pests, safety and security, water quality, noise, and lighting and views. ROI planning should also include continuous sensing and monitoring technologies for building systems that would enable them to display and record measures of these environmental attributes in real time, as well as communicate safety warnings. These mobile sensing technologies at the human and built environment interface would not only lead to minimizing risk, but also improve employee performance, and potentially reduce disease transmission, which in turn would positively impact ROI.

It is difficult to keep track of the rapidly changing field of mobile sensing; however, such technological innovations are essential to help employers prepare for the future. One key ROI strategy may be to appoint a point person such as a facilities manager, assisted by a task force to keep track of rapidly developing innovative health and safety solutions and implement them effectively. The ultimate goal of such interdisciplinary teams is to make workplace environments suitable for employees to thrive and not just survive.

Smart, Adaptive, and Responsive Workplaces

Combining Sensors and Automatic Countermeasures in the Workplace

Mobile sensing at the interface of humans and the built environment has exciting possibilities for the development of smart, responsive environments that respond to human needs for health and well-being. Once any number of disparate sensors can create a stream of real-time data, a countermeasure to offset the detrimental aspects of a particular issue may be automatically deployed by a built environment. As an example, if a CO_2 sensor were to detect a rising level of CO_2 in a worker's office, local ventilation could automatically be turned on to turn over the air and decrease the volume of CO_2.

If a noise sensor picks up sound over a certain decibel or identifies an intermittent noise that is out of the ordinary, sound dampening or noise cancellation via speakers could be deployed within these types of environments. Aside from understanding the level of noise in the environment and its impact on health, it is important to utilize acoustical sensing data for the development of safer and health-supporting workplaces. Acoustical sensing data collection can be used to eliminate risk of injury and accidents, provide automatic sound levels based on learned sound signatures, and quickly provide indoor mapping to facilitate better and more optimally designed workspaces. Utilizing these aspects of sound sensing will help facilitate a built environment that can support optimal health and well-being of personnel.

Lighting in windowless factories or in small, confined spaces like submarines could be altered to utilize light and lighting schedules that increase alertness at appropriate times and gradually transition lighting levels to assist in the work to rest transition. The data collected from environmental light sensors can inform the development of both natural and artificial lighting strategies that are optimal for regulating circadian rhythms, and other physiological and psychological benefits. These lighting systems could respond, change, and adapt in real time or could work according to a preset optimized schedule for workers.

Temperature and humidity comfort levels are particularly idiosyncratic, suggesting the value of technologies to create personalized temperature and humidity-controlled environments. A new method is even being developed to accomplish these environments using bioresponsive materials that can be applied to building systems and technologies (Aviv et al., 2020).

A common theme among these automated responsive systems is their local deployment to create individualized comfort zones. Such local solutions will both improve health outcomes on an individual basis and save energy, as one size in environmental comfort does not fit all.

Evidence-Based Design

A good example of smart and responsive design can be seen in newer passenger aircraft. Boeing launched the 787 "Dreamliner" in 2007 and incorporated various research findings on built environments into this aircraft. A carbon fiber composite was used to build parts of the airframe, therefore reducing weight, and allowing for a higher cabin pressurization that led to greater oxygen concentration in the blood of passengers. Additionally, cabin humidity level was increased to reduce dehydration, and ceiling lighting was altered to reflect the destination time zone and decrease the perception of jetlag (Hinninghofen & Enck, 2006).

Going forward, to move evidence-based workplace design forward, creating testbeds, termed *living labs*, of different scales and typologies provides a way to develop and test smart responsive environments (Hasan et al., 2018). Interdisciplinary research teams could identify specific typologies and locations for these testbeds. Human responses to different environmental conditions in carefully controlled workspaces, which include building materials, acoustics, temperature, humidity, daylight, layout, and furniture, would be measured. The health, behavioral, and performance data would then automatically inform environments at a local level (personal space, desk, chair, room) and trigger adaptive responses of local environments to optimize individual health, performance, and well-being. This could be accomplished by developing state-of-the-art materials, technologies, and systems to test human interactions and performance outcomes and by connecting them to the Internet of Things (IoT) continuously and in real time.

Outlook and Conclusion

Many of the technologies outlined in this chapter can be used to optimize built environment design and operations in a post-SARS-CoV-2 world. Most important for prevention of viral spread are ventilation systems powerful enough to provide frequent hourly fresh air turnover. However, all the features of the built environment described here that enhance both physical health and emotional well-being are important in helping passively reduce stress of building occupants, thereby helping them to remain resilient to more severe viral infections. Healthy sleep is particularly important in optimizing resilience, as are features that reduce stress, such as green spaces, views to nature, and places to meditate and contemplate. Individually responsive environments would also help optimize individual health.

Responsive built environments could soon comprise flexible environments that integrate multiple kinds of sensors and data streams that enhance human performance by collecting and tracking individual physiological, behavioral, and social responses and interactions in real time and combine these with environmental monitoring to create responsive systems within the workplace. Key indicators of human health, well-being, and performance, including stress responses, physical activity, cognitive performance, and sleep quality, can all be monitored and modified through evidence-based design of these types of spaces. Detection of subnormal health responses could then automatically signal building systems to adjust in real time to optimize health, including lowering stress responses and optimizing cognitive performance and comfort. Privacy issues will be a substantial hurdle that will need to be continually addressed for such automated systems to be put in place. Investing in the design and monitoring of health and subsequently creating more responsive occupational environments that enhance worker performance, increase safety and productivity, enhance worker satisfaction, and produce positive financial returns is of benefit to both organizations and their employees.

ACKNOWLEDGMENTS

We wish to acknowledge the following members of the General Services Administration's (GSA's) Wellbuilt for Wellbeing Project Team. Wellbuilt for Wellbeing is a multidisciplinary research project team (GSA Contract No. GS-00-H-14-AA-C-0094) consisting of the following members: Kevin Kampschroer, Judith Heerwagen, and Brian Gilligan of GSA; Esther Sternberg, Casey Lindberg, and Matthias Mehl of the University of Arizona Institute on Place, Wellbeing & Performance; Bijan Najafi, Javad Razjouyan, Hyoki Lee, and Hung Nguyen of the Baylor College of Medicine Interdisciplinary Consortium on Advanced Motion Performance (iCAMP); Sudha Ram, Faiz Curim, and Karthik Srinivasian of the University of Arizona INSITE Center for Business Intelligence and Analytics; Kelly Canada of LMI Inc.; Priya Saha, Rebecca Goldfinger-Fein, Alicia Darbishire, and Mills Wallace of the Federal Occupational Health Service; and Davida Herzl, Reuben Herzl, Melissa Lunden, Nicole Goebel, and Scott Andrews of Aclima Inc. We also thank the Andrew Weil Endowed Chair for Research in Integrative Medicine and Andrew Weil Center for Integrative Medicine for research support and the support of Esther M. Sternberg; Paula Cook and the Andrew Weil Center for Integrative Medicine staff for assistance with formatting and referencing; and the University of Arizona Institute on Place, Wellbeing & Performance and the University of Arizona BIO5 Institute for contributions to research.

REFERENCES

Adams, J. M. (2019). The value of worker well-being. *Public Health Reports, 134*(6), 583–586.

Ahrentzen, S., & Tural, E. (2015). The role of building design and interiors in ageing actively at home. *Building Research and Information: Physical Activity, Sedentary Behaviour and the Indoor Built Environment, 43*(5), 582–601.

Al Mamun, M. A., & Yuce, M. R. (2019). Sensors and systems for wearable environmental monitoring toward IoT-enabled applications: A review. *IEEE Sensors Journal, 19*(18), 7771–7788.

Allen, J. G., MacNaughton, P., Satish, U., Santanem, S., Vallerino, J. & Spengler, J. D. (2016). Associations of cognitive function scores with carbon dioxide, ventilation, and volatile organic compound exposures in office workers: A controlled exposure study of green and conventional office environments. *Environmental Health Perspectives, 124*(6), 805–812.

Allen, J. G., & Macomber, J. D. (2020, April). What makes an office building "healthy"? *Harvard Business Review, 29*. https://hbr.org/2020/04/what-makes-an-office-building-healthy

Altomonte, S., Allen, J., Bluyssen, P. M., Brager,

G., Heschong, L., Loder, A., et al. (2020). Ten questions concerning well-being in the built environment. *Building and Environment, 180*, 106949.

Aviv, D., Moradnejad, M., Ida, A., Wang, Z., Teitelbaum, E., & Meggers, F. (2020). Hydrogel-based evaporative and radiative cooling prototype for hot-arid climates. *Symposium on Simulation in Architecture+Urban Design (SimAUD)*, 273–280.

Basner, M., Babisch, W., Davis, A., Brink, M., Clark, C., Janssen, S., et al. (2014). Auditory and non-auditory effects of noise on health. *Lancet, 383*(9925), 1325–1332.

Bhatt, J. M., Bhattacharyya, N., & Lin, H. W. (2017). Relationships between tinnitus and the prevalence of anxiety and depression. *Laryngoscope, 127*(2), 466–469.

Brown, A. L., Gjestland, T., & Dubois, D. (2016). Acoustic environments and soundscapes. In J. Kang and B. Schulte-Fortkamp (Eds.), *Soundscape and the built environment* (pp. 1–16). CRC Press.

Conrad, P. (1988). Health and fitness at work: A participants' perspective. *Social Science and Medicine, 26*(5), 545–550.

Engineer, A. Gualano, R. A., Crocker, R. L., Smith, J. L., Maizes, V., Weil, A., & Sternberg, E. M. (2021). An integrative health framework for wellbeing in the built environment. *Building and Environment, 205*, 108253.

Figueiro, M. G. (2013). An overview of the effects of light on human circadian rhythms: implications for new light sources and lighting systems design. *Journal of Light and Visual Environment, 37*(2_3), 51–61.

Figueiro, M. G., Steverson, B., Heerwagen, J., Kampschroer, K., Hunter, C. M., Gonzales, K., et al. (2017). The impact of daytime light exposures on sleep and mood in office workers. *Sleep Health, 3*(3), 204–215.

Figueiro, M., Steverson, B., Heerwagen, J., Yucel, R., Roohan, C., Sahin, L., et al. (2019). Light, entrainment and alertness: A case study in offices. *Lighting Research and Technology 52*(6), 736–750.

Ghahramani, A., Pantelic, J., Lindberg, C., Mehl, M., Srinivasan, K., Gilligan, B., et al. (2018). Learning occupants' workplace interactions from wearable and stationary ambient sensing systems. *Applied Energy, 230*, 42–51.

Ghahramani, A., Pantelic, J., Vannucci, M., Pistore, L., Liu, S., Gilligan, B., et al. (2019). Personal CO2 bubble: Context-dependent variations and wearable sensors usability. *Journal of Building Engineering, 22*, 295–304.

Goel, R., Pham, A., Nguyen, H., Lindberg, C., Gilligan, B., Mehl, M. R., et al. (2021). Effect of workstation type on the relationship between fatigue, physical activity, stress, and sleep. *Journal of Occupational and Environmental Medicine, 63*(3), e103-e110.

Goines, L., & Hagler, L. (2007). Noise pollution: a modern plague. *Southern Medical Journal, 100*(3), 287–294.

Google. (n.d.). *Google nest protect 2nd generation.* https://store.google.com/us/product/nest_protect_2nd_gen

Hasan, S. S., Jamrozik, A., Campanella, C., Aristizabal, S., Zhang, R., & Clements, N. (2018). Living labs: Measuring human experience in the built environment. *CHI EA '18: Extended Abstracts of the 2018 CHI Conference on Human Factors in Computing Systems*, Paper No. W31, pp. 1–8.

Hawley, B., Cox-Ganser, J. M., & Cummings, K. J. (2017). Carbon monoxide exposure in workplaces, including coffee processing facilities. *American Journal of Respiratory and Critical Care Medicine, 196*(8), 1080–1081.

Heerwagen, J. H. (1990). Affective functioning, "light hunger," and room brightness preferences. *Environment and Behavior, 22*(5), 608–635.

Hinninghofen, H., & Enck, P. (2006). Passenger well-being in airplanes. *Autonomic Neuroscience, 129*(1–2), 80–85.

Hoge, C. W., Castro, C. A., Messer, S. C., McGurk, D., Cotting, D. I., & Koffman, R. L. (2004). Combat duty in Iraq and Afghanistan, mental health problems, and barriers to care. *New England Journal of Medicine, 351*(1), 13–22.

Jafari, M. J., Khosrowabadi, R., Khodakarim, S., & Mohammadian, F. (2019). The effect of noise exposure on cognitive performance and brain activity patterns. *Open Access Macedonian Journal of Medical Sciences, 7*(17), 2924–2931.

Kim, T., McFee, E., Olguin, D. O., Waber, B., & Pentland, A. S. (2012). Sociometric badges: Using sensor technology to capture new forms of collaboration. *Journal of Organizational Behavior, 33*(3), 412–427.

Konis, K., Mack, W. J., & Schnieder, E. L. (2018). Pilot study to examine the effects of indoor daylight exposure on depression and other neuropsychiatric symptoms in people living with dementia in long-term care communities. *Clinical Interventions in Aging, 13*, wley1071–77.

Kuo, F. E., & Sullivan, W. C. (2001). Environment and crime in the inner city: Does vegetation reduce crime? *Environment and behavior, 33*(3), 343–367.

Lee, H., Razjouyan, J., Lindburg, C., Srinivasan, K., Gilligan, B., Sharafkhaneh, A., et al. (2018). *Sensor-Based Sleep Quality Index (SB-SQI): A new metric to examine the association of office workstation type on stress and sleep.* https://www.preprints.org/manuscript/201808.0457/v1

Lindberg, C. M., Srinivasan, K., Gilligan, B., Razjouyan, J., Lee, H., Najafi, B., et al. (2018). Effects of office workstation type on physical activity and stress. *Occupational and Environmental Medicine, 75*(10), 689–695.

Majumder, S., Mondal, T., & Deen, M. (2017). Wearable sensors for remote health monitoring. *Sensors, 17*(1), 130.

Mehl, M. R. (2017). The electronically activated recorder (EAR): A method for the naturalistic observation of daily social behavior. *Current Directions in Psychological Science, 26*(2), 184–190.

Mehl, M. R., & Conner, T. S. (Eds.). (2012). *Handbook of research methods for studying daily life.* Guilford Press.

Misra, V., Bozkurt, A., Calhoun, B., Jackson, T., Jur, J., Lach, J., et al. (2015). Flexible technologies for self-powered wearable health and environmental sensing. *Proceedings of the IEEE, 103*(4), 665–681.

Occupational Safety and Health Administration. (2012). *Sampling and analytical methods: carbon dioxide in workplace atmospheres.* https://www.osha.gov/dts/sltc/methods/inorganic/id172/id172.html

Pantelic, J., Liu, S., Pistore, L., Licina, D., Vannucci, M., Sadrizadeh, S., et al. (2020). Personal CO_2 cloud: Laboratory measurements of metabolic CO_2 inhalation zone concentration and dispersion in a typical office desk setting. *Journal of Exposure Science and Environmental Epidemiology, 30*(2), 328–337.

Philips Actiwatch Spectrum: Activity Monitor. (n.d.). *Features.* https://www.usa.philips.com/healthcare/product/HC1046964/actiwatch-spectrum-activity-monitor

Razjouyan, J., Lee, H., Gilligan, B., Lindberg, C., Nguyen, H., Canada, K., et al. (2019). Wellbuilt for wellbeing: Controlling relative humidity in the workplace matters for our health. *Indoor Air, 30*(1), 167–179.

Rea, M. S., & Figueiro, M. G. (2018). Light as a circadian stimulus for architectural lighting. *Lighting Research and Technology, 50*(4), 497–510.

Rea, M. S., Figueiro, M. G., Bierman, A., & Bullough, J. D. (2010). Circadian light. *Journal of Circadian Rhythms*, 8(1), 1–10.

Rosati, R., & Jamesdaniel, S. (2020). Environmental exposures and hearing loss. *International Journal of Environmental Research and Public Health, 17*(13), 4879.

Rubin H. R. R., Owens A. J., & Golden G. (1998). *Investigation to determine whether the built environment affects patients' medical outcomes.* Center for Health Design. https://www.healthdesign.org/chd/research/investigation-determine-whether-built-environment-affects-patients-medical-outcomes

Satish, U., Mendell, M. J., Shekhar, K., Hotchi, T., Sullivan, D., Streufert, S., et al. (2012). Is CO2 an indoor pollutant? Direct effects of low-to-moderate CO2 concentrations on human decision-making performance. *Environmental health perspectives, 120*(12), 1671–1677.

Taylor, S., & Hugentobler, W. (2016). Is low indoor humidity a driver for healthcare-associated infections? *Indoor Air, 98*(340). www.isiaq.org/docs/Papers/Paper340.pdf

Thayer, J. F., & Sternberg, E. (2006). Beyond heart rate variability: Vagal regulation of allostatic systems. *Annals of the New York Academy of Sciences, 1088*, 361–372.

Thayer, J. F., Verkuil, B., Brosschotj, J. F., Kampschroer, K., West, A., Sterling, C., et al. (2010). Effects of the physical work environment on physiological measures of stress. *European Journal of Prevention Cardiology, 17*(4), 431–439.

Tung, Y.-C. (2018). *Acoustic sensing: Mobile applications and frameworks.* https://search-proquest-com.ezproxy2.library.arizona.edu/docview/2077235545?pq-origsite=summon

Ulrich, R. S. (1984). View through a window may influence recovery from surgery. *Science, 224*(4647), 420–421S.

U.S. Environmental Protection Agency. (1989). *Report to Congress on indoor air quality: Volume* 2 (EPA/400/1–89/001C). Author.

Veitch, J. A., Charles, K. E., Farley, K. M., & Newsham, G. R. (2007). A model of satisfaction with open-plan office conditions: COPE field findings. *Journal of Environmental Psychology,* 27(3), 177–189.

Velux. (n.d.). *Daylight calculations and measurements.* https://www.velux.com/deic/daylight/daylight-calculations-and-measurements

Williams, D. P., Koenig, J., Carnevali, L., Sgoifo, A., Jarczok, M. N., Sternberg, E. M., et al. (2019). Heart rate variability and inflammation: A meta-analysis of human studies. *Brain, Behavior, and Immunity, 80,* 219–226.

Zhou, B. (2019). *Acoustic sensing on mobiles: From indoor mapping, tracking, to user authentication.* Unpublished doctoral dissertation. https://search-proquest-com.ezproxy2.library.arizona.edu/docview/2316520540?pq-origsite=summon

CHAPTER 24

Emotion Detection with Mobile Sensing

Koen Niemeijer and Peter Kuppens

CHAPTER OVERVIEW

In this chapter, we examine the benefits, opportunities, and challenges of already existing applications that use mobile sensing to monitor emotions. We describe how mobile sensing enables a novel, unobtrusive method of studying people's emotions *in situ* that was previously not possible. Because of the multimodal nature of mobile sensing studies, there is a rich array of measurement options that relates to emotions. Illustrated by examples, we conclude that using mobile sensing to track moment-to-moment and daily average levels of emotions shows a lot of promise, but this promise has yet to be fulfilled. Moreover, because each study takes a different approach, there is currently no established corpus of literature on which to depend to reliably and validly measure emotions in daily life using mobile sensing. Even though obstacles remain, mobile sensing is a promising method that has the potential to play a valuable role in understanding and predicting emotions in the future.

Emotions play a large role in coloring people's lives and in determining their well-being. Measuring how people feel is therefore of great importance for improving our understanding of both healthy and unhealthy emotional functioning. Emotions can change quickly, however; a person can go from tears to smiling in mere seconds. This means that proper measurement of emotion cannot take the form of a global assessment of a person (like other more stable person characteristics such as personality or values), but rather should take place repeatedly over time. Mobile sensing, with its continuous and unobtrusive collection of data in daily life, holds considerable promise in this regard, yet the question is whether it can deliver on this promise.

In this chapter, we review the nascent field of research in which mobile sensing is used and evaluated as an indication of people's emotional states and/or functioning (both in health and abnormality). First, we start by briefly explaining a number of key concepts from the field of emotion research. Second, we give a short overview of existing methods with which emotions and their temporal dynamics have been studied in daily life in past research, along with their advantages and disadvantages. Next, we turn to how mobile sensing can be used to track people's emotions and emotional functioning. We will review research that has examined how and which sensors are related to various characteristics of people's emotional lives and summarize some of the key findings. Finally, this chapter concludes by discussing possible limitations, improvements, and opportunities in the field of mobile sensing when applied to the study of emotion.

Introduction

The study of emotions is as old as the study of psychology itself, as they assume a central place in people's experience and co-determine people's behavior, perception, decision, and ultimately, well-being. Emotions are generally considered to alert individuals of personally relevant environmental challenges and opportunities, and to motivate them to cope with the events. Emotions are therefore not stable characteristics of an individual, but they change over time (Frijda, 2007; Kuppens, Oravecz, & Tuerlinckx, 2010; Kuppens & Verduyn, 2015, 2017; Larsen, 2000). They are also multicomponential, consisting of experiential (how a person feels), physiological (changes on bodily reactions), and behavioral components (how one behaves). There is tremendous variation in the quality of emotional experience, and various theories exist to explain this variation. It is beyond the scope of this chapter to extensively review the different theoretical accounts of emotion causation and composition. For the present purpose, the most important element is probably how different views organize emotions into an overarching system.

Categorical approaches primarily divide the emotional universe into a number of (basic) emotions; an example is the often-used categorization by Ekman and colleagues (1987): anger, disgust, fear, happiness, surprise, and sadness. One can also combine several basic components to form new categorizations, for instance, compound emotions (Plutchik, 1980). Second, dimensional approaches primarily characterize emotions in terms of underlying dimensions such as valence and arousal in the circumplex model of affect (Russell, 2003) or positive and negative affect (Crawford & Henry, 2004; Watson, Clark, & Tellegen, 1988). Rather than forming separate categories, specific emotions are then considered to be positioned in specific regions of the space defined by the dimensions. Both approaches are used in emotion research, including when investigating emotions in daily life.

Studying Emotions in Daily Life

Aside from experimental studies examining emotions in the lab context, emotion research has made extensive use of *in situ* sampling involving collecting data in the wild, that is, in the context of people's normal daily lives. While this does not afford experimental control over one's circumstances, it has the large benefits that it is ecologically valid and that findings are representative of real life.

For decades, the primary method for tracking people's emotional experiences has been through the use of (daily) diaries or repeated reporting using pen-and-paper, tablet computers, and eventually smartphones. This method has been labeled the experience sampling method (ESM) or ecological momentary assessment (EMA) (Kahneman, Krueger, Schkade, Schwarz, & Stone, 2004). In a typical ESM study, people are prompted with a short questionnaire a few times per day to ask how they feel. Because participants evaluate their feelings in the moment instead of later in the day (as is the case in a diary study), recall bias is limited, which leads to higher ecological validity and more reliable data (Vachon, Rintala, Viechtbauer, & Myin-Germeys, 2018; Vachon, Viechtbauer, Rintala, & Myin-Germeys, 2019). Another advantage of ESM is that it captures a person's emotions multiple times a day and so allows researchers to look at moment-to-moment emotion fluctuations (Trull & Ebner-Priemer, 2020). These improvements over traditional methods have made ESM the gold standard for studying the behavior of emotions in daily life.

Despite its many advantages, ESM also has serious drawbacks. First and foremost, ESM is a large burden to participants, depending on the number of items in the survey, the number of prompts per day, and the length of the study (Rintala, Wampers, Myin-Germeys, & Viechtbauer, 2019). Prompting participants more times per day or having a longer study duration to get more fine-grained data quickly becomes infeasible because of reduced data quality, lower compliance, and participant dropout (De Vuyst, Dejonckheere, Van der Gucht, & Kuppens, 2019; Eisele et al., 2022). This also poses a problem for practical use outside a research setting. Because of this great burden, it is not easy to motivate people to use ESM by themselves without being in a study.

In addition to ESM being obtrusive, participants may also demonstrate reactivity to the method where taking part in such a study and repeatedly reporting on their emotions may alter their emotional experience to begin with (although research suggests that the extent to which this is the case is limited; De Vuyst et al., 2019). Also, participants may adapt their daily routine to make sure they do not miss any measurement occasions, thereby effectively interfering with their normal daily activities (Barta, Tennen, & Litt, 2012).

Yet another issue in using ESM for tracking emotions has to do with the nature of emotions themselves. Because emotions are inherently dynamic, it is essential to sample them on an appropriately fine-grained time scale. However, to do this with ESM is impractical because a very high-frequency sampling scheme even further increases burden and obtrusiveness. An additional concern is that we do not know what the "right" frequency is to gather data when it comes to studying emotional responses. In short, if a method is available that can provide information on people's emotions in daily life in a continuous, automatic, and unobtrusive way, this would mean a huge leap forward, for both research and potential applications.

An obvious way forward could be through the use of (passive) mobile sensing, employing smartphone sensors to capture (contextual) information on participants such as keyboard data; app usage; or phone calls, texts, and emails. The key question that arises, however, is to what extent do these sensors convey reliable and valid data about people's emotional state and functioning? In the field of mobile sensing and affective computing, most researchers have tried to infer several characteristics related to emotions, such as a person's diagnosis of or global risk for disorders related to emotions such as bipolar disorder (e.g., Palmius et al., 2017) or related constructs such as anxiety (e.g., Place et al., 2017), daily average of emotions (e.g., Sandstrom, Lathia, Mascolo, & Rentfrow, 2017), or sleep (e.g., Saeb, Cybulski, Kording, & Mohr, 2017), among others. Relatively fewer studies have focused on capturing and understanding moment-to-moment fluctuations in people's emotion-related experience, behavior, and physiology.

State of the Literature

The foundation of the mobile sensing research of emotion lies most likely with the work of Picard (1995), who defined the field of affective computing as follows: "Computing that relates to, arises from, or influences emotions" (p. 1). However, fewer means were available in 1995 than today to track participants' emotions ecologically and unobtrusively; hence the field made relatively little progress until about 2010 when smartphones became increasingly pervasive, allowing for both ESM and automatic data capture (i.e., mobile sensing).

Since then, contemporary mobile sensing has advanced to be an interdisciplinary field and is mainly undertaken from three disciplines: (1) psychology, (2) medicine/psychiatry, and (3) engineering and computer science. These disciplines have different approaches. In psychology and medicine, for example, research focuses primarily on understanding the underlying processes and takes a more theoretically driven approach (i.e., specifying how sensors should be a readout of emotionally relevant behavior) but often lacks statistical sophistication. In engineering or computer science, the focus lies on building optimal and sophisticated predictive models but less on advancing theoretical knowledge about emotion or its underlying mechanisms. Important to note is that in most research, self-report data on the experiential component of emotion obtained through ESM is used as the criterion or label to evaluate or compare mobile sensing data too. Such validation is typically done by bringing passive data on the same time scale as the ESM data and then using these self-reports as dependent variables to compare against. Alternatively, other passive data reflecting physiology or behavior (e.g., from wearables) may be used as ground truth, especially in sleep (Z. Chen et al., 2013; Cuttone et al., 2017) and stress (Lu et al., 2012) research.

In the rest of this chapter, we will provide an overview of the current literature studying emotion using mobile sensing. The goal here is not to provide an exhaustive list through a systematic literature review, but rather to detail some key findings which, in our view, characterize the field and give a good impression of current advancements. We will first discuss the specific relevance that a number of smartphone sensors could hold for detecting emotion, foremost in terms of predicting experiential emotional experience (though we also touch on research aimed primarily at detecting emotion-related physiology and behavior). Next, we will scrutinize a number of seminal studies that have made a significant contribution to the field of emotion research. Finally, we conclude this chapter by discussing future research and challenges and summarizing the most important points to take away from our overview.

Emotion-Relevant Smartphone-Sensed Context and Behavior Variables

In the following section, we describe a number of variables that are potentially relevant for emotion detection and are therefore often used in mobile sensing research on emotion. For clarity, we distinguish between behavior and context variables. Behavior-related variables concern everything that a participant does, either actively or passively, while context-related variables are about their surroundings, that is, either where they are or what is happening around them. Note that some sensors may be used for multiple variables; for example, GPS can be used for both location and physical activity.

Behavior

Physical Activity

It is well known that physical activity strongly impacts emotion (Kanning & Schlicht, 2010; Peluso & Andrade, 2005). For example, maintaining regular physical activity levels is known to decrease emotional instability (Bowen, Balbuena, Baetz, & Schwartz, 2013), and people who perform regular physical activity in nature (in woods or forest) have a lower risk of poor mental health (Mitchell, 2013). For this reason, physical activity is often included in mobile sensing studies since it could potentially be a strong predictor for changes in emotional state (see also Giurgiu & Bussman, Chapter 5, this volume, on physical activity).

Indeed, various studies which included some form of physical activity to predict emotions or well-being found a significant relationship between physical exercise and well-being (Asselbergs et al., 2016; LiKamWa, 2012; Zanna, King, Neal, & Canavan, 2019; X. Zhang, Li, Chen, & Lu, 2018). For instance, Zhu, Satizabal, Blanke, Perez-Uribe, and Troster (2016) (93 days, $N = 18$) extracted both physical activity and location to predict discrete within-person emotions. By modeling the circumplex model of affect (Russell, 2003) as a circle with one discrete emotion at every 45-degree angle (i.e., using the number of radians between emotions instead of distinct categories as outcome), they achieved an absolute error of 0.76 radians and a sensitivity of 41% when predicting emotions on a scale of 1–8, 61% on a scale of 1–4, and 88% when choosing between a positive and negative feeling. However, their method only barely outperformed a model that merely consisted of the participant's average emotional level. A similar result was obtained by Soleimaninejadian, Zhang, Liu, and Ma (2018) (25 days, $N = 6$), who used various activity features to achieve an accuracy of 77.97% with personalized C4.5 models (a decision-tree algorithm) when predicting binary arousal (feeling either high or low) and 84.58% when predicting binary valence (feeling either good or bad).

In two larger-scale studies, Morshed and colleagues (2019) (65 days, $N = 805$) used overall physical activity duration, indoor and outdoor mobility, conversation duration (inferred from audio fragments using a hidden Markov model), and sleep duration to predict within-person emotional instability scores. They found that indoor mobility correlated positively while the others related negatively to emotional instability. Additionally, Lathia, Sandstrom, Mascolo, and Rentfrow (2017) provided a substantial contribution (2017) (51 days, $N = 12{,}838$), Their study showed that physical activity and happiness are related within persons: lower happiness relates to less physical activity; on average, emotions seem to be more positive at social locations versus at home and when being at home versus at work, and personality may moderate the relationship between emotions and location.

Sleep

While sleep is not a directly measurable component of mobile sensing, it can be approximated through various sensors (for more details, see Giurgiu & Bussman, Chapter 5, this volume). Sleep plays an important role in people's emotions and risk of ill health, like depression, and it is an important factor for well-being. For example, subjective sleep quality has been linked to positive affect (Bower, Bylsma, Morris, & Rottenberg, 2010; Steptoe, O'Donnell, Marmot, & Wardle, 2008), negative affect (Minkel et al., 2012; Sonnentag & Binnewies, 2013), and depression (Riemann, Berger, & Voderholzer, 2001; Steiger & Kimura, 2010; Tsuno, Besset, & Ritchie, 2005).

While research on sleep monitoring "in the wild" through smartphones (excluding wearables) only has provided some positive findings, it still leaves potential for progress. Bai, Xu, Ma, Sun, and Zhao (2012) (30 days, N = 15), for example, made an initial attempt to measure within-person subjective sleep quality by utilizing location (GPS), physical activity (accelerometer), text and call logs, and contextual data via sound and light. Plugging this information into a factor graph model yielded an accuracy of 78%. However, a recent paper, based on a sensitivity analysis, showed that it is difficult to predict subjective sleep quality, negative affect, or depression from nightly data (R^2 of 0.35, 0.10, and 0.03, respectively) to achieve given various choices (e.g., preprocessing choices, various statistical models, different features; Niemeijer, Mestdagh, & Kuppens, 2022). Furthermore, Chen, He, Benesty, Khotilovich, and Tang (2015) (7 days, N = 8) developed a smartphone application that offers improved user experience and less perceived intrusiveness than wearables. Subsequently, Wang and colleagues (2014; 70 days, N = 48) found an important negative between-person correlation between sleep, depression, and stress. Despite this finding, Bhat and colleagues (2015; 6 days, N = 20) have not identified any significant connection between more objective sleep monitoring via polysomnography and a smartphone device. For the sake of emotion monitoring, it is essential to bring smartphone sensing accuracy to the same degree as wearable accuracy since wearables are not yet ubiquitous; therefore, smartphones are the least obtrusive option at present.

Device Activity

Except for sensors collecting data in the background without the involvement of the participant, there may also be a great deal of information in the way one uses their phone (also see Chapters 7, 8, and 9, this volume). This component of mobile sensing thus hypothesizes that the way a person uses their phone says something about their emotional state. Concretely, the most often-used subcomponents are communication (i.e., calls and short messaging services [SMS] texts), screen activity (i.e., screen on or off), and app usage. These activities make up for most of what a person can do with their phone. We will now go over each of these subcomponents and discuss how they are used in the context of emotions.

First, seemingly, the most often-used form of device activity is information about participants' calls and SMS texts (e.g., Bhat et al., 2015; Lathia et al., 2017; Morshed et al., 2019; Zanna et al., 2019; X. Zhang et al., 2018). This functionality was (naturally) the first to be added to mobile phones—even before they became "smart"—and is therefore relatively straightforward to collect. Features extracted from SMS text and call logs are the quantity, duration, and sometimes even the sender or recipient of the SMS text or call (Asselbergs et al., 2016; LiKamWa, 2012). Despite its ease of use, call or SMS text information is usually weak or even insignificant (Cai et al., 2018) predictor for emotions. Note that content (both what is typed and how it is typed) of the messages falls under keyboard sensing.

Second, screen changes reflect when the phone's screen gets turned on or off. From this we can also extract screen time, a variable that—when high—is known to be related to a higher risk of depression and anxiety (Feng, Zhang, Du, Ye, & He, 2014; Maras et al., 2015), poorer sleep quality (Feng et al., 2014; Hale & Guan, 2015), and lower well-being (Twenge, Martin, & Campbell, 2018). While mobile sensing has successfully used screen changes to predict all of these emotion disorders (Saeb et al., 2017; Sano et al., 2018; Xu et al., 2019), it has not yet linked screen changes to daily or momentary emotions. Such an effort has been made by X. Zhang and colleagues (2018) (29 days, N = 30) who, in their compound emotion (Plutchik, 1980) model, found that screen changes were one of the weakest predictors in their general (i.e., person-nonspecific) random forest model. However, when building participant-specific (i.e., within-person) models, screen changes were among the top six features (out of 110) for 9 out of 30 participants, possibly indicating that there are major differences between participants' device usage.

Finally, app usage refers to the frequency, duration, and type of apps that one uses on their phone throughout the day. There already exists a multitude of apps that allows an individual to track their app usage, demonstrating that the technology for collecting this information is readily available. One reason why app usage is of interest to emotions is that increased social media usage has been linked to the greater odds of having depression and anxiety (Kross et al., 2013; Maras et al., 2015; Woods & Scott, 2016), although this has also been disputed (Verduyn, Gugushvili, & Kross, 2021). When it comes to predicting the daily average level of emotions, app duration was the third most chosen predictor after Wi-Fi (indoor location) and the number of social contacts (X. Zhang et al., 2018), indicating that who people contact, where people have been, and which apps people use regularly have a significant effect on their emotional state.

Speech and Text

Keyboard Dynamics

Keyboard dynamics is a very promising subfield of mobile sensing (Müller et al., Chapter 7, this volume). This area of research involves analyzing typing dynamics, for example, how fast a person types or a person's regularity in keystrokes. For emotion research, keyboard dynamics is interesting since the way a person types has already been linked to their emotional state (Epp, Lippold, & Mandryk, 2011)—for example, that keystroke duration and latency is related to arousal (Lee, Tsui, & Hsiao, 2015) or that typing speed and keystroke latency are significantly correlated with perceived stress (Lim, Ayesh, & Stacey, 2015).

A pioneering keyboard dynamics study on emotion was conducted by Zualkernan, Aloul, Shapsough, Hesham, and El-Khorzaty (2017), who asked three participants to use a custom keyboard that tracked their typing behavior for 30 days. Every time a participant started typing, a logging session was initiated spanning 5 seconds during which the number of letters, number of backspaces, and acceleration were logged. At the start of each session, a bar appeared on top of the keyboard where a user could select one of four emotion categories: happy, angry, sad, and neutral. These responses were used as labels for the person-specific models. By combining keyboard dynamics features with an accelerometer, they achieved a 90% within person accuracy in distinguishing between one of the four emotional states. Furthermore, they found that it was easier to distinguish between especially angry and sad, while happy and neutral states were more difficult to detect.

Natural Language Processing

The field of natural language processing—a field that has received a lot of attention in the past decade—complements keyboard dynamics since it analyzes natural text from keyboards. That is, not only the form but also the content of what has been typed are of interest in emotion research because this may be a potent source that conveys a more nuanced emotional state of being. Especially when considering the dynamic nature of emotion, it is easy to imagine how a person can "type" their heart out when they are in an extreme (e.g., very happy or very angry) state. The discovery of affective states from naturally typed text is also the primary interest of sentiment analysis (Bao et al., 2012; Cambria, 2016; Yadollahi, Shahraki, & Zaiane, 2017), a subfield of natural language processing. For example, sentiment analysis on Facebook posts have been able to detect emotions with high accuracy on a within-person level, which has also been used for e-learning to improve adaptive personalized learning models (Ortigosa, Martín, & Carro, 2014).

Recorded Audio

Another way to acquire natural language data using mobile sensing is to record audio and then transcribe these recordings. The electronically activated recorder (EAR) is such a device that regularly captures audio fragments for post-hoc transcription and analysis (Mehl, Pennebaker, Crow, Dabbs, & Price, 2001). From this work, several studies have been published on how audio content (i.e., what is said) relates to emotions; for example, within-person positive affect is associated with more positive words (Cohen, Minor, Baillie, & Dahir, 2008) and within-person negative affect with more negative emotion and sadness-related words (Kahn, Tobin, Massey, & Anderson, 2007). More recent studies, however, found no or only weak correlations between typical emotion-associated words and positive or negative emotions (Carlier et al., 2022), though a higher total word count seems to be associated with more positive within- and between-person emotions (Sun, Schwartz, Son, Kern, & Vazire, 2020). We refer to Hebbar and colleagues, Chapter 10, this volume, for a global overview of using audio data in mobile sensing.

Physiology

Not only smartphones but also other wearable devices (e.g., smartwatches or activity trackers) have benefited from technological developments in hardware and software development as well as visual design. As a result, commercial wearables have become relatively commonplace, with 21% of American adults owning a smartwatch or fitness tracker, a trend that is likely to rise in the future (Pew Research Center, 2020). In terms of capabilities, photoplethysmography (PPG) and accelerometer-based movements are now used in even the most basic wearables, while higher-end wearables also incorporate electrocardiography (ECG), galvanic skin response (GSR), or skin temperature sensors. The growing adoption rate of these wearables has significantly reduced the barrier to scientific data collection—in terms not just of availability, but also user acceptance—allowing for large-scale monitoring of physiological and mobility factors in daily life.

Indeed, wearable technology has already been shown to be a valuable addition to the field of passive sensing. In comparison to smartphone sensors, accelerometer data generated from body-worn sensors gives considerably more accurate information on physical movements. Additional information regarding the intensity of the participant's physical activity can be obtained using the accelerometer or physiological indicators such as heart rate and breathing patterns (Treuth et al., 2004). A growing body of research is looking at the idea of employing passive sensing characteristics to predict distinct experience states, such as emotion. For example, physiological and mobility data acquired via wearable devices have been used to anticipate the occurrence of acute stress (Healey & Picard, 2005; Hovsepian et al., 2015; Sano & Picard, 2013; Smets et al., 2018). Although these machine learning models have yet to perform sufficiently in practice, they may in the future provide opportunities to estimate experience states without the participant's active participation, especially when combined with mobile sensing. For instance, Wang and colleagues (2018) used wearables to measure heart rate as an indicator of fatigue. When combined with mobile sensing data, their models could accurately track changing depression levels within students. We refer to Bettis, Burke, Nesi, and Liu (2021) for further discussion of how to use physiology (and other sensors) for tracking emotions and emotion regulation and to Chapter 6 (this volume) for physiology in general.

Context

Location

A widely used measure for emotion tracking is participants' physical location (also described in more details by Lautenbach et al., Chapter 4, this volume). It is used in research on emotion because it is considered that a person's location could reveal something about their emotional state. For example, a participant may feel more relaxed at home and tenser at work or, conversely, might be in a more positive mood in a social situation than at home or work (Sandstrom et al., 2017). Indeed, because physical location is known to relate to the daily average level of emotion and even moment-to-moment emotions, it is often incorporated in mobile sensing studies.

In a study by Cai and colleagues (2018), participants ($N = 220$) were asked for 14 days to rate both their positive and negative affect on a 100-point gliding scale six times per day. Among several sensors (physical activity, call and text log, location, time of day), only location and day of the week were significantly correlated with negative affect on a within-person level. Furthermore, being at a food place such as a restaurant led to a significantly lower average negative affect than when at home, as much as a 10-point drop in average momentary negative affect. This result mirrors previous results; for example, LiKamWa (2012) (60 days, $N = 32$) found that location features correlate with high pleasure. Also, in recreational areas, participants showed less negative affect than, for example, at a university campus. Cai and colleagues also noticed that there are individual differences; while some participants rated more negative affect at a university campus, this was not true for all participants in the study. This nonhomogeneous relation indicates that the participants' personal routines and preferences influence the spatial distribution of negatives.

Surroundings

Information about surroundings is not directly related to the participant but it helps place the other variables into context. In other words, the surroundings consist of directly measurable surrounding variables such as ambient noise, the amount of light captured by the phone, or the use of Bluetooth to detect how many people are in the vicinity of the participant (further described by Hebbar et al., Chapter 10, this volume). This information is important for emotions and emotion disorders. For example, more sunlight (and thus also vitamin D) has been found to have a positive between-person effect on depression (Benedetti, Colombo, Barbini, Campori, & Smeraldi, 2001; Berk et al., 2007), and people experience more positive emotions in social settings. Emotion predictions could therefore benefit from having this information. While various studies have been conducted that use environment sensors, no studies—to the best of our knowledge—have reported exact effects that tell us to what extent they relate to emotion. Only X. Zhang and colleagues (2018) reported that light intensity and ambient noise were the fourth and fifth most frequently selected sensor, respectively.

Another interesting possibility for mobile sensing to contribute to the context of surroundings is by capturing ambient noise. That is, audio recordings (or features thereof) could be predictive of emotion (Scherer, 1986). Distinguishing between distinct emotions can be accomplished to some extent solely through acoustic features (such as pitch, loudness, and tone; Laukka, Neiberg, & Elfenbein, 2014). However, neither multilevel nor machine learning models using acoustic features extracted from audio recordings—nor human coders—could determine the intensity of corresponding momentary emotions (N = 20,197) on a within-person level (Weidman et al., 2020). Determining emotion intensity from raw audio fragments directly may be possible when predicting abstract emotion dimensions like valence and arousal and more complex methods such as deep learning (Tang, Kuppens, Geurts, & van Waterschoot, 2021).

Examples of Emotion Research Using Mobile Sensing

In this section, we highlight three recent examples of research that use a combination of mobile sensors to study emotion. Our examples aim to shed insight into how such studies are conducted, which features are included, how many participants are involved, and their degree of success. Our goal is to analyze the kinds of specific issues that can be dealt with by measuring emotions intensively over time and by developing the technological strategy required to focus on the temporal aspect of these results.

MoodExplorer

A unique take on assessing emotions is the one proposed by X. Zhang and colleagues (2018), who posited that studying compound emotions—a mixture of basic emotions (Ekman et al., 1987; Plutchik, 1980)—could be a more effective way of detecting emotions. Their dataset revealed that in approximately 60% of recorded cases, participants selected two or more basic emotions, indicating that these are, in fact, composite (multidimensional) emotions.

X. Zhang and colleagues (2018) developed an Android app they called MoodExplorer. Every 5 minutes, the app collected the location from GPS, checked whether the screen was on or off, and noted the Wi-Fi status. Additionally, at every measurement moment, the accelerometer, compass, light sensor, microphone, and gyroscope were sampled for 15 seconds. MoodExplorer also registered app usage and sent and received SMS messages and phone calls. After developing the app, a study was launched involving 42 participants for a total period of 29 days. Participants were administered three beeps per day. After the data collection phase, only 30 participants were retained because of the requirement that they had to have more than 50 responses.

After extracting some second-order features, the six best features per person were selected and subsequently plugged into a personalized factor graph that accounted for the correlation between distinct categories of emotions. Overall, the most important features were related to social (call duration or SMS text frequency of a specific contact), (indoor) location (time spent using a particular Wi-Fi network), and smartphone behavior (specific app usage duration). When comparing this to other methods (i.e., a decision tree, support vector machine, and logistic regression), the personalized factor graph models performed decisively better at a 76% "exact match" versus around 72% for the other methods. Thus, X. Zhang and colleagues (2018) show that moment-to-moment emotions can be predicted reasonably well when using a sophisticated data-analytic strategy. Nevertheless, they admit that tracking emotion on a fine-grained level is hard, given that mobile sensing often produces coarse-grained data.

MoodCast

Besides trying to directly assess emotions by looking at participants' behavior, another approach is to look at indirect emotional relationships. More specifically, the notion that emotions are inherently connected to that of people in one's social network could be of great use. Such "emotional contagion" (Easterlin, 2003; Wilson, Meyers, & Gilbert, 2003) means that emotions can, to some degree, be transferred from one person to another and that other people can "catch" emotional states by observation after days or even weeks (Bolger, 2005; Larson & Richards, 1994; Scollon, Kim-Prieto, & Scollon, 2003). For example, Fowler and Christakis (2008) found that happiness can spread within social networks, such as to a co-resident spouse, a next-door neighbor, or a friend who lives within a mile. Hence, Y. Zhang, Tang, Sun, Chen, and Rao (2010) capitalized on this idea by including emotions of social connections as a factor in their model alongside several mobile sensing features. Their method, called MoodCast, comprised three aspects:

1. Temporal, that is, the relationship between emotion and its previous self.
2. Social, that is, the relationship between emotion and other people's emotion status in the same social network.
3. Attribute, that is, mobile sensing attributes that describe the environment (location, call log, SMS text) and physical activities.

These three aspects were then integrated into a dynamic, continuous factor graph model to predict one of three discrete emotional states (positive, negative, or neutral) that users assigned to a post. The MoodCast method was compared to two support vector machines and two naïve Bayes models, both one with and one without social and temporal information. All models were tested on a real-world dataset and a virtual Web-based network (LiveJournal).

MoodCast performed, on average, 8% better than the other models in terms of F1 score, ranging from 49.77% to 75.44% when predicting negative and neutral emotions, respectively, on a within-person level. Moreover, adding social network information clearly improved the models, more so with the Web-based network than with the real-life dataset. This is possibly because in the real-life dataset, participants only had 3.2 connections versus 49.6 connections in the Web-based dataset, showcasing the need for taking participants' social networks into account. While this is an early study, it shows the interesting notion of making a distinction between temporal, social, and participant-specific information and how including social network dynamics can add to the understanding of emotion.

EmotionSense

Finally, one of the largest mobile sensing studies carried out to date is the one from the University of Cambridge with an app called EmotionSense. Because the app was free to download in the Google Play store, the team was able to collect data from approximately 18,000 participants who had completed at least one self-report survey in a period of more than 3 years. Participants received two ESM notifications per day that measured valence and arousal, positive and negative affect, and happiness (Satisfaction with Life Scale; Diener, Emmons, Larsen, & Griffin, 1985). In the background, the app collected the location, physical activity as measured by the accelerometer, and ambient sound using the microphone. For each study, a slightly different subset of the data was used based on the research question.

From this massive dataset, Lathia and colleagues (2017) found that physical activity and happiness are positively related: Lower happiness relates to less physical activity. Related to this finding is that the momentary emotional state seems to be more positive at social locations versus when at home, and yet this emotional state is also more positive when being at home than when at work. Moreover, personality may moderate the relationship between emotion and location (Sandstrom et al., 2017).

When it comes to using EmotionSense data to predict emotion on a daily level, Servia-Rodríguez and colleagues (2017) used deep neural networks—a method that is feasible to use thanks to the large size of the dataset—to achieve an accuracy of 68% when predicting the valence of users who completed surveys on weekends and 65% on weekdays. For arousal, the predictive accuracy was lower, namely, 56% on weekends and around 60% on weekdays. The general noise level, location, physical activity, and sociability could also be related to the demographics of a person. For example, females tend to be less physically active than males but send and receive more text messages per day. In general, Servia-Rodríguez and colleagues found that people with similar demographics have similar usage patterns.

Tagging on to these deep-learning techniques, Spathis, Servia-Rodriguez, Farrahi, Mascolo, and Rentfrow (2019), using the same data, attempted to classify whether participants could be described as being more relaxed (i.e., being lower in arousal) only by looking at one-off questionnaires describing personality traits and mobile sensing data. A participant is considered to be relaxed/nonrelaxed based on the results of *k*-means clustering to find the groups. Through an extensive method for selecting both the best feature and model combination, they achieved an area under the curve of 0.749, with a logistic regression using both sensor and questionnaire information. The sensors on a daily level (instead of weekly) did not improve the results (Spathis et al., 2019).

These studies make clear a strong need for reliable longitudinal data from a large group of participants, although these samples sizes are usually not pervasive in mobile sensing studies. However, as stated at the beginning of this chapter, one of the challenges involved in tracking emotions is that they have a highly dynamic nature. It is therefore essential not only to track many participants for a longer amount of time, but also to do so at a high sample frequency.

Challenges

While every study has different strengths and weaknesses, there are some overlapping factors that hold back the field as a whole. A general challenge is to collect data such that they are (1) least invasive (in terms of privacy and battery drain), (2) both reliable and valid, and (3) gathered over a longer duration of time and of high frequency while still retaining an acceptable compliance rate. Especially for tracking emotions, high-frequency data are needed to capture these moment-to-moment events. While many other issues are keeping back the field, here we focus on three of the most necessary.

First, the number of participants in the studies is often quite low. Of course, this cannot be seen independently of the short existence of the field; that is, because most works are aimed toward discovering the best method to predict their target variable, they are of an explorative nature. Once a state-of-the-art method has been developed, sample sizes can be increased to strengthen the statistical power of the analyses. Growing the number of participants further benefits the creation of person-specific models through which, for example, emotions can be measured when communicating through personality.

Such a state-of-the-art method is hindered by a second limitation, namely, that technical difficulties are generally abundant and that it is therefore challenging to perform reliable measurements (Bähr et al., 2022; Niemeijer, Mestdagh, and Kuppens, 2023). Currently, most researchers build their own mobile applications to collect data, even though alternatives already exist. These alternatives are not used because they (1) are not open source or too expensive, (2) do not collect the right information, or (3) lack documentation to use them. This is why collaborative efforts need to be made and a common ground and strategy decided.

Finally, studies often lack rigor in their descriptions of their methods, to the point that they are hard to reproduce without inquiring into the research about their specific implementation (De Angel et al., 2022; Langener, Stulp, Kas, & Bringmann, 2023). Coincidentally, since the results of similar studies greatly vary, this often complicates pinpointing what makes some studies more successful than others. These and other challenges are based on the fact that there is currently no consensus on a method, model, or tool for detecting daily averaged or momentary emotion levels from mobile sensing data. The sector should see enormous success, and its influence should function to transform it into a widely agreed standard procedure.

Future Directions

Although mobile sensing has not yet lived up to its promise, the field has much to look forward to. Overall, mobile sensing is getting more important for society as high-quality mobile telephones are becoming more widespread. Furthermore, the increasing efficiency of the sensors and the mobile phones themselves will further boost both data and predictive quality. However, the greatest improvement could be achieved by a state-of-the-art method—specifically designed to track emotions—that has been verified and tested on a large population.

In terms of sensors, location and physical activity are two often used sensors, both because they are relatively easy to collect and because they have historically been known to have a strong relationship with emotion. Unsurprisingly, this promise holds up in mobile sensing studies. We therefore recommend including these sensors in a mobile sensing study for tracking emotions.

There are also opportunities with categories of sensors that—in contrast to location or physical activity—are not often used to predict emotion but that could be insightful. For example, natural typed text or spoken language is known to contain a wide spectrum of emotions (as showcased by the field of sentiment analysis; e.g., Bao et al., 2012; Cambria, 2016; Tang et al., 2021; Yadollahi et al., 2017), and yet it is frequently left out in mobile sensing studies for either privacy reasons or its technical complexity to collect and analyze. There are also novel information sources that have only started to be used recently in other contexts, such as image analysis (Darvariu, Convertino, Mehrotra, & Musolesi, 2020) and music choice analysis (Sarda, Halasawade, Padmawar, & Aghav, 2019).

REFERENCES

Asselbergs, J., Ruwaard, J., Ejdys, M., Schrader, N., Sijbrandij, M., & Riper, H. (2016). Mobile phone-based unobtrusive ecological momentary assessment of day-to-day mood: An explorative Study. *Journal of Medical Internet Research, 18*(3), e72.

Bai, Y., Xu, B., Ma, Y., Sun, G., & Zhao, Y. (2012). Will you have a good sleep tonight?: Sleep quality prediction with mobile phone. *Proceedings of the 7th International Conference on Body Area Networks*, pp. 124–130.

Bähr, S., Haas, G.-C., Keusch, F., Kreuter, F., & Trappmann, M. (2022). Missing Data and Other Measurement Quality Issues in Mobile Geolocation Sensor Data. *Social Science Computer Review, 40*(1), 212–235.

Bao, S., Xu, S., Zhang, L., Yan, R., Su, Z., Han, D., et al. (2012). Mining social emotions from affective text. *IEEE Transactions on Knowledge and Data Engineering, 24*(9), 1658–1670.

Barta, W. D., Tennen, H., & Litt, M. D. (2012). Measurement reactivity in diary research. In M. R. Mehl & T. S. Conner (Eds.), *Handbook of research methods for studying daily life* (pp. 108–123). Guilford Press.

Benedetti, F., Colombo, C., Barbini, B., Campori, E., & Smeraldi, E. (2001). Morning sunlight reduces length of hospitalization in bipolar depression. *Journal of Affective Disorders, 62*(3), 221–223.

Berk, M., Sanders, K. M., Pasco, J. A., Jacka, F. N., Williams, L. J., Hayles, A. L., et al. (2007). Vitamin D deficiency may play a role in depression. *Medical Hypotheses, 69*(6), 1316–1319.

Bettis, A. H., Burke, T. A., Nesi, J., & Liu, R. T. (2021). Digital technologies for emotion-regulation assessment and intervention: A conceptual review. *Clinical Psychological Science, 10*(1), 3–26.

Bhat, S., Ferraris, A., Gupta, D., Mozafarian, M., DeBari, V. A., Gushway-Henry, N., et al. (2015). Is there a clinical role for smartphone sleep apps? Comparison of sleep cycle detection by a smartphone application to polysomnography. *Journal of Clinical Sleep Medicine, 11*(7), 709–715.

Bolger, N. (2005). Using diary methods to study marital and family processes. *Journal of Family Psychology, 19*(1), 86–97.

Bowen, R., Balbuena, L., Baetz, M., & Schwartz, L. (2013). Maintaining sleep and physical activity alleviate mood instability. *Preventive Medicine, 57*(5), 461–465.

Bower, B., Bylsma, L. M., Morris, B. H., & Rottenberg, J. (2010). Poor reported sleep quality predicts low positive affect in daily life among healthy and mood-disordered persons. *Journal of Sleep Research, 19*(2), 323–332.

Cai, L., Boukhechba, M., Wu, C., Chow, P. I., Teachman, B. A., Barnes, L. E., et al. (2018). State affect recognition using smartphone sensing data. *Proceedings of the 2018 IEEE/ACM International Conference on Connected Health: Applications, Systems and Engineering Technologies*, pp. 120–125.

Cambria, E. (2016). Affective computing and sentiment analysis. *IEEE Intelligent Systems, 31*(2), 102–107.

Carlier, C., Niemeijer, K., Mestdagh, M., Bauwens, M., Vanbrabant, P., Geurts, L., et al.

(2022). In search of state and trait emotion markers in mobile-sensed language: A field study. *JMIR Mental Health, 9*(2), *e31724*.

Chen, T., He, T., Benesty, M., Khotilovich, V., & Tang, Y. (2015). Xgboost: Extreme gradient boosting. *R Package Version 0.4-2*, 1–4.

Chen, Z., Lin, M., Chen, F., Lane, N. D., Cardone, G., Wang, R., et al. (2013). Unobtrusive sleep monitoring using smartphones. *Proceedings of the 7th International Conference on Pervasive Computing Technologies for Healthcare*, pp. 145–152.

Cohen, A. S., Minor, K. S., Baillie, L. E., & Dahir, A. M. (2008). Clarifying the linguistic signature: Measuring personality from natural speech. *Journal of Personality Assessment, 90*(6), 559–563.

Crawford, J. R., & Henry, J. D. (2004). The Positive and Negative Affect Schedule (PANAS): Construct validity, measurement properties and normative data in a large non-clinical sample. *British Journal of Clinical Psychology, 43*(3), 245–265.

Cuttone, A., Bækgaard, P., Sekara, V., Jonsson, H., Larsen, J. E., & Lehmann, S. (2017). SensibleSleep: A Bayesian model for learning sleep patterns from smartphone events. *PLOS ONE, 12*(1), 1–20.

Darvariu, V.-A., Convertino, L., Mehrotra, A., & Musolesi, M. (2020). Quantifying the relationships between everyday objects and emotional states through deep learning based image analysis using smartphones. *Proceedings of the ACM on Interactive, Mobile, Wearable and Ubiquitous Technologies, 4*(1), 1–21.

De Angel, V., Lewis, S., White, K., Oetzmann, C., Leightley, D., Oprea, E., et al. (2022). Digital health tools for the passive monitoring of depression: A systematic review of methods. *Npj Digital Medicine, 5*(1), 1–14.

De Vuyst, H.-J., Dejonckheere, E., Van der Gucht, K., & Kuppens, P. (2019). Does repeatedly reporting positive or negative emotions in daily life have an impact on the level of emotional experiences and depressive symptoms over time? *PLoS One, 14*(6), e0219121.

Diener, E., Emmons, R. A., Larsen, R. J., & Griffin, S. (1985). The Satisfaction with Life Scale. *Journal of Personality Assessment, 49*(1), 71–75.

Easterlin, R. A. (2003). Explaining happiness. *Proceedings of the National Academy of Sciences, 100*(19), 11176–11183.

Eisele, G., Vachon, H., Lafit, G., Kuppens, P., Houben, M., Myin-Germeys, I., et al. (2022). The effects of sampling frequency and questionnaire length on perceived burden, compliance, and careless responding in experience sampling data in a student population. *Assessment, 29*(2), 136–151.

Ekman, P., Friesen, W. V., O'Sullivan, M., Chan, A., Diacoyanni-Tarlatzis, I., Heider, K., et al. (1987). Universals and cultural differences in the judgments of facial expressions of emotion. *Journal of Personality and Social Psychology, 53*(4), 712–717.

Epp, C., Lippold, M., & Mandryk, R. L. (2011). Identifying emotional states using keystroke dynamics. In *Proceedings of the 2011 Annual Conference on Human Factors in Computing Systems—CHI '11*, pp. 715–724.

Feng, Q., Zhang, Q., Du, Y., Ye, Y., & He, Q. (2014). Associations of physical activity, screentTime with depression, anxiety and sleep quality among Chinese college freshmen. *PLoS One, 9*(6), e100914.

Fowler, J. H., & Christakis, N. A. (2008). Dynamic spread of happiness in a large social network: Longitudinal analysis over 20 years in the Framingham Heart Study. *British Medical Journal, 337*, 1–9.

Frijda, N. H. (2007). *The laws of emotion*. Erlbaum.

Hale, L., & Guan, S. (2015). Screen time and sleep among school-aged children and adolescents: A systematic literature review. *Sleep Medicine Reviews, 21*, 50–58.

Healey, J. A., & Picard, R. W. (2005). Detecting stress during real-world driving tasks using physiological sensors. *IEEE Transactions on Intelligent Transportation Systems, 6*(2), 156–166.

Hovsepian, K., al'Absi, M., Ertin, E., Kamarck, T., Nakajima, M., & Kumar, S. (2015). cStress: Towards a gold standard for continuous stress assessment in the mobile environment. *Proceedings of the 2015 ACM International Joint Conference on Pervasive and Ubiquitous Computing—UbiComp '15*, pp. 493–504.

Kahn, J. H., Tobin, R. M., Massey, A. E., & Anderson, J. A. (2007). Measuring emotional expression with the Linguistic Inquiry and Word Count. *American Journal of Psychology, 120*(2), 263–286.

Kahneman, D., Krueger, A. B., Schkade, D. A.,

Schwarz, N., & Stone, A. A. (2004). A survey method for characterizing daily life experience: The day reconstruction method. *Science, 306*(5702), 1776–1780.

Kanning, M., & Schlicht, W. (2010). Be active and become happy: An ecological momentary assessment of physical activity and mood. *Journal of Sport and Exercise Psychology, 32*(2), 253–261.

Kross, E., Verduyn, P., Demiralp, E., Park, J., Lee, D. S., Lin, N., et al. (2013). Facebook use predicts declines in subjective well-being in young adults. *PLoS One, 8*(8), e69841.

Kuppens, P., Oravecz, Z., & Tuerlinckx, F. (2010). Feelings change: Accounting for individual differences in the temporal dynamics of affect. *Journal of Personality and Social Psychology, 99*(6), 1042–1060.

Kuppens, P., & Verduyn, P. (2015). Looking at emotion regulation through the window of emotion dynamics. *Psychological Inquiry, 26*(1), 72–79.

Kuppens, P., & Verduyn, P. (2017). Emotion dynamics. *Current Opinion in Psychology, 17*, 22–26.

Langener, A. M., Stulp, G., Kas, M. J., & Bringmann, L. F. (2023). Capturing the dynamics of the social environment through experience sampling methods, passive sensing, and egocentric networks: Scoping review. *JMIR Mental Health, 10*(1), e42646.

Larsen, R. J. (2000). Toward a science of mood regulation. *Psychological Inquiry, 11*(3), 129–141.

Larson, R., & Richards, M. H. (1994). *Divergent realities: The emotional lives of mothers, fathers, and adolescents.* Basic Books.

Lathia, N., Sandstrom, G. M., Mascolo, C., & Rentfrow, P. J. (2017). Happier people live more active lives: Using smartphones to link happiness and physical activity. *PLoS One, 12*(1), e0160589.

Laukka, P., Neiberg, D., & Elfenbein, H. A. (2014). Evidence for cultural dialects in vocal emotion expression: Acoustic classification within and across five nations. *Emotion, 14*(3), 445–449.

Lee, P.-M., Tsui, W.-H., & Hsiao, T.-C. (2015). The influence of emotion on keyboard typing: An experimental study using auditory stimuli. *PLoS One, 10*(6), e0129056.

LiKamWa, R. (2012). *MoodScope: Building a mood sensor from smartphone usage patterns.* Master's thesis, Rice University. https://scholarship.rice.edu/bitstream/handle/1911/64654/LI-KAM-WA-THESIS.pdf

Lim, Y. M., Ayesh, A., & Stacey, M. (2015). Using mouse and keyboard dynamics to detect cognitive stress during mental arithmetic. In K. Arai, S. Kapoor, & R. Bhatia (Eds.), *Intelligent systems in science and information 2014* (pp. 335–350). Springer.

Lu, H., Frauendorfer, D., Rabbi, M., Mast, M. S., Chittaranjan, G. T., Campbell, A. T., et al. (2012). StressSense: Detecting stress in unconstrained acoustic environments using smartphones. *Proceedings of the 2012 ACM Conference on Ubiquitous Computing - UbiComp '12*, pp. 351–360.

Maras, D., Flament, M. F., Murray, M., Buchholz, A., Henderson, K. A., Obeid, N., et al. (2015). Screen time is associated with depression and anxiety in Canadian youth. *Preventive Medicine, 73*, 133–138.

Mehl, M. R., Pennebaker, J. W., Crow, D. M., Dabbs, J., & Price, J. H. (2001). The electronically activated recorder (EAR): A device for sampling naturalistic daily activities and conversations. *Behavior Research Methods, Instruments, and Computers, 33*(4), 517–523.

Minkel, J. D., Banks, S., Htaik, O., Moreta, M. C., Jones, C. W., McGlinchey, E. L., et al. (2012). Sleep deprivation and stressors: Evidence for elevated negative affect in response to mild stressors when sleep deprived. *Emotion, 12*(5), 1015–1020.

Mitchell, R. (2013). Is physical activity in natural environments better for mental health than physical activity in other environments? *Social Science and Medicine, 91*, 130–134.

Morshed, M. B., Saha, K., Li, R., D'Mello, S. K., De Choudhury, M., Abowd, G. D., et al. (2019). Prediction of mood instability with passive sensing. *Proceedings of the ACM on Interactive, Mobile, Wearable and Ubiquitous Technologies, 3*(3), 1–21.

Niemeijer, K., Mestdagh, M., & Kuppens, P. (2022). Tracking subjective sleep quality and mood with mobile sensing: A multiverse study. *Journal of Medical Internet Research, 24*(3), e25643.

Niemeijer, K., Mestdagh, M., Verdonck, S., Meers, K., & Kuppens, P. (2023). Combining experience sampling and mobile sensing for digital phenotyping with m-path sense: Performance study. *JMIR Formative Research, 7*(1), e43296.

Ortigosa, A., Martín, J. M., & Carro, R. M. (2014). Sentiment analysis in Facebook and its application to e-learning. *Computers in Human Behavior, 31*, 527–541.

Palmius, N., Tsanas, A., Saunders, K. E. A., Bilderbeck, A. C., Geddes, J. R., Goodwin, G. M., et al. (2017). Detecting bipolar depression from geographic location data. *IEEE Transactions on Biomedical Engineering, 64*(8), 1761–1771.

Peluso, M. A. M., & Andrade, L. H. S. G. de. (2005). Physical activity and mental health: The association between exercise and mood. *Clinics, 60*(1), 61–70.

Pew Research Center. (2020, January 9). *About one-in-five Americans use a smart watch or fitness tracker.* www.pewresearch.org/fact-tank/2020/01/09/about-one-in-five-americans-use-a-smart-watch-or-fitness-tracker

Picard, R. W. (1995). *Affective computing* (Technical Report No. 321). MIT Media Laboratory. https://hd.media.mit.edu/tech-reports/TR-321.pdf

Place, S., Blanch-Hartigan, D., Rubin, C., Gorrostieta, C., Mead, C., Kane, J., et al. (2017). Behavioral indicators on a mobile sensing platform predict clinically validated psychiatric symptoms of mood and anxiety disorders. *Journal of Medical Internet Research, 19*(3), e75.

Plutchik, R. (1980). A general psychoevolutionary theory of emotion. In R. Plutchik & H. Kellerman (Eds.), *Theories of Emotion* (pp. 3–33). Academic Press.

Riemann, D., Berger, M., & Voderholzer, U. (2001). Sleep and depression—results from psychobiological studies: An overview. *Biological Psychology, 57*(1), 67–103.

Rintala, A., Wampers, M., Myin-Germeys, I., & Viechtbauer, W. (2019). Response compliance and predictors thereof in studies using the experience sampling method. *Psychological Assessment, 31*(2), 226–235.

Russell, J. A. (2003). Core affect and the psychological construction of emotion. *Psychological Review, 110*(1), 145–172.

Saeb, S., Cybulski, T. R., Kording, K. P., & Mohr, D. C. (2017). Scalable passive sleep monitoring using mobile phones: Opportunities and obstacles. *Journal of Medical Internet Research, 19*(4), e118.

Sandstrom, G. M., Lathia, N., Mascolo, C., & Rentfrow, P. J. (2017). Putting mood in context: Using smartphones to examine how people feel in different locations. *Journal of Research in Personality, 69*, 96–101.

Sano, A., & Picard, R. W. (2013). Stress recognition using wearable sensors and mobile phones. In *2013 Humaine Association Conference on Affective Computing and Intelligent Interaction*, pp. 671–676.

Sano, A., Taylor, S., McHill, A. W., Phillips, A. J., Barger, L. K., Klerman, E., et al. (2018). Identifying objective physiological markers and modifiable behaviors for self-reported stress and mental health status using wearable sensors and mobile phones: Observational study. *Journal of Medical Internet Research, 20*(6), e210.

Sarda, P., Halasawade, S., Padmawar, A., & Aghav, J. (2019). Emousic: Emotion and activity-based music player using machine learning. In S. K. Bhatia, S. Tiwari, K. K. Mishra, & M. C. Trivedi (Eds.), *Advances in computer communication and computational sciences* (pp. 179–188). Springer.

Scherer, K. R. (1986). Vocal affect expression: A review and a model for future research. *Psychological Bulletin, 99*(2), 143–165.

Scollon, C. N., Kim-Prieto, C., & Scollon, C. N. (2003). Experience sampling: Promises and pitfalls, strengths and weaknesses. *Journal of Happiness Studies, 4*(1), 5–34.

Servia-Rodríguez, S., Rachuri, K. K., Mascolo, C., Rentfrow, P. J., Lathia, N., & Sandstrom, G. M. (2017). Mobile sensing at the service of mental well-being: A large-scale longitudinal study. *Proceedings of the 26th International Conference on World Wide Web—WWW '17*, pp. 103–112.

Smets, E., Rios Velazquez, E., Schiavone, G., Chakroun, I., D'Hondt, E., De Raedt, W., et al. (2018). Large-scale wearable data reveal digital phenotypes for daily-life stress detection. *npj Digital Medicine, 1*(1), 1–10.

Soleimaninejadian, P., Zhang, M., Liu, Y., & Ma, S. (2018). Mood detection and prediction based on user daily activities. n *2018 First Asian Conference on Affective Computing and Intelligent Interaction (ACII Asia)*, pp. 1–6.

Sonnentag, S., & Binnewies, C. (2013). Daily affect spillover from work to home: Detachment from work and sleep as moderators.

Journal of Vocational Behavior, 83(2), 198–208.

Spathis, D., Servia-Rodriguez, S., Farrahi, K., Mascolo, C., & Rentfrow, J. (2019). Passive mobile sensing and psychological traits for large scale mood prediction. *Proceedings of the 13th EAI International Conference on Pervasive Computing Technologies for Healthcare*, pp. 272–281.

Steiger, A., & Kimura, M. (2010). Wake and sleep EEG provide biomarkers in depression. *Journal of Psychiatric Research, 44*(4), 242–252.

Steptoe, A., O'Donnell, K., Marmot, M., & Wardle, J. (2008). Positive affect, psychological well-being, and good sleep. *Journal of Psychosomatic Research, 64*(4), 409–415.

Sun, J., Schwartz, H. A., Son, Y., Kern, M. L., & Vazire, S. (2020). The language of well-being: Tracking fluctuations in emotion experience through everyday speech. *Journal of Personality and Social Psychology, 118*(2), 364–387.

Tang, D., Kuppens, P., Geurts, L., & van Waterschoot, T. (2021). End-to-end speech emotion recognition using a novel context-stacking dilated convolution neural network. *EURASIP Journal on Audio, Speech, and Music Processing, 2021*(1), 18.

Treuth, M. S., Schmitz, K., Catellier, D. J., McMurray, R. G., Murray, D. M., Almeida, M. J., et al. (2004). Defining accelerometer thresholds for activity intensities in adolescent girls. *Medicine and Science in Sports and Exercise, 36*(7), 1259–1266.

Trull, T. J., & Ebner-Priemer, U. W. (2020). Ambulatory assessment in psychopathology research: A review of recommended reporting guidelines and current practices. *Journal of Abnormal Psychology, 129*(1), 56–63.

Tsuno, N., Besset, A., & Ritchie, K. (2005). Sleep and depression. *The Journal of Clinical Psychiatry, 66*(10), 1254–1269.

Twenge, J. M., Martin, G. N., & Campbell, W. K. (2018). Decreases in psychological well-being among American adolescents after 2012 and links to screen time during the rise of smartphone technology. *Emotion, 18*(6), 765–780.

Vachon, H., Rintala, A., Viechtbauer, W., & Myin-Germeys, I. (2018). Data quality and feasibility of the Experience Sampling Method across the spectrum of severe psychiatric disorders: A protocol for a systematic review and meta-analysis. *Systematic Reviews, 7*(1), 7.

Vachon, H., Viechtbauer, W., Rintala, A., & Myin-Germeys, I. (2019). Compliance and retention with the experience sampling method over the continuum of severe mental disorders: Meta-analysis and recommendations. *Journal of Medical Internet Research, 21*(12), e14475.

Verduyn, P., Gugushvili, N., & Kross, E. (2021). The impact of social network sites on mental health: Distinguishing active from passive use. *World Psychiatry, 20*(1), 133–134.

Wang, R., Chen, F., Chen, Z., Li, T., Harari, G., Tignor, S., et al. (2014). StudentLife: Assessing mental health, academic performance and behavioral trends of college students using smartphones. *Proceedings of the 2014 ACM International Joint Conference on Pervasive and Ubiquitous Computing—UbiComp '14 Adjunct*, pp. 3–14.

Wang, R., Wang, W., daSilva, A., Huckins, J. F., Kelley, W. M., Heatherton, T. F., et al. (2018). Tracking depression dynamics in college students using mobile phone and wearable sensing. *Proceedings of the ACM on Interactive, Mobile, Wearable and Ubiquitous Technologies, 2*(1), 1–26.

Watson, D., Clark, L. A., & Tellegen, A. (1988). Development and validation of brief measures of positive and negative affect: The PANAS scales. *Journal of Personality and Social Psychology, 54*(6), 1063–1070.

Weidman, A. C., Sun, J., Vazire, S., Quoidbach, J., Ungar, L. H., & Dunn, E. W. (2020). (Not) hearing happiness: Predicting fluctuations in happy mood from acoustic cues using machine learning. *Emotion, 20*(4), 642–658.

Wilson, T. D., Meyers, J., & Gilbert, D. T. (2003). "How happy was I, anyway?": A retrospective impact bias. *Social Cognition, 21*(6), 421–446.

Woods, H. C., & Scott, H. (2016). #Sleepyteens: Social media use in adolescence is associated with poor sleep quality, anxiety, depression and low self-esteem. *Journal of Adolescence, 51*, 41–49.

Xu, X., Creswell, J. D., Mankoff, J., Dey, A. K., Chikersal, P., Doryab, A., et al. (2019). Leveraging routine behavior and contextually-filtered features for depression detection among college students. *Proceedings of the ACM on Interactive, Mobile, Wearable and Ubiquitous Technologies, 3*(3), 1–33.

Yadollahi, A., Shahraki, A. G., & Zaiane, O. R.

(2017). Current state of text sentiment analysis from opinion to emotion mining. *ACM Computing Surveys, 50*(2), 1–33.

Zanna, K., King, S., Neal, T., & Canavan, S. (2019). *Studying the impact of mood on identifying smartphone users.* http://arxiv.org/abs/1906.11960

Zhang, X., Li, W., Chen, X., & Lu, S. (2018). MoodExplorer: Towards compoundeEmotion detection via smartphone sensing. *Proceedings of the ACM on Interactive, Mobile, Wearable and Ubiquitous Technologies, 1*(4), 1–30.

Zhang, Y., Tang, J., Sun, J., Chen, Y., & Rao, J. (2010). MoodCast: Emotion prediction via dynamic continuous factor graph model. *2010 IEEE International Conference on Data Mining*, pp. 1193–1198.

Zhu, Z., Satizabal, H. F., Blanke, U., Perez-Uribe, A., & Troster, G. (2016). Naturalistic recognition of activities and mood using wearable electronics. *IEEE Transactions on Affective Computing, 7*(3), 272–285.

Zualkernan, I., Aloul, F., Shapsough, S., Hesham, A., & El-Khorzaty, Y. (2017). Emotion recognition using mobile phones. *Computers and Electrical Engineering, 60*, 1–13.

CHAPTER 25

Cognition on the Go

Opportunities and Challenges for Mobile Cognitive Health Research

Martin Sliwinski, Nelson Roque, and Karra Harrington

CHAPTER OVERVIEW

Advances in pervasive mobile technology have created new opportunities for high-precision measurement of cognitive function *in situ*. Mobile approaches can provide ecologically sensitive tools for exploring cognitive processes as they unfold in the context of time. This chapter focuses on the opportunities and challenges facing researchers who would use mobile technology for scientific research on human cognition. First, we describe unique advantages provided by mobile approaches to measuring cognitive function. Second, we provide a selective review of research that demonstrates the feasibility, validity, and utility of mobile cognitive testing. We conclude this chapter with a discussion of some challenges and potential solutions for researchers planning to use mobile devices to study human cognition.

Introduction

Cognitive abilities are vital to performing nearly every activity of daily life successfully and safely. Some cognitive failures, such as misplacing car keys or forgetting a recent acquaintance's name, can be frustrating or embarrassing. Others, such as attentional lapses while driving or forgetting to take a medication can have serious, even life-threatening, consequences. Despite the centrality of cognitive function for everyday life, researchers have primarily studied cognition in controlled laboratory or clinical settings. This approach places people in social situations and physical settings that are fundamentally dissimilar to their natural environment. Moreover, the financial and logistic costs imposed by requiring participants to visit a centralized testing location limits the size and diversity of research samples, as well constrains the frequency of repeated assessments necessary to track changes in cognitive function over time.

Advances in pervasive mobile technology have and will continue to change the way that researchers study cognitive function. Devices such as smartphones now possess sufficient computing power, high-resolution displays, and input sensors (e.g., touch screens, gyroscopes) that support deployment of an expansive array of digital tools for assessing cognition in naturalistic settings. Mobile cognitive assessment offers unique opportunities to overcome the limitations of conventional in-person cognitive assessment, but it also presents significant challenges to researchers. This chapter focuses on the opportunities and challenges facing researchers who adopt mobile technology for scientific research on human cognition. First, we describe some of the unique advantages provided by mobile approaches to measuring cognitive function. Second, we provide a selective review of research that demonstrates the feasibility, validity, and utility of mobile cognitive testing. And we conclude with a discussion of some challenges and potential solutions for researchers planning to use mobile devices to administer cognitive tests.

Rationale for Mobile Cognitive Assessment

Several reasons have motivated researchers to use pervasive mobile technology to study human cognition. First, by mitigating time, geographic, space, and personnel constraints imposed by in-person testing, mobile assessments provide new opportunities to conduct cognitive research at scale by obtaining large and geographically diverse samples that can enhance statistical power and inferential strength (Germine, Strong, Singh, & Sliwinski, 2021). Second, by allowing assessments to take place in the context of people's everyday lives, mobile approaches make it possible to explore temporal (e.g., diurnal rhythms) or social-contextual (e.g., recent activities) influences on cognitive functioning as people interact with the real-world environment (Moore, Swendsen, & Depp, 2017). And third, mobile cognitive assessments make possible frequent repeated assessments without imposing excessive participant burden and at minimal cost. Increasing the assessment frequency offers the dual benefit of providing more stable estimates of cognitive function than "single-shot" measurements as well as improved accuracy for detecting trends and relationships across time.

Scalability

In this context, "scalability" refers to the capability of research approaches to measure cognition at the scale necessary for population-based research and large cohort-based longitudinal studies. Logistical constraints faced by many studies of human cognition impose limits on the size of their samples. These limitations include limited numbers of testing rooms in a lab or clinic, limited personnel available to administer and oversee testing, and the cost in both time and money required for participants' travel to a central testing location. The result is an overreliance on small and homogeneous samples that may not generalize to the population of interest. This limitation is especially problematic for some research questions (e.g., examination of genome-wide associations) that require sample sizes well into the hundreds, thousands, or even tens of thousands to achieve adequate statistical power. More broadly, small and biased samples contribute to measurement error, which perpetuates the so-called replication crises in psychological and biomedical science (Loken & Gelman, 2017).

Shifting to remote cognitive testing that relies on mobile technology affords the opportunity to increase the size and diversity of samples, as well as to reach specialized study populations. Access to mobile technology is becoming increasingly pervasive. As of April 2021, the share of U.S. adults who owned smartphones was 85%, up from 35% in 2011 (Pew Research Center, 2021). Worldwide, current estimates (June 2021) are that 3.8 billion people (approximately 48% of the world's population) own a smartphone. One example of "scaling-up" comes from a study that used a commercial mobile application for the iPad to measure cognitive performance on more than 15,000 individuals (Lee et al., 2012) ranging in age from early childhood (<9 years) throughout adulthood (age 60+). Other examples of using mobile technology to measure cognition at scale involve targeting patient populations for longitudinal assessment. The mPower study of Parkinson's disease (PD) used a smartphone app to evaluate the feasibility of remotely collecting information about daily changes in symptoms and cognitive function (short-term visual working memory) in people with PD (Bot et al., 2016). Using completely remote "hands-off" recruitment and onboarding, the mPower study enrolled 6,805 participants, 1,087 of whom self-identified as having a diagnosis of PD. In another patient study (Pratap et al., 2020), investigators used a mobile app (elevateMS) to monitor symptoms, including cognitive performance on a voice-based variant of the Digit Symbol Substitution Test (DSST) and finger-tapping test, in 495 patients with multiple sclerosis (MS). These and other studies have demonstrated the feasibility of using mobile technology to measure cognitive performance in large numbers of people in lifespan studies, as well as in targeted patient groups. Their results also provide favorable evidence of measurement quality, replicating age gradients in cognitive performance typically observed in the literature (Lee et al., 2012), as well as showing expected relationships of cognitive performance with severity of neurological disease (Pratap et al., 2020).

Cognition in Context and Ecological Validity

In broad terms, ecological validity describes whether findings from a study are generalizable to real-life situations. Cognitive assessments have ecological validity to the extent that they accurately characterize how people function cognitively in real-world, naturalistic settings. To this end, neuropsychologists have mostly emphasized verisimilitude and veridicality, which refer to the face validity of task demands (e.g., stimuli and responses) and the predictive relationships between assessments and activities of daily living, respectively (Spooner & Pachana, 2006). Much less attention has been paid to the ecological validity of the assessment setting, which is especially important for examining the effects of contextual influences (e.g., mood, social setting) on cognitive function (Timmers et al., 2014). Performance in laboratory settings may be either elevated through social facilitation (Strauss, 2002) or hampered by unintended evaluative and stereotype threat (Schmader, Johns, & Forbes, 2008) in ways that obscure the broader contextual effects of people's social environment and mental health on their cognitive function. Regardless of the specific differences, the settings in which researchers typically measure cognitive abilities are very unlike the situations in which people typically use those abilities. Although in-person testing allows for good experimental control, this control provides no assurance that the performance observed in the lab reflects how people would perform in their natural settings.

Ecological momentary assessment (EMA) is a technique that involves frequent sampling of a person's thoughts, experiences, and behaviors in real time and in natural environments. Embedding brief cognitive tests into EMA can increase ecological validity and permit the study of microprocesses that reflect the co-influences among cognitive function, behaviors, and psychological or somatic states in real-world contexts (Shiffman, Stone, & Hufford, 2008). To the extent that EMA involves representative sampling of occasions, it can be used to characterize a person's average (or typical) cognitive performance over a wide variety of contexts in their daily lives. This approach to cognitive assessment differs from traditional assessment approaches that seek to create optimized environments in order to obtain an individual's maximum rather than their average performance. Attempting to measure an individual performance under optimal conditions might be ideal for certain purposes, such as aptitude testing. However, for other purposes, such as detecting the influence of social context or physical symptoms on cognitive function, a person's average or typical cognitive performance might be a better choice than their performance under optimized conditions (Moore et al., 2017; Sliwinski et al., 2018).

Temporal Precision

Traditional single-shot approaches to measuring cognition seek to obtain a person's best performance while being assessed under controlled and optimal conditions. However, imposing procedural control over testing cannot correct for a person having a bad night's sleep the evening before testing, nor can it correct for them feeling fatigued or stressed. Indeed, any single time-point estimate of cognitive performance is influenced by the peculiarities of a person's immediate physical environment, psychosocial context, and biological state. Therefore, results on any particular measurement occasion are influenced by both random and systematic within-person variability (good days/moments vs. bad days/moments). This is not a trivial issue; the amount of moment-to-moment and day-today within-person cognitive variability is substantial, and there is evidence of short-term variation in cognitive performance associated with recent stress (Sliwinski, Smyth, Hofer, & Stawski, 2006), positive and negative affect (Brose, Lövdén, & Schmiedek, 2014), recent social activities (Bielak, Mogle, & Sliwinski, 2019), and current motivational state (Brose, Schmiedek, Lövdén, & Lindenberger, 2012).

Ignoring short-term variability results in *temporal sampling error*, which refers to variability in measurement that reflects time-of-testing effects that can differ substantially from a person's average (Germine et al., 2021). That is, measuring cognition only once produces a point estimate that reflects a person's environment (e.g., noisy, distracting) and their psychological (e.g., stress) and somatic (e.g., fatigue) states at the time of testing. Temporal sampling error is highly relevant for longitudinal designs that rely on single-shot assessments separated by lengthy intervals. Figure 25.1 illustrates how testing an individual on a "bad" day (e.g., high stress, high fatigue) at baseline and a "good" day (e.g., low stress, low fatigue) at follow-up may suggest improvement that masks true long-term declines in *average* level of functioning. Thus, temporal sampling error can significantly impede longitudinal studies that must extract a very subtle signal (e.g., cognitive change in preclinical Alzheimer's disease) from the background of variations in performance associated with other variables (e.g., fatigue, stress) operating at a faster cadence. Temporal sampling error may be even *more* problematic for single-shot mobile assessments because they take place in naturalistic settings and thus are vulnerable to extrinsic (e.g., noise levels) as well as to intrinsic (e.g., fatigue, stress) sources of variability.

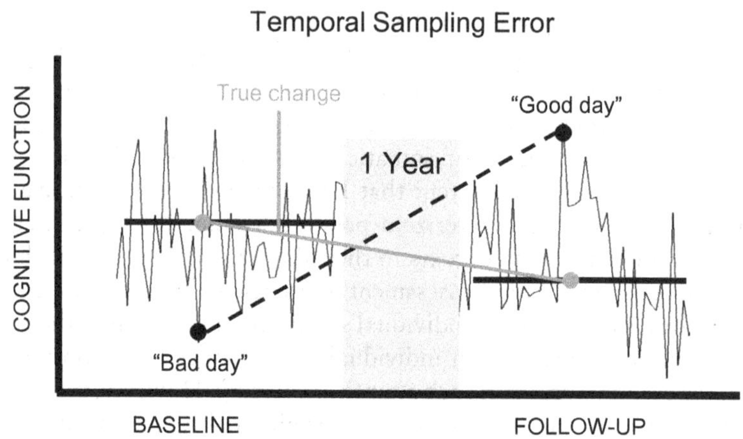

FIGURE 25.1. Temporal sampling error.

Embedding mobile cognitive assessments into intensive measurements designs, such as EMA or measurement bursts (Sliwinski, 2008), affords novel opportunities for the study of both short-term and long-term change. First, by aggregating across closely spaced repeated measurements, the effects of both random and systematic within-person variability can be "averaged out," improving the precision and reliability of cognitive scores (Hassenstab et al., 2020; Sliwinski et al., 2018). Second, variability in performance may not just be *noise* but can also be viewed as *signal*, a view consistent with recent conceptualizations of dynamic phenotypes, a term originally coined to refer to time-dependent observable characteristics of single cells (Bounab et al., 2020). Explicitly measuring and modeling short-term cognitive variability (i.e., performance changes observable across moments, hours, and days) may elucidate important processes and produce novel performance indicators that have prognostic value for predicting cognitive decline over the long term (Lövdén, Li, Shing, & Lindenberger, 2007).

Research in Mobile Cognitive Assessment

The incredible pace of scientific and technological advances in digital cognitive health will render any review of the literature hopelessly dated in short order. Therefore, we will provide a selective review of several key studies illustrating the validity and potential uses of mobile cognitive testing.

Supervised versus Unsupervised Cognitive Assessment

A key issue for mobile cognitive assessment is the degree to which unsupervised assessments can generate high-quality and valid cognitive performance data. Although relatively few studies directly compare supervised and unsupervised assessment using mobile devices, relevant evidence can be drawn from studies using unsupervised Web-based assessments administered via personal computers. Loss of control of stimuli presentation and of testing environment, as well as participant distraction and cheating, are key factors that have the potential to confound performance estimates and reduce data quality obtained in unsupervised cognitive assessments. A series of studies (Germine et al., 2012) examined this issue using a battery of cognitive tests that were likely to be particularly vulnerable to such confounding factors and comparing performance across unsupervised and traditional in-lab settings. They found no systematic difference in mean performance, reliability, or variance when comparing data from a self-selected Web-based sample that completed the tests unsupervised to data from samples tested in supervised lab settings.

Several additional studies using within-subject crossover designs also report no systematic within-person differences in mean performance, reliability, or variability for data obtained from most cognitive tests that were completed supervised in-lab and unsupervised (Cromer et al., 2015; Cyr, Romero, & Galin-Corini, 2021). The only exception was one study that reported slower reaction times during the unsupervised Web-based assessment, which they attributed to variations in computer hardware (Backx, Skirrow, Dente, Barnett, & Cormack, 2020). Taken together, these studies indicate that unsupervised administration of cognitive tests in uncontrolled environments can produce high-quality data that are comparable to that obtained in traditional supervised in-lab settings.

A further issue is the feasibility of conducting unsupervised cognitive assessments with populations who may have difficulty completing the assessment independently or who may be less familiar with the technology required to complete the assessment, such as older adults or clinical populations. Notably, two large studies (N = 6,463 and 1,594) that administered the Cogstate Brief Battery in an unsupervised online format to adults aged over 55 years demonstrated age associations with cognitive performance in the expected direction (slower reaction time, lower accuracy on learning and working memory), suggesting the validity of data collected within this context (Mackin et al., 2018; Perin et al., 2020).

Psychometrics and Validity

Due to the relative novelty of using mobile devices to study cognitive performance, much of the research in this area has focused on evaluating feasibility, validity, and psychometrics. In this section we review three illustrative studies that demonstrate the ways in which validation has been approached in three separate populations: healthy adults, school-age children, and patients with PD. Each of these studies took a different approach to validation, which highlights a range of approaches to demonstrating the validity of a mobile cognitive measure.

The approach to validation in an adult sample taken by Sliwinski and colleagues (2018) focuses on evaluating construct validity by examining patterns of *between-person* correlations among the mobile measures and "gold standard" cognitive tests administered in the lab. In this study a probability sample of 219 racially diverse adults (25–65 years, 66% female) completed a battery of traditional neuropsychological tests in-lab at the start of the study, followed by a 14-day measurement burst with five assessments per day completed on a study-provided smartphone. Each of the assessments during the measurement burst included a brief survey and three cognitive assessments that measured perceptual speed and working memory. Confirmatory factor analysis (CFA) supported a two-factor model (perceptual speed and working memory), with the mobile cognitive assessments loading on the appropriate factor with in-lab cognitive assessments of the same construct. Furthermore, the results were robust to practice effects across the study and invariant across age. Between-person reliability for the mobile cognitive assessments averaged across the 14 days was ≥.97.

Dirk and Schmiedek (2016) focus instead on *within-person* convergent validity in their study of working memory processes in school age children. Female grade 3 and 4 students (N =110, ages 8 to 11 years) completed assessments on study-provided smartphones three times per day for 31 consecutive days. The mobile cognitive assessments included two working memory updating tasks that had been adapted from tasks that had previously been used with school-age children. One task included numerical content and the other spatial content, and both tasks included two memory load conditions. Within-person convergent validity was assessed with correlation between daily aggregate scores for the four task conditions. Moderate within-person positive correlations (r's ranged from .33 to .58) were observed for the daily accuracy scores of the four task conditions. This provided evidence for convergent validity of the mobile cognitive assessments as measuring the same construct, as well as for the working memory fluctuations observed in the study.

Weizenbaum and colleagues (2021) also consider convergent validity, but focus on convergence with performance on traditional neuropsychological tests and subjective reports of cognitive dysfunction in a patient population. The study included 27 individuals (mean age 63.2 years, 48% female) with mild to moderate PD who did not meet criteria for dementia. Participants completed mobile assessments five times per day for 10 days, which included one measure of working memory and one measure of executive function. Prior to commencing the mobile assessments, participants underwent in-lab neuropsychological assessment that included a cognitive screening measure (the Montreal Cognitive Assessment), a measure of working memory (backward spatial span), and a measure of executive function (accuracy on Trailmaking Form B). Participants also completed a subjective questionnaire of executive dysfunction. Only performance on the working memory mobile cognitive assessment was significantly predicted by performance on each of the three traditional neuropsychological assessments. The subjective measure was not a significant predictor of performance on either of the mobile cognitive assessments. The authors note that there was limited variability in scores on the executive function mobile cognitive assessment and that performance on this measure was more closely related to measures of motor and tremor symptoms. This suggests that the measure had low validity for assessing executive function and instead was capturing variability related to psychomotor function. Furthermore, these results highlight the importance of careful test design when developing cognitive assessments for mobile devices, an issue we discuss further later in this chapter.

Two of the three studies reviewed above evaluated validity by correlating scores from mobile cognitive assessments with scores obtained from in-lab cognitive testing. This approach is common practice in neuropsychology for validation and useful for interpreting scores from new cognitive tests. However, it is also problematic because we expect mobile assessment to differ from in-person cognitive testing not only in ways that could negatively impact validity (e.g., distractions) but also in ways that could be beneficial (e.g., improved ecological validity, sensitivity to context). There is much interest in using mobile approaches to cognitive measurement as "digital biomarkers" that can be used to discriminate among clinical phenotypes, predict risk, and monitor progression of disease (Baker, Belachew, Gossens, & Lindemann, 2019; Ferrar et al., 2021; Lancaster et al.,

2020). For these clinical purposes, moderate or even low correlations with conventional in-person neuropsychological testing could indicate potential added value of mobile cognitive assessments, rather than their lack of validity. Given the growing evidence that remote and unsupervised cognitive testing can produce high-quality data, we suggest that mobile cognitive tests that have been developed based on established paradigms should enjoy some degree of presumptive construct validity. In such cases, simple manipulation checks, such as demonstrating reliable interference effects in a Stroop paradigm or set size effects in a working memory paradigm, should be sufficient.

Relationships between Contextual Factors and Cognition

A unique advantage of mobile cognitive assessments is that they can be embedded in intensive longitudinal designs, such as EMA, to explore microprocesses that reflect co-influences of cognition and contextual factors (e.g., affect, daily activities). By collecting frequent measurements across short periods of time, it is possible to model short-term within-person trends and fluctuations in cognitive performance, and to assess temporal sequences among theoretically connected variables. In this section, we review illustrative studies that have used mobile cognitive assessments to examine contextual factors, to explore interactions between psychological and physiological processes in real time, and to evaluate whether a person's current cognitive performance might predict future psychological states and behaviors.

Contextual Influences on Within-Person Variations in Cognitive Performance

Prior work has demonstrated that between-person differences in social contact are associated with cognitive decline and risk of dementia (Lara et al., 2019). However, from these studies it cannot be inferred how fluctuations in social interaction influence cognitive performance within an individual. An EMA study by Zhaoyang, Scott, Martire, and Sliwinski (2021) examined this question of within-person influences of social interaction on cognitive performance in a sample of 312 older adults (mean age 76.97 [4.85] years, 67% female). Participants completed five assessments per day for 16 days that included surveys on social interactions and cognitive assessments of processing speed, working memory, and memory binding. They demonstrated the frequency of social interactions on a given day, especially pleasant interactions or interactions with close friends or family, which were associated with better cognitive performance on the same day and across the following 2 days. Furthermore, they found that older adults who tended to have less frequent social interactions on average benefited the most in terms of improvement in cognitive performance on days where they had an increase above their usual amount of social interaction.

Daily experiences of stress have also been linked to within-person reductions in response time on tests of attention and working memory on the same day (Sliwinski et al., 2006). A recent study (Hyun, Sliwinski, & Smyth, 2019) used mobile cognitive testing to explore the temporal dynamics of the stress–cognition relationship in an EMA study that incorporated measures of anticipatory stress. Participants (N = 240, ages 25–65 years, 66% female) completed 2 weeks of EMA that included a morning assessment completed upon waking and five prompted assessments dispersed randomly across the day. Each prompted assessment included a measure of momentary stress and a spatial working memory task. An assessment completed upon waking each morning included a measure of anticipatory stress ("Overall, how stressful do you think today/tomorrow will be?"). Results demonstrated that stress anticipation upon waking was associated with poorer working memory performance later the same day and that this relationship was independent of whether stress was experienced later in the day.

In addition to being able to examine temporal dynamics and within-person processes of psychological and cognitive phenomena, mobile cognitive assessments can also be coupled with ambulatory measures of physiological function. Riediger and colleagues (2014) examined the temporal relationship between cognitive performance and physiological and psychological arousal across 24 hours. Participants ($N = 92$, mean age 42.4 [19.0] years, 55% female) wore an ambulatory biomonitoring system that recorded cardiac and physical activity, as well as completed seven momentary ambulatory assessments of tense arousal (feeling nervous), energetic arousal (feeling wide awake), and two trials of a working memory task. All participants had previously practiced the working memory task extensively and were familiar with the task requirements prior to the 24-hour study period. They found that tense arousal was associated with increased momentary heart rate, and that there was an age-moderated relationship between tense arousal and working memory performance such that middle-aged and older adults performed worse when feeling more nervous. They also found a similar age-moderated relationship between increased heart rate (physiological arousal) and working memory performance. Additionally, the relationship between tense arousal and working memory was no longer significant after controlling for physiological arousal. However, the relationship between physiological arousal and working memory persisted after controlling for tense arousal. This finding suggested that physiological arousal was the driving mechanism behind reduced working memory performance assessed in naturalistic settings.

Momentary Cognition as a Predictor of Symptoms and Behaviors

Using EMA designs with embedded mobile cognitive assessments can be used not only to identify contextual influences on cognitive performance, but also to evaluate whether short-term variations in cognitive performance predict health behaviors or other psychological states. For example, one study used a modified Stroop task embedded into an EMA protocol to measure attentional bias prior to and during temptation episodes (Waters, Marhe, & Franken, 2012) in heroin-dependent patients ($N = 68$, mean age 40.87 [7.72] years, 14.7% female). This study found that attentional bias to drug cues was elevated during assessments where the participant was experiencing temptation and that this elevation was evident one hour prior to the temptation episode. Another study examining the reciprocal relationships between pain and cognitive function in fibromyalgia (Whibley, Williams, Clauw, Sliwinski, & Kratz, 2021) found that a reduction in working memory performance preceded an increase in pain intensity. Over 7 days, participants (50 with fibromyalgia and 50 controls, mean age 45.1[13.9] years, 88% female) completed five assessments per day that included a survey of pain intensity and self-reported cognitive function, as well as cognitive assessments of processing speed and working memory. Pain intensity and working memory performance were unrelated at concurrent assessments, but errors on the working memory task predicted a subsequent increase in pain intensity 3–4.5 hours later for the fibromyalgia group. Thus, in both of these studies a change in cognitive performance functioned as a signal prior to a self-reported elevation in clinically relevant symptoms. Studies such as these may identify potential mechanisms (increased attentional bias, decreased working memory) as targets for "just-in-time" interventions (Nahum-Shani et al., 2017) designed to reduce the probability or severity of later symptoms (temptation episode, pain flare).

Challenges and Solutions

Several challenges face researchers who use mobile devices to study human cognition. The process of translating cognitive assessment paradigms designed for administration on large displays or paper forms for use on smartphones is not as straightforward as decreasing stimuli size and changing response style. Whether designing a brand-new "digital" cognitive assessment or adapting a conventional clinic-based neuropsychological test to a smartphone, the design process starts with consideration of the intended target audience (e.g., those with mild cognitive impairment [MCI]), device type (e.g., smartphone vs. tablet), and administration modality (e.g., with or without supervision; study-provided vs. participant-owned devices). Some of these challenges pertain to the design of tests and paradigms, which may require adapting testing procedures intended for administration on large displays to a smaller form factor. Others are associated with test administration, such as how to handle interruptions and specification of pause–resume rules that preserve test validity. In addition, some nontrivial technical considerations are associated with inter- and intra-device variability in hardware (e.g., touch screen sensitivity, screen resolution, and refresh rates) and operating system (e.g., iOS vs. Android). In this section, we outline several principles to consider when developing or adapting cognitive tests and paradigms for administration on mobile devices: (1) using cognitive tests that have intuitive task demands, (2) prioritizing brief administration times, and (3) designing tests with minimal technical requirements. We also describe recent work in "passive cognitive sensing" that does not require any explicit involvement or responses from participants (i.e., they do not "perform" a cognitive task), but rather relies on smartphone sensors to gather meaningful data in the background.

Intuitive Task Demands

In laboratory settings, a research technician is usually available to provide task instructions, monitor performance, and guide participants through complex cognitive paradigms by providing feedback and answering questions about task demands. Because mobile test administration is unsupervised, task demands should be intuitive so that participants clearly understand the requirements to perform for each step of the test, even if they have undergone in-person onboarding and instruction. This is important to ensure proper engagement with the task (i.e., participants are performing the task as intended) and its accessibility to individuals who vary in sociodemographic factors, health status, technology fluency, and sensorimotor function.

Certain types of paradigms are relatively simple and require a single type of operation from the participant (e.g., comparing two stimuli), whereas others are more complex, consisting of multiple stages. Figure 25.2 displays screen shots from a simple multiphase

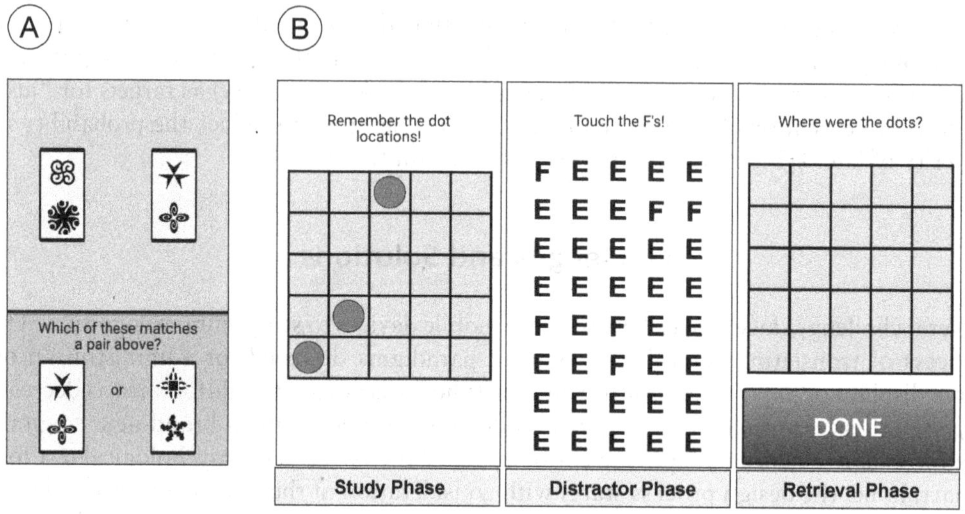

FIGURE 25.2. Examples of mobile cognitive tests.

mobile cognitive test that were designed to follow the principle of intuitive task demands (Sliwinski et al., 2018). The Symbol Match task (Figure 25.2A), which taps perceptual comparison speed, begins with an instruction screen encouraging participants to respond as quickly and accurately as they can, and each trial consists of a forced-choice response. A more complex task that measures spatial working memory is the Dot Memory task (Figure 25.2B), which consists of a study phase, a distractor phase, and a retrieval phase. Even though Dot Memory has three task phases (Figure 25.2B), requirements for each phase are clearly communicated by the interface design and a single-line instruction. We have found that single-line instructions accompanied by appropriate example images, demonstrations, and practice trials are more effective than lengthy, detailed instructions for mobile test administration. In addition, they are less likely to be confounded by factors related to age, education, cognitive status, and language abilities.

Brief Administration Times

Because mobile cognitive assessments take place in naturalistic settings, interruptions while performing a cognitive test can compromise the validity of test scores. For in-person assessments completed in the lab or clinic, efforts are made to reduce noise levels and overall distractibility of the environment. Mobile testing protocols can attempt to simulate these more controlled testing environments by providing instructions that encourage participants to proceed at a time and in a place that minimize distractibility. This approach, however, cannot eliminate the effect of frequent interruptions that are intrinsic to using a modern mobile device. These interruptions come in the form of app or operating system notifications (e.g., prompting software updates), text messages, and incoming phone calls. Tests that require several minutes of continuous performance to complete require specification of pause–resume rules and can create frustration in participants who are required to restart a test due to an interruption. Moreover, to the extent that mobile cognitive tests are embedded in experience sampling protocols, asking individuals to seek out optimal environments for testing could compromise estimation of the effects of momentary states, social contexts, and very recent events on performance.

We recommend a two-prong strategy for addressing interruptions during cognitive assessments taking place in naturalistic settings. The first is to keep administration times brief to reduce the likelihood that an interruption occurs during performance—experience sampling studies have used mobile cognitive tests that take a minute or less to complete (Hyun, Slwinski, & Smyth, 2019; Whibley et al., 2021). Second, we recommend collecting ancillary information by self-report and passive monitoring from smartphone sensors (e.g., ambient sound/light) to measure and statistically control for variations in the social and physical environment during each assessment.

Technical Requirements and Device "Robust" Tests

Although the computing power of modern mobile devices far exceeds the needs of most cognitive paradigms, mobile platforms impose inherent technical and procedural constraints. Some studies have given participants smartphones in order to provide a standardized hardware and software environment for testing. Because relying on investigator-provided mobile devices is expensive and inconvenient for participants who may be required to carry two mobile devices, studies are increasingly adopting a "bring-your-own-device" (BYOD) approach. Cognitive paradigms that require tight control over visual angle (stimulus size), auditory stimulus presentation, and open-ended input via voice responses are all susceptible to hardware and operating system differences inherent to BYOD studies. Small effects (e.g., Stroop or Flanker effects) or subtle differences in very fast response times may be overwhelmed by variability between devices (e.g., older vs. new smartphone models) and within devices (e.g., operating system updates, installation of other apps) over time. Thus, we recommend avoiding cognitive paradigms that rely highly on precise timing for stimulus presentation and speeded responses that exceed typical screen refresh and touch-sampling rates.

Variability across devices may not only introduce noise but may also be a source of bias if device preference, availability, and affordability systematically vary with people's characteristics (e.g., personality, geographic location, socioeconomic status) that are related to cognitive performance. Thus, an important technical challenge is to manage the influence of inter-device and intra-device variability with respect to screen refresh rate, tap registration latency, and usage of device RAM during a graphic-intensive mobile cognitive assessment. In general, most Web-based frameworks for delivering online experiments have "reasonable accuracy and precision for display duration and manual response time" (Anwyl-Irvine, Dalmaijer, Hodges, & Evershed, 2020, p. 1407), though less is known about app-based assessment approaches. When exploring individual differences, one strategy supported by the literature to mitigate potential biases in measurement due to technical variability involves juxtaposing participant performance across multiple conditions or manipulations (Pronk, Wiers, Molenkamp, & Murre, 2020). This approach to designing "device robust" tests rests on the reasonable assumption that any systematic differences across devices should be equivalent across task manipulations (e.g., varying the number of display items, distractor load, or response options). Thus, including "control" condition in mobile cognitive paradigms could be an effective strategy to correct for hardware and software variations in timings associated with response registration and stimulus presentation.

On the Horizon: Passive Cognitive Sensing

The technical simplification of collecting various sensor streams over the last decade, including development and validation of ready-to-use frameworks (Torous, Kiang, Lorme, & Onnela, 2016), has opened the door to novel work leveraging digital mobile tools in order to passively measure cognition and optimize the design of studies. Onboard most modern smartphones are a suite of sensors that are able to passively collect location (lifespace) measures via GPS sensors (Liddle et al., 2014; Parrish et al., 2020), gait and general activity patterns (via accelerometer and gyroscopes), as well as markers of social interaction (e.g., number of text messages received). As highlighted in a recent review, while the utilization of these rich data streams is on the rise, there remains extensive heterogeneity with respect to how they are leveraged, processed, and analyzed, (Piau, Rumeau, Nourhashemi, & Martin, 2019). In this section, we review a set of proof-of-concept studies that lay the foundation for the future of digital cognitive biomarkers in predicting cognitive state, status, neuropsychological function, and real-world outcomes (e.g., driving).

Predicting Cognitive State

One advancement made possible with ambulatory technologies is detecting cognitive states, such as alertness, from user-completed self-reported assessments and objective cognitive assessments. In a study by Abdullah and colleagues (2016), leveraging an ecological momentary assessment protocol, they asked participants to complete a psychomotor vigilance task (PVT), while passively collecting smartphone usage measures. Models predicting alertness from PVT performance, participant demographics, and usage patterns demonstrated high accuracy—highlighting the promise of this low-cost, passive-prediction approach.

Predicting Cognitive Status

An exploratory study of digital health assessment applied this passive sensing approach to predict cognitive status. For the 12-week study period, researchers offered participants (82 healthy controls and 31 individuals previously diagnosed with MCI or mild Alzheimer's disease [AD]) a set of mobile devices (i.e., iPhone and iPad) and wearables (i.e., Apple Watch) to use as their primary devices (Chen et al., 2019). By applying machine learning techniques to data collected from these devices, it was possible to predict cognitive status (controls vs. MCI vs. mild AD) with reasonable accuracy (area under the curve = 0.80).

Digital Biomarkers of Neuropsychological Outcomes/Function

Passive measures have also been demonstrated to be useful in predicting neuropsychological test scores. In a study by Dagum (2018), a stream of digital biomarkers from a smartphone application (e.g., keystroke and event patterns) were collected over the course of 7 days following a neuropsychological exam. In this study, passively collected digital biomarkers significantly predicted scores on neuropsychological assessments of working memory, language, dexterity, and memory, with correlations ranging from .62 to .83 (p's $< 10^{-4}$).

With respect to the assessment of memory using passive methods, several studies have employed the use of acoustic analysis and natural language processing (NLP; Haas et al., 2022; Polsinelli, Moseley, Grilli, Glisky, & Mehl, 2020; Wank et al., 2020) to better understand the relationship between typical assessments of memory function and biomarkers from everyday life. In a sample of 91 adults (53 younger adults, ages 19–32; 38 older adults, ages 60–81), Haas and colleagues investigated the relationship between three approaches to memory assessments: (1) a prospective memory task, administered by an experimenter, (2) a daily diary approach following up on intentionally set plans, and (3) unobtrusively sampled audio recordings of spontaneous speech production (electronically activated recorder [EAR]). Results demonstrated that age deficits were not apparent in experimenter-driven tasks, but older adults completed more self-assigned intentions (in daily diaries) compared with younger adults. Wank and colleagues (2020) also leveraged the EAR for assessment of autobiographical memory in older adults. Interestingly, this study replicated typical age effects on autobiographical memory that are expected on laboratory tasks (less details with increased age), with passively assessed indicators of cognition from spontaneous voice samples. Of note, the passively assessed indicators of autobiographical memory did not correlate with data from traditional list learning paradigms. This showed that passively assessed indicators do not always behave in the same ways we would expect constructs to behave in the lab (e.g., we would expect a correlation between in-lab memory tasks). Evaluating how the semantics of natural language using the EAR relate to executive functioning, Polsinelli and colleagues (2020) characterized the recordings of participants with respect to analytic language, emotional tone, and other constructs (e.g., health, home). This study demonstrated that higher executive functioning was related to increased use of analytical language. Altogether, digital biomarkers of speech samples (i.e., the decomposition into acoustic, semantic, and higher-level cognitive properties, e.g., minutes spent in analytical language) are a promising way forward in the study of cognition in daily life and may even challenge our understanding of cognition from decades of laboratory work.

Digital Biomarkers of Functional Activities of Daily Living

In addition to predicting cognitive state, status, and neuropsychological outcomes, recent work has paved the way with respect to monitoring functional activities, such as driving. In a proof-of-concept study, Seelye and colleagues (2017) unobtrusively monitored the driving activities of older adults (n = 21, with intact cognition; n = 7 with MCI) for 6 months. In addition to participants' general acceptance of this technology, Seelye and colleagues (2017) provided evidence of feasibility, noting that this technology allowed for the discovery of patterning that is associated with MCI (e.g., fewer miles driven, less highway driving, less day-to-day fluctuation in habits). The novelty of this approach is the ability to monitor subtle variations in driving behavior (e.g., hard breaks), the time of use (e.g., night driving), and situations (e.g., highway driving), all with a single sensor stream (i.e., a sensor that plugs into the OBD-2 port on most modern vehicles).

Integrating Active and Passive Assessments

Regardless of which sensor (or collection of features) is used, with this approach comes the perspective that we might be able to leverage the *signal* in the features of various sensor streams (e.g., acoustic features of voice samples, daily aggregates of activity monitoring via GPS and accelerometer, patterns of touchscreen typing), in order to *predict* who might be experiencing atypical cognitive functioning (Ntracha et al., 2020). From a public health perspective, capitalizing on *passively sensed* behaviors that correlate with clinical phenotypes and outcomes could be immensely valuable due to its scalability and minimal respondent burden. However, there is no guarantee that passively sensed behaviors, even if they are strongly correlated with cognitive outcomes such as dementia, would prove useful for monitoring *changes* in risk status, disease progression, or intervention effects. That is, some passively measured cognitive behaviors may capture relatively stable, nonmalleable individual differences that convey lifelong risk and thus may be less sensitive to subtle changes in specific cognitive processes. An important and exciting area of new research involves developing approaches that can integrate and co-validate passive and active approaches to cognitive sensing to improve not only prediction of important outcomes but our ability to measure cognitive functioning in everyday life.

Concluding Remarks and Future Directions

Although researchers have only recently begun to explore the potential uses of mobile cognitive assessments, a rapidly growing body of evidence points to their added value as a complementary tool to traditional in-person assessment methods. For example, mobile methods provide a scalable solution to cognitive assessment that can enhance ecological validity and improve measurement precision, particularly in the context of longitudinal designs. Studies to date have also provided strong evidence that mobile testing can produce measurements that are reliable, valid, and appropriate for use with individuals from across a wide age range, including clinical populations. And mobile testing allows for rapid and repeatable assessments, which researchers can leverage to explore antecedents (e.g., stress, social activity) and consequents (e.g., pain, cravings) of variations in cognitive function as they unfold in real time and in naturalistic settings. In the near future, mobile cognitive assessments could be used to monitor disease progression, rapidly identify acute adverse reactions (or benefits) to therapeutics, and assist patients and clinicians in self-management and in providing patient-centered care. Indeed, using mobile technology to assess cognition "anytime, anyplace" holds tremendous potential to transform biomedical and behavioral research that depends on the sensitive detection and accurate monitoring of cognitive variability and change.

ACKNOWLEDGMENTS

This work was supported in part by the National Institute on Aging under Grant Nos. P01AG003949 and U2CAG060408.

REFERENCES

Abdullah, S., Murnane, E. L., Matthews, M., Kay, M., Kientz, J. A., Gay, G., et al. (2016). Cognitive rhythms: unobtrusive and continuous sensing of alertness using a mobile phone.

Proceedings of the 2016 ACM International Joint Conference on Pervasive and Ubiquitous Computing, pp. 178–189.

Anwyl-Irvine, A., Dalmaijer, E. S., Hodges, N., & Evershed, J. K. (2020). Realistic precision and accuracy of online experiment platforms, Web browsers, and devices. *Behavior Research Methods, 53*(4), 1407–1425.

Backx, R., Skirrow, C., Dente, P., Barnett, J. H., & Cormack, F. K. (2020). Comparing Web-based and lab-based cognitive assessment using the Cambridge Neuropsychological Test Automated Battery: A within-subjects counterbalanced study. *Journal of Medical Internet Research, 22*(8), e16792.

Baker, M., Belachew, M., Gossens, C., & Lindemann, M. (2019). *Digital biomarkers for cognition and movement diseases or disorders.* Patent No. US 2019/0200915 A1.

Bielak, A. A. M., Mogle, J., & Sliwinski, M. J. (2019). What did you do today?: Variability in daily activities is related to variability in daily cognitive performance. *Journals of Gerontology. Series B, Psychological Sciences and Social Sciences, 74*(5), 764–771.

Bot, B. M., Suver, C., Neto, E. C., Kellen, M., Klein, A., Bare, C., et al. (2016). The mPower study, Parkinson disease mobile data collected using ResearchKit. *Scientific Data, 3*, 160011.

Bounab, Y., Eyer, K., Dixneuf, S., Rybczynska, M., Chauvel, C., Mistretta, M., et al. (2020). Dynamic single-cell phenotyping of immune cells using the microfluidic platform DropMap. *Nature Protocols, 15*(9), 2920–2955.

Brose, A., Lövdén, M., & Schmiedek, F. (2014). Daily fluctuations in positive affect positively co-vary with working memory performance. *Emotion, 14*(1), 1–6.

Brose, A., Schmiedek, F., Lövdén, M., & Lindenberger, U. (2012). Daily variability in working memory is coupled with negative affect: The role of attention and motivation. *Emotion, 12*(3), 605–617.

Chen, R., Jankovic, F., Marinsek, N., Foschini, L., Kourtis, L., Signorini, A., et al. (2019). Developing measures of cognitive impairment in the real world from consumer-grade multimodal sensor streams. *Proceedings of the 25th ACM SIGKDD International Conference on Knowledge Discovery & Data Mining*, pp. 2145–2155.

Cromer, J. A., Harel, B. T., Yu, K., Valadka, J. S., Brunwin, J. W., Crawford, C. D., et al. (2015). Comparison of cognitive performance on the Cogstate Brief Battery when taken in-clinic, in-group, and unsupervised. *The Clinical Neuropsychologist, 29*(4), 542–558.

Cyr, A.-A., Romero, K., & Galin-Corini, L. (2021). Web-based cognitive testing of older adults in person versus at home: Within-subjects comparison study. *JMIR Aging, 4*(1), e23384.

Dagum, P. (2018). Digital biomarkers of cognitive function. *npj Digital Med, 1*, 10.

Dirk, J., & Schmiedek, F. (2016). Fluctuations in elementary school children's working memory performance in the school context. *Journal of Educational Psychology, 108*(5), 722–739.

Ferrar, J., Griffith, G. J., Skirrow, C., Cashdollar, N., Taptiklis, N., Dobson, J., et al. (2021). Developing digital tools for remote clinical research: How to evaluate the validity and practicality of active assessments in field settings. *Journal of Medical Internet Research, 23*(6), e26004.

Germine, L., Nakayama, K., Duchaine, B. C., Chabris, C. F., Chatterjee, G., & Wilmer, J. B. (2012). Is the Web as good as the lab?: Comparable performance from Web and lab in cognitive/perceptual experiments. *Psychonomic Bulletin and Review, 19*(5), 847–857.

Germine, L., Strong, R. W., Singh, S., & Sliwinski, M. J. (2021). Toward dynamic phenotypes and the scalable measurement of human behavior. *Neuropsychopharmacology, 46*(1), 209–216.

Haas, M., Mehl, M., Ballhausen, N., Zuber, Z., Kliegel, M., & Hering, A. (2022). The sounds of memory: Extending the age-prospective memory paradox to everyday behavior and conversations. *Journals of Gerontology Series B: Psychological Sciences and Social Sciences, 77*(44), 695–703.

Hassenstab, J., Aschenbrenner, A. J., Balota, D. A., McDade, E., Lim, Y. Y., Fagan, A. M., et al. (2020). Remote cognitive assessment approaches in the Dominantly Inherited Alzheimer Network (DIAN). *Alzheimer's and Dementia, 16*(S6), e038144.

Hyun, J., Sliwinski, M. J., & Smyth, J. M. (2019). Waking up on the wrong side of the bed: The effects of stress anticipation on working memory in daily life. *Journals of Gerontology: Series B, 74*(1), 38–46.

Lancaster, C., Koychev, I., Blane, J., Chinner, A., Wolters, L., & Hinds, C. (2020). Evaluating the feasibility of frequent cognitive assessment using the Mezurio smartphone app: Observational and interview study in adults with elevated dementia risk. *JMIR MHealth and UHealth, 8*(4), e16142.

Lara, E., Martín-María, N., De la Torre-Luque, A., Koyanagi, A., Vancampfort, D., Izquierdo, A., et al. (2019). Does loneliness contribute to mild cognitive impairment and dementia?: A systematic review and meta-analysis of longitudinal studies. *Ageing Research Reviews, 52*, 7–16.

Lee, H., Baniqued, P. L., Cosman, J., Mullen, S., McAuley, E., Severson, J., et al. (2012). Examining cognitive function across the lifespan using a mobile application. *Computers in Human Behavior, 28*(5), 1934–1946.

Liddle, J., Ireland, D., McBride, S. J., Brauer, S. G., Hall, L. M., Ding, H., et al. (2014). Measuring the lifespace of people with Parkinson's disease using smartphones: Proof of principle. *JMIR mHealth and uHealth, 2*(1), e13.

Loken, E., & Gelman, A. (2017). Measurement error and the replication crisis. *Science, 355*(6325), 584–585.

Lövdén, M., Li, S.-C., Shing, Y. L., & Lindenberger, U. (2007). Within-person trial-to-trial variability precedes and predicts cognitive decline in old and very old age: Longitudinal data from the Berlin Aging Study. *Neuropsychologia, 45*(12), 2827–2838.

Mackin, R. S., Insel, P. S., Truran, D., Finley, S., Flenniken, D., Nosheny, R., et al. (2018). Unsupervised online neuropsychological test performance for individuals with mild cognitive impairment and dementia: Results from the Brain Health Registry. *Alzheimer's and Dementia: Diagnosis, Assessment and Disease Monitoring, 10*, 573–582.

Moore, R. C., Swendsen, J., & Depp, C. A. (2017). Applications for self-administered mobile cognitive assessments in clinical research: A systematic review. *International Journal of Methods in Psychiatric Research, 26*(4), e1562.

Nahum-Shani, I., Smith, S. N., Spring, B. J., Collins, L. M., Witkiewitz, K., Tewari, A., et al. (2017). Just-in-time adaptive interventions (JITAIs) in mobile health: Key components and design principles for ongoing health behavior support. *Annals of Behavioral Medicine, 52*(6), 446–462.

Ntracha, A., Iakovakis, D., Hadjidimitriou, S., Charisis, V. S., Tsolaki, M., & Hadjileontiadis, L. J. (2020). Detection of mild cognitive impairment through natural language and touchscreen typing processing. *Frontiers in Digital Health, 2*.

Parrish, E. M., Kamarsu, S., Harvey, P. D., Pinkham, A., Depp, C. A., & Moore, R. C. (2020). Remote ecological momentary testing of learning and memory in adults with serious mental illness. *Schizophrenia Bulletin, 224*, 67–73.

Perin, S., Buckley, R. F., Pase, M. P., Yassi, N., Lavale, A., Wilson, P. H., et al. (2020). Unsupervised assessment of cognition in the Healthy Brain Project: Implications for Web-based registries of individuals at risk for Alzheimer's disease. *Alzheimer's and Dementia: Translational Research and Clinical Interventions, 6*(1), e12043.

Pew Research Center. (2021). *Demographics of mobile device ownership and adoption in the United States.* www.pewresearch.org/internet/fact-sheet/mobile

Piau, A., Rumeau, P., Nourhashemi, F., & Martin, M. S. (2019). Information and communication technologies, a promising way to support pharmacotherapy for the behavioral and psychological symptoms of dementia. *Frontiers in Pharmacology, 10*, 1122.

Polsinelli, A. J., Moseley, S. A., Grilli, M. D., Glisky, E. L., & Mehl, M. R. (2020). Natural, everyday language use provides a window into the integrity of older adults' executive functioning. *Journals of Gerontology. Series B, Psychological Sciences and Social Sciences, 75*(9), e215–e220.

Pratap, A., Grant, D., Vegesna, A., Tummalacherla, M., Cohan, S., Deshpande, C., et al. (2020). Evaluating the utility of smartphone-based sensor assessments in persons with multiple sclerosis in the real-world using an app (elevateMS): Observational, prospective pilot digital health study. *JMIR mHealth and uHealth, 8*(10), e22108.

Pronk, T., Wiers, R. W., Molenkamp, B., & Murre, J. (2020). Mental chronometry in the pocket?: Timing accuracy of Web applications on touchscreen and keyboard devices. *Behavior Research Methods, 52*(3), 1371–1382.

Riediger, M., Wrzus, C., Klipker, K., Müller, V., Schmiedek, F., & Wagner, G. G. (2014). Outside of the laboratory: Associations of working-memory performance with psychological and physiological arousal vary with age. *Psychology and Aging, 29*(1), 103–114.

Schmader, T., Johns, M., & Forbes, C. (2008). An integrated process model of stereotype threat effects on performance. *Psychological Review, 115*(2), 336–356.

Seelye, A., Mattek, N., Sharma, N., Witter, P., Brenner, A., Wild, K., et al. (2017). Passive assessment of routine driving with unobtrusive sensors: A new approach for identifying and monitoring functional level in normal aging and mild cognitive impairment. *Journal of Alzheimer's Disease, 59*(4), 1427–1437.

Shiffman, S., Stone, A. A., & Hufford, M. R. (2008). Ecological momentary assessment. *Annual Review of Clinical Psychology, 4*(1), 1–32.

Sliwinski, M. J. (2008). Measurement-burst designs for social health research. *Social and Personality Psychology Compass, 2*(1), 245–261.

Sliwinski, M. J., Mogle, J. A., Hyun, J., Munoz, E., Smyth, J. M., & Lipton, R. B. (2018). Reliability and validity of ambulatory cognitive assessments. *Assessment, 25*(1), 14–30.

Sliwinski, M. J., Smyth, J. M., Hofer, S. M., & Stawski, R. S. (2006). Intraindividual coupling of daily stress and cognition. *Psychology and Aging, 21*(3), 545–557.

Spooner, D., & Pachana, N. (2006). Ecological validity in neuropsychological assessment: A case for greater consideration in research with neurologically intact populations. *Archives of Clinical Neuropsychology, 21*(4), 327–337.

Strauss, B. (2002). Social facilitation in motor tasks: A review of research and theory. *Psychology of Sport and Exercise, 3*(3), 237–256.

Timmers, C., Maeghs, A., Vestjens, M., Bonnemayer, C., Hamers, H., & Blokland, A. (2014). Ambulant cognitive assessment using a smartphone. *Applied Neuropsychology: Adult, 21*, 136–142.

Torous, J., Kiang, M. V., Lorme, J., & Onnela, J.-P. (2016). New tools for new research in psychiatry: A scalable and customizable platform to empower data driven smartphone research. *JMIR Mental Health, 3*(2), e16.

Wank, A. A., Mehl, M. R., Andrews-Hanna, J. R., Polsinelli, A. J., Moseley, S., Glisky, E. L., et al. (2020). Eavesdropping on autobiographical memory: A naturalistic observation study of older adults' memory sharing in daily conversations. *Frontiers in Human Neuroscience, 14*, 238.

Waters, A. J., Marhe, R., & Franken, I. H. A. (2012). Attentional bias to drug cues is elevated before and during temptations to use heroin and cocaine. *Psychopharmacology, 219*(3), 909–921.

Weizenbaum, E. L., Fulford, D., Torous, J., Pinsky, E., Kolachalama, V. B., & Cronin-Golomb, A. (2022). Smartphone-based neuropsychological assessment in Parkinson's disease: Feasibility, validity, and contextually driven variability in cognition. *Journal of the International Neuropsychological Society, 28*(4), 401–413.

Whibley, D., Williams, D. A., Clauw, D. J., Sliwinski, M., & Kratz, A. L. (2021). Within-day rhythms of pain and cognitive function in people with and without fibromyalgia: Synchronous or syncopated? *Pain, 163*(3), 474–482.

Zhaoyang, R., Scott, S. B., Martire, L. M., Sliwinski, M. J. (2021). Daily social interactions related to daily performance on mobile cognitive tests among older adults. *PLOS One, 16*(8), e0256583.

CHAPTER 26

Mobile Sensing in Developmental Science
A Practical Guide for Researchers

Kaya de Barbaro and Caitlin M. Fausey

CHAPTER OVERVIEW

Wearable sensors that travel with learners—whether young or old—can provide unique access to the rich experiences available to shape their development. The increasing availability of devices and algorithms for activity recognition is a boon for researchers interested in understanding the everyday processes of development. At the same time, the varied opportunities provided by these tools can be overwhelming, opening a floodgate of unconstrained practical decisions. In this chapter, we share practicalities and principles to guide researchers as they pursue "the next right thing" in their research program: (1) less is more, (2) more is more, and (3) harness tradeoffs. We highlight how each of these strategies are well suited to yield advances for developmentalists and sensing innovators alike.

Sampling the Rich Structure of Everyday Experiences

Everyday experiences drive developmental change (e.g., Aslin, 2017; Hensch, 2005; Scott, Pascalis, & Nelson, 2007; Werker & Hensch, 2015). However, theories of development are traditionally based on sampling learners' activity in researcher-structured paradigms. Free-flowing, unscripted interactions taking place in children's everyday home environments are rich with unique features that shape children's experiences. For example, in everyday interactions, children's activity occurs in the context of a particular home, with a particular set of objects, people, and musical tastes. There are mealtimes, bedtimes, and diaper changes. There are often multiple caregivers or social partners present, each with their own needs and responsibilities, including care of other siblings or leisure activities. More broadly, the extended space and time scales of home environments have implications for both children's and caregivers' activity: creating distinct possibilities for lulls in conversation, moments of distance as well as closeness, or the accumulation of stressors across the many hours of the day (see review by de Barbaro & Fausey, 2022). Recent advances in computing and hardware, including miniaturizing sensors, batteries, and storage, mean that these devices can provide researchers access to the rich everyday experiences available to shape learners' development. Additionally, by capturing changes in learners' adaptive functioning as they vocalize, do, and move in everyday settings, sensors can capture the changing tasks of development.

The use of sensors to study child development in context began over a decade ago, with the first publications of infant-worn video and audio recorders capturing what's in view (and earshot) of learners (Fausey, Jayaraman, & Smith, 2016; Zimmerman et al., 2009), and Deb Roy outfitting his entire house with video recorders to capture the first 3 years of his child's life (Roy, Frank, DeCamp, Miller, & Roy, 2015). This now burgeoning literature is gaining widespread traction with recent publications providing theoretical motivations for, and technical, ethical, and logistical possibilities of, incorporating sensors into developmental science research (Cychosz et al., 2020; de Barbaro, 2019; Levin et al., 2021). A recently published review (de Barbaro & Fausey, 2022) summarizes the last decade of research using sensors to capture infants' everyday experiences, highlighting both the variability and structure of infants' everyday experience and what it means for the next generation of theories about development.

Two features of sensors make them ideally suited to characterize the processes of developmental change. First, sensors can capture everyday multimodal activity in context (see Table 26.1). Common wearable devices with video, audio, motion, and physiological sensors can capture features of individual behavior and experiences, including everyday sights and sounds, postures, and affect. They can capture features of social interactions, including patterns of proximity, physical contact, or caregiver sensitivity. Sensors can also capture features of the broader ecological contexts, including household chaos, air quality, and access to nearby resources. Next, with batteries that can last from hours to weeks and protocols that make it possible for participants to recharge or replace sensors without additional researcher contact, these devices can capture the real-time dynamics of everyday activities for hours, days, or even weeks and months at a time. This means that researchers can examine rising and falling quantities across multiple modalities as they cohere into recognizable, everyday activities, such as playing, mealtimes, or bedtimes, as well as changes in those quantities over repeated instances on both short and longitudinal time scales.

By capturing infants' activity in their natural home settings, sensing research centers on everyday tasks as a driver of learning. By capturing features of infants' environments, including first-person sensory access or activity of their social partners, sensing research provides access to input for learning and potential sources of systematic individual differences. And insofar as researchers can use sensors to access multimodal data streams across nested time scales, they can gain access to the processes of change by which learners develop and individual trajectories of learning take shape (de Barbaro, 2019).

Practical Considerations

A developmental scientist who takes to heart the desiderata to sample multimodal behaviors densely and continuously over extended periods of everyday life might abort their

TABLE 26.1. Examples of Everyday Activities Captured by Sensors

Level of analysis	Dimensions of everyday activity	Sensors used	Example citations
Individual			
Internal physiology	Physiological stress and regulation[1,2,3]; vagal activity[3]	Electrodermal sensors[1,2]; heart rate[3]	Goodwin et al. (2019)[1]; Han et al. (2021)[2]; Madden-Rusnak et al. (2022)[3]
Sensory inputs and experiences	Prevalence of faces, hands, or objects in view[1]; presence of TV noise[2]; daily tasks[3]	Wearable cameras[1] and audio recorders[2,3]	Fausey et al. (2016)[1]; Zimmerman et al. (2009)[2]; Soderstrom & Wittebolle (2013)[3]
Embodied activity and affect	Sleep[1]; physical activity[2]; posture[3]; infant distress[4]	Motion sensors[1,2,3]; video or audio recorders[4]	Sadeh et al. (1995)[1]; Buss (1981)[2]; Franchak et al. (2021)[3]; Micheletti et al. (2022)[4]
Cognition and internal states	Parent-reported child activity[1,2]; caregiver activity[2]; stress, mental health symptoms[4]	Ecological momentary assessments[1,2,3,4]	Franchak (2019)[1]; Do et al. (2020)[2]; de Barbaro et al. (2022b)[3]
Social or interpersonal	Proximity[1,2]; holding[3]; caregiver sensitivity[4]; conflict[5]; annoyance with partner[6]	Radio frequency[1]; Bluetooth[2]; motion sensors[3]; audio recorders[4,5,6]	Messinger et al. (2019)[1]; Salo et al. (2021)[2]; Yao et al (2019)[3]; de Barbaro et al. (2022a)[4]; Han et al. (2021)[5]
Ecological	Household "chaos"[1]; air quality[2]; access to greenspace[3] or other resources[4] by location	Audio recorders[1]; particle detection[2]; GPS[3,4]	Khante et al. (2022)[1]; Schultz et al. (2020)[2]; Ward, Duncan, Jarden, & Stewart (2016)[3]; Dunton et al. (2014)[4]

Note. Sensed activity is organized according to individual, interpersonal, and ecological levels of the developmental system. Superscript numerals link example citations in each row to the dimensions of activity they capture and the sensors used to do so.

mission in the face of seemingly unconstrained practical decisions. For many research questions, there is no gold-standard agreed-upon approach, in part because there is so much we do not yet know. We encourage researchers to adopt a mindset in which they pursue "the next right thing" on the route to chipping away at unknown answers to their primary research question. We suggest three lenses to consider as you articulate your rationale for which options you implement: (1) less is more, (2) more is more, and (3) harness tradeoffs. Astute readers will note that some of the advice across these lenses is in conflict; this is, of course, by design. Optimizing for one set of outcomes often causes tension with another—equally valid—set of outcomes. As such, our lenses represent different approaches to sensing that researchers may usefully consider.

Lens 1: Less Is More

No single developmental mobile sensing study can or needs to quantify every modality and time scale. Here, we emphasize the priority of your primary research question and known realities, as well as discuss feasibility considerations like reducing participant burden, shortening timelines to initial discoveries, and satisficing with existing expertise and tools.

Selecting Modalities of Interest

Know Thy Question

Although everyday experiences are multimodal, theorists need not always sample all modalities in all studies. Theorists can often build on prior evidence to strategically select which modality to sample in order to answer their primary research question. For example, if you are interested in understanding the nature of play or joint attention across development, then you are faced with decisions about sampling everyday experiences by using video and/or audio, capturing overhead and/or egocentric (caregiver and/or child) views, eye gaze and/or hands and/or heads, and more. If your primary question is about dynamics within play episodes, then prior research motivates using video rather than audio because of known dynamics in gaze and manual activity (Deak, Krasno, Triesch, Lewis, & Sepeta, 2014; Yu & Smith, 2013). Prior research also informs how you might choose how many and which kinds of cameras to use. For example, because we know that caregivers' gaze alternates between the child and manipulated objects, you might not need to capture the caregivers' point of view per se with a dedicated camera and instead infer their gaze locations over time from another camera. Similarly, because eye gaze is centered within head direction (Smith, Yu, Yoshida, & Fausey, 2015) and eyes and hands are coordinated (Yu & Smith, 2013), cameras optimized to detect hands-on-objects will yield informative dynamics. In some cases, a well-placed overhead camera could be sufficient to infer gaze directions, given these existing findings. If your primary question about play is about how opportunities for play change across development, then detecting everyday instances of play throughout a day could be optimized by using longform audio recordings (e.g., Soderstrom & Wittebolle, 2013).

Single-Modality Insights

Often, a productive route to new discoveries is as straightforward as adding one sensor to sample a previously unsampled modality of everyday activities. If you are interested in attachment, then a sensor capturing proximity or physical contact could provide insight into patterns of caregiver and child co-regulation (e.g., Salo et al., 2021; Yao, Johnson, Ploetz, & de Barbaro, 2019). If you are interested in sleep, then a sensor capturing daily fluctuations in light or in experienced chaos could provide relevant predictors for children's sleep outcomes (e.g., Khante, Thomaz, & de Barbaro et al., 2023; Lungarella, Pegors, Bulwinkle, & Sporns, 2005). Given the broad relevance of attachment and sleep to many developmental trajectories (e.g., attention, executive function, emotion regulation, and more; for reviews, see Mason, Lokhandwala, Riggins, & Spencer, 2021; Ranson & Urichuk, 2008), these single-modality sensors could open the floodgates of insights into within- and between individual variation that is meaningful for multiple routes of developmental change.

Reduce Participant and Researcher Burden

Practically speaking, fewer sensors eases burdens for both participants and researchers. Each additional sensor means another device that needs charging and upkeep on its own timeline, with its own instructions and its own manual for what can go wrong. Additional sensors also necessitate increasingly complex synchronization protocols (see de Barbaro,

2019, for considerations). Reducing participant burdens benefits recruitment and retention, and simpler protocols mean less training and effort for research staff. These issues can be nontrivial when sampling everyday experiences in hard-to-reach populations and/or repeatedly over longitudinal time.

Lower Fidelity Sensors Get the Job Done

Researchers must motivate how many and what fidelity sensors to use when sampling everyday experiences. For many research questions, high-fidelity data such as video and audio that preserve rich, human-interpretable records of experiences are required. Lower fidelity sensors, however, can often get the job done for many questions. For example, motion sensors can detect sleep and activity (Bussman & Ebner-Priemer, 2012; see also Giurgiu & Bussman, Chapter 5, this volume) that can provide insight into individual differences in motor activity, temperament, or cognition (Buss, 1981; Franchak, Scott, & Luo., 2021; Mason et al., 2021; Worobey, 2014). Physiological sensors that capture changes in heart rate or electrodermal activity can detect momentary arousal changes related, for example, to instances of an infant crying (Madden-Rusnak, Micheletti, & de Barbaro, 2023) or the presence of a supportive partner (Han et al., 2021), or they can predict upcoming aggressive episodes (Goodwin, Mazefsky, Ioannidis, Erdogmus, & Siegel, 2019). Daily surveys known as ecological momentary assessments can also quantify caregiver experience and behaviors, such as maternal support of fruit and vegetable consumption (Do et al., 2020) and caregiver-reported child behaviors such as posture and manual activity over the course of days and weeks (e.g., Franchak, 2019) in order to test hypotheses about developmentally changing rates and coordination among these variables.

Low-fidelity sensing has many benefits. For one thing, low-fidelity sensors are often more comfortable for participants, such as heart rate sensors worn on the wrist rather than higher-resolution chest-worn or electrode-based sensors. By virtue of being less interpretable, families are generally more comfortable using low-fidelity sensors to record home activity. Recruiting more, and more diverse, families is therefore facilitated (Levin et al., 2021). Datafiles from low-fidelity sensors are also typically smaller, making storage capacity less likely to limit the length of sensing and making weak or unstable access to Wi-Fi less likely to be a barrier to participation. Inclusive, representative mobile sensing is similarly well served by low-fidelity sensors because such sensors are often less expensive than high-fidelity sensors. Cost effectiveness means any single study can use more sensors across more families and for longer sampling periods in which families use multiple sensors over time.

Determining How Much to Sample

Everything Is a Sample, and Short Recordings Reveal More Than No Recordings

In principle, one could sample three continuous years of everyday experiences (e.g., Roy et al., 2015). Three years is "a lot" relative to typical developmental study durations but "a little" relative to typical lifespans. We suggest that it is productive to consider one's sample relative to what is and is not known, rather than any atheoretical impression of "a lot." Currently, very little is known about most everyday experiences in human infancy, and so even relatively short samples can yield important insights. For example, play in laboratory settings is typically sampled for 5 to 15 minutes. A similar duration sampled from everyday life will yield new insights, including potential similarities between laboratory and home contexts. Extending sampling durations even a few-fold beyond current knowledge also yields theory-relevant insights, such as rhythms of interleaved speech and silence when recording for 45 minutes (Tamis-LeMonda, Kuchirko, Luo, Escobar, & Bornstein, 2017). Furthermore, cross-sectional approaches in which shorter samples across many families yield large corpora of previously unobserved everyday experiences often generate guideposts for subsequent longitudinal studies in which longer durations are sampled per individual (e.g., Fausey et al., 2016; Long, Kachergis, Agrawal, & Frank, 2020). Finally, sample durations are often constrained by available technologies that will also evolve over time. For example, longform audio recordings (e.g., using LENA; Ford, Baer, Xu, Yapanel, & Gray, 2008) are sometimes lauded for their "day-long" extent, yet their 16-hour capacity is driven by battery life and might reasonably be recast as "day-short." There is unlikely to be one optimal sampling route to discovery, and we encourage theorists to push whatever the frontiers may be at each moment in the long game of science (see Mendoza & Fausey, 2021a, for discussion).

Know Thy Base Rates

Extant literature often provides anchors to guide sample duration, including hourly, daily, or weekly regularities about your target phenomenon. For example, caregiver surveys had long indicated that children encounter music daily, and so audio sampling one waking day was likely to—and indeed, did—capture everyday instances of music (Mendoza & Fausey, 2021b). Many everyday activities have a diurnal rhythm, including infant crying and adult speech (Johnson, Andres, Micheletti, Yao, & de Barbaro, 2020). Others have weekly rhythms, including affect and sleep (Larsen & Kasimatis, 1990; Szymczak, Jasińska, Pawlak, & Zwierzykowska, 1993). Accounting for these known rhythms can make it possible to detect hypothesized relationships between the everyday phenomena that you sample. For example, only after accounting for time-of-day effects in adult speech rhythms did an effect of mood on speech become apparent (Johnson et al., 2020). Thus, we encourage theorists to ground sampling and analytic decisions in existing knowledge about the base rates of everyday phenomena where possible and to publish these values as they are discovered.

Sample Short Bursts Repeatedly

For everyday behaviors that happen often, continuous sampling may not be necessary to capture many, and varied, instances of these behaviors. For example, many short samples can reveal the nature of tasks such as walking, object play, and interpersonal interactions in everyday life. Short bursts can be scheduled, such as capturing 1.5 hours of video twice per week (e.g., Sullivan, Mei, Perfors, Wojcik, & Frank, 2022) or 10 activity queries per day, 4 days per week (e.g., Kadooka, Caufield, Fausey, & Franchak, 2021). Practically, short bursts minimize burdens of longitudinal protocols given the battery and storage limitations of some sensors. Collecting short bursts can be facilitated by inviting caregivers into the empirical endeavor by requesting that they sample particular activities of interest or even everyday challenges such as bedtime routines or walking up stairs.

Such repeated short samples may yield important insights about the nature of pervasive behaviors.

Downsample

Even when a sampling window is long, it is not always necessary to sample everyday behaviors continuously within the window. Some sensors allow researchers to downsample at the point of data collection, including options for both sound (e.g., 30–90 seconds per hour; Mehl, 2017) and sights (e.g., one photo per 30 seconds; Casillas, Brown, & Levinson, 2020) data. Researchers can also record everyday experiences continuously and then downsample the captured streams before annotating and analyzing them (e.g., Fausey et al., 2016).

Recent analyses have begun to shed light on downsampling schemes that yield enough data to reliably estimate rates of everyday behaviors. For example, downsampling randomly for short durations of time approximates a population mean distribution for everyday behaviors with medium or high base rates of occurrence (Micheletti et al., 2020). If every participant in a study exceeds a minimum base rate of activity, such downsampling can also be used to reliably assess individual differences among participants (Micheletti et al., 2020). Similarly, sampling 1.5 hours' worth of audio distributed randomly in 30-second audio clips throughout a day yields stable estimates of the proportion of everyday speech that is adult-directed, child-directed, and in each of two available languages (Cychosz, Villanueva, & Weisleder, 2021). Behaviors that happen rarely will likely be missed by downsampling, and thus, other strategies may be required to identify them. For example, Khante and colleagues (2023) used existing models trained to detect everyday sound classes, including car horns, dishes clanking, and dogs barking, to detect segments that have a high likelihood of containing highly chaotic sounds. Annotating these selected segments reduced coding time necessary to detect positive samples of high chaos by a factor of nine. Event-based downsampling, that is, annotating segments identified to be interesting by automated algorithms, can also yield theory-relevant insights about everyday behaviors. For example, Romeo and colleagues (2018) annotated word counts in the hour detected to have the greatest number of conversational turns in a day of sampled audio and found that annotated word counts correlated with individual differences in verbal skill. And new insights about everyday experiences have been discovered by characterizing the nature of episodes like mealtimes (e.g., Clerkin, Hart, Rehg, Yu, & Smith, 2017) or pre-sleep (e.g., Teti, Kim, Mayer, & Countermine, 2010) from within longer recordings.

Detecting and Annotating Data

Identifying developmentally relevant units within data streams captured using mobile sensors can sometimes be accomplished using existing automatic algorithms; more often, manual annotation of rich everyday behaviors is the most straightforward approach.

Off-the-Shelf Algorithms

For some everyday behaviors, existing algorithms can provide robust and reliable annotations of raw data using commercial devices and tools. For audio data captured using digital language processors by LENA, software can automatically segment captured sounds into adult and child voices, TV, silence, and more (Ford et al., 2008). From speech-like segments, this software also estimates the number of adult words, child vocalizations, and conversational turns at centisecond resolution. From wrist-worn motion and physiology sensors, the detection of sleep–wake cycles is also robust and can be reliably measured with children (e.g., Bélanger, Bernier, Paquet, Simard, & Carrier, 2013; Sadeh, Acebo, Seifer, Aytur, & Carskadon, 1995). Thus, developmental theorists can take advantage of these easy-to-use tools to speed data processing and, therefore, discoveries when their research questions center on these constructs. Note that any algorithm, as well as industry-standard thresholds of reliability, can (and should) change over time (e.g., Cristia et al., 2020; Ferjan Ramírez, Hippe, & Kuhl, 2021), so researchers will benefit from mindful use of these tools in the context of their main research questions.

Manual Annotation

Rigorous, reliable manual annotation of rich everyday data has been the workhorse of developmental psychology for decades (Adolph, 2020; Bakeman & Gottman, 1997), and this long history has yielded sophisticated protocols for researchers. Because automatic algorithms are not yet up to the challenge of reliably annotating most kinds of everyday data, leaning into this hard-won manual annotation expertise is often more cost-effective in time and money than attempting to build bespoke new algorithms de novo (though see below for one contrasting "more is more" lens). Recent discoveries about everyday language (e.g., Bergelson & Aslin, 2017; Weisleder & Fernald, 2013), music (e.g., Mendoza & Fausey, 2021b), and visual objects (e.g., Fausey et al., 2016; Sugden, Mohamed-Ali, & Moulson, 2014) have all been achieved by manually annotating data captured from sensors worn by young infants in everyday life. Several open-source tools facilitate systematic manual annotation, including Datavyu (https://datavyu.org) and ELAN (Wittenburg, Brugman, Russel, Klassmann, & Sloetjes, 2006). These tools have large user bases and therefore community support in training research team members. Detailed schemes for manually annotating everyday data are increasingly published as protocol papers and/or shared as coding manuals on Open Science Framework (*https://osf.io*; e.g., Mendoza & Fausey, 2020; Soderstrom et al., 2021; see Mendoza & Fausey, 2021a, for general principles), making road-tested scalable schemes easy to find and use. One ongoing endeavor even brings together experts across many domains of development to craft and share manual annotation protocols for structure in everyday play (Adolph, Gilmore, & Soska, 2019). Manual annotation is also a productive way to make the most of existing raw data that primary researchers have shared in repositories such as HomeBank (VanDam et al., 2016), CHILDES (MacWhinney, 2000), and Databrary (databrary.org; Gilmore, Kennedy, & Adolph, 2018).

Analyzing Everyday Data

Atemporal Everyday Statistics

Statistical summaries like frequency distributions quantify the availability and variability of what young learners sample as they build knowledge over time. Foundational questions such as how many minutes of music per day are available to constrain early musical enculturation (Mendoza & Fausey, 2021b), how many and how diverse are the everyday faces that help to develop infants' early perception (Jayaraman, Fausey, & Smith, 2015; Sugden et al., 2014), and how many and how repetitive are everyday objects that are early identified (Clerkin et al., 2017), are answerable by quantifying encountered frequency distributions. These distributions serve to constrain computational theories of developmental change by providing ecologically valid parameters for dimensions such as frequency, similarity, and diversity that are relevant for nearly every model of learning and memory. Summaries of such daily behaviors can also be considered over longitudinal time to provide insight into learning inputs across development. For example, the persistence of faces-in-view declines over the first year of infancy (Jayaraman & Smith, 2018). They can also be included as inputs in common correlation or regression analyses to examine how individual differences in daily experiences relate to developmental achievements. For example, quantities of child-directed speech matter for speech processing speed and subsequent vocabulary (e.g., Weisleder & Fernald, 2013) and maternal emotional availability at bedtime is associated with higher infant sleep quality (Teti et al., 2010). Straightforward analytic techniques can thus provide relevant, valuable insight into the structure of everyday experiences (see also Adolph, 2019).

Lens 2: More Is More

"More is more" is a lens best suited for goals of building capacity in the long game of advancing developmental theory. Taking on expansive everyday data collection, annotation, and/or analyses demands considerable resources initially, but the rewards extend far beyond a single project. Large up-front investments are sometimes the only way to get started on a truly new path of discovery, since by definition no evidence provides a rationale for any particular sensor, sampling scheme, or analytic approach. "The next right thing" may be to disrupt "looking only where the light is" disciplinary habits and to shine a light elsewhere.

Capturing, Annotating, and Detecting Data

Capture More Than Your Target Behavior

In order to characterize everyday behaviors that may be infrequent, unpredictable, and/or of varying durations, it is worthwhile to sample continuously for extended periods of time. For example, sampling a whole day allows theorists to later detect toddler tantrum episodes, their full duration, as well as insight into what triggered them and how they get resolved. A sparser record of everyday behaviors would likely miss these quantitative insights. One reward of capturing dense, continuous everyday behaviors is the very high likelihood for data reuse and further insights (Adolph, 2020; Nastase, Goldstein, & Hasson, 2020).

Manually Annotate Your Captured Data

Manually annotating everyday recordings requires massive amounts of person-hours. For example, transcribing language is estimated to require 8 hours for every hour of speech captured (MacWhinney, 2000). Recent discoveries about everyday music based on 35 day-long audio recordings required approximately 6,400 person-hours of manual annotation (Mendoza & Fausey, 2021b). Automated algorithms currently fall short of the rigor required to advance developmental theory, and so manual annotation is often key to discovery. The payoff, however, is enormous when researchers share their painstaking manual annotation efforts (see above). Other researchers can analyze the annotations in new ways and/or combine them with new annotations of the same shared data. Carefully developed annotation schemes and associated documentation facilitate aggregation that makes it possible to quantify the structure of everyday experiences more representatively and robustly sampled across the world's individuals (e.g., Adolph et al., 2019; Soderstrom et al., 2021). Finally, annotated data can also serve as training and evaluation sets in the process of developing automated algorithms (e.g., Räsänen et al., 2019).

BUILD BESPOKE DETECTION MODELS

Eventually, someone will develop automated algorithms to parse everyday data, and that someone could be you. Intrepid researchers who make the most of collaborations with engineers and computer scientists provide real value to multiple areas of inquiry relevant for advancing developmental theory. The process of building bespoke activity recognition models has been described elsewhere (de Barbaro, 2019; Lara & Labrador, 2013) and can be applied to any raw sensing data, including audio, video, and physical motion. Developing these models goes hand-in-hand with manual annotation and indeed may require more, and finer-grained, annotation than would otherwise be required to answer your primary research question.

It is essential to train models with annotated everyday datasets that are representative of the contexts, time scales, individuals, and populations to which the model will eventually be applied. A common source of poor model performance is having been trained on "sanitized" laboratory behaviors rather than richer everyday behaviors that also vary a lot across families (Alameda-Pineda, Ricci, & Sebe, 2019; Cristia, Ganesh, Casillas, & Ganapathy, 2018; Yao, Micheletti, Johnson, Thomaz, & de Barbaro, 2022). Interdisciplinary teams with technical and theoretical expertise have produced algorithms specifically developed and validated with the goal of providing large-scale uptake by the developmental science community. These algorithms include detection of crying, holding, and proximity, as well as speaker diarization (Messinger et al., 2019; Räsänen et al., 2021; Salo et al., 2021; Yao et al., 2019, 2022), with promising ongoing efforts for face and object detection as well (Long et al., 2020; Tsutsui, Zhi, Reza, Crandall, & Yu, 2019).

Expansive Possibilities for Analyzing Everyday Data

Longform high-density data provide an abundance of riches in terms of modalities and time scales. Sometimes your primary research question may center on a particular modality or time scale, but your recordings make it possible to annotate and analyze others. Other times, your primary research question is itself about multimodal and/or multiscalar structure. Here, we discuss some options for analyses that go beyond commonly used descriptive summaries.

Leverage Descriptive Summaries

Descriptive summaries can be analyzed with more complex statistical analyses to derive important insights. For example, rather than just considering population means, person- or population-specific approaches can be used to understand subgroups of individuals within a population whose behaviors may differ qualitatively from others (Molenaar & Campbell, 2009). For example, descriptive analyses of individual adolescents' cell phone use revealed unique patterns of interaction on daily, weekly, and moment-by-moment time scales (Ram et al., 2020). In developmental domains, related analyses have been used with laboratory data and could easily transfer to data collected in everyday settings. For example, patterns of synchronous locomotion in mother–infant dyads revealed two clusters in a free-flowing lab play session: one cluster of dyads in which mothers tended to track infants, and another in which lead–follow relations were more varied (Hoch, Ossmy, Cole, Hasan, & Adolph, 2021). In the case of longitudinally sampled everyday behaviors, descriptive summaries can be incorporated into models that consider change over time. For example, vector autoregressive (VAR) models that consider mutual influences between interacting partners over time have revealed dynamics like how mothers' responses to boys' versus girls' everyday motor achievements differ and matter for motor development (Eason, Carver, Kelty-Stephen, & Fausto-Sterling, 2020, written as an introductory tutorial to VAR).

Embrace Variability

Environments and learners are not static, and there is much to discover about patterns of variability in everyday data from hour-to-hour, day-to-day, month-to-month, and more (e.g., Anderson & Fausey, 2019; d'Apice, Latham, & von Stumm, 2019; de Barbaro, Madden-Rusnak, & Momin, 2022). Collecting multiple samples, or splitting data into multiple samples, allows theorists to assess the stability versus dynamic shifting of sampled behaviors using measures such as intraclass correlations (aka test–retest reliability; Bolger & Laurenceau, 2013), multistage coefficient of variation (e.g., Abney, Kello, & Balasubramaniam, 2017), and others. Within-person variability may be a critical measure in its own right. For example, sleep variability is a key predictor of symptom severity in children with autism (Bangerter et al., 2020). High-density sensor data can also be used to model predictors of within-person variability over time, key to accessing developmental processes at the individual level (Hamaker & Wichers, 2017; Ram, Brose, & Molenaar, 2013; for an introduction, see Bolger & Laurenceau, 2013). For example, multilevel models have been used to characterize how within-person variability in maternal mental health is predicted by changes in day-by-day and hour-by-hour exposure to infant crying (de Barbaro, Micheletti, et al., 2023).

Embrace Real-Time Dynamics

Time series created from sensor data streams can be used to characterize the temporal structure of uni- or multimodal everyday data. For example, in everyday language, certain sequences of infant and adult vocalizations relate to vocabulary development (Lopez, Walle, Pretzer, & Warlaumont, 2020). And dynamic properties of infants' motor and verbal behavior as quantified by recurrence quantification analysis or the Allan factor relate to developmental milestones (Abney, Warlaumont, Haussman, Ross, & Wallot, 2014). Time-series analyses have been employed in laboratory settings to characterize moment-by-moment influences between and within individuals (e.g. Cohn & Tronick, 1988). In everyday settings, extended recording allows for windowing approaches or change-point analyses that can identify state-changes and nonlinearities in the data (Behrens, Moulder, Boker, & Kret, 2020; Olthof et al., 2020) such as changes in children's heart rate variability over the course of an episode of distress (Buhler-Wassman & Hibel, 2021; Madden-Rusnak, Micheletti, & de Barbaro, 2023). Tutorials and analysis code for these techniques are increasingly available (e.g., Xu, de Barbaro, Abney, & Cox, 2020).

Model Dynamic Systems

Dynamic systems analyses by definition require multiple modalities and multiple time scales of data. To pursue these analyses, theorists must identify an observable activity (e.g., breastfeeding) that involves the coordination of different dimensions of the system. They must capture that activity—with all relevant dimensions—multiple times, over shorter time scales as well as over longitudinal time (e.g., multiple times per day or week, over weeks to months). Visualizations and analyses that characterize the real-time multimodal temporal dynamics of these events reveal variation in the emergent configurations over short and longitudinal time scales. We point interested readers to previously published work focused on such analyses (e.g., de Barbaro, Johnson, Forster, & Deak, 2013; Granic, Hollenstein, & Lichtwarck-Aschoff, 2016; Spencer, Perone, & Buss, 2011; Thelen & Smith, 1994). Modeling dynamic systems is a counterpoint to a "less is more" single modality, lower fidelity sensor, downsampled empirical approach. Dynamic systems analyses often reveal how very small differences in timing can change the qualitative or emergent nature of activity. The importance of such differences in timing is highlighted by constructs such as synchrony or contingency and can be the difference between a successful or unsuccessful step, reach, or wink. As such, everyday mobile sensing that can capture multimodal activity at the resolution of milliseconds over extended periods of time will be required to answer many questions of interest to developmental scientists.

Lens 3: Harness Tradeoffs

The "less is more" and "more is more" lenses pull in opposing directions. We suggest that theorists can productively lean into the complexities of sampling everyday life by strategically harnessing tradeoffs between these lenses. For example, if your rationale demands "more is more" for one part of your research, then opting for "less is more" in other parts may dramatically increase the chances of reaching meaningful insights in doable time frames. Harnessing tradeoffs is familiar territory for any empiricist; here, we provide some examples of such decision making in the context of everyday mobile sensing.

High Volume versus High Burden

If your focus is on getting high volumes of data, whether for continuous recordings or repeated samples over longitudinal time, then it may benefit you to prioritize easing burdens on participants. This could mean selecting a more comfortable but lower-resolution sensor (see above). By contrast, if you need high-fidelity or multimodal data from which many dimensions of activity can be derived, you will likely need to sacrifice some data volume in order to make it feasible for your participants.

Exhaustive Modalities versus Exhaustive Contexts

When your question demands high-density, multimodal, repeated samples of everyday data, limiting recording to a restricted physical space where specific interactions are likely to occur will ease burdens on families. For example, an overhead camera placed over a playmat can capture caregiver–child play episodes. Similarly, an audio recorder can be positioned to capture dinner interactions in which speech as well as caregiver–child conflict are likely to occur. Caregivers can also be involved in sampling particular activities or even everyday challenges, such as walking up the stairs. As such, context-specific sampling can facilitate rich microdynamic analyses that would be otherwise difficult to capture in home settings. Alternatively, if you need a more exhaustive set of contexts to answer your research question, then you might consider using fewer and/or lower fidelity sensors.

Video versus Audio

If your research question does not require sampling a particular modality per se (e.g., everyday interaction dynamics when much is not yet known), then you must decide whether to use video and/or audio sensors. Video data provide unmatched multimodal access into complex behavior, making it the modality of choice for many developmentalists (e.g., Adolph, 2020). However, audio records have many benefits for home recordings. Many audio sensors are omnidirectional, capturing events occurring in all directions rather than only what is captured by a video lens itself. On average, parents report feeling more comfortable sharing audio rather than video data of their family interactions, but differences in comfort are relatively small and not significant (Levin et al., 2021). However, in many jurisdictions, audio records are not considered to be identifiable data (unless the person is famous), whereas video data are. Finally, at full frame rates necessary to capture contingency and synchrony, most commercially available wearable video sensors achieve only 1 to 2 hours of data, while similarly sized audio sensors achieve 24 to 72 hours of continuous data without need to charge batteries. Thus, when an unobtrusive setup or high-fidelity data for long periods of time is important, audio may be advantageous. For other research priorities, video may permit richer discoveries.

Go It Alone versus Collaborate

The technical and computational skills required to work with high-density data can pose challenges to traditionally trained psychologists. One way to minimize such challenges is to use methods that do not demand entirely new skill sets (see "Less Is More"). Another option is to collaborate with colleagues who have skills that you do not (e.g., computer scientists and engineers, among many others). Because cross-disciplinary teams can get tangled in webs of competing priorities, we suggest starting with light touch collaborations that evolve over time. For example, engineers often prioritize projects that push the bounds of computation and development of new algorithmic structures or techniques, while applied social scientists often prioritize tried-and-true techniques that can provide known results (e.g., Abowd, 2019). In the worst case, competing priorities will stall progress in all directions and sink a project. In the best case, each team will compromise to identify projects that are technically appealing and advance developmental theory. Mindful construction of research teams, including students conducting time-limited projects, can cohere into these best cases.

Rapid versus Delayed Theoretical Gratification

All theorists want to discover meaningful answers to important questions. Using everyday mobile sensing, rich insights about developmental tasks and trajectories are now achievable with enormous time and effort, including collecting many hours of continuous recordings plus multimodal manual annotations modeled as dynamic systems. Embarking on a multiyear endeavor with many unknowns, however, could be an untenable commitment of resources, and so satisficing calls for more constrained implementation. Such implementation can still advance theory as long as any limitations are acknowledged. For example, while few automated algorithms can currently robustly detect everyday activities, many "proof-of-concept" algorithms are available. These algorithms have typically been built using data from a few individuals in few situations, and so their accuracy suffers when used at scale in everyday settings. However, leveraging an imperfect solution may still shift a theoretical needle forward. This is particularly true in cases where very little is known about a phenomenon. We suggest that theorists carefully assess and clearly state any limitations of imperfect implementations, while highlighting the potential benefits even given those limitations (see also Cristia et al., 2020). Alternatively, if you and your team are well positioned to do so, capacity-building projects will be an investment yielding manyfold returns.

Next-Generation Developmental Theory and Mobile Sensing

Theories of developmental change demand models of both learners and their learning environments (e.g., Smith & Slone, 2017). Models grounded in evidence from the tasks and trajectories of everyday learners are likeliest to account for real developmental change. Mobile sensing, in which theorists sample rather than script experiences, can now serve as an essential tool in developmentalists' toolkit en route to understanding the multimodal and multiscalar structure of everyday experiences as learners and their environments change over time.

We see three opportunities for real breakthroughs in a future of continued synergy between developmental theorists and mobile sensing: (1) expanding our understanding of the experiences of learners the world over, making theories of developmental process more honestly parameterized across variation in languages, resources, sociopolitical ecosystems, and more; (2) accelerating automated measurement protocols that successfully detect and quantify important features of everyday experiences, with applications deployed in real life, including adaptive tutoring, strengths-based parenting supports, just-in-time risk mitigation, and more; and (3) tuning models of adaptive intelligences to detailed individual experiences, with an emphasis on the multiple pathways, complexities, and flexibilities of development.

REFERENCES

Abney, D., Kello, C., & Balasubramaniam, R. (2017). Introduction and application of the multiscale coefficient of variation analysis. *Behavior Research Methods, 49*(5), 1571–1581.

Abney, D. H., Warlaumont, A. S., Haussman, A., Ross, J. M., & Wallot, S. (2014). Using nonlinear methods to quantify changes in infant limb movements and vocalizations. *Frontiers in Psychology, 5*, 771.

Abowd, G. (2019, January). *Confessions of an applied computer scientist.* Georgia Tech GVU Center Brown Bag Seminar. https://gvu.gatech.edu/event/brown-bag-archive/gregory-abowd-confessions-applied-computer-scientist

Adolph, K. E. (2019). An ecological approach to learning in (not and) development. *Human Development, 63*, 180–201.

Adolph, K. E. (2020). Oh, behave! Presidential address. *Infancy, 25*, 347–392.

Adolph, K. E., Gilmore, R. O. & Soska, K. (2019). Play and Learning Across a Year (PLAY) Project—Protocols and documentation. *Databrary.*

Alameda-Pineda, X., Ricci, E., & Sebe, N. (2019). Multimodal behavior analysis in the wild: An introduction. In X. Alameda-Pineda, E. Ricci, & N. Sebe (Eds.), *Multimodal behavior analysis in the wild* (pp. 1–8). Academic Press.

Anderson, H., & Fausey, C. M. (2019). *Modeling non-uniformities in infants' everyday speech environments.* Paper presented at the 2019 biennial meeting of the Society for Research in Child Development.

Aslin, R. N. (2017). Statistical learning: a powerful mechanism that operates by mere exposure. *Wiley Interdisciplinary Reviews: Cognitive Science, 8*(1–2), e1373.

Bakeman, R., & Gottman, J. (1997). *Observing interaction: An introduction to sequential analysis.* Cambridge University Press.

Bangerter, A., Chatterjee, M., Manyakov, N. V., Ness, S., Lewin, D., Skalkin, A., et al. (2020). Relationship between sleep and behavior in autism spectrum disorder: Exploring the impact of sleep variability. *Frontiers in Neuroscience, 14*, 211.

Behrens, F., Moulder, R. G., Boker, S. M., & Kret, M. (2020). *Quantifying physiological synchrony through windowed cross-correlation analysis: Statistical and theoretical considerations.* www.biorxiv.org/content/biorxiv/early/2020/08/28/2020.08.27.269746.full.pdf

Bélanger, M. È., Bernier, A., Paquet, J., Simard, V., & Carrier, J. (2013). Validating actigraphy as a measure of sleep for preschool children. *Journal of Clinical Sleep Medicine, 9*(7), 701–706.

Bergelson, E., & Aslin, R. N. (2017). Nature and origins of the lexicon in 6-mo-olds. *Proceedings of the National Academy of Sciences, 114*(49), 12916–12921.

Bolger, N., & Laurenceau, J. P. (2013). *Intensive longitudinal methods: An introduction to diary and experience sampling research.* Guilford Press.

Buhler-Wassmann, A. C., & Hibel, L. C. (2021). Studying caregiver-infant co-regulation in dynamic, diverse cultural contexts: A call to action. *Infant Behavior and Development, 64*, 101586

Buss, D. M. (1981). Predicting parent–child interactions from children's activity level. *Developmental Psychology, 17*(1), 59.

Bussmann, J., & Ebner-Priemer, U. (2012). Ambulatory assessment of movement behavior: Methodology, measurement, and application. In M. R. Mehl & T. S. Conner (Eds.), *Handbook of research methods for studying daily life* (pp. 235–250). Guilford Press.

Casillas, M., Brown, P., & Levinson, S. C. (2020). Early language experience in a Tseltal Mayan village. *Child Development, 91*(5), 1819–1835.

Clerkin, E. M., Hart, E., Rehg, J. M., Yu, C., & Smith, L. B. (2017). Real-world visual statistics and infants' first-learned object names. *Philosophical Transactions of the Royal Society B: Biological Sciences, 372*(1711), 20160055.

Cohn, J. F., & Tronick, E. Z. (1988). Mother–infant face-to-face interaction: Influence is bidirectional and unrelated to periodic cycles in either partner's behavior. *Developmental Psychology, 24*(3), 386.

Cristia, A., Ganesh, S., Casillas, M., & Ganapathy, S. (2018, October). Talker diarization in the wild: The case of child-centered daylong audio-recordings. *Proceedings of Interspeech 2018*, pp. 2583–2587.

Cristia, A., Lavechin, M., Scaff, C., Soderstrom, M., Rowland, C., Räsänen, O., et al. (2020). A thorough evaluation of the Language Environment Analysis (LENA) system. *Behavior Research Methods, 53*(2), 467–486.

Cychosz, M., Romeo, R., Soderstrom, M., Scaff, C., Ganek, H., Cristia, A., et al. (2020). Long-form recordings of everyday life: Ethics for best practices. *Behavior Research Methods, 52*, 1951–1969.

Cychosz, M., Villanueva, A., & Weisleder, A. (2021). Efficient estimation of children's language exposure in two bilingual communities. *Journal of Speech, Language, and Hearing Research, 64*(10), 3843–3866.

d'Apice, K., Latham, R. M., & von Stumm, S. (2019). A naturalistic home observational approach to children's language, cognition, and behavior. *Developmental Psychology, 55*(7), 1414–1427.

Deak, G. O., Krasno, A. M., Triesch, J., Lewis, J., & Sepeta, L. (2014). Watch the hands: Infants can learn to follow gaze by seeing adults manipulate objects. *Developmental Science, 17*(2), 270–281.

de Barbaro, K. (2019). Automated sensing of daily activity: A new lens into development. *Developmental Psychobiology, 61*(3), 444–464.

de Barbaro, K., & Fausey, C. M. (2022). Ten lessons about infants' everyday experiences. *Current Directions in Psychological Science, 31*(1), 28–33.

de Barbaro, K., Johnson, C. M., Forster, D., & Deak, G. O. (2013). Methodological considerations for investigating the micro-dynamics of social interaction development. *IEEE Transactions on Autonomous Mental Development, 5*(3), 258–270.

de Barbaro, K., Madden-Rusnak, A., & Momin, N. (2022, July). *Maternal sensitivity "in the wild" is highly variable and systematically varies across contexts.* Paper presented at the International Conference on Infant Studies, Ottawa, Canada.

de Barbaro, K., Micheletti, M., Yao, X., Khante, P., Johnson, M., & Goodman, S. (2023) Infant crying predicts real-time fluctuations in maternal mental health in ecologically valid home settings. *Developmental Psychology, 59*(4), 733–744.

Do, B., Yang, C. H., Lopez, N. V., Mason, T. B., Margolin, G., & Dunton, G. F. (2020). Investigating the momentary association between maternal support and children's fruit and vegetable consumption using ecological momentary assessment. *Appetite, 150*, 104667.

Dunton, G. F., Dzubur, E., Kawabata, K., Yanez, B., Bo, B., & Intille, S. (2014). Development of a smartphone application to measure physical activity using sensor-assisted self-report. *Frontiers in Public Health, 2*, 12.

Eason, E. G., Carver, N. S., Kelty-Stephen, D. G., & Fausto-Sterling, A. (2020). Using vector autoregression modeling to reveal bidirectional relationships in gender/sex-related interactions in mother–infant dyads. *Frontiers in Psychology, 11*, 1507.

Fausey, C. M., Jayaraman, S., & Smith, L. B. (2016). From faces to hands: Changing visual input in the first two years. *Cognition, 152*, 101–107.

Ferjan Ramírez, N., Hippe, D. S., & Kuhl, P. K. (2021). Comparing automatic and manual measures of parent–infant conversational turns: A word of caution. *Child Development, 92*(2), 672–681.

Ford, M., Baer, C. T., Xu, D., Yapanel, U., & Gray, S. (2008). *The LENA™ language environment analysis system: Audio specifications of the DLP-0121.* www.lenafoundation.org/wp-content/uploads/2014/10/LTR- 03-2_Audio_Specifications.pdf

Franchak, J. M. (2019). Changing opportunities for learning in everyday life: Infant body position over the first year. *Infancy, 24*(2),187–209.

Franchak, J. M., Scott, V., & Luo, C. (2021). A contactless method for measuring full-day, naturalistic motor behavior using wearable inertial sensors. *Frontiers in Psychology, 12*, 4632.

Gilmore, R. O., Kennedy, J. L., & Adolph, K. E. (2018). Practical solutions for sharing data and materials from psychological research. *Advances in Methods and Practices in Psychological Science, 1*(1), 121–130.

Goodwin, M. S., Mazefsky, C. A., Ioannidis, S., Erdogmus, D., & Siegel, M. (2019). Predicting aggression to others in youth with autism using a wearable biosensor. *Autism Research, 12*(8), 1286–1296.

Granic, I., Hollenstein, T., & Lichtwarck-Aschoff, A. (2016). A survey of dynamic systems methods for developmental psychopathology. In D. Cicchetti (Ed.), *Developmental psychopathology*. Wiley.

Hamaker, E. L., & Wichers, M. (2017). No time like the present: Discovering the hidden dynamics in intensive longitudinal data. *Current Directions in Psychological Science, 26*(1), 10–15.

Han, S. C., Schacter, H. L., Timmons, A. C., Kim, Y., Sichko, S., Pettit, C., et al. (2021). Romantic partner presence and physiological responses in daily life: Attachment style as a moderator. *Biological Psychology, 161*, 108082.

Hensch, T. K. (2005). Critical period plasticity in local cortical circuits. *Nature Reviews Neuroscience, 6*(11), 877–888.

Hoch, J., Ossmy, O., Cole, W. G., Hasan, S., & Adolph, K. E. (2021). "Dancing" together: Infant-mother locomotor synchrony. *Child Development, 92*(4), 1337–1353.

Jayaraman, S., Fausey, C. M., & Smith, L. B. (2015). The faces in infant-perspective scenes change over the first year of life. *PLoS One, 10*(5), e0123780.

Jayaraman, S., & Smith, L. B. (2018). Faces in early visual environments are persistent not just frequent. *Vision Research, 157*, 213–221.

Johnson, M. L., Andres, L., Micheletti, M., Yao, X., & de Barbaro, K. (2020, July). *Who talks to babies? Multimodal ambulatory assessments predict hour-by-hour fluctuations in caregiver speech.* Paper presented at the International Conference on Infant Studies, Glasgow, Scotland.

Kadooka, K., Caufield, M., Fausey, C. M., & Franchak, J. (2021). *Visuomotor learning opportunities are nested within infants' everyday activities.* Paper presented at the Society for Research in Child Development.

Khante, P., Thomaz, E., & de Barbaro, K. (2023). *Detecting auditory household chaos in child-worn real-world audio.* Manuscript under review.

Lara, O. D., & Labrador, M. A. (2013). A survey on human activity recognition using wearable sensors. *IEEE Communications Surveys and Tutorials, 15*(3), 1192–1209.

Larsen, R. J., & Kasimatis, M. (1990). Individual differences in entrainment of mood to the weekly calendar. *Journal of Personality and Social Psychology, 58*(1), 164–171.

Levin, H. I., Egger, D., Andres, L., Johnson, M., Bearman, S. K., & de Barbaro, K. (2021). Sensing everyday activity: Parent perceptions and feasibility. *Infant Behavior and Development, 62*, 101511.

Long, B., Kachergis, G., Agrawal, K., & Frank, M. C. (2020). *Detecting social information in a dense dataset of infants' natural visual experience.* https://psyarxiv.com/z7tdg

Lopez, L. D., Walle, E. A., Pretzer, G. M., & Warlaumont, A. S. (2020). Adult responses to infant prelinguistic vocalizations are associated with infant vocabulary: A home observation study. *PloS One, 15*(11), e0242232.

Lungarella, M., Pegors, T., Bulwinkle, D., & Sporns, O. (2005). Methods for quantifying the informational structure of sensory and motor data. *Neuroinformatics, 3*(3), 243–262.

MacWhinney, B. (2000). *The CHILDES Project: Tools for analyzing talk* (3rd ed.). Erlbaum.

Madden-Rusnak, A., Micheletti, M., & de Barbaro, K. (2023). *Spontaneous infant crying modulates vagal activity in real time.* Manuscript under review.

Mason, G. M., Lokhandwala, S., Riggins, T., & Spencer, R. M. (2021). Sleep and human cognitive development. *Sleep Medicine Reviews, 57*, 101472.

Mehl, M. R. (2017). The electronically activated recorder (EAR): A method for the naturalistic observation of daily social behavior. *Current Directions in Psychological Science, 26*(2), 184–190.

Messinger, D. S., Prince, E. B., Zheng, M., Martin, K., Mitsven, S. G., Huang, S., et al. (2019). Continuous measurement of dynamic classroom social interactions. *International Journal of Behavioral Development, 43*(3), 263–270.

Mendoza, J. K., & Fausey, C. M. (2020). Everyday music in infancy. *Open Science Framework, 24*(6), e13122.

Mendoza, J. K., & Fausey, C. M. (2021a). Quantifying everyday ecologies: Principles for manual annotation of many hours of infants' lives. *Frontiers in Developmental Psychology, 12*, 710636.

Mendoza, J. K., & Fausey, C. M. (2021b). Everyday music in infancy. *Developmental Science, 24*(6), e13122.

Micheletti, M., de Barbaro, K., Fellows, M. D., Hixon, J. G., Slatcher, R. B., & Pennebaker,

J. W. (2020). Optimal sampling strategies for characterizing behavior and affect from ambulatory audio recordings. *Journal of Family Psychology, 34*(8), 980–990.

Molenaar, P. C., & Campbell, C. G. (2009). The new person-specific paradigm in psychology. *Current Directions in Psychological Science, 18*(2), 112–117.

Nastase, S. A., Goldstein, A., & Hasson, U. (2020). Keep it Real: Rethinking the primacy of experimental control in cognitive neuroscience. *NeuroImage, 222*, 117254.

Olthof, M., Hasselman, F., Strunk, G., van Rooij, M., Aas, B., Helmich, M. A., et al. (2020). Critical fluctuations as an early-warning signal for sudden gains and losses in patients receiving psychotherapy for mood disorders. *Clinical Psychological Science, 8*(1), 25–35.

Ram, N., Brose, A., & Molenaar, P. C. (2013). Dynamic factor analysis: Modeling person-specific process. In *The Oxford handbook of quantitative methods* (Vol. 2, pp. 441–457). Oxford University Press.

Ram, N., Yang, X., Cho, M. J., Brinberg, M., Muirhead, F., Reeves, B., et al. (2020). Screenomics: A new approach for observing and studying individuals' digital lives. *Journal of Adolescent Research, 35*(1), 16–50.

Ranson, K. E., & Urichuk, L. J. (2008). The effect of parent–child attachment relationships on child biopsychosocial outcomes: A review. *Early Child Development and Care, 178*(2), 129–152.

Räsänen, O., Seshadri, S., Karadayi, J., Riebling, E., Bunce, J., Cristia, A., et al. (2019). Automatic word count estimation from daylong child-centered recordings in various language environments using language-independent syllabification of speech. *Speech Communication, 113*, 63–80.

Räsänen O., Seshadri S., Lavechin M., Cristia A., & Casillas M. (2021). ALICE: An open-source tool for automatic measurement of phoneme, syllable, and word counts from child-centered daylong recordings. *Behavior Research Methods, 53*(2), 818–835.

Romeo, R. R., Leonard, J. A., Robinson, S. T., West, M. R., Mackey, A. P., Rowe, M. L., et al. (2018). Beyond the 30-million-word gap: Children's conversational exposure is associated with language-related brain function. *Psychological science, 29*(5), 700–710.

Roy, B. C., Frank, M. C., DeCamp, P., Miller, M., & Roy, D. (2015). Predicting the birth of a spoken word. *Proceedings of the National Academy of Sciences, 112*(41), 12663–12668.

Sadeh, A., Acebo, C., Seifer, R., Aytur, S., & Carskadon, M. A. (1995). Activity-based assessment of sleep–wake patterns during the 1st year of life. *Infant Behavior and Development, 18*, 329–337

Salo, V. C., Pannuto, P., Hedgecock, W., Biri, A., Russo, D. A., Piersiak, H. A., et al. (2021). Measuring naturalistic proximity as a window into caregiver-child interaction patterns. *Behavior Research Methods*, 1–15.

Scott, L. S., Pascalis, O., & Nelson, C. A. (2007). A domain-general theory of the development of perceptual discrimination. *Current Directions in Psychological Science, 16*(4), 197–201.

Schultz, A. A., Malecki, K., Olson, M. M., Selman, S. B., Olaiya, O. I., Spicer, A., et al. (2020). Investigating cumulative exposures among 3-to 4-year-old children using wearable ultrafine particle sensors and language environment devices: A pilot and feasibility study. *International Journal of Environmental Research and Public Health, 17*(14), 5259.

Smith, L. B., & Slone, L. K. (2017). A developmental approach to machine learning? *Frontiers in Psychology, 8*, 2124.

Smith, L. B., Yu, C., Yoshida, H., & Fausey, C. M. (2015). Contributions of head-mounted cameras to studying the visual environments of infants and young children. *Journal of Cognition and Development, 16*(3), 407–419.

Soderstrom, M., Casillas, M., Bergelson, E., Rosemberg, C. R., Alam, F., Warlaumont, A. S., et al. (2021). Developing a cross-cultural annotation system and metacorpus for studying infants' real world language experience. *Collabra: Psychology*, 7(1), 23445.

Soderstrom, M., & Wittebolle, K. (2013). When do caregivers talk?: The influences of activity and time of day on caregiver speech and child vocalizations in two childcare environments. *PloS One, 8*, e80646.

Spencer, J. P., Perone, S., & Buss, A. T. (2011). Twenty years and going strong: A dynamic systems revolution in motor and cognitive development. *Child Development Perspectives, 5*(4), 260–266.

Sugden, N. A., Mohamed-Ali, M. I., & Moulson,

M. C. (2014). I spy with my little eye: Typical, daily exposure to faces documented from a first-person infant perspective. *Developmental Psychobiology, 56*(2), 249–261.

Sullivan, J., Mei, M., Perfors, A., Wojcik, E. H., & Frank, M. C. (2022). SAYCam: A large, longitudinal audiovisual dataset recorded from the infant's perspective. *Open Mind, 5*, 20–29.

Szymczak, J. T., Jasińska, M., Pawlak, E., & Zwierzykowska, M. (1993). Annual and weekly changes in the sleep-wake rhythm of school children. *Sleep, 16*(5), 433–435.

Tamis-LeMonda, C. S., Kuchirko, Y., Luo, R., Escobar, K., & Bornstein, M. H. (2017). Power in methods: Language to infants in structured and naturalistic contexts. *Developmental Science, 20*(6), e12456.

Teti, D., Kim, B.-R., Mayer, G., & Countermine, M. (2010). Maternal emotional availability at bedtime predicts infant sleep quality. *Journal of Family Psychology, 24*(3), 307–315.

Thelen, E., & Smith, L. B. (1994*). A dynamic systems approach to the development of cognition and action*. MIT Press.

Tsutsui, S., Zhi, D., Reza, M. A., Crandall, D., & Yu, C. (2019). *Active object manipulation facilitates visual object learning: an egocentric vision study*. arXiv Preprint.

VanDam, M., Warlaumont, A. S., Bergelson, E., Cristia, A., Soderstrom, M., De Palma, P., et al. (2016). HomeBank: An online repository of daylong child-centered audio recordings. *Seminars in Speech and Language, 37*(2), 128–142.

Ward, J. S., Duncan, J. S., Jarden, A., & Stewart, T. (2016). The impact of children's exposure to greenspace on physical activity, cognitive development, emotional wellbeing, and ability to appraise risk. *Health and Place, 40*, 44–50.

Weisleder, A. & Fernald, A. (2013). Talking to children matters: Early language experience strengthens processing and builds vocabulary. *Psychological Science, 24*(11), 2143–2152.

Werker, J. F., & Hensch, T. K. (2015). Critical periods in speech perception: New directions. *Annual Review of Psychology, 66*, 173–196.

Wittenburg, P., Brugman, H., Russel, A., Klassmann, A., & Sloetjes, H. (2006). ELAN: A professional framework for multimodality research. *5th International Conference on Language Resources and Evaluation (LREC 2006)*, pp. 1556–1559.

Worobey, J. (2014). Physical activity in infancy: developmental aspects, measurement, and importance. *American Journal of Clinical Nutrition, 99*(3), 729–733.

Xu, T. L., de Barbaro, K., Abney, D. H., & Cox, R. F. (2020). Finding structure in time: visualizing and analyzing behavioral time series. *Frontiers in Psychology, 11*, 1457.

Yao, X., Johnson, M., Ploetz, T., & de Barbaro, K. (2019). Automated detection of infant holding using wearable sensing: Implications for developmental science and intervention. *Proceedings of the ACM on Interactive, Mobile, Wearable and Ubiquitous Technologies, 3*(2), 64.

Yao, X., Micheletti, M., Johnson, M., Thomaz, E., & de Barbaro, K. (2022). *Infant crying detection in real-world environments*. https://arxiv.org/abs/2005.07036.

Yu, C., & Smith, L. B. (2013). Joint attention without gaze following: Human infants and their parents coordinate visual attention to objects through eye-hand coordination. *PLoS One, 8*(11), e79659.

Zimmerman, F. J., Gilkerson, J., Richards, J. A., Christakis, D. A., Xu, D., Gray, S., et al. (2009). Teaching by listening: The importance of adult-child conversations to language development. *Pediatrics, 124*(1), 342–349.

CHAPTER 27

Mobile Sensing in Aging Research

Birthe Macdonald, Melanie Becker,
Mike Martin, and Christina Röcke

CHAPTER OVERVIEW

Mobile sensing provides unique opportunities to examine functional ability as a key indicator of healthy aging. Functional ability includes mobility as well as physical, social, and cognitive activities that older adults exhibit in their daily life environments. Sensing approaches facilitate the inclusion of older adults with varying levels and profiles of health, including those who are no longer able to actively report on their behavior. In addition, novel sensing tools such as smartphones, GPS trackers, accelerometers, and audio recorders can provide information on a diverse set of contexts that interact with person-level variables to shape individual functional ability trajectories. Research has provided promising results on late-life mobility, physical activity, and sleep derived from GPS and accelerometry in relation to well-being and cognition, as well as social and cognitive activity derived from naturally occurring speech and smartphone applications. The chapter closes with an outlook on design considerations and future directions for successful sensing in older adults.

Mobile Sensing in Aging: The Why and the What

It is expected that by 2050, the proportion of people over 60 years of age worldwide will have doubled from 2020 to approximately 20% (World Health Organization [WHO], 2020), life expectancy will increase, and chronic multimorbidity will be increasingly prevalent. In essence, one can anticipate that an increasing proportion of longer-living individuals will contract multiple chronic diseases who, at the same time, will be able to maintain high levels of functioning. Therefore, the WHO (2015) has now redefined healthy aging not as the absence of disease but as "the process of developing and maintaining the functional ability that enables well-being in older age" (p. 13). In this context, functional ability is understood as an individual's ability to *be and do* what they have reason to value. Thus, an individual's social, cognitive, or physical activities are defining features of the healthy aging concept. In fact, they represent the interactions of individual characteristics with society and environment, including building and maintaining social relationships, learning, being mobile, and being an active member of society. In line with this view, reliable ways of assessing, contextualizing, analyzing, and interpreting daily life activities are needed to improve our understanding of healthy aging.

Novel ways to collect data in the context of individuals' daily lives provide important improvements to healthy aging research in at least three ways. First, they go beyond cross-sectional, laboratory-based, and long-term longitudinal designs by capturing microlongitudinal and ecologically valid developmental trajectory data. These are amenable to the study of processes related to development and aging, including functional ability in essential life domains. Second, when used to collect introspective data, those methods reduce retrospective memory biases affecting traditional questionnaire methods. This use of ambulatory assessment (AA) approaches to aging research has predominantly included active mobile assessment methods such as electronically based experience sampling (for review, see Brose & Ebner-Priemer, 2015; Hoppmann & Riediger, 2009; Ebner-Priemer & Santangelo Chapter 13, this volume). As outlined in these reviews, AA-based experience sampling approaches have provided knowledge that enables researchers to understand age-related differences in a variety of everyday competencies. This includes emotional-motivational processes, both independently and in relation to social interactions, daily events and stress, as well as first insights into health and physiological processes and activities. Third, the measurement of high-density activity data contributes a new type of information for healthy aging research. Note that some activities related to healthy aging occur on time scales of milliseconds or seconds (e.g., affective responses or the unfolding of social interactions). These patterns are not predicted by stable person or environment characteristics, as they represent behavioral choices or adaptations across situations and contexts. Objectively capturing essential activity patterns and their interpretation-relevant situational contexts can provide the evidence needed to justify situation- and context-aware interventions. Furthermore, these patterns are often not accessible to self-report despite their relation to healthy aging (e.g., see the complexity of physical activity states; Paraschiv-Ionescu, Perruchoud, Buchser, & Aminian, 2012). Accordingly, this chapter, in line with the overall theme of this book, focuses on passive mobile sensing approaches, for we believe these approaches deserve increasing attention in aging research to help address important open issues. To complement this focus, we add a short section on AA of cognitive, social, and emotional activities at the end of this chapter.

Understanding Aging Inclusively and in Context: The Role of Mobile Sensing

Research on the context of healthy aging has mostly been conducted using self-report questionnaires. For example, social networks and interactions, representing an important context for development and aging, can be investigated by using questionnaires such as the convoy model (Antonucci, 1986; Antonucci, Ajrouch, & Birditt, 2014) and the Rochester Interaction Record (Reis & Wheeler, 1991). Questionnaire approaches also exist to assess the characteristics of a person's built neighborhood (i.e., neighborhood walkability; Saelens, Sallis, Black, & Chen, 2003). Mobility, as a behavioral reflection of one's exposure to and use of the built environment, can be measured with map-based questionnaires such as VERITAS (Chaix et al., 2012) or the Life Space Questionnaire (Fillekes, Röcke, Katana, & Weibel, 2019). However, due to the retrospective nature of these questionnaires as well as the cognitive abilities required to complete them, this type of data collection can be subject to reporting and population biases. Passive mobile sensing information combined with traditional experience sampling methods offer one way to overcome this limitation. Lin and Moudan (2010) pointed out that objective measures of the built environment provided higher associations with physical activity (i.e., walking) than self-reports. Therefore, utilizing mobile sensing methods will enable researchers to include older adults of a wide age range and with a variety of functional capabilities. In addition, being able to objectively and passively capture a proportion of participants' daily lives allows researchers to investigate some of the contextual factors that provide insights into environmental opportunities that represent daily life contexts in which aging and functional ability unfold, such as physical, social, and cognitively relevant context characteristics (e.g., Wolf, Seifert, Martin, & Oswald, 2021). Table 27.1 provides ideas on which patterns of context variables can be extracted from mobile sensing data.

This chapter reviews key examples of how mobile sensing technologies are implemented in aging research. It also suggests ways in which mobile sensing methods might be used in the future to further advance research methods and suggests some practical implications of monitoring older adults' functional ability in their day-to-day lives. Finally, this chapter will highlight issues that should be considered when using mobile sensing technologies with older adults. The most commonly used passive mobile sensing technologies to investigate aging-related phenomena are accelerometry and GPS tracking, the collection of audio samples to obtain natural speech data, and the passive sensing features in smartphones. (These methods are explained in more detail in the chapters in Part II of this volume.)

Studying Older Adults' Functional Ability in Their Daily Life Contexts

The WHO regards healthy aging as the functional ability "to be and to do what older individuals have reason to value" (WHO, 2015, p. 13). Thus, while the likelihood of having to adapt to changes due to disease and disability (both mental and physical) increases with age, this does not necessarily result in impaired functional ability that lasts for the remainder of an individual's life nor does it impact all aspects of a person's life. Even with degenerative diseases, decline can be domain-specific and progress at varying speeds. In addition, even when individuals receive (major) support, there are often ways in which they can maintain their functional ability. This is possible, for instance, when individuals find meaningful ways of engagement in selected areas of their lives, as indicated by relatively high and well-maintained levels of well-being and satisfaction with life until old age (Kunzmann, Richter, & Schmukle, 2013; Röcke &

TABLE 27.1. Examples of Variability in Context and Time Scale That Can Be Used for Between-Person and Within-Person Predictor Models

Context types	Examples of person-level characteristics and assessment (cross-sectional)	Examples of day-level patterns (within-person daily)	Examples of situation-level patterns (within-person momentary)
Physical context	Type of housing (apartment, house) Type of area (urban vs. rural) Neighborhood walkability Distance to closest park/ green recreational area Distance to closest blue area (e.g., river, lake) Proportion of time spent in blue and green versus other built environmental spaces	Number of places visited Daily lifespace Variety of place types visited Daily time spent out of home Daily time spent in blue/ green spaces	Type of place in current situation (public vs. private, outdoor vs. indoor, green vs. blue vs. neither) Place classification Place of interest Location of current social interaction
Social context	Marital status Number of children Living with someone	Number of persons interacted with Variety of social partners interacted with	Presence of others Type of others present Number of others present
Cognitive demands as context	Number of novel places visited on average Spatial orientation demands inferred from typical mobility behavior	Number of novel places visited daily Number of new routes taken (that are not part of usual mobility routines) daily	Type of interaction partner (e.g., familiar vs. unfamiliar) Type of current activity (e.g., cognitively complex vs. passive leisure)

Lachman, 2008; Wettstein, Schilling, Reidick, & Wahl, 2015). Thus, while participants might not be able to complete "traditional" pen-and-paper questionnaires or physical tasks and are, therefore, excluded from experiments or surveys, they might maintain their functional ability by "doing what they have reason to value" and engaging in a variety of activities in accordance with their abilities, as agents of their own development (Freund, 2008). Mobile sensing technology can facilitate the investigation of older adults' everyday activities and functional ability in passive ways, requiring little to no active effort from participants. This creates opportunities to study the heterogeneity of aging by being able to include the full range of aging and expand researchers' and society's view of life at advanced age. With increasing smartphone use in the older adult population, particularly the so-called young–old, a new opportunity for useful research implementations using mobile sensing of a wide range of activities (e.g., physical, social, cognitive) also in later life (Seifert, 2021) has arisen.

In the following, we briefly review selected studies that have used (passive) mobile sensing technologies to gain a new understanding of the heterogeneity of aging. We cover three major daily life domains that can be inferred from mobile sensing devices: spatial context, including mobility and physical activity; sensor-based assessments of social activities; and more active ways of investigating older adults' cognitive performance or cognitive activities and their correlates in daily life.

Spatial Context, Mobility, and Physical Activity

An early utilization of mobile sensing methods in research of age-related physical and spatial activity was to investigate frailty and predict falls using accelerometers (devices that record acceleration and orientation). Accelerometers can be used as devices by themselves, or they can be embedded in smartphones (Harari, Müller, Aung, Rentfrow, 2017). As falls are the leading cause of accidental death and injuries in older adults (Rubenstein, 2006), they constitute a major threat to functional ability maintenance, with significant physical and psychological consequences. A study by Klenk and colleagues (2015), for example, predicted falls from physical activity in the context of the Activity and Function in the Elderly in Ulm (ActiFE Ulm) study and found that participants with low physical activity and slow walking speed at baseline experienced the most falls per 100 hours walked over the next year. This might also be indicative of prior mobility issues and health problems associated with a higher risk of experiencing falls. Nevertheless, a recent review (Gillain et al., 2018) concluded that the literature on accelerometer-based fall detection is encouraging, but further studies are needed to highlight the cross-sectional and, more importantly, longitudinal relationships between gait parameters and falls in older adults. In addition to falls, accelerometers can also be used to investigate sleep in older adults to determine frailty and individuals' risk for becoming frail in the future (Ensrud et al., 2009, 2012). Researchers determined that a higher number of sleep disruptions was predictive of both current frailty status (Ensrud et al., 2009) and frailty status in male samples at follow-up 3 to 4 years later (Ensrud et al., 2012). Combining sleep assessment with physical activity assessment, Razjouyan and colleagues (2020) were able to predict not only physical frailty status but also cognitive frailty status in a sample of older adults over the age of 60 from their sleep patterns (sleeping position, time spent in bed, sleep onset latency, and total sleep time), as well as physical activity (time spent in sedentary activities, standing, walking, or doing moderate-to-vigorous exercise, as well as step counts). Using accelerometer data in this way might not only facilitate valid, inclusive research on older adults' cognitive and physical status, but might also enable clinicians to monitor patients and predict, to a certain extent, their prospective physical and cognitive trajectories.

In addition to the investigation of falls in relation to cognitive and physical decline, smartphones offer an additional relevant sensor, namely, GPS (satellite connections that track individuals' position in geographical space). GPS can be used in addition to and in combination with accelerometer sensors to examine facilitating conditions and environmental contexts related to older adults' activities. Determining conditions that facilitate functional ability in older adults include investigating individuals' spatial contexts, that is, their neighborhoods and places they visit, as well as their daily mobility, i.e., whether and how they move between destinations, including the level of physical activity they engage in (Harari, Green, Zelber-Sagi, 2015). Using multiples of these data sources jointly increases the predictive power of machine learning approaches to support analysis of activity data from young and older adults (e.g., Allahbakhshi, Röcke, & Weibel, 2021).

Neighborhood characteristics can influence the independence of older adults in a multitude of ways, including recovery from illness, physical activity, as well as the ability to perform activities of daily living (Beard et al., 2016; Cannuscio, Block, & Kawachi, 2003; Mendes de Leon et al., 2009; Wen & Christakis, 2005). However, lifespace, which "refers to the area within which a person moved over a specific period of time" (Fillekes,

Giannouli, Kim, Zijlstra, & Weibel, 2019, p. 3) is typically defined by "residential buffers" (the space immediately surrounding individuals' place of residence), and spaces older adults move in that fall outside of their immediate environment can be missed. Using data from the "Walk the Talk" study, researchers investigated different ways to characterize lifespace in older adults in Vancouver (Hirsch, Winters, Ashe, Clarke, & McKay, 2016; Hirsch, Winters, Clarke, & McKay, 2014). They found that lifespace was better defined by GPS data than by residential buffers. Specifically, older adults' lifespace was defined by key destinations they might visit regularly, such as supermarkets or post offices. In addition, a larger number of destinations on participants' routine walking or cycling routes was associated with higher physical activity. The same was found in a study of older Belgian adults: Those who lived in neighborhoods that included a larger number of destinations in a walkable distance showed higher levels of physical activity as indicated by accelerometer data (Van Holle et al., 2014). This suggests that living close to spaces that combine a number of facilities that need to be visited regularly might facilitate walking or cycling instead of using the car. Similarly, older adults in New York City also regularly moved outside of their immediate environment (York Cornwell & Cagney, 2017), with 25% of participants spending more than 50% of their time outside of their immediate residential area. Interestingly, use of public transport has also been found to be associated with increased physical activity in older adults (Mikolaizak, Klenk, Rothenbacher, Denkinger, & Rapp, 2019; Voss et al., 2016). This means access to public transport may contribute to older adults' prolonged functional ability in two ways: Having access to public transport in walking distance facilitates physical activity, as does continued engagement in activities that can be accessed by public transport.

In contrast to older adults living in urban environments who have access to public transport, older adults in rural areas often tend to be highly reliant on their cars. Hanson and Hildebrand (2011) found that nonaccess to a vehicle was associated with reduced activities—older adults indicated that they would not take trips for which they did not have access to a car or friends or family to assist them. This challenge likely differs by global region, with rural public transport infrastructure being much higher in Switzerland versus the United States, for example. The urban–rural comparison, however, highlights, how rural and urban environments typically represent life contexts that provide different opportunities and obstacles for older adults, and it suggests a need for specific, older-adult-focused solutions to allow nondriving individuals in particular to continue to live an active life.

GPS-derived lifespace has been found to be associated with cognitive abilities in older adults. Increasing levels of cognitive impairment are typically associated with growing difficulties orienting, navigating, and completing different activities outside of the home (Petersen et al., 2001; Petersen & Morris, 2003). These difficulties might significantly reduce the number of activities older adults with beginning cognitive impairments feel confident they can engage in, thereby reducing their independence.

Wettstein, Wahl, Shoval, Oswald, and colleagues (2015) assessed out-of-home activities using combined GPS and questionnaire data and classified it at different levels of complexity (i.e., analyzing out-of-home walking distance, duration, and speed; global indicators of out-of-home mobility; duration and number of locations visited; and specific out-of-home activities, e.g., number and frequency of physically and cognitively demanding activities). Aiming to investigate whether cognitive status (cognitively healthy [CH] versus mild cognitive impairment [MCI] versus early-stage Alzheimer's-type dementia

[AD]) could be predicted from these activities, they found that the AD group could be distinguished from CH and MCI when considering activities at a medium complexity level (total amount of time spent outside individuals' homes). Significant differences between all three groups could only be detected when the total number of cognitively demanding activities outside of home during the study period was considered, that is, when GPS data was enriched with meaningful questionnaire data.

In support of the idea that mobility is an important predictor of well-being in older adults, the same group also found that older adults with more severe cognitive (Alzheimer's-type dementia) or physical difficulties showed reduced mobility compared to healthier older adults (Wettstein, Wahl, Shoval, Auslander, et al., 2015). However, it is important to note here that sociodemographic and physical health indicators were more predictive of mobility in this group of older adults than cognitive status. Alzheimer's dementia has also been associated with smaller lifespace in older adults, which in turn, is related to reduced physical function and increased apathy and depression (Tung et al., 2014).

From a within-person perspective, mobile assessment can provide a major improvement in the type of studies examining population trends for cross-context mobility measures. As an example, despite the significant difference in orientation ability between persons diagnosed with cognitive impairment versus nonimpaired, Schaat, Koldrack, Yordanova, Kirste, and Teipel (2020), using high-density movement data, showed that individuals with cognitive impairment behaved in an oriented manner in up to 99% of all observed real-life situations. Thus, investing in the development and testing of individual and contextualized predictor models to detect instances of orientation or other functional ability-defining activities seems a highly useful approach. In fact, there is increasing interest in finding reliable and valid ways of assessing physical activity and mobility "in the wild" in addition to controlled clinical settings, and to understanding the relation between the two types of assessments, particularly in the movement sciences (see, e.g., Allahbakhshi et al., 2021; Soltani, Dejnabadi, Savary, & Aminian, 2020; Warmerdam et al., 2020).

In addition to the association between mobility and cognitive status, longitudinal studies assessing self-reported physical activity also showed that reduced mobility might be a risk factor for cognitive decline and dementia (Abbott et al., 2004; Buchman et al., 2012; Weuve et al., 2004). On the other hand, more time spent outside or in physical activities was associated not only with better physical functioning but also with more positive affective outcomes (Kerr et al., 2012; Mollenkopf et al., 2004; Mollenkopf, Marcellini, Ruoppilla, Széman, & Tacken, 2005). Interestingly, the benefits of physical activity for mood vary across the week: Weekend activities have a greater effect than midweek activities (Kaspar, Oswald, Wahl, Voss, & Wettstein, 2015). This highlights how continuous data collection can uncover such within-person variations.

Physical activity has also been shown to be related to social aspects of older adults' lives. Social support and social network size were found to be important facilitating factors for physical activity in older adults, suggesting that interventions to encourage older adults to engage in physical activity might benefit from a social component, such as when they join a walking group (Beenackers, Kamphuis, Mackenbach, Burdorf, & van Lenthe, 2013; Carlson et al., 2012). Furthermore, Herbolsheimer, Mosler, and Peter (2017) combined accelerometer data with self-reported social isolation and activity diaries and showed that low levels of indoor physical activity were associated with isolation from kin networks, while low levels of outdoor activity were associated with isolation from nonkin networks. Similarly, it has been shown that spending time with a greater number of loose social ties was associated with higher overall physical activity (Fingerman, Huo, Charles, & Umberson, 2020); explaining findings by studies showing the physical benefits of older adults moving within a diverse social network (Baker, Cahalin, Gerst, & Burr, 2005; Litwin & Shiovitz-Ezra, 2006). In contrast, Mikolaizak and colleagues (2019) found that social contacts increased time spent out-of-home but decreased physical activity. However, this finding might be due to participants' engaging in sedentary activities with their social contacts.

These diverse findings illustrate how social networks are intertwined with physical activity, suggesting one mechanism in which social context might influence older adults' physical health. The pattern of different relations also illustrates the benefits of combining continuous mobile sensing data with self-report data. This will facilitate a full understanding of the implications and functional correlation and consequences, and thus provide meaningful insights into factors that might facilitate functional health.

GPS and accelerometry are thus valuable ways to assess older adults' physical living conditions, which are related to a number of functional health aspects such as cognition, mental health, and physical activity. These mobile sensing methods have enabled researchers to accurately track older adults' movements to determine environmental characteristics that facilitate mobility and physical activity. Furthermore, associations have been drawn suggesting that cognitive decline is a limiting factor for mobility, possibly due to growing disorientation and resulting insecurities in navigating the environment. Sensor-based activity and mobility data can be quantified beyond mean levels to identify more in-depth time-based activity and mobility patterns (e.g., indicators of complexity of the behavior; see Zhang et al., 2018). In addition, physical activity has also been found to be related to mood. In the future, researchers might be able to suggest measures that alleviate these issues and help older adults maintain their independence for longer periods of time, which, in turn, might positively influence older adults' cognitive performance. The successful use of GPS and accelerometer data to assess lifespaces in older adults with reduced cognitive capacity shows its potential to assess activities and functional capabilities in a variety of individuals, including the "oldest-old." This population is currently underresearched, partly because of the incidence of cognitive and physical limitations.

Social Context and Activities: Speech-Based Analysis of Healthy Aging

Given the importance of social connectedness and activities for health and concerns of growing loneliness particularly in later life, mobile sensing has also been used to examine various characteristics of social interactions in older adults' daily lives (for a review, see Fingerman, Birditt, & Umberson, 2020). In the past, this study was mainly done by using active sensing via smartphone-assessed self-reports. However, smartphones also include a wide range of embedded sensors that provide a wide array of passive assessments of social activities, such as the use of microphone, phone, and social networking and communication apps to infer interpersonal activities (Harari et al., 2017). With increasing smartphone use by the older segments of the population (Anderson & Perrin, 2017; Seifert, 2020; Seifert & Schelling, 2015), these approaches yield new ways to gain insights into older adults' social activities. In addition, ambient sound recordings can also inform about (social) environments such as participants' location or activities, for example, whether participants are at home or out of home and whether they are working, watching TV, or doing housework (Mehl & Robbins, 2012). Thus, employing such a technique has the potential to inform researchers about aspects of older adults' daily lives independently of their functional ability and enables them to infer a multitude of aspects such as social connectedness, formal or informal help. Nevertheless, most of the research employing this method focuses on specific aspects of social interactions, such as content and style of interaction (e.g., what the interactions are about and whether they contain specific emotion words or temporal aspects), often in relation to emotional expressions, as well as aspects of general language use within interactions (Brianza & Demiray, 2019; Demiray, Mehl, & Martin, 2018; Herbette & Rimé, 2004; Polsinelli, Moseley, Grilli, Glisky, & Mehl, 2020; Wank et al., 2020).

A recent study, however, utilized the EAR (electronically activated recorder; Mehl, 2017) method to investigate the frequency of older adults' daily interaction frequency and mood and to compare married to divorced and widowed individuals (Ng, Huo, Han, Birditt, & Fingerman, 2021). The researchers found that while married older adults had the highest number of daily conversations, divorced participants had more conversations through contact with friends than married participants. Higher interaction frequency was associated with improved mood across groups, but this effect was stronger in widowed than in married participants.

Studies in younger populations reveal promising strategies to analyze affective expressions with or without an interaction partner: In a study on chronic pain, Herbette and Rimé (2004) found that patients' psychological adjustment hinged not only on their physical well-being but also on how well they could communicate their health problems to others: Psychological adjustment correlated negatively with patients' belief that talking about their health problem would strain others and with the perception of others' disbelief toward their health problem. Although this study did not employ passive sensing methods, the results underline the relevance of investigating social contextual factors to improve coping with the increasing number of health issues as individuals age. In a similar fashion to the investigation of expressions of age-related difficulties, ambient sound recordings could be used to examine positive expressions such as laughter to gain further insights into the contexts that enhance older adults' mood, activity, and health. Recently, Sun, Schwartz, Son, Kern, and Vazire (2020) suggested a novel method to analyze EAR data that allows inferences about daily fluctuations in emotions. They rely not only on language markers suggested in linguistic programs but also on exploration of other language variables derived from open-vocabulary approaches (clusters of data-driven semantically related words). Sentiment analysis is yet another approach to extracting information on emotion semantics from naturally occurring texts (even in combination with georeference information about spatial locations), such as those in social media use (e.g., Shaughnessy et al., 2018; Sykora, Jackson, O'Brien, & Elayan, 2013). These novel ways to analyze EAR and nonspeech text data are paving the way for a more in-depth investigation of affective processes in older adults' lives.

In addition to specific aspects of affective expressions and experience, the EAR-derived general quality of social interactions (small talk vs. substantive conversations) is also associated with life satisfaction and happiness (Milek et al., 2018; Sun, Harris, & Vazire, 2020). Especially when facing age-related losses, older adults can be at risk of social isolation and loneliness. Therefore, employing passive sensing to investigate the quantity and quality of older adults' daily interactions without relying on potentially biased self-reports will be a valuable focus of future research.

Thus, passive sensing of ambient sounds is a promising tool in the study of aging, as it allows researchers to investigate psychologically interesting aspects of functional ability in older adults' daily lives, such as affect, as well as aspects of social interactions and networks. Furthermore, it can add to GPS- and accelerometer-derived location and activity data or as a method to link daily activity data and contexts to social activities. Alternatively, it can be used to infer cognitive functions from daily interactions, as highlighted in the following section.

Sensing of Daily Life Cognitive Activities and Performance

Cognitive functioning outside of the lab has been examined using ambulatory cognitive tasks developed on the basis of their psychometric laboratory-based versions and by passive sensing methods utilizing smartphones or ambient sound recordings. Sliwinski and colleagues (2018) have introduced a battery of AA cognitive tests administered on smartphones for use in daily life research, measuring perceptual speed, executive functioning, and working memory. A subset of these has been used, for example, to investigate the association between EMA-derived social interactions and cognitive performance in older adults (Zhaoyang, Scott Martire, & Sliwinski, 2021). The authors examined different features of older adults' daily social interactions (i.e., frequency, quality, and partner types) in relation to fluctuations in cognitive performance throughout the day. Their results indicated that more frequent, particularly pleasant, social interactions were related to same-day cognitive performance; this relation also held for performance over the following 2 days. This association was most pronounced for older adults with overall lower mean levels of social interactions. No evidence was found for the opposite direction of cognitive performance predicting social interaction fluctuations.

Using a combination of the same ambulatory cognition tasks, combined with sleep measures derived from actigraphy, Derby, Zhaoyang, Jiao, Sliwinski, and Buxton (2020) showed that poorer sleep quality (e.g., waking after onset of sleep) was related to worse performance in working memory, memory binding, and processing speed, on both the between-person and within-person level. Sleep duration, however, showed no such associations with daily life cognition. Other researchers used another smartphone-based ambulatory working memory task (i.e., numerical or visual updating) in samples of children as well as young and older adults (e.g., Galeano Weber, Dirk, & Schmiedek, 2018; Riediger et al., 2014; Röcke et al., 2023) to examine associations between daily fluctuations in cognition, affect, and sleep. Traditional laboratory-based cognitive tests have thus successfully been implemented in novel mobile versions and applications.

In addition to these ambulatory cognitive tasks that mimic their laboratory counterparts, an alternative passive data source for daily cognitive sensing is naturally occurring speech data obtained with the EAR. It can be used to analyze language markers as indicators of cognitive activity. Polsinelli and colleagues (2020) utilized the Linguistic Inquiry and Word Count (LIWC; Pennebaker, Francis, & Booth, 2001) to analyze individuals' language use and found that executive function was positively associated with higher levels of analytic language use, the use of more complex words (words of more than six letters) and numbers. In addition, better executive function was also related to a less positive verbal tone and to the use of more swear and sexual words. Working memory capacity mainly drove those effects, and participants with higher working memory capacity also showed less verbal present focus in the content of their speech.

The focus on past, present, or future in older adults' everyday language use was examined in other studies employing the EAR method (Brianza & Demiray, 2019; Demiray et al., 2018; Demiray, Mischler, & Martin, 2019). Demiray and colleagues (2018) found that young and older adults did not differ in their "conversational time travel"—the extent to which they talked about the past or the future—with past-oriented utterances being significantly more frequent than future-oriented utterances in both age groups. To further investigate temporal referencing in older adults' utterances, Demiray and colleagues (2019) focused on older adults' reminiscence, the recall of meaningful past experiences, in social interactions. They found variability in the frequency of reminiscing in older adults ranging from 0 to 29% of utterances. Depending on the interlocutor, reminiscing served different functions, mostly for conversational purposes, but also to give advice to others (especially when talking to their children) or for identity affirmation (when talking with their partner or children). Reminiscing for these three purposes was generally positively related to life satisfaction.

Recently, Wank and colleagues (2020) investigated older adults' sharing of autobiographical memories compared to a younger group of adults. They found that older adults generally shared fewer episodic and semantic autobiographical memories. In contrast, they found less robust effects for the sharing of future thoughts, although the sharing of semantic future thoughts was also negatively associated with age. These examples highlight that cognitive activities cannot only be assessed by means of active momentary assessment methods using established test batteries, but that passive sensing can provide information about cognition on a situational level.

Complementing mobile cognitive test applications and speech and language markers of cognition, a third and very recent development in sensing research focuses on smartphone-derived data on human–computer interactions (e.g., swipes, taps, and keystroke events). These interactions have been proposed as digital biomarkers (i.e., passive sensing) of cognitive functioning in a small sample of young adults, with reliable associations to standard psychometric tests of a range of cognitive abilities, including working memory, memory, executive functioning, and verbal fluency (Dagum, 2018). This approach could provide a promising avenue for research on cognitive aging as well. In a similar vein, machine learning has been used increasingly to analyze the intensive longitudinal data streams obtained from sensing to predict cognitive abilities from a wide range of data. This includes at-home mobility tracking applied to predicting broader cognitive functioning in older adults with and without cognitive impairments (Botros et al., 2022); naturally occurring speech to predict social reminiscence behavior (Ferrario, Demiray, Yordanova, Luo, & Martin, 2020); and machine learning used to identify real world situations of adequate spatial orientation or disorientation in later life (Schaat et al., 2020).

Design Considerations and Future Directions for Successful Mobile Sensing in Older Adult Samples

One central advantage of using mobile sensing technologies in psychological research, especially in aging research, is that these technologies enable researchers to collect data relatively unobtrusively, without the need for much active involvement of individuals.

This paves the way to involve individuals who are not yet routinely included in aging research, for example, those who would no longer be able to complete pen-and-paper questionnaires due to reduced cognitive or physical abilities. Nevertheless, mobile sensing requires more technical knowledge from both the researcher and the participant (Seifert, Hofer, & Allemand, 2018). Therefore, additional resources and training regimes to familiarize participants (or caretakers) with the use and operation of the sensors are needed to support participants during data collection, for example, reminding them to charge the device if necessary or to wear the device throughout the day. It is therefore recommended that research assistants be on call for participants to support them with potentially malfunctioning hard- or software. Most of the data that have been used during the studies reviewed here could be collected on participants' own smartphones, which reduces the strain on participants somewhat if they routinely carry a phone on them. However, data quality might be reduced if participants carry their phone in their pockets rather than (openly) on their waist. In addition, some of the individuals who are routinely excluded from scientific studies (as outlined above) might not own a smartphone or may not remember to charge it regularly and to carry it on their person due to physical or cognitive impairments (Dagum, 2018). However, the situation is likely to change in future generations of older adults for whom smartphone usage and possession are likely to be much more common. It is also important to employ and develop sensors that can easily and reliably capture a variety of functional ability domains to avoid the need to use multiple sensors (e.g., a state-of-the-art accelerometer and state-of-the-art GPS tracker in addition to a smartphone) which could be especially taxing for older adults. One attempt to develop such a sensor and obtain multidomain real-life activity and context data was recently made in the Mobility, Activity, and Social Interaction Study (MOASIS; Röcke et al., 2023). In this study, a custom-built sensor assessed continuous GPS data, continuous accelerometer data, and audio recordings in a predefined schedule for 90-second windows every 18 minutes over 30 days (following EAR recommendations by Mehl & Robbins, 2012). A mute button was provided for moments that participants wanted to keep out of the study. These sensing data were complemented by experience sampling and mobile cognitive tests carried out on a smartphone multiple times a day over the first 2 weeks of the month-long study period.

Similarly, combining mobile sensing methodology with information obtained through traditional questionnaires can supply researchers with important additional insights. One study identified highly active older adults from their self-reported and accelerometer data to investigate factors that older adults themselves saw as facilitating for physical activity. This revealed both internal (e.g., self-control) and external aspects of their living context. The living context corresponded to some of the GPS studies: social connections and a facilitating environment (shops, the post office in walking distance; available green spaces) were seen as important determinants of activity (Franke, Tong, Ashe, McKay, & Sims-Gould, 2013). This illustrates the informative value of using mobile sensing technologies and shows the added value of combining it with additional information (see also Shoval et al., 2010; Wettstein, Wahl, Shoval, Oswald et al., 2015).

Fillekes, Röcke, and colleagues (2019) also showed that both self-report and sensor data sources can provide distinct types of information in a direct comparison between self-reported and sensor-assessed mobility information in community-dwelling older adults (those not institutionalized) age 65 and older. Whereas moderate to high within-person correlations between the two data sources were obtained overall, suggesting that both roughly capture comparable information if only one source is available, there were some indicator-specific distinctions. For example, lifespace self-reports slightly underestimated mobility compared to GPS assessments. In contrast, when asked about their active and passive modes of transport, that is, getting from A to B via car or public transport versus walking or cycling, older adults greatly overestimated their mobility when reporting it compared to the sensor-based measures.

Similarly, Bayat and colleagues (2020) developed an algorithm to infer outdoor destinations and activity types directly from GPS data, and they compared it with participants' self-report. Although the algorithm was fairly accurate in classifying destinations and activities, the authors noted that this might depend on neighborhood characteristics such as destination density and walkability (i.e., participants' ability to walk between destinations vs. dependence on a car). Therefore, algorithm accuracy might differ between rural and urban areas, and passively collected mobile sensing data alone might not yet be informative without individual subjective classification (as is often the case in psychological research).

Thus, although the use of mobile sensing methods has a promising future, the addition of subjective self-report data, for example, in the form of traditional experience sampling, remains essential to classify and semantically annotate passive mobile sensing data and advance research on healthy aging in context, including the oldest-old.

Conclusions

The first important steps in aging research have been undertaken to investigate daily life experiences and functioning in later life more closely. A wide range of research has been done on socioemotional, cognitive, and self-related processes captured through repeated laboratory assessments, diary methods, and paper-based and mobile experience sampling (e.g., Birditt, Fingerman, & Almeida, 2005; Huo, Fuentecilla, Birditt, & Fingerman, 2019; Röcke, Li, & Smith, 2009). These self-report approaches often lack a clear focus on incorporating information on functional ability within environmental contexts beyond social interactions, and they still require an active response by participants (i.e., active sensing). More recently, novel mobile sensing approaches have been introduced to aging research. These approaches provide unique opportunities to include a wider range of the aging population (i.e., also individuals with greater difficulties in providing valid self-reports); to obtain information less intrusively and potentially in a more reliable way (i.e., certain time-based estimates about one's activities have proven difficult to make; e.g., Fillekes, Röcke, et al., 2019; Wrzus & Mehl, 2015); and to capture a diverse range of functional ability indicators in daily life contexts as important indicators of healthy aging. Despite the fact that as a society we are living to more advanced ages than ever before, adults are often seen as one homogeneous group once they reach 65. This is particularly apparent when it comes to health advice. More often than not, age is seen as the defining risk factor for certain diseases. For example, during the COVID-19 pandemic, individuals older than 65 were warned to strictly socially distance because it was assumed that they were universally at risk of more severe outcomes from the virus. However, it has also been shown that social distancing bears the risk of increased loneliness and negative affect (González-Sanguino et al., 2020; Losada-Baltar et al., 2020;

Macdonald & Hülür, 2021; Zacher & Rudolph, 2021). In addition, it is likely that other aspects of individuals' life spaces and activities, and not chronological age by itself, influence well-being and functional ability (see also the classic writings of Wohlwill, 1970). It is, therefore, vital to gain a better understanding of the systematic heterogeneity and across-situation variability within this group so that more targeted recommendations can be made and personalized and context-sensitive interventions can be developed that consider the diversity of individuals and daily life situations (e.g., Nahum-Shani et al., 2018). Furthermore, the WHO (2015) defined the improvement of aging research and monitoring to be more inclusive of diverse global aging populations as a key action for the Decade of Healthy Aging 2020–2030. As outlined in this chapter, we believe that mobile sensing technologies can be one step on the way toward meeting that goal and in providing real-life contextualized information on many functional ability domains that cannot be directly assessed via active sensing tools.

ACKNOWLEDGMENTS

The preparation of parts of this chapter was supported by Swiss National Science Foundation Grant No. CRS115_186239 (to Birthe Macdonald and Melanie Becker) and Velux Stiftung Grant No. 917 (to Mike Martin and Christina Röcke), and by the European Union's Horizon 2020 research and innovation program under Grant Agreement No. 769643 (to Christina Röcke).

REFERENCES

Abbott, R. D., White, L. R., Ross, G. W., Masaki, K. H., Curb, J. D., & Petrovitch, H. (2004). Walking and dementia in physically capable elderly men. *The Journal of the American Medical Association, 292*(12), 1447–1453.

Allahbakhshi, H., Röcke, C., & Weibel, R. (2021). Assessing the transferability of physical activity type detection models: Influence of age group is underappreciated. *Frontiers in Physiology, 12*, 1–15.

Anderson, M., & Perrin, A. (2017, May 17). *Tech adoption climbs among older Americans.* Pew Research Center. www.pewresearch.org/internet/2017/05/17/tech-adoption-climbs-among-older-adults.

Antonucci, T. C. (1986). Hierarchical mapping technique. *Generations: Journal of the American Society on Aging, 10*(4), 10–12.

Antonucci, T. C., Ajrouch, K. J., & Birditt, K. S. (2014). The convoy model: Explaining social relations from a multidisciplinary perspective. *The Gerontologist, 54*(1), 82–92.

Baker, L. A., Cahalin, L. P., Gerst, K., & Burr, J. A. (2005). Productive activities and subjective well-being among older adults: The influence of number of activities and time commitment. *Social Indicators Research, 73*(3), 431–458.

Bayat, S., Naglie, G., Rapoport, M. J., Stasiulis, E., Chikhaoui, B., & Mihailidis, A. (2020). Inferring destinations and activity types of older adults from GPS data: Algorithm development and validation. *JMIR Aging, 3*(2), 1–14.

Beard, J. R., Officer, A., de Carvalho, I. A., Sadana, R., Pot, A. M., Michel, J.-P., et al. (2016). The World report on ageing and health: A policy framework for healthy ageing. *Lancet, 387*(10033), 2145–2154.

Beenackers, M. A., Kamphuis, C. B. M., Mackenbach, J. P., Burdorf, A., & van Lenthe, F. J. (2013). Why some walk and others don't: Exploring interactions of perceived safety and social neighborhood factors with psychosocial cognitions. *Health Education Research, 28*(2), 220–233.

Birditt, K. S., Fingerman, K. L., & Almeida, D. M. (2005). Age differences in exposure and reactions to interpersonal tensions: A daily diary study. *Psychology and Aging, 20*(2), 330–340.

Botros, A., Schütz, N., Röcke, C., Weibel, R., Martin, M., Müri, R., et al. (2022). Eigenbehaviour as an indicator of cognitive abilities. *Sensors*, 22(7):2769.

Brianza, E., & Demiray, B. (2019). Future time perspective and real-life utterances about the future in young and older adults. *Journal of Gerontopsychology and Geriatric Psychiatry, 32*(4), 161–173.

Brose, A., & Ebner-Priemer, U. W. (2015). Ambulatory assessment in the research on aging: Contemporary and future applications. *Gerontology, 61*(4), 372–380.

Buchman, A. S., Boyle, P. A., Yu, L., Shah, R. C., Wilson, R. S., & Bennett, D. A. (2012). Total daily physical activity and the risk of AD and cognitive decline in older adults. *Neurology, 78*(17), 1323–1329.

Cannuscio, C., Block, J., & Kawachi, I. (2003). Social capital and successful aging: The role of senior housing. *Annals of Internal Medicine, 139*(5, Pt. 2), 395–399.

Carlson, J. A., Sallis, J. F., Conway, T. L., Saelens, B. E., Frank, L. D., Kerr, J., et al. (2012). Interactions between psychosocial and built environment factors in explaining older adults' physical activity. *Preventive Medicine, 54*(1), 68–73.

Chaix, B., Kestens, Y., Perchoux, C., Karusisi, N., Merlo, J., & Labadi, K. (2012). An interactive mapping tool to assess individual mobility patterns in neighborhood studies. *American Journal of Preventive Medicine, 43*(4), 440–450.

Dagum, P. (2018). Digital biomarkers of cognitive function. *npj Digital Medicine, 1*(10), 1–3.

Demiray, B., Mehl, M. R., & Martin, M. (2018). Conversational time travel: Evidence of a retrospective bias in real life conversations. *Frontiers in Psychology, 9*, 1–18.

Demiray, B., Mischler, M., & Martin, M. (2019). Reminiscence in everyday conversations: A naturalistic observation study of older adults. *Journals of Gerontology: Series B, 74*(5), 745–755.

Derby, C. A., Zhaoyang, R., Jiao, J. L., Sliwinski, M. J., & Buxton, O. M. (2020). Within and between person effects of sleep quality on daily cognitive performance: Data from the Einstein Aging Study (EAS). *Alzheimer's and Dementia, 16*(S10), 596–608.

Ensrud, K. E., Blackwell, T. L., Ancoli-Israel, S., Redline, S., Cawthon, P. M., Paudel, M. L., et al. (2012). Sleep disturbances and risk of frailty and mortality in older men. *Sleep Medicine, 13*(10), 1217–1225.

Ensrud, K. E., Blackwell, T. L., Redline, S., Ancoli-Israel, S., Paudel, M. L., Cawthon, P. M. et al. (2009). Sleep disturbances and frailty status in older community-dwelling men. *Journal of the American Geriatrics Society, 57*(11), 2085–2093.

Ferrario, A., Demiray, B., Yordanova, K., Luo, M., & Martin, M. (2020). Social reminiscence in older adults' everyday conversations: Automated prediction using natural language processing and machine learning. *Journal of Medical Internet Research, 22*(9), e19133.

Fillekes, M. P., Giannouli, E., Kim, E.-K., Zijlstra, W., & Weibel, R. (2019). Towards a comprehensive set of GPS-based indicators reflecting the multidimensional nature of daily mobility for applications in health and aging research. *International Journal of Health Geographics, 18*, 1–20.

Fillekes, M. P., Röcke, C., Katana, M., & Weibel, R. (2019). Self-reported versus GPS-derived indicators of daily mobility in a sample of healthy older adults. *Social Science and Medicine, 220*, 193–202.

Fingerman, K. L., Birditt, K. S., & Umberson, D. J. (2020). Use of technologies for social connectedness and well-being and as a tool for research data collection in older adults. In National Academies of Sciences, Engineering, Medicine (Eds.), *Mobile technology for adaptive aging: Proceedings of a workshop* (pp. 67–84). National Academies Press.

Fingerman, K. L., Huo, M., Charles, S. T., & Umberson, D. J. (2020). Variety is the spice of late life: Social integration and daily activity. *Journals of Gerontology: Series B, 75*(2), 377–388.

Franke, T., Tong, C., Ashe, M. C., McKay, H., & Sims-Gould, J. (2013). The secrets of highly active older adults. *Journal of Aging Studies, 27*(4), 398–409.

Freund, A. M. (2008). Successful aging as management of resources: The role of selection, optimization, and compensation. *Research in Human Development, 5*(2), 94–106.

Galeano Weber, E. M., Dirk, J., & Schmiedek, F. (2018). Variability in the precision of children's spatial working memory. *Journal of Intelligence, 6*(1), 1–19.

Gillain, S., Boutaayamou, M., Beaudart, C., Demonceau, M., Bruyère, O., Reginster, J. Y., et al. (2018). Assessing gait parameters with accelerometer-based methods to identify older adults at risk of falls: A systematic review. *European Geriatric Medicine, 9*(4), 435–448.

González-Sanguino, C., Ausín, B., Castellanos, M. Á., Saiz, J., López-Gómez, A., Ugidos, C., et al. (2020). Mental health consequences during the initial stage of the 2020 Coronavirus pandemic (COVID-19) in Spain. *Brain, Behavior, and Immunity, 87*, 172–176.

Hanson, T. R., & Hildebrand, E. D. (2011). Can rural older drivers meet their needs without a car? Stated adaptation responses from a GPS travel diary survey. *Transportation, 38*(6), 975–992.

Harari, G., Green, M. S., & Zelber-Sagi, S. (2015). Combined association of occupational and leisure-time physical activity with all-cause and coronary heart disease mortality among a cohort of men followed-up for 22 years. *Occupational and Environmental Medicine, 72*(9), 617–624.

Harari, G. M., Müller, S. R., Aung, M. S., & Rentfrow, P. J. (2017). Smartphone sensing methods for studying behavior in everyday life. *Current Opinion in Behavioral Sciences, 18*, 83–90.

Herbette, G., & Rimé, B. (2004). Verbalization of emotion in chronic pain patients and their psychological adjustment. *Journal of Health Psychology, 9*(5), 661–676.

Herbolsheimer, F., Mosler, S., & Peter, R. (2017). Relationship between social isolation and indoor and outdoor physical activity in community-dwelling older adults in Germany: Findings from the ActiFE study. *Journal of Aging and Physical Activity, 25*(3), 387–394.

Hirsch, J. A., Winters, M., Ashe, M. C., Clarke, P. J., & McKay, H. A. (2016). Destinations that older adults experience within their GPS activity spaces: Relation to objectively measured physical activity. *Environment and Behavior, 48*(1), 55–77.

Hirsch, J. A., Winters, M., Clarke, P., & McKay, H. (2014). Generating GPS activity spaces that shed light upon the mobility habits of older adults: A descriptive analysis. *International Journal of Health Geographics, 13*, 1–14.

Hoppmann, C. A., & Riediger, M. (2009). Ambulatory assessment in lifespan psychology: An overview of current status and new trends. *European Psychologist, 14*(2), 98–108.

Huo, M., Fuentecilla, J. L., Birditt, K. S., & Fingerman, K. L. (2019). Older adults' empathy and daily support exchanges. *Journal of Social and Personal Relationships, 36*(11–12), 3814–3834.

Kaspar, R., Oswald, F., Wahl, H.-W., Voss, E., & Wettstein, M. (2015). Daily mood and out-of-home mobility in older adults: Does cognitive impairment matter? *Journal of Applied Gerontology, 34*(1), 26–47.

Kerr, J., Marshall, S., Godbole, S., Neukam, S., Crist, K., Wasilenko, K., et al. (2012). The relationship between outdoor activity and health in older adults using GPS. *International Journal of Environmental Research and Public Health, 9*(12), 4615–4625.

Klenk, J., Kerse, N., Rapp, K., Nikolaus, T., Becker, C., Rothenbacher, D., et al. (2015). Physical activity and different concepts of fall risk estimation in older people: Results of the ActiFE-Ulm study. *PloS One, 10*(6), 1–11.

Kunzmann, U., Richter, D., & Schmukle, S. C. (2013). Stability and change in affective experience across the adult life span: Analyses with a national sample from Germany. *Emotion, 13*(6), 1086–1095.

Lin, L., & Moudon, A. V. (2010). Objective versus subjective measures of the built environment, which are most effective in capturing associations with walking? *Health and Place, 16*(2), 339–348.

Litwin, H., & Shiovitz-Ezra, S. (2006). Network type and mortality risk in later life. *The Gerontologist, 46*(6), 735–743.

Losada-Baltar, A., Jiménez-Gonzalo, L., Gallego-Alberto, L., Pedroso-Chaparro, M. del S., Fernandes-Pires, J., & Márquez-González, M. (2020). "We are staying at home." Association of self-perceptions of aging, personal and family resources, and loneliness with psychological distress during the lock-down period of COVID-19. *Journals of Gerontology: Series B, 76*(2), e10–e16.

Macdonald, B. & Hülür, G. (2021). Well-being and loneliness in Swiss older adults during the COVID-19 pandemic: The role of social relationships. *The Gerontologist, 61(2)*, 240–250.

Mehl, M. R. (2017). The electronically activated recorder (EAR): A method for the naturalistic observation of daily social behavior. *Current*

Directions in Psychological Science, 26(2), 184–190.

Mehl, M. R., & Robbins, M. L. (2012). Naturalistic observation sampling: the electronically activated recorder (EAR). In M. R. Mehl & T. S. Conner (Eds.), *Handbook of research methods for studying daily life* (pp. 176–192). Guilford Press.

Mendes de Leon, C. F., Cagney, K. A., Bienias, J. L., Barnes, L. L., Skarupski, K. A., Scherr, P. A., et al. (2009). Neighborhood social cohesion and disorder in relation to walking in community-dwelling older adults: A multilevel analysis. *Journal of Aging and Health, 21*(1), 155–171.

Mikolaizak, A. S., Klenk, J., Rothenbacher, D., Denkinger, M. D., & Rapp, K. (2019). Purpose, frequency, and mode of transport by which older adults leave their home—A cross-sectional analysis. *Journal of Aging and Physical Activity, 27*(5), 688–695.

Milek, A., Butler, E. A., Tackman, A. M., Kaplan, D. M., Raison, C. L., Sbarra, et al. (2018). "Eavesdropping on happiness" revisited: A pooled, multisample replication of the association between life satisfaction and observed daily conversation quantity and quality. *Psychological Science, 29*(9), 1451–1462.

Mollenkopf, H., Marcellini, F., Ruoppila, I., Széman, Z., & Tacken, M. (Eds.). (2005). *Enhancing mobility in later life: Personal coping, environmental resources and technical support. The out-of-home mobility of older adults in urban and rural regions of five European countries.* IOS Press.

Mollenkopf, H., Marcellini, F., Ruoppila, I., Széman, Z., Tacken, M., & Wahl, H.-W. (2004). Social and behavioural science perspectives on out-of-home mobility in later life: Findings from the European project MOBILATE. *European Journal of Ageing, 1*(1), 45–53.

Nahum-Shani, I., Smith, S. N., Spring, B. J., Collins, L. M., Witkiewitz, K., Tewari, A., et al. (2018). Just-in-time adaptive interventions (JITAIs) in mobile health: Key components and design principles for ongoing health behavior support. *Annals of Behavioral Medicine, 52*(6), 446–462.

Ng, Y. T., Huo, M., Han, S. H., Birditt, K. S., & Fingerman, K. L. (2021). Older adult's marital status, conversation frequency, and well-being in everyday life. *Journals of Gerontology: Series B, 77*(3), 499–512.

Paraschiv-Ionescu, A., Perruchoud, C., Buchser, E., & Aminian, K. (2012). Barcoding human physical activity to assess chronic pain conditions. *PLoS One, 7*(2), 1–12.

Pennebaker, J. W., Francis, M. E., & Booth, R. J. (2001). *Linguistic inquiry and word count (LIWC).* Erlbaum.

Petersen, R. C., Doody, R., Kurz, A., Mohs, R. C., Morris, J. C., Rabins, P. V., et al. (2001). Current concepts in mild cognitive impairment. *Archives of Neurology, 58*(12), 1985–1992.

Petersen, R. C., & Morris, J. C. (2003). Clinical features. In R. C. Petersen (Ed.), *Mild cognitive impairment: Aging to Alzheimer's disease* (pp. 15–40). Oxford University Press.

Polsinelli, A. J., Moseley, S. A., Grilli, M. D., Glisky, E. L., & Mehl, M. R. (2020). Natural, everyday language use provides a window into the integrity of older adults' executive functioning. *Journals of Gerontology: Series B, 75*(9), e215–e220.

Razjouyan, J., Najafi, B., Horstman, M., Sharafkhaneh, A., Amirmazaheri, M., Zhou, H., et al. (2020). Toward using wearables to remotely monitor cognitive frailty in community-living older adults: An observational study. *Sensors, 20*(8), 1–15.

Reis, H. T., & Wheeler, L. (1991). Studying social interaction with the Rochester Interaction Record. *Advances in Experimental Social Psychology, 24*, 269–318.

Riediger, M., Wrzus, C., Klipker, K., Müller, V., Schmiedek, F., & Wagner, G. G. (2014). Outside of the laboratory: Associations of working-memory performance with psychological and physiological arousal vary with age. *Psychology and Aging, 29*(1), 103–114.

Röcke, C., & Lachman, M. E. (2008). Perceived trajectories of life satisfaction across past, present, and future: Profiles and correlates of subjective change in young, middle-aged, and older adults. *Psychology and Aging, 23*(4), 833–847.

Röcke, C., Li, S.-C., & Smith, J. (2009). Intraindividual variability in positive and negative affect over 45 days: Do older adults fluctuate less than young adults? *Psychology and Aging, 24*(4), 863–878.

Röcke, C., Luo, M., Bereuter, P., Katana, M.,

Fillekes, M., Gehriger, V., et al. (2023). Charting everyday activities in later life: Study protocol of the Mobility, Activity, and Social Interactions Study (MOASIS). *Frontiers in Psychology, 13*, 1011177.

Rubenstein, L. Z. (2006). Falls in older people: Epidemiology, risk factors and strategies for prevention. *Age and Ageing, 35*(Suppl. 2), ii37–ii41.

Saelens, B. E., Sallis, J. F., Black, J. B., & Chen, D. (2003). Neighborhood-based differences in ohysical activity: An environment scale evaluation. *American Journal of Public Health, 93*(9), 1552–1558.

Schaat, S., Koldrack, P., Yordanova, K., Kirste, T., & Teipel, S. (2020). Real-time detection of spatial disorientation in persons with mild cognitive impairment and dementia. *Gerontology, 66*(1), 85–94.

Seifert, A. (2020). Smartwatch use among older adults: Findings from two large surveys. In Q. Gao & J. Zhou (Eds.), *Human aspects of IT for the aged population: Technologies, design and user experience* (pp. 372–385). Springer.

Seifert, A. (2021). Digitale Transformation in den Haushalten älterer Menschen [Digital transformation in the households of older people]. *Zeitschrift für Gerontologie und Geriatrie, 55*, 305–311.

Seifert, A., Hofer, M., & Allemand, M. (2018). Mobile data collection: Smart, but not (yet) smart enough. *Frontiers in Neuroscience, 12*, 1–4.

Seifert, A., & Schelling, H. R. (2015). Mobile seniors: Mobile use of the Internet using smartphones or tablets by Swiss people over 65 years. *Gerontechnology, 14*(1), 57–62.

Shaughnessy, K., Reyes, R., Shankardass, K., Sykora, M., Feick, R., Lawrence, H., et al. (2018). Using geolocated social media for ecological momentary assessments of emotion: Innovative opportunities in psychology science and practice. *Canadian Psychology/Psychologie Canadienne, 59*(1), 47–53.

Shoval, N., Auslander, G., Cohen-Shalom, K., Isaacson, M., Landau, R., & Heinik, J. (2010). What can we learn about the mobility of the elderly in the GPS era? *Journal of Transport Geography, 18*(5), 603–612.

Sliwinski, M. J., Mogle, J. A., Hyun, J., Munoz, E., Smyth, J. M., & Lipton, R. B. (2018). Reliability and validity of ambulatory cognitive assessments. *Assessment, 25*(1), 14–30.

Soltani, A., Dejnabadi, M., Savary, M., & Aminian, K. (2020). Real-world gait speed estimation using wrist sensor: A personalized approach. *IEEE Journal of Biomedical and Health Informatics, 24*(3), 658–668.

Sun, J., Harris, K., & Vazire, S. (2020). Is well-being associated with the quantity and quality of social interactions? *Journal of Personality and Social Psychology, 119*(6), 1478–1496.

Sun, J., Schwartz, H. A., Son, Y., Kern, M. L., & Vazire, S. (2020). The language of well-being: Tracking fluctuations in emotion experience through everyday speech. *Journal of Personality and Social Psychology, 118*(2), 364–387.

Sykora, M. D., Jackson, T. W., O'Brien, A., & Elayan, S. (2013). Emotive ontology: Extracting fine-grained emotions from terse, informal messages. *IADIS International Journal on Computer Science and Information Systems, 8*(2), 106–118.

Tung, J. Y., Rose, R. V., Gammada, E., Lam, I., Roy, E. A., Black, S. E., et al. (2014). Measuring life space in older adults with mild-to-moderate Alzheimer's disease using mobile phone GPS. *Gerontology, 60*(2), 154–162.

Van Holle, V., Van Cauwenberg, J., Van Dyck, D., Deforche, B., Van de Weghe, N., & De Bourdeaudhuij, I. (2014). Relationship between neighborhood walkability and older adults' physical activity: Results from the Belgian Environmental Physical Activity Study in Seniors (BEPAS Seniors). *International Journal of Behavioral Nutrition and Physical Activity, 11*, 1–9.

Voss, C., Sims-Gould, J., Ashe, M. C., McKay, H. A., Pugh, C., & Winters, M. (2016). Public transit use and physical activity in community-dwelling older adults: Combining GPS and accelerometry to assess transportation-related physical activity. *Journal of Transport and Health, 3*(2), 191–199.

Wank, A. A., Mehl, M. R., Andrews-Hanna, J. R., Polsinelli, A. J., Moseley, S., Glisky, E. L., et al. (2020). Eavesdropping on autobiographical memory: A naturalistic observation study of older adults' memory sharing in daily conversations. *Frontiers in Human Neuroscience, 14*, 1–14.

Warmerdam, E., Hausdorff, J. M., Atrsaei, A., Zhou, Y., Mirelman, A., Aminian, K., et al. (2020). Long-term unsupervised mobility assessment in movement disorders. *Lancet Neurology, 19*(5), 462–470.

Wen, M., & Christakis, N. A. (2005). Neighborhood effects on posthospitalization mortality: A population-based cohort study of the elderly in Chicago. *Health Services Research, 40*(4), 1108–1127.

Wettstein, M., Schilling, O. K., Reidick, O., & Wahl, H.-W. (2015). Four-year stability, change, and multidirectionality of well-being in very-old age. *Psychology and Aging, 30*(3), 500–516.

Wettstein, M., Wahl, H.-W., Shoval, N., Auslander, G., Oswald, F., & Heinik, J. (2015). Identifying mobility types in cognitively heterogeneous older adults based on GPS-tracking: What discriminates best? *Journal of Applied Gerontology, 34*(8), 1001–1027.

Wettstein, M., Wahl, H.-W., Shoval, N., Oswald, F., Voss, E., Seidl, U., et al. (2015). Out-of-home behavior and cognitive impairment in older adults: Findings of the SenTra Project. *Journal of Applied Gerontology, 34*(1), 3–25.

Weuve, J., Kang, J. H., Manson, J. E., Breteler, M. M. B., Ware, J. H., & Grodstein, F. (2004). Physical activity, including walking, and cognitive function in older women. *Journal of the American Medical Association, 292*(12), 1454–1461.

Wohlwill, J. F. (1970). The age variable in psychological research. *Psychological Review, 77*(1), 49–64.

Wolf, F., Seifert, A., Martin, M., & Oswald, F. (2021). Considering situational variety in contextualized aging research—Opinion about methodological perspectives. *Frontiers in Psychology, 12*, 1–5.

World Health Organization. (2015). *Summary—World report on aging and health.* Author.

World Health Organization. (2020). *Decade of healthy ageing: Baseline report.* Author.

Wrzus, C., & Mehl, M. R. (2015). Lab and/or field? Measuring personality processes and their social consequences. *European Journal of Personality, 29*(2), 250–271.

York Cornwell, E., & Cagney, K. A. (2017). Aging in activity space: Results from smartphone-based GPS-tracking of urban seniors. *Journals of Gerontology: Series B, 72*(5), 864–875.

Zacher, H., & Rudolph, C. W. (2021). Individual differences and changes in subjective wellbeing during the early stages of the COVID-19 pandemic. *The American Psychologist, 76*(1), 50–62.

Zhang, W., Schwenk, M., Mellone, S., Paraschiv-Ionescu, A., Vereijken, B., Pijnappels, M., et al. (2018). Complexity of daily physical activity is more sensitive than conventional metrics to assess functional change in younger older adults. *Sensors, 18*(7), 1–12.

Zhaoyang, R., Scott, S. B., Martire, L. M., & Sliwinski, M. J. (2021). Daily social interactions related to daily performance on mobile cognitive tests among older adults. *PLoS One, 16*(8), 1–16.

CHAPTER 28

mHealth Interventions for Health Behaviors

Christine Vinci, Brian Gonzalez, Darla Kendzor,
Michael Businelle, and Santosh Kumar

CHAPTER OVERVIEW

The use of mHealth to address modifiable health risk factors has increased exponentially in recent years. This chapter focuses on how mHealth has been used to intervene in substance use disorders and insomnia, with a specific focus on short messaging service (SMS) interventions, smartphone applications, and sensor-based technology. Brief descriptions of mHealth interventions for physical activity, medication management, and glucose monitoring are also provided. Recommendations for future research are provided throughout, and the chapter concludes by emphasizing the need for continued technological advancement, new conceptual models of behavior change, large-scale randomized controlled trials, interdisciplinary collaborations, and innovative funding opportunities.

Introduction

This chapter describes how mobile technologies have been used to intervene in substance use disorders (SUDs) and insomnia. Although this chapter focuses primarily on these two specific health behaviors, research in these areas can inform treatment for other disorders and health behaviors not discussed in this chapter (e.g., cardiovascular disease, anxiety), and the potential for generalizability is discussed when applicable. A brief overview of mHealth interventions for physical activity, medication management, and glucose monitoring is also presented toward the end of the chapter. The chapter concludes with recommendations for future research.

Substance Use Disorders

In 2018, findings from the National Survey on Drug Use and Health indicated that 20.3 million American adults (6% of the population) met the diagnostic criteria for an SUD (Substance Abuse and Mental Health Services Administration, 2019). The abuse of tobacco, alcohol, and other illicit substances costs over $740 billion annually due to treatment costs and indirect costs such as crime and decreased work productivity (National Institute on Drug Abuse, 2017). Unfortunately, less than 15% of diagnosed individuals receive treatment (Grant et al., 2015). mHealth technologies can increase access to SUD treatments. This section will focus on the role of SMS interventions, smartphone-based interventions (e.g., apps), and sensor-based technology for the treatment of SUDs.

SMS Interventions (Text Messaging Interventions)

According to the Pew Research Center (2021), 97% of U.S. adults overall reported owning a cell phone in 2021. Thus, mobile phone interventions offer a means to overcome many barriers to treatment, as well as to reach individuals across settings and situations. Broadly speaking, SMS interventions involve sending brief text messages to the user to aid in behavior change (Bock et al., 2015). Key benefits of SMS interventions include high scalability and reach, as SMS interventions can operate on nearly all cell phones (i.e., a smartphone is not required). To date, the majority of SUD-related SMS interventions have been implemented for smoking cessation (Abroms et al., 2017; Christofferson, Hertzberg, Beckham, Dennis, & Hamlett-Berry, 2016; Naughton et al., 2017; Spohr et al., 2015; Whittaker, McRobbie, Bullen, Rodgers, & Gu, 2016) and have demonstrated efficacy (Whittaker et al., 2016). Here, we provide information on the most efficacious components of SMS interventions, with a focus on tobacco and alcohol use, which have received the most attention. That said, note that SMS interventions for marijuana use (Shrier, Rhoads, Burke, Walls, & Blood, 2014) and general drug use (Liang, Han, Du, Zhao, & Hser, 2018) have been examined in pilot studies.

Smoking Cessation

A recent meta-analysis of SMS interventions for smoking cessation revealed that interventions are most effective when they are tailored to the user in the moment and have a fixed schedule of message delivery (Spohr et al., 2015). Ideally, when participants respond to specific questions (e.g., How many cigarettes have you smoked today?), text messages may be immediately tailored to the participant's response (Haug, Schaub, Venzin, Meyer, & John, 2013). Regarding the frequency of intervention messages, various schedules have been examined. For instance, a higher frequency of messages may be delivered around the quit day and will then decrease in frequency over time (Naughton, Prevost, Gilbert, & Sutton, 2012). Other studies have kept a fairly fixed schedule of messages (Haug et al., 2013), which seems to be the most effective approach (Spohr et al., 2015). SMS interventions may also include on demand components for which the user can text a keyword to receive a message. For instance, in one intervention, participants could text CRAVE when they experienced a craving, and this triggered a text message offering a craving coping strategy. Interacting with the system in this way was associated with an increased likelihood of biochemically confirmed tobacco abstinence (Abroms, Boal, Simmens, Mendel, & Windsor, 2014).

Alcohol Use

SMS interventions developed for alcohol have focused on multiple topics, including motivating readiness to change drinking (Mason, Benotsch, Way, Kim, & Snipes, 2014), reducing/eliminating current alcohol use (Suffoletto et al., 2014, 2015; Thomas, Linderoth, Bendtsen, Bendtsen, & Müssener, 2016), relapse prevention (Haug, Lucht, John, Meyer, & Schaub, 2015), and alcohol use comorbidities such as depression (Agyapong, McLoughlin, & Farren, 2013). Alcohol use tends to vary based on day of the week, holidays, special occasions/events, and age (Neighbors et al., 2011; Riordan, Conner, Flett, & Scarf, 2015). Thus, SMS interventions have attempted to address these unique aspects of alcohol use, including 21st-birthday alcohol consumption (Bernstein et al., 2018), days leading into the weekend (Suffoletto et al., 2014, 2015), and college student use (Bock et al., 2016; Mason et al., 2014; Riordan, Scarf, & Conner, 2015). Overall, although published results have tended to be preliminary with small sample sizes, findings have been promising and suggest that the efficacy of text messaging interventions that target alcohol use warrant continued investigation.

Smartphone Applications

As of 2021, 85% of U.S. adults overall and 76% of low-income adults reported owning a smartphone (Pew Research Center, 2021). However, less than 1% of commercially available SUD apps available in the iTunes and Google Play stores used evidence-based approaches to reduce use (Tofighi, Chemi, Ruiz-Valcarcel, Hein, & Hu, 2019). (*Note:* This review did not include smoking cessation apps.) When rating apps using the Mobile App Rating Scale (MARS), most apps were rated low for engagement, functionality, aesthetics, information, and satisfaction (Tofighi et al., 2019). A systematic review of smoking cessation smartphone applications revealed that 4% (N = 2) had scientific support (Haskins, Lesperance, Gibbons, & Boudreaux, 2017). Thus, although many individuals own smartphones, few empirically validated applications for substance use treatment are currently available. Similar to SMS interventions, published research on SUD-focused smartphone applications have focused primarily on the treatment of tobacco and alcohol use, so we focus on these specific substances below.

Smoking Cessation

Smartphone ownership and use among smokers are similar to that of the general U.S. population, and smokers who are motivated to quit have high rates of smartphone ownership (Borrelli, Bartlett, Tooley, Armitage, & Wearden, 2015; Oliver et al., 2018). Nonetheless, experience with smoking cessation apps is infrequent (Oliver et al., 2018), suggesting that strategies to increase awareness of these types of applications should be investigated. Among smokers interested in quitting, appealing smartphone features include: adaptive and personalized content, rewards, gaming features (particularly among younger smokers), tracking of progress, and social support (Hartzler, BlueSpruce, Catz, & McClure, 2016). Among smokers not yet ready to quit, appealing features include security, tracking of behaviors related to smoking (e.g., spending), adaptive content, ability to request social support, rewards, and information on quitting smoking and managing withdrawal and mood (McClure, Heffner, Hohl, Klasnja, & Catz, 2017). Features that may be reported as desirable are not always the most frequently used when made available in smartphone applications (Heffner, Vilardaga, Mercer, Kientz, & Bricker, 2015).

The literature on the efficacy of smartphone applications for smoking cessation is limited. Although a handful of teams have conducted randomized controlled trials to evaluate the efficacy of fully developed apps, most research is in the developmental phase. Ortis, Caponnetto, Polosa, Urso, and Battiato (2020) recently published a report that described several quit smoking applications based on their ratings in the app stores. The reader is directed to that article for a more comprehensive review. Craving to Quit is a mindfulness-based smartphone application that was compared to a control group among 325 individuals interested in quitting smoking (Garrison et al., 2020). Results indicated that both groups demonstrated a reduction in smoking and craving from baseline to 6 months; however, groups did not significantly differ on biochemically confirmed abstinence at 6 months. Bricker and colleagues (2014) compared SmartQuit, a smartphone application that delivers acceptance and commitment therapy, to QuitGuide, the National Cancer Institute's application for smoking cessation. Results indicated that among 196 randomized to the two groups, individuals in SmartQuit had a self-reported abstinence rate of 13% versus 7% in QuitGuide. A revised version of the app has since been developed and tested (Bricker et al., 2017).

Businelle and colleagues (2016) have used ecological momentary assessment (EMA) data to develop a novel smoking lapse risk estimator that has been integrated into the Smart-Treatment app (Smart-T). Early work (Businelle, Ma, Kendzor, Frank, Wetter, et al., 2016) showed that six EMA variables predicted 80% of smoking lapses within 4 hours of the lapse (false-positive rate = 17%). The Smart-T app incorporates on-demand features (e.g., tips on coping with stress) and the lapse risk estimator to deliver tailored messages based on a person's momentary risk for smoking lapse. The Smart-T feasibility study showed that this intervention was feasible, with 97% reporting that they would like to use the app in the future if they were to relapse and 85% indicating that they would refer their friends who smoke to use the app (Businelle, Ma, Kendzor, Frank, Vidrine, et al., 2016). Analyses of EMA data revealed that urges to smoke were significantly reduced when tailored urge messages were delivered by the app, as opposed to instances where nontailored messages were delivered (Hébert et al., 2018). A total of 20% of participants were biochemically confirmed abstinent at 12 weeks post-quit (Businelle, Ma, Kendzor, Frank, Vidrine, et al., 2016). Project Smart-T2, a 12-week pilot randomized controlled trial compared smoking cessation rates for those randomized to the Smart-T app, the National Cancer Institute (NCI) QuitGuide app, or clinic-based smoking cessation treatment. Participants completed 84% of five daily EMAs (over 5 weeks), and 12 weeks post-quit biochemically confirmed that 7-day point prevalence abstinence rates were as follows: Smart-T2 = 22.2%, QuitGuide = 14.8%, in-clinic counseling = 14.8% (Hébert et al., 2020). These preliminary results suggest that smartphone-based smoking cessation interventions may perform as well as traditional in-person interventions. A fully powered randomized clinical trial comparing the efficacy of the Smart-T3 app to the NCI QuitGuide app is ongoing.

Several other teams are in the process of developing and/or conducting preliminary work on other smartphone applications (Baskerville, Struik, & Dash, 2018; Brandon et al., 2021; Hernandez, Wetter, Kumar, Sutton, & Vinci, 2021; Iacoviello et al., 2017; Kendzor et al., 2020; Tombor et al., 2019; Vinci, Brandon, Kleinjan, Hernandez, et al., 2020). Many of these applications are tailored to certain populations, such as Learn to Quit for smokers with serious mental illness (Vilardaga et al., 2018), Crush the Crave for young adult smokers (Baskerville et al., 2018), and SmokeFreeBaby for pregnant smokers (Tombor et al., 2019). Others are modifying theoretically based approaches that are traditionally delivered in the clinic (e.g., cue exposure treatment) by leveraging cutting-edge technology to enhance real-world application (Brandon et al., 2021; Vilardaga et al., 2018; Vinci, Brandon, Kleinjan, & Brandon, 2020; Vinci, Brandon, Kleinjan, Hernandez, et al., 2020).

Alcohol Use

Similar to smoking cessation apps, the app stores contain hundreds of apps related to alcohol use, albeit the majority have no scientific evidence of efficacy (Crane, Garnett, Brown, West, & Michie, 2015). A paper examining peer-reviewed publications on alcohol use reduction apps found that six apps met review criteria of having published feasibility or efficacy data (Meredith, Alessi, & Petry, 2015). Of those six, two apps demonstrated efficacy in reducing self-reported alcohol use (A-CHESS and LBMI-A), two did not reduce alcohol use (Promillekoll & PartyPlanner), and two required further evaluation (HealthCalls and Chimpshop). We describe A-CHESS and LBMI-A here in more detail.

Arguably, the most well-researched and efficacious app for alcohol reduction is A-CHESS (Alcohol-Comprehensive Health Enhancement Support System), which is a relapse prevention app for individuals recently discharged from residential treatment for alcohol dependence (Gustafson et al., 2014; McTavish, Chih, Shah, & Gustafson, 2012). In a trial evaluating the effectiveness of the app, participants (N = 349) were randomized to either A-CHESS or treatment as usual. A-CHESS utilized a just-in-time adaptive intervention (JITAI) framework to deliver intervention content based on participant behavior. For example, if the participant entered a high-risk location (such as a place where alcohol use had been consumed frequently in the past), the app would send a message to the participant inquiring whether they wanted to be in that location. The app also has static educational and relaxation content on the phone that the user can use on-demand, along with weekly assessments of alcohol use that could be available to their counselor. Overall, A-CHESS participants self-reported significantly fewer risky drinking days through the 4-month posttreatment follow-up than those in the treatment as usual group.

LBMI-A (Location-Based Monitoring and Intervention for Alcohol Use Disorders) utilizes cognitive-behavioral strategies combined with interventions delivered in real time when the participant enters a high-risk location (Dulin, Gonzalez, & Campbell, 2014; Gonzalez & Dulin, 2015). LBMI-A was compared to DCU (Drinker's Checkup), an internet-based brief motivational intervention supplemented with bibliotherapy. Although the sample size was small (N = 54), LBMI-A increased the percentage of days of self-reported abstinence, whereas DCU did not. Both groups demonstrated reductions in self-reported percent heavy drinking days and drinks per week (Gonzalez & Dulin, 2015).

Many recent apps have focused on addressing problematic alcohol use and/or alcohol dependence (Bertholet, Godinho, & Cunningham, 2019; Crane, Garnett, Michie,

West, & Brown, 2018; Harder, Musau, Musyimi, Ndetei, & Mutiso, 2020; Mellentin et al., 2019; You et al., 2017). For instance, Smart-T Alcohol (an app similar to Smart-T for smoking described above) is currently being investigated (Businelle et al., 2020; Walters et al., 2021). Other apps have focused on specific populations, such as youth and young adults (Gajecki et al., 2017; Hides et al., 2018) and men who have sex with men (Wray, Kahler, Simpanen, & Operario, 2019). Although findings from some of these studies are promising, additional research is needed with larger sample sizes and active comparison conditions to determine efficacy and effectiveness.

Sensor-Based Technology

The development of wearable wireless sensors and accompanying machine learning algorithms that can detect behavior automatically and unobtrusively and use this information to inform novel treatments has led to advancements in health care delivery in recent years. Examples include algorithms that can passively detect smoking (Saleheen et al., 2015), alcohol use (Selvam, Muthukumar, Kamakoti, & Prasad, 2016), visits to tobacco outlets and smoking spots (Chatterjee et al., 2020), and stress (Hovsepian et al., 2015). Data from these sensors can provide a more nuanced understanding of relationships between biopsychosocial mechanisms and behavior (e.g., the role of stress in relapse). Such technology lends itself to the development of JITAIs, wherein real-time detection of physiologically identified risk factors can trigger adaptation and delivery of intervention content developed by the researcher (Nahum-Shani et al., 2014; Spruijt-Metz & Nilsen, 2014). Since JITAIs may be tailored to the needs of a particular individual and the surrounding context, leveraging data collected via wearable sensors and using that information to deploy intervention content is ideal.

Sensor-Based Detection of Smoking Behavior

Various scientific teams have been developing and testing technology to automatically detect smoking behavior (Dar, 2018; Parate, Chiu, Chadowitz, Ganesan, & Kalogerakis, 2014; Saleheen et al., 2015; Sazonov, Metcalfe, Lopez-Meyer, & Tiffany, 2011; Wu, Hsieh, Cheng, Cheng, & Tseng, 2010). A recent report on smoking detection sensors describes various technologies in detail (Ortis et al., 2020), a few of which we highlight here. *puffMarker*, a model that uses a machine learning algorithm based on data collected from wrist sensor accelerometers and a chest band that tracks respiration to detect smoking episodes, has demonstrated a sensitivity rate of 96.9% and a false-positive rate of 1.1% for smoking detection (Saleheen et al., 2015). Other teams have solely used wrist sensors that detect the motion of smoking behavior (Chen et al., 2018; Cole, Anshari, Lambert, Thrasher, & Valafar, 2017; Senyurek, Imtiaz, Belsare, Tiffany, & Sazonov, 2019). For example, RisQ showed a 95.7% accuracy rating in overall gesture recognition for smoking and a 91% precision rate in detecting smoking gestures (Parate et al., 2014). Other examples include inconspicuous and noninvasive devices such as a radio-frequency-based hand gesture sensor to detect distance between the hand and chest when smoking (Lopez-Meyer, Patil, Tiffany, & Sazonov, 2013; Sazonov et al., 2011) and visual interaction cues (e.g., color, shape) of the cigarette being smoked via video (Wu et al., 2010).

The detection of smoking via wearable sensors has enabled researchers to passively identify situations in which smoking occurs (e.g., at a bar, after meals, lunchtime at work) in order to assess risk for imminent smoking (Chatterjee et al., 2020). Thus, future interventions may anticipate and intervene when a person is in a risky context, without requiring the individual to self-report this elevated risk. In the context of smoking cessation interventions, this type of passive data collection may ultimately allow treatments to more accurately target precipitants of smoking lapse, prevent relapse, and aid in long-term abstinence. Although several ongoing studies are evaluating the efficacy of providing smoking cessation interventions based on data collected via sensors, no outcome papers have been published yet. Nonetheless, protocol papers describing these studies have been published (Chen et al., 2018; Dar, 2018; Hernandez et al., 2021). For example, Hernandez and colleagues (2021) are testing whether mindfulness-based strategies, sent to the participant's smartphone when sensors indicate certain levels of negative affect and smoking, can increase tobacco abstinence among those making an active quit attempt.

Portable and low-cost breath carbon monoxide (CO) sensors are now widely available and can assist with the detection of smoking and verification of abstinence outside of the laboratory. For example, Kendzor and colleagues (2020) described the development of an automated, mobile approach to contingency management for smoking cessation that included remote sensor-based smoking status assessment and identity verification. Wong and colleagues (2019) compared the Bedfont iCO Smokerlyzer to the piCO+ Smokerlyzer and found that expired CO values were highly correlated between the devices and that first and second readings were highly correlated for both devices. Other smoking cessation intervention research that utilizes the Smokerlyzer iCO as part of a smartphone-based intervention strategy is underway (Martinez et al., 2020).

Sensor-Based Detection of Alcohol Use

Over the past several years, a number of biosensors have been developed to passively detect alcohol use in the natural environment (for a recent review, see Piasecki, 2019). For instance, biosensors can provide a continuous estimate of blood alcohol concentration (BAC) based on the concentration of alcohol in perspiration on the skin (Hawthorne & Wojcik, 2006; Leffingwell et al., 2013; Rash, Petry, Alessi, & Barnett, 2019; Swift, 1993, 2003). The device with the most extensive evaluation is the SCRAM bracelet (Alcohol Monitoring Systems, Littleton, CO), which is worn on the ankle. SCRAM has an electrochemical sensor that samples the vapor near the skin every 30 minutes for ethanol and stores readings for later retrieval. In a recent study, 93% of self-reported heavy drinking episodes of five or more drinks were detected with the SCRAM device (Barnett, Meade, & Glynn, 2014). New technologies like the BACtrack Skyn (a winner of the National Institute on Alcohol Abuse and Alcoholism wearable alcohol biosensor challenge for a novel passive alcohol use detection sensor) have promise, without the stigma that may accompany wearing an ankle bracelet. However, lack of rigorous tamper-proofing features and high failure rates during the initial testing of this device have tempered excitement for this technology (Fairbairn & Kang, 2019).

Alessi and Petry (2013) and others have used portable alcohol monitors with smartphone cameras to verify alcohol use in the real world (Alessi & Petry, 2013; Koffarnus, Bickel, & Kablinger, 2018). Typically, these studies involve compensating participants for completing prompted alcohol breath tests as part of contingency management interventions. Alessi and Petry (2013) compensated participants for uploading videos of themselves blowing into a portable alcohol breathalyzer. Koffarnus and colleagues (2018) compensated participants for completing breath tests using the Soberlink SL2 breathalyzer, which automatically takes and uploads pictures of the participant while they provide the breath sample. Study findings indicated that these methods are feasible (e.g., 88–95% of requested samples were submitted on time) and acceptable to participants who take part in research studies.

Recently, sensors embedded within standard mobile phones have been used in conjunction with machine learning to identify drinking events (Bae, Chung, Ferreira, Dey, & Suffoletto, 2018; Piasecki, 2019). Bae and colleagues (2018) showed that variables such as typing speed, call duration, and movement patterns were useful in correctly classifying alcohol use in the individual's natural environment. Other groups have used smartphones to assess gait during prompted walking tasks to estimate levels of alcohol intoxication. Much of this technology has only recently been developed and tested, and there is a need to further investigate the value of such sensors within alcohol intervention research.

Sensors That Detect Correlates of Substance Use Behaviors

Location

Global Positioning System (GPS) provides a unique opportunity to know when an individual enters a "high-risk" location for substance use. For example, prior research has indicated that there are neighborhood-level contextual precipitants to smoking lapse, including proximity to smoking outlets (Kendzor et al., 2012; Ma, Businelle, Balis, & Kendzor, 2015; Reitzel et al., 2012). The detection of location via GPS may support the creation of novel interventions that can automatically intervene when an individual enters a high-risk situation or environment (Chatterjee et al., 2020; Gustafson et al., 2014; Naughton et al., 2016). For example, the A-CHESS application intervened in high-risk situations for alcohol use (Gustafson et al., 2014). Businelle and colleagues (2020) are currently investigating an intervention for homeless adults with alcohol use disorder that combines data collected via GPS, transdermal alcohol sensor, and EMA to provide treatment messages that will address drinking-related risk factors.

The *SmokingOpp* model was recently developed to detect not only general smoking locations (e.g., bars), but also personal smoking spots (i.e., "micro-locations") that are unique to a given individual such as in one's home and outside one's office building (Chatterjee et al., 2020). These "micro-locations" are personal smoking places that are not easily captured via traditional means (e.g., GPS-indicated bars or convenience stores where many people smoke). Micro-locations are identified by occurrence of smoking as detected by puffMarker and combining it with self-reported information on smoking allowance and cigarette availability. GPS data of these locations are recorded during prequit, which is then used to reidentify any visitation to these spots during the abstinence period, by only using the GPS data (i.e., proximity of real-time GPS data to previously recorded locations of smoking micro-locations). These micro-locations may actually be some of the most important places to target when someone is quitting smoking. Initial testing of the *SmokingOpp* model found that the combination of cigarette availability (whether someone has current access to a cigarette) and smoking allowance (whether smoking is permitted in that location) predicted future cigarettes smoked (Chatterjee et al., 2020). During a smoking quit attempt, this model could be used to send an intervention strategy (e.g., "You are about to enter a location where you commonly smoke!

Consider finding another route."). As noted by the authors, similar models can be developed to detect "opportunity contexts" for other adverse behaviors, including binge drinking, overeating, and gambling.

Stress

The experience of stress/negative affect is strongly associated with risk for relapse in the context of addictive behaviors (Sinha, 2001, 2007). If stress can be detected via wearable sensors, scientists may be able to develop ways to intervene during high-stress moments, prior to lapse occurring. Several teams have been developing and testing technologies to capture stress unobtrusively through various methods (Gimpel, Regal, & Schmidt, 2015; Gjoreski, Gjoreski, Lusterk, & Gams, 2016; Hovsepian et al., 2015; Kostopoulos, Kyritsis, Deriaz, & Konstantas, 2017; Suk & Prabhakaran, 2014; Yoon, Sim, & Cho, 2016). Importantly, stress detection via wearable sensors may have applicability to other mental and physical health outcomes aside from addiction (e.g., anxiety, depression, cardiovascular disease).

Sensor-based detection of stress has advanced to the point that sensors can passively detect physiological responses (e.g., heart rate), behaviors (e.g., social interaction, facial recognition), and sounds (e.g., airplanes, traffic, and other high decibel sounds). For example, *cStress* is a machine learning model of stress detection that uses physiological stress data collected via a chest band—specifically, electrocardiogram and respiration data (Hovsepian et al., 2015; Sarker et al., 2016, 2017). Wrist-worn devices have also been used to detect stress via heart rate, galvanic skin response, and accelerometer data (Gjoreski et al., 2016). Yoon and colleagues (2016) have developed a flexible stress monitoring patch that is about the size of a stamp and worn on the wrist. This patch collects and integrates skin temperature, skin conductance, and arterial pulsewave data to monitor stress.

Other teams have been working to detect stress from subtle behaviors, as well as sounds in the environment (collected primarily via smartphone). Examples of these technologies include smartphone-based facial recognition to identify basic emotions (Suk & Prabhakaran, 2014); daily smartphone usage (e.g., sleeping patterns, social interactions, physical activity) to estimate stress (Kostopoulos et al., 2017); and usage of other smartphone sensors and data (e.g., calendar events, notifications, weather, audio frequency/amplitude) to passively estimate stress levels (Gimpel et al., 2015). Moving forward, behavioral scientists could leverage such technologies when designing mHealth interventions in order to more effectively intervene in stress when it occurs and before it contributes to SUD lapse/relapse.

Insomnia

Insomnia is the most prevalent sleep disorder (American Academy of Sleep Medicine, 2014) and is associated with over $150 billion in direct and indirect costs in the United States (Reynolds & Ebben, 2017). Insomnia may be particularly amenable to mHealth interventions, and there is a critical unmet need for delivering such treatments. Numerous meta-analyses have indicated that cognitive-behavioral therapy for insomnia (CBT-I) is efficacious and safe for the general population (Koffel, Koffel, & Gehrman, 2015) as well as specific subgroups (e.g., older adults, cancer survivors; Irwin, Cole, & Nicassio, 2006; Johnson et al., 2016; Wu, Appleman, Salazar, & Ong, 2015). Although the American

College of Physicians recommends CBT-I as *first-line* care for insomnia (Qaseem, Kansagara, Forciea, Cooke, & Denberg, 2016), patients are not typically referred for CBT-I (Conroy & Ebben, 2015). This is due in part to physicians' and patients' lack of understanding of the risks and benefits of behavioral treatment as compared to pharmacological treatment (Conroy & Ebben, 2015; Koffel, Bramoweth, & Ulmer, 2018; Ulmer et al., 2017) and to a lack of providers trained to administer CBT-I (Thomas, Grandner, et al., 2016). Several groups have developed mHealth treatments for insomnia to address this unmet need (Zachariae, Lyby, Ritterband, & O'Toole, 2016).

Measuring Sleep and Sleep Quality

Polysomnography (PSG), commonly referred to as a "sleep study," is considered the "gold standard" for assessment of sleep. PSG uses several physiologic parameters (e.g., electroencephalogram, pulse oximetry) to collect data on time spent asleep, time spent in various stages of sleep, and factors necessary for diagnosing and/or ruling out sleep disorders (e.g., obstructive sleep apnea). The high cost, patient burden, and restricted access of PSG limit its uptake in research settings. Thus, research has increasingly used wearable sensors and patient-reported outcomes to test behavioral interventions for insomnia. A large and growing literature supports the validity of assessing sleep using research-grade, wrist-worn accelerometers (Smith et al., 2018). These devices use patients' activity data to estimate time spent awake versus asleep. With additional data on bedtime and rising time from patient sleep logs, these data can also be used to determine additional data elements (e.g., time to sleep onset, number of awakenings). A recent meta-analysis found that accelerometers are valid for assessing important outcomes in patients with insomnia, such as time to fall asleep and time spent awake after initial sleep onset (Smith et al., 2018). One drawback of research-grade accelerometers is that data on these devices are typically accessed only after users return them to the clinic or laboratory so that their data can be uploaded to a desktop computer. This limits the ability of investigators to develop JITAIs that incorporate real-time or recent data to adjust guidance based on recent sleep, as is routinely done in CBT-I. However, at least one manufacturer (e.g., Actigraph Corp.) markets accelerometers that allow ongoing data collection by sending data to a telemetry device that pushes these data onto the manufacturer's servers. These data can then be accessed manually via a Web dashboard or automatically via an application programming interface (API).

Consumer-grade wearable sensors may support further development of mHealth interventions for insomnia. Devices manufactured by companies such as Fitbit have demonstrated validity for measuring sleep parameters. Because some consumer-grade devices include a heart rate sensor, unlike research-grade accelerometers, these devices may be able to estimate time spent in various stages of sleep. Typically, these devices send data to a smartphone/tablet, which processes the data and/or uploads to the manufacturer's servers for processing. This process makes access to sleep data faster than is typical for research-grade accelerometers, facilitating the use of sleep data in mHealth-based JITAIs. One important limitation of consumer-grade devices is the opacity of the raw data processing steps taken by manufacturers of these devices. Another limitation is that whereas some research-grade actigraphs have up to 30 days of battery life, consumer-grade devices may need to be recharged several times during a 30-day assessment period. Despite these limitations, consumer-grade wearables should be considered for measuring sleep in mHealth studies.

mHealth Interventions

There has been a recent increase in the development of mHealth interventions to reduce insomnia. This is not only due to the great unmet need for behavioral interventions for insomnia, but also because the main components of CBT-I are all amenable to standardization and delivery via an app. Somryst (Ritterband et al., 2017) and Sleepio (Espie et al., 2012) are two empirically supported mHealth apps for insomnia that allow users to receive intervention components at their convenience. Both have strong empirical support, and both include the main components of CBT-I. Interactive educational components instruct patients on the etiology of insomnia, stimulus control (i.e., restricting the use of the bed for only sleep and sex), cognitive restructuring (i.e., counteracting maladaptive thoughts and beliefs regarding sleep), and sleep restriction (i.e., consolidating the sleep period by reducing amount of time in bed). Sleep restriction requires that patients be provided a "prescription" for when they should get into bed each night and rise from bed each morning. This "prescription" relies on factors that are unique to each patient; therefore, both apps solicit data from patients such as when they need to arise each morning (e.g., for work). Users of Somryst and Sleepio complete sleep diaries to help customize this prescription, but Sleepio also allows users to import data from Fitbit devices (Cowie, Bower, Gonzalez, & Alfano, 2018). One observational study found that integrating wearable data with Sleepio did not affect efficacy or engagement (Luik, Machado, & Espie, 2018). Somryst is currently available with a prescription (PEAR Therapeutics, 2021), and Sleepio is available through agreements with employers (Big Health, n.d.).

Numerous other mHealth apps are available on smartphone app stores that purport to treat insomnia; however, a recent review found that few use evidence-based principles shown to reduce it (Yu, Kuhn, Miller, & Taylor, 2019). Of the nine unique apps identified and tested, most were free to download and use, including CBT-I Coach, and two had a fee for download and/or to use certain features. Each app was rated based on its adherence to seven empirically supported principles (e.g., stimulus control, sleep restriction, cognitive restructuring) and ease of use on a scale of 0 (not applicable) to 3 (adherent and very easy to use). CBT-I Coach demonstrated the greatest adherence to empirically supported principles and ease of use with an average score of 2.85. The remaining eight apps showed large differences in adherence and usability, with apps like Somnology earning a score of 2.00 and others earning scores as low as 0.14 (Yu et al., 2019). Thus, there is wide variability in the adherence to empirical supported principles for publicly available mHealth apps, which creates confusion regarding which apps are evidenced-based for insomnia.

Additional Innovative Uses of mHealth for Health Behaviors

Physical Activity Interventions

Recent estimates indicate that only 54.2% (Centers for Disease Control and Prevention, 2018) of adults are achieving the recommended levels of physical activity. With increasing rates of smartphone (Pew Research Center, 2019) and wearable smartwatch/fitness tracker ownership (Vogels, 2020), mHealth interventions have the potential to broadly influence physical activity across settings. As such, interest in mobile interventions focused on promoting physical activity and decreasing sedentary behavior has increased dramatically, as evidenced by the proliferation of published reviews (Buckingham, Williams, Morrissey, Price, & Harrison, 2019; Elavsky, Knapova, Klocek, & Smahel, 2019; Hardeman, Houghton, Lane, Jones, & Naughton, 2019; Hosseinpour & Terlutter, 2019; McCallum, Rooksby, & Gray, 2018; Schoeppe et al., 2016) and meta-analyses on this topic over the past 5 years (Brickwood, Watson, O'Brien, & Williams, 2019; Direito, Carraça, Rawstorn, Whittaker, & Maddison, 2017; Eckerstorfer et al., 2018; Flores Mateo, Granado-Font, Ferré-Grau, & Montaña-Carreras, 2015; Hodkinson et al., 2019; Romeo et al., 2019; Silva, Simões, Queirós, Rocha, & Rodrigues, 2020; Yerrakalva, Yerrakalva, Hajna, & Griffin, 2019).

Recent reviews have indicated that mobile physical activity interventions commonly include behavior change techniques such as self-monitoring through manual logging or automated physical activity tracking, goal-setting, feedback about activity in relation to goals, social comparisons among users, and rewards (Buckingham et al., 2019; Elavsky et al., 2019; Hardeman et al., 2019; Hosseinpour & Terlutter, 2019). The inclusion of self-monitoring, goal-setting, and feedback, in particular, appear to have a significant positive impact on physical activity (Eckerstorfer et al., 2018; Hosseinpour & Terlutter, 2019). Mobile interventions that have included a wearable physical activity tracker to objectively monitor activity have produced greater increases in physical activity than interventions that did not include a tracker (Brickwood et al., 2019). Combining wearable activity trackers with in-person counseling may have a greater impact on physical activity than the trackers alone (Ash et al., 2021; Hodkinson et al., 2019). Overall, meta-analyses have concluded that mHealth interventions have a small positive effect on activity, particularly daily step count, relative to no treatment or traditional interventions, though the longer-term effects are less favorable (Direito et al., 2017; Eckerstorfer et al., 2018; Flores Mateo et al., 2015; Romeo et al., 2019; Silva et al., 2020; Yerrakalva et al., 2019). However, the limited number and quality of studies limits certainty about the efficacy of mHealth interventions for physical activity. Large-scale randomized controlled trials are needed to investigate the impact of mHealth interventions on physical activity in both the short term and long term.

Medication Monitoring Interventions

Patient nonadherence to medication regimens is common (Cheen, Tan, Oh, Wee, & Thumboo, 2019), and often leads to poor health outcomes (Walsh et al., 2019). mHealth interventions, including smartphone apps and electronic reminder interventions (text messages, reminder devices), offer a means to support adherence remotely; recent reviews have tentatively concluded that these interventions improve medication adherence (Peng et al., 2020; Vervloet et al., 2012; Wong, Siy, Da Silva Lopes, & Georgiou, 2020). Common mobile intervention features include education, adherence monitoring (personal and external), medication reminders/alerts, and the ability to communicate with caregivers (Ahmed et al., 2018; Peng et al., 2020; Wong et al. 2020). Smartphone apps that aim to increase medication adherence are widely available, though most are not evidence-based (Ahmed et al., 2018). Electronic reminder interventions have shown short-term efficacy for improving medication adherence across studies (Vervloet et al., 2012). However, a more recent large-scale randomized controlled trial evaluated the impact of three types of reminder devices: (1) pill bottle strip with toggles (i.e., take-n-slide attaches to the pill bottle, and daily switch is pushed to the right after medication is taken each day);

(2) digital timer cap (displays time elapsed since medication was last taken); and (3) a standard pillbox (plastic box with compartments for each day of the week) on medication adherence among nonadherent patients relative to a no-device control group. No benefit of the devices was found over the 12-month follow-up period (Choudhry et al., 2017). Overall, similar to many other areas of mHealth, the available evidence for mHealth interventions focused on medication adherence is limited. Randomized controlled trials examining the outcomes of medication adherence interventions are needed, as outcomes may vary widely, depending on the specific population, medical condition, and medication type under study.

Diabetes Management Interventions

In 2018, 34.2 million people were diagnosed with diabetes in the United States, which is 10.5% of the population (Centers for Disease Control and Prevention, 2020). Management of this chronic disease is complex, and poor management can lead to adverse health outcomes. Mobile health interventions can simplify diabetes management, and they often take the form of mobile apps, text messaging, portable monitoring devices, pedometers, or a combination (Wang et al., 2020). Interventions commonly offer self-monitoring, education, reminders/alerts, feedback, social support, and counseling (Wang et al., 2020), typically with a focus on insulin management (i.e., calculating insulin bolus, insulin titration), glucose tracking (e.g., via glucose meters), and lifestyle modification (e.g., physical activity, diet, sleep; Shan, Sarkar, & Martin, 2019). Shan and colleagues (2019) offered a detailed review of specific apps, notably the BlueStar mobile diabetes coach (Quinn et al., 2008, 2011), which became the first type 2 diabetes app available by prescription. With the BlueStar app, individuals enter their monitored values on a mobile phone (e.g., glucose, carbohydrate intake, medications) and receive tailored educational, motivational, and behavioral messages based on the data they entered. The BlueStar app has demonstrated efficacy for improving glycemic control in randomized controlled trials (Quinn et al., 2008, 2011).

Overall, mHealth interventions have shown a positive impact on health indicators, primarily glycemic control for individuals diagnosed with either type 1 or type 2 diabetes (Greenwood, Gee, Fatkin, & Peeples, 2017; Wang et al., 2019, 2020) even within socioeconomically disadvantaged and vulnerable populations (Mayberry et al., 2019). Additional studies with rigorous designs are needed to identify effective tailoring strategies based on age, sex, type of diabetes, health literacy, and other individual factors.

Future Directions and Conclusions

The development and testing of mHealth interventions for health behaviors is arguably in its infancy. Opportunities for research in this area are numerous, and in addition to those described earlier in this chapter, we highlight several more here. First, leveraging scalable technologies that address multiple health behaviors concurrently would be beneficial. For example, continued alcohol use while trying to quit smoking presents an increased risk of relapse to smoking (Businelle, Ma, Kendzor, Frank, Wetter, & Vidrine, 2016; Kahler, Spillane, & Metrik, 2010; Lam et al., 2014), and interventions that address alcohol use during a quit smoking attempt are needed. An intervention could enable location monitoring to allow for the delivery of a JITAI when entering high-risk situations for smoking and drinking, as well as integrate wearable wireless sensors to quickly intervene if smoking or drinking does occur. Addressing the nuanced relationship between smoking and alcohol use could also be a target for novel treatments. For instance, if alcohol use is detected, a notification could be delivered to advise the individual to be mindful of their elevated risk for smoking lapse. Another example would be an intervention that targets both sleep and stress concurrently. Here, it may be possible for the same device (wrist sensor) to detect both sleep and stress, reducing participant burden by requiring them to wear a single device. Feedback on improvements in sleep and stress would be possible via graphs in a phone app, and intervention content could be pushed and available on demand.

Second, although JITAIs may allow for the delivery of an intervention at just the right moment, we first need to understand exactly when to deliver an intervention, the conditions under which delivery makes sense, and what content is best to deliver. As such, microrandomized trials (MRTs; Klasnja et al., 2015) that enable the randomization of moments in which participants will receive intervention content, or not, are well positioned to help identify the active ingredients of a multicomponent JITAI. For example, although we know that stress is a potent predictor of substance use relapse, we do not have good data on exactly when and how stress should be targeted on a daily/weekly basis. Thus, an MRT might test whether delivering intervention content via smartphone at certain times of the day is more/less beneficial than delivering intervention content at other times of the day. For instance, Hernandez and colleagues (2021) are conducting an MRT that provides mindfulness strategies at key moments during a quit smoking attempt. A better understanding of the nuanced relationships among such variables has application not only to treatment development, but also to existing theoretical models of behavior change.

Third, our conceptualization of behavior change and intervention delivery may need to be modified as technology advances. For instance, as technology allows for interventions to occur in real time, existing models of behavior change will likely need to be updated and/or new models developed. EMAs may improve our understanding of complex relationships between the environment, thoughts, feelings, and behaviors. To date, most theoretical models have not considered the impact of intervention content on proximal and distal health behaviors, likely because prior to recent years, the ability to intervene in this manner was not possible (i.e., most interventions have been delivered in-person on a once weekly basis).

Fourth, research is needed to determine how to best modify what we already know works (e.g., CBT) to fit mHealth technology. For example, do we need to integrate in-person counseling within mHealth interventions, or can mHealth interventions stand alone? One important future direction in the area of mHealth interventions for insomnia is to test and disseminate stepped-care interventions. This pragmatic approach currently in use for therapist-led CBT-I (Reynolds et al., 1997) is aimed at improving access to CBT-I, increasing efficiency in the use of clinic resources, and providing a low-intensity intervention that is efficacious in treating insomnia (Cheung, Jarrin, Ballot, Bharwani, & Morin, 2019; Wong, Chung, & Au, 2021). One stepped-care model showed that about 46% of patients experienced a remission of insomnia after the self-administered intervention, and the overall stepped-care model dramatically increased efficiency in use of clinic resources (i.e., more patients were treated). Similar models are under examination among subpopulations, such as cancer survivors (Zhou, Michaud, & Recklitis, 2020). However, future studies should further examine the benefits of incorporating mHealth interventions into stepped-care approaches for insomnia and other health behaviors.

Fifth, interdisciplinary partnerships are necessary to advance mHealth interventions for health behaviors. Collaboration among computer scientists, engineers, and behavioral scientists is needed to fully leverage the potential of evolving technology. For example, although there have been great advances in the detection of stress via wearable sensors, very little research has been conducted to evaluate the efficacy of these technologies regarding behavior change. Implementation and dissemination in this area are also greatly lacking. The National Institutes of Health (2022) has recently urged the scientific community to bridge the science-to-practice gap by conducting studies focused on how to best implement and disseminate evidence-based interventions in real-world settings. Although many mHealth interventions are designed to be automated, understanding how to increase the uptake of such treatments for health behaviors is warranted. Scientific collaboration with hospitals, practitioners, and other public health leaders may be required.

Sixth, the costs and timelines for mHealth intervention development and testing often differ from what is traditionally offered via funding mechanisms (e.g., 5-year ROI). Budgets often involve greater costs that not only include development and testing of the mHealth intervention itself, but also increased costs associated with data storage and interdisciplinary collaborations. Once funding ends, many mHealth treatments need to be maintained, and it is often unclear who should oversee this and how the funding will be sustained (e.g., source of funding). The National Institutes of Health does offer Small Business Innovation Research (SBIR) and Small Business Technology Transfer (STTR) grant funding, which can facilitate mHealth interventions. Nonetheless, these mechanisms are not applicable to all mHealth projects. There is a need for federal funding mechanisms that support rapid, iterative data collection that may vary from the traditional funding mechanisms in scope, costs, and time frame. Additionally, funding opportunities are needed that can expedite the translation of effective interventions into real-world practice.

In conclusion, the current landscape of mobile interventions for health behaviors is vast. Opportunities for research in this area are numerous, including: continued technology development, evaluation of technology on specific health behaviors (and on targeting health behaviors concurrently), and new conceptualizations of behavior change. Large-scale randomized controlled trials are needed to rigorously evaluate the efficacy and real-world effectiveness of health-focused apps. Finally, interdisciplinary collaborations and innovative funding opportunities will be a key factor in moving the science of mHealth for health behaviors forward.

REFERENCES

Abroms, L. C., Boal, A. L., Simmens, S. J., Mendel, J. A., & Windsor, R. A. (2014). A randomized trial of Text2Quit: A text messaging program for smoking cessation. *American Journal of Preventive Medicine, 47*(3), 242–250.

Abroms, L. C., Johnson, P. R., Leavitt, L. E., Cleary, S. D., Bushar, J., Brandon, T. H., et al. (2017). A randomized trial of text messaging for smoking cessation in pregnant women. *American Journal of Preventive Medicine, 53*(6), 781–790.

Agyapong, V. I. O., McLoughlin, D. M., & Farren, C. K. (2013). Six-months outcomes of a randomised trial of supportive text messaging for depression and comorbid alcohol use disorder. *Journal of Affective Disorders, 151*(1), 100–104.

Ahmed, I., Ahmad, N. S., Ali, S., Ali, S., George, A., Saleem Danish, H., et al. (2018). Medication adherence apps: Review and content analysis. *JMIR mHealth and uHealth, 6*(3), 1–13.

Alessi, S. M. & Petry, N. M. (2013). A randomized study of cellphone technology to reinforce alcohol abstinence in the natural environment. *Addiction, 108*(5), 900–909.

American Academy of Sleep Medicine. (2014). Chronic insomnia disorder. In *International classification of sleep disorders* (3rd ed., pp. 21–40). Author.

Ash, G. I., Stults-Kolehmainen, M., Busa, M. A., Gaffey, A. E., Angeloudis, K., Muniz-Pardos, B., et al. (2021). Establishing a global standard for wearable devices in sport and exercise medicine: Perspectives from academic and industry stakeholders. *Sports Medicine, 51*(11), 2237–2250.

Bae, S., Chung, T., Ferreira, D., Dey, A. K., & Suffoletto, B. (2018). Mobile phone sensors and supervised machine learning to identify alcohol use events in young adults: Implications for Just-in-Time Adaptive Interventions. *Addictive Behaviors, 83*, 42–47.

Barnett, N. P., Meade, E., & Glynn, T. R. (2014). Predictors of detection of alcohol use episodes using a transdermal alcohol sensor. *Experimental and Clinical Psychopharmacology, 22*(1), 86–96.

Baskerville, N. B., Struik, L. L., & Dash, D. (2018). Crush the crave: Development and formative evaluation of a smartphone app for smoking cessation. *JMIR mHealth and uHealth, 6*(3), 1–14.

Bernstein, M. H., Stein, L. A., Neighbors, C., Suffoletto, B., Carey, K. B., Ferszt, G., et al. (2018). A text message intervention to reduce 21st birthday alcohol consumption: Evaluation of a two-group randomized controlled trial. *Psychology of Addictive Behaviors, 32*(2), 149–161.

Bertholet, N., Godinho, A., & Cunningham, J. A. (2019). Smartphone application for unhealthy alcohol use: Pilot randomized controlled trial in the general population. *Drug and Alcohol Dependence, 195*, 101–105.

Big Health. (n.d.). *Sleepio is a revolutionary digital therapeutic for insomnia.* www.bighealth.com/sleepio

Bock, B. C., Barnett, N. P., Thind, H., Rosen, R., Walaska, K., Traficante, R., et al. (2016). A text message intervention for alcohol risk reduction among community college students: TMAP. *Addictive Behaviors, 63*, 107–113.

Bock, B. C., Rosen, R. K., Barnett, N. P., Thind, H., Walaska, K., Foster, R., et al. (2015). Translating behavioral interventions onto mHealth platforms: Developing text message interventions for smoking and alcohol. *JMIR mHealth and uHealth, 3*(1), 1–9.

Borrelli, B., Bartlett, Y. K., Tooley, E., Armitage, C. J., & Wearden, A. (2015). Prevalence and frequency of mHealth and eHealth use among US and UK smokers and differences by motivation to quit. *Journal of Medical Internet Research, 17*(7), 1–15.

Brandon, K. O., Vinci, C., Kleinjan, M., Hernandez, L. M., Sawyer, L. E., Sutton, S. K., et al. (2021). Testing augmented reality for eliciting cue-provoked urges to smoke: Toward moving cue-exposure into the real world. *Nicotine and Tobacco Research, 23*(5), 861–865.

Bricker, J. B., Copeland, W., Mull, K. E., Zeng, E. Y., Watson, N. L., Akioka, K. J., et al. (2017). Single-arm trial of the second version of an acceptance & commitment therapy smartphone application for smoking cessation. *Drug and Alcohol Dependence, 170*, 37–42.

Bricker, J. B., Mull, K. E., Kientz, J. A., Vilardaga, R., Mercer, L. D., Akioka, K. J., et al. (2014). Randomized, controlled pilot trial of a smartphone app for smoking cessation using acceptance and commitment therapy. *Drug and Alcohol Dependence, 143*, 87–94.

Brickwood, K.-J., Watson, G., O'Brien, J., & Williams, A. D. (2019). Consumer-based wearable activity trackers increase physical activity participation: Systematic review and meta-analysis. *JMIR mHealth and uHealth, 7*(4), 1–20.

Buckingham, S. A., Williams, A. J., Morrissey, K., Price, L., & Harrison, J. (2019). Mobile health interventions to promote physical activity and reduce sedentary behaviour in the workplace: A systematic review. *Digit Health, 5*, 1–50.

Businelle, M. S., Ma, P., Kendzor, D. E., Frank, S. G., Vidrine, D. J., & Wetter, D. W. (2016).

An ecological momentary intervention for smoking cessation: Evaluation of feasibility and effectiveness. *Journal of Medical Internet Research, 18*(12), 1–13.

Businelle, M. S., Ma, P., Kendzor, D. E., Frank, S. G., Wetter, D. W., & Vidrine, D. J. (2016). Using intensive longitudinal data collected via mobile phone to detect imminent lapse in smokers undergoing a scheduled quit attempt. *Journal of Medical Internet Research, 18*(10), 1–10.

Businelle, M. S., Walters, S. T., Mun, E.-Y., Kirchner, T. R., Hébert, E. T., & Li, X. (2020). Reducing drinking among people experiencing homelessness: Protocol for the development and testing of a Just-in-Time Adaptive Intervention. *JMIR Research Protocols, 9*(4), 1–15.

Centers for Disease Control and Prevention. (2018). *Trends in meeting the 2008 physical activity guidelines, 2008–2018.* www.cdc.gov/physicalactivity/downloads/trends-in-the-prevalence-of-physical-activity-508.pdf

Centers for Disease Control and Prevention. (2020). *National diabetes statistics report 2020: Estimates of diabetes and its burden in the United States.* www.cdc.gov/diabetes/pdfs/data/statistics/national-diabetes-statistics-report.pdf

Chatterjee, S., Moreno, A., Lizotte, S. L., Akther, S., Ertin, E., Fagundes, C. P., et al. (2020). SmokingOpp: Detecting the smoking "opportunity" context using mobile sensors. *Proceedings of the ACM on Interactive, Mobile, Wearable and Ubiquitous Technologies, 4*(1), 1–26.

Cheen, M. H. H., Tan, Y. Z., Oh, L. F., Wee, H. L., & Thumboo, J. (2019). Prevalence of and factors associated with primary medication non-adherence in chronic disease: A systematic review and meta-analysis. *International Journal of Clinical Practice, 73*(6), 1–18.

Chen, T., Zhang, X., Jiang, H., Asaeikheybari, G., Goel, N., Hooper, M. W., et al. (2018). Are you smoking?: Automatic alert system helping people keep away from cigarettes. *Smart Health, 9–10,* 158–169.

Cheung, J. M. Y., Jarrin, D. C., Ballot, O., Bharwani, A. A., & Morin, C. M. (2019). A systematic review of cognitive behavioral therapy for insomnia implemented in primary care and community settings. *Sleep Medicine Reviews, 44,* 23–36.

Choudhry, N. K., Krumme, A. A., Ercole, P. M., Girdish, C., Tong, A. Y., Khan, N. F., et al. (2017). Effect of reminder devices on medication adherence: The REMIND randomized clinical trial. *JAMA Internal Medicine, 177*(5), 624–631.

Christofferson, D. E., Hertzberg, J. S., Beckham, J. C., Dennis, P. A., & Hamlett-Berry, K. (2016). Engagement and abstinence among users of a smoking cessation text message program for veterans. *Addictive Behaviors, 62,* 47–53.

Cole, C. A., Anshari, D., Lambert, V., Thrasher, J. F., & Valafar, H. (2017). Detecting smoking events using accelerometer data collected via smartwatch technology: Validation study. *JMIR mHealth and uHealth, 5*(12), 1–11.

Conroy, D. A., & Ebben, M. R. (2015). Referral practices for cognitive behavioral therapy for insomnia: A survey study. *Behavioural Neurology, 2015,* 1–4.

Cowie, J., Bower, J. L., Gonzalez, R., & Alfano, C. A. (2018). Multimedia field test: Digitalizing better sleep using the Sleepio program. *Cognitive and Behavioral Practice, 25*(3), 442–448.

Crane, D., Garnett, C., Brown, J., West, R., & Michie, S. (2015). Behavior change techniques in popular alcohol reduction apps: Content analysis. *Journal of Medical Internet Research, 17*(5), e118.

Crane, D., Garnett, C., Michie, S., West, R., & Brown, J. (2018). A smartphone app to reduce excessive alcohol consumption: Identifying the effectiveness of intervention components in a factorial randomised control trial. *Scientific Reports, 8,* 1–11.

Dar, R. (2018). Effect of real-time monitoring and notification of smoking episodes on smoking reduction: A pilot study of a novel smoking cessation app. *Nicotine and Tobacco Research, 20*(12), 1515–1518.

Direito, A., Carraça, E., Rawstorn, J., Whittaker, R., & Maddison, R. (2017). mHealth technologies to influence physical activity and sedentary behaviors: Behavior change techniques, systematic review and meta-analysis of randomized controlled trials. *Annals of Behavioral Medicine, 51*(2), 226–239.

Dulin, P. L., Gonzalez, V. M., & Campbell, K. (2014). Results of a pilot test of a self-administered smartphone-based treatment system for alcohol use disorders: Usability and early outcomes. *Substance Abuse, 35*(2), 168–175.

Eckerstorfer, L. V., Tanzer, N. K., Vogrincic-Haselbacher, C., Kedia, G., Brohmer, H., Dinslaken, I., et al. (2018). Key elements of mHealth interventions to successfully increase physical activity: Meta-regression. *JMIR mHealth and uHealth, 6*(11), 1–18.

Elavsky, S., Knapova, L., Klocek, A., & Smahel, D. (2019). Mobile health interventions for physical activity, sedentary behavior, and sleep in adults aged 50 years and older: A systematic literature review. *Journal of Aging and Physical Activity, 27*(4), 565–593.

Espie, C. A., Kyle, S. D., Williams, C., Ong, J. C., Douglas, N. J., Hames, P., et al. (2012). A randomized, placebo-controlled trial of online cognitive behavioral therapy for chronic insomnia disorder delivered via an automated media-rich Web application. *Sleep, 35*(6), 769–781.

Fairbairn, C. E., & Kang, D. (2019). Temporal dynamics of transdermal alcohol concentration measured via new-generation wrist-worn biosensor. *Alcoholism: Clinical and Experimental Research, 43*(10), 2060–2069.

Flores Mateo, G., Granado-Font, E., Ferré-Grau, C., & Montaña-Carreras, X. (2015). Mobile phone apps to promote weight loss and increase physical activity: A systematic review and meta-analysis. *Journal of Medical Internet Research, 17*(11), 1–11.

Gajecki, M., Andersson, C., Rosendahl, I., Sinadinovic, K., Fredriksson, M., & Berman, A. H. (2017). Skills training via smartphone app for university students with excessive alcohol consumption: A randomized controlled trial. *International Journal of Behavioral Medicine, 24*(5), 778–788.

Garrison, K. A., Pal, P., O'Malley, S. S., Pittman, B. P., Gueorguieva, R., Rojiani, R., et (2020). Craving to quit: A randomized controlled trial of smartphone app–based mindfulness training for smoking cessation. *Nicotine and Tobacco Research, 22*(3), 324–331.

Gimpel, H., Regal, C., & Schmidt, M. (2015). myStress: Unobtrusive smartphone-based stress detection. *Proceedings of the 23th European Conference on Information Systems (ECIS 2015)*, pp. 1–12.

Gjoreski, M., Gjoreski, H., Luštrek, M., & Gams, M. (2016, August 31–September 2). *Demo for continuous live stress monitoring with a wristband.* Paper presented at Prestigious Applications of Intelligent Systems Conference 2016, The Hague, The Netherlands.

Gonzalez, V. M., & Dulin, P. L. (2015). Comparison of a smartphone app for alcohol use disorders with an Internet-based intervention plus bibliotherapy: A pilot study. *Journal of Consulting and Clinical Psychology, 83*(2), 335–345.

Grant, B. F., Goldstein, R. B., Saha, T. D., Chou, S. P., Jung, J., Zhang, H., et al. (2015). Epidemiology of DSM-5 alcohol use disorder: Results from the National Epidemiologic Survey on Alcohol and Related Conditions III. *JAMA Psychiatry, 72*(8), 757–766.

Greenwood, D. A., Gee, P. M., Fatkin, K. J., & Peeples, M. (2017). A systematic review of reviews evaluating technology-enabled diabetes self-management education and support. *Journal of Diabetes Science and Technology, 11*(5), 1015–1027.

Gustafson, D. H., McTavish, F. M., Chih, M.-Y., Atwood, A. K., Johnson, R. A., Boyle, M. G., et al. (2014). A smartphone application to support recovery from alcoholism: A randomized clinical trial. *JAMA Psychiatry, 71*(5), 566–572.

Hardeman, W., Houghton, J., Lane, K., Jones, A., & Naughton, F. (2019). A systematic review of Just-in-Time Adaptive Interventions (JITAIs) to promote physical activity. *International Journal of Behavioral Nutrition and Physical Activity, 16*(1), 1–21.

Harder, V. S., Musau, A. M., Musyimi, C. W., Ndetei, D. M., & Mutiso, V. N. (2020). A randomized clinical trial of mobile phone motivational interviewing for alcohol use problems in Kenya. *Addiction, 115*(6), 1050–1060.

Hartzler, A. L., BlueSpruce, J., Catz, S. L., & McClure, J. B. (2016). Prioritizing the mHealth design space: A mixed-methods analysis of smokers' perspectives. *JMIR mHealth and uHealth, 4*(3), 1–16.

Haskins, B. L., Lesperance, D., Gibbons, P., & Boudreaux, E. D. (2017). A systematic review of smartphone applications for smoking cessation. *Translational Behavioral Medicine, 7*(2), 292–299.

Haug, S., Lucht, M. J., John, U., Meyer, C., & Schaub, M. P. (2015). A pilot study on the feasibility and acceptability of a text message-based aftercare treatment programme among alcohol outpatients. *Alcohol and Alcoholism, 50*(2), 188–194.

Haug, S., Schaub, M. P., Venzin, V., Meyer, C., & John, U. (2013). Efficacy of a text message-based smoking cessation intervention for young people: A cluster randomized controlled trial. *Journal of Medical Internet Research, 15*(8), 1–14.

Hawthorne, J. S., & Wojcik, M. H. (2006). Transdermal alcohol measurement: A review of the literature. *Canadian Society of Forensic Science Journal, 39*(2), 65–71.

Hébert, E. T., Ra, C. K., Alexander, A. C., Helt, A., Moisiuc, R., Kendzor, D. E., et al. (2020). A mobile Just-in-Time Adaptive Intervention for smoking cessation: Pilot randomized controlled trial. *Journal of Medical Internet Research, 22*(3), 1–14.

Hébert, E. T., Stevens, E. M., Frank, S. G., Kendzor, D. E., Wetter, D. W., Zvolensky, M. J., et al. (2018). An ecological momentary intervention for smoking cessation: The associations of just-in-time, tailored messages with lapse risk factors. *Addictive Behaviors, 78*, 30–35.

Heffner, J. L., Vilardaga, R., Mercer, L. D., Kientz, J. A., & Bricker, J. B. (2015). Feature-level analysis of a novel smartphone application for smoking cessation. *American Journal of Drug and Alcohol Abuse, 41*(1), 68–73.

Hernandez, L. M., Wetter, D. W., Kumar, S., Sutton, S. K., & Vinci, C. (2021). Smoking cessation using wearable sensors: Protocol for a microrandomized trial. *JMIR Research Protocols, 10*(2), 1–14.

Hides, L., Quinn, C., Cockshaw, W., Stoyanov, S., Zelenko, O., Johnson, D., et al. (2018). Efficacy and outcomes of a mobile app targeting alcohol use in young people. *Addictive Behaviors, 77*, 89–95.

Hodkinson, A., Kontopantelis, E., Adeniji, C., van Marwijk, H., McMillan, B., Bower, P., et al. (2019). Accelerometer- and pedometer-based physical activity interventions among adults with cardiometabolic conditions: A systematic review and meta-analysis. *JAMA Network Open, 2*(10), 1–16.

Hosseinpour, M., & Terlutter, R. (2019). Your personal motivator is with you: A systematic review of mobile phone applications aiming at increasing physical activity. *Sports Medicine, 49*(9), 1425–1447.

Hovsepian, K., al'Absi, M., Ertin, E., Kamarck, T., Nakajima, M., & Kumar, S. (2015). cStress: Towards a gold standard for continuous stress assessment in the mobile environment. *Proceedings of the 2015 ACM International Joint Conference on Pervasive and Ubiquitous Computing*, pp. 493–504.

Iacoviello, B. M., Steinerman, J. R., Klein, D. B., Silver, T. L., Berger, A. G., Luo, S. X., et al. (2017). Clickotine, a personalized smartphone app for smoking cessation: Initial evaluation. *JMIR mHealth and uHealth, 5*(4), 1–15.

Irwin, M. R., Cole, J. C., & Nicassio, P. M. (2006). Comparative meta-analysis of behavioral interventions for insomnia and their efficacy in middle-aged adults and in older adults 55+ years of age. *Health Psychology, 25*(1), 3–14.

Johnson, J. A., Rash, J. A., Campbell, T. S., Savard, J., Gehrman, P. R., Perlis, M., et al. (2016). A systematic review and meta-analysis of randomized controlled trials of cognitive behavior therapy for insomnia (CBT-I) in cancer survivors. *Sleep Medicine Reviews, 27*, 20–28.

Kahler, C. W., Spillane, N. S., & Metrik, J. (2010). Alcohol use and initial smoking lapses among heavy drinkers in smoking cessation treatment. *Nicotine and Tobacco Research, 12*(7), 781–785.

Kendzor, D. E., Businelle, M. S., Waring, J. J., Mathews, A. J., Geller, D. W., Barton, J. M., et al. (2020). Automated mobile delivery of financial incentives for smoking cessation among socioeconomically disadvantaged adults: Feasibility study. *JMIR mHealth and uHealth, 8*(4), 1–13.

Kendzor, D. E., Reitzel, L. R., Mazas, C. A., Cofta-Woerpel, L. M., Cao, Y., Ji, L., et al. (2012). Individual- and area-level unemployment influence smoking cessation among African Americans participating in a randomized clinical trial. *Social Science and Medicine, 74*(9), 1394–1401.

Klasnja, P., Hekler, E. B., Shiffman, S., Boruvka, A., Almirall, D., Tewari, A., et al. (2015). Micro-randomized trials: An experimental design for developing just-in-time adaptive interventions. *Health Psychology, 34S*, 1220–1228.

Koffarnus, M. N., Bickel, W. K., & Kablinger, A. S. (2018). Remote alcohol monitoring to facilitate incentive-based treatment for alcohol use disorder: A randomized trial. *Alcoholism: Clinical and Experimental Research, 42*(12), 2423–2431.

Koffel, E., Bramoweth, A. D., & Ulmer, C. S.

(2018). Increasing access to and utilization of cognitive behavioral therapy for insomnia (CBT-I): A narrative review. *Journal of General Internal Medicine, 33*(6), 955–962.

Koffel, E., Koffel, J. B., & Gehrman, P. R. (2015). A meta-analysis of group cognitive behavioral therapy for insomnia. *Sleep Medicine Reviews, 19*, 6–16.

Kostopoulos, P., Kyritsis, A. I., Deriaz, M., & Konstantas, D. (2017). Stress detection using smart phone data. In K. Giokas, L. Bokor, & F. Hopfgartner (Eds.), *eHealth 360°* (pp. 340–351). Springer.

Lam, C. Y., Businelle, M. S., Aigner, C. J., McClure, J. B., Cofta-Woerpel, L., Cinciripini, P. M., et al. (2014). Individual and combined effects of multiple high-risk triggers on postcessation smoking urge and lapse. *Nicotine and Tobacco Research, 16*(5), 569–575.

Leffingwell, T. R., Cooney, N. J., Murphy, J. G., Luczak, S., Rosen, G., Dougherty, D. M., et al. (2013). Continuous objective monitoring of alcohol use: Twenty-first century measurement using transdermal sensors. *Alcoholism: Clinical and Experimental Research, 37*(1), 16–22.

Liang, D., Han, H., Du, J., Zhao, M., & Hser, Y.-I. (2018). A pilot study of a smartphone application supporting recovery from drug addiction. *Journal of Substance Abuse Treatment, 88*, 51–58.

Lopez-Meyer, P., Patil, Y., Tiffany, S., & Sazonov, E. (2013). Detection of hand-to-mouth gestures using a RF operated proximity sensor for monitoring cigarette smoking. *Open Biomedical Engineering Journal, 7*, 41–49.

Luik, A. I., Machado, P. F., & Espie, C. A. (2018). Delivering digital cognitive behavioral therapy for insomnia at scale: Does using a wearable device to estimate sleep influence therapy? *NPJ Digital Medicine, 1*(3), 1–6.

Ma, P., Businelle, M. S., Balis, D. S., & Kendzor, D. E. (2015). The influence of perceived neighborhood disorder on smoking cessation among urban safety net hospital patients. *Drug and Alcohol Dependence, 156*, 157–161.

Martinez, S. A., Quaife, S. L., Hasan, A., McMillan, K. A., Beebe, L. A., & Muirhead, F. (2020). Contingency management for smoking cessation among individuals with type 2 diabetes: Protocol for a multi-center randomized controlled feasibility trial. *Pilot and Feasibility Studies, 6*(82), 1–10.

Mason, M., Benotsch, E. G., Way, T., Kim, H., & Snipes, D. (2014). Text messaging to increase readiness to change alcohol use in college students. *Journal of Primary Prevention, 35*(1), 47–52.

Mayberry, L. S., Lyles, C. R., Oldenburg, B., Osborn, C. Y., Parks, M., & Peek, M. E. (2019). mHealth interventions for disadvantaged and vulnerable people with type 2 diabetes. *Current Diabetes Reports, 19*(12), 1–15.

McCallum, C., Rooksby, J., & Gray, C. M. (2018). Evaluating the impact of physical activity apps and wearables: Interdisciplinary review. *JMIR mHealth and uHealth, 6*(3), 1–20.

McClure, J. B., Heffner, J., Hohl, S., Klasnja, P., & Catz, S. L. (2017). Design considerations for mHealth programs targeting smokers not yet ready to quit: Results of a sequential mixed-methods study. *JMIR mHealth and uHealth, 5*(3), 1–15.

McTavish, F. M., Chih, M.-Y., Shah, D., & Gustafson, D. H. (2012). How patients recovering from alcoholism use a smartphone intervention. *Journal of Dual Diagnosis, 8*(4), 294–304.

Mellentin, A. I., Nielsen, B., Nielsen, A. S., Yu, F., Mejldal, A., Nielsen, D. G., et al. (2019). A mobile phone app featuring cue exposure therapy as aftercare for alcohol use disorders: An investigator-blinded randomized controlled trial. *JMIR mHealth and uHealth, 7*(8), 1–16.

Meredith, S. E., Alessi, S. M., & Petry, N. M. (2015). Smartphone applications to reduce alcohol consumption and help patients with alcohol use disorder: A state-of-the-art review. *Advanced Health Care Technologies, 1*, 47–54.

Nahum-Shani, I., Smith, S. N., Tewari, A., Witkiewitz, K., Collins, L. M., Spring, B., et al. (2014). *Just-in-Time Adaptive Interventions (JITAIs): An organizing framework for ongoing health behavior support* (The Methodology Center Tech. Report No. 14–126, pp. 1–37).

National Institute on Drug Abuse. (2017). *Trends and statistics.* from https://archives.drugabuse.gov/trends-statistics/costs-substance-abuse#supplemental-references-for-economic-costs

National Institutes of Health. (2022). *Dissemination and implementation (D&I) research.* https://prevention.nih.gov/research-priorities/dissemination-implementation

Naughton, F., Cooper, S., Foster, K., Emery, J., Leonardi-Bee, J., Sutton, S., et al. (2017). Large multi-centre pilot randomized controlled trial testing a low-cost, tailored, self-help smoking cessation text message intervention for pregnant smokers (MiQuit). *Addiction, 112*(7), 1238–1249.

Naughton, F., Hopewell, S., Lathia, N., Schalbroeck, R., Brown, C., Mascolo, C., et al. (2016). A context-sensing mobile phone app (Q sense) for smoking cessation: A mixed-methods study. *JMIR mHealth and uHealth, 4*(3), 1–13.

Naughton, F., Prevost, A. T., Gilbert, H., & Sutton, S. (2012). Randomized controlled trial evaluation of a tailored leaflet and SMS text message self-help intervention for pregnant smokers (MiQuit). *Nicotine and Tobacco Research, 14*(5), 569–577.

Neighbors, C., Atkins, D. C., Lewis, M. A., Lee, C. M., Kaysen, D., Mittmann, A., et al. (2011). Event-specific drinking among college students. *Psychology of Addictive Behaviors, 25*(4), 702–707.

Oliver, J. A., Hallyburton, M. B., Pacek, L. R., Mitchell, J. T., Vilardaga, R., Fuemmeler, B. F., et al. (2018). What do smokers want in a smartphone-based cessation application? *Nicotine and Tobacco Research, 20*(12), 1507–1514.

Ortis, A., Caponnetto, P., Polosa, R., Urso, S., & Battiato, S. (2020). A report on smoking detection and quitting technologies. *International Journal of Environmental Research and Public Health, 17*(7), 1–18.

Parate, A., Chiu, M.-C., Chadowitz, C., Ganesan, D., & Kalogerakis, E. (2014). RisQ: Recognizing smoking gestures with inertial sensors on a wristband. *MobiSys '14: Proceedings of the 12th Annual International Conference on Mobile Systems, Applications, and Services*, pp. 149–161.

PEAR Therapeutics. (2021). *Somryst.* www.somryst.com

Peng, Y., Wang, H., Fang, Q., Xie, L., Shu, L., Sun, W., et al. (2020). Effectiveness of mobile applications on medication adherence in adults with chronic diseases: A systematic review and meta-analysis. *Journal of Managed Care and Specialty Pharmacy, 26*(4), 550–561.

Pew Research Center. (2019). *Mobile technology and home broadband 2019.* www.pewresearch.org/internet/2019/06/13/mobile-technology-and-home-broadband-2019

Pew Research Center. (2021). *Mobile fact sheet.* www.pewresearch.org/internet/fact-sheet/mobile

Piasecki, T. M. (2019). Assessment of alcohol use in the natural environment. *Alcoholism: Clinical and Experimental Research, 43*(4), 564–577.

Qaseem, A., Kansagara, D., Forciea, M. A., Cooke, M., & Denberg, T. D. (2016). Management of chronic insomnia disorder in adults: A clinical practice guideline from the American College of Physicians. *Annals of Internal Medicine, 165*(2), 125–133.

Quinn, C. C., Shardell, M. D., Terrin, M. L., Barr, E. A., Ballew, S. H., & Gruber-Baldini, A. L. (2011). Cluster-randomized trial of a mobile phone personalized behavioral intervention for blood glucose control. *Diabetes Care, 34*(9), 1934–1942.

Quinn, C. C., Sysko Clough, S., Minor, J. M., Lender, D., Okafor, M. C., & Gruber-Baldini, A. (2008). WellDoc mobile diabetes management randomized controlled trial: Change in clinical and behavioral outcomes and patient and physician satisfaction. *Diabetes Technology and Therapeutics, 10*(3), 160–168.

Rash, C. J., Petry, N. M., Alessi, S. M., & Barnett, N. P. (2019). Monitoring alcohol use in heavy drinking soup kitchen attendees. *Alcohol, 81*, 139–147.

Reitzel, L. R., Vidrine, J. I., Businelle, M. S., Kendzor, D. E., Cao, Y., Mazas, C. A., et al. (2012). Neighborhood perceptions are associated with tobacco dependence among African American smokers. *Nicotine and Tobacco Research, 14*(7), 786–793.

Reynolds, C. F., Frank, E., Houck, P. R., Mazumdar, S., Dew, M. A., Cornes, C., et al. (1997). Which elderly patients with remitted depression remain well with continued interpersonal psychotherapy after discontinuation of antidepressant medication? *American Journal of Psychiatry, 154*(7), 958–962.

Reynolds, S. A., & Ebben, M. R. (2017). The cost of insomnia and the benefit of increased access to evidence-based treatment: Cognitive behavioral therapy for insomnia. *Sleep Medicine Clinics, 12*(1), 39–46.

Riordan, B. C., Conner, T. S., Flett, J. A., & Scarf, D. (2015). A brief orientation week ecological momentary intervention to reduce university student alcohol consumption. *Journal of Studies on Alcohol and Drugs, 76*(4), 525–529.

Riordan, B. C., Scarf, D., & Conner, T. S. (2015). Is orientation week a gateway to persistent alcohol use in university students? A preliminary investigation. *Journal of Studies on Alcohol and Drugs, 76*(2), 204–211.

Ritterband, L. M., Thorndike, F. P., Ingersoll, K. S., Lord, H. R., Gonder-Frederick, L., Frederick, C., et al. (2017). Effect of a Web-based cognitive behavior therapy for insomnia intervention with 1-year follow-up: A randomized clinical trial. *JAMA Psychiatry, 74*(1), 68–75.

Romeo, A., Edney, S., Plotnikoff, R., Curtis, R., Ryan, J., Sanders, I., et al. (2019). Can smartphone apps increase physical activity?: Systematic review and meta-analysis. *Journal of Medical Internet Research, 21*(3), 1–14.

Saleheen, N., Ali, A. A., Hossain, S. M., Sarker, H., Chatterjee, S., Marlin, B., et al. (2015). puffMarker: A multi-sensor approach for pinpointing the timing of first lapse in smoking cessation. *UbiComp '15: Proceedings of the 2015 ACM International Joint Conference on Pervasive and Ubiquitous Computing*, pp. 999–1010.

Sarker, H., Hovsepian, K., Chatterjee, S., Nahum-Shani, I., Murphy, S. A., Spring, B., et al. (2017). From markers to interventions: The case of just-in-time stress intervention. In J. M. Rehg, S. A. Murphy, & S. Kumar (Eds.), *Mobile health* (pp. 411–433). Springer.

Sarker, H., Tyburski, M., Rahman, M. M., Hovsepian, K., Sharmin, M., Epstein, D. H., et al. (2016). Finding significant stress episodes in a discontinuous time series of rapidly varying mobile sensor data. *CHI '16: Proceedings of the 2016 CHI Conference on Human Factors in Computing Systems*, pp. 4489–4501.

Sazonov, E., Metcalfe, K., Lopez-Meyer, P., & Tiffany, S. (2011). RF hand gesture sensor for monitoring of cigarette smoking. *2011 Fifth International Conference on Sensing Technology*, pp. 426–430.

Schoeppe, S., Alley, S., Van Lippevelde, W., Bray, N. A., Williams, S. L., Duncan, M. J., et al. (2016). Efficacy of interventions that use apps to improve diet, physical activity and sedentary behaviour: A systematic review. *International Journal of Behavioral Nutrition and Physical Activity, 13*(1), 1–26.

Selvam, A. P., Muthukumar, S., Kamakoti, V., & Prasad, S. (2016). A wearable biochemical sensor for monitoring alcohol consumption lifestyle through Ethyl glucuronide (EtG) detection in human sweat. *Scientific Reports, 6*, 1–11.

Senyurek, V. Y., Imtiaz, M. H., Belsare, P., Tiffany, S., & Sazonov, E. (2019). Smoking detection based on regularity analysis of hand to mouth gestures. *Biomedical Signal Processing and Control, 51*, 106–112.

Shan, R., Sarkar, S., & Martin, S. S. (2019). Digital health technology and mobile devices for the management of diabetes mellitus: State of the art. *Diabetologia, 62*(6), 877–887.

Shrier, L. A., Rhoads, A., Burke, P., Walls, C., & Blood, E. A. (2014). Real-time, contextual intervention using mobile technology to reduce marijuana use among youth: A pilot study. *Addictive Behaviors, 39*(1), 173–180.

Silva, A. G., Simões, P., Queirós, A., Rocha, N. P., & Rodrigues, M. (2020). Effectiveness of mobile applications running on smartphones to promote physical activity: A systematic review with meta-analysis. *International Journal of Environmental Research and Public Health, 17*(7), 1–16.

Sinha, R. (2001). How does stress increase risk of drug abuse and relapse? *Psychopharmacology, 158*(4), 343–359.

Sinha, R. (2007). The role of stress in addiction relapse. *Current Psychiatry Reports, 9*(5), 388–395.

Smith, M. T., McCrae, C. S., Cheung, J., Martin, J. L., Harrod, C. G., Heald, J. L., et al. (2018). Use of actigraphy for the evaluation of sleep disorders and circadian rhythm sleep-wake disorders: An American Academy of Sleep Medicine systematic review, meta-analysis, and GRADE assessment. *Journal of Clinical Sleep Medicine, 14*(7), 1209–1230.

Spohr, S. A., Nandy, R., Gandhiraj, D., Vemulapalli, A., Anne, S., & Walters, S. T. (2015). Efficacy of SMS text message interventions for smoking cessation: A meta-analysis. *Journal of Substance Abuse Treatment, 56*, 1–10.

Spruijt-Metz, D. & Nilsen, W. (2014). Dynamic models of behavior for Just-in-Time Adaptive Interventions. *IEEE Pervasive Computing, 13*(3), 13–17.

Substance Abuse and Mental Health Services Administration. (2019). *Key substance use and mental health indicators in the United States: Results from the 2018 national survey on drug use and health.* www.samhsa.gov/data/sites/default/files/cbhsq-reports/NSDUHNationalFindingsReport2018/NSDUHNationalFindingsReport2018.pdf

Suffoletto, B., Kristan, J., Callaway, C., Kim, K. H., Chung, T., Monti, P. M., et al. (2014). A text message alcohol intervention for young adult emergency department patients: A randomized clinical trial. *Annals of Emergency Medicine, 64*(6), 664–672.

Suffoletto, B., Kristan, J., Chung, T., Jeong, K., Fabio, A., Monti, P., et al. (2015). An interactive text message intervention to reduce binge drinking in young adults: A randomized controlled trial with 9-month outcomes. *PloS One, 10*(11), 1–12.

Suk, M., & Prabhakaran, B. (2014). Real-time mobile facial expression recognition system—A case study. *Proceedings of the 2014 IEEE Conference on Computer Vision and Pattern Recognition Workshops (CVPRW)*, pp. 132–137.

Swift, R. (1993). Transdermal measurement of alcohol consumption. *Addiction, 88*(8), 1037–1039.

Swift, R. (2003). Direct measurement of alcohol and its metabolites. *Addiction, 98*(Suppl. 2), 73–80.

Thomas, A., Grandner, M., Nowakowski, S., Nesom, G., Corbitt, C., & Perlis, M. L. (2016). Where are the behavioral sleep medicine providers and where are they needed?: A geographic assessment. *Behavioral Sleep Medicine, 14*(6), 687–698.

Thomas, K., Linderoth, C., Bendtsen, M., Bendtsen, P., & Müssener, U. (2016). Text message-based intervention targeting alcohol consumption among university students: Findings from a formative development study. *JMIR mHealth and uHealth, 4*(4), 1–11.

Tofighi, B., Chemi, C., Ruiz-Valcarcel, J., Hein, P., & Hu, L. (2019). Smartphone apps targeting alcohol and illicit substance use: Systematic search in in commercial app stores and critical content analysis. *JMIR mHealth and uHealth, 7*(4), 1–12.

Tombor, I., Beard, E., Brown, J., Shahab, L., Michie, S., & West, R. (2019). Randomized factorial experiment of components of the SmokeFree Baby smartphone application to aid smoking cessation in pregnancy. *Translational Behavioral Medicine, 9*(4), 583–593.

Ulmer, C. S., Bosworth, H. B., Beckham, J. C., Germain, A., Jeffreys, A. S., Edelman, D., et al. (2017). Veterans affairs primary care provider perceptions of insomnia treatment. *Journal of Clinical Sleep Medicine, 13*(8), 991–999.

Vervloet, M., Linn, A. J., van Weert, J. C., de Bakker, D. H., Bouvy, M. L., & van Dijk, L. (2012). The effectiveness of interventions using electronic reminders to improve adherence to chronic medication: A systematic review of the literature. *Journal of the American Medical Informatics Association, 19*(5), 696–704.

Vilardaga, R., Rizo, J., Zeng, E., Kientz, J. A., Ries, R., Otis, C., et al. (2018). User-centered design of learn to quit, a smoking cessation smartphone app for people with serious mental illness. *JMIR Serious Games, 6*(1), 1–19.

Vinci, C., Brandon, K. O., Kleinjan, M., & Brandon, T. H. (2020). The clinical potential of augmented reality. *Clinical Psychology: Science and Practice, 27*(3), 1–8.

Vinci, C., Brandon, K. O., Kleinjan, M., Hernandez, L. M., Sawyer, L. E., Haneke, J., et al. (2020). Augmented reality for smoking cessation: Development and usability study. *JMIR uHealth and mHealth, 8*(12), 1–13.

Vogels, E. A. (2020, January 9). *About one-in-five Americans use a smart watch or fitness tracker.* Pew Research Center. www.pewresearch.org/fact-tank/2020/01/09/about-one-in-five-americans-use-a-smart-watch-or-fitness-tracker.

Walsh, C. A., Cahir, C., Tecklenborg, S., Byrne, C., Culbertson, M. A., & Bennett, K. E. (2019). The association between medication non-adherence and adverse health outcomes in ageing populations: A systematic review and meta-analysis. *British Journal of Clinical Pharmacology, 85*(11), 2464–2478.

Walters, S. T., Businelle, M. S., Suchting, R.,

Li, X., Hébert, E. T., & Mun, E.-Y. (2021). Using machine learning to identify predictors of imminent drinking and create tailored messages for at-risk drinkers experiencing homelessness. *Journal of Substance Abuse Treatment, 127*, 1–27.

Wang, X., Shu, W., Du, J., Du, M., Wang, P., Xue, M., et al. (2019). Mobile health in the management of type 1 diabetes: A systematic review and meta-analysis. *BMC Endocrine Disorders, 19*(1), 1–10.

Wang, Y., Min, J., Khuri, J., Xue, H., Xie, B., Kaminsky, L. A., et al. (2020). Effectiveness of mobile health interventions on diabetes and obesity treatment and management: Systematic review of systematic reviews. *JMIR mHealth and uHealth, 8*(4), 1–12.

Whittaker, R., McRobbie, H., Bullen, C., Rodgers, A., & Gu, Y. (2016). Mobile phone-based interventions for smoking cessation (Review). *Cochrane Database of Systematic Reviews, 4*, 1–45.

Wong, H. Y., Subramaniyan, M., Bullen, C., Siddiq, A. A., Danaee, M., & Yee, A. (2019). The mobile-phone-based iCOTM Smokerlyzer®: Comparison with the piCO+ Smokerlyzer® among smokers undergoing methadone-maintained therapy. *Tobacco Induced Diseases, 17*, 1–5.

Wong, K.-Y., Chung, K.-F., & Au, C.-H. (2021). Low-intensity cognitive behavioral therapy for insomnia as the entry of the stepped-care model in the community: A randomized controlled trial. *Behavioral Sleep Medicine, 19*(3), 378–394.

Wong, Z. S., Siy, B., Da Silva Lopes, K., & Georgiou, A. (2020). Improving patients' medication adherence and outcomes in non-hospital settings through eHealth: A systematic review of randomized controlled trials. *Journal of Medical Internet Research, 22*(8), 1–14.

Wray, T. B., Kahler, C. W., Simpanen, E. M., & Operario, D. (2019). A preliminary randomized controlled trial of game plan, a web application to help men who have sex with men reduce their HIV risk and alcohol use. *AIDS and Behavior, 23*(6), 1668–1679.

Wu, J. Q., Appleman, E. R., Salazar, R. D., & Ong, J. C. (2015). Cognitive behavioral therapy for insomnia comorbid with psychiatric and medical conditions: A meta-analysis. *JAMA Internal Medicine, 175*(9), 1461–1472.

Wu, P., Hsieh, J.-W., Cheng, J.-C., Cheng, S.-C., & Tseng, S.-Y. (2010). Human smoking event detection using visual interaction clues. *2010 20th International Conference on Pattern Recognition*, pp. 4344–4347.

Yerrakalva, D., Yerrakalva, D., Hajna, S., & Griffin, S. (2019). Effects of mobile health app interventions on sedentary time, physical activity, and fitness in older adults: Systematic review and meta-analysis. *Journal of Medical Internet Research, 21*(11), 1–13.

Yoon, S., Sim, J. K., & Cho, Y.-H. (2016). A flexible and wearable human stress monitoring patch. *Scientific Reports, 6*, 1–11.

You, C.-W., Chen, Y.-C., Chen, C.-H., Lee, C.-H., Kuo, P.-H., Huang, M.-C., et al. (2017). Smartphone-based support system (SoberDiary) coupled with a Bluetooth breathalyser for treatment-seeking alcohol-dependent patients. *Addictive Behaviors, 65*, 174–178.

Yu, J. S., Kuhn, E., Miller, K. E., & Taylor, K. (2019). Smartphone apps for insomnia: Examining existing apps' usability and adherence to evidence-based principles for insomnia management. *Translational Behavioral Medicine, 9*(1), 110–119.

Zachariae, R., Lyby, M. S., Ritterband, L. M., & O'Toole, M. S. (2016). Efficacy of internet-delivered cognitive-behavioral therapy for insomnia—A systematic review and meta-analysis of randomized controlled trials. *Sleep Medicine Reviews, 30*, 1–10.

Zhou, E. S., Michaud, A. L., & Recklitis, C. J. (2020). Developing efficient and effective behavioral treatment for insomnia in cancer survivors: Results of a stepped care trial. *Cancer, 126*(1), 165–173.

CHAPTER 29

Sensing in Clinical Psychology

Geneva K. Jonathan and Dror Ben-Zeev

CHAPTER OVERVIEW

Sensing technologies offer unique opportunities to address some of the long-standing challenges in diagnosing and treating mental illnesses. With a particular focus on severe mental illness, this chapter draws attention to behavioral features such as location, physical activity, social functioning, speech, medication adherence, and sleep that can be assessed by sensors to detect and monitor symptoms of mental illness. This chapter also provides examples of how these sensors, if applied within a mental health setting, may help mental health care providers prevent, intervene, and treat these illnesses as well as further understand illness features and trajectory. The chapter concludes with a discussion of the implications of using sensors in mental health care, the ongoing challenges within the scope of research, and potential future directions for the continued integration of sensors within clinical psychology.

Background

Mental illness affects one in four individuals across a lifetime (Vigo, Thornicroft, & Atun, 2016). Psychopathology, ranging from mild to severe, is a leading cause of years lost to disability globally and can result in significant symptom burden, high rates of medical morbidity, and premature mortality (Eaton, Anthony, Mandel, & Garrison, 1990; Judd et al., 2003). Effective management of mental illness requires intensive symptom monitoring, face-to-face clinical assessment, and timely clinical intervention. Early recognition of symptoms is critical in lessening the impact of long-term psychological distress and cognitive and social impairment (Elshahawi et al., 2011; Morrison, O'Carroll, & McCreadie, 2006). However, the management, treatment, and prognosis of these illnesses are contingent on access to and utilization of treatment, which is not without its challenges. Many individuals with mental illness cannot access treatment due to financial barriers, societal stigma, limited availability of trained mental health professionals, and lack of mental health education and awareness (Mojtabai et al., 2011; Rowan, McAlpine, & Blewett, 2013). Furthermore, to diagnose, inform, and shape the treatment of a mental illness, providers rely on clinical interviews and self-report information, although these forms of information gathering are often subjective and susceptible to recall inaccuracies and reporting bias (Ben-Zeev & Young, 2010). As such, there have been increased efforts to develop tools for early detection and monitoring of mental health problems.

Sensing technologies offer unique solutions to address the limitations and challenges of diagnosis, treatment, and prevention in mental health care. These technologies can be leveraged to provide important contextual and behavioral insights. First, sensors are easy to access as they are typically embedded in commonly used, portable devices. A recent study on mobile device ownership demonstrated that most individuals with serious mental illness (schizophrenia, major depression, and bipolar disorders) own a mobile phone, with the majority owning a smartphone (Young et al., 2020). The accessibility and mobility of sensors offer individuals an alternative to direct, face-to-face, often stigmatized, interaction with clinic-based services. Second, sensors can automatically generate in-the-moment, objective information and reduce social desirability and recall biases that may impact clinical case conceptualization and treatment planning. The automatic collection of data not only is less intrusive of an individual's daily activities but also minimizes the risk of nonengagement with daily monitoring due to its limited demand on the end user. Finally, sensing may provide opportunities for mental health screening that can alert individuals to seek out services before or during a mental health crisis and reduce costs to health care systems by preventing severe cases from getting worse.

Here, we describe the current state of sensing within the scope of clinical psychology research and mental health practice. This chapter aims to provide a detailed description of how sensors can be used for monitoring behavioral features that correlate with the symptomatology of psychopathology, emphasizing serious mental illnesses. We conclude this chapter with a brief description of implications for practice, limitations, challenges, and future directions.

Recent Sensing Work and Its Application in Clinical Psychology

Mobile devices such as smartphones can be leveraged as an easy and inexpensive tool to continuously and electronically self-monitor subjective information about illness activity and objective data such as calls, text messages, and social media activities. In conjunction with phone use data, remote sensors can collect data passively, including location, physical activity, and patterns in speech or sleep. These data can be interpreted to detect the presence of anxiety, stress, mood, and psychotic symptoms (Seppälä et al., 2019). At the core of psychopathology is a shift in the extant pattern of dysfunctional thoughts and feelings. This shift may affect any number of features about a person's external presentation, such as location, physical activity, social functioning, communication style, medication nonadherence, and sleep. In the following section, we describe how sensing technologies can track behavior and psychological states and how they can be uniquely applied to the field of clinical psychology.

Location and Mobility

Individuals with mental illness, particularly those with serious mental illness, often experience isolation and lack opportunities to engage in meaningful activities in their communities (McCormick, Funderburk, Lee, & Hale-Fought, 2005). This lack of community engagement is compounded by the fact that 85% of individuals with serious mental illness are unemployed and lack educational and leisure activities (Bond, Salyers, Rollins, Rapp, & Zipple, 2004). Although research typically focuses on an individual's functioning as a measure of community engagement, an emerging body of work focuses on the role of place and movement within communities as an indication of illness severity and recovery outcomes (Townley, Kloos, & Wright, 2009). Physical presence in a community is operationalized as the cumulative frequency of self-initiated participation in community activities and use of community resources (Aubry & Myner, 1996). In remote sensing, physical presence (location) and movement within a location (mobility) can be tracked continuously and leveraged to identify community engagement. Location and mobility information is primarily gathered through cellular networks, Bluetooth and Wi-Fi connections, and Global Positioning System (GPS) data. The most common digital biomarkers using these sensors are the number of locations visited, entropy (indications of regularity or routine), mobility (patterns of movement between locations), and, though not typical, activity (shopping or playing sports).

To successfully predict the symptomatology of mental illnesses, researchers have used self-report questionnaires to contextualize GPS data. This approach has found strong associations between geolocation and various self-report questionnaires. For example, higher entropy, or the more locations at which an individual spent time, is correlated with a better mood (Rohani, Faurholt-Jepsen, Kessing, & Bardram, 2018). In contrast, individuals were more likely to score high on a depressed mood scale the more they remained at home (Doryab, Min, Wiese, Zimmerman, & Hong, 2014; Saeb, Lattie, Schueller, Kording, & Mohr, 2016). In schizophrenia, individuals were less likely to visit new places when symptomatic (Wang et al., 2016). Additionally, less GPS mobility is associated with greater negative symptom severity and diminished motivation (Depp et al., 2019). Meanwhile, greater GPS mobility has been weakly associated with more community functioning (Depp et al., 2019). Among individuals with bipolar disorder, researchers have found a positive correlation between mood and the percentage of time spent outdoors (Sabatelli, Osmani, Mayora, Gruenerbl, & Lukowicz, 2014). Recent work has utilized passive sensing to predict relapse in individuals with schizophrenia, and preliminary findings have suggested that location patterns can identify which individuals are more likely to relapse (Ben-Zeev et al., 2017; Wang, Wang, Aung, et al., 2018; Wang, Wang, et al., 2020).

Location and mobility data may also provide context about how individuals with mental illness engage with their communities. Identifying the specific baseline patterns of an individual's engagement with locations and their community might offer an alternative way to detect prodromal symptoms. For instance, if individuals spend too much sedentary time at home, they may be slipping into a depressive state, and mental health providers can be activated to respond. Not all individuals with mental illness that experience the same condition have similar manifestations of symptomatology. For example, due to diagnostic criteria for bipolar disorder, one might assume that affective states, like mania, where individuals may experience increased social behavior, hypersexuality, and euphoria, are associated with increased locations visited and mobility. However, the literature suggests that mobility in manic individuals decreases when they are experiencing a manic state (Beiwinkel et al., 2016). Differences across studies indicate that modeling using location and mobility data may have to be personalized to the individual's locations, activities, and social roles rather than the population.

Physical Activity

Mental health is related to physical health and activity. Individuals with mental illness are more likely to be physically inactive and to experience challenges in attainment and maintenance of fitness and weight loss due to the impact of symptoms on motivation, lack of affordable options for exercise, the metabolic effects of psychoactive medications, and poor diet (Bartels et al., 2013). The lack of physical activity in this population, combined with a high prevalence of unhealthy behaviors such as smoking, increases the risk of comorbid medical conditions and reduces life expectancy (Colton & Manderscheid, 2006). In the general population, activity tracking using basic devices like pedometers is an effective technique for supporting health promotion efforts (Burke et al., 2015). Among individuals with mental illness, outpatients have indicated that they feel comfortable using smartphone sensors for characterizing their activity patterns (Ben-Zeev et al., 2016). Preliminary studies have demonstrated that the use of passive data to encourage health promotion efforts in this population is acceptable and feasible (Naslund, Aschbrenner, & Bartels, 2016). Beyond physical health, the amount by which an individual is physically active can indicate deterioration in mental health status. For example, depression is marked by decreased daytime motor activity compared with improved (euthymic) or manic mood states (Wolff, Putnam, & Post, 1985). Sensing can remotely measure changes in activity level using accelerometry and gyroscope data to measure different types of activity (walking versus running), duration of time spent sedentary, duration of physical activity, as well as the intensity of movement.

Several studies have utilized physical activity data to identify the features of mental illness (Rohani et al., 2018; Seppälä et al., 2019). Individuals with bipolar and unipolar disorders have been found to have lower levels of acceleration, fitness, and energy expenditure (Faurholt-Jepsen et al., 2012). When adjusted for symptom severity, bipolar disorder was associated with significantly lower and different daily acceleration patterns (e.g., a greater range of activity between 6:00 A.M. and 12:00 P.M.) and expenditure compared to unipolar disorders (Faurholt-Jepsen et al., 2012). A similar study found that individuals with bipolar disorder, even when asymptomatic, were still significantly more sedentary than the general population (Janney et al., 2014). Among individuals with schizophrenia, reduced physical activity is also associated with increased symptom severity (Walther et al., 2015). Step count is positively correlated with positive, disorganized, and excited measures on a positive and negative syndrome scale, but not with negative and depressed factors (Tron, Resheff, Bazhmin, Peled, & Weinshall, 2017). Efforts have also been made to utilize sensing data for interventional purposes, such as evaluating the impact of physical activity on mood states. For instance, among depressed alcohol-dependent individuals, increased activity levels were associated with reductions in anxiety and depression symptoms (Abrantes et al., 2017).

Physical activity can improve the quality of life among individuals with mental illness by improving their physical health while also alleviating their psychiatric and social disabilities. Regular physical activity has been shown to improve quality of life and emotional well-being even in the absence of objective diagnostic treatment (Faulkner & Biddle, 1999). There is a serious need to promote physical activity in this population, given their heightened risk for comorbid health conditions, high obesity rates, and the gap in mortality. Lifestyle interventions promoting physical activity among individuals with mental illness have shown substantial promise for improving cardiovascular health and contributing to weight loss (Bartels et al., 2013, 2015). Passively collected physical activity data could be integrated into these lifestyle interventions as summary reports or feedback to reinforce positive health behaviors. Finally, reinforcement and encouragement to engage in physical activity from passive sensing data could play a role in reducing social isolation. This aspect of physical activity is still not well understood, although some studies suggest that physical activity can engage individuals in mental health services and offer safer opportunities for social interaction (Faulkner & Sparkes, 1999).

Social Functioning

Social functioning or the extent to which individuals can occupy functional social roles and actively contribute to their community is often impaired in people with mental illness. Understanding social functioning within this population provides insights into an individual's severity of symptoms and their capacity to live independently. Recovery and quality of life outcomes often consider recovery from mental illness as an improvement not just of symptoms but also of individuals' interaction with their respective environment (Bartels & Pratt, 2009). Even after complete remission of psychopathology, however, residual impairments tend to remain. Social functioning can be studied using a multidimensional approach that evaluates behavioral (network size, time and frequency of social activities, and frequency of perceived social support) and affective (loneliness, affiliation, perceived social disability) indicators (Santini, Koyanagi, Tyrovolas, Mason, & Haro, 2015). These indicators translate to remote sensing activities in a complex way and often require referencing a combination of passively collected data such as communication patterns (number of in/out phone calls, duration of calls, number of in/out text messages), smartphone usage (application use such as Facebook, Twitter, Instagram), face-to-face conversations (microphone), sleep patterns (accelerometer, ambient light, and sound), mobility (accelerometer), physical activities (accelerometer), and semantic location (GPS coordinates associated with frequently visited places).

Initial sensing studies have evaluated the connection between communication patterns and illness states. In individuals with bipolar disorder, fewer outgoing text messages were associated with increased depressive symptoms, whereas an increase in calls was associated with manic symptoms (Beiwinkel et al., 2016). Furthermore, fewer outgoing calls, as well as the duration of incoming and outgoing calls, were correlated with depressive symptoms (Faurholt-Jepsen et al., 2015). Among individuals with schizophrenia, self-reported positive attributes (e.g., calm, hopeful, sleeping well) were associated with fewer phone calls, conversations, and text messages (Wang et al., 2016). On the other hand, negative attributes were associated with having fewer conversations but making more phone calls and sending more text messages (Wang et al., 2016). Building on this body of work, one study found that communication patterns could be used to identify oncoming relapse among individuals with schizophrenia. Before relapse, individuals placed fewer, shorter outgoing phone calls and sent and received fewer text messages (Buck et al., 2019). Communication patterns have also been used to identify meaningful relationships in an individual's network. Longer calls were typically from family and friends and were determined by the frequency of text messages during the week (Min, Wiese, Hong, & Zimmerman, 2013). Work contacts were characterized by when calls were received (during the work week instead of over the weekend) and fewer text messages (Min et al., 2013).

Social information can also be remotely gathered through social media platforms where individuals engage with others and share their activities, thoughts, and photos. A large body of literature has demonstrated that specific words that include negative and positive emotions can be used to make inferences about affect and mood (Rude, Gortner, & Pennebaker, 2004). Several studies have utilized data from Twitter, Facebook, Reddit, and other Web forums to detect the presence of depression (Guntuku, Yaden, Kern, Ungar, & Eichstaedt, 2017). However, few studies integrate social media data collection with structured clinical interviews to determine how they may impact the screening and assessment of mental illnesses. Though not directly tied to clinical interviews, online language may predict mental illness prior to a formal diagnosis. In a study that examined words on Reddit, individuals with depression used terms related to sadness, life problems, medications, ugliness, and harm, among other topics (Thorstad & Wolff, 2019). These findings suggest that it may be valuable to examine the content of remotely collected text messages and social media posts to gain more insight into social functioning and mental health symptomatology.

Automated sensing tools provide the capacity to understand patterns, individual differences, and community-specific information that may help researchers understand varying levels of social functioning. Sensing information specific to the respective community in which an individual resides would allow interventions to be more personally relevant as well as help individuals address community-specific challenges in social functioning. Objective information about social functioning may also provide a clearer understanding of mechanisms, skills, and strategies that individuals with higher functioning have found useful in their day-to-day lives to benefit those with lower social capacities who may continue to struggle with community engagement. Objective sensor-derived information about social functioning could also be provided to the end user through an intervention to help them develop self-awareness and insight into their successes and failures in social interaction. One critical consideration for assessing social functioning in individuals with mental illness is multimodal sensing. Often, one or two sensors on their own are not enough to gather context-specific information and classify distinct features (Wang, Mirjafari, et al., 2020). For example, depressed college students may engage in more social activities and programming to meet requirements for school. In contrast, a same-aged young adult outside a school setting may appear to be lower in functioning because they do not have access to community-organized social events. Researchers must incorporate context-specific information about the individual before interpreting these data at the individual level and in a sample.

Language and Speech Patterns

Deficits or abnormalities in speech and communication are common among people with mental illness. These deficits are chronic, resistant to medications, and associated with poor outcomes (Kirkpatrick, Buchanan, Ross, & Carpenter, 2001). Language is considered a biologically relevant phenotype of mental illnesses (Arevian et al., 2020). Although patterns in speech have been identified as instrumental in understanding the underlying pathophysiological processes of the disease, there is limited knowledge about their course (Insel et al., 2010). One common barrier to studying speech pathology is its reliance on interviewer-based rating scales and observational, face-to-face treatment settings that cannot examine these deficits over long periods (Kirkpatrick et al., 2011). With advances in technology, researchers can measure voice features such as sound, quality, frequency, as well as conversation frequency and duration from a smartphone or wearables' microphone.

Voice data have been used to classify manic and depressive states as well as suicide risk in individuals with bipolar disorder and depression (Cummins et al., 2015; Karam et al., 2014). Arevian and colleagues (2020) evaluated the domains of affective words as well as complexity and acoustic properties of longitudinal voice data from individuals with serious mental illness and found that they were able to predict self-harm and depression using self-report measures. In depression, paralinguistic elements of voice have been associated with depressive symptoms and response to treatment (Hashim, Wilkes, Salomon, Meggs, & France, 2017; Mundt, Vogel, Feltner, & Lenderking, 2012). Acoustic pitch variability and changes in pause time between words have also been significantly correlated with depression (Mundt, Snyder, Cannizzaro, Chappie, & Geralts, 2007). More broadly, conversational patterns have been linked to perceived stress—individuals proximally close to more frequent and longer conversations are less likely to feel stressed (Wang et al., 2014). Thus far, no studies have found significant associations between relapse and speech duration. However, this may be because speech duration as a standalone variable may not have enough variability to significantly relate to relapse (Buck et al., 2019).

Speech patterns are an essential secondary measure of social functioning. However, the current measurement of speech among individuals with mental illness is limited in its capacity to determine how speech deficits vary within and across individuals, as well as how they are related to cognitive, pathophysiological, and genetic variables (Insel, 2017). Advances in our knowledge about how sensors might identify speech pathology shifts throughout illness could clarify how speech pathology relates to the severity of symptoms and cognitive impairment. For example, in an individual with bipolar disorder who experienced pressured speech in a manic phase and slowed, disorganized speech when depressed, exploration of their shift in speech pattern may provide insights about their illness trajectory. Regarding social functioning, sensors can offer an opportunity to evaluate how disorganized speech in the wild affects the ability to attain and maintain societal roles.

Medication Adherence

Nonadherence to medications or, the extent to which an individual follows a medication regime prescribed by a doctor, is a widespread public health issue (Sabaté, 2003). Approximately 50% of chronically ill individuals do not adhere to their medications, although among individuals with mental illness, nonadherence rates can reach up to 89% (Schulze et al., 2019). Nonadherence can be intentional and related to an individual's dissatisfaction with taking psychotropic medications in the long term or unintentionally, including forgetting to take the correct dose at the right time, failing to fill or refill a prescription, or discontinuing medication before completion of the recommended dose. Regardless of intention, nonadherence can lead to an exacerbation of symptoms, rehospitalization, poor quality of life outcome, and increased risk of suicide (Rana & Ayub, 2002). Several technological solutions have been studied, such as smartphone interventions that provide reminders and pill containers that record the number of times opened (Steinkamp et al., 2019). The challenge posed by these newer technologies is that they do not confirm that the individual ingested the medication once obtained. On this occasion, an ingestible sensor may make a clinically meaningful difference.

In a preliminary feasibility and safety study of ingestible sensors among individuals with schizophrenia and bipolar disorder using a placebo pill, average medication adherence was 74% (Kane et al., 2013). Following this study, in 2017, the U.S. Food and Drug Administration (FDA) approved a version of a second-generation antipsychotic embedded with a sensor that activates in the stomach, communicates ingestion to a wearable sensor (a patch), and then records adherence on a smartphone application and Web portal. In a multicenter, open-label study, the average medication adherence with the ingestible sensor was 73.9%, and most individuals expressed satisfaction with the sensor's associated technology (Peters-Strickland et al., 2016). An initial challenge that arose was that ingestion of the pill could only be detected if the patch was worn, ultimately depending on an individual's ability to regularly replace the patch and pair it with the smartphone application. Only 55% of the study's participants could replace the patch and connect it to their smartphone without help. However, this number increased to 81% when participants were assisted by a remote human support coach, indicating that minimal assistance may improve usability (Peters-Strickland et al., 2016). A replication study reported 88.6% medication adherence and found that individuals with schizophrenia needed more support with the technology (Kopelowicz et al., 2017).

Despite the availability of interventions designed to address medication nonadherence among individuals with mental illness, high rates of nonadherence persist (Steinkamp et al., 2019). An ingestible sensor embedded in a psychotropic medication would provide a way for providers and end users, for the first time, to get real-time, accurate information about adherence to identify and intervene if medication nonadherence begins. A recent survey of mental health care experts indicated that they believe a notification about medication nonadherence after three consecutively missed days would be helpful for interventional purposes (Hatch, Docherty, Carpenter, Ross, & Weiden, 2017). Additionally, this type of technology could encourage an individual to develop insight about the relationship between discontinuation of psychiatric medications and symptom exacerbation, as well as create an opportunity for an open dialogue between providers, supports, and end users about challenges with adherence. For individuals who experience persistent, residual symptoms between psychiatric episodes, real-time evaluation of adherence could help distinguish between partial efficacy of medication due to nonadherence versus lack of effectiveness due to nonrespondence of the psychoactive component (Hatch et al., 2017). Out of all the behaviors sensors monitor, the least is known about the efficacy of ingestible sensors on improving outcomes. Currently, the FDA has approved only one sensor-embedded psychotropic medication. The generalizability and relevance of this technology to the effective long-term management of mental health conditions are unknown. More research is also needed to address whether these sensors can address some of the current challenges facing nonadherence and their connection to treatment outcomes.

Sleep

Abnormalities in sleep behavior are commonly reported in the general population (Singleton, Bumpstead, O'Brien, Lee, & Meltzer, 2003). The prevalence of sleep dysfunction is substantially higher in people with serious mental illness (Harvey, Murray, Chandler, & Soehner, 2011). Changes in sleep behaviors are a primary biological symptom of depression (Berk, 2009), an indicator of relapse in bipolar disorder (Harvey, 2008), and present in approximately 90% of those with psychotic illnesses (Wulff, Dijk, Middleton, Foster, & Joyce, 2012). Accordingly, monitoring sleep behaviors can provide information about an individual's clinical status. Four measures of sleep obtained by sensors are key in the treatment of mental illnesses: sleep efficiency (quality), total sleep duration (amount of time slept), sleep onset latency (bedtime), and wake after sleep onset (rise time). Actigraphy and accelerometers have been used as a long-standing measure for sleep duration, efficiency, and circadian rhythms in the general population, though only recently have they been used to evaluate these measures in mentally ill populations.

Many researchers have aligned sensor data from wearables to self-report measures for mental health problems to predict sleep disturbances. In a recent assessment of sleep quality among individuals with schizophrenia, accelerometer data were moderately correlated with participants; self-reported daily sleep duration (Staples et al., 2017). Objectively measured sleep duration is also significantly associated with the severity of depressive symptoms (Ben-Zeev, Scherer, Wang, Xie, & Campbell, 2015; Wang et al., 2014). In other words, individuals who are more depressed tend to sleep more. Among college students, sensors indicated that students with depression slept for shorter periods, woke up later, and generally had more irregular sleep schedules (Wang, Wang, DaSilva, et al., 2018).

Beyond comparison to self-report assessments, sleep efficiency, duration, and bedtime/rise times have been estimated from device activity patterns. Phone usage patterns—specifically screen lock and unlock patterns—can be used to detect and predict individual daily variations indicative of sleep duration, efficiency, and timing of bedtime and rise time (Abdullah, Matthews, Murnane, Gay, & Choudhury, 2014). Inferences about sleep can also be made through the use of silence/do-not-disturb mode, ambient light, and the length of time the phone sits stationary. However, these device activity findings have not been replicated among individuals with mental illnesses. Finally, some researchers suggest that the standalone feature detection of sleep leads to weak predictions, whereas when multiple features are combined, the accuracy of sleep duration and prediction is much more robust (Chen et al., 2013). For instance, several features, including sleep disturbance, computed from individuals' environmental audio, as potential correlates of anxiety and depression symptomatology, were, in fact, strongly associated with depression (Di Matteo et al., 2020).

Sleep directly impacts daily functioning. For individuals with mental illnesses, sleep disturbances are associated with poor clinical outcomes (Waite, Sheaves, Isham, Reeve, & Freeman, 2020); however, the impact of these disturbances remains poorly understood (Jagannath, Peirson, & Foster, 2013). Sensors' ability to measure circadian inputs provides an opportunity to identify how sleep disturbances impact individuals' presentation of illness differently and advance the knowledge around this symptom. The length of time that sensors can monitor sleep behaviors allows researchers to examine sleep comprehensively over a long-term period, which would allow more insight into how sleep evolves throughout a psychiatric episode. Additionally, given the connection between sleep disturbance and psychotic features, remote monitoring may provide an opportunity to better understand how psychotic experiences are linked to sleep dysfunction. From a relapse prevention perspective, deterioration in functioning can often start with abnormal sleep behaviors, so remote monitoring and the ability to characterize sleep continuously may encourage a prompter response to psychiatric emergencies. In detecting sleep features, it is important to remember the varying differences in a disturbance between the general population and individuals with mental illnesses, Thus, when studying this behavioral feature, researchers should acknowledge the limits to generalizability if it is purely studied in a nonclinical sample.

Research Challenges and Future Directions

This chapter discusses currently available health and activity monitoring sensors that can measure important behavioral parameters present in mental illnesses. The current state of the field demonstrates that sensing technologies, which can remotely monitor an individual's clinical status, are well positioned to improve mental health care as they offer a novel way to address many of the current problems in the field. Although these technologies are innovative, exciting, and filled with promise, significant research is still needed to help advance these tools from research to implementation and dissemination.

Standardization and Replicability

Most existing studies are based on nonrandomized, nonblinded, proof-of-concept studies that utilize a limited clinical sample. While a growing number of studies have begun to replicate the findings of preliminary studies, there is a widespread tendency to glamorize the novelty of these technologies and underestimate the value of reproducibility in real-world settings where end users may be dealing with the challenges of homelessness, poverty, and cognitive impairment that would make using these tools difficult. Of the studies that replicate prior findings regarding the severity of symptoms or behavioral markers, there is a lack of standardization and regulation between self-assessment measures and sensors, making it difficult to draw comparisons between studies. There are hundreds of smartphone versions, wearable devices, and sensors across various operating systems. It is challenging to draw confirmatory conclusions on how these tools may be helpful in mental health care when the generalizability of these approaches is limited. (For details, see Giurgiu & Bussman Chapter 5, this volume, on physical behavior data.) In the same fashion, many self-assessment surveys are used to diagnose and assess symptomatology that have been used to classify and predict behavioral features, again making it hard to compare findings across studies.

Feature Detection

To successfully categorize and identify specific mood, anxiety, and psychotic features, one must also consider symptom-specific details such as intensity, frequency, and variability that can significantly differ between individuals. Existing work on predicting mood states using sensors typically focuses on identifying generic behavioral features to predict or map onto a self-assessment scale. Additionally, of the existing studies, many use short assessment periods, such as 3 months, to assess relapse and to detect features (Ebner-Priemer et al., 2020). It is naïve to believe that these studies accurately detect variations in illness that typically occur over more extended periods such as 6 to 12 months.

Moving forward, it is critical to shift beyond the detection of generic behavioral features to accommodate specificities in the day-to-day lives of those with mental illnesses. Although many studies demonstrate a clinically significant association between symptomatology and sensor findings, this link has yet to transition into a clinically meaningful prediction parameter. On this note, it is equally important that sensors align or function within research models such as the Research Domain Criteria (RDoC), a conceptual framework introduced by the National Institute of Mental Health that integrates various modalities of information (behavior, physiology, and self-report) to understand and treat mental illnesses (Insel et al., 2010). For example, Wang, Wang, DaSilva, and colleagues (2018) designed a set of behavioral features to capture the unique characteristics of a college student (e.g., going to class, working in study areas, socializing in a campus setting), while also monitoring for RDoC depressive symptomatology. Other researchers have proposed guidelines for reporting electronic mood data to enhance interpretation, reproducibility, and future meta-analyses of these technologies (Faurholt-Jepsen et al., 2019). Future work should pay particular attention to data collection, feature extraction, and any existing guidelines, as well as self-reported questionnaires and surveys used to assess the severity of symptoms so that comparison with prior work is possible.

Privacy and Confidentiality

Among the most prominent concerns about utilizing sensors to collect mental health care data are privacy and confidentiality. As is true of any technology, users are at risk of having their clinical information exposed through data breaches. Concerns also exist about this field's ethical and societal impact due to the implications of collecting 24/7, large-scale, mental health-related data. Although sensors offer a new horizon of possibility for illness monitoring and continuity of care, these same sensors could also be used for unethical purposes, such as discrimination by potential employers to reduce the risk of insurance payouts. With ingestible sensors specifically, there is some concern that private insurers might incentivize their use—for example, by providing discounted copayments—but also mandate digital medicine as a requirement for parole or release from a psychiatric facility (Belluck, 2017). More efforts are needed to develop and ensure data privacy and information security. One viable suggestion would be to anonymize health data before their synthesis to ensure confidentiality and compliance with health information privacy regulations (El Emam, Rodgers, & Malin, 2015). It may also be helpful to include an option for individuals to modify the frequency of monitoring or to turn it off entirely. Alternatively, some individuals may appreciate more transparency, such as reviewing the tangible metrics of processed raw data on the device before sharing it with mental health care professionals.

Continuity of Care and Integration of the Data

Finally, it is unclear how the data from these sensing technologies can be integrated into face-to-face clinical services to provide a more comprehensive clinical picture. Given that mental health care is already overwhelmed by clinician burnout and overextended providers (Morse, Salyers, Rollins, Monroe-DeVita, & Pfahler, 2012), researchers must strive to develop visualizations and summaries that transform sensor data into easy-to-read summaries and insights. An emerging body of work alongside the proliferation of clinical technologies is the addition of human support roles or clinical technologists (Jonathan, Pivaral, & Ben-Zeev, 2017; Mohr, Cuijpers, & Lehman, 2011). In essence, individuals familiar with the range of digital health resources would fulfill these support roles. They could assess end users' needs and preferences to match them with the tools most likely to be relevant, while also assisting with technical support. Finally, it is essential to consider how sensing information might coexist with, corroborate. or inform preexisting information about the mental health condition of the end user. Although most research presents innovative findings, sensing in real-world settings is rare, and few studies integrate sensing data into clinical settings or intervention tools to measure or report changes in clinical outcomes. Existing studies that monitor users' well-being and various clinical states rely heavily on correlation analysis to understand how well-being connects to different sensors and users' smartphone interactions. More experimental work is needed to uncover the causal links between affective states, smartphone interactions, and context modalities. Understanding the effectiveness of providing end-user facing feedback from the sensors would readily allow integration of these tools into effective behavior interventions and study of their impact on clinical outcomes.

Conclusion

A number of studies have examined the use of multimodal sensors for gathering and monitoring objective behavioral patterns, with some promising applications to the assessment and treatment of mental illness. Multimodal sensors can create a rich, context-specific picture of an individual's mental health status and thus provide more personalized and clinically relevant care. Although this body of work offers exciting prospects for the future of mental health care, a considerable amount of work remains to be done before we can understand how sensing can be integrated into the current mental health care system, to the greatest benefit of both providers and individuals using these tools.

REFERENCES

Abdullah, S., Matthews, M., Murnane, E. L., Gay, G., & Choudhury, T. (2014). Towards circadian computing: "Early to bed and early to rise" makes some of us unhealthy and sleep deprived. *Proceedings of the 2014 ACM International Joint Conference on Pervasive and Ubiquitous Computing*, pp. 673–684.

Abrantes, A. M., Blevins, C. E., Battle, C. L., Read, J. P., Gordon, A. L., & Stein, M. D. (2017). Developing a Fitbit-supported lifestyle physical activity intervention for depressed alcohol dependent women. *Journal of Substance Abuse Treatment, 80*, 88–97.

Arevian, A. C., Bone, D., Malandrakis, N., Martinez, V. R., Wells, K. B., Miklowitz, D. J., et al. (2020). Clinical state tracking in serious mental illness through computational analysis of speech. *PLoS One, 15*(1), 1–17.

Aubry, T., & Myner, J. (1996). Community integration and quality of life: A comparison of persons with psychiatric disabilities in housing programs and community residents who are neighbours. *Canadian Journal of Community Mental Health, 15*(1), 5–20.

Bartels, S. J., & Pratt, S. I. (2009). Psychosocial rehabilitation and quality of life for older adults with serious mental illness: Recent findings and future research directions. *Current Opinion in Psychiatry, 22*(4), 381–385.

Bartels, S. J., Pratt, S. I., Aschbrenner, K. A., Barre, L. K., Jue, K., Wolfe, R. S., et al. (2013). Clinically significant improved fitness and weight loss among overweight persons with serious mental illness. *Psychiatric Services, 64*(8), 729–736.

Bartels, S. J., Pratt, S. I., Aschbrenner, K. A., Barre, L. K., Naslund, J. A., Wolfe, R., et al. (2015). Pragmatic replication trial of health promotion coaching for obesity in serious mental illness and maintenance of outcomes. *American Journal of Psychiatry, 172*(4), 344–352.

Beiwinkel, T., Kindermann, S., Maier, A., Kerl, C., Moock, J., Barbian, G., et al. (2016). Using smartphones to monitor bipolar disorder symptoms: A pilot study. *JMIR Mental Health, 3*(1), 1–15.

Belluck, P. (2017, November 13). First digital pill approved to worries about biomedical "big brother." *New York Times.* www.nytimes.com/2017/11/13/health/digital-pill-fda.html

Ben-Zeev, D., Brian, R., Wang, R., Wang, W., Campbell, A. T., Aung, M. S., et al. (2017). CrossCheck: Integrating self-report, behavioral sensing, and smartphone use to identify digital indicators of psychotic relapse. *Psychiatric Rehabilitation Journal, 40*(3), 266–275.

Ben-Zeev, D., Scherer, E. A., Wang, R., Xie, H., & Campbell, A. T. (2015). Next-generation psychiatric assessment: Using smartphone sensors to monitor behavior and mental health. *Psychiatric Rehabilitation Journal, 38*(3), 218–226.

Ben-Zeev, D., Wang, R., Abdullah, S., Brian, R., Scherer, E. A., Mistler, L. A., et al. (2016). Mobile behavioral sensing for outpatients and inpatients with schizophrenia. *Psychiatric Services, 67*(5), 558–561.

Ben-Zeev, D., & Young, M. A. (2010). Accuracy of hospitalized depressed patients' and healthy controls' retrospective symptom reports: An experience sampling study. *Journal of Nervous and Mental Disease, 198*(4), 280–285.

Berk, M. (2009). Sleep and depression—theory and practice. *Australian Family Physician, 38*(5), 302–304.

Bond, G. R., Salyers, M. P., Rollins, A. L., Rapp, C. A., & Zipple, A. M. (2004). How evidence-based practices contribute to community integration. *Community Mental Health Journal, 40*(6), 569–588.

Buck, B., Scherer, E., Brian, R., Wang, R., Wang, W., Campbell, A., et al. (2019). Relationships between smartphone social behavior and relapse in schizophrenia: A preliminary report. *Schizophrenia Research, 208*, 167–172.

Burke, L. E., Ma, J., Azar, K. M., Bennett, G. G., Peterson, E. D., Zheng, Y., et al. (2015). Current science on consumer use of mobile health for cardiovascular disease prevention: A scientific statement from the American Heart Association. *Circulation, 132*(12), 1157–1213.

Chen, Z., Lin, M., Chen, F., Lane, N. D., Cardone, G., Wang, R., et al. (2013). Unobtrusive sleep monitoring using smartphones. *Proceedings of the 2013 7th International Conference on Pervasive Computing Technologies for Healthcare and Workshops*, pp. 145–152.

Colton, C. W., & Manderscheid, R. W. (2006). Congruencies in increased mortality rates, years of potential life lost, and causes of death among public mental health clients in eight states. *Preventing Chronic Disease, 3*(2), 1–14.

Cummins, N., Scherer, S., Krajewski, J., Schnieder, S., Epps, J., & Quatieri, T. F. (2015). A review of depression and suicide risk assessment using speech analysis. *Speech Communication, 71*, 10–49.

Depp, C. A., Bashem, J., Moore, R. C., Holden, J. L., Mikhael, T., Swendsen, J., et al. (2019). GPS mobility as a digital biomarker of negative symptoms in schizophrenia: A case control study. *NPJ Digital Medicine, 2*(1), 1–7.

Di Matteo, D., Fotinos, K., Lokuge, S., Yu, J., Sternat, T., Katzman, M. A., et al. (2020). The relationship between smartphone-recorded environmental audio and symptomatology of anxiety and depression: Exploratory study. *JMIR Formative Research, 4*(8), e18751.

Doryab, A., Min, J. K., Wiese, J., Zimmerman, J., & Hong, J. (2014, July). Detection of behavior change in people with depression. *Proceedings of Workshops at the Twenty-Eighth AAAI Conference on Artificial Intelligence*, pp. 12–16.

Eaton, W. W., Anthony, J. C., Mandel, W., & Garrison, R. (1990). Occupations and the prevalence of major depressive disorder. *Journal of Occupational Medicine, 32*(11), 1079–1087.

Ebner-Priemer, U. W., Mühlbauer, E., Neubauer, A. B., Hill, H., Beier, F., Santangelo, P. S., et al. (2020). Digital phenotyping: Towards replicable findings with comprehensive assessments and integrative models in bipolar disorders. *International Journal of Bipolar Disorders, 8*(1), 1–9.

El Emam, K., Rodgers, S., & Malin, B. (2015). Anonymising and sharing individual patient data. *British Medical Journal, 350*, 1–6.

Elshahawi, H. H., Essawi, H., Rabie, M. A., Mansour, M., Beshry, Z. A., & Mansour, A. N. (2011). Cognitive functions among euthymic bipolar I patients after a single manic episode versus recurrent episodes. *Journal of Affective Disorders, 130*(1–2), 180–191.

Faulkner, G., & Biddle, S. (1999). Exercise as an adjunct treatment for schizophrenia: A review of the literature. *Journal of Mental Health, 8*(5), 441–457.

Faulkner, G., & Sparkes, A. (1999). Exercise as therapy for schizophrenia: An ethnographic study. *Journal of Sport and Exercise Psychology, 21*(1), 52–69.

Faurholt-Jepsen, M., Brage, S., Vinberg, M., Christensen, E. M., Knorr, U., Jensen, H. M., et al. (2012). Differences in psychomotor activity in patients suffering from unipolar and bipolar affective disorder in the remitted or mild/moderate depressive state. *Journal of Affective Disorders, 141*(2–3), 457–463.

Faurholt-Jepsen, M., Geddes, J. R., Goodwin, G. M., Bauer, M., Duffy, A., Kessing, L. V., et al. (2019). Reporting guidelines on remotely collected electronic mood data in mood disorder (eMOOD): Recommendations. *Translational Psychiatry, 9*(1), 1–10.

Faurholt-Jepsen, M., Vinberg, M., Frost, M., Christensen, E. M., Bardram, J. E., & Kessing, L. V. (2015). Smartphone data as an electronic biomarker of illness activity in bipolar disorder. *Bipolar Disorders, 17*(7), 715–728.

Guntuku, S. C., Yaden, D. B., Kern, M. L., Ungar, L. H., & Eichstaedt, J. C. (2017). Detecting depression and mental illness on social media: An integrative review. *Current Opinion in Behavioral Sciences, 18*, 43–49.

Harvey, A. G. (2008). Sleep and circadian rhythms in bipolar disorder: Seeking synchrony, harmony, and regulation. *American Journal of Psychiatry, 165*(7), 820–829.

Harvey, A. G., Murray, G., Chandler, R. A., & Soehner, A. (2011). Sleep disturbance as transdiagnostic: Consideration of neurobiological mechanisms. *Clinical Psychology Review, 31*(2), 225–235.

Hashim, N. W., Wilkes, M., Salomon, R., Meggs, J., & France, D. J. (2017). Evaluation of voice acoustics as predictors of clinical depression scores. *Journal of Voice, 31*(2), 256.

Hatch, A., Docherty, J. P., Carpenter, D., Ross, R., & Weiden, P. J. (2017). Expert consensus survey on medication adherence in psychiatric patients and use of a digital medicine system. *Journal of Clinical Psychiatry, 78*(7), e803–812.

Insel, T. R. (2017). Digital phenotyping: Technology for a new science of behavior. *Journal of the American Medical Association, 318*(13), 1215–1216.

Insel, T., Cuthbert, B., Garvey, M., Heinssen, R., Pine, D. S., Quinn, K., et al. (2010). Research Domain Criteria (RDoC): Toward a new classification framework for research on mental disorders. *American Journal of Psychiatry, 167*(7), 748–751.

Jagannath, A., Peirson, S. N., & Foster, R. G. (2013). Sleep and circadian rhythm disruption in neuropsychiatric illness. *Current Opinion in Neurobiology, 23*(5), 888–894.

Janney, C. A., Fagiolini, A., Swartz, H. A., Jakicic, J. M., Holleman, R. G., & Richardson, C. R. (2014). Are adults with bipolar disorder active? Objectively measured physical activity and sedentary behavior using accelerometry. *Journal of Affective Disorders, 152–154*, 498–504.

Jonathan, G. K., Pivaral, L., & Ben-Zeev, D. (2017). Augmenting mHealth with human support: Notes from community care of people with serious mental illnesses. *Psychiatric Rehabilitation Journal, 40*(3), 336–338.

Judd, L. L., Schettler, P. J., Akiskal, H. S., Maser, J., Coryell, W., Solomon, D., et al. (2003). Long-term symptomatic status of bipolar I vs. bipolar II disorders. *International Journal of Neuropsychopharmacology, 6*(2), 127–137.

Kane, J. M., Perlis, R. H., DiCarlo, L. A., Au-Yeung, K., Duong, J., & Petrides, G. (2013). First experience with a wireless system incorporating physiologic assessments and direct confirmation of digital tablet ingestions in ambulatory patients with schizophrenia or bipolar disorder. *Journal of Clinical Psychiatry, 74*(6), 533–540.

Karam, Z. N., Provost, E. M., Singh, S., Montgomery, J., Archer, C., Harrington, G., et al. (2014, May). Ecologically valid long-term mood monitoring of individuals with bipolar disorder using speech. *Proceedings-ICASSP, IEEE International Conference on Acoustics, Speech and Signal Processing*, pp. 4858–4862.

Kirkpatrick, B., Buchanan, R. W., Ross, D. E., & Carpenter, W. T. (2001). A separate disease within the syndrome of schizophrenia. *Archives of General Psychiatry, 58*(2), 165–171.

Kirkpatrick, B., Strauss, G. P., Nguyen, L., Fischer, B. A., Daniel, D. G., Cienfuegos, A., et al. (2011). The Brief Negative Symptom Scale: Psychometric properties. *Schizophrenia Bulletin, 37*(2), 300–305.

Kopelowicz, A., Baker, R. A., Zhao, C., Brewer, C., Lawson, E., & Peters-Strickland, T. (2017). A multicenter, open-label, pilot study evaluating the functionality of an integrated call center for a digital medicine system to optimize monitoring of adherence to oral aripiprazole in adult patients with serious mental illness. *Neuropsychiatric Disease and Treatment, 13*, 2641–2651.

McCormick, B. P., Funderburk, J. A., Lee, Y., & Hale-Fought, M. (2005). Activity characteristics and emotional experience: Predicting boredom and anxiety in the daily life of community mental health clients. *Journal of Leisure Research, 37*(2), 236–253.

Min, J.-K., Wiese, J., Hong, J. I., & Zimmerman, J. (2013). Mining smartphone data to classify life-facets of social relationships. *Proceedings of the 2013 Conference on Computer Supported Cooperative Work*, pp. 285–294.

Mohr, D., Cuijpers, P., & Lehman, K. (2011). Supportive accountability: A model for providing human support to enhance adherence to eHealth interventions. *Journal of Medical Internet Research, 13*(1), 1–11.

Mojtabai, R., Olfson, M., Sampson, N. A., Jin, R., Druss, B., Wang, P. S., et al. (2011). Barriers to mental health treatment: Results from the National Comorbidity Survey Replication. *Psychological Medicine, 41*(8), 1751–1761.

Morrison, G., O'Carroll, R., & McCreadie, R. (2006). Long-term course of cognitive impairment in schizophrenia. *British Journal of Psychiatry, 189*(6), 556–557.

Morse, G., Salyers, M. P., Rollins, A. L., Monroe-DeVita, M., & Pfahler, C. (2012). Burnout in mental health services: A review of the problem and its remediation. *Administration and Policy in Mental Health and Mental Health Services Research, 39*(5), 341–352.

Mundt, J. C., Snyder, P. J., Cannizzaro, M. S., Chappie, K., & Geralts, D. S. (2007). Voice acoustic measures of depression severity and treatment response collected via interactive voice response (IVR) technology. *Journal of Neurolinguistics, 20*(1), 50–64.

Mundt, J. C., Vogel, A. P., Feltner, D. E., & Lenderking, W. R. (2012). Vocal acoustic biomarkers of depression severity and treatment response. *Biological Psychiatry, 72*(7), 580–587.

Naslund, J. A., Aschbrenner, K. A., & Bartels, S. J. (2016). Wearable devices and smartphones for activity tracking among people with serious mental illness. *Mental Health and Physical Activity, 10*, 10–17.

Peters-Strickland, T., Pestreich, L., Hatch, A., Rohatagi, S., Baker, R. A., Docherty, J. P., et al. (2016). Usability of a novel digital medicine system in adults with schizophrenia treated with sensor-embedded tablets of aripiprazole. *Neuropsychiatric Disease and Treatment, 12*, 2587–2594.

Rana, N. H., & Ayub, M. (2002). Non-compliance to medication in psychiatric patients. *Pakistan Journal of Medical Sciences, 18*(1), 52–54.

Rohani, D. A., Faurholt-Jepsen, M., Kessing, L. V., & Bardram, J. E. (2018). Correlations between objective behavioral features collected from mobile and wearable devices and depressive mood symptoms in patients with affective disorders: Systematic review. *JMIR mHealth and uHealth, 6*(8), 1–21.

Rowan, K., McAlpine, D., & Blewett, L. (2013). Access and cost barriers to mental health care by insurance status, 1999 to 2010. *Health Affairs (Project Hope), 32*(10), 1723–1730.

Rude, S., Gortner, E.-M., & Pennebaker, J. (2004). Language use of depressed and depression-vulnerable college students. *Cognition and Emotion, 18*(8), 1121–1133.

Sabaté, E. (2003). *Adherence to long-term therapies: Evidence for action*. World Health Organization.

Sabatelli, M., Osmani, V., Mayora, O., Gruenerbl, A., & Lukowicz, P. (2014). Correlation of significant places with self-reported state of bipolar disorder patients. *Proceedings of the 2014 4th International Conference on Wireless Mobile Communication and Healthcare—Transforming Healthcare through Innovations in Mobile and Wireless Technologies (MOBIHEALTH)*, pp. 116–119.

Saeb, S., Lattie, E. G., Schueller, S. M., Kording, K. P., & Mohr, D. C. (2016). The relationship between mobile phone location sensor data and depressive symptom severity. *PeerJ, 4*, 1–15.

Santini, Z. I., Koyanagi, A., Tyrovolas, S., Mason, C., & Haro, J. M. (2015). The association between social relationships and depression: A systematic review. *Journal of Affective Disorders, 175*, 53–65.

Schulze, L. N., Stentzel, U., Leipert, J., Schulte, J., Langosch, J., Freyberger, H. J., et al. (2019). Improving medication adherence with telemedicine for adults with severe mental illness. *Psychiatric Services, 70*(3), 225–228.

Seppälä, J., De Vita, I., Jämsä, T., Miettunen, J., Isohanni, M., Rubinstein, K., et al. (2019). Mobile phone and wearable sensor-based mHealth approaches for psychiatric disorders and symptoms: Systematic review. *JMIR Mental Health, 6*(2), 1–14.

Singleton, N., Bumpstead, R., O'Brien, M., Lee, A., & Meltzer, H. (2003). Psychiatric morbidity among adults living in private households, 2000. *International Review of Psychiatry, 15*(1–2), 65–73.

Staples, P., Torous, J., Barnett, I., Carlson, K., Sandoval, L., Keshavan, M., et al. (2017). A comparison of passive and active estimates of sleep in a cohort with schizophrenia. *NPJ Schizophrenia, 3*(1), 1–6.

Steinkamp, J. M., Goldblatt, N., Borodovsky, J. T., LaVertu, A., Kronish, I. M., Marsch, L. A., et al. (2019). Technological interventions for medication adherence in adult mental health and substance use disorders: A systematic review. *JMIR Mental Health, 6*(3), 1–24.

Thorstad, R., & Wolff, P. (2019). Predicting future mental illness from social media: A big-data approach. *Behavior Research Methods, 51*(4), 1586–1600.

Townley, G., Kloos, B., & Wright, P. A. (2009). Understanding the experience of place: Expanding methods to conceptualize and measure community integration of persons with serious mental illness. *Health Place, 15*(2), 520–531.

Tron, T., Resheff, Y. S., Bazhmin, M., Peled, A., & Weinshall, D. (2017). Real-time schizophrenia monitoring using wearable motion sensitive devices. In P. Perego, A. M. Rahmani, & N. TaheriNejad (Eds.), *Wireless Mobile Communication and Health, 7th International Conference, MobiHealth 2017, Proceedings* (pp. 242–249). Springer.

Vigo, D., Thornicroft, G., & Atun, R. (2016). Estimating the true global burden of mental illness. *Lancet Psychiatry, 3*(2), 171–178.

Waite, F., Sheaves, B., Isham, L., Reeve, S., & Freeman, D. (2020). Sleep and schizophrenia: From epiphenomenon to treatable causal target. *Schizophrenia Research, 221*, 44–56.

Walther, S., Stegmayer, K., Horn, H., Razavi, N., Müller, T. J., & Strik, W. (2015). Physical activity in schizophrenia is higher in the first episode than in subsequent ones. *Frontiers in Psychiatry, 5*, 1–5.

Wang, R., Aung, M. S., Abdullah, S., Brian, R., Campbell, A. T., Choudhury, T., et al. (2016). CrossCheck: Toward passive sensing and detection of mental health changes in people with schizophrenia. In *Proceedings of the 2016 ACM International Joint Conference on Pervasive and Ubiquitous Computing*, pp. 886–897.

Wang, R., Chen, F., Chen, Z., Li, T., Harari, G., Tignor, S., et al. (2014). StudentLife: Assessing mental health, academic performance and behavioral trends of college students using smartphones. *Proceedings of the 2014 ACM International Joint Conference on Pervasive and Ubiquitous Computing*, pp. 3–14.

Wang, R., Wang, W., Aung, M. H., Ben-Zeev, D., Brian, R., Campbell, A. T., et al. (2018). Predicting symptom trajectories of schizophrenia using mobile sensing. *GetMobile: Mobile Computing Communications, 22*(2), 32–37.

Wang, R., Wang, W., DaSilva, A., Huckins, J. F., Kelley, W. M., Heatherton, T. F., et al. (2018). Tracking depression dynamics in college students using mobile phone and wearable sensing. *Proceedings of the ACM on Interactive, Mobile, Wearable and Ubiquitous Technologies, 2*(1), 1–26.

Wang, R., Wang, W., Obuchi, M., Scherer, E., Brian, R., Ben-Zeev, D., et al. (2020). On predicting relapse in schizophrenia using mobile sensing in a randomized control trial. *Proceedings of the 2020 IEEE International Conference on Pervasive Computing and Communications (PerCom).*

Wang, W., Mirjafari, S., Harari, G., Ben-Zeev, D., Brian, R., Choudhury, T., et al. (2020). Social sensing: Assessing social functioning of patients living with schizophrenia using mobile phone sensing. *CHI '20: Proceedings of the 2020 CHI Conference on Human Factors in Computing Systems*, pp. 1–15.

Wolff, E. A., Putnam, F. W., & Post, R. M. (1985). Motor activity and affective illness: The relationship of amplitude and temporal distribution to changes in affective state. *Archives of General Psychiatry, 42*(3), 288–294.

Wulff, K., Dijk, D.-J., Middleton, B., Foster, R. G., & Joyce, E. M. (2012). Sleep and circadian rhythm disruption in schizophrenia. *British Journal of Psychiatry, 200*(4), 308–316.

Young, A. S., Cohen, A. N., Niv, N., Nowlin-Finch, N., Oberman, R. S., Olmos-Ochoa, T. T., et al. (2020). Mobile phone and smartphone use by people with serious mental illness. *Psychiatric Services, 71*(3), 280–283.

CHAPTER 30

Smart Interventions

Inbal Nahum-Shani

CHAPTER OVERVIEW

Advances in mobile and wireless devices hold tremendous potential for adapting interventions to the unique and changing needs of individuals over time. An adaptive intervention is an intervention design in which dynamic information about the individual is used to recommend whether and how to intervene. A just-in-time adaptive intervention (JITAI) is a form of an adaptive intervention that leverages powerful mobile and sensing technologies to obtain dynamically changing information about the individual's internal state and context, and use this information to recommend whether and how to intervene in real time, in the individual's natural environment. This chapter is intended to provide a brief introduction to adaptive interventions and JITAIs in mobile health. Different examples of adaptive intervention and JITAIs from various domains of behavior change are used to discuss opportunities and challenges for harnessing digital technology to adapt interventions and to highlight directions for future research.

Introduction

Mobile health (mHealth) tools hold tremendous potential for helping people achieve and sustain behavior change (e.g., to increase physical activity, adopt a healthier diet, manage psychological distress). Intervention components are considered to be mHealth when they employ mobile and wireless devices (e.g., tablets, smartphones, wearables) to promote people's health and well-being (Kumar et al., 2013). The widespread use, acceptability, and convenience of mobile and wireless devices can help reduce certain societal and structural barriers (Amico, 2015) and facilitate scalability across geographic locations (Muessig, LeGrand, Horvath, Bauermeister, & Hightow-Weidman, 2017), including within resource-limited (Haberer et al., 2017) and hard-to-reach (McInnes et al., 2014) settings. Smartphones and tablet computers can host a wide variety of applications (apps) with therapeutic content and engaging features such as social networking and gaming that can be harnessed for health promotion purposes (Mohr, Burns, Schueller, Clarke, & Klinkman, 2013). Mobile devices can also give round-the-clock, real-time reminders, prompts, and feedback. Using these technologies to deliver interventions whenever and wherever they are needed can mitigate the logistical challenges associated with traditional in-person health care, such as scheduling conflicts, travel to treatment facilities, and social distancing constraints.

Because mHealth interventions can be disseminated conveniently with potential to promote behavior change at low cost, they may have particular utility in the initial phases of stepped-care strategies—staged systems comprising a hierarchy of interventions, ranging from the least to the most costly/intensive, matched to the individual's needs (Sobell & Sobell, 2000). In a stepped-care strategy, minimal support (i.e., relatively inexpensive and/or low-burden intervention components) is offered initially, and then more resource-intensive components are offered only to those who need it most (e.g., those showing early signs of nonresponse), whereas less resource-intensive components can be offered to individuals who show adequate response to minimal support. The goal is to enhance resource efficiency by stepping up and down the intensity or cost of interventions based on early signs of progress. Such a stepped-care strategy is a form of an adaptive intervention—an intervention delivery framework that leverages ongoing (i.e., time-varying) information about the individual's progress in the course of the intervention (e.g., early signs of nonresponse or nonadherence) to decide whether and how to modify the type, dosage, intensity, or delivery modality of an intervention.

Adaptive interventions are motivated to address the changing needs of individuals over time, while minimizing cost, effort, and burden. This is done by providing the most appropriate intervention only to those who need it, and only when they need it, therefore minimizing the provision of unnecessary interventions (Collins, Murphy, & Bierman, 2004; Murphy, Lynch, Oslin, McKay, & TenHave, 2007). mHealth tools also offer novel opportunities for delivering just-in-time adaptive interventions (JITAIs). A JITAI is an adaptive intervention that harnesses powerful mobile and sensing technologies to obtain dynamically changing information about the individual's internal state (e.g., craving, stress), and context (e.g., physical location) and use this information to recommend whether and how to deliver interventions in real time, in the individual's natural environment. JITAIs are motivated to address the rapidly changing needs of individuals, while minimizing participant effort, burden, and habituation (Nahum-Shani, Hekler, & Spruijt-Metz, 2015; Nahum-Shani, Smith, et al., 2018).

The present chapter provides a brief introduction to adaptive interventions and JITAIs in mHealth. Different examples of adaptive intervention and JITAIs from various domains of behavior change are used to discuss opportunities and challenges for leveraging digital technology to adapt interventions and to highlight directions for future research.

Adaptive Interventions in mHealth

What Is an Adaptive Intervention?

An adaptive intervention is a protocolized sequence of individualized intervention options that use ongoing information about the individual's progress to decide which intervention option to offer (Collins et al., 2004). An intervention can be considered "adaptive" if (1) ongoing (time-varying) information is used to make intervention decisions and (2) there is a clear protocol describing how to make these decisions in practice in order to enhance intervention replicability in research and real-world implementation (Nahum-Shani & Almirall, 2019).

As an example, consider the following adaptive intervention for promoting weight loss among overweight/obese adults (Ghosh, Nahum-Shani, Spring, & Chakraborty, 2020; Pfammatter et al., 2019). At program entry, a weight loss mobile app is offered to all individuals; this app is designed to support the self-monitoring of weight, dietary intake, and physical activity. The individual's response status is assessed at weeks 2, 4, and 8 based on the amount of weight-loss measures via a wireless scale. If the individual does not lose at least 0.5 pound on average per week, they are classified as a nonresponder; otherwise the individual is classified as a responder. At the first time point when an individual is classified as a nonresponder, the mobile app is augmented with supportive messaging (delivered via push notifications within the app) and weekly coaching sessions (delivered by trained coaches via 10- to 15-minute phone calls). As long as the individual is responsive, they continue with the mobile app alone. This intervention is adaptive because (1) it uses ongoing information about the individual's progress over time (i.e., weight loss measured by home Wi-Fi scale) to decide how to intervene (i.e., whether to continue with minimal mHealth support or step up with more burdensome/costly components) and (2) it is clearly protocolized to guide its implementation in practice.

Adaptive interventions can be protocolized with decision rules. For example, the decision rule illustrated in Figure 30.1 protocolizes the weight-loss adaptive intervention described above:

The decision rule includes four key components:

1. ***Decision points***, namely, points in time in which treatment decisions should be made. In the weight-loss program, decisions are first made at program entry and then every several weeks (i.e., weeks 2, 4, and 8).

2. ***Tailoring variables***, namely, information about the individual used to decide whether and how to modify the intervention. In the weight-loss program, the tailoring variable is the participant's average weekly weight loss, measured based on daily monitoring via the wireless scale.

3. ***Intervention options,*** namely, different intervention types, intensities, dosages, tactics, or delivery modalities that are under consideration at each decision point. The

At program entry,

First-stage intervention option = mobile app alone

Then, at weeks 2, 4, and 8,

IF average weekly weight loss < 0.5 pound

THEN, second-stage intervention option = add supportive messaging and coaching (and stop assessing response status)

ELSE, continue with app alone (and continue assessing response status until week 8)

FIGURE 30.1. Example of a decision rule for protocolizing an adaptive intervention.

weight-loss program offers two intervention options, which represent two alternative tactics: either add supportive messaging and coaching (and stop monitoring response status) or continue with the mobile app alone.

4. ***Thresholds*** or levels of the tailoring variable that differentiate between conditions in which one intervention option should be delivered versus another. In the weight-loss program, the threshold is < 0.5 pound. Specifically, the decision rule specifies that additional support in the form of messaging and coaching should be offered when average weekly weight loss is suboptimal, that is, below 0.5 pound. As long as this threshold is not met, additional support is not required.

The adaptation is operationalized via the tailoring variables, their thresholds/levels, and the intervention options. Here, adaptation refers to a process in which the individual is monitored to obtain information about the tailoring variable(s), thresholds/levels of the tailoring variable(s) are used to decide which intervention option to offer, and the appropriate intervention options are delivered to the individual. This adaptation process is triggered at decision points and is guided by the goal of achieving a prespecified distal outcome (e.g., 5% weight loss by month 12) by impacting proximal outcomes. Proximal outcomes are the short-term goals of the adaptation, typically reflecting key mechanisms of change through which the distal outcome can be achieved (e.g., ongoing weight loss in the course of the program, intervention engagement).

Why Are Adaptive Interventions Needed?

Adaptive interventions are intended to increase the number of participants who benefit from an intervention while minimizing cost, effort, and burden. To clarify this, consider the weight-loss adaptive intervention described above. Coaching is an effective, yet relatively costly and burdensome, weight-loss intervention component (Appel et al., 2011). Text messages are a less costly component, yet participant burden and message fatigue (leading to disengagement) are potential drawbacks (Griffin et al., 2018). The mobile app may be less burdensome, yet low participant engagement with the app can undermine efficacy (Dounavi & Tsoumani, 2019). Still, given empirical evidence indicating that mobile apps can support weight loss at relatively low cost (Pellegrini, Pfammatter, Conroy, & Spring, 2015), a mobile app may be a suitable component to initiate a weight-loss intervention. However, empirical evidence suggests that not all individuals benefit sufficiently from using a mobile app to lose weight; about 50% are unlikely to achieve clinically meaningful weight loss in the long term. Importantly, empirical evidence suggests that these individuals can be identified early, based on the extent of weight loss achieved during the first few weeks of a mobile intervention (Pfammatter et al., 2019). Specifically, existing empirical evidence indicates that those who lose less than 0.5 pound on average per week during the first 2 weeks of a mobile intervention are unlikely to lose 5% of their body weight by month 6. Hence, providing additional support in the form of messaging and coaching to those who lose less than 0.5 pound on average during the first 2 weeks of a mobile intervention has the potential to increase the rate of individuals who achieve a clinically meaningful weight loss by month 6. As long as the individual is meeting the 0.5-pound threshold during the first few weeks, they are likely to achieve a clinically meaningful weight loss by month 6. Hence, continuing with the least costly and burdensome component (i.e., mobile app alone) would be a resource-efficient decision. Overall, this adaptive intervention is motivated to increase the number of individuals who benefit ultimately from a mobile-based weight-loss intervention, while efficiently allocating scarce resources to those who need it most. The next section provides three additional examples of adaptive interventions from different areas of behavior change. These examples highlight the various ways in which digital technology can be leveraged to deliver adaptive interventions.

Examples of Adaptive Interventions Using Digital Technology

Example 1. An Adaptive Intervention for Youth Cannabis Use

Stanger and colleagues (2019) conducted a study to inform the development of an adaptive intervention for reducing drug use among youth with cannabis use disorder attending intensive outpatient programs. The following describes one of the adaptive interventions considered in this study: First, youth received standard contingency management (financial incentives for documented abstinence) with technology-based working memory training (a commercially available digital training program to improve working memory for youth, involving 25 sessions with eight training tasks per session). Drug use was monitored weekly via urinalysis and alcohol breathalyzer tests over 14 weeks. Second, at week 4, if the individual tested positive or did not provide drug tests, they were offered enhanced (i.e., higher magnitude) incentives; otherwise the individual continued with the initial intervention.

Example 2. An Adaptive Adherence Intervention for Youth Living with HIV

Belzer and colleagues (2018) conducted a study to inform the development of an adaptive intervention for improving adherence to antiretroviral therapy (ART) in youth living with HIV. The following describes one of the adaptive interventions considered in this study: First, youth were offered daily personalized but automated text messaging (short messaging service [SMS] support). Participants were able to choose the timing and the wording of these daily adherence reminders and were asked to respond by texting back whether they had taken their ART medications. Second, at month 3, if the individual had viral load ≥200 copies/milliliter or was unable to provide documented viral load results, they were offered incentivized SMS support (i.e., financial incentives for responding to the text messages). Otherwise individuals were offered a tapered intervention whereby the frequency of the text messages was reduced to 2 days per week.

Example 3. An Adaptive Prevention Intervention for High-Risk Drinking in College

Patrick and colleagues (2020) conducted a study to inform the development of an adaptive preventive intervention to reduce high-risk drinking among first-year college students. The following describes one of the adaptive interventions considered in this study. First, before the start of the fall semester, students were offered Web-based personalized normative feedback[1] combined with bi-weekly technology-supported self-monitoring of alcohol use. Second, if students' self-monitoring indicated (1) two or more occasions of consuming 4/5+ drinks for women/men in the past 2 weeks (i.e., binge drinking) or (2) one or more occasions of consuming 8/10+ drinks for women/men in the past 2 weeks (i.e., high-intensity drinking), then self-monitoring stopped and emails were delivered, providing information about available online and in-person treatment resources. Otherwise (i.e., if the student did not report binge or high-intensity drinking or they did not respond to the self-monitoring survey), self-monitoring continued until the end of the semester.

Key Similarities and Differences between Example Adaptive Interventions

In this section, we discuss similarities and differences between the three examples described in the previous section as well as the weight-loss adaptive intervention described earlier in order to highlight the various ways technology can be integrated in adaptive interventions.

Technology Can Be Used in Different Components of an Adaptive Intervention

The weight-loss adaptive intervention discussed earlier, as well as the adaptive intervention in Example 3, use digital technology as part of the first- and second-stage intervention options, as well as to assess the tailoring variable. However, in Example 2, technology (i.e., text messaging) is used as part of the first- and the second-stage intervention options, but not to measure the tailoring variable, and in Example 1 technology is used only in the first-stage intervention option (i.e., to deliver working memory training). Moreover, technology-based components vary in terms of the extent to which they involve human support. For example, the first-stage intervention option in Example 3 (i.e., personalized normative feedback) is entirely technology-based, involving sending students a link to a website where they view the feedback (Patrick et al., 2020). However, the first-stage intervention option in Example 1 (i.e., technology-based working memory training) was completed by youth in the clinic, with staff supervising the training and providing feedback and motivational support (Stanger et al., 2019).

Technology and Measuring the Tailoring Variable

Adaptive interventions may or may not use mobile and/or wireless technology to measure the tailoring variables. As discussed earlier, while both Example 3 and the weight-loss adaptive intervention rely on mobile and/or wireless technology to measure the tailoring variable, Examples 1 and 2 use other tools. Specifically, in Example 1 the tailoring variable was measured via once-weekly onsite urine testing and alcohol breath tests (Stanger et al., 2019). In Example 2, the tailoring variable (viral load) was obtained from participants or their care provider, or via blood sample provided by participants for a study-sponsored viral load assay (Belzer et al., 2018). Moreover, adaptive interventions that use technology to assess the tailoring variable may employ different measurement tools. For example, the adaptive weight-loss program relies on sensor-based assessments (i.e., weight loss measured via a wireless scale) to measure the tailoring variable. Example 3, on the other hand, relies on self-reports obtained via technology-based self-monitoring of alcohol use, possibly because mobile sensor-based approaches for detecting alcohol use are still in the early stages of development (Piasecki, 2019).

Measuring the Tailoring Variable May Have a Dual Purpose

In many adaptive interventions, the measurement of the tailoring variable is intended to not only guide intervention decisions, but also to facilitate behavior change. In Examples 1 and 2, the tailoring variable is measured primarily to inform intervention decisions, that is, for use in deciding whether and how to modify the intervention. However, in Example 3 the tailoring variable is measured for two reasons: both to inform intervention decisions and to facilitate behavior change by prompting reflection and self-awareness (Swendeman et al., 2015). Indeed, systematic reviews indicate that self-monitoring is an effective self-regulation strategy and that interventions designed to increase the frequency of monitoring are likely to promote behavior change, especially when self-monitoring is combined with feedback on performance (Harkin et al., 2016; Michie, Abraham, Whittington, McAteer, & Gupta, 2009). Hence, while sensor-based assessments can be integrated in adaptive interventions to unobtrusively measure the tailoring variables for the purpose of informing intervention decisions, careful consideration should be given to whether relying on sensor-based assessments (vs. self-reports) is consistent with the therapeutic goals of the intervention.

Frequency of Measuring the Tailoring Variable

Adaptive interventions can vary in terms of how frequently the tailoring variables are measured. Practically, this frequency can be similar to or greater than the frequency of decision points in the adaptive intervention. In Example 2, the tailoring variable (viral load) was measured once and used at a single decision point (month 3). In Example 1, the tailoring variable was measured weekly, but this information was summarized and used at a single decision point (week 4). In Example 3, the tailoring variable was measured every 2 weeks, and this information was used in each of the bi-weekly decision points. Note that the weight-loss adaptive intervention discussed above employs daily assessments to measure the tailoring variable. At each of the week 2, 4, and 8 decision points, a summary based on this daily information is used to make intervention decisions. Overall, in Examples 2 and 3, the frequency of assessing the tailoring variable is similar to the frequency of decision points. However, in Example 1 and in the weight-loss adaptive intervention, the tailoring variable is assessed more frequently compared to the frequency of decision points. In general, the frequency of the decision points should be based primarily on how fast the conditions the intervention is intended to address are likely to change over time (see Nahum Shani, Smith, et al., 2018). For example, in the weight-loss adaptive intervention, there are decision points at weeks 0, 2, 4, and 8 because this intervention is designed to address conditions that likely unfold every several weeks (i.e., insufficient weight loss, which indicates early nonresponse to a mobile-based intervention). The frequency of measuring the tailoring variables, on the other hand, should be based on several considerations, including the frequency of the decision points (to ensure that at each decision point, the information needed to make intervention decisions was obtained), the validity and reliability of the measurement (Collins et al., 2004), practical feasibility, and participant burden.

Handling Missing Data on the Tailoring Variable

Adaptive interventions vary in how missing data on the tailoring variable are handled. In both Examples 1 and 2, participants who did not provide information on the tailoring variable (i.e., drug tests in Example 1 and viral load results in Example 2) were offered additional support. The underlying assumption is that missing data on the tailoring variable are informative, capturing early signs of nonresponsiveness to the initial intervention. In Example 3 students who did not provide information about the tailoring variable (i.e., did not self-monitor) continued with self-monitoring (i.e., the initial stage of the adaptive intervention) and were not offered additional support. Here, the underlying assumption is that missing data on the tailoring variable do not necessarily indicate nonresponsiveness to the initial intervention. In general, an adaptive intervention should include a concrete prespecified plan for how to handle situations when information about the tailoring variable is missing, in order to enhance intervention replicability.

JITAIs in mHealth

What Is a JITAI?

A JITAI is a form of an adaptive intervention intended to address the rapidly changing needs of individuals. As an example, consider the following simplified description of Sense2Stop (Battalio et al., 2021; Spring, 2018), a JITAI designed to provide support for smoking cessation. This JITAI is based on evidence suggesting that if smokers who are attempting to quit experience stress (a state characterized by high arousal and displeasure; see Kristensen, 1996; Posner, Russell, & Peterson, 2005), then this experience is likely lead to a lapse (an isolated smoking episode), which in turn likely leads to a full relapse (Lam et al., 2014). To prevent stress episodes from leading to full relapse, in Sense2Stop smokers attempting to quit wear AutoSense (Ertin et al., 2011)—a collection of sensors that monitor their physiology continuously. An algorithm on the mobile device (Hovsepian et al., 2015) uses this data to determine, for every given minute, whether or not the person is experiencing stress. Every minute, if the person is experiencing stress, and the person is receptive (i.e., they are not driving a car and did not receive an intervention in the past 60 minutes), the mobile device prompts the individual to engage in a stress regulation exercise (recommending one of three apps on the mobile device). Similar to adaptive interventions, JITAIs are protocolized with decision rules to enhance replicability. For example, the decision rule illustrated in Figure 30.2 protocolizes the simplified version of Sense2Stop described above:

Similar to standard adaptive interventions, JITAIs include decision points, tailoring variable(s), intervention options, and thresholds that link the tailoring variable(s) to

Every minute,

IF Stress = Yes; and minutes since last intervention >60; and driving = No

THEN, intervention option = Deliver a prompt recommending a stress-regulation exercise

ELSE, intervention option = No Prompt

FIGURE 30.2. Example of a decision rule for protocolizing a JITAI.

intervention options. In Sense2Stop, the decisions are made every minute; the tailoring variables are stress (determined based on passive sensing of the participant's physiology), minutes since previous intervention prompt, and driving; the intervention options include delivering a prompt recommending a stress-regulation exercise or no prompt. The thresholds and levels of the tailoring variables in Sense2Stop specify the conditions in which a prompt should be delivered (i.e., when the person experiences stress, did not receive an intervention prompt in the past 60 minutes, and is not driving a car), as well as the conditions in which a prompt should not be delivered (i.e., when stress is not experienced, or an intervention prompt was delivered in the past 60 minutes, or when the person is driving a car).

Compared to standard adaptive interventions, where decision points are set in relatively long intervals (e.g., every several weeks or months), JITAIs utilize rapid decision points (e.g., every minute, every several hours, or every day). This is because the adaptation process in JITAIs is intended to address conditions that change rapidly. In the simplified version of Sense2Stop described above, the adaptation process includes monitoring individuals continuously to obtain information about their stress, driving, and minutes since last intervention prompt; using the prespecified thresholds/levels of these tailoring variables to decide whether a prompt should be delivered; and triggering (or not) an intervention prompt based on this decision. Because this adaptation process is designed to address conditions that change rapidly (e.g., every minute the individual may transition from experiencing no stress to experiencing stress), it is initiated every minute via the decision points. This adaptation process is guided by the need to achieve a distal outcome (smoking abstinence) by impacting proximal outcomes (e.g., reducing the probability of a lapse in the next 2 hours, reducing the probability of experiencing a stress episode in the next 2 hours).

Why Are JITAIs Needed?

JITAIs are motivated by the need to address conditions that change rapidly, in the person's natural environment (Nahum-Shani et al., 2015; Nahum-Shani, Smith, et al., 2018). These conditions can represent vulnerability (high risk) in terms of the proximal outcome, as in the simplified version of Sense2Stop (where the key assumption is that stress represents a state of vulnerability for a lapse), or alternatively they may represent opportunity in terms of the proximal outcome. For example, a JITAI for promoting step count in the next 30 minutes as the proximal outcome in order to promote 5% weight loss by month 12 (as the distal outcome) can use information about the person's location to identify when they are close to a park or a recreational facility to trigger a recommendation for the person to take a walk. Here, proximity to a park or a recreational facility represents a state of opportunity for promoting the proximal outcome rather than a state of vulnerability in terms of the proximal outcome.

Stress episodes are expected to occur rapidly (e.g., every minute a person can transition from experiencing no-stress to experiencing stress), and in the person's natural environment (e.g., stress can happen at home as a result of family-related demands or at work due to job-related demands). Hence, addressing such conditions requires the capabilities to continuously monitor the person's state and context (e.g., in order to identify when stress occurs, as soon as it occurs), as well as to deliver interventions outside of standard treatment settings. Advances in mobile and wireless devices provide these capabilities.

Sense2Stop capitalizes on sensors to monitor the person's physiology continuously in order to identify episodes of stress. This JITAI also uses smartphones to host a collection of apps with stress-regulation exercises and deliver a prompt to engage the person in these activities as soon as stress is identified, in the person's natural environment.

Finally, because JITAIs attempt to address conditions that emerge rapidly and "in the wild," where multiple demands compete for the person's time, effort, and attention, these interventions are also motivated to minimize participant effort, burden, and habituation. This is done by delivering an intervention only when the person is receptive, namely, able and willing to receive, process, and utilize a particular intervention (Nahum-Shani, Smith, et al., 2018). In Sense2Stop, a prompt recommending a stress-regulation exercise is delivered only when the person (1) is experiencing stress, (2) did not receive an intervention in the past 60 minutes, and (3) is not driving a car. The first condition (stress) represents a state of vulnerability in terms of the proximal outcome, whereas the second (no intervention received in the past 60 minutes) and third (not driving) conditions represent a state of receptivity to a prompt recommending a stress-regulation exercise. It is assumed that if the person is driving a car, an intervention prompt could be distracting, and the person should not engage with the stress-regulation exercises on the phone. Moreover, it is assumed that if the person has already received an intervention prompt in the past 60 minutes, their ability to attend to the prompt and their willingness to utilize the recommended exercise would be undermined due to habituation and burden, respectively. Note that in this simplified description of Sense2Stop it is also assumed that individuals are generally receptive to the prompt when they experience stress, although it is possible that cognitive interferences during stress episodes hinder receptivity to intervention (see Battalio et al., 2021).

While the difference between states of vulnerability to an adverse proximal outcome and states of receptivity to just-in-time interventions seems rather straightforward, the difference between states of opportunity for positive changes and states of receptivity to a just-in-time adaptive intervention is often more challenging to grasp. Consider a JITAI that focuses on increasing physical activity in the next 30 minutes (the proximal outcome) by delivering a prompt encouraging the individual to walk when they are close to a park or a recreational facility. Here, proximity to a park or a recreational facility is a state of opportunity in terms of the proximal outcome. However, an individual may be close to a park or a recreational facility, but they may not be receptive to the prompt. For example, the person may be engaged in a conversation with someone and may not pay attention to the prompt. It follows that similar to states of vulnerability, states of opportunity are defined in relation to the primary proximal outcome motivating the JITAI (e.g., increasing physical activity in the next 30 minutes following a decision point). Receptivity to just-in-time intervention, on the other hand, is intervention-specific (i.e., it describes a state that relates to a particular just-in-time intervention option, such as a prompt encouraging the person to take a walk), and it is defined in relation to a proximal pathway/mediator that captures the investment of effort in a specific just-in-time intervention. For example, an individual may be receptive to the prompt under conditions in which they can pay attention to the recommendation (e.g., when they are not in the presence of other people). Here, paying attention to the content delivered via the prompt is viewed as a pathway through which this just-in-time intervention option can improve the primary proximal outcome (i.e., an increase in physical activity in the next 30 minutes). Overall, even when individuals are in a state of vulnerability (to an adverse proximal outcome such as smoking lapse) or opportunity (to promote a beneficial proximal outcome, such as physical activity), they may not necessarily be receptive to a specific just-in-time intervention.

The next section provides three additional examples of JITAIs from different areas of behavior change to highlight various characteristics of JITAIs.

Examples of JITAIs

Example 4. JITAIs to Promote Fluid Intake

sip^{IT} is a JITAI to support patients with kidney stones in their efforts to develop a habit for regular fluid intake (Conroy, West, Brunke-Reese, Thomaz, & Streeper, 2020). Decision points were set for every 30 minutes outside of a user-defined do-not-disturb period. The tailoring variable was fluid intake since the last decision point, measured by combining manual (e.g., self-monitoring via an app) with automated (e.g., connected water bottles, gesture detection) tracking methods. The intervention options included sending the patient a notification message (via smartphone) reminding them to drink or not sending a notification. The decision rule specifies that a reminder notification should not be delivered if the patient exceeded a prespecified threshold corresponding to drinking volume or drinking gesture frequency since the last decision point; otherwise, a reminder notification should be delivered.

Example 5. A JITAI to Improve Physical Activity in Individuals with Spinal Cord Injury

Hiremeth and colleagues (2019) developed a JITAI to improve physical activity levels in individuals with spinal cord injury. Here, decision points were set for every minute. The tailoring variable was wheelchair-based physical activity, monitored passively via a smartwatch and a wheel rotation monitor. The intervention options included personalized feedback prompts delivered through the smartphone (audio and/or vibration: based on participants' choice) and smartwatch (vibration) or no feedback prompt. The decision rule specified that a prompt should be delivered when the participant performed a bout (at least 3 continuous minutes) of moderate-intensity (or higher) physical activity; otherwise no feedback prompt should be delivered.

Example 6. A JITAI for Reducing Sedentary Behavior

B-MOBILE is a JITAI for reducing sedentary behavior (i.e., activities that require very low-energy expenditure and occur during waking hours while sitting or lying down) in overweight/obese individuals (Thomas & Bond, 2015). Here, we describe one of the decision rules investigated by Thomas and Bond (2015) for inclusion in B-MOBILE. Decision points were set for every minute. The tailoring variable was sedentary behavior measured via an Android smartphone and a software app that automatically monitored and categorized participants' behavior as either sedentary or not sedentary in one-minute epochs using the onboard accelerometer and a validated algorithm. The intervention options included sending (via smartphone) a prompt encouraging a 6-minute walking break, or not sending a prompt. The decision rule specifies sending a prompt after 60 continuous minutes of sedentary behavior; otherwise, a prompt for walking should not be delivered.

Key Similarities and Differences between the Example JITAIs

The Primary Motivation of the JITAI

JITAIs can be designed primarily to address states of vulnerability or opportunity, or both. Compared to Sense2Stop, which was designed mainly to address states of vulnerability (in this simplified example), Examples 4 and 6 focus on addressing states that represent both vulnerability for an adverse proximal outcome and opportunity for positive change, whereas Example 5 focuses primarily on addressing states of opportunity. Specifically, the JITAI in Example 4 delivers a notification message reminding the patient to drink if they did not exceed a prespecified threshold for fluid intake. The assumption is that patients with kidney stones who do not meet this prespecified threshold are at risk for not achieving standard clinical guidelines for preventing a recurrence of stones; these guidelines recommend increasing fluid consumption enough to produce greater than 2.0–2.5 liters of urine daily (Conroy et al., 2020). Similarly, the JITAI in Example 6 delivered a prompt encouraging overweight/obese individuals to take a 6-minute walking break if they have been sedentary for 60 or more continuous minutes. The assumption is that individuals who exhibit 60 or more continuous minutes of sedentary behavior are at risk for prolonged periods of sedentary behavior, which is linked to adverse health outcomes (e.g., poor cardiometabolic health) and mortality (see Thomas & Bond, 2015). Hence, a message is delivered to interrupt prolonged periods of sedentary behavior. While the primary motivation for the JITAIs in Examples 4 and 6 is to address states of vulnerability, in both cases these states are also viewed as an opportunity for habit formation—to promote automaticity by strengthening habits for fluid consumption (Conroy et al., 2020)—or for breaking bouts of sedentary behavior—so that individuals can learn to perform these behaviors on their own without the requiring a prompt. The JITAI in Example 5, on the other hand, focuses primarily on addressing states of opportunity to increase physical activity in individuals with spinal cord injury. The assumption is that performing a bout of moderate (or higher) intensity physical activity represents a state of opportunity to positively reinforce the behavior (by delivering feedback and congratulation messages) in order to increase future physical activity (Hiremath et al., 2019).

Measurement of the Tailoring Variable

Given that they involve rapid decision points, JITAIs typically leverage mobile and wireless technology to measure the tailoring variables, but different measurement tools may be utilized. All three JITAI examples described above, as well as the Sense2Stop JITAI discussed earlier, rely on sensor-based assessments to measure the tailoring variable. However, Example 4 integrates sensor-based assessments (i.e., a connected water bottle and gesture-detection app in a watch) with self-reported assessments via a mobile app. Although self-reported assessments involve a data-entry burden on the participant, they are highly useful in the absence of valid sensor-based assessments for measuring the tailoring variable. Specifically, although passive assessments via contemporary smartphones (i.e., mobile phones with computational capacities) or wearable sensors represent a less burdensome alternative to self-reported data collection, research using sensors in behavioral health sciences is still in its infancy. Moreover, it is unclear whether the types of behavioral data collected with sensors could serve as meaningful indicators of vulnerability/opportunity and receptivity to just-in-time interventions. More work is needed to develop robust and clinically tested algorithms to identify states of vulnerability/

opportunity and receptivity based on data from smartphone and wearable physiological sensors. In the absence of valid unobtrusive methods for measuring the tailoring variables, relying solely on or integrating self-reported assessments with sensor-based assessment may be a suitable option despite the data-entry burden.

The Inclusion of a No Intervention Option

JITAIs typically include an intervention option that provides no intervention at a decision point. This was the case in Examples 4, 5, and 6 described above, as well as in Sense2Stop. Because JITAIs are motivated to minimize participant effort, burden, and habituation, this intervention option is included to ensure that an intervention prompt is delivered only when it is needed: that is, only when the person is vulnerable or is experiencing a window of opportunity for positive changes. An intervention option that provides no intervention is also useful in addressing conditions that represent unreceptivity to a particular intervention. For example, in Sense2Stop a "no prompt" intervention option is initiated when the individual is driving a car or when they received an intervention prompt in the past 60 minutes. Similarly, in Example 4, a notification was not delivered during a user-defined do-not-disturb period.

Tailoring the Intervention Options versus Tailoring within an Intervention Option

In addition to *tailoring intervention options* for the purpose of deciding which intervention option to deliver, JITAIs may involve *tailoring within an intervention option* for the purpose of making the content more relevant and appealing to the individual. The JITAIs in Examples 4, 5, and 6, as well as in Sense2Stop used rapidly collected information to tailor the intervention options, that is, to decide which intervention option to deliver at a particular decision point. However, the JITAI in Example 5 also used this information to tailor the content inside one of the intervention options. Specifically, in Example 5 information about wheelchair-based physical activity (monitored passively via a smartwatch and a wheel rotation monitor) was used to decide whether or not to deliver a personalized feedback prompt, meaning that this information was used as a tailoring variable in the JITAI decision rule. However, this information was also used to "personalize" the feedback prompt. For example, based on the number of physical activity minutes completed, the message stated: "Good Job! 5 minutes completed; 30 minutes remaining to complete the daily goal."

Challenges and Directions for Future Research

Adaptive interventions and JITAIs are intervention delivery frameworks that have tremendous potential in leveraging mobile and wearable devices to deliver the right intervention options, at the right time, while minimizing drawbacks such as participant burden and cost. However, several challenges warrant additional research to facilitate the development of effective and practical technology-based adaptive interventions and JITAIs.

First, the use of technology-based interventions offers tremendous opportunities for leveraging intensive longitudinal data from the mobile device (e.g., app usage), ecological momentary assessments (EMAs), and sensor-based assessments to construct sophisticated tailoring variables for use in identifying early signs of nonresponsiveness. The decision rule in the weight-loss adaptive intervention example uses the same threshold of average weekly weight loss (i.e., 0.5 pound) at each decision point (i.e., week 2, 4, and 8) to differentiate between those who need more support and those who should continue with the minimal mHealth intervention. However, in practice, different thresholds may be needed at different points in time. For example, it is possible that while at week 2 losing less than 0.5 pound on average per week would be indicative of need for further support (i.e., predictive of failure to achieve a clinically meaningful weight loss by month 6; see Pfammatter et al., 2019), in later weeks this threshold might be lower as average weekly weight loss may decline over time even among individuals who succeed in the long term. Moreover, in this example, only a single kind of measurement (weekly weight loss measured via daily monitoring with the wireless scale) was used to differentiate between those who should receive more support and those who should continue with the minimal mHealth intervention. However, it may be beneficial to combine multiple sources and types of intensive longitudinal data (e.g., information about mobile app usage with weekly weight loss) to form more powerful tailoring variables.

Existing data-analytic approaches used to empirically inform the inclusion of tailoring variables in adaptive interventions, such as those using logistic regression models with receiver operating characteristic (ROC) curve analyses (Czyz, Yap, King, & Nahum-Shani, 2020; Steidtmann et al., 2013), are not suitable for constructing dynamic tailoring variables in which different types of information and/or thresholds are used at each decision point. Additionally, while black box machine learning models (e.g., neural networks and deep learning) have been recently used for prediction with intensive longitudinal data (E. Choi, Schuetz, Stewart, & Sun, 2016; Mei & Eisner, 2017), their interpretability remains a major challenge to their application in constructing tailoring variables that integrate multiple sources and types of intensive longitudinal data. New data-analytic methods are needed to leverage the rich, intensive longitudinal data afforded by emerging technologies to systematically develop dynamic and more comprehensive tailoring variables. Importantly, while wearable technologies offer tremendous potential for (near) real-time adaptation of interventions in real-world settings, their validity in measuring the construct(s) of interest across a variety of activities, settings, and populations remains a critical challenge. More research is needed and better algorithms have to be developed to use wearable devices in JITAIs with confidence (Puterman, Pauly, Ruissen, Nelson, & Faulkner, 2021).[2]

Second, critical to the development of efficacious JITAIs is evidence concerning what constitutes receptivity to specific just-in-time interventions and how fast receptivity is expected to change over time. However, receptivity is measured differently in different studies. For example, Sarker and colleagues (2014) measured it in terms of time taken to respond to an EMA prompt, whereas Kramer and colleagues (2019) measured receptivity in terms of whether or not the individual responded to a notification from a chatbot-based mobile health intervention for increasing physical activity and the time between notification and response. Chan and colleagues (Chan, Sapkota, Mathews, Zhang, & Nanayakkara, 2020) measured three dimensions of receptivity: (1) how prompts from a conversational memory coach were handled (e.g., whether the individual ignored the prompt and whether they elected to start the training then or later), (2) response time, and (3) participant subjective ratings on how appropriate the timings of the prompts were. Moreover, various terms are used to describe constructs that are different from, yet related to, receptivity. These terms include interruptibility, which is defined as a person's ability to immediately take action to open and view the content of a real-time notification (W. Choi, Park, Kim, Lim, & Lee, 2019), and availability, which refers to conditions in which it is feasible and appropriate to deliver a just-in-time intervention at a decision point (Klasnja et al., 2015). Defining receptivity in terms of an individual's ability and willingness to receive, process, and utilize a just-in-time intervention (Nahum-Shani, Smith, et al., 2018) suggests that an individual may be interruptible and/or available, but not necessarily receptive. For example, when an individual is not driving a car, it may be appropriate and feasible to deliver a prompt recommending a stress-regulation exercise (i.e., the individual is available), and the likelihood that the individual will open and view the content may be high (i.e., the individual is interruptible), but due to various demands on their time and effort the individual may not be able to cognitively process the suggested recommendation (i.e., the individual is not receptive). Future research should focus on clearly differentiating between receptivity and other related constructs and on developing tools and procedures for measuring receptivity to just-in-time interventions.

Third, while mobile technology holds great potential in terms of intervention adaptation, accessibility and scalability, the law of attrition (Eysenbach, 2005)—a phenomenon in digital health where users abandon a technology shortly after use—remains a major barrier that hinders the effectiveness of digital interventions. For example, in a survey of veterans who had attended an appointment relating to a mental health concern at a single Department of Veterans Affairs facility, Lipschitz and colleagues (2019) found that access and interest in using mobile apps for mental illness outpaced their actual use. Specifically, while nearly 80% reported owning smart devices (of those, nearly 90% reported that they use apps), and over 70% expressed interest, only 1 in 10 participants used apps for mental illness. In a systematic engine search using Google Play to identify Android apps with 10,000 installs or more targeting anxiety, depression, or emotional well-being, Baumel, Muench, Edan, and Kane (2019) found that despite the high number of app installs and daily active minutes of use, only a small portion of users actually used the apps for long periods of time. Specifically, the median percentage of daily active users was 4%, and the medians of retention rates over 15 and 30 days were 3.9% and 3.3%, respectively. Finally, in a systematic review of physical activity mobile apps, Peterson and colleagues (Petersen, Prichard, & Kemps, 2019) found that interventions incorporating physical activity apps alone demonstrated a decline in app engagement over time, whereas those integrating physical activity apps with existing Web-based social networking platforms showed increased and sustained engagement. Overall, these findings are consistent with conceptual frameworks highlighting the importance of human support in prompting engagement in digital interventions by generating accountability—"the implicit or explicit expectation that an individual may be called upon to justify his or her actions or inactions" (the section "Accountability" in Mohr, Cuijpers, & Lehman, 2011; Schueller, Tomasino, & Mohr, 2017). It follows that incorporating human support in digital interventions involves a tradeoff between benefits to effectiveness (via increased engagement) and drawbacks in the form of greater cost and potential burden. More work is needed to systematically investigate how to best integrate, sequence, and adapt digital interventions and human support so as to maximize effectiveness with minimal cost and burden (Nahum-Shani, Dziak, et al., 2022; 2023). Furthermore, while in recent years increased research attention has been given to understanding stable and dynamic predictors of engagement in digital interventions (e.g., Buck, Chander, & Ben-Zeev, 2020;

Perski, Watson, Mull, & Bricker, 2021; Psihogios et al., 2021), the absence of agreed upon definitions and operationalizations of engagement in mobile health represent critical barriers to advancing the field. Integrating theories and empirical evidence across multiple scientific fields, we define engagement as "a state of energy investment involving physical, affective, and cognitive energies directed toward a focal stimulus or task" (Nahum-Shani, Shaw, et al., 2022), and we provide a framework that explains how in-the-moment engagement unfolds in digital interventions (Nahum-Shani, Shaw, et al., 2022).

Finally, existing empirical evidence and theories lack the temporal specificity needed to guide the development of effective adaptive interventions and JITAIs (Nahum-Shani et al., 2015, 2018). In many areas of behavior change, little is known about how fast risk and protective factors change over time. Even when the dynamic nature of mechanisms such as affect and coping is acknowledged, it remains unclear how rapidly these mechanisms might change over time in a way that indicates the need for an intervention and what type of intervention should be delivered to address this need. Open scientific questions may concern how to best intervene at different decision points, how to tailor the intervention options, how to measure the tailoring variables, and how often intervention decisions should be made. Various types of experimental approaches exist to help investigators address different types of scientific questions about the construction of adaptive interventions and JITAIs. These include the sequential multiple assignment randomized trial (SMART; Lavori & Dawson, 2000, 2014; Murphy, 2005; Nahum-Shani et al., 2012); the singly randomized trial (Almirall, Nahum-Shani, Wang, & Kasari, 2018); the factorial design (Collins, 2018; Collins, Dziak, & Li, 2009; Dziak, Nahum-Shani, & Collins, 2012; Nahum-Shani, Dziak, & Collins, 2018); the microrandomized trial (Liao, Klasnja, Tewari, & Murphy, 2016; Qian et al., 2022); the hybrid experimental design (Nahum-Shani, Dziak, et al., 2022, 2023); and the standard randomized controlled trial (Collins, 2018). Each experimental approach can be used to address different types of scientific questions relating to building and evaluating adaptive interventions and JITAIs. However, some of these designs are relatively new; hence, most researchers are not exposed to these methodologies as part of their formal training. New pragmatic frameworks are needed to help researchers better understand the connection between these experimental approaches and decide which experimental tool and data-analytic methods are most appropriate given their scientific questions (Nahum-Shani, Dziak, & Wetter, 2022).

ACKNOWLEDGMENTS

I would like to thank John Dziak for his helpful comments and suggestions, and I acknowledge support from National Institutes of Health Grant Nos. P50 DA054039, U01 CA229437, R01 DA039901, R01 CA224537, R01 AA026574, R01 DK108678; and from Patient-Centered Outcomes Research Institute Grant No. PCS-2017C2-7613

Notes

1. An intervention that targets individuals' perceptions of peer alcohol use, by contrasting their perceptions with their own alcohol use and the actual normative behavior for their peer group; see Patrick et al. (2020).
2. Approval by the U.S. Food and Drug Administration/Medical Device Recording might be necessary for some of these studies.

REFERENCES

Almirall, D., Nahum-Shani, I., Wang, L., & Kasari, C. (2018). Experimental designs for research on adaptive interventions: Singly and sequentially randomized trials. In L. M. Collins & K. C. Kugler (Eds.), *Optimization of behavioral, biobehavioral, and biomedical interventions* (pp. 89–120). Springer.

Amico, K. R. (2015). Evidence for technology interventions to promote ART adherence in adult populations: A review of the literature 2012–2015. *Current HIV/AIDS Reports, 12*(4), 441–450.

Appel, L. J., Clark, J. M., Yeh, H.-C., Wang, N.-Y., Coughlin, J. W., Daumit, G., et al. (2011). Comparative effectiveness of weight-loss interventions in clinical practice. *New England Journal of Medicine, 365*(21), 1959–1968.

Battalio, S. L., Conroy, D. E., Dempsey, W., Liao, P., Menictas, M., Murphy, S., et al. (2021). Sense2Stop: A micro-randomized trial using wearable sensors to optimize a just-in-time-adaptive stress management intervention for smoking relapse prevention. *Contemporary Clinical Trials, 109*, 106534.

Baumel, A., Muench, F., Edan, S., & Kane, J. M. (2019). Objective user engagement with mental health apps: Systematic search and panel-based usage analysis. *Journal of Medical Internet Research, 21*(9), e14567.

Belzer, M. E., MacDonell, K. K., Ghosh, S., Naar, S., McAvoy-Banerjea, J., Gurung, S., et al. (2018). Adaptive antiretroviral therapy adherence interventions for youth living with HIV through text message and cell phone support with and without incentives: Protocol for a sequential multiple assignment randomized trial (SMART). *JMIR Research Protocols, 7*(12), e11183.

Buck, B., Chander, A., & Ben-Zeev, D. (2020). Clinical and demographic predictors of engagement in mobile health vs. clinic-based interventions for serious mental illness. *Journal of Behavioral and Cognitive Therapy, 30*(1), 3–11.

Chan, S. W., Sapkota, S., Mathews, R., Zhang, H., & Nanayakkara, S. (2020). Prompto: investigating receptivity to prompts based on cognitive load from memory training conversational agent. *Proceedings of the ACM on Interactive, Mobile, Wearable and Ubiquitous Technologies, 4*(4), 1–23.

Choi, E., Schuetz, A., Stewart, W. F., & Sun, J. (2016). Using recurrent neural network models for early detection of heart failure onset. *Journal of the American Medical Informatics Association, 24*(2), 361–370.

Choi, W., Park, S., Kim, D., Lim, Y.-k., & Lee, U. (2019). Multi-stage receptivity model for mobile just-in-time health intervention. *Proceedings of the ACM on Interactive, Mobile, Wearable and Ubiquitous Technologies, 3*(2), 1–26.

Collins, L. M. (2018). *Optimization of behavioral, biobehavioral, and biomedical interventions: The multiphase optimization strategy (MOST)*. Springer.

Collins, L. M., Dziak, J. J., & Li, R. (2009). Design of experiments with multiple independent variables: A resource management perspective on complete and reduced factorial designs. *Psychological Methods, 14*(3), 202.

Collins, L. M., Murphy, S. A., & Bierman, K. L. (2004). A conceptual framework for adaptive preventive interventions. *Prevention Science, 5*(3), 185–196.

Conroy, D. E., West, A. B., Brunke-Reese, D., Thomaz, E., & Streeper, N. M. (2020). Just-in-time adaptive intervention to promote fluid consumption in patients with kidney stones. *Health Psychology, 39*(12), 1062.

Czyz, E. K., Yap, J. R., King, C. A., & Nahum-Shani, I. (2020). Using intensive longitudinal data to identify early predictors of suicide-related outcomes in high-risk adolescents: Practical and conceptual considerations. *Assessment, 28*(8), 1949–1959.

Dounavi, K., & Tsoumani, O. (2019). Mobile health applications in weight management: A systematic literature review. *American Journal of Preventive Medicine, 56*(6), 894–903.

Dziak, J. J., Nahum-Shani, I., & Collins, L. M. (2012). Multilevel factorial experiments for developing behavioral interventions: Power, sample size, and resource considerations. *Psychological Methods, 17*(2), 153.

Ertin, E., Stohs, N., Kumar, S., Raij, A., Al'Absi, M., & Shah, S. (2011). *AutoSense: Unobtrusively wearable sensor suite for inferring the onset, causality, and consequences of stress in the field.* Paper presented at the 9th ACM Conference on Embedded Networked Sensor Systems.

Eysenbach, G. (2005). The law of attrition. *Journal of Medical Internet Research, 7*(1), e11.

Ghosh, P., Nahum-Shani, I., Spring, B., & Chakraborty, B. (2020). Noninferiority and equivalence tests in sequential, multiple assignment, randomized trials (SMARTs). *Psychological Methods, 25*(2), 182.

Griffin, J. B., Struempler, B., Funderburk, K., Parmer, S. M., Tran, C., & Wadsworth, D. D. (2018). My Quest, an intervention using text messaging to improve dietary and physical activity behaviors and promote weight loss in low-income women. *Journal of Nutrition Education and Behavior, 50*(1), 11–18.e11.

Haberer, J. E., Sabin, L., Amico, K. R., Orrell, C., Galárraga, O., Tsai, A. C., et al. (2017). Improving antiretroviral therapy adherence in resource-limited settings at scale: A discussion of interventions and recommendations. *Journal of the International AIDS Society, 20*(1), 21371.

Harkin, B., Webb, T. L., Chang, B. P., Prestwich, A., Conner, M., Kellar, I., et al. (2016). Does monitoring goal progress promote goal attainment?: A meta-analysis of the experimental evidence:. *Psychological Bulletin, 142*(2), 198.

Hiremath, S. V., Amiri, A. M., Thapa-Chhetry, B., Snethen, G., Schmidt-Read, M., Ramos-Lamboy, M., et al. (2019). Mobile health-based physical activity intervention for individuals with spinal cord injury in the community: A pilot study. *PloS One, 14*(10), e0223762.

Hovsepian, K., Al'Absi, M., Ertin, E., Kamarck, T., Nakajima, M., & Kumar, S. (2015). *cStress: towards a gold standard for continuous stress assessment in the mobile environment.* Paper presented at the 2015 ACM International Joint Conference on Pervasive and Ubiquitous Computing.

Klasnja, P., Hekler, E. B., Shiffman, S., Boruvka, A., Almirall, D., Tewari, A., et al. (2015). Microrandomized trials: An experimental design for developing just-in-time adaptive interventions. *Health Psychology, 34*(S), 1220.

Kramer, J.-N., Künzler, F., Mishra, V., Presset, B., Kotz, D., Smith, S., et al. (2019). Investigating intervention components and exploring states of receptivity for a smartphone app to promote physical activity: Protocol of a microrandomized trial. *JMIR Research Protocols, 8*(1), e11540.

Kristensen, T. S. (1996). Job stress and cardiovascular disease: A theoretic critical review. *Journal of Occupational Health Psychology, 1*(3), 246.

Kumar, S., Nilsen, W. J., Abernethy, A., Atienza, A., Patrick, K., Pavel, M., et al. (2013). Mobile health technology evaluation: The mHealth evidence workshop. *American Journal of Preventive Medicine, 45*(2), 228–236.

Lam, C. Y., Businelle, M. S., Aigner, C. J., McClure, J. B., Cofta-Woerpel, L., Cinciripini, P. M., et al. (2014). Individual and combined effects of multiple high-risk triggers on postcessation smoking urge and lapse. *Nicotine and Tobacco Research, 16*(5), 569–575.

Lavori, P. W., & Dawson, R. (2000). A design for testing clinical strategies: Biased adaptive within-subject randomization. *Journal of the Royal Statistical Society: Series A (Statistics in Society), 163*(1), 29–38.

Lavori, P. W., & Dawson, R. (2014). Introduction to dynamic treatment strategies and sequential multiple assignment randomization. *Clinical Trials, 11*(4), 393–399.

Liao, P., Klasnja, P., Tewari, A., & Murphy, S. A. (2016). Sample size calculations for microrandomized trials in mHealth. *Statistics in Medicine, 35*(12), 1944–1971.

Lipschitz, J., Miller, C. J., Hogan, T. P., Burdick, K. E., Lippin-Foster, R., Simon, S. R., et al. (2019). Adoption of mobile apps for depression and anxiety: Cross-sectional survey study on patient interest and barriers to engagement. *JMIR Mental Health, 6*(1), e11334.

McInnes, D. K., Sawh, L., Petrakis, B. A., Rao, S. R., Shimada, S. L., Eyrich-Garg, K. M., et al. (2014). The potential for health-related uses of mobile phones and Internet with homeless veterans: Results from a multisite survey. *Telemedicine and e-Health, 20*(9), 801–809.

Mei, H., & Eisner, J. M. (2017). *The neural Hawkes process: A neurally self-modulating multivariate point process.* Paper presented at the Advances in Neural Information Processing Systems Conference.

Michie, S., Abraham, C., Whittington, C., McAteer, J., & Gupta, S. (2009). Effective techniques in healthy eating and physical activity interventions: A meta-regression. *Health Psychology, 28*(6), 690.

Mohr, D., Cuijpers, P., & Lehman, K. (2011). Supportive accountability: A model for providing human support to enhance adherence to eHealth interventions. *Journal of Medical Internet Research, 13*(1), e30.

Mohr, D. C., Burns, M. N., Schueller, S. M., Clarke, G., & Klinkman, M. (2013). Behavioral intervention technologies: Evidence review and recommendations for future research in mental health. *General Hospital Psychiatry, 35*(4), 332–338.

Muessig, K. E., LeGrand, S., Horvath, K. J., Bauermeister, J. A., & Hightow-Weidman, L. B. (2017). Recent mHealth interventions to support medication adherence among HIV-positive men who have sex with men. *Current Opinion in HIV and AIDS, 12*(5), 432.

Murphy, S. A. (2005). An experimental design for the development of adaptive treatment strategies. *Statistics in Medicine, 24*(10), 1455–1481.

Murphy, S. A., Lynch, K. G., Oslin, D., McKay, J. R., & TenHave, T. (2007). Developing adaptive treatment strategies in substance abuse research. *Drug and Alcohol Dependence, 88*, S24-S30.

Nahum-Shani, I., & Almirall, D. (2019). *An introduction to adaptive interventions and SMART designs in education* (NCSER 2020–001). National Center for Special Education Research.

Nahum-Shani, I., Dziak, J. J., Venera, H., Pfammatter, A. F., Spring, B., & Dempsey, W. (2023). Design of experiments with sequential randomizations on multiple timescales: The hybrid experimental design. *Behavior Research Methods.*

Nahum-Shani, I., Dziak. J. J., Walton, M. A., & Dempsey, W. (2022). Hybrid experimental designs for intervention development: What, why, and how. *Advances in Methods and Practices in Psychological Science*, 5(3).

Nahum-Shani, I., Dziak, J. J., & Collins, L. M. (2018). Multilevel factorial designs with experiment-induced clustering. *Psychological Methods, 23*(3), 458.

Nahum-Shani, I., Dziak, J. J., & Wetter, D. W. (2022). MCMTC: A pragmatic framework for selecting an experimental design to inform the development of digital interventions. *Frontiers in Digital Health, 4*, 798025.

Nahum-Shani, I., Hekler, E. B., & Spruijt-Metz, D. (2015). Building health behavior models to guide the development of just-in-time adaptive interventions: A pragmatic framework. *Health Psychology, 34*(Suppl.), 1209.

Nahum-Shani, I., Qian, M., Almirall, D., Pelham, W. E., Gnagy, B., Fabiano, G., et al. (2012). Experimental design and primary data analysis for developing adaptive interventions. *Psychological Methods, 17*(4), 457–477.

Nahum-Shani, I., Shaw, S., Carpenter, S. M., Murphy, S. A., & Yoon C. (2022). Engagement in digital interventions. *American Psychologist, 77*(7), 836–852.

Nahum-Shani, I., Smith, S. N., Spring, B. J., Collins, L. M., Witkiewitz, K., Tewari, A., et al. (2018). Just-in-Time Adaptive Interventions (JITAIs) in Mobile health: Key components and design principles for ongoing health behavior support. *Annals of Behavioral Medicine, 52*, 446–462.

Patrick, M. E., Boatman, J. A., Morrell, N., Wagner, A. C., Lyden, G. R., Nahum-Shani, I., et al. (2020). A sequential multiple assignment randomized trial (SMART) protocol for empirically developing an adaptive preventive intervention for college student drinking reduction. *Contemporary Clinical Trials, 96*, 106089.

Pellegrini, C. A., Pfammatter, A. F., Conroy, D. E., & Spring, B. (2015). Smartphone applications to support weight loss: current perspectives. *Advanced Health Care Technologies, 1*, 13.

Perski, O., Watson, N. L., Mull, K. E., & Bricker, J. B. (2021). Identifying content-based engagement patterns in a smoking cessation website and associations with user characteristics and cessation outcomes: A sequence and cluster analysis. *Nicotine and Tobacco Research, 23*(7), 1103–1112.

Petersen, J. M., Prichard, I., & Kemps, E. (2019). A comparison of physical activity mobile apps with and without existing web-based social networking platforms: Systematic review. *Journal of Medical Internet Research, 21*(8), e12687.

Pfammatter, A. F., Nahum-Shani, I., DeZelar, M., Scanlan, L., McFadden, H. G., Siddique, J., et al. (2019). SMART: Study protocol for a sequential multiple assignment randomized controlled trial to optimize weight loss management. *Contemporary Clinical Trials, 82*, 36–45.

Piasecki, T. M. (2019). Assessment of alcohol

use in the natural environment. *Alcoholism: Clinical and Experimental Research, 43*(4), 564–577.

Posner, J., Russell, J. A., & Peterson, B. S. (2005). The circumplex model of affect: An integrative approach to affective neuroscience, cognitive development, and psychopathology. *Development and Psychopathology, 17*(3), 715.

Psihogios, A. M., King-Dowling, S., O'Hagan, B., Darabos, K., Maurer, L., Young, J., et al. (2021). Contextual predictors of engagement in a tailored mHealth intervention for adolescent and young adult cancer survivors. *Annals of Behavioral Medicine, 55*(12), 1220–1230.

Puterman, E., Pauly, T., Ruissen, G., Nelson, B., & Faulkner, G. (2021). Move more, move better: A narrative review of wearable technologies and their application to precision health. *Health Psychology, 40*(11), 803–810.

Qian, T., Walton, A. E., Collins, L. M., Klasnja, P., Lanza, S. T., Nahum-Shani, I., et al. (2022). The micro-randomized trial for developing digital interventions: Experimental design and data analysis considerations. *Psychological Methods, 27*(5), 874–894.

Sarker, H., Sharmin, M., Ali, A. A., Rahman, M. M., Bari, R., Hossain, S. M., et al. (2014). Assessing the availability of users to engage in just-in-time intervention in the natural environment. *Proceedings of the 2014 ACM International Joint Conference on Pervasive and Ubiquitous Computing.*

Schueller, S. M., Tomasino, K. N., & Mohr, D. C. (2017). Integrating human support into behavioral intervention technologies: The efficiency model of support. *Clinical Psychology: Science and Practice, 24*(1), 27–45.

Sobell, M. B., & Sobell, L. C. (2000). Stepped care as a heuristic approach to the treatment of alcohol problems. *Journal of Consulting and Clinical Psychology, 68*(4), 573.

Spring, B. (2018). *Sense2Stop: Mobile sensor data to knowledge.* ClinicalTrials.gov.

Stanger, C., Scherer, E. A., Vo, H. T., Babbin, S. F., Knapp, A. A., McKay, J. R., & et al. (2019). Working memory training and high magnitude incentives for youth cannabis use: A SMART pilot trial. *Psychology of Addictive Behaviors, 34*(1), 31.

Steidtmann, D., Manber, R., Blasey, C., Markowitz, J. C., Klein, D. N., Rothbaum, B. O., et al. (2013). Detecting critical decision points in psychotherapy and psychotherapy + medication for chronic depression. *Journal of Consulting and Clinical Psychology, 81*(5), 783–792.

Swendeman, D., Ramanathan, N., Baetscher, L., Medich, M., Scheffler, A., Comulada, W. S., et al. (2015). Smartphone self-monitoring to support self-management among people living with HIV: Perceived benefits and theory of change from a mixed-methods, randomized pilot study. *Journal of Acquired Immune Deficiency Syndromes (1999), 69*(01), S80.

Thomas, J. G., & Bond, D. S. (2015). Behavioral response to a just-in-time adaptive intervention (JITAI) to reduce sedentary behavior in obese adults: Implications for JITAI optimization. *Health Psychology, 34*(S), 1261.

CHAPTER 31

Mobile Technologies for Behavior Change

Jean Costa, Pablo Paredes, and Tanzeem Choudhury

CHAPTER OVERVIEW

Many mobile technologies have been designed to help users change their behaviors. By leveraging sensors from mobile devices, it is now possible to unobtrusively infer various behavioral patterns, including physical activities, eating, sleep, and social interactions. Similarly, new mobile interventions have emerged that collect and present personally relevant information to help users self-reflect and take appropriate actions. Despite the advance of mobile technologies for behavior change, many challenges remain to be addressed. In this chapter, we present an overview of existing theories, models, and mobile technologies for behavior change, and we discuss some barriers that compromise the effectiveness of these technologies. Based on these barriers, we introduce a novel closed-loop model to design behavior change technologies, and we present suggestions and examples that show how to design technological interventions that are unobtrusive, effortless, and adaptive.

Introduction

The topic of behavior change has received significant attention in social psychology and health psychology, with numerous papers presenting theories and findings discussing how or why people change their behaviors. In parallel, many technologies have been designed and deployed for behavior change, including mobile sensing systems that encourage users to exercise more (Consolvo et al., 2008), eat healthier foods (Chi, Chen, Chu, & Lo, 2008), sleep better (Bauer et al., 2012), and keep more sustainable habits (Froehlich et al., 2009). These technologies are known by many names, including persuasive technologies (Fogg, 1998), behavior change support systems (Oinas-Kukkonen, 2013), personal informatics (Li, Dey, & Forlizzi, 2010), ecological momentary interventions (Heron & Smyth, 2010), and just-in-time adaptive interventions (Nahum-Shani, Hekler, & Spruijt-Metz, 2015). But regardless of the name used, the goal is often the same: to provide relevant information to users so that they can change their behaviors to reach specific goals.

Despite the advances mobile technologies have made in behavior change, some challenges remain. One of the main challenges is that the technologies often lead to just short-term adoption and changes in behavior (Shih, Han, Poole, Rosson, & Carroll, 2015). In a previous study, it was found that more than half of the individuals who own activity trackers do not use them anymore, and a third of the users stopped using their trackers within 8 months (Ledger & McCaffrey, 2014). People have many reasons to abandon these technologies, one of the main reasons being the high level of attention and effort required (Lazar, Koehler, Tanenbaum, & Nguyen, 2015).

In this chapter, we present an overview of existing theoretical and technological models of behavior change, provide examples of mobile technologies designed to help users change their behaviors, and discuss some barriers that compromise the usage and effectiveness of behavior change technologies. Based on these barriers, we introduce a novel closed-loop model to design technologies for behavior change, and show how this model can be used to guide the design of technological interventions that are unobtrusive, effortless, and adaptive.

Technologies for Behavior Change

One of the first researchers to propose the design of technologies for behavior change was BJ Fogg, who introduced the concept of persuasive technologies. Persuasive technologies are defined as systems designed to change people's attitudes and/or behavior toward an issue, object, or action (Fogg, 1998). Many strategies have been used to design persuasive technologies, including self-monitoring, conditioning, surveillance, reduction, tunneling, tailoring, and suggestion (Fogg, 2002).

Among the strategies used to design persuasive technologies, one of the most popular is conditioning, which is often achieved by providing positive or negative reinforcement (Klasnja, Consolvo, & Pratt, 2011). For example, the mobile application UbiFit rewards users for meeting their physical activity goals by using an aesthetic representation of physical activities on the background screen (wallpaper) (Consolvo et al., 2008). Another popular design strategy is social influence. One example in which this strategy has been applied can be found in the mobile sensing application Houston (Consolvo, Everitt, Smith, & Landay, 2006), which was designed to encourage physical activity by allowing users to share their step count with friends. Finally, another widely used strategy is self-monitoring (Klasnja et al., 2011), which allows users to monitor and reflect about their behaviors and take actions accordingly. Systems designed with this strategy are often called personal informatics systems.

Personal informatics systems are defined as systems that "help people collect personally relevant information for the purpose of self-reflection and gaining self-knowledge" (Li et al., 2010, p. 558). With the development of mobile sensing technologies, personal informatics tools can be used to monitor a myriad of personal information, including physical activities, eating behavior, and sleep. These technologies use different ways of providing feedback. The most common approach is to present quantitative information, such as calories burned and hours slept per night, but the feedback can also be provided using abstract representations. In the mobile application BeWell (Lane et al., 2011), for instance, the wallpaper of the user's mobile phone changes based on the inferred sleep, exercise, and social interactions of the user.

Another class of technologies for behavior change is called just-in-time adaptive interventions (JITAIs), which are "interventions that adapt over time to an individual's time-varying status, with the goal to address the individual's changing needs for support" (Nahum-Shani et al., 2015, p. 1209). Systems based on JITAIs have been used for many behavioral health issues, including alcohol use, smoking cessation, and mental health disorders.

Behavioral Theories and Models

One of the most frequently used theories to guide the design of behavior change technologies is goal-setting theory. This theory states that both the difficulty and specificity of goals influence task performance. If the person commits to a goal, has the ability to achieve it, and does not have conflicting goals, then there should be a positive and linear relationship between goal difficulty and task performance (Locke & Latham, 2006). Examples of technologies that were designed based on this theory include the mobile application UbiFit, which allows users to set their own primary and alternate weekly physical goals (Consolvo, Klasnja, McDonald, & Landay, 2009), and the app presented by Gasser and colleagues (2006), in which users have a daily goal of earning "lifestyle points" by doing moderate/vigorous physical activity or by consuming one serving of fruit or vegetables.

Another common model used to design behavior change technologies is the transtheoretical model (TTM; Prochaska & Velicer, 1997). The model posits that behavior change occurs through six temporal stages: precontemplation, contemplation, preparation, action, maintenance, and termination. One way in which the model is often used is by following the TTM stages of change to personalize the interaction with the user. For instance, Bickmore, Schulman, and Sidner used the TTM stages to adjust how an automated health counselor agent promotes physical activity and fruit/vegetable consumption (Bickmore et al., 2013).

In addition to guiding the design and implementation of specific features, behavioral theories and models can also be used to guide the recruitment of participants for studies. For this purpose, the TTM is one of the most often used models. For instance, in the study that described the wearable device Pediluma (Lim, Shick, Harrison, & Hudson, 2010), a shoe accessory designed to encourage opportunistic physical activity, the researchers administered the Sample Physical Activity Questionnaire in the beginning of the study, aiming to recruit participants at various stages of the TTM.

Finally, theories and models of behavior are also used to guide the evaluation of the technologies. For instance, in the work from Schneider, Moser, Butz, and Alt (2016), the authors used the core elements of the theory of planned behavior to evaluate the intention of users to work out using the mobile fitness app Freeletics. Similarly, Grimes, Kantroo, and Grinter (2010) used the TTM to guide the qualitative evaluation of the mobile game OrderUp!, which helps players make healthier meal choices. The authors found that playing OrderUp! helped users engage in four processes of change of the TTM.

Technological Models

Behavioral theories from psychology help to explain the factors that influence behavior and why a behavior occurs, and they can also be used to guide efforts to change behaviors. However, these theories are often inadequate for guiding the design of behavior change technologies as the interventions become more interactive and adaptive (Klasnja et al., 2015; Riley et al., 2011). For this reason, different models have been proposed to help researchers design technological interventions for behavior change.

The Fogg behavior model (FBM) is one of the most frequently used models in the design of persuasive technologies (Fogg, 2009). According to this model, a person will perform a target behavior only if he or she is sufficiently motivated, has the necessary abilities to perform the behavior, and receives a "trigger" to perform the behavior. The model was proposed to help designers systematically think about the elements of motivation, simplicity, and the strategies used for triggering behavior.

Other models have been proposed specifically for personal informatics systems. The first and most often used model is the stage-based model of personal informatics, which consists of five stages: *preparation*, which concerns people's motivation to collect personally relevant information; *collection*, which refers to people's collection of information about themselves; *integration*, which concerns the processing and transformation of information; *reflection*, which refers to the user's reflection of the information obtained; and finally *action*, in which users decide what they will do with the new information obtained about themselves (Li et al., 2010). Epstein, Ping, Fogarty, and Munson (2015) extended this model and proposed the Lived Informatics Model, which adds more elements to characterize the challenges that users face when using self-tracking tools, including how users lapse and resume their goals, switch between tools, and adjust their tracking goals. One emerging design for behavior change technologies is JITAIs, which aim to provide the right type of support, at the right time, by adapting to the individual's state (Nahum-Shani et al., 2018). Mobile systems with JITAIs can leverage data collected from the individual and the environment and offer personalized interventions that are delivered when the user needs it most and it is most likely to be receptive (Nahum-Shani et al., 2018). Mobile technologies based on this approach have targeted smoking cessation (Naughton et al., 2017), alcohol use (Gustafson et al., 2014), physical inactivity (Consolvo et al., 2008), and many other behaviors and health conditions.

Barriers of Behavior Change Technologies

Although mobile technologies for behavior change are becoming increasingly available, there are many barriers that can compromise their effectiveness. Previous research shows that users often abandon these technologies after a short amount of time (Lazar et al., 2015), and the behavioral changes are also short-lived (Shih et al., 2015). In this section, we discuss some of the reasons associated with these barriers.

Reliance on Reflective and Conscious Processes

Many behavior change technologies have been designed based on behavioral models such as the theory of planned behavior and the TTM. However, some have argued that existing behavioral models are inadequate even for interventions that do not involve technology (Riley et al., 2011); studies have shown that these models are not very effective in predicting and changing health behavior (Webb & Sheeran, 2006).

One of the main criticisms of existing behavior models such as the TTM is that they focus solely on reflective action and conscious processes, and changing a person's conscious cognition is enough to cause significant changes in behavior (Sheeran, Gollwitzer, & Bargh, 2013). More recent models explain behavior by considering both conscious and automatic processes, often using dual-process theories (Sheeran et al., 2013). However, there is still a lack of models to guide the design of behavior change technologies using both conscious and automatic processes. For example, in both the stage-based model and the lived informatics model of personal informatics, engagement with the technologies involves the use of reflection, which requires the conscious engagement of the user.

Behavior Change as a Long-Term Process

Traditional theories and models of behavior, such as the TTM, focus on behavior change as a long-term process, which can take several months or even years to truly "stick" (Carver & Scheier, 1982; Prochaska & Velicer, 1997). One reason why behavior change is seen as a lengthy process is that the human capacity for self-control is limited, so behavior change setbacks can always occur, especially when a person is stressed or under high cognitive load (Klasnja et al., 2011). Since designers of behavior change technologies often leverage these models to design interventions, the technologies are often designed with a long-term focus.

Although it is important to keep the focus on long-term goals, proximal outcomes can be mediators to achieve distal outcomes (Nahum-Shani et al., 2015). Thus, successfully performing single activities can help individuals to remain on track to achieve their long-term goals. Furthermore, in many situations a single performance can have major consequences for the individual. For example, a driver who is urged to slow down may avoid a car accident, and a person who adjusts his or her behavior during a job interview can create a better first impression (Adams, Costa, Jung, & Choudhury, 2015).With a major focus on long-term goals, designers can neglect important design considerations that would make behavior change technologies more effective in the short term.

Obtrusiveness of Behavior Change Technologies

The effectiveness of behavior change technologies can be compromised by the level of engagement required. For example, many personal informatics tools present data that enable users to reflect and change their behavior if needed. This approach requires users to consciously interact and evaluate the information presented, which may not be feasible when users are busy or have low cognitive capacity (e.g., under stress).

In addition to the availability issue, self-reflecting about the current state can also be distracting and compromise people's ability to focus on ongoing activities (Adams et al., 2015). In particular, when a person starts to perform a task automatically and without thinking, such as riding a bike, the conscious thought about the task can be detrimental to the performance, which has been known as the "centipede effect" (Colman, 2015). In these situations, a different approach needs to be used to help people adjust their behaviors in-the-moment.

So how do we develop behavior change technologies that address the aforementioned barriers? The core idea of this chapter is that it is possible to mitigate existing barriers of behavior change technologies by designing technological interventions that are unobtrusive, effortless, and adaptive. For this purpose, in the next section we introduce the closed-loop model and show how this model can be used to guide the design of behavior change technologies.

Closed-Loop Model

In this section, we introduce the closed-loop model (CLM), a simple model to design closed-loop technologies for behavior change inspired by the feedback loop from Carver and Scheier (1982). Figure 31.1 shows a graphical description of the model.

The CLM has the following elements: perception, evaluation, goal/reference, and response. The model can be used to consider the user perspective (user-centered) or the system perspective (system-centered). For the user, the elements represent how the user perceives stimuli (perception), evaluates the information (evaluation), based on a goal or reference standard (goal/reference), and initiates a response (response). For the system, the elements represent how the system collects or senses data (perception), processes the data collected, and evaluates the need to intervene (evaluation), based on user's goals or a certain trigger condition (goal/reference), and finally provides feedback or triggers the intervention (response).

The output of the CLM's response stage leads to a change in the person or the environment, which starts a new feedback loop. From the user perspective, the person satisfied with the changes based on his or her goals may keep the same strategy as before. If not, a different response may be initiated. From the system perspective, the system can use a specific measure to identify whether or not the intervention was effective (e.g., step

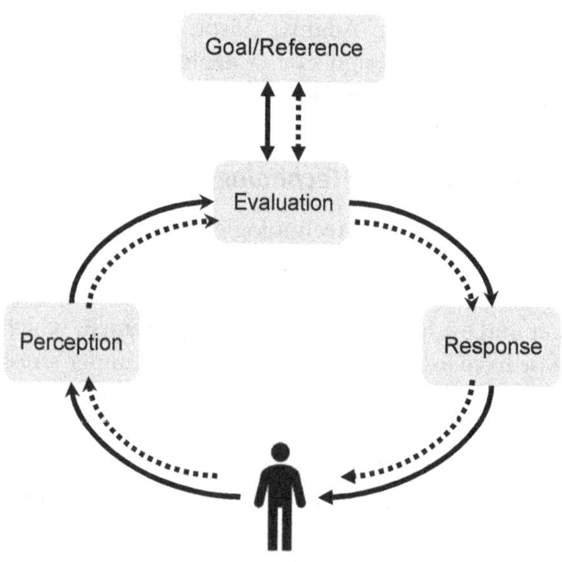

FIGURE 31.1. The closed-loop model for designing behavior change technologies.

count). If not, the parameters of the behavioral intervention could change for the next feedback loop, or a completely different behavioral strategy could be applied.

Another characteristic of the CLM is that there are two parallel pathways for each stage: the effortful path and the effortless path. In the effortful path, the user is consciously aware of the inputs and outputs. For instance, a person who installs a mobile health application to lose weight may continuously check the graphs shown in the app to monitor their calories burned over time (perception). If this person concludes (evaluation) that his or her goal of calories burned (goal/reference) is not being achieved, changes in the diet or a plan to do more exercise (response) may be in order.

In the effortless path, the inputs and outputs of the model require little or no attention and effort from individuals. In this path, events can be triggered automatically because of innate programming, learning, or habit (Baumeister & Heatherton, 1996). One typical example of automaticity is the driving activity. Experienced drivers perceive what happens on the road (perception), automatically evaluate the need to slow down, break, or take another action (evaluation) to ensure that they will reach their destination safely (goal), and quickly and mindlessly start the actions (action). Such persons are still aware that they are driving, but they do not need to be consciously aware of all their actions, unless they want to or if a new event happens. For instance, a roadblock may force the driver to decide on a new direction to take, which would require the effortful path to be engaged.

Behavior change technologies can be designed to leverage the effortful path, the effortless path, or both. If the technology acts peripherally and requires little or no effort from users, then the technology is leveraging the effortless path. On the other hand, if a technology requires manual input, provides feedback for the user to reflect, or requires a high level of engagement, then the technology is leveraging the effortful path.

Stages of the CLM

In this section, we describe the elements present in the CLM: perception, evaluation and goal/reference, and response. The section also includes examples of design features and mobile sensing technologies based on these elements. In the beginning of each subsection, we include specific questions to guide the design of relevant strategies centered on the system or user of the system.

Perception

System-centered: How will the system collect or sense relevant data from the user?

User-centered: How is the user expected to perceive the information provided by the system?

During the behavior change process, we constantly notice cues from our body or the environment that can suggest whether or not our behavior is changing. Similarly, systems can collect and detect relevant behavior and emotions from users by leveraging sensors in mobile or wearable devices (e.g., accelerometer, heart rate monitor). This represents the process of perception from the user and system perspective, respectively.

System-Centered Perspective

From the system perspective, a mobile system designed for behavior change can collect sensor and usage data to detect the target behavior and other relevant activities and engagement measures. This unobtrusive data collection can also be combined with self-report and ecological momentary assessment (EMA), which can provide richer information about users' behaviors, emotions, and attitudes.

Depending on the target behavior that is to change, some sensing capabilities may more appropriately be included in a mobile system. For instance, mobile systems designed to improve eating behavior can leverage the motion sensors available in smartwatches or utensils to detect when and how people eat (Thomaz, Essa, & Abowd, 2015). One example is the Sensing Fork and Hungry Panda application, which was designed to encourage children to eat balanced meals and concentrate while eating (Kadomura, Li, Tsukada, Chu, & Siio, 2014).

In addition to motion sensors, GPS signals and GSM cell tower data can be used to detect indoor and outdoor mobility patterns. In the mobile application UbiGreen, for instance, it is possible to infer when a participant is traveling by vehicle by collecting GSM data, and this information is used to provide visual feedback to encourage green transportation habits (Froehlich et al., 2009). It can also be useful to identify location-based data when users are near a location that may lead to relapse. The A-CHESS application, for instance, alerts users with alcohol dependence when they are approaching high-risk locations, such as a bar that the patient once visited (Gustafson et al., 2014).

Another sensor that has been used in mobile systems designed for behavior change is the microphone. The mobile application BeWell, for instance, uses a privacy-preserving method to detect ambient conversations using the smartphone's microphone (Lane et al., 2011); this information is processed to provide visual feedback about people's social interactions. A similar approach is used in the mobile application SociableSense, which leverages both microphone and Bluetooth data to capture and provide feedback about people's interaction and co-location patterns (Rachuri, Mascolo, Musolesi, & Rentfrow, 2011).

User-Centered Perspective

After mobile systems sense and process data collected from users, they can intervene and provide feedback about users' behavior and progress. The output of the mobile system then becomes the input of the user. One way of distinguishing how users can perceive the feedback provided by mobile systems is to determine whether they notice it through a push or pull mechanism.

Push feedback, such as notifications and alerts, is provided whether the user wants it or not, and it is often designed to draw the user's attention (Cauchard et al., 2019). One example is the "Stand Up" reminder provided by some smartwatch applications to prevent sedentary behavior. Although Push feedback can be a useful mechanism to intervene at the right time, users may miss the information or decide to ignore it, especially if they are physically or cognitively engaged in another task, such as during a meeting at work.

With pull feedback, the information is available for the user to look at whenever the user wants (Cauchard et al., 2019). The feedback can be designed to be easily perceived, such as by using simple quantitative information (e.g., step count, calories burned), or it can be designed to encourage exploration and self-reflection, such as by using charts or abstract representations of user's behavior (e.g., flowers, sea life). One limitation of pull feedback is that users may not perceive it if they do not have the ability or motivation to voluntarily look at the information.

Given that users may not notice the information provided by a mobile system, it is important to include measures of engagement to identify if users are interacting with the mobile system as intended. Examples of measures that can be useful include the following: number of times the user opens the app within a certain time period (e.g., 1 day), number of times the user notices the feedback provided by the app, and how long users interact with the app.

Evaluation and Goal/Reference

System-centered: How will the system process the data and evaluate the need to intervene?

User-centered: How is the user expected to evaluate the information?

Although we are constantly receiving perceptual input from the environment and from our bodies, it is ultimately how we evaluate that information that defines how we will respond. In many situations, we carefully evaluate the information received (effortful path), but since we have limited capacity to evaluate all the perceptual information that we are exposed to, we also rely on heuristics and automatic processes to make quick judgments (effortless path). Behavior change technologies can play a role by guiding us to evaluate information (effortful path) or by automatically evaluating information for us (effortless path), often by using machine learning algorithms to make inferences about our current state.

System-Centered Perspective

Mobile systems can help during the evaluation process by automatically defining or suggesting goals or reference standards for the users and by evaluating the users' progress over time. For instance, the wearable device FitBit can evaluate users' progress toward their health and fitness goals, such as by tracking the number of minutes spent exercising and the number of hours slept per night.

Mobile systems can also use algorithms to identify the best way of presenting the information to the user or the best time to intervene. For example, the mobile application BreakSense encourages workers to do short and playful physical activities, but only when the application detects that the users left their work area, thereby reducing the chances of work interruptions (Cambo, Avrahami, & Lee, 2017). Another example is the mobile library InterruptMe, which uses data collected from smartphone sensors and self reports, such as activity, location, and emotions, to identify the most opportune moments to intervene (Pejovic & Musolesi, 2014).

User-Centered Perspective

Mobile systems often present information about the evaluation of users' behaviors to the users, so that they can have a better understanding of their progress and how close they are from reaching their goals. The way the information is presented can lead users to evaluate their behavior in a way that they normally would not without a technology, so it is important that researchers and designers carefully consider how users may evaluate the feedback provided.

Even if users notice the information presented by a mobile system, they might not know how to make sense of the information. In a previous paper that discussed why users abandon smart devices, researchers found that unprocessed data were not considered useful for users, since users did not know how to analyze the data or if the numbers representing their behavior were supposed to be within one range or another (Lazar et al., 2015).

Another important consideration is that users may assess the evaluation presented by the mobile system in a way that is more harmful than helpful. For instance, previous research has found that mobile applications that allow users to self-monitor their emotions can end up increasing negative emotional states (Faurholt-Jepsen et al., 2015). This is especially relevant for individuals with mood disorders, since they are more likely to interpret ambiguous stimuli negatively (Joorman, Waugh, & Gotlib, 2015).

To identify barriers in the evaluation stage, it is important to obtain self-report information from users about their perceived behavior, mood, or cognition. Potential issues could be identified by comparing people's self-perception with quantitative data collected automatically from the mobile system. For example, if a person continuously reports dissatisfaction with an activity level, but the system detects significant physical activity based on mobile sensor data, this could be a sign that the person is not evaluating their own behavior accurately.

Response

System-centered: How will the system provide feedback or trigger the intervention?

User-centered: How is the user expected to respond?

The response phase represents the output of the feedback loop. For the user, this response can be behavioral (e.g., walking), mental (e.g., reframe a thought), or physiological (e.g., increased heart rate; Gross, 2015). For the system, the response is any form of intervention or feedback to the user, such as sending notifications, showing data visualizations, or triggering haptic or audio cues.

System-Centered Perspective

Although intervening or presenting feedback to users is not a requirement for many mobile sensing technologies, it is a crucial feature of mobile sensing technologies designed for behavior change. Two main aspects must be considered when designing how to intervene: (1) the presentation modality and (2) the level of engagement required.

For the presentation modality, a mobile technology can intervene by using visual, auditory, or haptic feedback. The visual feedback is the most common modality, and it leverages graphical displays present in mobile devices to present visual information, such as persuasive messages, pictures, and data visualizations. The use of visual feedback often requires users to voluntarily interact with the interfaces, which involves use of the effortful path in the closed-loop model. However, technologies can also intervene in using the effortless path, such as by triggering subtle and peripheral audio or haptic cues to make users perceive their current behavioral (Cauchard et al., 2019) or emotional state

(Costa, Guimbretière, Jung, & Choudhury, 2019). One example is the smartwatch application ActiVibe, which uses vibrotactile icons to communicate users' progress toward their goals (Cauchard et al., 2019).

In addition to the presentation modality, designers should consider how long users are expected to interact with the technology to process all the information. For example, a mobile application can present a glanceable display or haptic cue to make users quickly aware of their current state (Cauchard et al., 2019; Gouveia, Pereira, Karapanos, Munson, & Hassenzahl, 2016), or it can present graphs with historical activity data, which would require a longer time commitment to notice and make sense of the information presented.

User-Centered Perspective

When a person is consciously controlling a response, such as deciding whether to eat a very caloric meal, the person may perform an action to reduce discrepancies between their perception of the current state and their desired state (Carver & Scheier, 1982). In some situations, however, a response may be activated without the person's conscious intention, such as increased heart rate under stress.

In many behavioral models, the output phase of the feedback loop is an "action." In the model presented in this chapter, we intentionally named the output phase as "response" to make clear that a response may involve not only an action, but also cognitive and physiological changes. In this way, designers can use cognitive or emotion-regulation strategies to achieve a behavioral outcome. Although the idea of helping individuals to change their behaviors by also focusing on their cognition and emotions is not novel, and it is in fact well established through cognitive-behavioral therapy, surprisingly few technologies for behavior change also incorporate cognitive and emotion-regulation strategies (Costa et al., 2019).

Barriers in the response stage can be identified using self-report and passive sensing methods to verify if people are changing their behaviors and making progress toward their goals. For this purpose, it is important to measure both distal and proximal outcomes. The distal outcome is the major goal of the behavior change technology (e.g., losing 50 pounds), while proximal outcomes refer to short-term goals that can be mediators of the distal outcome (e.g., running 30 minutes per day; Nahum-Shani et al., 2015). In the closed-loop model, the end of the response stage leads to a proximal outcome, and many iterations of closed loops can lead to a distal outcome.

It is crucial to continuously evaluate the proximal outcomes to verify if people are on track to achieve their long-term goals. However, it is also important to measure additional physical, emotional, and/or cognitive responses that may help to identify existing barriers. For example, a person may continuously fail to achieve his or her daily productivity goal due to stress, so including measures of stress can help to identify this barrier.

Addressing Barriers of Behavior Change Technologies

As discussed previously in this chapter, many barriers may compromise the effectiveness of behavior change technologies. To mitigate these barriers, in this section we present some guidelines and examples of mobile technologies for behavior change that are unobtrusive, effortless, and adaptive.

Unobtrusive and Effortless

There are many examples of methods that will make people's interaction with behavior change technologies less obtrusive. In this section, we present some guidelines and examples for each stage of the CLM.

Perception

One common approach used in behavior change technologies is to use "pull" interfaces that users can access whenever they wish (Cauchard et al., 2019). Although this kind of feedback is helpful, people need to be available and motivated to engage with the interfaces (Nahun-Shani et al., 2015). One way of making users unobtrusively engage with "pull" interfaces is to make them visible in a place where users already tend to look quite often. For instance, in UbiFit (Consolvo et al., 2008), UbiGreen (Froehlich et al., 2009), and Zuki (Murnane et al., 2020), the wallpaper of the smartphone changes depending on the user's physical activities or pro-environmental behaviors. Since many people check their phones several times a day, they can see information about their activities without having to manually open an application.

"Push" feedback reduces the user's effort by automatically sending information when a trigger condition is met. However, this kind of feedback can be disruptive if the information is sent at a time when users are not available or receptive. For example, a smartwatch application that sends reminders for users to stand up can be distracting if users are busy and unable to follow the prompt, such as during an important meeting.

One way to make push feedback less obtrusive is to use algorithms that infer the best moments to send the push information. In this way, if users are busy and unavailable to attend to the technology or to follow the prompts, the system can recognize that and send the push notification at a more appropriate time later. This is the approach used in just-in-time adaptive interventions (Nahum-Shani et al., 2015).

Another approach to make push feedback less obtrusive is to automatically change the user's perception of stimuli, either by making some stimuli more salient or by overriding the perceptual input. For instance, Novak and Novak (2006) developed a wearable device that provides haptic feedback on the soles of the feet in synchrony with the user's steps. They found that this enhanced sensory feedback can make people with Parkinson's disease walk more steadily. Another example is the work from Tajadura-Jimenez and colleagues (2015), who developed a shoe-based wearable prototype that provides a modified sound feedback as the user walks. The researchers manipulated the feedback to make it sound as if it was being produced by a lighter or heavier body, and they found that this manipulation changed not only participants' perception of their body weight, but also their gait pattern.

Effortless push features can also be designed to influence a user's feelings and physiological signals, which in turn can lead to behavioral changes. For example, Costa, Adams, Jung, Guimbretière, and Choudhury (2016) presented the wearable device EmotionCheck, shown in Figure 31.2, which is a watch-like device that can override a user's perception of their own heart rate by providing subtle haptic feedback that resembles slow heartbeats. The results of a laboratory experiment revealed that participants believed that the slow haptic feedback represented their own heart rate, and, as a consequence, they felt calmer during a stressful task. This intervention was used in a follow-up study in which participants had to take math tests under high pressure (Costa et al.,

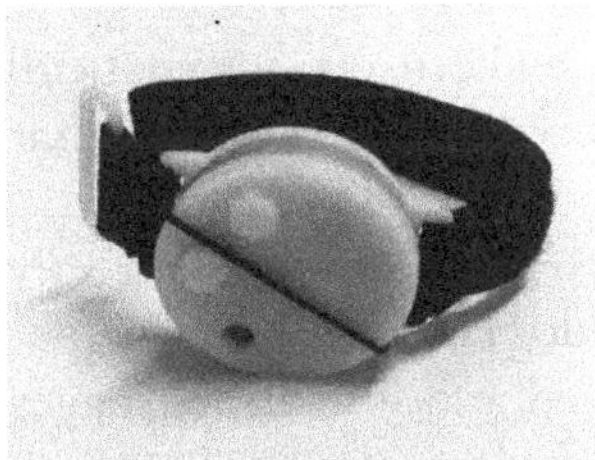

FIGURE 31.2. The EmotionCheck device, which can make users feel calmer using subtle haptic feedback. From Costa et al. (2016). Reprinted with permission from the Association for Computing Machinery.

2019); the findings indicate that this intervention can not only make people feel calmer, but it can also reduce physiological arousal and improve cognitive performance.

Evaluation and Goal/Reference

In addition to presenting information to users, interfaces can also guide users to evaluate their performance. One way of guiding this evaluation unobtrusively is to show simple visualizations that allow users to quickly evaluate their progress or to see how close they are from reaching their goals. For example, using this approach, Gouveia and colleagues (2016) designed prototypes of glanceable displays for smartwatches. The results of an in-the-wild study revealed the strong effects of these glanceable displays on individuals' behaviors.

Interventions can also help users evaluate whether or not they are reaching their goals by providing subtle sound feedback using mobile technologies. A great example is the sonification approach presented by Newbold, Bianchi-Berthouze, Gold, Tajadura-Jiménez, and Williams (2016). These authors investigated how sound feedback triggered by body movements could be used as an implicit mechanism to avoid overdoing motor movements, and also to facilitate progress during stretching exercises. They conducted a study in which they sonified the target goal of a stretch exercise to encourage either the end of a motor movement (using a musically stable sound) or the continuation of the exercise (using a musically unstable sound). The results show that the musically stable sound feedback led participants to continue the exercise beyond the target goal, while the unstable sound feedback led to a smoother stop close to the target point.

Response

One approach that can be used to reduce the effort required by users to perform certain actions is designing technologies that directly actuate user movements. A great example is the LiftWare device, which is an electronic handle with attachments for utensils (e.g., a spoon). The device uses motion sensors and actuators to sense and counteract hand tremors while the user is eating. In this way, people with disorders that affect their hand movements, such as Parkinson's disease, can eat more easily. Electrical muscle stimulation (EMS) is another way to intervene in the user's movements automatically. In one example of EMS usage, Lopes, Jonell, and Baudisch (2015) proposed extending the affordance of objects by allowing them to actuate directly on the user's muscles during the interaction. This approach can make users automatically perform specific movements while approaching an object or even avoiding objects that should not be touched, such as dangerous materials.

In addition to actuating users' movements directly, technologies can learn what activities are easier for users to do. For instance, the mobile app MyBehavior (shown in Figure 31.3) presents personalized and low-effort suggestions of physical activities and meals based on the user's past behavior. The goal of the application is to provide tailored health suggestions that users would be more confident in following (Rabbi, Aung, Zhang, & Choudhury, 2015). Another example is the mobile application PopTherapy. The application repurposes popular applications and websites as stress management interventions and provides suggestions using a recommendation system that learns how to match interventions to individuals over time (Paredes et al., 2014).

Adaptive

A key challenge in the design of behavior change technologies is ensuring that the interventions continue being effective over time. For this purpose, mobile technologies can

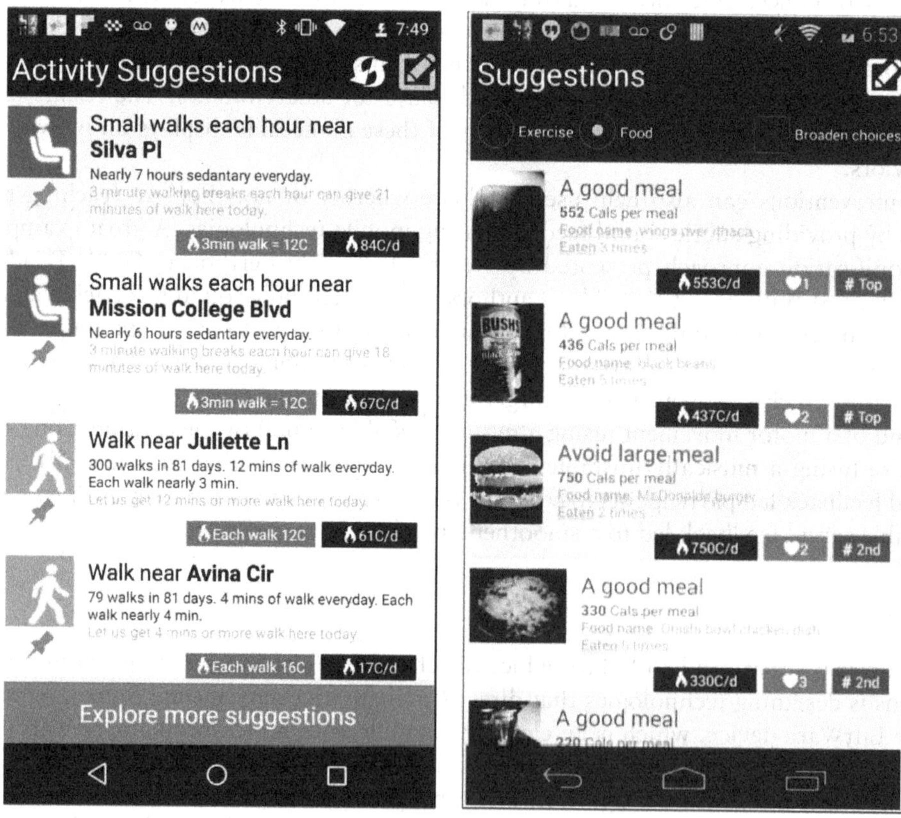

FIGURE 31.3. The MyBehavior app, which provides low-effort suggestions of physical activities and meals. From Rabbi et al. (2015). Reprinted with permission from the Association for Computing Machinery.

leverage JITAIs to learn users' context, personal traits, preferences, and behaviors, and adapt the interventions accordingly.

Existing frameworks for the design of JITAIs highlight four components that have to be taken into account: (1) decision points, which refer to the times when the decisions to intervene are made; (2) intervention points, which refer to the possible interventions that can be used at a decision point; (3) tailoring variables, which is the information about the person used to select the appropriate intervention; and (4) decision rules, which are the rules that connect the options of interventions and tailoring variables in a systematic way (Nahum-Shani et al., 2018).

One important consideration is how designers should select the possible interventions that can be provided to users. How to write the persuasive message? What actions should be suggested? These are some of the questions that designers may need to answer. One approach to creating the interventions is to leverage the knowledge of domain experts and design the interventions based on existing strategies that demonstrated positive results in previous studies. Another approach is to leverage applications, websites, or other resources that users may have access to and repurpose them as behavioral or stress management interventions. In PopTherapy, for instance, users are urged to use popular applications and websites to manage their stress. For instance, a notification can be shown to the user with the prompt "Find an example on your Facebook timeline that showcases one of your strengths" (Paredes et al., 2014).

One approach to determine the best intervention to the user at a given time is to use reinforcement learning algorithms, which make a sequence of decisions in a dynamic environment by learning through trial and error (Kaelbling, Littman, & Moore, 1996). Multi-armed bandit (MAB) is an example of reinforcement learning algorithms with an exploration–exploitation trade-off; its goal is to maximize the expected gains by either trying new options that might give higher payoffs in the future (exploration) or continuing with the option that gave the highest gains in the past (exploitation; Bubeck & Cesa-Bianchi, 2012). In the application PopTherapy, for instance, the researchers used MAB to maximize stress reduction using different stress management interventions, such as somatic relaxation, positive psychology, and cognitive-behavioral therapy (Paredes et al., 2014). In the mobile application MyBehavior, MAB was used to maximize the chances of achieving calorie loss goals by suggesting a combination of frequent and infrequent healthy behaviors (Rabbi et al., 2015). Based on users' responses, the MAB continuously adapts and picks the most useful interventions to users, while discarding the ones that are not useful.

A challenge regarding the formulation of adaptive systems is to optimize for both short-term and long-term outcomes. Users who find interventions useful and practice them constantly may still stop using them or reduce their usage over time. On the one hand, they may grow tired of using the same interventions, even if they are being effective. On the other hand, they may learn the mechanics from the repeated practice, and so they may no longer need support from the system. One possibility to address this issue is to provide additional rewards to a learning agent to guide the learning process, a tactic known as reward shaping. In this case, the rewards could balance both short-term and long-term outcomes, and they could include measures of efficacy, adherence, learning effects, and health outcomes. Measures of efficacy and adherence can be obtained passively using mobile sensors based on users' behaviors and interactions, and learning effects and health outcomes would require the use of psychometrics administered less frequently (i.e., weekly or monthly measurements).

Overall, the implementation of adaptive interventions is a promising area, but many challenges remain, and there are still open questions that require further research and development. Practitioners and researchers interested in this approach must move away from "one-size-fits-all" solutions and commit themselves to launching a system that continuously learns and adapts over time. In this way, they can take full advantage of the learning process provided by the algorithms.

Conclusion

The development of mobile and ubiquitous technologies has increased opportunities to help users monitor and change their behaviors. With the advance of sensors and passive sensing methods, it is now possible to collect a vast amount of behavioral, cognitive, and emotional information unobtrusively. The information collected is often presented to the users, prompting them to self-reflect and take appropriate actions. Although this approach works well when users are motivated and have high cognitive capacity, it can fail when self-control resources are drained by demands in other areas of one's life, such as when a person is stressed or under high cognitive load.

In this chapter, we have discussed how to design mobile technologies for behavior change that are unobtrusive, effortless, and adaptive. We presented for the first time a closed-loop model that can be used to guide the design of technologies that leverage both conscious and effortless processes for behavior change, and we offered some suggestions and examples of interventions that are unobtrusive, effortless, and adaptive. Many challenges still need to be addressed in this area. However, this research direction offers exciting opportunities for designing mobile technologies that can easily blend into people's lives and help them accomplish their goals.

REFERENCES

Adams, A. T., Costa, J., Jung, M. F., & Choudhury, T. (2015, September). Mindless computing: designing technologies to subtly influence behavior. *Proceedings of the 2015 ACM International Joint Conference on Pervasive and Ubiquitous Computing*, pp. 719–730.

Bauer, J. S., Consolvo, S., Greenstein, B., Schooler, J., Wu, E., Watson, N. F., et al. (2012, May). ShutEye: encouraging awareness of healthy sleep recommendations with a mobile, peripheral display. *Proceedings of the SIGCHI Conference on Human Factors in Computing Systems*, pp. 1401–1410.

Baumeister, R. F., & Heatherton, T. F. (1996). Self-regulation failure: An overview. *Psychological Inquiry, 7*(1), 1–15.

Bickmore, T. W., Schulman, D., & Sidner, C. (2013). Automated interventions for multiple health behaviors using conversational agents. *Patient Education and Counseling, 92*(2), 142–148.

Bubeck, S., & Cesa-Bianchi, N. (2012). Regret analysis of stochastic and nonstochastic multi-armed bandit problems. *Foundations and Trends in Machine Learning, 5*(1), 1–122.

Cambo, S. A., Avrahami, D., & Lee, M. L. (2017, May). BreakSense: Combining physiological and location sensing to promote mobility during work-breaks. *Proceedings of the 2017 CHI Conference on Human Factors in Computing Systems*, pp. 3595–3607.

Carver, C. S., & Scheier, M. F. (1982). Control theory: A useful conceptual framework for personality–social, clinical, and health psychology. *Psychological Bulletin, 92*(1), 111–135.

Cauchard, J. R., Frey, J., Zahrt, O., Johnson, K., Crum, A., & Landay, J. A. (2019). The positive impact of push vs pull progress feedback: A 6-week activity tracking study in the wild. *Proceedings of the ACM on Interactive, Mobile, Wearable and Ubiquitous Technologies, 3*(3), 1–23.

Chi, P. Y. P., Chen, J. H., Chu, H. H., & Lo, J. L. (2008). Enabling calorie-aware cooking in a smart kitchen. In H. Oinas-Kukkonen, P. Hasle, M. Harjumaa, K. Segerstahl, & P. Ohrstrom (Eds.), *Persuasive technology* (pp. 116–127). Springer.

Colman, A. M. (2015). *A dictionary of psychology*. Oxford University Press.

Consolvo, S., Everitt, K., Smith, I., & Landay, J. A. (2006, April). Design requirements for technologies that encourage physical activity. *Proceedings of the SIGCHI Conference on Human Factors in Computing Systems*, pp. 457–466.

Consolvo, S., Klasnja, P., McDonald, D. W., & Landay, J. A. (2009, April). Goal-setting considerations for persuasive technologies that encourage physical activity. In *Proceedings of the 4th International Conference on Persuasive Technology*, pp. 1–8.

Consolvo, S., McDonald, D. W., Toscos, T., Chen, M. Y., Froehlich, J., Harrison, B., et al. (2008, April). Activity sensing in the wild: a field trial of UbiFit garden. *Proceedings of the SIGCHI Conference on Human Factors in Computing Systems*, pp. 1797–1806.

Costa, J., Adams, A. T., Jung, M. F., Guimbretière, F., & Choudhury, T. (2016, September). EmotionCheck: Leveraging bodily signals and false feedback to regulate our emotions. *Proceedings of the 2016 ACM International Joint Conference on Pervasive and Ubiquitous Computing*, pp. 758–769.

Costa, J., Guimbretière, F., Jung, M. F., & Choudhury, T. (2019). Boostmeup: Improving cognitive performance in the moment by unobtrusively regulating emotions with a smartwatch. *Proceedings of the ACM on Interactive, Mobile, Wearable and Ubiquitous Technologies, 3*(2), 1–23.

Epstein, D. A., Ping, A., Fogarty, J., & Munson, S. A. (2015, September). A lived informatics model of personal informatics. *Proceedings of the 2015 ACM International Joint Conference on Pervasive and Ubiquitous Computing*, pp. 731–742.

Faurholt-Jepsen, M., Frost, M., Ritz, C., Christensen, E. M., Jacoby, A. S., Mikkelsen, R. L., et al. (2015). Daily electronic self-monitoring in bipolar disorder using smartphones—the MONARCA I trial: A randomized, placebo-controlled, single-blind, parallel group trial. *Psychological Medicine, 45*(13), 2691–2704.

Fogg, B. J. (1998, January). Persuasive computers: Perspectives and research directions. *Proceedings of the SIGCHI Conference on Human Factors in Computing Systems*, pp. 225–232.

Fogg, B. J. (2002, December). Persuasive technology: Using computers to change what we think and do. *Ubiquity, 2002*, 2.

Fogg, B. J. (2009, April). A behavior model for persuasive design. *Proceedings of the 4th International Conference on Persuasive Technology*, pp. 1–7.

Froehlich, J., Dillahunt, T., Klasnja, P., Mankoff, J., Consolvo, S., Harrison, B., et al. (2009, April). UbiGreen: Investigating a mobile tool for tracking and supporting green transportation habits. *Proceedings of the SIGCHI Conference on Human Factors in Computing Systems*, pp. 1043–1052.

Gasser, R., Brodbeck, D., Degen, M., Luthiger, J., Wyss, R., & Reichlin, S. (2006, May). Persuasiveness of a mobile lifestyle coaching application using social facilitation. In *International Conference on Persuasive Technology* (pp. 27–38). Springer.

Gouveia, R., Pereira, F., Karapanos, E., Munson, S. A., & Hassenzahl, M. (2016, September). Exploring the design space of glanceable feedback for physical activity trackers. *Proceedings of the 2016 ACM International Joint Conference on Pervasive and Ubiquitous Computing*, pp. 144–155.

Grimes, A., Kantroo, V., & Grinter, R. E. (2010, September). Let's play!: Mobile health games for adults. *Proceedings of the 12th ACM International Conference on Ubiquitous Computing*, pp. 241–250.

Gross, J. J. (2015). Emotion regulation: Current status and future prospects. *Psychological Inquiry, 26*(1), 1–26.

Gustafson, D. H., McTavish, F. M., Chih, M. Y., Atwood, A. K., Johnson, R. A., Boyle, M. G., et al. (2014). A smartphone application to support recovery from alcoholism: A randomized clinical trial. *JAMA Psychiatry, 71*(5), 566–572.

Heron, K. E., & Smyth, J. M. (2010). Ecological momentary interventions: Incorporating mobile technology into psychosocial and health behaviour treatments. *British Journal of Health Psychology, 15*(1), 1–39.

Joormann, J., Waugh, C. E., & Gotlib, I. H. (2015). Cognitive bias modification for interpretation in major depression: Effects on memory and stress reactivity. *Clinical Psychological Science, 3*(1), 126–139.

Kadomura, A., Li, C. Y., Tsukada, K., Chu, H. H., & Siio, I. (2014, September). Persuasive technology to improve eating behavior using a sensor-embedded fork. *Proceedings of the 2014 ACM International Joint Conference on Pervasive And Ubiquitous Computing*, pp. 319–329.

Kaelbling, L. P., Littman, M. L., & Moore, A. W. (1996). Reinforcement learning: A survey. *Journal of Artificial Intelligence Research, 4*, 237–285.

Klasnja, P., Consolvo, S., & Pratt, W. (2011, May). How to evaluate technologies for health behavior change in HCI research. *Proceedings of the SIGCHI Conference on Human Factors in Computing Systems*, pp. 3063–3072.

Klasnja, P., Hekler, E. B., Shiffman, S., Boruvka, A., Almirall, D., Tewari, A., et al. (2015). Microrandomized trials: An experimental design for developing just-in-time adaptive interventions. *Health Psychology, 34*(Suppl.), 1220–1228.

Lane, N. D., Mohammod, M., Lin, M., Yang, X., Lu, H., Ali, S., et al. (2011, May). BeWell: A smartphone application to monitor, model and promote wellbeing. *Proceedings of the 5th International ICST Conference on Pervasive Computing Technologies for Healthcare, 10.*

Lazar, A., Koehler, C., Tanenbaum, J., & Nguyen, D. H. (2015, September). Why we use and abandon smart devices. *Proceedings of the 2015 ACM International Joint Conference on Pervasive and Ubiquitous Computing*, pp. 635–646.

Ledger, D., & McCaffrey, D. (2014). Inside wearables: How the science of human behavior change offers the secret to long-term engagement. *Endeavour Partners, 200*(93), 1.

Li, I., Dey, A., & Forlizzi, J. (2010, April). A stage-based model of personal informatics systems. *Proceedings of the SIGCHI Conference on Human Factors in Computing Systems*, pp. 557–566.

Lim, B. Y., Shick, A., Harrison, C., & Hudson, S. E. (2010, January). Pediluma: Motivating physical activity through contextual information and social influence. *Proceedings of the Fifth International Conference on Tangible, Embedded, and Embodied Interaction*, pp. 173–180.

Locke, E. A., & Latham, G. P. (2006). New directions in goal-setting theory. *Current Directions in Psychological Science, 15*(5), 265–268.

Lopes, P., Jonell, P., & Baudisch, P. (2015, April). Affordance++ Allowing objects to communicate dynamic use. *Proceedings of the 33rd Annual ACM Conference on Human Factors in Computing Systems*, pp. 2515–2524.

Murnane, E. L., Jiang, X., Kong, A., Park, M., Shi, W., Soohoo, C., et al. (2020, April). Designing ambient narrative-based interfaces to reflect and motivate physical activity. *Proceedings of the 2020 CHI Conference on Human Factors in Computing Systems*, pp. 1–14.

Nahum-Shani, I., Hekler, E. B., & Spruijt-Metz, D. (2015). Building health behavior models to guide the development of just-in-time adaptive interventions: A pragmatic framework. *Health Psychology, 34*, 1209–1219.

Nahum-Shani, I., Smith, S. N., Spring, B. J., Collins, L. M., Witkiewitz, K., Tewari, A., et al. (2018). Just-in-time adaptive interventions (JITAIs) in mobile health: Key components and design principles for ongoing health behavior support. *Annals of Behavioral Medicine, 52*(6), 446–462.

Naughton, F. (2017). Delivering "just-in-time" smoking cessation support via mobile phones: current knowledge and future directions. *Nicotine and Tobacco Research, 19*(3), 379–383.

Newbold, J. W., Bianchi-Berthouze, N., Gold, N. E., Tajadura-Jiménez, A., & Williams, A. C. (2016, May). Musically informed sonification for chronic pain rehabilitation: Facilitating progress and avoiding over-doing. *Proceedings of the 2016 CHI Conference on Human Factors in Computing Systems*, pp. 5698–5703.

Novak, P., & Novak, V. (2006). Effect of step synchronized vibration stimulation of soles on gait in Parkinson's disease: A pilot study. *Journal of Neuroengineering and Rehabilitation, 3*(1), 9.

Oinas-Kukkonen, H. (2013). A foundation for

the study of behavior change support systems. *Personal and Ubiquitous Computing, 17*(6), 1223–1235.

Paredes, P., Gilad-Bachrach, R., Czerwinski, M., Roseway, A., Rowan, K., & Hernandez, J. (2014, May). PopTherapy: Coping with stress through pop-culture. In *Proceedings of the 8th International Conference on Pervasive Computing Technologies for Healthcare* (pp. 109–117). Institute for Computer Sciences, Social-Informatics and Telecommunications Engineering.

Pejovic, V., & Musolesi, M. (2014, September). InterruptMe: Designing intelligent prompting mechanisms for pervasive applications. *Proceedings of the 2014 ACM International Joint Conference on Pervasive and Ubiquitous Computing*, pp. 897–908.

Prochaska, J. O., & Velicer, W. F. (1997). The transtheoretical model of health behavior change. *American Journal of Health Promotion, 12*(1), 38–48.

Rabbi, M., Aung, M. H., Zhang, M., & Choudhury, T. (2015, September). MyBehavior: automatic personalized health feedback from user behaviors and preferences using smartphones. *Proceedings of the 2015 ACM International Joint Conference on Pervasive and Ubiquitous Computing*, pp. 707–718.

Rachuri, K. K., Mascolo, C., Musolesi, M., & Rentfrow, P. J. (2011, September). Sociablesense: exploring the trade-offs of adaptive sampling and computation offloading for social sensing. *Proceedings of the 17th Annual International Conference on Mobile Computing and Networking*, pp. 73–84.

Riley, W. T., Rivera, D. E., Atienza, A. A., Nilsen, W., Allison, S. M., & Mermelstein, R. (2011). Health behavior models in the age of mobile interventions: Are our theories up to the task? *Translational Behavioral Medicine, 1*(1), 53–71.

Schneider, H., Moser, K., Butz, A., & Alt, F. (2016, May). Understanding the mechanics of persuasive system design: A mixed-method theory-driven analysis of freeletics. *Proceedings of the 2016 CHI Conference on Human Factors in Computing Systems*, pp. 309–320.

Sheeran, P., Gollwitzer, P. M., & Bargh, J. A. (2013). Nonconscious processes and health. *Health Psychology, 32*(5), 460–473.

Shih, P. C., Han, K., Poole, E. S., Rosson, M. B., & Carroll, J. M. (2015). Use and adoption challenges of wearable activity trackers. *iConference 2015 Proceedings.*

Tajadura-Jiménez, A., Basia, M., Deroy, O., Fairhurst, M., Marquardt, N., & Bianchi-Berthouze, N. (2015, April). As light as your footsteps: Altering walking sounds to change perceived body weight, emotional state and gait. *Proceedings of the 33rd Annual ACM Conference on Human Factors in Computing Systems*, pp. 2943–2952.

Thomaz, E., Essa, I., & Abowd, G. D. (2015, September). A practical approach for recognizing eating moments with wrist-mounted inertial sensing. *Proceedings of the 2015 ACM International Joint Conference on Pervasive and Ubiquitous Computing*, pp. 1029–1040.

Webb, T. L., & Sheeran, P. (2006). Does changing behavioral intentions engender behavior change?: A meta-analysis of the experimental evidence. *Psychological Bulletin, 132*(2), 249–268.

CHAPTER 32

Mobile Sensing in Neuroscience

Predicting Brain Functional Connectivity Using Smartphone Data

Mikio Obuchi, Jeremy Huckins, Weichen Wang,
Arvind Pillai, and Andrew Campbell

CHAPTER OVERVIEW

Neuroscientists have found that mental health is associated with connectivity between specific brain regions. In this chapter, we investigate whether sensing data from mobile phones can predict brain functional connectivity; specifically, connectivity between the ventromedial prefrontal cortex (vmPFC) and the amygdala that is known to be associated with mental illness, such as anxiety and depression. Here, we report the insights gained from our NeuroSense exploratory study of 105 first-year university students across a 10-week semester using neuroimaging, mobile sensing, and self-reports. Several behavioral features from students' phones correlate with vmPFC–amygdala connectivity; for example, two important features are conversation duration ($r = .365$, $p < .001$) and sleep onset time ($r = .299$, $p < .001$). We train a support vector classifier to predict whether students have higher or lower vmPFC–amygdala connectivity purely based on mobile sensing data with an F1 score (harmonic mean of sensitivity and precision) of .793. We show for the first time that brain functional connectivity can be predicted using passive sensing data from phones, potentially offering a continuous and cost-effective alternative to functional magnetic resonance imaging (fMRI).

Introduction

Mental illness impacts one in four people worldwide, affecting mood, perception, thinking, and behavior (Anxiety and Depression Association of America, https://adaa.org).

Two of the most common types of mental illness are (1) the spectrum of depressive disorders, which is characterized by persistently depressed mood or loss of interest in activities, causing significant impairment in daily life, and (2) anxiety disorder, which is characterized by feelings of worry, anxiety, or fear that are strong enough to interfere with one's daily activities. College-age students are more prone to experience their first mental health episode at this time than at any other time in their lives, with their brains continuing to develop into their mid-20s (Sowell, Thompson, Tessner, & Toga, 2001). The transition from home, with its familiar support networks, to college can be challenging for teens. Adapting to academic pressures, new environments and living conditions, social pressures, erratic sleep habits, and other worries and stressors present challenges even for the healthiest and most resilient individuals. Among college students, 46% and 39% seek counseling for anxiety and depression, respectively (Reetz, Krylowicz, & Mistler, 2014).

Neuroscientists believe that abnormalities in how particular brain circuits function are related to mental illness; that is, mental illness relates to brain functioning. Therefore, measuring a person's brain activity is a natural approach to understanding the neural correlates of mental health. With the advent of brain-imaging techniques such as fMRI, researchers can measure brain activity and functional connectivity in increasing detail. Through use of neuroimaging, brain functions associated with various mental illnesses have been widely studied (Dickstein et al., 2010; Kaiser, Andrews-Hanna, Wager, & Pizzagalli, 2015; Kim et al., 2011). Neuroscientists have found that mental illness is associated with brain circuit functioning and connectivity between specific regions of the brain resulting in abnormal mood, perception, and behavior. They have used resting-state functional connectivity (RSFC) as one method to explore the network structure of the brain and its association with mental illness through temporal synchronization. Resting-state captures the synchrony between brain regions when no explicit task is conducted by the person being scanned.

Additionally, computer scientists working in mobile sensing have found correlates and predictors of individual differences associated with sensing data from phones and wearables. Mobile sensing, ecological momentary assessment (EMA; Shiffman, Stone, & Hufford, 2008), and machine learning allow researchers to infer complex human behavior (e.g., physical activity, sleep state) and context (e.g., social interaction, places visited) using passive sensing data from phones and wearables. Recently, Huckins and colleagues (2019) published the first findings from a study on brain imaging and mobile sensing in the neuroscience literature. The authors found correlations between smartphone usage from a group of college students and their fMRI scans. They scanned 257 students at Dartmouth College and computed RSFC for the subgenual cingulate cortex (sgCC), a brain region related to depression. Motivated by these insights, we performed an exploratory study of 105 first-year college students using neuroimaging, mobile sensing, and ecological momentary assessment across one semester (Obuchi et al., 2020). In addition to correlating distinct mobile sensing features that contribute to functional connectivity, we go one important step further and demonstrate for the first time that mobile behavioral features can predict the connectivity between brain regions. In this chapter, we describe the outcomes and insights about combining fMRI data with mobile sensing from our published NeuroSense study (Obuchi et al., 2020).

Background on Brain Imaging and Mental Health

In this section, we introduce the neuroscience basics necessary for researchers in the mobile sensing community to best understand our work. The human brain is roughly 1.4 kilograms of tissue containing roughly 86 billion neurons to perform the complex processing tasks that humans perform every day (von Bartheld, Bahney, & Herculano-Houzel, 2016). Interaction among an enormous number of neurons in the brain allows us to learn, remember, recognize, and think as humans. Neuroscientists have found some localization of brain functions; the role of specific brain regions is well studied. For instance, a region called the visual cortex plays a role in processing the information from vision. Similar to a node in a neural network that is discussed in the context of computer science, a neuron transmits information to another neuron. Communication between specific parts of the brain have been observed to be related to individual differences in behaviors or mental states.

fMRI is used to measure changes in blood flow related to brain activity (Ogawa et al., 1992). Temporal changes in blood oxygenation in different regions of the brain closely mirror brain activity. By measuring the change in blood oxygenation after neural activity, the brain regions that are actively working during a particular period can be determined. In short, fMRI captures the dynamic changes in blood flow as a proxy for neuronal activity. Researchers frequently use fMRI to study cognitive and affective processes, in both healthy subjects and subjects with conditions, such as mental disorders (Kaiser et al., 2015, 2016; Kim, Gee, Loucks, Davis, & Whalen, 2010; Moran et al., 2013).

A more recent trend is to take a network approach to studying the brain, namely, RSFC, which observes the temporal relationship between distinct brain regions over time when no explicit task is conducted by the person being scanned. The general idea is that these networks have developed over time and depict a lasting history of activating and deactivating together. RSFC is often done using Pearson's correlation between the fMRI signal of different regions. While general brain organization measured with RSFC is similar across thousands of different individuals (Biswal et al., 2010) and is stable and robust over both the short term (hourly) and the long term (monthly; Shehzad et al., 2009), there are small individual differences in connectivity, which can be reliably observed across time. Finally, another advantage of resting brain scans is that individuals who have difficulty performing certain tasks typically can complete resting-state fMRI scans.

Moreover, RSFC between the ventromedial prefrontal cortex (vmPFC) and the amygdala is shown to be associated with anxiety (Davidson, 2002; Ganella, Barendse, Kim, & Whittle, 2017; Gold, Morey, & McCarthy, 2015; Kim et al., 2011; Kim & Whalen, 2009) and depression (Connolly et al., 2017). Figure 32.1 shows the locations of vmPFC and amygdala in the brain. The vmPFC is reported to be related to decision making (Bechara, Damasio, Damasio, & Lee, 1999; Hare, Camerer, & Rangel, 2009), reward evaluation (Rushworth, Noonan, Boorman, Walton, & Behrens, 2011), morality (Greene, Sommerville, Nystrom, Darley, & Cohen, 2001), and emotion regulation (Etkin, Egner, & Kalisch, 2011; Hänsel & von Känel, 2008). In contrast, the amygdala is a more evolutionarily conserved part of the brain, which responds to fear (LeDoux, 1998; Öhman, 2005), threat (Fox, Oler, Tromp, Fudge, & Kalin, 2015; Gunduz-Cinar et al., 2013), facial expressions (e.g., fearful faces; Morris et al., 1998), and emotional processing (Aggleton, 1993; LeDoux, 1998). Researchers have shown that the vmPFC and

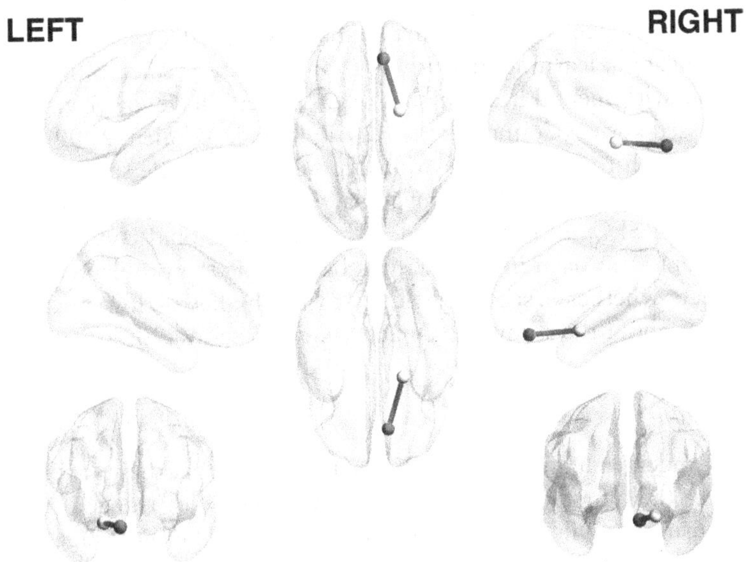

FIGURE 32.1. Location of vmPFC (black) and right amygdala (white). The functional connectivity between these regions is known to be associated with various aspects of mental health. The Montreal Neurological Institute coordinates are (8, 36, –18) and (20, –3, –15) for the right vmPFC and amygdala, respectively.

amygdala play a particularly important role in human anxiety (Davidson, 2002; Ganella et al., 2017; Gold et al., 2015; Kim et al., 2010, 2011; Kim & Whalen, 2009). The vmPFC inhibits the amygdala's reaction to fear or threats that make people anxious.

NeuroSense Study

Materials and Methods

In our study, we used the important neurological insight that *higher functional connectivity defined by the synchronization of neural activity between the vmPFC and amygdala regions is inversely correlated with anxiety. In other words, stronger connectivity relates to lower anxiety and vice versa*. Therefore, the goal of our study is threefold: (1) to investigate if human behavior inferred from mobile phones is associated with the RSFC between the vmPFC and amygdala, which is known to relate to mental health (e.g., anxiety); (2) to study various machine learning models to determine if we can coarsely predict the brain activity between the vmPFC and amygdala regions (i.e., higher connectivity relates to lower anxiety and vice versa) using mobile phone sensing as a pragmatic starting point for this exploratory study; and (3) to stimulate discussion on this new topic in the ubiquitous computing and neuroscience communities, potentially opening the way for new research at the intersection of neuroimaging and mobile sensing.

Our analysis consists of two parts: an exploratory correlation analysis and a performance evaluation of machine learning models. The exploratory correlation analysis allows us to identify sensing features that show a relationship with vmPFC–amygdala

RSFC. In the performance evaluation part of analysis, a predictive model is trained using eight different machine learning algorithms to investigate predictability. Research indicates that people with mental health issues (e.g., anxiety) have lower vmPFC–amygdala RSFC, as discussed above (Connolly et al., 2017; Kim & Whalen, 2009). As part of our preliminary approach to study the relationship between mobile sensing data and functional connectivity between vmPFC–amygdala, we split participants into two groups for analysis based on RSFC: a "higher" and a "lower" functional connectivity group. We have taken a simple approach in our analysis by treating the problem as a classification task that predicts whether a student belongs to the higher or lower RSFC group. For additional details about the study, see Obuchi and colleagues (2020).

Cohort Description

We recruit 105 undergraduate students (75 female, 30 male) at the start of the fall semester as they enter their first year at Dartmouth College, with the goal of investigating mental health using mobile sensing and brain imaging. The mean age of participants at the beginning of the study is 18.2 years (standard deviation of 0.63). Among the participants, the majority are Caucasian (56%), 21% are Asian, 16% are multiracial, 3% are African, 1% are Hispanic, and the rest 2% answer that they belong to other or unknown ethnicity group. After the subjects consent to participate in the study, two types of data are collected: brain connectivity using fMRI and mobile sensing data captured using the students' own phones. We use a Siemens MAGNETOM Prisma 3-Tesla scanner (Siemens, 2019) for brain imaging the participants during the start of the fall semester when all subjects are scanned. The study is approved by the study institution's Institutional Review Board, and the students receive monetary compensation for participating in the study.

Ground Truth: fMRI Data

We use the fMRI data collected from scanning the subjects as ground truth for correlation and predictive analysis using mobile sensing features, which we discuss in the "Analysis" section. During scanning, participants view a white fixation cross on a black background. The scanner collects both anatomical images of the brain and the fMRI signal that represents the proxy of neural activity. Figure 32.2 shows anatomical brain images centered at the positions of the vmPFC and right amygdala of a coauthor. With our scanner, we can collect the fMRI signal with a 2.4-millimeter × 2.4-millimeter in-plane resolution. The complete functional brain image is collected roughly every 1.2 seconds, acquiring a total of 605 volumes for 12 minutes of data acquisition. For more details regarding the neuroimaging data collection, please see Huckins and colleagues (2019). Functional connectivity between the vmPFC and amygdala is calculated using the Pearson's correlation (*r*) of the fMRI signal of these two regions over time. Only subjects with 5 minutes or more of low-motion data are included in the analysis to minimize the influence of motion. Ultimately, in terms of the data quality criteria, of the 105 students consenting to be part of the study, only 92 opted to be scanned at the start of the semester. In addition, only 75 of the 92 scanned subjects met the mobile sensing data quality criteria (R. Wang, Harari, Hao, Zhou, & Campbell, 2015) of 18 hours of sensing data per day for a minimum of 14 days across the term. As there is no existing

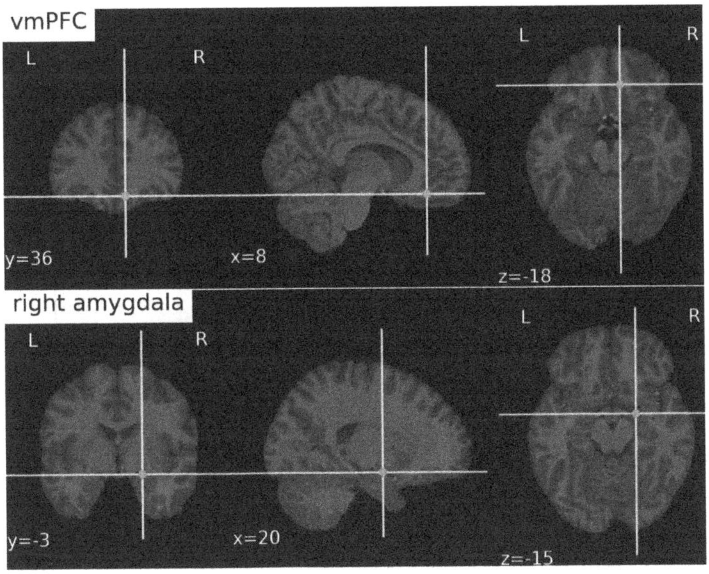

FIGURE 32.2. An anatomical brain image of a coauthor. The crosshairs are centered over the right vmPFC and amygdala.

literature on splitting RSFC into groups, we decided to use the median after discussions with domain experts. Although we applied the RSFC median split before filtering the participants, the number of higher RSFC and lower RSFC subjects is well balanced (i.e., 38 students in the higher RSFC group and 37 in the lower group). Furthermore, we did not have any clinical screening procedures to recruit participants, as this study involved a nonclinical population (university students). Consequently, identifying correlations between RSFC and clinical assessments related to mental health (anxiety, depression, etc.) was not possible.

Figure 32.3 represents the distribution of vmPFC–amygdala RSFC of all subjects who are scanned. The average value of RSFC is 0.12, with the median of 0.14, and the vertical line denotes the median.

Mobile Sensing

System

We use a smartphone application to continuously collect students' sensing and behavioral data from their phones over one semester as predictive variables for the study. The passive sensing app records a variety of data from sensors on the students' phone, subsequently transferring them to a secure server for offline analysis. The application works on both iOS and Android phones. We use GPS data to estimate a subject's location on campus, which is in a college town where all first-year students live on a compact campus. Thus, we compute semantic location data by creating a dictionary table that links campus buildings to several different location categories; for example, the libraries are categorized as "study area" locations, while cafeterias are categorized as a "food" location. To compute their "home" location, we infer the student's dormitory. The "Greek" location category

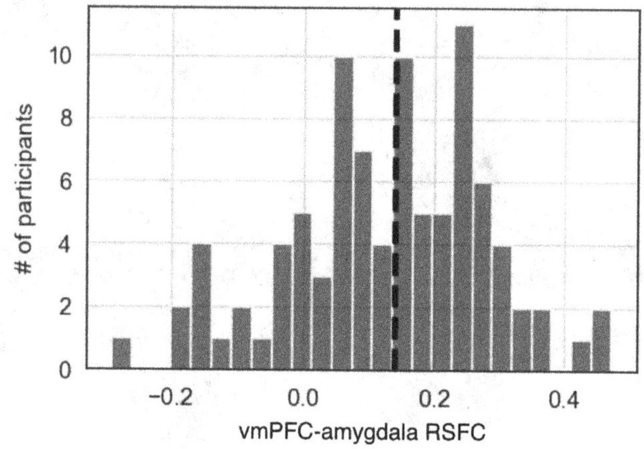

FIGURE 32.3. Distribution of vmPFC-amygdala resting-state functional connectivity among participants.

denotes Greek Letter Organization Houses (i.e., fraternities and sororities). Furthermore, our application detects sleep (Z. Chen et al., 2013) and speech/conversation data (Lane et al., 2011; Rabbi, Ali, Choudhury, & Berke, 2011) by incorporating pretrained classifiers. The application does not record raw audio data in order to protect the users' privacy. We cannot be completely sure if the subject is actively involved in the conversation; the inference of conversation is associated with the subject being around conversation. We use this as a proxy for social engagement or isolation.

Features

In our study, we design behavioral features from mobile sensing data inspired by our previous research on mobile sensing (R. Wang et al., 2014, 2015). Table 32.1 shows the list

TABLE 32.1. Features Generated from Mobile Sensing Data

Sensing type	Features
Activity (Wang et al., 2014)	• Duration of still, walking, and running
Location (Wang et al., 2014)	• Time spent at home (dorm), other dorms, study, food, social, Greek, religious, and workout areas • Number of places visited • Distance traveled
Phone usage (Wang et al., 2014)	• Unlock duration • Number of unlocks
Microphone (Lane et al., 2011; Rabbi et al., 2011)	• Audio amplitude • Conversation duration • Number of conversations • Ratio of voice (speed)
Sleep (Chen et al., 2013)	• Sleep start time • Sleep end time • Sleep duration

of features computed in our study. To increase the interpretability of features and to better understand students' behavior, we divided time across the day into three epochs (R. Wang et al., 2015). Epoch 0 represents the entire 24-hour day. Epochs 1, 2, and 3 denote day (9 A.M.–6 P.M.), evening (6 P.M.–0 A.M.), and night (0 A.M.–9 A.M.), respectively. As a basic strategy, we compute the average value (e.g., how many hours a user uses the phone) and the count (e.g., how many times a user unlocks the phone) within the epochs 0–3 for each sensor. Furthermore, we compute the standard deviations to estimate the variability of a student's behavior (R. Wang et al., 2018; W. Wang et al., 2018). This measure attempts to capture the variability of their week and ultimately across the semester. Similarly, we compute the regularity index for each sensing feature using negation of approximate entropy (Pincus, 1991). The regularity feature differs from the variability since it considers the unpredictability of changes over time-series data.

Analysis

A key goal of our exploratory study is to investigate the relationship between mobile sensing features and vmPFC–amygdala RSFC and predict that connectivity. In what follows, we describe our analysis, and then in the next section we review our results. For data quality reasons and to prevent distortion of data caused by missing data, we set some criteria based on prior data quality insights associated with mobile phone sensing (R. Wang et al., 2018). Specifically, we exclude data with less than 18 hours of data per day and less than 14 days of data during the term (R. Wang et al., 2018; W. Wang et al., 2018). As described in the "Ground Truth" section, our final cohort size is 75 participants.

Correlation Analysis

We compute Spearman's correlation to investigate the relationship between each mobile sensing feature and vmPFC–amygdala RSFC. Although the correlation coefficient does not explain the cause–effect relationship, we can examine the monotonic relationship in the observed data. Because the number of comparisons is high (i.e., >100), the result may have multiple testing problems: including more false-positive errors. To avoid this issue, we use the Benjamini-Hochberg procedure (Benjamini & Hochberg, 1995), which regulates the false discovery rate (FDR) in our exploratory analysis. The statsmodels package (Seabold & Perktold, 2010) with 165 extracted features was used for the correction procedure. We report correlation along with FDR-adjusted p-values and standard p-values.

Prediction Analysis

A key aim of our study is to evaluate the performance of various machine learning models, trained to predict vmPFC–amygdala RSFC from mobile sensing features. We formulate this research problem as a simple binary classification problem as a starting point for analysis and perform a median split on the RSFC data into higher or lower RSFC groups; that is, those subjects with higher and lower resting state functional connectivity between the vmPFC–amygdala regions. We then train our model to predict if a person is in the higher or lower RSFC group. All sensing features are standardized before training, transforming the data distribution to have a mean of 0 and a standard deviation of 1. We evaluate eight machine learning algorithms based on their ability to classify RFSC groups.

Each machine learning algorithm has its own hyperparameters, which are variables that the user controls to guide the training process. To identify the optimal hyperparameters for classification performance, we use a grid search strategy that iterates through all possible hyperparameters. Descriptions of the machine learning algorithms are beyond the scope of this chapter; for specific details, see the resources provided in Table 32.2, which shows algorithms evaluated and the hyperparameters selected for tuning. We use a nested cross-validation (CV) scheme to prevent overfitting, to build a generalized model, and to restrict hyperparameters from being solely adapted to the training data (see Figure 32.4). The outer cross-validation for evaluating the performance of the machine learning model is tenfold, and the inner CV for hyperparameter tuning is threefold. We do not include the same individual's data on both training and testing set while doing record-wise cross-validation.

Furthermore, for each algorithm and CV scheme, we evaluate 20 models using different random seeds when training each model and average the score to prevent bias from the initial seed selection. We apply the sequential forwarding selection (Jain & Zongker, 1997) as the feature selection method. For readers interested in additional information regarding analysis, we refer to our paper (Obuchi et al., 2020).

Results

Correlation: Mobile Sensing and Neuroimaging

The correlation between each feature generated from mobile sensing data and vmPFC–amygdala RSFC is shown in Table 32.3. The physical activity of subjects correlates with vmPFC–amygdala RSFC. Specifically, we observe four regularity features (i.e., running/walking during the entire day, running during the daytime, and walking in the evening) correlates to vmPFC–amygdala RSFC. All results show the same direction: participants

TABLE 32.2. Machine Learning Algorithms and Hyperparameters

Algorithm	Hyperparameter	Values
KNN (Taunk et al., 2019)	n_neighbors	1, 3, 5, 7, 9
Linear SVC (Burges, 1998)	C	0.1, 1, 10
SVC (RBF kernel) (Burges, 1998)	C Gamma	0.1, 1, 10 0.01, 0.1, 1, 10
Gaussian naïve Bayes (Rish, 2001)	No hyperparameter	
Bernoulli naïve Bayes (Rish, 2001)	No hyperparameter	
Logistic regression (Sperandei, 2014)	C Penalty	0.1, 1, 10 l1, l2
Random forest (Breiman, 2001)	max_depth max_sample_split	3, 5, 7 3, 5
XGBoost (Chen & Guestrin, 2016)	max_depth min_child_weight Gamma	3, 5, 7 1, 3, 5, 0.01, 0.1, 1, 10

Note. These algorithms were implemented using scikit-learn. For information regarding the specific hyperparameters, see Pedregosa et al. (2011).

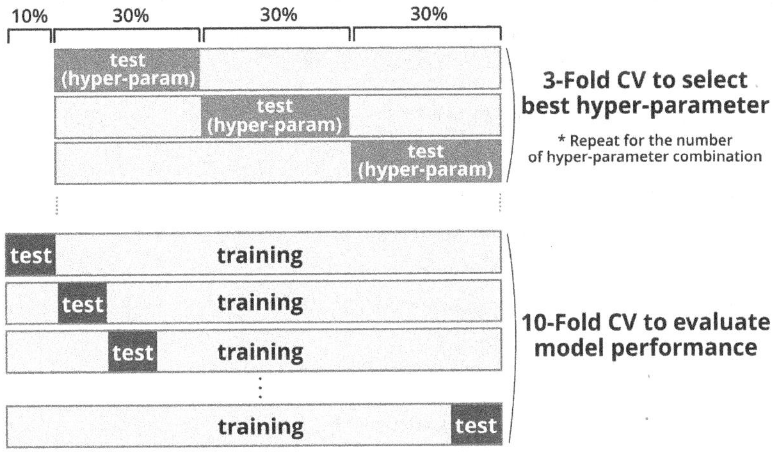

FIGURE 32.4. Overview of nested cross-validation. We set an inner threefold CV to select the best combination of hyperparameters for training a model in the outer fold. The outer 10-fold CV is used to evaluate the generalizability of the model.

with higher physical activity are more likely to have higher RSFC. Among the five sensor types shown in Table 32.1, the microphone demonstrates several significant correlations, as shown in Table 32.3. The result suggests that RSFC is higher for subjects who have more frequent and longer conversations; this is inferred using the microphone that captures when a person is "around" conversation. This could be a social encounter or a class lecture, we do not know for sure. We consider the inference of conversation frequency (i.e., the number of conversations per day) and duration (i.e., the length of each conversation) as a proxy for social engagement or isolation. The dynamics of these conversational features change over the term as students engage in increased workload and exams, and so on. Furthermore, the variability of conversation duration shows a significant correlation, as shown in Table 32.3. Considering location features, the time spent at "social" places shows a positive correlation (see Table 32.3). Similar to conversational features, our results confirm that students who spend more time in social areas, where conversations are more likely, have a higher RSFC. We do not observe a significant relationship with spending time at "religious" places (RSFC: $r = .045$, $p = .703$), in contrast to existing literature (Huang et al., 2016; Saeb, Lattie, Schueller, Kording, & Mohr, 2016) (i.e., spending time at "religious" locations negatively correlates with anxiety). The regularity of time spent at other students' dorms demonstrates the most significant correlation among location-based features, as shown in Table 32.3. This result suggests that the regular pattern of visiting friends' dorm rooms is associated with a higher RSFC. We find that correlation associated with smartphone usage relates to the unlock duration between time epoch of 0 A.M.–9 A.M. During the same epoch, we also observe that the number of unlocks positively correlates with RSFC.

Finally, sleep onset time shows the most significant and only correlation among sleep features, implying that RSFC is higher for students that go to sleep later at night. On academically challenging college campuses, many students have poor sleep habits, going to bed late into the night. Surprisingly, we do not find significant correlations for sleep

TABLE 32.3. Correlation between Sensing Data and vmPFC-Amygdala RSFC

Sensor	Feature	Spearman's rho
Activity	Regularity of running (24 hr)	0.231
	Regularity of running (9 A.M.–6 P.M.)**	**0.362**
	Regularity of walking (24 hr)	0.229
	Regularity of walking (6 P.M.–0 A.M.)	0.285
Microphone	Audio amplitude (9 A.M.–6 P.M.)	−0.251
	Conversation duration (24 hr)**	**0.365**
	Conversation duration (0–9 A.M.)**	**0.330**
	Conversation duration (9 A.M.–6 P.M.)*	**0.312**
	Conversation duration (6 P.M.–0 A.M.)**	**0.363**
	Number of conversations (24 hr)**	**0.360**
	Number of conversations (0–9 A.M.)*	**0.314**
	Number of conversations (9 A.M.–6 P.M.)	0.255
	Number of conversations (6 P.M.–0 A.M.)**	**0.366**
	Ratio of voice (24 hr)**	**0.365**
	Ratio of voice (0–9 A.M.)*	**0.293**
	Ratio of voice (9 A.M.–6 P.M.)	0.246
	Ratio of voice (6 P.M.–0 A.M.)**	**0.348**
	Variability of conversation duration (24 hr)**	**0.368**
	Variability of conversation duration (0–9 A.M.)*	**0.318**
	Variability of conversation duration (9 A.M.–6 P.M.)**	**0.355**
	Variability of conversation duration (6 P.M.–0 A.M.)	0.281
	Variability of number of conversations (24 hr)**	**0.358**
	Variability of number of conversations (0–9 A.M.)**	**0.339**
	Variability of number of conversations (6 P.M.–0 A.M.)	0.243
	Variability of number of ratio of voice (24 hr)*	**0.318**
	Variability of number of ratio of voice (0–9 A.M.)	0.278
	Regularity of number of conversation (24 hr)	−0.261
Location	Distance traveled (0–9 A.M.)	−0.245
	Time spent at "social" location	0.236
	Regularity of number of places visited (24 hr)	0.278
	Regularity of number of places visited (6 P.M.–0 A.M.)	0.255
	Regularity of time spent at "other dorms" location *	**0.321**
Phone usage	Unlock duration (0–9 A.M.)	0.276
	Number of unlock (0–9 A.M.)	0.253
	Variability of number of unlock (24 hr)	0.260
Sleep	Sleep start time*	**0.299**

Note. Standard $p < .05$; bold standard $p < .01$; *FDR-adjusted $p < 0.1$; **FDR-adjusted $p < .05$.

duration ($r = -.161$, $p = .168$) and sleep variability features in our study. While there is an error of +/– 30 minutes in the sleep classifier used in Z. Chen and colleagues (2013), the trends remain accurate.

Classification: Higher and Lower RSFC

In this section, we analyze the ability of the eight machine algorithms to classify students in higher or lower RSFC groups. We use the F1 score, a composite metric of the harmonic mean between precision and recall (sensitivity), to compare the performance. Among the algorithms, the support vector classifier (SVC) with radial basis function (RBF) kernel using 23 features achieves the highest F1 score of .793. Generally, RBF kernels can capture nonlinear features when dealing with a smaller feature set (23 features in our case) to increase performance; we observe the improved performance when compared to a linear SVC (see Table 32.4). Although some research finds that tree-based boosting and bagging algorithms (i.e., random forest, XGBoost) improve the performance when compared to other machine learning algorithms, they are unsuitable for our dataset because of its relatively small sample size. Although random forest and XGBoost have more hyperparameters to be tuned, requiring more training time than others, the SVC using 23 features performed best when classifying students into higher (i.e., stronger) or lower RSFC (i.e., weaker) connectivity groups. A model can achieve high precision and high recall by reducing the number of false positives and false negatives, respectively. We observe that the SVC RBF F1 score strikes an even balance between precision and recall. The 23 features are listed in Table 32.5. Note that the accuracy is .791, precision is .798, recall is .788, and the area under the receiving operator characteristic (AUROC) is .811. Figure 32.5 and Figure 32.6 show the confusion matrix and ROC curve, respectively. Regarding the variance of the 20 models of the best SVC, the standard deviation of the F1 score is 0.03, and the mean of the standard deviation of 10-fold cross-validation is 0.17. Readers interested in the machine learning algorithms and implementation can refer to Breiman (2001); Burges (1998); T. Chen and Guestrin (2016); Pedregosa and colleagues (2011); Rish (2001); Sperandei (2014); and Taunk, De, Verma, and Swetapadma (2019).

TABLE 32.4. F1 Score among Eight Machine Learning Algorithms Using Feature Selection

Algorithm	F1 score
KNN	.756
Linear SVC	.644
SVC (RBF kernel)	.793
Gaussian naïve Bayes	.654
Bernoulli naïve Bayes	.736
Logistic regression	.672
Random forest	.672
XGBoost	.641

TABLE 32.5. The 23 Features Selected by Sequential Forwarding Selection for Support Vector Classifier

K	Accumulated features	F1
1	Audio amplitude (24 hr)	.657
2	Audio amplitude (6 P.M.–0 A.M.)	.655
3	Variability of time spent at "religious" location	.642
4	Distance traveled (24 hr)	.668
5	Variability of activity "walking" duration (6 P.M.–0 A.M.)	.680
6	Number of places visited (6 P.M.–0 A.M.)	.710
7	Variability of activity "still" duration (6 P.M.–0 A.M.)	.775
8	Variability of number of places visited (24 hr)	.698
9	Variability of audio amplitude (24 hr)	.718
10	Number of unlock (0–9 A.M.)	.719
11	Regularity of time spent at "religious" location	.727
12	Variability of audio amplitude (0–9 A.M.)	.719
13	Regularity of activity "running" duration (0–9 A.M.)	.746
14	Activity "still" duration (6 P.M.–0 A.M.)	.743
15	Time spent at "religious" location	.747
16	Variability of conversation duration (24 hr)	.762
17	Distance traveled (0–9 A.M.)	.789
18	Variability of distance traveled (24 hr)	.777
19	Activity "walking" duration (24 hr)	.772
20	Regularity of time spent at "Greek" location	.759
21	Conversation duration (0–9 A.M.)	.766
22	Variability of number of unlocks (6 P.M.–0 A.M.)	.764
23	Regularity of number of unlocks (6 P.M.–0 A.M.)	.793

Note. K indicates an iteration number in feature selection.

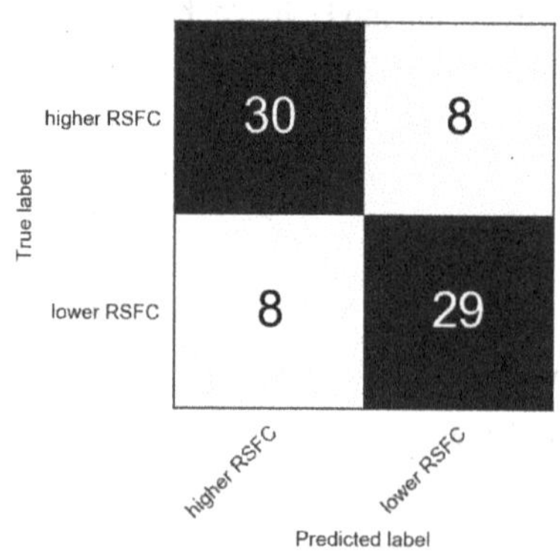

FIGURE 32.5. Confusion matrix of support vector classifier using 23 features. F1 score is 0.793.

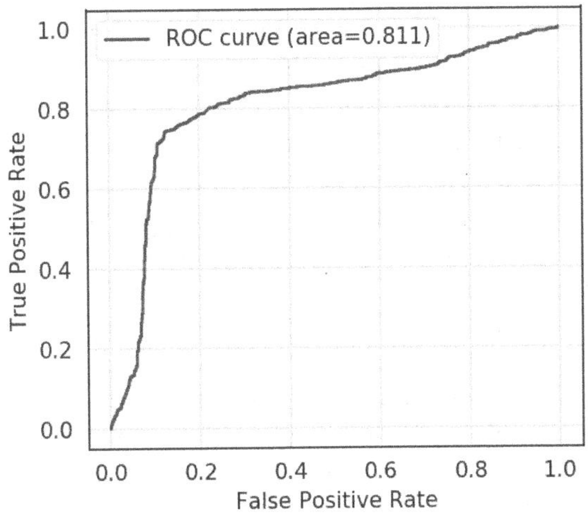

FIGURE 32.6. ROC curve of support vector classifier using 23 features.

Discussion

In summary, our study makes the following contributions: (1) We are the first group to use behavioral features from mobile sensing to study the brain functioning of 105 first-year college students over one semester. Specifically, we propose to use mobile sensing to predict functional connectivity between brain regions, (2) We have discovered a set of mobile sensing features that relate to brain functional connectivity. Specifically, we find that behavioral features from students' mobile phones correlate with functional connectivity between vmPFC and amygdala shown in Figure 32.1, including the conversation duration a student is around ($r = .365, p < .001$), their sleep onset time ($r = .299, p < .001$) and the number of phone unlocks ($r = .299, p = .029$) they initiate. (3) We train eight different machine learning algorithms to predict whether a student belongs to the higher or lower vmPFC–amygdala RSFC group. The higher connectivity group relates to lower anxiety and vice versa. After applying a 10-fold nested cross-validation with hyperparameter tuning, the support vector classifier achieves an F1 score of .793.

Correlated Mobile Sensing Features

Among all different categories of mobile sensing features, the conversational features from phones are the most correlated ones with vmPFC–amygdala functional connectivity. The StudentLife study found that social engagement made students feel more connected, less lonely, and more resilient with better mental well-being, positive emotions, and potentially better academic performance (R. Wang et al., 2014, 2015). Additionally, our results indicate that people with higher vmPFC–amygdala RSFC tend to be around a conversation (i.e., ambient speech was collected using the microphone) or spend more time in social or working locations where they typically engage with other students (e.g., they spend time at friends' dorms). Moreover, these results are consistent with previous studies indicating that people who have substantial social connection tend to have better psychological well-being (George, Blazer, Hughes, & Fowler, 1989). Also, our results show that subjects with higher functional connectivity tend to be more socially engaged. As discussed in the "Background" section, several neuroscientists find that higher vmPFC–amygdala functional connectivity is correlated with lower depression and anxiety (Connolly et al., 2017; Kim et al., 2010). Based on these findings, we can hypothesize that more social engagement and stronger functional connectivity (as found in our study) are likely to be related to better mental well-being among students.

Regarding phone usage, vmPFC–amygdala RSFC correlates with the number of phone unlocks and unlock duration between 0 A.M. and 9 A.M., but not with the other time epochs. We hypothesize that phone usage with social apps (e.g., texting) might be an important behavior that positively correlates with RSFC. During the night, we presume that most students rely on their phones to interact with their friends instead of face-to-face interaction. As proof, we would need to understand which specific apps users interact with on their phones. Some apps are clearly more socially potent than others. We would also need to better understand the context of the conversational interaction: sitting through an hour-long lecture (which would likely be inferred as a single conversation of 1 hour by our sensing platform) is different from a 1-hour conversation with close friends. We do not have this contextual information in our study.

In terms of sleep, previous studies (Feng, Becker, Feng, & Zheng, 2018; Yoo, Gujar, Hu, Jolesz, & Walker, 2007) found that sleep deprivation is related to weaker vmPFC–amygdala RSFC. Our analysis indicates that vmPFC–amygdala RSFC is higher (i.e., stronger) when students go to sleep later. We do not have any further data on why students go to sleep later, but the two most common reasons discussed in the StudentLife study (R. Wang et al., 2014) are academic demands such as assignment due dates and exams and social events such as hanging out with friends and parties. Without the specific reasons, we cannot fully interpret if late sleep is motivated by work or social life, or both (e.g., students working together on joint assignments). We could interpret our result along several lines. By linking it to behavior at night before sleep; for example, students attending social events (e.g., party, drinking) at night may result in positive mental well-being. In this study, we have used a phone-based sleep algorithm (Z. Chen et al., 2013) that is described as a "best effort" estimator for sleep onset and duration. In a future study, we would use wearables for sleep stage analysis. Having deeper sleep data and more contextual information about the behavior before sleep would lead to better insights. Also, four regularity features correlate with vmPFC–amygdala RSFC in our dataset. Students who regularly walk or run are prone to have higher RSFC. It is widely accepted that frequent aerobic exercise (i.e., running) plays a vital role in improving mental well-being (Sharma, Madaan, & Petty, 2006).

Classification

Although our goal to predict neural activity from mobile sensing is challenging, we consider the model that we trained as robust. In our analysis, we make our best effort to prevent overfitting or to bias training data. As a drawback of machine learning, we need to sacrifice some interpretability. The SVC with RBF kernel using 23 features has the best performance among all the models, but we cannot easily comprehend why the model selects those specific features. Note that the sequential forward selection features differ from the rankings of feature importance because the sequential forward selection is accumulating a feature that improves a model on the stacked features (i.e., audio amplitude in the first place) over each iteration. Interestingly, the time spent at religious locations is selected for all types of feature calculation (i.e., mean, variability, and regularity). We do not see a relationship with vmPFC–amygdala RSFC in the correlation analysis; however, visits to religious places have been shown to have an association with mental well-being (i.e., anxiety) (Huang et al., 2016; Saeb, Lattie, Kording, & Mohr, 2017).

In terms of performance, SVC results in the highest F1 score (.793) using 23 features, whereas using the six or seven features results in an F1 score of .710 and .775, respectively. Considering our dataset size, a smaller number of features may be more robust and generalizable. We assume that the performance of our machine learning model (i.e., SVC) is reliable. Our model exceeds the 50% baseline, which is relevant to random prediction, reasoning that mobile sensing contains a signal for predicting brain activity. We believe that our classifier performance could be improved by increasing the number of subjects in the dataset. We consider we have good power, but increasing the number would be the next step as well as studying the replicability of our results at higher scale.

Limitations

Although we succeeded in training a model to predict the functional connectivity using mobile sensing data, we recognize some limitations of our work. First, all the subjects who participated in our study are first-year undergraduate, mostly female, students at Dartmouth College. Therefore, our results cannot be broadly generalized (e.g., age, gender, socioeconomics, nationality). We do not screen for students with mental health conditions. Future work needs to examine a more diverse set of subjects and incorporate demographic information to train a generalized machine learning model.

Furthermore, we must be careful when identifying the function at a specific brain localization. In other words, we have to be aware that a particular brain region is not playing a single role. Based on prior research in neuroscience, we assume that vmPFC–amygdala RSFC is associated with mental health—anxiety, in the current study. However, the physiological phenomenon or mechanism that forms anxiety has not yet been elucidated. We may need to focus not only on a particular localization of the brain but also on the "representation" that the entire network forms.

Conclusion

This chapter discussed an exploratory study to examine how brain imaging and mobile sensing from phones are associated. In particular, we studied the brain connectivity between the vmPFC and amygdala, which relates to multiple mental health aspects. We believe our work opens a new research area by showing a first example of how mobile sensing can give in-depth longitudinal human behavioral data that provides further contextual information when analyzing costly neuroimaging data. Our experiment assessed brain connectivity using fMRI and collected behavioral data using a continuous sensing smartphone app over one academic semester at Dartmouth College. We identified a set of behaviors that correlate with vmPFC–amygdala connectivity. We also trained and evaluated the performance of machine learning models to predict if a student belongs to a higher or lower connectivity group using mobile sensing features. The support vector classifier produced the best performance (F1 score of .793). We successfully illustrated the feasibility of predicting people's brain functioning by linking mobile sensing and fMRI data.

REFERENCES

Aggleton, J. P. (1993). The contribution of the amygdala to normal and abnormal emotional states. *Trends in Neurosciences, 16*(8), 328–333.

Bechara, A., Damasio, H., Damasio, A. R., & Lee, G. P. (1999). Different contributions of the human amygdala and ventromedial prefrontal cortex to decision-making. *Journal of Neuroscience, 19*(13), 5473–5481.

Benjamini, Y., & Hochberg, Y. (1995). Controlling the false discovery rate: A practical and powerful approach to multiple testing. *Journal of the Royal Statistical Society: Series B (Methodological), 57*(1), 289–300.

Biswal, B. B., Mennes, M., Zuo, X.-N., Gohel, S., Kelly, C., Smith, S. M., et al. (2010). Toward discovery science of human brain function. *Proceedings of the National Academy of Sciences of the USA, 107*(10), 4734–4739.

Breiman, L. (2001). Random forests. *Machine Learning, 45*(1), 5–32.

Burges, C. J. (1998). A tutorial on support vector machines for pattern recognition. *Data Mining and Knowledge Discovery, 2*(2), 121–167.

Chen, T., & Guestrin, C. (2016). XGBoost: A scalable tree boosting system. *Proceedings of the 22nd ACM SIGKDD International Conference on Knowledge Discovery and Data Mining*, pp. 785–794.

Chen, Z., Lin, M., Chen, F., Lane, N. D., Cardone, G., Wang, R., et al. (2013). Unobtrusive sleep monitoring using smartphones. *Proceedings of the 7th International Conference on Pervasive Computing Technologies for Healthcare*, pp. 145–152.

Connolly, C. G., Ho, T. C., Blom, E. H., LeWinn, K. Z., Sacchet, M. D., Tymofiyeva, O., et al. (2017). Resting-state functional connectivity of the amygdala and longitudinal changes in depression severity in adolescent depression. *Journal of Affective Disorders, 207*, 86–94.

Davidson, R. J. (2002). Anxiety and affective style: Role of prefrontal cortex and amygdala. *Biological Psychiatry, 51*(1), 68–80.

Dickstein, D. P., Gorrostieta, C., Ombao, H., Goldberg, L. D., Brazel, A. C., Gable, C. J., et al. (2010). Fronto-temporal spontaneous resting state functional connectivity in pediatric bipolar disorder. *Biological Psychiatry, 68*(9), 839–846.

Etkin, A., Egner, T., & Kalisch, R. (2011). Emotional processing in anterior cingulate and medial prefrontal cortex. *Trends in Cognitive Sciences, 15*(2), 85–93.

Feng, P., Becker, B., Feng, T., & Zheng, Y. (2018). Alter spontaneous activity in amygdala and vmPFC during fear consolidation following 24 h sleep deprivation. *NeuroImage, 172*, 461–469.

Fox, A. S., Oler, J. A., Tromp, D. P., Fudge, J. L., & Kalin, N. H. (2015). Extending the amygdala in theories of threat processing. *Trends in Neurosciences, 38*(5), 319–329.

Ganella, D. E., Barendse, M. E. A., Kim, J. H., & Whittle, S. (2017). Prefrontal-amygdala connectivity and state anxiety during fear extinction recall in adolescents. *Frontiers in Human Neuroscience, 11*, 587.

George, L. K., Blazer, D. G., Hughes, D. C., & Fowler, N. (1989). Social support and the outcome of major depression. *British Journal of Psychiatry, 154*(4), 478–485.

Gold, A. L., Morey, R. A., & McCarthy, G. (2015). Amygdala–prefrontal cortex functional connectivity during threat-induced anxiety and goal distraction. *Biological Psychiatry, 77*(4), 394–403.

Greene, J. D., Sommerville, R. B., Nystrom, L. E., Darley, J. M., & Cohen, J. D. (2001). An fMRI investigation of emotional engagement in moral judgment. *Science, 293*(5537), 2105–2108.

Gunduz-Cinar, O., MacPherson, K. P., Cinar, R., Gamble-George, J., Sugden, K., Williams, B., et al. (2013). Convergent translational evidence of a role for anandamide in amygdala-mediated fear extinction, threat processing and stress-reactivity. *Molecular Psychiatry, 18*(7), 813.

Hänsel, A., & von Känel, R. (2008). The ventro-medial prefrontal cortex: A major link between the autonomic nervous system, regulation of emotion, and stress reactivity? *BioPsychoSocial Medicine, 2*(1), 21.

Hare, T. A., Camerer, C. F., & Rangel, A. (2009). Self-control in decision-making involves modulation of the vmPFC valuation system. *Science, 324*(5927), 646–648.

Huang, Y., Xiong, H., Leach, K., Zhang, Y., Chow, P., Fua, K., et al. (2016). Assessing social anxiety using Gps trajectories and point-of-interest Data. *Proceedings of the 2016 ACM International Joint Conference on Pervasive and Ubiquitous Computing*, pp. 898–903.

Huckins, J. F., DaSilva, A. W., Wang, R., Wang, W., Hedlund, E. L., Murphy, E. I., et al. (2019). Fusing mobile phone sensing and brain imaging to assess depression in college students. *Frontiers in Neuroscience, 13*, 248.

Jain, A., & Zongker, D. (1997). Feature selection: Evaluation, application, and small sample performance. *IEEE Transactions on Pattern Analysis and Machine Intelligence, 19*(2), 153–158.

Kaiser, R. H., Andrews-Hanna, J. R., Wager, T. D., & Pizzagalli, D. A. (2015). Large-scale network dysfunction in major depressive disorder: A meta-analysis of resting-state functional connectivity. *JAMA Psychiatry, 72*(6), 603–611.

Kaiser, R. H., Whitfield-Gabrieli, S., Dillon, D. G., Goer, F., Beltzer, M., Minkel, J., et al. (2016). Dynamic resting-state functional connectivity in major depression. *Neuropsychopharmacology, 41*(7), 1822–1830.

Kim, M. J., Gee, D. G., Loucks, R. A., Davis, F. C., & Whalen, P. J. (2010). Anxiety dissociates dorsal and ventral medial prefrontal cortex functional connectivity with the amygdala at rest. *Cerebral Cortex, 21*(7), 1667–1673.

Kim, M. J., Loucks, R. A., Palmer, A. L., Brown, A. C., Solomon, K. M., Marchante, A. N., et al. (2011). The structural and functional connectivity of the amygdala: From normal emotion to pathological anxiety. *Behavioural Brain Research, 223*(2), 403–410.

Kim, M. J., & Whalen, P. J. (2009). The structural integrity of an amygdala prefrontal pathway predicts trait anxiety. *Journal of Neuroscience, 29*(37), 11614–11618.

Lane, N. D., Mohammod, M., Lin, M., Yang, X., Lu, H., Ali, S., et al. (2011). Bewell: A smartphone application to monitor, model and promote wellbeing. *Proceedings of the 5th International ICST Conference on Pervasive Computing Technologies for Healthcare*, pp. 23–26.

LeDoux, J. (1998). *The emotional brain: The mysterious underpinnings of emotional life.* Simon & Schuster.

Moran, L. V., Tagamets, M. A., Sampath, H., O'Donnell, A., Stein, E. A., Kochunov, P., et al. (2013). Disruption of anterior insula modulation of large-scale brain networks in schizophrenia. *Biological Psychiatry, 74*(6), 467–474.

Morris, J. S., Friston, K. J., Büchel, C., Frith, C. D., Young, A. W., Calder, A. J., et al. (1998). A neuromodulatory role for the human amygdala in processing emotional facial expressions. *Brain: A Journal of Neurology, 121*(1), 47–57.

Obuchi, M., Huckins, J. F., Wang, W., daSilva, A., Rogers, C., Murphy, E., et al. (2020). Predicting brain functional connectivity using mobile sensing. *Proceedings of the ACM on Interactive, Mobile, Wearable and Ubiquitous Technologies, 4*(1), 1–22.

Ogawa, S., Tank, D. W., Menon, R., Ellermann, J. M., Kim, S. G., Merkle, H., et al. (1992). Intrinsic signal changes accompanying sensory stimulation: Functional brain mapping with magnetic resonance imaging. *Proceedings of the National Academy of Sciences the USA, 89*(13), 5951–5955.

Öhman, A. (2005). The role of the amygdala in human fear: Automatic detection of threat. *Psychoneuroendocrinology, 30*(10), 953–958.

Pedregosa, F., Varoquaux, G., Gramfort, A., Michel, V., Thirion, B., Grisel, O., et al. (2011). Scikit-learn: Machine learning in Python. *Journal of Machine Learning Research, 12*, 2825–2830.

Pincus, S. M. (1991). Approximate entropy as a measure of system complexity. *Proceedings of the National Academy of Sciences of the USA, 88*(6), 2297–2301.

Rabbi, M., Ali, S., Choudhury, T., & Berke, E. (2011). Passive and in-situ assessment of mental and physical well-being using mobile sensors. *Proceedings of the 13th International Conference on Ubiquitous Computing*, pp. 385–394.

Reetz, D. R., Krylowicz, B., & Mistler, B. (2014). The association for university and college counseling center directors annual survey. *Aurora, 51*, 60506.

Rish, I. (2001). An empirical study of the naive Bayes classifier. *IJCAI 2001 Workshop on Empirical Methods in Artificial Intelligence, 3*(22), 41–46.

Rushworth, M. F., Noonan, M. P., Boorman, E. D., Walton, M. E., & Behrens, T. E. (2011). Frontal cortex and reward-guided learning and decision-making. *Neuron, 70*(6), 1054–1069.

Saeb, S., Lattie, E. G., Kording, K. P., & Mohr, D. C. (2017). Mobile phone detection of semantic location and its relationship to depression and anxiety. *JMIR MHealth and UHealth, 5*(8), e112.

Saeb, S., Lattie, E. G., Schueller, S. M., Kording, K. P., & Mohr, D. C. (2016). The relationship between mobile phone location sensor data and depressive symptom severity. *PeerJ, 4*, e2537.

Seabold, S., & Perktold, J. (2010). Statsmodels: Econometric and statistical modeling with python. *Proceedings of the 9th Python in Science Conference, 57*, 61.

Sharma, A., Madaan, V., & Petty, F. D. (2006). Exercise for mental health. *Primary Care Companion to the Journal of Clinical Psychiatry, 8*(2), 106.

Shehzad, Z., Kelly, A. C., Reiss, P. T., Gee, D. G., Gotimer, K., Uddin, L. Q., et al. (2009). The resting brain: Unconstrained yet reliable. *Cerebral Cortex, 19*(10), 2209–2229.

Shiffman, S., Stone, A. A., & Hufford, M. R. (2008). Ecological momentary assessment. *Annual Review of Clinical Psychology, 4*, 1–32.

Siemens. (2019). *MAGNETOM Prisma.* www.siemens-healthineers.com/en-us/magnetic-resonance-imaging/3t-mri-scanner/magnetom-prisma

Sowell, E. R., Thompson, P. M., Tessner, K. D., & Toga, A. W. (2001). Mapping continued brain growth and gray matter density reduction in dorsal frontal cortex: Inverse relationships during postadolescent brain maturation. *Journal of Neuroscience, 21*(22), 8819–8829.

Sperandei, S. (2014). Understanding logistic regression analysis. *Biochemia Medica*, 12–18.

Taunk, K., De, S., Verma, S., & Swetapadma, A. (2019). A brief review of nearest neighbor algorithm for learning and classification. *Proceedings of the 2019 International Conference on Intelligent Computing and Control Systems (ICCS)*, pp. 1255–1260.

von Bartheld, C. S., Bahney, J., & Herculano-Houzel, S. (2016). The search for true numbers of neurons and glial cells in the human brain: A review of 150 years of cell counting. *Journal of Comparative Neurology, 524*(18), 3865–3895.

Wang, R., Chen, F., Chen, Z., Li, T., Harari, G., Tignor, S., et al. (2014). StudentLife: Assessing mental health, academic performance and behavioral trends of college students using smartphones. *Proceedings of the 2014 ACM International Joint Conference on Pervasive and Ubiquitous Computing*, pp. 3–14.

Wang, R., Harari, G., Hao, P., Zhou, X., & Campbell, A. T. (2015). SmartGPA: How smartphones can assess and predict academic performance of college students. *Proceedings of the 2015 ACM International Joint Conference on Pervasive and Ubiquitous Computing*, pp. 295–306.

Wang, R., Wang, W., daSilva, A., Huckins, J. F., Kelley, W. M., Heatherton, T. F., et al. (2018). Tracking depression dynamics in college students using mobile phone and wearable sensing. *Proceedings of the ACM on Interactive, Mobile, Wearable and Ubiquitous Technologies, 2*(1), 1–26.

Wang, W., Harari, G. M., Wang, R., Müller, S. R., Mirjafari, S., Masaba, K., et al. (2018). Sensing behavioral change over time: Using within-person variability features from mobile sensing to predict personality traits. *Proceedings of the ACM on Interactive, Mobile, Wearable and Ubiquitous Technologies, 2*(3), 141.

Yoo, S.-S., Gujar, N., Hu, P., Jolesz, F. A., & Walker, M. P. (2007). The human emotional brain without sleep—A prefrontal amygdala disconnect. *Current Biology, 17*(20), R877–R878.

PART V

Conclusions and Future Directions

CHAPTER 33

Mobile Sensing in Psychology

Where We Are and Where We Might Go from Here

Matthias R. Mehl, Michael Eid, Cornelia Wrzus,
Gabriella M. Harari, and Ulrich W. Ebner-Priemer

CHAPTER OVERVIEW

In this concluding chapter to the *Handbook*, we highlight central lessons learned from the first wave of mobile sensing research in psychology and reflect on current challenges, open questions, and future directions. Mobile sensing is an exciting new methodology for studying daily life, and, in psychological science, its trajectory is at a critical inflection point in terms of uptake and potential. At the same time, at this moment, mobile sensing is still best thought of as in its infancy with respect to challenges around the ease of implementation, the lack of knowledge, consensus, and standardization around important procedures and practices, and the realization of sound psychometric measurement, particularly in the context of consequential psychological (e.g., diagnostic) assessment. Because of its ability to capture daily (digital) behavior passively, continuously, and comprehensively, mobile sensing offers unique opportunities for studying person–environment interactions ecologically and at scale. At the same time, it raises unprecedented new questions about participant privacy and data confidentiality, ownership, and stewardship. Also, as mobile sensing expands its capabilities and reach, the potential synergies and tensions of conducting mobile sensing research in academic and/or corporate environments must be considered.

Introduction

The idea for this handbook originated in 2018, when four of the editors of this handbook met in Berlin, Germany, as part of a working group tasked to provide recommendations for best practices when using new technologies for data collection (e.g., pertaining to data quality, data management, research ethics, and data protection; RatSWD, 2020). The

Zeitgeist at that time was the following: Psychologists had emerged from what the American Psychological Association had labeled as the "Decade of Behavior" (2000–2010; cf. Ebner & Kubiak, 2010), humbled by the realization that the field's overreliance on survey and simple lab measures had been stifling progress in actually studying real-world behavior (Baumeister, Vohs, & Funder, 2007; Cialdini, 2009; Furr, 2009; Rozin, 2009). Many psychologists were fueled with a desire to find novel methods that could help with studying actual behavior in the context of people's daily lives (e.g., Mehl & Conner, 2012; Reis & Gosling, 2010). Around this time, the field also found itself thrown into a profound and painful self-questioning of methodological standards and research practices as a result of the replicability crisis (Nosek et al., 2022). Among other realizations, this questioning resulted in the key insight that efforts must be made to "scale up" to achieve sample sizes (and measurement occasions) that would yield replicable and generalizable findings. Such changes to the field's methodological standards were in stark contrast to what had long been deemed sufficient—and feasible—for conducting research about human behavior in psychology (Nelson, Simmons, & Simonsohn, 2018; Shrout & Rodgers, 2018; Vazire, Schiavone, & Bottesini, 2022).

Psychologists recognized the need for much larger samples, extended measurements, and real-world behavioral measures, and were thus thrilled that it seemed "help was on its way" from the neighboring fields of computer science and electrical engineering (e.g., Eagle Pentland, & Lazer, 2009; Lane et al., 2010; Macias, Suarez, & Lloret, 2013). And, not just help but, rather, provide exactly the solution they were looking for: The development of a new set of methods to track behavior directly (i.e., without having to rely on a proxy), passively (i.e., without the need for a participant response), objectively (i.e., without a subjective/reflective component), automatically (i.e., without the need for human processing), and at-scale (i.e., with the potential to yield "Big Data") within the natural flow of daily life, via mobile sensors and event logs produced by consumer smartphones (Harari et al., 2016; Miller, 2012; Schödel & Mehl, in press), wearables (Brown, Blake, & Sherman, 2017; Schmid Mast et al., 2015), and smart home devices (Nelson & Allen, 2018). These methods were initially conceived in the 1990s within the fields of ubiquitous, mobile, and pervasive computing (Krumm, 2018), but they experienced a major developmental thrust as smartphones became widespread for their ability to facilitate communication and many other activities in daily life (e.g., media consumption, travel, shopping). Ultimately, these methods came to be known as "sensing" methods, with the vast majority of research using this method to date being conducted with "mobile sensing" devices such as smartphones and wearables.

In this concluding chapter, we highlight and reflect on some central lessons and current challenges, open questions, and future directions for mobile sensing research in psychological science. First, we consider the key lessons learned from mobile sensing research in psychology so far. Next, we turn to the question of where psychological measurement based on mobile sensing currently stands. Finally, we consider the potential synergies and tension of mobile sensing research conducted in academic and corporate environments.

Lessons Learned from Mobile Sensing Research in Psychology

A couple of key lessons are evident to the editorial team as we conclude this handbook project. These lessons are based on the chapter submissions as well as our own experiences and reflections on conducting mobile sensing research. We share them in an effort to answer the most pressing question: How can psychologists thrive, conducting research on human behavior using mobile sensing methods?

The first, and most important, lesson is that mobile sensing is not a panacea for all methodological challenges facing the field of psychology. We hope it is clear by now that mobile sensing holds considerable promise for measuring human behavior naturally and directly in daily life. However, we also hope it is clear that a lot of work remains to be done before this method can be considered an established "standard" tool in the psychologist's methodological toolkit. These are still the early days of mobile sensing, particularly with respect to its use in the social (relative to computer) sciences. As such, this is a particularly exciting time to be developing, employing, and evaluating these methods. One opportunity to come of this lesson is the realization that we need improved standards and agreed-upon guidelines for collecting, processing, and analyzing mobile sensing data. For example, what is the right sampling rate to use when collecting data from mobile sensors or event logs, and how should this be decided? How should one go about creating variables (or "features") from mobile sensing data? When and how should top-down or bottom-up approaches be used to reduce complexity in multimodal datasets and to make decisions with regard to modeling strategies? How should one go about evaluating the reliability and validity of mobile sensing measurements? These are just some of the questions that come to the forefront of our minds when we think of what remains to be thoroughly investigated and established.

We believe the chapters in this handbook are the first steps toward providing a foundation for such guidelines. However, this is ultimately a comprehensive research task, akin to the process of evaluating self-reports as a methodology and developing best practices for scale construction and validation. Therefore, what has been done so far can only be the basic foundation and beginning of the discussion, and we anticipate that a great deal of progress will be made to establish important "how-tos" around this method in the years to come. In the following section, we discuss some of the advantages and limitations that are unique to measurement based on mobile sensing in the context of two assessment examples (for personality and clinical psychology) to render some of these points more concrete.

The second lesson is that it "takes a village," and an interdisciplinary one, to conduct mobile sensing research in psychology today. We anticipate this will change to some extent as the methodology matures, and in particular as more commercial software platforms become available to facilitate both the collection and processing of mobile sensing data. However, at the time of writing this chapter and wrapping up this handbook project, it seems that mobile sensing research in psychology is still, and will continue to be for some time, profoundly an interdisciplinary effort. Most of the research teams working on mobile sensing studies include a blend of social scientists working with researchers or staff with more technical and computational expertise (e.g., computer scientists, engineers, data scientists).

At present, such interdisciplinary collaborations can be instrumental to ensuring that data collection proceeds smoothly (e.g., without running into inexplicable software crashes or bugs) and that the data processing and/or analyses are being carried out systematically and correctly (and ideally in ways that are transparent and reproducible). However, as mobile sensing becomes more mainstream, we expect that we will see parallels to how the field of experience sampling has developed over time. There, in the early days, experience sampling was done via various researcher-developed software (e.g., the

ESP program; Barrett & Barrett, 2001). Today few of those programs exist, and the implementation is largely accomplished via commercial app platforms. A parallel gradual move toward providing access to mobile sensing platforms as a (commercial) service would, we suspect, reduce the need for interdisciplinary team efforts to conduct mobile sensing research in psychology. On the other hand, it could also bring new challenges (e.g., increased cost, less flexibility). We discuss some of the issues around academic versus corporate mobile sensing research in the section "How Will Mobile Sensing Research in the Academic versus Corporate Environment Inform Psychological Science?."

What Are We Actually Measuring with Mobile Sensing?

Mobile sensing offers psychological science (and neighboring disciplines) novel ways of measuring *in situ* behavior directly, and it also holds promise for measuring *in situ* thoughts and feelings indirectly. We want to highlight some advantages of measurement based on mobile sensing by considering two examples from personality and clinical assessment. We will then discuss some limitations and desiderata for future research.

Personalized Assessment of Personality

In the domain of personality assessment, several studies have demonstrated that Big Five personality traits can be predicted from aggregate indicators derived from mobile sensing data with varying levels of accuracy (for an overview, see Peltonen et al., 2020). More work is needed before such an assessment approach can become useful in applied domains. However, another relatively unexplored area of research for more personalized personality assessment lies in identifying behavioral signatures.

In a prominent theory of personality, Mischel and Shoda (1995) characterized personality signatures as "intra-individually stable, if . . . then, situation behavior relations" (i.e., behavioral signatures; p. 248). The *if* component refers to the situations a person is in, and the *then* component refers to the individual's responses to the situation. Mobile sensing allows researchers to assess the *if* and the *then* components in a passive, more comprehensive, and ecologically valid way compared to what has been possible so far. For example, situations can be assessed *in situ* in real life, and they can be characterized by their temporal-spatial context (e.g., time, location, climate) as well as the social context using complex measurement approaches (e.g., GPS data, videos, pictures, Bluetooth measures, self-reports; Harari, Müller, & Gosling, 2020). Moreover, the *then* component could be more comprehensively assessed using multimethod data (e.g., physiological responses, activity data, behavior in social networks, self-report). This not only allows testing basic assumptions about the situation–behavior link, but it also offers new possibilities for analyzing the development of personality. From this theoretical perspective, the change of the behavior per se (e.g., an individual shows more conscientious behavior with increasing age) seems to be less important than analyzing the stability and change of the situation–behavior link. If this link does not change over time, but the frequency of situations does, an increase of conscientious behavior might not indicate a change in personality signatures but rather a change in the occurrence of situations encountered over time. Such behavior changes would need to transfer to different situations (i.e., new if–then contingencies developed) for the changes to be considered personality development, and not simply a result of persistent environmental demands (Wrzus & Roberts, 2017). By combining sophisticated longitudinal designs with multimethod mobile sensing assessments, researchers can analyze hypotheses about the facets and development of personality in new ways that were not possible in previous research with more traditional assessment strategies.

Personalized Assessment of Psychopathology

In clinical psychology, personalized models of psychopathology are being widely discussed. According to Wright and Woods (2020), "the personalized approach of psychopathology conceptualizes mental disorders as a complex system of contextualized dynamic processes that is non-trivially specific to each individual, and it seeks to develop formal idiographic statistical models to represent these individual processes" (p. 49). For clinical assessment, the context is also gaining increasing importance for understanding individual psychopathological processes, and this requires a different type of clinical assessment (e.g., Sewall & Wright, 2021). As is true of the example of personality assessment, mobile sensing can contribute to personalized clinical assessment by providing critical information about the relationship between the context of behavior and feelings in daily life.

Clinical interventions can also be tailored to contexts by taking the individual meaning of a context for an individual into account, and they can be directly presented and evaluated on the smartphone as needed (Nahum-Shani, Chapter 30, this volume; Nahum-Shani et al., 2018). Advanced statistical modeling methods such as those featured in Part III of the *Handbook* (e.g., machine learning, deep learning, Big Data dimensionality reduction methods, dynamic network models, dynamic structural equation models) can be applied to analyze this type of data, to develop new models of assessment, and to evaluate their psychometric qualities (e.g., Lane et al., 2019).

Challenges of Measurement Based on Mobile Sensing

These two examples from personality and clinical assessment illustrate some advantages that mobile sensing methods can provide in psychology (see other chapters of the *Handbook* for additional examples), but they also reveal some important challenges.

Meaning of Measurements

The richness of mobile sensing data and the automated way in which they can be passively obtained via ubiquitous mobile technology can tempt researchers to preemptively ascribe them the status of "objective measurements" and to equate objectivity with validity. However, the many chapters in this handbook have shown that the interpretation of mobile sensing data is not as simple as it may seem at first glance. For example, if one is interested in measuring smartphone behavior (such as application use from event logs), then the measurements seem quite valid at face value, and the challenge lies in deciding how to categorize or interpret the observations. However, other—and effectively most— forms of mobile sensing data are more complex, such as activity data, which require the assessment of additional information such as the context or experience to imbue them with psychological meaning. Otherwise, the dormancy of the device may well be mistaken as inactivity of the owner. Thus, mobile sensing should not substitute existing measures in psychology, but it can complement them in meaningful ways—and vice versa (Ebner-Priemer & Santangelo, Chapter 13, this volume).

Let's be more specific, using the prime example in clinical research: predicting upcoming episodes in bipolar disorder. Why is this often considered the prime example? Simply because symptomatology of interest (activity, social interaction, sleep) is connatural to smartphone sensing (GPS tracking, tracking of phone calls and social media use, tracking alarm clock, acceleration, rest mode) and prediction of new episodes is a major treatment goal (Ebner-Priemer & Santangelo, 2020). Although we highlighted in our introduction that mobile sensing offers the possibility to measure behavior directly, without relying on proxies, we are ultimately again dependent on proxies, as we are interested in activity rather than in mere GPS coordinates. In addition, pure mobile sensing data alone is useless for this kind of research, as heightened intraindividual physical activity in patients with bipolar disorder might also be caused by new running shoes, the move into a more walkable neighborhood, retirement, medical advice, and so on—all issues entirely unrelated to an ostensibly oncoming bipolar episode. To train machine learning models, we need labeled data (ground truth; e.g., exact information about on what days a patient experienced a depressive episode), which calls for integrating classical psychological daily life research methods such as experience sampling or daily diaries (Mehl & Conner, 2012). In other words, for quite a while, mobile sensing will not replace traditional ambulatory assessment methods. Rather, traditional ambulatory assessment methods will continue to be needed and critical for elevating mobile sensing to higher psychometric grounds.

The validity of the (diagnostic) inference is crucial (Eid & Holtmann, Chapter 14, this volume; Mohr, Zhang, & Schueller, 2017). Just taking mobile sensing variables as "proxies" of established psychological constructs might be too simplistic, and it goes against the principles of multimethod measurement and triangulation, as well as against the importance of an integrative understanding of the complex phenomena of the social and behavioral sciences. The psychological meaning and construct validity of mobile sensing measures might be less important in cases where prediction instead of explanation is in the focus of research (Yarkoni & Westfall, 2017). Recent advances in modern modeling methods such as machine learning might strengthen the tendency to value prediction over explanation. However, the intelligent application of machine learning methods does not take place in a theoretical vacuum, and it requires a theoretical understanding of the phenomenon under investigation (Brandmaier, Chapter 17, this volume). Fruitfully integrating mobile sensing into psychological science therefore requires studies that not only focus on technological feasibility but also carefully consider the psychometric properties of the derived measures (e.g., construct validity). And such "holistic" endeavors need appropriate funding for research programs that do not inherently equate mobile sensing with objective measurement but, rather, harness the power of mobile sensing in the spirit of and with an eye on sound psychometric measurement.

Development of New Theories

In psychology, the emergence of new methods is often followed by the development of new theories (about behavior and measurement). One reason for this is the fact that method effects are rather strong in psychology (e.g., Eid & Diener, 2006). If novel methods fail to converge with established methods, it often points to the new methods, in fact, measuring (at least partially) a different/new construct. Methods effects are not "the serpent in psychologist's Eden" (Cronbach, 1995, p. 145); rather, they often capture meaningful differences in substantive aspects of constructs. For example, the development of implicit attitude measures (e.g., Hofmann, Gawronski, Gschwendner, Le, & Schmitt, 2005) spurred the development of attitude theories and the importance of the distinction between implicit and explicit attitudes. It is likely—and desirable—that the full arrival of mobile sensing in psychology will spur the refinement of existing theories and development of new ones. In this regard, we think mobile sensing has the potential to ultimately cause a paradigm shift (Kuhn, 1962) in psychological science. This type of shift requires openness to challenge established theories and the courage to leave known methodological and theoretical paths behind.

How Will Mobile Sensing Research in the Academic versus Corporate Environment Inform Psychological Science?

Mobile sensing research is conducted in both academia and industry, and some collaboration occurs between the two domains. Academics use industry-developed apps, tools, and data, and industry builds on academic research and draws hires from university-based teams, suggesting a largely synergistic coexistence. At the same time, mobile sensing in academia differs from corporate research in at least three aspects: (1) resources, (2) regulations, and (3) aims. All three of these differences affect the progress and societal implications of mobile sensing research.

Resources

Even with the best funded project and research program, academic mobile sensing researchers have by a factor less financial and human resources compared to technology companies. And, increasingly so these days, even if an academic project is well-funded, it encounters difficulties in finding suitable doctoral, postdoctoral, staff, or faculty researchers because industry is often offering substantially more attractive "package deals" (e.g., with respect to pay, benefits, schedules, and the ability to choose where to live and work). Financial and personnel resources impact the progress that can be made with any given project. While developing an app or analyzing mobile sensing data might take months if one developer or doctoral/postdoctoral student works on it alone, large(r) industry teams can achieve so much more in a much shorter time. In addition, major tech companies accrue immense amounts of mobile sensing data as a natural product of their business activity. For example, whereas collecting objective sleep and activity (actigraphy) data on a few hundred participants constitutes a multiyear research project for an academic team, major technology companies accrue these data naturally and continuously, day after day, for millions of people. Therefore, answering, for example, the question whether physical activity promotes a good night of sleep is, for academic mobile sensing researchers, a matter of years, whereas, for corporate researchers, it amounts to metaphorically not much more than a press of a button. This might lead to academics asking themselves (or, as in our personal experience, being asked by funders) if or how they could ever compete with companies doing this type of research.

Regulations

Academic researchers are well aware of the many regulations they have to adhere to: Ethical guidelines ensure that scientific studies do not cause harm to the mental or physical well-being of participants. This concerns immediate effects, such as too much distress or harmful behavior, as well as long-term effects that might arise if private, sensitive information becomes public. The protection of personal information as mundane as birth date and as sensitive as medical conditions is additionally ruled by laws in many countries, most recently with the European General Data Protection Regulation ("Data Protection in the EU," 2022) or the Federal Trade Commission Act and several state-level acts in the United States. Still, many countries do not possess such legal regulations (Woodward, 2021).

Of course, in many countries, corporations are also subject to these kinds of legal regulations, and yet countless examples exist where companies fail to adhere to them (e.g., Venturini & Rogers, 2019). Similarly, research was carried out by companies, or in cooperation with companies, that demonstrates the ethical sensitivities and responsibilities of mobile sensing research. For example, when girls and women have a higher probability to develop body image problems after viewing social media content related to thinness (WSJ noted, 2021); when consumers buy more goods after viewing personality-tailored advertisements (Matz, Kosinski, Nave, & Stillwell, 2017); and when algorithms detect political or sexual orientation from social media pictures (Kosinski, 2021; Wang & Kosinski, 2018). The last named is especially problematic in countries where political opposition is suppressed or homosexuality is amerceable, and yet even in democratic countries this information might be misused. While ethics boards of academic institutions seek to prevent unethical and harmful research, and perhaps fail in some cases, problems are compounded if such studies are carried out with millions of customers.

An additional complication arises from confidentiality agreements that companies arrange with employees or academic collaborators. Public information (WSJ noted, 2021) and personal communication with researchers reveal that companies can and do restrict what is published outside of their company. Presumably, this applies to results that might threaten the company's profit or reputation, whereas favorable results are more likely published. Science has taught us for decades that this kind of publication bias impedes balanced evaluation of scientific knowledge (e.g., Ferguson & Brannick, 2011). Some tension between open-science standards in academia (e.g., Nosek et al., 2015) and the protection of company knowledge through confidentiality and patents in industry is comprehensible. It will be interesting to see how cooperation between open-science-oriented academic researchers and profit-oriented corporations will develop in the future (King & Persily, 2018).

Aims

It is not a political statement to proclaim that a company's central aim is to reap profit. This aim is certainly legitimate (up to a certain point), but technology end users have to be aware that making money is the driving force behind commercial technology, and making consumers' lives easier via their products, apps, and services is either a nice side effect or an "epiphenomenon." As many articles have highlighted (e.g., Matz et al., 2017; Venturini & Rogers, 2019; WSJ noted, 2021), conflicts of interest can arise when people use technology, although it harms their health, relationships, or finances. At the same time, it is hard to imagine how companies could sustainably prioritize consumer well-being over financial benefit.

In contrast, the academic ideal of psychological science is about understanding human behavior, thoughts, and feelings. Although money in the form of sufficient funding is relevant, profit is irrelevant to the scientific endeavor. This allows academic researchers to follow discoveries without censoring results, depending on how marketable they are. In our opinion, this highlights a unique advantage of academia. Still, academia sometimes has to defend this important advantage to university administration and funding agencies that can (some would say have to) approach academia with more of a business mindset (Forschung & Lehre, 2018).

Overall, it would be preferable to be more optimistic about the synergistic coexistence and collaboration of academia and industry. Yet several examples and conversations with colleagues paint (to us) a somewhat sober picture—at least at this moment in time. While resources and regulations seem to disadvantage academic research, freedom of research and independence of discovery are the hallmarks of science, and we are well advised to uphold and defend them. Undoubtedly, individual researchers might at times also operate under bias (e.g., to maximize publication impact or funding); yet the scientific community and its debates (ideally) act as checks-and-balances to counteract individual researcher bias. For example, the scientific debates surrounding the risks and benefits of computer games (e.g., Granic, Lobel, & Engels, 2014) led to a better understanding and more nuanced picture than the (lopsided) evaluation by the gaming industry. Unbiased research—or, in more idealistic terms, "unraveling the truth"—is only possible with sufficient funding and motivated researchers who subscribe to this scientific ideal. To the extent that these two conditions are met, there should be no shortage of motivated researchers in our scientific community.

Conclusions

The assessment of behavior directly, passively, objectively, and at-scale in the natural environment by mobile sensing, together with neuroscientific developments, is one of the most important revolutions in psychological assessment. Many of the existing psychological assessment methods are ultimately refinements and further developments of methods that were already available 100 years ago. These established methods, of course, continue to be important. However, mobile sensing offers a completely new and unique access to human behavior (as well as thoughts and feelings indirectly), and its technical capabilities are bound to dramatically increase over the next years. Also, statistical methods for analyzing these data are bound to co-develop at an accelerated rate in the years to come.

From purely technical perspectives, many of the challenges around and limitations of the current generation approaches will gradually, and possibly more rapidly than one anticipates, disappear. However, what makes the field of mobile sensing so intriguing for researchers in the social and behavioral sciences is not the overcoming of the technical limitations but, rather, the solving of the fascinating, broader methodological and theoretical issues that this emerging approach highlights. How can the validity of inferences drawn on the basis of mobile sensing data be proved? How can the incremental validity beyond traditional methods be demonstrated? How can quality standards be established and open-science standards be fulfilled? In which way can results of mobile sensing studies be explained by current theories, and in what ways do theories need to be adapted? How can theories of behavior, feelings, attitudes, physiology, personality, sociality, and environments be integrated into our understanding of thoughts, feelings, and behavior in daily life? And how can these theories be validly tested with the use of mobile sensing methods? Getting answers to these questions requires large-scale interdisciplinary research programs that critically examine this emerging field, drawing on theories and methodological concepts from the behavioral and social sciences. We hope that the chapters of this handbook help social and behavioral scientists further their understanding of mobile sensing methods and ultimately ignite the spark to see how they can use them to enrich their own research programs.

REFERENCES

Barrett, L. F., & Barrett, D. J. (2001). An introduction to computerized experience sampling in psychology. *Social Science Computer Review, 19*(2), 175–185.

Baumeister, R. F., Vohs, K. D., & Funder, D. C. (2007). Psychology as the science of self-reports and finger movements: Whatever happened to actual behavior? *Perspectives on Psychological Science, 2*(4), 396–403.

Brown, N. A., Blake, A. B., & Sherman, R. A. (2017). A snapshot of the life as lived: Wearable cameras in social and personality psychological science. *Social Psychological and Personality Science, 8*(5), 592–600.

Cialdini, R. B. (2009). We have to break up. *Perspectives On Psychological Science, 4*(1), 5–6.

Cronbach, L. J. (1995). Giving method variance its due. In P. E. Shrout & S. T. Fiske (Eds.), *Personality research, methods, and theory: A festschrift honoring Donald W. Fiske* (pp. 145–160). Erlbaum.

Data protection in the EU. (2022, July 15). https://ec.europa.eu/info/law/law-topic/data-protection/data-protection-eu_en

Eagle, N., Pentland, A., & Lazer, D. (2009). Inferring friendship network structure by using mobile phone data. *Proceedings of the National Academy of Sciences, 106*(36), 15274–15278.

Ebner-Priemer, U. W., & Kubiak, T. (2010). The decade of behavior revisited: Future prospects for ambulatory assessment. *European Journal of Psychological Assessment, 26*(3), 151–153.

Ebner-Priemer, U., & Santangelo, P. (2020). Digital phenotyping: hype or hope? *The Lancet Psychiatry, 7*(4), 297–299.

Eid, M. & Diener, E. (Eds.) (2006). *Handbook of multimethod measurement in psychology.* American Psychological Association.

Ferguson, C. J., & Brannick, M. T. (2011). Publication bias in psychological science: Prevalence, methods for identifying and controlling, and implications for the use of meta-analyses. *Psychological Methods, 17*(1), 120–128.

Forschung & Lehre. (2018). *Studie: Zielvereinbarung hat keine motivierende Wirkung.* www.forschung-und-lehre.de/management/studie-zielvereinbarung-hat-keine-motivierende-wirkung-525

Furr, R. M. (2009). Personality psychology as a truly behavioural science. *European Journal of Personality, 23*(5), 369–401.

Granic, I., Lobel, A., & Engels, R. C. (2014). The benefits of playing video games. *American Psychologist, 69*(1), 66–78.

Harari, G. M., Lane, N. D., Wang, R., Crosier, B. S., Campbell, A. T., & Gosling, S. D. (2016). Using smartphones to collect behavioral data in psychological science: Opportunities, practical considerations, and challenges. *Perspectives on Psychological Science, 11*(6), 838–854.

Harari, G. M., Müller, S. R., & Gosling, S. D. (2020). Naturalistic assessment of situations using mobile Sensing methods. In J. F. Rauthmann, R. Sherman, & D. C. Funder (Eds.), *The Oxford handbook of psychological situations* (pp. 299–311). Oxford University Press.

Hofmann, W., Gawronski, B., Gschwendner, T., Le, H., & Schmitt, M. (2005). A meta-analysis on the correlation between the implicit association test and explicit self-report measures.

Personality and Social Psychology Bulletin, 31, 1369–1385.
King, G., & Persily, N. (2018). A new model for industry-academic partnerships. *PS: Political Science and Politics, 53*(4), 703–709.
Kosinski, M. (2021). Facial recognition technology can expose political orientation from naturalistic facial images. *Scientific Reports, 11*(1), 1–7.
Krumm, J. (Ed.). (2018). *Ubiquitous computing fundamentals*. CRC Press.
Kuhn, T. S. (1962). *The structure of scientific revolutions*. University of Chicago Press.
Lane, N. D., Miluzzo, E., Lu, H., Peebles, D., Choudhury, T., & Campbell, A. T. (2010). A survey of mobile phone sensing. *IEEE Communications Magazine, 48*(9), 140–150.
Lane, S. T., Gates, K. M., Pike, H. K., Beltz, A. M., & Wright, A. G. (2019). Uncovering general, shared, and unique temporal patterns in ambulatory assessment data. *Psychological Methods, 24*(1), 54–69.
Laurila, J. K., Gatica-Perez, D., Aad, I., Bornet, O., Do, T. M. T., Dousse, O., et al. (2012). The mobile data challenge: Big data for mobile computing research. *Pervasive Computing*, No. EPFL-CONF-192489.
Macias, E., Suarez, A., & Lloret, J. (2013). Mobile sensing systems. *Sensors, 13*(12), 17292–17321.
Matz, S. C., Kosinski, M., Nave, G., & Stillwell, D. J. (2017). Psychological targeting as an effective approach to digital mass persuasion. *Proceedings of the National Academy of Sciences, 114*(48), 12714–12719.
Mehl, M. R., & Conner, T. S. (Eds.). (2012). *Handbook of research methods for studying daily life*. Guilford Press.
Miller, G. (2012). The smartphone psychology manifesto. *Perspectives on Psychological Science, 7*, 221–237.
Mischel, W., & Shoda, Y. (1995,). A cognitive-affective system theory of personality: Reconceptualizing situations, dispositions, dynamics, and invariance in personality structure. *Psychological Review, 102*, 246–268.
Mohr, D. C., Zhang, M., & Schueller, S. M. (2017). Personal sensing: Understanding mental health using ubiquitous sensors and machine learning. *Annual Review of Clinical Psychology, 13*, 23–47.
Nahum-Shani, I., Smith, S. N., Spring, B. J., Collins, L. M., Witkiewitz, K., Tewari, A., & Murphy, S. A. (2018). Just-in-time adaptive interventions (JITAIs) in mobile health: key components and design principles for ongoing health behavior support. *Annals of Behavioral Medicine, 52*(6), 446–462.
Nelson, B. W., & Allen, N. B. (2018). Extending the passive-sensing toolbox: Using smart-home technology in psychological science. *Perspectives on Psychological Science, 13*(6), 718–733.
Nelson, L. D., Simmons, J., & Simonsohn, U. (2018). Psychology's renaissance. *Annual Review of Psychology, 69*, 511–534.
Nosek, B. A., Alter, G., Banks, G. C., Borsboom, D., Bowman, S. D., Breckler, S. J., et al. (2015). Promoting an open research culture: Author guidelines for journals could help to promote transparency, openness, and reproducibility. *Science, 348*(6242), 1422–1425.
Nosek, B. A., Hardwicke, T. E., Moshontz, H., Allard, A., Corker, K. S., Dreber, A., et al. (2022). Replicability, robustness, and reproducibility in psychological science. *Annual Review of Psychology, 73*, 719–748.
Peltonen, E., Sharmila, P., Opoku Asare, K., Visuri, A., Lagerspetz, E., & Ferreira, D. (2020). When phones get personal: Predicting Big Five personality traits from application usage. *Pervasive and Mobile Computing, 69*.
RatSWD [German Data Forum]. (2020). *Data collection using new information technology. Recommendations on data quality, data management, research ethics, and data protection*. RatSWD Output 6 (6). German Data Forum (RatSWD). https://doi.org/10.17620/02671.51.
Reis, H. T., & Gosling, S. D. (2010). Social psychological methods outside the laboratory. In S. Fiske, D. Gilbert, & G. Lindzey (Eds.), *Handbook of social psychology* (5th ed., Vol. 1, pp. 82–114). Wiley.
Rozin, P. (2009). What kind of empirical research should we publish, fund, and reward?: A different perspective. *Perspectives on Psychological Science, 4*(4), 435–439.
Schmid Mast, M., Gatica-Perez, D., Frauendorfer, D., Nguyen, L., & Choudhury, T. (2015). Social sensing for psychology: Automated interpersonal behavior assessment. *Current Directions in Psychological Science, 24*(2), 154–160.
Schödel, R. & Mehl, M. R. (in press). Mobile sensing methods. In: H. T. Reis, T. West, & C. M. Judd (Eds.), *Handbook of research meth-*

ods in social and personality psychology (3rd ed.). Cambridge University Press.

Sewall, C. J., & Wright, A. G. (2021). Personalizing suicidology. *Crisis, 42*(6), 405–410.

Shrout, P. E., & Rodgers, J. L. (2018). Psychology, science, and knowledge construction: Broadening perspectives from the replication crisis. *Annual Review of Psychology, 69*, 487–510.

Vazire, S., Schiavone, S. R., & Bottesini, J. G. (2022). Credibility beyond replicability: Improving the four validities in psychological science. *Current Directions in Psychological Science, 31*(2), 162–168.

Venturini, T., & Rogers, R. (2019). "API-based research" or how can digital sociology and digital journalism studies learn from the Facebook and Cambridge Analytica breach. *Digital Journalism, 7*(4), 532–540.

Wang, Y., & Kosinski, M. (2018). Deep neural networks are more accurate than humans at detecting sexual orientation from facial images. *Journal of Personality and Social Psychology, 114*(2), 246.

WSJ noted. (2021, September 29). How Instagram is hurting teen girls. www.wsj.com/articles/how-instagram-is-hurting-teen-girls-11632940937

Woodward, M. (2021). *16 countries with GDPR-like data privacy laws.* https://security-scorecard.com/blog/countries-with-gdpr-like-data-privacy-laws

Wright, A. G. C., & Woods, W. C. (2020). Personalized models of psychopathology. *Annual Review of Clinical Psychology, 16*, 49–74.

Wrzus, C., & Roberts, B. W. (2017). Processes of personality development in adulthood: The TESSERA framework. *Personality and Social Psychology Review, 21*(3), 253–277.

Yarkoni, T., & Westfall, J. (2017). Choosing prediction over explanation in psychology: Lessons from machine learning. *Perspectives on Psychological Science, 12*, 1100–1122.

Author Index

Subject Index

Note. *f* or *t* following a page number indicates a figure or a table.

About the Editors

Matthias R. Mehl, PhD, is Professor of Psychology at the University of Arizona. He is a social and personality psychologist interested in the conceptualization and measurement of how everyday social processes affect health and well-being. He employs mobile sensing methods for studying real-world social interactions and has pioneered a method that involves the unobtrusive sampling of ambient sounds via a smartphone app (the Electronically Activated Recorder, or EAR). Dr. Mehl has published extensively and given workshops on mobile sensing and other real-world psychological research methods. He is a Fellow of the Association for Psychological Science and the Society for Personality and Social Psychology.

Michael Eid, PhD, is Professor of Methods and Evaluation at the Free University of Berlin in Germany. His research focuses on measurement theory, in particular, the development of psychometric models for longitudinal and multimethod research. His more applied research contributions are in the areas of subjective well-being, mood regulation, and health psychology. With respect to mobile sensing, Dr. Eid is especially interested in the psychometric foundation of multimethod mobile sensing research strategies and the modeling of intensive longitudinal data. Widely published, he has served as editor of several journals in the area of methodology and assessment.

Cornelia Wrzus, PhD, is Professor of Psychological Aging Research at the Ruprecht-Karls University of Heidelberg, Germany, where she founded the Daily Life Lab. Her research focuses on socioemotional and personality development across the entire adult lifespan. Dr. Wrzus has published many articles on personality development, emotional processes, and social dynamics in daily life, using experience sampling, ambulatory physiological assessments, and mobile sensing. One particular concern is the integration of both open science standards and privacy protection in ambulatory assessment research of people's daily lives. She has served on the editorial boards of several personality journals and is president-elect of the Society for Ambulatory Assessment.

Gabriella M. Harari, PhD, is Assistant Professor in the Department of Communication at Stanford University, where she directs the Media and Personality Lab. Her research focuses on everyday behavior and its relationship to personality and well-being. She takes an ecological approach to conducting her research, emphasizing the importance of studying people in their natural physical and digital contexts. Over the last decade, Dr. Harari has published extensively on mobile sensing and given workshops about using the method for studying daily life.

Ulrich W. Ebner-Priemer, PhD, is Professor of Psychology and Chair of the Mental mHealth (mobile health) Lab at the Karlsruhe Institute of Technology in Germany. His work is characterized by its methodological focus on ambulatory assessment, investigating phenomena of interest in everyday life and real time. He is particularly interested in a multimodal operationalization of phenomena of interest, combining e-diaries with wearables, and digital phenotypes; real-time analyses and real-time feedback; and analysis of dynamic processes. Dr. Ebner-Priemer provides the technological mHealth framework for studies on a broad range of mental disorders. He is former president of the Society for Ambulatory Assessment and current Chair of the ECNP Digital Health Network.

Contributors

Mathias Allemand, PhD, Dynamics of Healthy Aging University Research Priority Program, University of Zürich, Zürich, Switzerland

Cara J. Arizmendi, PhD, Department of Population Health Sciences, Duke University School of Medicine, Durham, North Carolina

Mohammad Atari, PhD, Department of Psychological and Brain Sciences, University of Massachusetts Amherst, Amherst, Massachusetts

Emorie D. Beck, PhD, Feinberg School of Medicine, Northwestern University, Chicago, Illinois; Department of Psychology, University of California, Davis, Davis, California

Melanie Becker, MSc, Department of Psychology (Gerontopsychology and Gerontology), University of Zürich, Zürich, Switzerland

Felix Beierle, PhD, National Institute of Informatics, Tokyo, Japan; Institute of Clinical Epidemiology and Biometry, University of Würzburg, Würzburg, Germany

Dror Ben-Zeev, PhD, Department of Psychiatry and Behavioral Sciences, University of Washington, Seattle, Washington

Andreas M. Brandmaier, PhD, Center for Lifespan Psychology, Max Planck Institute for Human Development, and Department of Psychology, MSB Medical School Berlin, Berlin, Germany

Michael Businelle, PhD, Department of Family and Preventive Medicine, University of Oklahoma Health Sciences Center, The University of Oklahoma, Oklahoma City, Oklahoma

J. B. J. (Hans) Bussmann, PhD, Department of Rehabilitation Medicine, Erasmus MC University Medical Center Rotterdam, Rotterdam, The Netherlands

Andrew Campbell, PhD, Department of Computer Science, Dartmouth College, Hanover, New Hampshire

Tanzeem Choudhury, PhD, Department of Information Science, Cornell Tech, New York, New York

Aaron Cohen, MA, Written World Consulting, Biddeford, Maine

Jean Costa, PhD, Toyota Research Institute, Los Altos, California

Alexander F. Danvers, PhD, Department of Psychology, University of Arizona, Tucson, Arizona

Kaya de Barbaro, PhD, Department of Psychology, The University of Texas at Austin, Austin, Texas

Munmun De Choudhury, PhD, Georgia Institute of Technology, Atlanta, Georgia

Eco J. C. de Geus, PhD, Department of Biological Psychology, Vrije Universiteit Amsterdam, Amsterdam, The Netherlands

Morteza Dehghani, PhD, Department of Psychology and Computer Science, University of Southern California, Los Angeles, California

Mariella Dimiccoli, PhD, Institut de Robòtica i Infomàtica Industrial, Universitat Politècnica de Catalunya, Barcelona, Spain

Ulrich W. Ebner-Priemer, PhD, Institute of Sports and Sports Sciences, Karlsruhe Institute of Technology, Karlsruhe, Germany

Michael Eid, PhD, Department of Psychology and Education, Division of Methods and Evaluation, Freie Universität Berlin, Berlin, Germany

Marcel Enge, MSc, Department of Differential Psychology, Personality Psychology, and Psychological Assessment, Bielefeld University, Bielefeld, Germany

Altaf Engineer, PhD, College of Architecture, Planning, and Landscape Architecture, University of Arizona, Tucson, Arizona

Caitlin M. Fausey, PhD, Department of Psychology, University of Oregon, Eugene, Oregon

Tiantian Feng, MS, Viterbi School of Engineering, University of Southern California, Los Angeles, California

Kathleen M. Gates, PhD, Department of Psychology, University of North Carolina at Chapel Hill, Chapel Hill, North Carolina

Martin J. Gevonden, PhD, Department of Biological Psychology, Vrije Universiteit Amsterdam, Amsterdam, The Netherlands

Marco Giurgiu, PhD, Institute of Sports and Sports Sciences, Karlsruhe Institute of Technology, Karlsruhe, Germany

Brian Gonzalez, PhD, Department of Health Outcomes and Behavior, Moffitt Cancer Center, Tampa, Florida

Gabriella M. Harari, PhD, Department of Communication, Stanford University, Stanford, California

Karra Harrington, PhD, College of Health and Human Development, The Pennsylvania State University, State College, Pennsylvania

Rajat Hebbar, MS, Viterbi School of Engineering, University of Southern California, Los Angeles, California

Jana Holtmann, PhD, Wilhelm Wundt Institute for Psychology, Leipzig University, Leipzig, Germany

Jason I. Hong, PhD, Human Computer Interaction Institute, School of Computer Science, Carnegie Mellon University, Pittsburgh, Pennsylvania

Andrea B. Horn, PhD, Dynamics of Healthy Aging University Research Priority Program, Center for Gerontology, Department of Psychology, University of Zürich, Zürich, Switzerland

Jeremy Huckins, PhD, Department of Psychological and Brain Sciences, Dartmouth College, Hanover, New Hampshire

Jacob N. Hyde, PsyD, Warfighter Consulting, Scottsdale, Arizona, and Department of Family and Community Medicine, University of Arizona, Tucson, Arizona

Arindam Jati, PhD, Viterbi School of Engineering, University of Southern California, Los Angeles, California

Geneva K. Jonathan, PhD, Department of Psychiatry, Massachusetts General Hospital/ Harvard Medical School, Cambridge, Massachusetts

Martina Kanning, PhD, Department of Sports Sciences, University of Konstanz, Konstanz, Germany

Farzan Karimi-Malekabadi, MA, Department of Psychology, University of Southern California, Los Angeles, California

Darla Kendzor, PhD, University of Oklahoma Health Sciences Center, The University of Oklahoma, Oklahoma City, Oklahoma

Beth Kramer, MPH, Mel and Enid Zuckerman College of Public Health, University of Arizona, Tucson, Arizona

Lara Kroencke, MSc, Department of Psychological Assessment and Personality Psychology, University of Münster, Münster, Germany

Santosh Kumar, PhD, Department of Computer Science, University of Memphis, Memphis, Tennessee

Peter Kuppens, PhD, Faculty of Psychology and Educational Sciences, KU Leuven, Leuven, Belgium

Sven Lautenbach, PhD, GIScience Research Group, Institute of Geography, Heidelberg University, Heidelberg, Germany

Casey M. Lindberg, PhD, Institute on Place and Wellbeing, University of Arizona, Tucson, Arizona

Sarah Lohr, MS, Potsdam Institute for Climate Impact Research, Potsdam, Germany

Birthe Macdonald, PhD, Department of Psychology (Gerontopsychology and Gerontology), University of Zürich, Zürich, Switzerland

Mike Martin, PhD, Department of Psychology (Gerontopsychology and Gerontology and Health Longevity Center, University of Zürich, Zürich, Switzerland

Sandra C. Matz, PhD, Management Division, Columbia Business School, New York, New York

Matthias R. Mehl, PhD, Department of Psychology, University of Arizona, Tucson, Arizona

Sandrine R. Müller, PhD, Google LLC, New York, New York

Inbal Nahum-Shani, PhD, Institute for Social Research, University of Michigan, Ann Arbor, Michigan

Shrikanth S. Narayanan, PhD, Viterbi School of Engineering, University of Southern California, Los Angeles, California

Koen Niemeijer, MS, Faculty of Psychology and Educational Sciences, KU Leuven, Leuven, Belgium

Mikio Obuchi, MS, Department of Computer Science, Dartmouth College, Hanover, New Hampshire

Pablo Paredes, PhD, Department of Computer Science, University of Maryland, College Park, College Park, Maryland

Arvind Pillai, MS, Department of Computer Science, Dartmouth College, Hanover, New Hampshire

John F. Rauthmann, PhD, Department of Differential Psychology, Personality Psychology, and Psychological Assessment, Bielefeld University, Bielefeld, Germany

Markus Reichert, PhD, Department of eHealth and Sports Analytics, Faculty of Sport Science, Ruhr University Bochum, Bochum, Germany

Ramon Reyes, Department of Psychology, University of Arizona, Tucson, Arizona

Christina Röcke, PhD, Dynamics of Healthy Aging University Research Priority Program, Center for Gerontology and Health Longevity Center, University of Zürich, Zürich, Switzerland

Nelson Roque, PhD, Department of Human Development and Family Studies, Penn State University, State College, Pennsylvania

Johnny R. Runyon, PhD, Department of Environmental Science, University of Arizona, Tucson, Arizona

Koustuv Saha, PhD, Department of Computer Science, University of Illinois at Urbana–Champaign, Champaign, Illinois

Philip Santangelo, PhD, Institute of Sports and Sports Sciences, Karlsruhe Institute of Technology, Karlsruhe, Germany

Ramona Schoedel, PhD, Department of Psychology, Ludwig-Maximilians-Universität München, Munich, Germany

Martin Sliwinski, PhD, College of Health and Human Development, The Pennsylvania State University, State College, Pennsylvania

Serena Soh, MA, Department of Communication, Stanford University, Stanford, California

Clemens Stachl, PhD, Institute of Behavioral Science and Technology, School of Management, University of St. Gallen, St. Gallen, Switzerland

Esther M. Sternberg, MD, Andrew Weil Center for Integrative Medicine, University of Arizona, Tucson, Arizona

Larissa Sust, MSc, Department of Psychology, Ludwig-Maximilians-Universität München, Munich, Germany

Sanaz Talaifar, PhD, Graduate School of Business, Stanford University, Stanford, California

Stuti Thapa, BS, Industrial–Organizational Psychology Program, Department of Psychology, University of Tulsa, Tulsa, Oklahoma

Edison Thomaz, PhD, Department of Electrical and Computer Engineering, The University of Texas at Austin, Austin, Texas

Adela C. Timmons, PhD, Department of Psychology, The University of Texas at Austin, Austin, Texas

Christopher J. Urban, MS, Department of Psychology, University of North Carolina at Chapel Hill, Chapel Hill, North Carolina

Kristof Van Laerhoven, PhD, Ubiquitous Computing–ETI, University of Siegen, Siegen, Germany

Christine Vinci, PhD, Department of Health Outcomes and Behavior, Moffitt Cancer Center, Tampa, Florida

Weichen Wang, MS, Department of Computer Science, Dartmouth College, Hanover, New Hampshire

Cornelia Wrzus, PhD, Department of Psychological Aging Research, Institute of Psychology, Heidelberg University, Heidelberg, Germany